THE FREUD ENCYCLOPEDIA
Theory, Therapy, and Culture

THE FREUD ENCYCLOPEDIA
Theory, Therapy, and Culture

EDITOR
EDWARD ERWIN

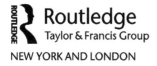

Routledge
Taylor & Francis Group

NEW YORK AND LONDON

Published in 2002 by
Routledge
711 Third Avenue,
New York, NY 10017

Published in Great Britain by
Routledge
2 Park Square, Milton Park,
Abingdon, Oxfordshire OX14 4RN

First issued in paperback 2016

Routledge is an imprint of the Taylor and Francis Group, an informa business

Library of Congress Cataloging-in-Publication Data

The Freud encyclopedia : theory, therapy, and culture / Edward Erwin, editor.
    p.cm
    Includes bibliographical references and index.
    ISBN 0-415-93677-2 (alk. paper)
    1. Psychoanalysis—Encyclopedias. 2. Freud, Sigmund, 1856–1939—Encyclopedias. I.
Erwin, Edward, 1937–

BF173.F6176 2001
150.19'52'092—dc21   2001048448

ISBN 13: 978-0-415-76233-5 (pbk)
ISBN 13: 978-0-415-93677-4 (hbk)

To Patricia Guarino Erwin

CONTENTS

ALPHABETICAL LIST OF ENTRIES   ix

PREFACE   xiii

ACKNOWLEDGMENTS   xvii

CONTRIBUTORS   xix

THE ENCYCLOPEDIA   1

INDEX   603

ALPHABETICAL LIST OF ENTRIES

Abraham, Karl
Abreaction
Abstinence, Rule of
Acting Out
Adler, Alfred
Aesthetics and Psychoanalysis
Affect
Africa, and Psychoanalysis
Aggression
Ambivalence
Anaclitic Object
Anal Character
Analyzability
Andreas-Salomé, Lou
Anna O.
Anthropology, and Psychoanalysis
Anxiety and Defense
Anxiety Neurosis
Aphasia
Argentina, and Psychoanalysis
Australia, and Psychoanalysis
Autoerotism
Autonomy

Baginsky, Adolf
Behaviorism, and Psychoanalysis
Belgium, and Psychoanalysis
Binding
Biography, Psychoanalysis and
Biology, and Psychoanalysis
Bonaparte, Marie
Brain Science, and Psychoanalysis
Brazil, and Psychoanalysis
Brentano, Franz
Breuer, Josef

Canada, and Psychoanalysis
Castration Anxiety
Catharsis

Cathexis
Character
Character Neurosis
Charcot, Jean-Martin
Child Psychoanalysis
Childhood Neurosis
Chile, and Psychoanalysis
China, and Psychoanalysis
Cinema, and Psychoanalysis
Clinical Theory
Cognitive Psychology, and Psychoanalysis
Committee, the Secret
Compulsion and Obsession
Confidentiality
Conflicts, Theory of
Consciousness
Conversion
Creativity
Criminality, Psychoanalysis
Critique of Psychoanalysis
Czech Republic, and Psychoanalysis

Defense Mechanisms
Delusions
Denial
Denmark, and Psychoanalysis
Depression
Deutsch, Helene
Developmental Theory
Displacement
Dissociation
Dora
Dreams, Theory of
Drive Theory

Education, and Analysts
Ego
Ego Psychology
Eissler, Kurt

Eitingon, Max
Electra Complex
Elizabeth von R.
Ellis, Havelock
Envy
Ethics, Clinical
Existentialism
Experimental Evidence, Freudian

Family Romance
Fantasy (Phantasy)
Fechner, Gustav Theodor
Feminism, and Psychoanalysis
Fenichel, Otto
Ferenczi, Sándor
Finland, and Psychoanalysis
Fliess, Wilhelm
France, and Psychoanalysis
Free Association
Free Will
Freud, Anna
Freud, Sigmund
Freud's Family
Fromm, Erich

Genetics, and Psychoanalysis
Geniality, Theories of
Germany, and Psychoanalysis
Glover, Edward
Goethe Prize
Great Britain, and Psychoanalysis
Greece, and Psychoanalysis
Groddeck, Georg
Guilt

Hallucinations
Hartmann, Heinz
Herbart, Johann Friedrich
Hermeneutics, and Psychoanalysis
Homosexuality, Psychoanalytic Theories of
Horney, Karen
Humanities, and Psychoanalysis
Hysteria

Id
Identification
Incest

India, and Psychoanalysis
Infantile Sexuality
Insight, Role in Therapy
Intellectualization
Interpretation
Irrationality
Isolation
Italy, and Psychoanalysis

Janet, Pierre
Japan, and Psychoanalysis
Jokes and Humor
Jones, Ernest
Judaism and Freud
Jung, Carl

Kassowitz Institute
Klein, Melanie
Kleinian Theory
Korea, and Psychoanalysis
Krafft-Ebing, Richard von
Kris, Ernst

Lacan, Jacques
Lay Analysis
Libido Theory
Literature, and Psychoanalysis
Little Hans

Marxism, and Freudianism
Masochism and Sadism
Metapsychology
Meaning, and Psychoanalysis
Mexico, and Psychoanalysis
Mind and Body
Modernism, Postmodernism, and Psychoanalysis
Morality, and Psychoanalysis
Multiple Personality (Dissociative Personality Disorder)
Myths

Narcissism
Netherlands, and Psychoanalysis
Neurasthenia
Neuroses
Nietzsche, Friedrich
Nineteenth-Century Philosophy Precursors of Freud
Norway, and Psychoanalysis

Object Relations Theory
Object
Obsessive Phenomena
Occult, and Freud
Oedipus Complex
Oral Character
Overdetermination

Paranoia
Penis Envy
Peru, and Psychoanalysis
Perversions
Pfister, Oskar
Philosophy and Psychoanalysis
Philippines, The, and Psychoanalysis
Piaget, Jean
Pleasure Principle
Preconscious
Primal Scene
Project for a Scientific Psychology
Projection
Projective Techniques
Pseduo-Science, and Psychoanalysis
Psychiatry, and Psychoanalysis
Physical Determinism
Psychoanalysis, Origin and History of
Psychoanalytic Movement
Psychoanalytic Technique and Process
Psychoanalytically Oriented Psychotherapy
Psychohistory
Psychopathology

Rank, Otto
Rat Man
Reaction Formation
Reality Testing
Reception of Freud's Ideas
Regression
Reich, Wilhelm
Reik, Theodor
Religion, and Psychoanalysis
Repetition Compulsion
Repression
Research on Psychoanalysis
Resistance
Return of the Repressed
Russia/Soviet Union and Psychoanalysis

Sachs, Hanns
Schizophrenia
Schopenhauer, Arthur
Schreber, Daniel Paul
Scientific Tests of Freud's Theories and Therapy
Screen Memories
Seduction Theory
Self Psychology
Self-analysis
Self-deception
Sexology
Shame
Sleep
Slips, Theory of
Sociobiology, and Psychoanalysis
Spielrein, Sabina
Splitting the Ego
Stekel, Wilhelm
Strachy, James
Structural Theory
Sublimation
Suggestion
Suicide
Sullivan, Harry Stack
Superego
Sweden, and Psychoanalysis
Symbiosis
Symbolism

Taboos
Tausk, Victor
Therapeutic Alliance
Toilet Training
Transference
Traumatic Neurosis

Unconscious, The
United States, and Psychoanalysis

Vaginal and Clitoral Orgasm
Venezuela, and Psychoanalysis
Vienna, and Psychoanalysis
Virginity

War Neurosis
Wednesday Society
Wolf Man
Working Through

PREFACE

We live in an age when some scholars seriously question the value of truth. Inquire of a theory, it is said, not whether it is true or false, but whether it is "insightful," "useful," "profound," "brilliant," or "penetrating." This way of thinking about theories was not congenial to Sigmund Freud. On a number of occasions, Einstein expressed admiration for Freud's "brilliant achievement" but refused to say that any of his theories were true. In response to one such congratulatory letter from Einstein, written to honor Freud's eightieth birthday, Freud replied: "But I have often asked myself what indeed there is to admire about them [his theories] if they are not true—i.e. if they do not contain a high degree of truth" (Grubrich-Simitis, 1995).

If the correctness of his ideas is what ultimately matters, however, then there is a problem in explaining why Freud is still worth taking seriously. Critics will point out that in the last thirty years, Freud's theories have been shown to be pseudo-scientific, or basically mistaken, or at the very least largely unproven. If these critics are right, why invite hundreds of expert scholars from around the world to devote so much time and effort to writing articles on Freud's work and influence? And why should a reader care? These questions deserve an answer.

As someone who has published a book skeptical about Freud's ideas (Erwin, 1996) but who has also spent much of the last nine years, together with his co-editors, putting together this encyclopedia, I would answer that despite the critiques, there are still very good reasons to care about Freud and what he created. One reason concerns *the degree* of truth in Freudian theory.

To What Extent Was Freud Right?

Many contemporary supporters of Freud argue not that he was mostly right, but that some of his theories contain deep insights and have received a reasonable amount of empirical support. Assuming that this is a credible viewpoint, there is still an important question to be answered: Exactly which parts of Freudian theory are at least approximately true and which are not? On this issue, scholars are still deeply divided.

If there have been impressive critiques of Freud's arguments and theories, there have also been impressive defenses. Some scholars argue that Freud's critics presuppose such high evidential standards that almost all psychological theories, including those we take for granted in our commonsense theorizing about human behavior, would fail to meet their requirements. Some argue that central parts of Freudian theory have been empirically confirmed by Freudian experimental studies; others appeal to recent work in biology, neuroscience, and linguistics; still others argue that newer versions of psychoanalytic theory, based partly on Freud's ideas and findings, have been empirically confirmed by recent scientific research.

On this question of exactly how much truth there is in Freud's work, some of the best arguments pro and con can be found in this volume (*see* Biology, and Psychoanalysis; Brain Science, and Psychoanalysis; Critique of Psychoanalysis; Dreaming, Theory of; Experimental Evidence, Freudian; Research on Psychoanalysis; Scientific Tests of Freud's Theories and Therapy; Sleep; and Slips, Theory of).

Freud's Influence

Suppose that Freud's theories fail to contain, as he put it, "a high degree of truth." If that were so, would that be a good reason not to read him? That depends partly on what happened after his theories entered the public domain. Some of his contemporaries, such as his friend

Wilhelm Fliess and his onetime follower Wilhelm Reich, introduced speculative theories, such as the theory of orgon energy, that were briefly taken seriously and then ignored; the effects of their theorizing quickly decayed and vanished. That clearly has not been the fate of Freudian theorizing.

Consider that even as late as approximately ten years ago, a survey of citation indexes concluded that of all the works that had ever been published, not counting the Bible, Freud's books and articles were still being cited more than those of any other author except for four people: Plato, Aristotle, Lenin, and Shakespeare (Friman et al., 1993). Pointing this out does not by itself explain why Freud's works are still worth contemplating, but if a high degree of truth is the only criterion, then why read Plato or Aristotle, or their philosophic successors such as Aquinas, Hume, Kant, Hegel, or Nietzsche? How many of *their* theories have been shown to be true? Very few. Yet if one wants to understand recent philosophic work, and the spillover effects into other disciplines, one cannot reasonably ignore all that has gone before on the grounds that the earlier philosophic theories are either untrue or unproven.

The same argument applies to Freud. A careful survey of twentieth-century intellectual developments will reveal the obvious marks of Freudian theorizing in art, literature, biography, history, cinema, psychiatry, clinical psychology, religion, anthropology, sociology, and, to a lesser degree, philosophy. Is there, in fact, any thinker of the last century whose intellectual influence was greater?

Central Characters

Not all that is of interest to Freud scholars directly concerns his theories or therapy. There is an intellectual drama that began early in the nineteenth century, if not before, with a cast of philosophers, psychologists, and others who thought deeply about many of the same problems that interested Freud and who developed theories in varying degrees similar to his theories. The work of some of these thinkers has been treated in recent decades, except by a few specialists, as if it had never come into being; it has been largely forgotten or ignored. How many of us have read the philosophic works of, say, Johann Herbart, who anticipated in great detail much of Freud's psychoanalytic theorizing? How many realize the degree to which Schopenhauer and Nietzsche, whose works are better known, anticipated Freud's theories not just in some vague fashion but in quite specif-

ic ways? The extent to which they influenced Freud is, of course, a separate issue (see the entries on each of these figures, and Nineteenth Century Philosophy Precursors of Freud: An Integrative Review).

Besides Freud's predecessors, there were his contemporaries and those who came to prominence after he died. Some who were in some way or other connected with psychoanalysis, such as Gustav Fechner, Havelock Ellis, and Richard von Krafft-Ebing, were not Freudians, but they made important intellectual contributions in their own right. Others, such as Alfred Adler, Carl Jung, and Wilhelm Reich, were psychoanalysts who clashed with Freud and who eventually started their own intellectual movements with their own followers. Some, such as Karl Abraham, Sándor Ferenczi, and Victor Tausk, remained loyal to Freud, and played an important part in the Freudian movement, while developing their own distinctive psychoanalytic theories, and others, such as Melanie Klein, Heinz Hartmann, and Jacques Lacan, moved Freudian theorizing in a very different direction, perhaps to a point where it ceased to be recognizably Freudian. All of these people and others played important roles in the psychoanalytic movement or in intellectual currents that ran counter to it.

Centers of Psychoanalysis

One can also think about psychoanalysis in terms not of specific people but of geographic locations. Freudianism originated in Vienna, but its influence spread after 1910 to other intellectual centers, such as Berlin, London, Paris, Oslo, and New York. In these cities and elsewhere, some of the great intellectual collisions of the twentieth century took place between psychoanalytic ideas and socialism, behaviorism, Marxism, fascism, and Catholicism, but collaborations also occurred as some thinkers tried to reduce Freud's ideas to those of Watson's or Pavlov's, or to blend them with Marxism, socialism, structuralism, phenomenology, hermeneutics, and various other theories.

The impact of the psychoanalytic movement has not been limited to Western Europe and the United States. Its influence may not have been as great in other locales, but it has still been significant in such countries as Argentina, Australia, Brazil, Chile, Poland, Hungary, and the Czech Republic. Many of the intellectual developments in these countries in the twentieth century were in some way or other connected with, or in opposition to, psychoanalysis. Much of the history of these developments has only recently become known outside of the countries where they occurred. Even less has been written about psychoanalytic developments in other regions. Yet, in varying degrees, Freud's ideas have also had an impact in Africa, Russia, Korea, Japan, India, China, the Philippines, and elsewhere, including Finland, Norway, the Netherlands, Sweden, Peru, Belgium, Venezuela, Italy, and Greece. Whether or not Freud's theories contain a high degree of truth, they have been intertwined, for better or worse, with much of the theorizing that has occurred around the world in the past one hundred years and more.

In this volume, references to Freud's works are generally to *The Standard Edition of the Complete Psychological Works of Sigmund Freud*, 24 volumes, James Strachey (Translator); London: Hogarth Press, 1953–1974. As Strachey points out in the General Preface to Volume

1 of the *Standard Edition*, there has been some confusion about the spelling of the technical Freudian term "phantasy." Some writers use Strachey's recommended spelling, "phantasy," but others prefer "fantasy." We have used both spellings, depending on the wishes of each author.

REFERENCES

E. Erwin (1996). *A Final Accounting: Philosophical and Empirical Issues in Freudian Psychology*. Cambridge, Mass.: Cambridge University Press.

Friman, P., Allen, K., Kerwin, M., and Larzelere, R. (1993). Changes in modern psychology. *American Psychologist*, 48: 658–664.

Grubrich-Simitis, I. (1995). "No greater, richer, more mysterious subject [. . .] than the life of the mind": An early exchange of letters between Freud and Einstein. *International Journal of Psycho-Analysis*, 76: 115–122.

EDWARD ERWIN

ACKNOWLEDGEMENTS

I would like to thank all of the members of my Advisory Board, especially Robert Holt, who was very helpful in many ways, as was Rosemarie Sand and Adolf Grünbaum.

I would also like to thank my Associate Editor, James Walkup, and a former Associate Editor, Michael Moskowitz, who were responsible for devising the structure of the encyclopedia and for useful suggestions about other matters. During the course of the project, graduate students in the philosophy department at the University of Miami worked for brief periods as editorial assistants. These include: Fredrick Altieri, David Anderson, Richard Billings, Robert Lane, Michael McCracken, Samantha Moody, Rick Morrell, Michael Shaffer, Matthew Schuh, Ansana Singh, and Lugan Yan. I would also like to thank present and former staff members of the philosophy department, including Jackie Binns, Alex Puentes, Bertha Danon, and Lianne Dookie, as well as my philosophical colleagues.

Were it not for the excellent analytical and editorial skills of Lowell Kleiman and Sidney Gendin, both co-editors and friends, the encyclopedia would have taken longer to complete and would have been a poorer product. The work of my editor at Routledge, Richard Steins, has been superb. I would also like to thank Gary Kuris, formerly of Garland Publishing, who began the project and invited me to serve as editor. I am grateful to Peter Swales, who gave me excellent advice about many matters.

It has been a pleasure to work with the more than two hundred Freud scholars who contributed essays. I thank them all.

Most of all I would like to thank Sidney Gendin for all he has done and for my wife Patricia Erwin, for her excellent advice and much else.

CONTRIBUTORS

D. Wilfred Abse
University of Virginia
(Conversion; Hysteria; Multiple Personality
[Dissociative Identity Disorder])

Salman Akhtar
Jefferson Medical College
Philadelphia, Pa.
(Psychoanalysis in India; Splitting of the Ego)

George H. Allison
Seattle Psychoanalytic Society and Institute, and
University of Washington
Seattle, Wash.
(United States and Psychoanalysis)

André Alsteens
Deceased
(Belgium, and Psychoanalysis)

George Awad
The Hospital for Sick Children
Toronto, Canada
(Canada, and Psychoanalysis; Rat Man; Wolf Man)

Christopher Badcock
London School of Economics
University of London
(Incest; Libido Theory; Sociobiology)

Eva Bänninger-Huber
University of Zurich
Zurich, Switzerland
(Envy; Guilt)

Francis Baudry
New York Psychoanalytic Institute
New York, N.Y.
(Character)

Brenda Bauer
Medical College of Wisconsin
Milwaukee, Wisc.
(Ego Psychology; Transference)

Martin S. Bergmann
New York University
(Kris, Ernst)

Emanuel Berman
University of Haifa
Haifa, Israel
(Dora)

Mark J. Blechner
William Alanson White Institute
New York
(Delusions; Hallucinations)

Geoffrey H. Blowers
University of Hong Kong
(China, and Psychoanalysis; Japan, and Psychoanalysis;
Korea, and Psychoanalysis; The Philippines, and
Psychoanalysis)

Philip K. Bock
The University of New Mexico
(Taboo)

Stanley Bone
Columbia University
(Paranoia)

Carlo Bonomi
University of Florence
Florence, Italy
(Baginsky, Adolf; Kassowitz Institute)

Jennifer M. Bonovitz
Philadelphia Psychoanalytic Institute
Philadelphia, Pa.
(Abstinence, Rule of; Agression)

Brigitte Boothe
University of Zurich
Zurich, Switzerland
(Oedipus Complex)

Miroslav Borecky
Prague, Czech Republic
(Czech Republic, and Psychoanalysis)

Robert Bornstein
Gettysburg College
Gettysburg, Pa.
(Free Association)

Ira Brenner
The Institute of Pennsylvania Hospital
Philadelphia, Pa.
(Dissociation)

Andrew Brook
Carleton University, Ottawa
Ontario, Canada
(Schopenhauer, Arthur)

Paul Brown
The Pierre Janet Centre
Melbourne, Australia
(Catharsis; Traumatic Neurosis; War Neurosis)

Vern L. Bullough
University of Southern California
(Sexology)

Daniel Burston
Duquesne University
Pittsburgh, Pa.
(Fromm, Erich)

L. S. Carrier
University of Miami
Coral Gables, Fla.
(Consciousness)

Allan Casebier
University of Miami
Coral Gables, Fla.
(Cinema, and Psychoanalysis)

Pietro Castelnuovo-Tedesco
Desceased
(Anna O.; Breuer, Josef; Psychoanalytic Movement;
Stekel, Wilhelm)

Marcia Cavell
Berkeley, Calif.
(Self-Deception; Irrationality)

Fidias R. Cesio
Buenos Aries, Argentina
(Argentina, and Psychoanalysis)

George L. Christie
Melbourne, Australia
(Jokes and Humor)

Aviva Cohen
Dublin City University
Dublin, Ireland
(Brentano, Franz)

Calvin A. Colarusso
University of California, San Diego
(Toilet Training)

Steven H. Cooper
Brookline, Mass.
(Conflict, Theory of)

Allan Compton
University of California, Los Angeles
(Anxiety and Defense; Structural Theory)

Christopher Cordess
The University of Sheffield
Sheffield, United Kingdom
(Criminality, and Psychoanalysis)

Phebe Cramer
Williams College
Williamstown, Mass.
(Denial; Projection)

Chiquit Crisanto-Estrada
Research Institute of Psychopathology
The Philippines
(The Philippines, and Psychoanalysis)

Karina Davidson
University of Alabama, Tuscaloosa
(Reaction Formation; Sublimation)

Giuseppe Di Chiara
Milan, Italy
(Italy, and Psychoanalysis)

Ilham Dilman
University of Wales, Swansea
Swansea, Wales
United Kingdom
(Infantile Sexuality)

Lance M. Dodes
Harvard Medical School
(Compulsion and Obsession)

Morris Eagle
Derner Institute of Advanced Psychological Studies
Adelphi University
Garden City, N.Y.
(Repression)

Alan Elms
University of California, Davis
(Biography, and Psychoanalysis)

Edward Erwin
University of Miami
Coral Gables, Fla.
(Castration Anxiety; Experimental Evidence, Freudian;
Fliess, Wilhelm; Free Will; The Id; Little Hans;
Meaning, and Psychoanalysis; Mind and Body;
Pseudoscience, and Psychoanalysis)

Philip J. Escoll
Philadelphia, Pa.
(Analyzability; Therapeutic Alliance)

Aaron H. Esman
Cornell University Medical College
New York, N.Y.
(Childhood Neurosis)

Allen Esterson
Southwark College
London, Great Britain
(Fantasy [Phantasy]; Seduction Theory)

John Farrell
Claremont McKenna College
Claremont, Calif.
(Literature, and Psychoanalysis)

John Fiscalini
New York University
(Sullivan, Harry Stack)

Seymour Fisher
Deceased
(Scientific Tests of Freud's Theories and Therapy)

David A. Freedman
Baylor College of Medicine (Emeritus)
Houston, Tex.
(Obsessional Phenomena)

Rhoda S. Frenkel
University of Texas Southwestern Medical Center
Dallas, Tex.
(Vaginal and Clitoral Orgasm)

Judith Kegan Gardiner
The University of Illinois at Chicago
(Feminism, and Psychoanalysis)

Sidney Gendin
Ann Arbor, Mich.
(Ellis, Havelock; Hartmann, Heinz; Kraft-Ebbing,
Richard)

Alfonso Gisbert S.
Caracas, Venezuela
(Venezuela, and Psychoanalysis)

Robert A. Glick
College of Physicians and Surgeons
Columbia University
(Pleasure Principle)

Clark Glymour
Carnegie Mellon University
Pittsburgh, Pa.
and University of California, San Diego
(Philosophy, and Psychoanalysis)

Jerrold R. Gold
Long Island University
Brooklyn, N.Y.
(Insight, Role of in Therapy)

Herbert L. Gomberg
Dallas, Tex.
(Self-Analysis)

Michael L. Good
Harvard Medical School
(Abraham, Karl)

George Graham
University of Alabama, Birmingham
(Behaviorism, and Psychoanalysis)

Roger P. Greenberg
State University of New York Health Science Center
Syracuse, N.Y.
(Scientific Tests of Freud's Theories and Therapy)

Joanne M. Greer
Loyola College in Maryland
Baltimore, Md.
(Return of the Repressed)

Alexander Grinstein
Wayne State University School of Medicine
Detroit, Mich.
(Symbolism)

Leendert F. Groenendijk
Vrije University
Amsterdam, The Netherlands
(Neurasthenia)

Han Groen-Prakken
Amsterdam, The Netherlands
(The Netherlands, and Psychoanalysis)

George E. Gross
New York Psychoanalytic Institute
New York, N.Y.
(Clinical Theory)

Lee Grossman
San Francisco Psychoanalytic Institute
San Francisco, Calif.
(Reality Testing)

Adolf Grünbaum
University of Pittsburgh
(Critique of Psychoanalysis)

Peter Hartocollis
University of Patras School of Medicine
Patras, Greece
(Greece, and Psychoanalysis)

Robert Hinshelwood
University of Essex
Colchester, Great Britain
(Klein, Melanie)

Axel Hoffer
Harvard Medical School
(Ferenczi, Sándor)

Leon Hoffman
New York Psychoanalytic Institute
(Adler, Alfred; Child Psychoanalysis)

Robert R. Holt
New York University (Emeritus)
(Metapsychology)

Deanna Holtzman
Wayne State University
Detroit, Mich.
(Virginity)

Philip S. Holzman
Harvard Medical School
(Psychopathology)

Thomas M. Horner
University of Michigan
(Symbiosis)

Athol Hughes
London, Great Britain
(Great Britain, and Psychoanalysis)

Juan Pablo Jiménez
University of Chile
Santiago, Chile
(Chile, and Psychoanalysis)

Per Magnus Johansson
Gothenburg University, Sweden
(Sweden, and Psychoanalysis)

Adrian Johnston
State University of New York at Stony Brook
(Lacan, Jacques)

David Joravsky
Northwestern University
Evanston, Ill.
(Russia, and Psychoanalysis)

Brett Kahr
Regent's College
London, Great Britain
(Bonaparte, Marie; Eitingon, Max; Family Romance;
Projective Techniques; Sachs, Hanns)

Betram P. Karon
Michigan State University
East Lansing, Mich.
(Schizophrenia)

William Kerrigan
University of Massachussetts
Amherst, Mass.
(Humanities, and Psychoanalysis)

Patricia Kitcher
Columbia University
(Cognitive Psychology, and Psychoanalysis)

Paul Kline
Deceased
(Defense Mechanisms)

Danielle Knafo
Long Island University
Brookville, N.Y.
(Creativity; Primal Scene)

Nathan M. Kravis
Cornell University Medical College
New York, N.Y.
(Identification)

Nancy Kulish
Wayne State University
Detroit, Mich.
(Virginity)

Edith Kurzweil
Boston University
(Eissler, Kurt; Reception of Freud's Ideas)

Peter Kutter
J. W. Goethe–University of Frankfurt on Main
Germany
(Germany, and Psychoanalysis)

Robert Langs
Mount Sinai School of Medicine
New York, N.Y.
(Biology, and Psychoanalysis)

Kim Larsen
University of Oslo
Oslo, Norway
(Tausk, Victor)

Richard Lasky
New York University
(Ego; Superego)

Ruth F. Lax
Cornell Medical School
(Character Neurosis)

Ronald Lehrer
Brooklyn College
City University of New York
(Nietzsche, Friedrich Wilhelm)

Mark Levey
Abraham Lincoln School of Medicine
University of Illinois
Chicago, Ill.
(Working Through)

Frederic J. Levine
University of Miami School of Medicine
Miami, Fla.
(Penis Envy)

Joseph E. Lifschutz
Oakland, Calif.
(Confidentiality)

Stephen W. Link
McMaster University
Hamilton
Ontario, Canada
(Fechner, Gustav Theodor)

Alexander C. Lo
Hong Kong Adventist Hospital
Hong Kong
(Suicide)

Karen L. Lombardi
Derner Institute of Advanced Psychological Studies
Adelphia University
Garden City, N.Y.
(Preconscious)

Zvi Lothane
Mount Sinai School of Medicine
New York, N.Y.
(Schreber, Daniel Paul)

Michael Wm. MacGregor
Dalhousie University
Halifax
Nova Scotia, Canada
(Reaction Formation; Sublimation)

Malcolm Macmillan
Monash University
Clayton
Victoria, Australia
(Charcot, Jean-Martin; Janet, Pierre)

Patrick Mahony
University of Montreal (Emeritus)
Quebec, Canada
(Goethe Prize)

Franklin G. Maleson
Philadelphia, Pa.
(Masochism and Sadism)

David W. Mann
Harvard Medical School
(Lay Analysis; Repetition Compulsion)

Ney Couto Marinho
Rio de Janeiro, Brazil
(Brazil, and Psychoanalysis)

Reginald T. Martin
Hunters Hill
New South Wales, Australia
(Australia, and Psychoanalysis)

Joseph Masling
State University of New York at Buffalo (Emeritus)
Buffalo, N.Y.
(Anal Character; Oral Character)

Edith R. McNutt
University of New Mexico School of Medicine
Alburquerque, N.M.
(Autonomy; Shame)

Purnima Mehta
Michigan Psychoanalytic Institute
(Anaclitic Object; Electra Complex)

William Meissner, S.J.
Boston College
(Religion, and Psychoanalysis)

Gerald A. Melchiode
Dallas Psychoanalytic Institute
Dallas, Tex.
(Neuroses)

Roy M. Mendelsohn
St. Louis, Mo.
(Acting Out)

Jon K. Meyer
Medical College of Wisconsin
Milwaukee, Wisc.
(Ego Psychology; Transference)

Burness E. Moore
Emory University School of Medicine (Emeritus)
(Narcissim)

Nancy K. Morrison
University of New Mexico School of Medicine
Albuquerque, N.M.
(Autonomy; Shame)

John Morton
La Trobe University
Bundoora
Victoria, Australia
(Myths)

Michael T. Motley
University of California, Davis
(Slips, Theory of)

Elke Mühlleitner
Gieben-Berlin, Germany
(Fenichel, Otto; Marxism, and Freudianism; Reich,
Wilhelm; Vienna, and Psychoanalysis; Wednesday
Society)

Jerome Neu
University of California, Santa Cruz
(Perversions)

Peter B. Neubauer
New York University
(Displacement)

Darius Ornston
School of Medicine
University of South Carolina
Greenville, S.C.
(Cathexis)

Henning Paikin
Copenhagen, Denmark
(Denmark, and Psychoanalysis)

Stanley R. Palombo
Washington, D.C.
(Dreams, The Theory of)

Bernard J. Paris
University of Florida (Emeritus)
Gainsville, Fla.
(Horney, Karen)

Karl Peltzer
University of the North
Sovenga, South Africa
(Africa, and Psychoanalysis)

Saúl Peña K
Lima, Peru
(Peru, and Psychoanalysis)

Mark F. Poster
Harvard Medical School
(Groddeck, Georg)

Karl Pribram
Stanford University (Emeritus)
(Project for a Scientific Psychology: Freud's Theory of
Neuronal Excitation, Conveyance, and Discharge)

John D. Rainer
Deceased
(Genetics, and Psychoanalysis)

Moss L. Rawn
New York Freudian Society
New York, N.Y.
(Education, and Analysts)

Johannes Reichmayr
University of Klagenfurt
Klagenfurt, Austria
(Africa, and Psychoanalysis; Fenichel, Otto; Marxism,
and Freudianism; Reich, Wilhelm; Vienna, and
Psychoanalysis; Wednesday Society)

Morton F. Reiser
Yale University
(Brain Science, and Psychoanalysis)

Joseph Reppen
Institute for Psychoanalytic Training and Research
New York, N.Y.
(Reik, Theodor)

Emanuel Rice
Mt. Sinai School of Medicine
New York, N.Y.
(Judaism, and Freud)

Arlene K. Richards
New York, N.Y.
(Psychoanalytic Technique and Process)

Arnold D. Richards
Journal of the American Psychoanalytic Association
(Editor) and the New York Psychoanalytic Institute
(Psychoanalytic Technique and Process)

Ana María Rizzuto
Brookline, Mass.
(Affect; Aphasia; Object)

Paul Roazen
Cambridge, Mass.
(Freud's Family; Glover, Edward; Pfister, Oskar)

Esa Roos
Helsinki, Finland
(Finland, and Psychoanalysis)

Gilbert J. Rose
Yale Medical School (Emeritus)
(Aesthetics, and Psychoanalysis)

Milton Rosenbaum
University of New Mexico School of Medicine
Albuquerque, N.M.
(Screen Memories)

Daria Rothe
Ann Arbor, Mich.
(Andreas-Salomé, Lou)

Elisabeth Roudinesco
University of Paris VII
Paris, France
(France, and Psychoanalysis)

Isaiah A. Rubin
New York Psychoanalytic Institute,
New York, N.Y.
(Clinical Theory)

Peter L. Rudnytsky
University of Florida
Gainsville, Fla.
(Freud, Sigmund; Rank, Otto)

Melvin Sabshin
University of Maryland School of Medicine
Baltimore, Md.
(Psychiatry, and Psychoanalysis)

Rosemarie Sand
Institute for Psychoanalytic Training and Research
White Plains, N.Y.
(Herbart, Johann)

Louis A. Sass
Rutgers University
(Modernism, Postmodernism, and Freudianism)

Janet Sayers
University of Kent at Canterbury
Kent, Great Britain
(Deutsch, Helene)

Jill Savege Scharff
International Institute of Object Relations Therapy
Chevy Chase, Md.
and Georgetown University
(Object Relations Theory)

Jean G. Schimek
Institute for Psychoanalytic Training and Research
New York, N.Y.
(Elizabeth von R.)

Herbert Schlesinger
New School for Social Research
New York, N.Y.
(Isolation; Intellectualization)

Clarence G. Schulz
Washington Psychoanalytic Institute
Towson, Md.
(Ambivalence)

Beth J. Seelig
Emory University School of Medicine
Atlanta, Ga.
(Psychoanalytically Oriented Psychotherapy)

Hanna Segal
London, Great Britain
(Kleinian Theory)

Sally K. Severino
University of New Mexico School of Medicine
Albuquerque, N.M.
(Autonomy; Shame)

Thedore Shapiro
Cornell University Medical Center
New York, N.Y.
(Developmental Theory; Research in Psychoanalysis)

Karl Sieg
Nova Southeastern University
Fort Lauderdale, Fla.
(Project for a Scientific Psychology: Freud's Theory of Neuronal Excitation, Conveyance, and Discharge)

Martin A. Silverman
New York University Medical Center
(Anxiety Neurosis)

Barry Silverstein
William Patterson University
Wayne, N.J.
(Psychoanalysis, Origin and History of)

David Livingstone Smith
University of New England
Biddeford, Maine
(Auto-Erotism; Binding; Existentialism; Genitality, Theories of; Occult, and Freud; Psychic Determinism; Suggestion; The Unconscious)

Charles W. Socarides
Albert Einstein College of Medicine/Montefiore Medical Center
New York, N.Y.
(Homosexuality, Psychoanalytic Theory of)

Mark Solms
St. Bartholomew's & Royal London School of Medicine
London, Great Britain
(Sleep)

Donald Spence
Robert Wood Johnson Medical School
New Brunswick, N.J.
(Interpretation)

Martha Stark
Boston Psychoanalytic Institute
(Resistance)

Jeff D. Stein
Derner Institute of Advanced Psychological Studies
Garden City, N.Y.
(Drive Theory)

Ricardo Steiner
London, Great Britain
(Jones, Ernest; Strachey, James)

Carlos Strenger
Tel-Aviv University
Israel
(Hermeneutics, and Psychoanalysis)

Jacques Szaluta
U.S. Merchant Marine Academy
Kings Point, N.Y.
(Psychohistory)

Eugene Taylor
Harvard University
(Jung, Carl)

Michael A. Teixeira
Michigan State University
East Lansing, Mich.
(Schizophrenia)

David Titelman
Karolinska Institutet
Stockholm, Sweden
(Sweden, and Psychoanalysis)

Saul Tuttman
Albert Einstein College of Medicine
New York, N.Y.
(Regression)

Onno van der Hart
Utrecht University
Utrecht, The Netherlands
(Abreaction; Traumatic Neurosis; War Neurosis)

Sverre Varvin
Norwegian Psychoanalytic Institute
Oslo, Norway
(Norway, and Psychoanalysis)

Fernando Vidal
Max Planck Institute for the History of Science
(Piaget, Jean; Spielrein, Sabina)

Jaime F. Ayala Villarreal
México D.F., Mexico
(Mexico, and Psychoanalysis)

Edwin R. Wallace, IV
University of South Carolina
Columbia, S.C.
(Anthropology, and Psychoanalysis)

Ernest Wallwork
Syracuse University
Syracuse, N.Y.
(Ethics, Clinical; Morality, and Psychoanalysis)

Joel Weinberger
Derner Institute of Advanced Psychological Studies
Adelphi University
Garden City, N.Y.
(Drive Theory)

David S. Werman
Duke University (Emeritus)
Durham, N.C.
(Depression)

Christine Widmer
University of Zurich
Zurich, Switzerland
(Envy; Guilt)

Gerhard Wittenberger
Kasseler Psychoanalytic Institute
Kassel, Germany
(Committee, The Secret)

Ernest S. Wolf
Northwestern University Medical School
(Self Psychology)

Christopher Young
Cornell University
Ithaca, N.Y.
(Schopenhauer, Arthur)

Elisabeth Young-Bruehl
New York, N.Y.
(Freud, Anna)

Emily Zakin
Miami University
Oxford, Ohio
(Overdetermination)

Marcel R. Zentner
University of Geneva
Geneva, Switzerland
(Nineteenth-Century Precursor's of Freud)

Abraham, Karl (1877-1925)

The first German to practice psychoanalysis and the founder of the Berlin Psychoanalytic Society, Karl Abraham was one of the earliest and most loyal of Freud's adherents. Considered by many to be second only to Freud in the history of the psychoanalytic movement, he made a number of original contributions to psychoanalytic thinking.

Family and Early Life

The second of two sons, Karl Abraham was born into an established but not well-to-do Orthodox Jewish family in Bremen, Germany, on May 3, 1877—three days short of twenty-one years after Freud's birth. His father, Nathan Abraham (1842–1915), a teacher of Jewish religion and law, in 1873 opened a wholesale drapery business in order to earn enough to marry (Hartman, 1976). His mother, Ida (née Oppenheimer), and his father were first cousins. According to his daughter, Hilda Abraham, there probably were other intermarriages in the family, and she concluded that Abraham's papers "The Significance of Intermarriage Between Close Relatives" (1909a) and "On Neurotic Exogamy" (1913b) are partly autobiographical.

Abraham showed an early interest in, and talent for, languages. However, when the time came to consider schooling beyond the *Gymnasium*, he was urged to study for a career in dentistry (which did not require university training). Instead, he agreed to study dental medicine, which did require a university degree. In 1895 he entered the University of Würzburg, but after one semester he switched to medical studies, which he pursued in Berlin and Freiburg im Breisgau. In Berlin, Abraham met his future wife, Hedwig Burgner (b. 1878), who shared his interest in languages. They were married January 23, 1906, while Abraham was working in Zurich. They had a daughter, Hilda (1906–1971), who edited and translated her father's works, and was a physician and training psychoanalyst in the British Psychoanalytical Society. A son was born in 1910.

Career

Abraham received his M.D. degree in June 1901. Because of emphysema, he was excused from military service. He took a position under Wilhelm Liepmann at the Berlin municipal mental hospital at Dalldorf, but he did not care for the neuropathological approach used there. He resigned in the spring of 1904, hoping to work at the Burghölzli Mental Hospital in Zurich, under Eugen Bleuler and Carl Jung. On December 8, 1904, Abraham was appointed to a position at Burghölzli, where Jung introduced him to Freud's work. Abraham studied the works of Freud and began corresponding with him in the late spring of 1907. By October 1907, his hope of promotion in Zurich had not been fulfilled, so Abraham moved to Berlin, where he began a practice in psychiatry and psychoanalysis. His first meeting with Freud took place in Vienna in December 1907 (Hartman, 1976). Their psychoanalytic relationship and friendship lasted for eighteen years.

For a number of years, Abraham was the only psychoanalyst in Berlin. He held weekly meetings in his home for those interested in psychoanalysis, like the Wednesday night meetings in Vienna. This Berlin group became the Berlin Psychoanalytic Society in 1910, and was the first group to join the International Psychoanalytic Association (IPA). Following Jung's resignation,

Abraham became the acting president (1914–1918) of the IPA, and he was elected president in 1924 and 1925.

Following the outbreak of World War I, Abraham was drafted and made a surgeon, serving initially near Berlin and then at Allenstein, East Prussia, in 1915. In 1916 he was able to form a military psychiatric unit, which made possible his contributions to the study of war neurosis (Abraham, 1921).

After World War I, Abraham was active in organizing the first psychoanalytic training institute, which opened on February 14, 1920, as the Berlin Polyclinic and was renamed the Berlin Institute in 1924. Max Eitingon was a financial backer and administrator of the new training facility, and Hanns Sachs was the first training analyst (Hartman, 1976).

Although Abraham himself was not analyzed (H. Abraham, 1974), he analyzed a number of eminent psychoanalysts, including Helene Deutsch, Robert Fliess, Edward Glover, Karen Horney, Melanie Klein, Theodor Reik, Sándor Radó, Ella Freeman Sharpe, and Alix Strachey (Falzeder, 1994).

Abraham's Ideas

Abraham was an early, energetic, and enthusiastic adherent of Freud and the evolving theories of psychoanalysis. He had an interest in embryology, neurology, and development, and, like Freud, had written on aphasia. Even after Freud had turned his attention away from the seduction theory of neurosogenesis, Abraham sought to investigate child sexual trauma further. Abraham initially agreed that the roots of hysterical symptoms lay in constitutional factors. He tried to demonstrate that infantile sexual trauma is not so much the cause of hysteria and dementia praecox as a determinant of the form of the disorders and the content of the patient's ideation. Even though Abraham's career revealed his capacity for deep psychological insights, his early emphasis on constitution exemplified the strong biological perspective in his education and training that he shared with Freud (Good, 1995).

In 1907, Abraham published his first psychoanalytic papers, "On the Significance of Sexual Trauma in Childhood for the Symptomatology of Dementia Praecox" and "The Experiencing of Sexual Traumas as a Form of Sexual Activity" (Abraham, 1907a, 1907b). In these two articles, among the very first articles on child sexual molestation, Abraham proposed that sexual abuse was particularly common among neurotic and psychotic patients as a result of what he termed a "traumatophilic diathesis," a tendency to repeat traumatic experiences. This concept anticipated Freud's pivotal concept of the repetition compulsion, a principle Freud did not introduce as such until 1914, in "Remembering, Repeating, and Working-Through" (Freud, 1914), and developed more fully in "Beyond the Pleasure Principle" (Freud, 1920).

Although Abraham was extensively occupied with his psychoanalytic activities in Berlin and with his military service in World War I, he managed to publish over two dozen more articles between 1907 and 1920, none of which addressed the seduction issue more extensively. A partial exception is an unpublished paper, "Incest and Incest Fantasies in Neurotic Families. Case Contributions Concerning Actual Sexual Relations Within Neurotic Families and Symptoms of Illness Based on Incest Fantasies," delivered at Berlin in 1910. It was a timely title on the fantasy-versus-reality issue, but unfortunately the paper apparently was lost (Simon, 1992; Good, 1995).

Abraham's published papers are in his *Selected Papers* (1927a/1979) and *Clinical Papers and Essays on Psycho-Analysis* (1927b/1955). Although he wrote some papers on technique (e.g., "Should Patients Write Down Their Dreams?" [1913a]), he is best known clinically for his writings on pregenital phases of development (especially the oral stage), his early contributions to the topic of manic-depression and other psychoses (e.g., paranoia), and his linking of developmental phases to character formation. He divided the oral stage into sucking and biting phases, the anal stage into destructive-expulsive and mastering-retaining phases, and the phallic period into early and mature stages. He was the first psychoanalyst to study manic-depressive illness.

In his writings, Freud made many references to Abraham's contributions, citing the influence of Abraham on his own ideas on several occasions. Interesting exceptions to Freud's acknowledging Abraham's work include Abraham's 1912 paper on Amenhotep IV, in which some of Freud's conclusions about Moses and monotheism are prefigured (Shengold, 1993, pp. 62–65; Good, 1995), and the influence of Abraham's traumatophilic diathesis on Freud's conception of the repetition compulsion (Good, 1995).

According to his daughter (H. Abraham, 1974), herself a physician and psychoanalyst, Abraham sublimated a good deal through his psychoanalytic writings. For him the mark of maturity was overcoming ambivalence, thus making reaction formation unnecessary and increasing the capacity for sublimation (Grotjahn, 1966). He was quite inclined to write about theoretical matters undisguisedly derived from his own family experience, for example, his papers on intermarriage (1909a) and on neurotic exogamy (1913b). Similarly, his seemingly repressed opposition to paternal authority in the person of Freud, who apparently resembled Abraham's father (H. Abraham, 1974, p. 20), may have found partial, sublimated expression in his writing on Prometheus in "Dreams and Myths" (1909b) and Amenhotep IV (1912).

Although Abraham was one of Freud's most gifted and favorite pupils, and among the staunchest of his supporters, he was not an idolater. Freud sometimes found Abraham "too Prussian" (Jones, 1955, p. 159; Gay, 1988, p. 461). Abraham disagreed with the master, for example, in supporting the idea of a film on psychoanalysis (Good, 1995). On theoretical matters, however, Abraham apparently did not differ with Freud. Near the end of his life, he remarked that the only differences he had with Freud pertained to judgments of personality (e.g., regarding Abraham's view of the situation between Jung and Freud) (H. Abraham and E. L. Freud, 1965).

Illness and Death

In May 1925, Abraham apparently choked on a fish bone, and it lodged in his lung. It caused a pulmonary abscess, septic bronchopneumonia, and a terminal subphrenic abscess from which he died on December 25, 1925 (H. Abraham and E. L. Freud, 1965, p. 382; Hartman, 1976; Roazen and Swerdloff, 1995). Some believe that he may have had lung cancer (Schur, 1972). Freud was deeply upset at the loss of his devoted friend and colleague (S. Freud, 1926; H. Abraham and E. L. Freud, 1965, pp. 399–400; Jones, 1926). Abraham's mother, wife, and children fled from the Nazis. His brother, Max, and his wife died in Poland in the Holocaust (Hartman, 1976).

REFERENCES

Abraham, H. C. (1974). Karl Abraham: An unfinished biography. *International Review of Psychoanalysis* 1: 17–72.

Abraham, H. C., and Freud, E. L. (eds.). (1965). *A Psycho-Analytic Dialogue: The Letters of Sigmund Freud and Karl Abraham*. New York: Basic Books.

Abraham, K. (1907a). On the significance of sexual trauma in childhood for the symptomatology of dementia praecox. In his *Clinical Papers and Essays on Psycho-Analysis*. New York: Basic Books, 1955, pp. 13–20.

———. (1907b). The experiencing of sexual traumas as a form of sexual activity. In *Selected Papers of Karl Abraham*. New York: Brunner/Mazel, 1979, pp. 47–63. (Reprint of 1927 edition published by Hogarth Press.)

———. (1909a). The significance of intermarriage between close relatives in the psychology of the neuroses. In his *Clinical Papers and Essays on Psycho-Analysis*. New York: Basic Books, 1955, pp. 21–28.

———. (1909b). Dreams and myths. IV. The analysis of the Prometheus myth. In his *Clinical Papers and Essays on Psycho-Analysis*. New York: Basic Books, 1955, pp. 172–176.

———. (1912). Amenhotep IV: A psycho-analytical contribution towards the understanding of his personality and of the monotheistic cult of Aton. In his *Clinical Papers and Essays on Psycho-Analysis*. New York: Basic Books, 1955, pp. 262–290.

———. (1913a). Should patients write down their dreams? In his *Clinical Papers and Essays on Psycho-Analysis*. New York: Basic Books, 1955, pp. 33–35.

———. (1913b). On neurotic exogamy: A contribution to the similarities in the psychic life of neurotics and of primitive man. In his *Clinical Papers and Essays on Psycho-Analysis*. New York: Basic Books, 1955, pp. 48–50.

———. (1921). Psycho-analysis and the war neuroses. In his *Clinical Papers and Essays on Psycho-Analysis*. New York: Basic Books, 1955, pp. 59–67.

———. (1927a). *Selected Papers of Karl Abraham, M.D.* London: Hogarth Press and the Institute of Psycho-analysis. 2nd ed., New York: Brunner/Mazel, 1979.

———. (1927b). *Clinical Papers and Essays on Psycho-Analysis*. New York: Basic Books, 1955.

Decke, B. (1997). Karl Abraham: Familie, kindheit und jugend in Bremen. *Zeitschrift zur Geschichte der Psychoanalyse* 10: 7–63.

Falzeder, E. (1994). The threads of psychoanalytic filiations or psychoanalysis taking effect. *Cahiers Psychiatriques Genevois* spec. iss., pp. 169–194.

———. (ed.). (2000). *The Complete Correspondence of Sigmund Freud and Karl Abraham*. Translated by C. Schwarzacher and C. Trollope. London: Karnac.

Freud, S. (1914). *Remembering, Repeating, and Working-Through*. S.E. 12: 145–156.

———. (1920). *Beyond the Pleasure Principle*. S.E. 18: 1–64.

———. (1926). Karl Abraham. S.E. 20: 277–278.

Gay, P. (1988). *Freud: A Life for Our Time*. New York: Norton.

Good, M. I. (1995) Karl Abraham, Sigmund Freud, and the fate of the seduction theory. *Journal of the American Psychoanalytic Association* 43: 1137–1167.

Grosskurth, P. (1991). *The Secret Ring: Freud's Inner Circle and the Politics of Psychoanalysis*. Reading, Mass.: Addison-Wesley.

Grotjahn, M. (1968). Karl Abraham, the first German psychoanalyst. In F. Alexander, S. Eisenstein, and M. Grotjahn (eds.), *Psychoanalytic Pioneers*. New York: Basic Books, pp. 1–13.

A

Hartman, F. R. (1976). Biographical sketches: Karl Abraham (1877–1925). In M. S. Bermann and F. R. Hartman (eds.), *The Evolution of Psychoanalytic Technique.* New York: Columbia University Press, pp. 42–45.

Jones, E. (1926). Karl Abraham, 1877–1925. *International Journal of Psycho-analysis.* 7: 155–189.

Pines, N. (1972). Hilda Abraham (1906–1971). *International Journal of Psycho-analysis.* 53: 331.

Roazen, P., and Swerdloff, B. (1995). Abraham's death. In P. Roazen and B. Swerdloff, *Heresy: Sandor Rado and the Psychoanalytic Movement.* Northvale, N.J.: Jason Aronson, pp. 87–95.

Schur, M. (1972). *Freud: Living and Dying.* New York: International Universities Press.

Shengold, L. (1993). Fliess, Karl Abraham, and Freud. In L. Shengold, *The Boy Will Come to Nothing! Freud's Ego Ideal and Freud as Ego Ideal.* New Haven, Conn.: Yale University Press, pp. 59–94.

Simon, B. (1992). Incest—see under Oedipus complex: The history of an error in psychoanalysis. *Journal of the American Psychoanalytic Association* 40: 955–988.

MICHAEL I. GOOD

Abreaction

Abreaction is an emotional release or discharge after recalling a painful experience that had been repressed because it was consciously intolerable. A therapeutic effect sometimes occurs through partial discharge or desensitization of the painful emotions and increased insight (American Psychiatric Association, 1980, p. 1).

This definition reflects Josef Breuer and Freud's (1893–1895) original view of abreaction, developed with regard to Breuer's treatment of Anna O. On this view, the discharge of excess emotional excitation developed during traumatic experiences is the essential ingredient in the treatment of hysteria. However, it has been noted that Breuer's view was actually one of "talking things out" rather than ventilating emotions per se (Brown et al., 1998).

Freud (1892) explained the effect of abreaction by referring to the quasi-neurological principle of constancy, according to which excessive buildup of post-traumatic emotional excitation is discharged and returns the organism to an appropriate emotional balance point. When Freud, in "Beyond the Pleasure Principle" (1920), reconsidered the constancy principle, he argued that affects owe their etiological importance to the concomitant production of large quantities of excitation, which in turn call for discharge. Traumatic experiences become pathogenic when they produce large quantities of exci-

tation beyond a normal coping capacity. Treatment of traumatic memories by abreaction (i.e., the cathartic method) is based upon this more fundamental principle of constancy.

It should be noted that in addition to abreaction, Breuer and Freud originally advocated the principle of therapeutic integration. This was alluded to in Freud's statement: "If we can succeed in bringing such a memory entirely into normal consciousness, it ceases to be capable of producing attacks" (1892, p. 151). However, the final abreactive model, widely used in the treatment of war neuroses during World Wars I and II, regarded the release of pent-up emotions as essential to the resolution of trauma-related symptoms (Brown et al., 1998; Van der Hart and Brown, 1992). In the early 1920s, this approach was the subject of a major professional debate in the *British Journal of Medical Psychology.* The British psychiatrist William Brown advocated emotional discharge, whereas his colleagues Charles Myers and William McDougall, as well as Carl Jung, emphasized "reintegration" of traumatic memories (i.e., a dissociation-integration rather than a repression-abreaction model of treatment). McDougall remarked that the emphasis on emotional expression had, in many cases, resulted in an increase, rather than relief, of symptoms.

In recent years, the consensus among experts treating traumatized patients is reflected in phase-oriented therapeutic approaches. Treatment consists of (1) emotional (or psychological) stabilization and symptom reduction, (2) assimilation of traumatic memories, and (3) personality reintegration and rehabilitation. The emphasis is on integration of emotional, cognitive, and sensory aspects of traumatic memories, not on emotional discharge per se. Thus, the majority no longer rely on the concept of abreaction. Nevertheless, a minority still uses the concept (e.g., when referring to "spontaneous abreactions" as flashback experiences, or "controlled or planned abreactions" as controlled therapeutic reactivation aimed at mastery and integration). By way of contrast, during the second treatment phase, the majority aim for integration rather than an emotional release of traumatic material into personal consciousness (Brown et al., 1997).

REFERENCES

American Psychiatric Association. (1980). *A Psychiatric Glossary.* 5th ed. Washington, D.C.: APA.

Breuer, J., and Freud, S. (1893–1895). *Studies on Hysteria.* S.E. 2.

Brown, D., Scheflin, A. W., and Hammond, D. C. (1998). *Memory, Trauma Treatment, and the Law.* New York: Norton.

Brown, P., Macmillan, M. B., Meares, R., and Van der Hart, O. (1996). Janet and Freud: Revealing the roots of dynamic psychiatry. *Australian and New Zealand Journal of Psychiatry* 30: 480–491.

Freud, S. (1892) Sketches for the 'Preliminary communication' of 1893 (1940–41 [1892]). S.E. 1: 147–151.

———. (1920). *Beyond the Pleasure Principle.* S.E. 18: 7–64.

Van der Hart, O., and P. Brown (1992). Abreaction re-evaluated. *Dissociation* 5: 127-140.

ONNO VAN DER HART

Abstinence, Rule of

Freud first mentioned the rule of abstinence in his technique paper "Observations on Transference Love" (1915). He noted that the phenomenon of the woman patient falling in love with her doctor occurs without fail, and urged that the analyst recognize that this phenomenon is induced by the analytic situation, and must not be attributed to his personal charms. The patient's love is an expression of resistance and has to be analyzed.

Posing the question "But how is the analyst to behave in order not to come to grief over this situation?," Freud replied that the treatment must be carried out in abstinence (1915, p. 165). Correct analytic technique requires that the doctor both deny satisfaction of the patient's cravings and at the same time allow them to persist so as to bring into consciousness what has been deeply hidden in the patient's erotic life. Only then may she know, and bring under her control, the infantile roots of her love and the fantasies wound around it.

Freud noted that the analytic approach to transference love has no model in real life. The patient in love with her doctor lacks regard for reality, and has little concern about the untoward consequences either for her or for the object of her love; the responsibility for abstaining from gratification lies solely with the analyst. It is in part from his example that the patient learns to "give up a satisfaction which lies at hand" (1915, p. 170), in favor of a future satisfaction in her love life outside of the analytic situation. Freud did not address the issue of transference love between the male patient and the female analyst.

In this same paper (1915), Freud wrote that the fundamental principle of the treatment being carried out in abstinence extends far beyond the case of transference love. He elucidated this statement in his Budapest Congress paper (1919), in which he related the principle of abstinence to his theory of pathogenesis and cure. He reminded the reader that it was a frustration of instinctual wishes that made the patient ill, and that neurotic symptoms serve as substitutive satisfactions. The treatment is in danger of achieving only insignificant or temporary changes if the patient's suffering ends prematurely with symptom relief, thus removing motivation for deeper analytic work. The analyst is charged with the task of first detecting these new substitutive satisfactions, whatever diverse forms they may take, and then requiring the patient to relinquish them. Freud gave as an example the patient's premature attachment to a marriage partner resulting in an unhappy marriage, which will then serve to gratify the unconscious need for punishment for the imagined transgressions of infantile libidinal life.

In particular the patient will seek substitutive gratifications in the transference relationship with the analyst. Freud acknowledged that it is necessary at times, depending upon the patient, to make some concessions, but he warned against the error of giving too much. He cited the example of nonanalytic institutions which go out of their way to make everything pleasant for the patient, but in doing so fail in the task of increasing the capacities to deal with the exigencies of everyday life. Again the path the analyst must take, in the interests of helping the patient, is to abstain from "all such spoiling." Indeed, the patient "must be left with unfulfilled wishes in abundance" (1919, p. 164), so that the energy required to conduct a more thorough analytic treatment is not dissipated.

It should be noted that Freud's written words on the subject of abstinence do not coincide with what he did in his clinical practice. Contemporary analysts tend to agree that wishes that are derivatives of the libidinal and aggressive drives should not be gratified. Gratification of other motivational factors, however, such as the need for object relatedness, is not only permitted but regarded as essential to the therapeutic process.

REFERENCES

Freud, S. (1915). Observations on transference love. S.E. 14: 163–170.

———. (1919). Advances in psychoanalytic therapy. S.E. 17: 162–164.

JENNIFER BONOVITZ

A

Acting Out

The concept of acting out has undergone considerable revision since it was first formulated by Freud (1914). Acting out was originally conceived of as the patient not remembering what had been repressed but "reproducing" the memory by acting it out; acting out was thus equated with transference behavior, which was also a repetition. The greater the resistance, the more extensively acting out would replace remembering.

Gradually the concept was expanded to encompass a wide variety of behaviors, with a subtle shift in emphasis being placed on unconscious conflicts and hidden messages contained in the behaviors, as well as their communicative aspects. By virtue of keeping these communicative functions clearly in mind, the specific characteristics of actions associated with acting out could be determined with greater discrimination (Robertiello, 1965; Rexford, 1966).

Widening the concept of acting out, however, created confusion as to how it should be defined, and consequently how manifestations of acting out could be understood and responded to therapeutically (A. Freud, 1971; Rangell, 1968; Boesky, 1982). The underlying psychic structure of any given behavior had to be identified as clearly as possible, for there were differing implications as to how therapeutic influence could be effective.

When acting out is functioning as a defense against recalling painful memories, as is often the case in the neurotically structured personality, the therapeutic task involves the use of interpretive interventions to call attention to and to elicit what has remained repressed. When acting out is primarily a way of communicating psychic contents having no other avenue of expression, as is often the case in a narcissistically structured personality where infantile trauma is a major factor in the pathology, the initial focus is on translating the unconscious communication embedded in the particular behavior. Afterward, whatever is required to enhance symbolization and verbalization can be offered. When acting out is a reflection of a developmental deficit, arrest, or gap in psychic functioning, usually created by early preverbal traumas, an opportunity must be presented for achieving new solutions to impossible infantile dilemmas accompanied by reconstructions of the original events. This may include modifications in the conditions of the treatment until interpretive interventions can be reestablished as the primary therapeutic instrument (Mendelsohn, 1991).

In addition, acting out may be instigated by, and mirror, a therapist's pathological attributes or lapses in empathy. In this case, it can be received as necessary information, aiding the therapist in the process of self-examination when exploring the source of any obstacle to therapeutic progress. The identification of a counter-transference-based barrier is the first step toward alleviating the problem, leading to its correction and an interpretation of its specific effects. Similarly, acting out may be a response to a therapist's colluding with a patient's pathological defenses, carrying with it the potential for unearthing just how this misalliance has taken place. A disruptive experience can then be turned to therapeutic advantage.

The increasing realization that preverbal experiences are in fact capable of being revived through the vehicle of transference has opened the door to recognizing their manifestations, primarily in behavior (Loewald, 1970). Along with this development, controversy has emerged as to whether interventions can reverse the harmful impact of these previously inarticulatable mental impressions (A. Freud, 1971). This controversy about whether the disturbances are reversible, or reflect the bedrock beyond which no therapeutic influence can be brought, is ongoing (Freedman, 1981).

There is also uncertainty as to how much and in what ways the treatment must be modified. Some clinicians advocate a rigorous handling of the transference in a secure treatment framework, believing that the pressure exerted to alter these conditions must be interpreted (Loewald, 1960; Bott-Spillius, 1983). They believe it possible to analyze these early conflicts without resorting to active therapy or controlled regression. Others consider these early conflicts to be analyzable only by changing the technique, using concrete experiences of involvement to replace interpretations as the primary therapeutic instrument (Winnicott, 1963; Balint, 1968; Gedo, 1984). These clinicians believe that serious failures in early development demand technical changes because only concrete experiences can alleviate them. Interpretations, being symbolic acts, can never reach what has not been symbolized.

Both approaches appear to have validity, since a firm therapeutic framework is essential for any treatment and the conditions must be flexible enough not to limit the range of regressive experiences that can be expressed. However, an exclusively interpretive mode of communication assumes that all regressive reenactments are capable of being represented, and that words can be utilized constructively (Kinston and Coen, 1986).

Thus, when preverbal traumas are embedded in unconscious wishes, any modification would serve only to strengthen repressive forces, and work in opposition to their integration. Furthermore, if psychic contents are transformed into actions to avoid remembering, to gain the therapist's participation in living out an unconscious fantasy, or to reinforce a pathological defense, containing influences of a well-managed treatment framework are required if the meaning of the behavior is to be understood well enough to offer appropriate interpretations. Yet the therapeutic relationship must also have room for creative, noninterpretive interventions when they are called for. In most instances, these would involve preverbal experiences requiring unique conditions in order to be reenacted.

REFERENCES

Balint, M. (1968). *The Basic Fault: Therapeutic Aspects of Regression.* London: Tavistock.

Boesky, D. (1982). Acting out: A reconsideration of the concept. *International Journal of Psycho-analysis* 63: 39–55.

Bott-Spillius, E. (1983). Some developments from the work of Melanie Klein. *International Journal of Psycho-analysis* 64: 321–332.

Freedman, D. A. (1981). The effect of sensory and other deficits in children on their experiences with people. *Journal of the American Psychoanalytic Association* 24: 831–867.

Freud, A. (1971). *The Writings of Anna Freud,* vol. III, pp. 124–156. New York: International Universities Press.

Freud, S. (1914). Remembering, repeating, and working through. S.E. 12: 145–156.

Gedo, J. (1984). *Psychoanalysis and Its Discontents.* New York: Guilford.

Kinston, W., and Coen, J. (1986). Primal repression: Clinical and theoretical aspects. *International Journal of Psycho-analysis* 67: 337–355.

Loewald, H. (1960). The therapeutic action of psychoanalysis. *International Journal of Psycho-analysis* 41: 16–33.

———. (1970). Psychoanalytic theory and the psychoanalytic process. *Psychoanalytic Study of the Child* 25: 45–67.

Mendelsohn, R. (1991). *Leaps: Facing Risks in Offering a Constructive Therapeutic Response When Unusual Measures Are Necessary.* Northvale, N.J.: Jason Aronson.

Rangell, L. (1968). Symposium: A point of view on acting out. *International Journal of Psycho-analysis* 49: 195–201.

Rexford, E. (1966). *A Developmental Approach to Problems of Acting Out.* New York: International Universities Press.

Robertiello, R. C. (1965). "Acting out" or "working through." In L. E. Abt and S. L. Weissman (eds.), *Acting Out,* New York: Grune and Stratton, pp. 247–274.

Winnicott, D. W. (1963). Dependence in infant-care, in child care, and in the psychoanalytic setting. In *The Maturational Process and the Facilitating Environment.* London: Hogarth Press, 1965, pp. 83–92.

ROY M. MENDELSOHN

Actual Neurosis See NEURASTHENIA; NEUROSES.

Adler, Alfred (1870–1937)

Alfred Adler was renowned for his individual psychology, a socially oriented theory of personality development and a system of psychotherapy in which a person strove to overcome a sense of inferiority. He became a frequent public speaker and prolific writer for the general public.

Understanding of the significance of Adler to psychoanalysis and his unacknowledged significant influence on the development of psychoanalytic theory comes through close examination of his interactions with Freud, fourteen years his senior. Freud invited him to join the Vienna Psychoanalytic Society in 1902; Adler separated from him in 1911.

In "On The History of the Psychoanalytic Movement" (1914), in the midst of a devastating polemic against Adler's and Carl Jung's attempts to diminish the centrality of infantile sexuality, Freud states: "Adler's investigation brought us something new to psychoanalysis—a contribution to the psychology of the ego— and then expected us to pay too high a price for this gift . . . so in the same way Jung and his followers paved the way for their fight against psychoanalysis by presenting it with a new acquisition. They traced in detail (as Pfister did before them) the way in which material of sexual ideas belonging to the family-complex and incestuous object-choice is made use of in representing highest ethical and religious interests of man" (1914, p. 61).

Adler essentially focused on the impact of external factors on the individual, and Jung, on a monistic, nonsexual libido. In his attempts to confront and rebut their challenges, Freud incorporated some of their ideas into his intrapsychic tripartite model. Greenberg and Mitchell state that Freud's responses to Adler's and Jung's dissents led to major revisions which advanced the original psychoanalytic model generating "a richer, more textured view of the nature of human experience" (1983, pp. 51–52). This textured richness contrasted with Adler's and Jung's theories, which would have led to a premature closure of understanding (Andreas-Salomé, 1964).

The debate between Freud and Adler and Jung has been repeated in various incarnations throughout the last eight decades of the twentieth century. A recent version of the debate involves so-called modern conflict theorists and relational analysts. In the current debate, the relational theorists, like Adler, relegate the role of infantile sexuality to a subsidiary position, and consider interactions with the external objects to be the primary motivators for mental development. For example, Greenberg and Mitchell, in discussing what they consider to be a new psychoanalytic paradigm, describe a strategy in which "relations with others constitute the fundamental building blocks of mental life. The creation, or re-creation, of specific modes of relatedness with others replaces drive discharge as the force motivating human behavior" (1983, p. 3).

Adler's earliest theoretical ideas are dramatically similar to subsequent theories which stress the primacy of interpersonal relationships, to the exclusion of sexual and aggressive drives, in human development. In 1924, Adler stated: "Individual Psychology has brought evidence to show that the line of movement of human striving originates in the blending of social interest with the striving for personal superiority. Both basic factors appear to be social formulations: the first [social interest], is innate and strengthens human society; the second, the product of education, is an obvious general temptation which constantly endeavors to exploit society for one own's prestige" (Ansbacher and Ansbacher, 1956, pp. 144–145).

Although Adler is an acknowledged forerunner of relational theoreticians, the centrality of his contribution does not seem to have been sufficiently appreciated. Some have observed that Karen Horney, Erich Fromm, Harry Stack Sullivan, Clara Thompson, and other so-called neo-Freudians should have been called neo-Adlerians because they were indebted to Adler "for his keen awareness of the reality of the influence of the total environment upon personality" (Ansbacher and Ansbacher, 1956, p. 17). In 1933, Adler himself complained that "today everyone speaks of community and social interest. We are not the very first, but we are the first to have strongly emphasized the basic nature of social interest" (Ansbacher and Ansbacher, 1956, p. 140).

Freud was both critical and admiring of Adler: "I do not consider these Adlerian doctrines insignificant and would like to predict that they will make a great impression, at first damaging psychoanalysis very much. The great impression has two sources: (1) it is obvious that a remarkable intellect with a great talent for writing is working on these matters, (2) the whole doctrine . . . instead of [dealing with] the psychology of the unconscious it concerns surface phenomena, that is, ego psychology. Finally, it deals with general psychology rather than the psychology of libido—sexuality. . . . It is ego psychology deepened by knowledge of the psychology of the unconscious. Therein lies the strength and weakness of Adler's presentation" (Nunberg and Federn, 1974, p. 147; Ansbacher and Ansbacher, 1956, pp. 70–71).

Reading these words almost a century later, one realizes that Freud and other psychoanalysts eventually did subsume many of Adler's ideas within a more comprehensive psychoanalytic theory. These concepts included aggression, repression as just one of many defenses, transformations of drives, elimination of the concept of ego drives, and the importance of the reality principle. Thus, it is no wonder that Ansbacher and Ansbacher state that "Adler was the adversary whom Freud heeded most" (1956, p. xvi).

In the case of Little Hans, for example, Freud (1909, pp. 140–141) spelled out his ambivalent disagreement with Adler's idea of an aggressive instinct. On the one hand, he maintained that Little Hans's analysis confirmed Adler's hypothesis that a patient's anxiety was caused by the repression of aggressive propensities. On the other hand, he decried the idea of such an instinct, preferring to conceptualize a pressing character for all instincts (i.e., their capacity for initiating movement). When Freud acknowledged the need for an aggressive instinct in psychoanalytic theory, he differentiated his instinct from Adler's by calling it the destructive or death instinct (1909, p. 140, note). In *Inhibitions, Symptoms, and Anxiety*, Freud (1926, p. 102) eventually did come to stress the role of defense against aggression in the development of Hans's phobia. Furthermore, the 1911 discussions at the Vienna Psychoanalytic Society demonstrate that Adler's challenge was likely a proximate cause for the change from the first to the second anxiety theory and to the development of the structural theory. For example, Freud stated that "the core of a neurosis is the anxiety of the ego confronted by libido, and Adler's expositions have merely strengthened *this view*" (Nunberg and Federn, 1974, p. 149; Ansbacher and Ansbacher, 1956, p. 71).

For Freud, the importance of libido was the major point of divergence. Adler moved the sexual drive to a subsidiary position, maintaining in 1908, for example, that the aggressive drive was the primary drive (Ansbacher and Ansbacher, 1956, pp. 34ff.), and in 1911 that "the libido cannot in any way be regarded uniformly as the driving factor" (Nunberg and Federn, 1974, pp. 102 ff.). A major thrust of Freud's work included attempts to integrate Adler's ideas about the role of the environment within a theoretical frame that continued to acknowledge the importance of drives.

Adler's direct, unacknowledged influence can be seen in Freud's work leading to the development of the reality principle and the concept of narcissism. In "Formulations on the Two Principles of Mental Functioning" (1911), the conception of the reality and pleasure principles allowed Freud to theoretically include the impact of the object (i.e., of the external world, which Adler stressed) on the mental life of the individual as well as the relationship between instincts and objects. In the 1915 revisions to the *Three Essays* (1905, pp. 125–245), Freud introduced many notions concerning objects and their connection to instincts, including, for the first time, the significance of the oral phase and the idea of incorporation (p. 198), an antecedent to identification. The extension of the theory to include narcissism allowed him to conceptualize that the ego, like an external love object, can be cathected with libido (Laplanche, 1976, p. 73). In other words, the concept of narcissism was intimately intertwined with the concept of objects, that is, narcissism was connected both to drive issues and to object relations issues (Freud, 1914, p. 76). The importance of the real world to the development of the individual is Adler's legacy to psychoanalysis.

REFERENCES

Andreas-Salomé, L. (1964). *The Freud Journal.* Translated by S. A. Leavy. London and New York: Quartet Encounters, 1987.

Ansbacher, H. L., and Ansbacher, R. R. (eds. and comps.). (1956). *The Individual Psychology of Alfred Adler.* New York: Harper and Row, 1964.

Freud, S. (1905). Three essays on the theory of sexuality. S.E. 7: 126–243.

———. (1909). Analysis of a phobia in a five-year-old boy. S.E. 10: 5–147.

———. (1911). Formulations on the two principles of mental functioning. S.E. 12: 213–226.

———. (1914). On the history of the psychoanalytic movement. S.E. 14: 7–66.

———. (1926). Inhibitions, symptoms, and anxiety. S.E. 20: 87–124.

Greenberg, J. (1991). *Oedipus and Beyond: A Clinical Theory.* Cambridge, Mass.: Harvard University Press.

Greenberg, J. R., and Mitchell, S. A. (1983). *Object Relations in Psychoanalytic Theory.* Cambridge, Mass.: Harvard University Press.

Laplanche, J. (1976). *Life and Death in Psychoanalysis.* Baltimore and London: Johns Hopkins University Press, 1985.

Nunberg, H., and Federn, E. (eds.) (1974). *Minutes of the Vienna Psychoanalytic Society,* Vol. 3, 1910–1911. New York: International Universities Press.

LEON HOFFMAN

Aesthetics, and Psychoanalysis

The traditional approach of psychoanalysis to aesthetics has been to discover the hidden, unconscious meaning behind the surface appearances of art, and to translate this hidden meaning into words. The same unconscious motivations were found embedded in psychological symptoms, dreams, mythology, literature, and visual art. However, what is artistic about nonverbal art is precisely what gets lost in translation into cognitive verbal content. How, then, can justice be done to what is uniquely creative about art, namely, that it restores fullness to the bleached-out experience of everyday life by invigorating thought and perception with the coloration of feeling? The answer is, by focusing on form rather than content.

The "meaning" of a picture is like the meaning of a poem: it lies less in the content of the ideas that can be extracted and served up than in the form in which physical sounds and irregular accents of words play across the regular beat of the meter. Nonverbal art deals with the transmutation of external arrangements of color, line, tone, and rhythm into internal emotional meanings.

Accordingly, a new approach to psychoanalytic aesthetics (Rose, 1980, 1987, 1996) shifts the primary focus from content to form, and from motivation to reality and perception. It views art as evolving within a more or less fluid reality where perception is engaged in the constant task of mixing and sorting the intermingling currents of objective knowledge and subjective imagination.

Classical descriptions by aestheticians commonly point out certain characteristics of the mounting feeling associated with the aesthetic experience: they note the coexistence of feelings of hyperacuity and tranquillity, simultaneous force and calm, vitality and ease, energy and repose. This boils down to a common dynamic in the structure of art and the emotional response to it: tension and release.

From the side of art, a visual artist, like a musical composer, knows how to enhance the expressive qualities inherent in ordinary perception, expressing it more energetically and clearly in order to highlight the dramatics of everyday experience. The core dynamic has to do with patterns of tension and release (e.g., in art, oblique lines, or rectangular or oval shapes, are more tension-producing; horizontal or vertical lines, or square or spherical shapes, are more stable and tension-releasing).

From the side of the viewer of art, a sensitivity and responsiveness to patterns of tension and release is the most elementary attribute of perception. This capacity for having an immediate emotional gut reaction—sensitivity to expressiveness—is rooted in a biological necessity: an organism must make an on-the-spot appraisal of the outside world's perceived hostility or friendliness in order to know whether to advance, withdraw, or wait and see. Affective perception is the first and most basic response to the dynamic aspects of reality, that is, its perceived qualities of tension and release, and the interpretation placed on these qualities in the light of knowledge and imagination.

What constitutes the emotional response to art? The congruence between the virtual tension and release that have been built into the aesthetic structure, on the one hand, and each observer's resonating response, on the other, with actual tension and release in the core dynamic of his or her personal feelings (this is not to be confused with any "communication" by the artist of his or her own feelings).

Susan Langer points out that art offers an objective image of the subjective experience of human feelings. "The establishment and organization of tensions is the basic technique in projecting the image of feeling, the artist's idea, in any medium. . . . [It leads to] an isomorphy of actual organic tensions and . . . virtual created tensions . . ." (Langer, 1967, p. 164).

The near-perfect fit between the attunement of art to one's own feelings and one's responsive resonance to aesthetic forms leads to an interplay between self and other, between the internal and the external. In this regard, several considerations are notable.

First, the correspondence between objective aesthetic forms and internal feelings is so close that it allows the viewer of art to create a preconscious illusion that art provides a responsive, witnessing presence. As in any intimate encounter (treatment, for example), the viewer

is licensed to feel more consciously what was always latent but unformed and inexpressible.

Second, such implicit "permission" amplifies emotional responses. They range from the present back to the remote past. Among the most significant of the latter is the experience of affective signaling that takes place between parent and infant. Ideally, this is geared toward the buildup and resolution of tension in a finely tuned dance of the mother's attunement and the infant's responsiveness. This promotes a graded differentiation of feelings in the very beginnings of a sense of self.

Third, since art, too, provides a reliably balanced tension and release, this allows affects to build up with intensity and offers the opportunity for further differentiation. In this way, art continues a biological function of early mothering: it elaborates transformations of affect, on higher, abstract levels, of the same resonating emotional responsiveness that existed in the beginning.

REFERENCES

Langer, S. (1967). *Mind: An Essay on Human Feeling.* Baltimore: Johns Hopkins University Press.

Rose, R. J. (1980). *The Power of Form. Psychoanalytic Approachs to Aesthetic Form.* Rev. ed., New York: International Universities Press, 1992.

———. (1987). *Trauma and Mastery in Life and Art.* New Haven, Conn.: Yale University Press. Rev. ed., Branford, Conn.: International Universities Press, 1996.

———. (1996). *Necessary Illusion: Art as Witness.* Branford, Conn.: International Universities Press.

GILBERT ROSE

Affect

As understood in psychoanalysis, "affect" expresses a metapsychological concept used to describe the topographical, economic, and dynamic organization of processes in psychic functioning. This technical use of the term should be contrasted with its use in nonpsychoanalytic psychology, where it is often used synonymously with "feeling," "emotion," or "mood." In psychoanalysis, the term denotes the same items, but it also refers to the dynamic processes—conscious, preconscious, and unconscious—that cause conscious feelings or the defensive processes that suppress their emergence.

Psychoanalysis and Freud's theory of affect are almost synonymous. Josef Breuer's momentous discovery that a hysterical symptom "immediately and permanently disappeared" when the patient described in detail the memory of the original disturbing event and its affect (Breuer and Freud, 1893-1895) offered the first clinical observation of a cure effected by verbalization of a painful past experience. Freud found such a clinical event to be "of so fundamental a nature" (1925, p. 21) that he repeated Breuer's investigations with his own patients and "worked at nothing else" (1925, p. 21), thus creating, through successive revisions, psychoanalytic technique and a complex metapsychology to give it theoretical foundations.

Freud's efforts led him to develop psychoanalytic concepts aimed at understanding the dynamic participation of affect in the psychoanalytic cure. The concepts of repression, drive, defenses, representation (idea), and pleasure-seeking were first developed to explain the vicissitudes of memories, representations, and affect in neurosis. Later, the formulation of the two principles of mental functioning (Freud, 1911); the pleasure principle and the reality principle, the examination of the vicissitudes of pleasure in psychic conflict (Freud, 1920); the structural theory of the tripartite mental apparatus (Freud, 1923); and the description of the signal function of affect (Freud, 1926) added dynamic complexity to the understanding of the emergence of affect as conscious subjective feelings, as well as the psychic price paid for the continuous suppression of affect.

On Freud's theory, feelings result from complex intrapsychic elaborations of memories, representations, fantasies, and wishes. What one feels, can be partially expressed to another, but its intrapsychic and interpersonal meaning can be determined only by a detailed analysis of its component elements. A concrete experienced feeling finds its origin in broad dynamic affective sources that condition its conscious emergence.

Feelings (affects) can be categorized as "pleasurable" or "unpleasurable." At a given moment, a somatic *source* acquires a *psychic representation* in the form of a *drive* which moves the psyche in the direction of seeking pleasurable *satisfaction* of its *aim* in an object capable of offering it. If satisfaction is achieved, a feeling of pleasure is experienced, and the psyche registers the particular experience of satisfaction as a *mnemic image* "which remains associated thenceforward with the memory trace of the excitation produced by the need" (Freud, 1900, pp. 565). The next time a need arises, the psyche "will seek to re-cathect the mnemic image of the perception . . . to re-establish the situation of the origi-

nal satisfaction. . . . The aim of this first psychical activity was to produce a 'perceptual identity'—a repetition of the perception which was linked with the satisfaction of need" (Freud, 1900, p. 566). The converse is true for the avoidance of the experience of unpleasure. To avoid unpleasure, every defensive measure must be undertaken to stop it at its inception.

The affective process begins in some somatic excitation composed of a representation of it and a quota of affect. They generally appear together as a psychic representative of the drive, but they need not be bound together. If they function together and reach their aim in an adequate object, the quota of affect is discharged and affect (feeling) is experienced. This is the optimal situation. If there is a threat of oncoming unpleasure, the psyche must defend against it. The ego's signal anxiety (affect) prompts it to stop the process of discharge to avoid massive anxiety or unpleasure. The ego does this by employing ego defenses. The two components of the drive representative are treated differently by the defenses (Freud, 1915).

Once the drive acquires psychic representation, the quota of affect present in it must either be repressed at once or find its proper processing and discharge. At this point, however, the components of the drive representative may split apart. The defenses may block awareness of the representation, which, however, remains active in the unconscious as a memory trace. The quota of affect, in this situation, may be discharged and experienced as diffuse anxiety (exchange of original affect by anxiety). If not, it may follow several vicissitudes. It may find a substitute idea (representation) for displacement that is connected to the previous one by associations; the affect is then linked to a phobic object, and phobia is the result. Or, by condensation of representations, it may attach itself to a bodily part while no feelings are experienced (transformation of affect), resulting in hysteria. Or it may find a substitute by displacement in other representations while, by a transformation of the ego, the affect shows reaction formation; this maneuver does not succeed in suppressing the tendency of the original drive representative to find its proper discharge of affect; but rather, it results in obsessional neurosis.

Freud's model of affect emergence describes the great complexity of affective processes and the continuous efforts of the psyche to seek satisfaction through dynamic reorganization of its drive representatives. The model has two pillars. The first is that psychic economic

A

processes of activation and stimulation must find pleasurable feelings in their proper discharge. The second is the persistence of memory traces of past experiences that are easily and continuously linked to past moments of pleasure or unpleasure. The dynamic organization of character structure in each individual is, in psychoanalytic terms, the structural recording of the psychic response to past moments of drive excitation and of having, or failing to have, obtained satisfaction of its aims in adequate drive objects in the human objects that are normally able to offer fulfillment.

This description of Freud's conception of affect brings to focus present-day infant observation research on the role of affect in development. These research efforts, in combination with those of object relations theorists, have moved the focus of the Freudian theory of affect from its economic center toward the great significance of the human object. Most analysts of various convictions converge today on this point. Nevertheless, the dynamic organization of affect should not be neglected by this change of focus. As valuable and illuminating as the investigations of the role of affect in development are, the results need to be translated, if possible, into the dynamic language of the intrapsychic organization of affect and representation (memory traces) if we are to understand the subjective registration of externally well documented events.

Many psychoanalytic theories about affect have emerged, but in the end, when it comes to the technical analysis of the emergence of affect in the clinical situation, they still need Freud's understanding of its dynamic organization. Intersubjective or interpersonal conceptualization of affective experience cannot bypass the subjects' need to process consciously perceived or preconscious communication through the dynamic organization of their own minds.

Finally, psychoanalysis cannot produce a comprehensive theory of affect. The neurological, chemical (neurotransmitters), and hormonal determinants of affect exceed the scientific scope of analytic theory. The unique and exclusive contribution of psychoanalysis to the understanding of affect is its ability to trace the intrapsychic determinants of the emergence of feelings.

REFERENCES

Basch, M. F. (1976). The concept of affect. *Journal of the American Psychoanalytic Association*, 24: 759–777.

Breuer, J., and Freud, S. (1895). *Studies on Hysteria*. S.E. 2: 19–305.

Freud, S. (1900). *The Interpretation of Dreams*. S.E. 4-5: 1–621.
———. (1911). Formulations on the two principles of mental functioning. S.E. 12: 213–226.
———. (1915). Repression. S.E. 14: 146–158.
———. (1920). *Beyond the Pleasure Principle*. S.E. 18: 1–64.
———. (1923). *The Ego and the Id*. S.E. 19: 12–59.
———. (1925). *An Autobiographical Study*. S.E. 20: 1–74.
———. (1926). *Inhibitions, Symptoms and Anxiety*. S.E. 20: 87–122.

Green, A. (1977). Conceptions of affect. *International Journal of Psycho-Analysis* 58: 129–157.

Lester, E. (1980). New directions in affect theory. *Journal of the American Psychoanalytic Association* 28: 197–211.

Sandler, J., and Sandler, A. M. (1978). On the development of object relations and affects. *International Journal of Psychoanalysis* 59: 285–296.

ANA-MARÍA RIZZUTO

Africa, and Psychoanalysis

Psychoanalysis has not yet taken root in Africa, except in South Africa, some North African countries, and Senegal.

During Africa's so-called colonial period, roughly 1900–1975, psychoanalysis did not have much impact, but traces of it can be found in the work of such people as René Laforgue and Octave Mannoni. Laforgue, a French psychoanalyst who settled in Morocco at the beginning of the 1950s, elaborated, using psychoanalytic terminology, on the allegedly inferior mental status of Arabic people (Bennani, 1997). Mannoni was a secondary school teacher in Madagascar from 1925 to 1945. In 1950 he published, *Prospero et Caliban: Psychologie de la Colonization* (Mannoni, 1985), in which he uses psychoanalytic concepts in analyzing the relationship between the colonist and the colonized. In *Peau Noir, Masques Blancs* (Fanon, 1952), Frantz Fanon, the most important theoretical figure of the African anticolonial liberation struggle, criticizes what he takes to be the racism of Mannoni's book.

In contrast to North and South America, the fertilization of psychoanalysis on the African continent was hindered by colonial immigration policies. Psychoanalysts who fled Fascism and National Socialism in Europe could not enter African countries due to the restrictive refugee and asylum policies of the colonial powers. An exception was South Africa, the only African country to accept a number of German-speaking (mostly Jewish) immigrants (Wojak, 1998, p. 402).

Some of the roots of psychoanalysis in South Africa were planted before World War II. In the 1930s, the president of the International Psychoanalytic Association (IPA), Ernest Jones, developed a plan to found a psychoanalytic group in South Africa with the Viennese psychoanalyst Richard Sterba as its director (Fenichel, 1998, p. 1846; Sterba, 1982, pp. 166f.). In seeking to help establish this group, the French psychoanalyst Marie Bonaparte, who was a family friend of Freud's, spent the period from 1941 to 1944 in South Africa (Bertin, 1982).

Fritz Perls, the founder of Gestalt therapy, trained as a psychoanalyst in Berlin and Vienna before emigrating to South Africa, and lived there from 1933 to 1946. Erich Heilbrun, a member of the Viennese Psychoanalytic Society after World War II, also emigrated from Berlin to South Africa. The Dutch psychoanalyst Johann H. W. van Ophuijsen worked in South Africa in 1935 before settling in the United States (Fenichel, 1998, p. 258). In 1933 the Berlin-based psychoanalyst Erich Simenauer (1961/1962) migrated via Cyprus to Tanganyika (today Tanzania), where he practiced as a physician and undertook psychoanalytic studies from 1941 to 1957. He then returned to Berlin.

Wulf Sachs, the pioneer of psychoanalysis in South Africa, moved to Johannesburg in 1922. In 1929, he began his psychoanalytic training with Theodor Reik in Berlin, and in 1934 became a member of the British Psychoanalytic Society. In 1935, the South African group became affiliated with the London Psychoanalytic Society, and in 1949 Sachs founded the first South African Psychoanalytic Society (Gillespie, 1992). His pioneering work is documented in his book *Black Hamlet: The Mind of an African Negro Revealed by Psychoanalysis*, first published in 1937 (Sachs 1947, 1996). The book is a biography of his client, a black Zimbabwean traditional healer named John Chavafambira, and is the first known report of psychoanalysis conducted with an African. In writing it, Sachs was going against prejudices and taboos characteristic of Christian European ethnocentrism and racism. Part of this racism held that blacks and "savages" (as well as children, women, and the mentally ill) were only animals, and did not have a soul. This ideology informed European colonial expansion as well as the slave trade. To credit a black African with an internal world was to go against the creeds not just of explicit racism but also of medical science (Rose, 1998, p. 334). Thus the contribution by Sachs is, in this context, significant. The psychoanalytic

group he founded disbanded shortly after his death in 1949. The installation of the apartheid system in South Africa prevented the further institutionalization of psychoanalysis until the Psychoanalytic Study Group was founded in 1979.

In the period of decolonization, the example of Senegal shows how psychoanalytic thinking became an integral part of modern social psychiatry in collaboration with traditional healers. A pioneer of this approach, the French psychiatrist Henri Collomb, who also trained in psychoanalysis, established and directed a psychiatric center in Dakar-Fann and founded the journal *Psychopathologie Africaine* in 1965 (Martino, 1989). The Dakar-Fann clinic became a center for psychoanalytic studies such as the work of Marie-Cécile and Edmond Ortigues, *Oedipe Africain*, based on their psychoanalytic experiences there from 1962 to 1966 (Ortigues and Ortigues, 1966). The Swiss psychoanalyst Lise Tripet (1990) has also reported from Senegal on the only psychoanalytic treatments of African patients known to have occurred anywhere on the continent.

The anthropologist Vincent Crapanzano conducted two ethnopsychoanalytic field studies in Morocco in which he combined theory and research methodology with psychoanalysis. In his book *Waiting: The Whites of South Africa* (1985), he emphasized the importance of the dialogical nature of the relationship between the researcher and the subject of the study. In this view, such a relationship would lead—as part of the research process—to a better understanding of the phenomena under study.

There was also an initiative by the retired American psychoanalyst Marie Nelson to establish psychoanalysis in Nairobi, Kenya, at the end of the 1980s. Some Kenyan professionals were trained in affiliation with the Philadelphia Psychoanalytic Institute, but progress came to a standstill when she left the country (Nelson, 1987).

In the area of developmental psychology, a number of researchers have undertaken studies from a psychoanalytic perspective. For example, M. D. S. Ainsworth (1967) wrote on attachment theories in Uganda, and R. A. LeVine (1992) wrote on the self in African culture. However, investigations of this kind are well covered in the journal *American Imago*, in an issue of volume 55 (1998) devoted exclusively to southern African topics presented from a psychoanalytic perspective.

If we reverse the question and ask what important traces Africa has left on psychoanalysis (besides the metaphoric usage of the term "dark continent" by Sigmund Freud), we will basically find an answer in the development of ethnopsychoanalysis. This subject can be seen as the most important application and development of German-speaking psychoanalysis after World War II. The pioneering achievements of the Swiss psychoanalysts Paul Parin, Goldy Parin-Matthèy, and Fritz Morgenthaler lay in their first application of the psychoanalytic technique as a research tool for the investigation of people belonging to two different traditional West African societies. By conducting ethnopsychoanalytic studies among the Dogon of Mali and the Agni of the Ivory Coast in the 1950s and 1960s, they were able to prove that psychoanalysis was practically and theoretically useful for studying and understanding the unconscious dynamics of people who had grown up and lived in non-European societal formations.

The ethnopsychoanalytic observations and studies made between 1954 and 1971 in West Africa led to insights into hitherto unrecognized and very revealing relationships between social institutions and unconscious processes. One major finding was that the primary influences at work on the individual are societal, with biological determinants being only secondary. Further ethnopsychoanalytic findings were: (1) normality is dependent on culture; (2) every defense mechanism (including the pathological) is most likely ego-syntonic; (3) not only early childhood experiences but also, to a large extent, adolescence and society strongly determine the personality and behavior of the adult; (4) the analyst's own role expectations and projections have to be taken into account so that transference can optimally unfold and develop in analysis; and (5) sufficient emotional openness develops only if the analyst observes the above factors (Reichmayr, 1995).

In the late 1990s, there were several indicators pointing to the future relevance of psychoanalysis in Africa. A number of clinical psychologists and psychiatrists who trained in Europe or North America and had been practicing psychotherapy in Africa for years adopted psychoanalysis in theory and practice. Some were teaching psychoanalysis at academic institutions, and at the same time were familiar with those African realities of psychotherapy in which traditional forms of psychotherapy are dominant.

Rapid societal change and urbanization in African societies seem to create the need for Western forms of psychotherapy, including psychoanalysis (Peltzer, 1995,

1998). The activities of psychotherapy societies such as those in Nigeria (Ebigbo et al., 1995) and the African chapter of the World Council for Psychotherapy play a major role by exchanging and promoting experiences with traditional healers at conferences (Madu et al., 1996). Psychoanalysis is recognized and taught in university departments of psychology, clinical psychology, and psychiatry (Peltzer and Ebigbo, 1989).

As can be seen in the example of the refounding of psychoanalytic study groups in South Africa in the late 1970s, African-born psychoanalysts, trained in Europe or North America, have played a major role in the spread of psychoanalysis in Africa (e.g., Joseph Sandler, Sadie Gillespie, Anne Hayman, Malcolm Pines, Max and Wally Joffe, Mark Solms). This has also led to an affiliation between a South African Psychoanalytic Study Group and the British Psychoanalytic Society, with a view to establishing a psychoanalytic training institute and society in South Africa.

REFERENCES

Ainsworth, M. D. S. (1967). *Infancy in Uganda: Infant Care and the Growth of Love*. Baltimore: John Hopkins University Press.

Bennani, J. (1997). *La Psychanalyse au Pays des Saints: Les Débuts de la Psychiatrie et de la Psychanalyse au Maroc*. Casablanca: Editions Le Fennec.

Bertin, C. (1982). *La Dernière Bonaparte*. Paris: Perrin.

Crapanzano, V. (1985). *Waiting: The Whites of South Africa*. New York: Random House.

Ebigbo, P. O., Oluka, J., Ezenwa, M., Obidigbo, and Okwaraji, F. (1995). *The Practice of Psychotherapy in Africa*. Enugu: International Federation for Psychotherapy.

Fanon, F. (1952). *Peau Noire, Masques Blancs*. Paris: Seuil.

Fenichel, O. (1998). *119 Rundbriefe 1934–1945*. Frankfurt am Main: Stroemfeld.

Gillespie, S. (1992). Historical notes on the first South African psychoanalytical society. *Psycho-analytic Psychotherapy in South Africa* 1: 1–7.

LeVine, R. A. (1992). The self in African culture. In D. H. Spain, (ed.), *Psychoanalytic Anthropology After Freud*, pp. 37–48. New York: Psyche Press.

Madu, S. N., Baguma, P. K. and Pritz, A. (eds.). (1996). *Psychotherapy in Africa: First investigations*. Vienna: World Council for Psychotherapy.

Mannoni, O. (1985). *Prospero et Caliban: Psychologie de la Colonisation*. Paris: Editions Universitaires.

Martino, P. (1989). Henri Collomb, 1913-1979. In *Psychiatrie Française* 20: 41–47.

Nelson, M. C. (1987). Immunization factors in development of the African personality: Preliminary observations. *Psychoanalytic Review* 74: 233–237.

Ortigues, M. C., and Ortigues, E. (1966). *Oedipe Africain*. Paris: Plon.

Peltzer, K. (1995). *Psychology and Health in African Cultures: Examples of Ethnopsychotherapeutic Practice.* Frankfurt am Main: IKO Verlag.

———. (1998). Psychology and health in sub-Saharan Africa. *Journal of Psychology in Africa* 8: 142–170.

Peltzer, K., and Ebigbo, P. O. (eds.). (1989). *Clinical Psychology in Africa.* Frankfurt am Main: IKO Verlag.

Reichmayr, J. (1995). *Einführung in die Ethnopsychoanalyse.* Frankfurt am main: Fischer Taschenbuch Verlag.

Rose, J. (1998). Wulf Sachs's *Black Hamlet.* In C. Lane (ed.), *The Psychoanalysis of Race,* pp. 333–352. New York: Columbia University Press.

Sachs, W. (1947). *Black Anger.* New York: Grove Press.

———. (1996). *Black Hamlet.* With new introductions by Saul Dubow and Jaqueline Rose. Baltimore: John Hopkins University Press.

Simenauer, E. (1961/1962) Ödipus-konflikt und neurosebedingungen bei den Bantu Ostafrikas. *Jahrbuch der Psychoanalyse* 2: 41–62.

Sterba, Richard F. (1982). *Reminiscences of a Viennese Psychoanalyst.* Detroit: Wayne State University Press.

Tripet, L. (1990). Wo steht das verlorene Haus meines Vaters? In *Afrikanische Analysen.* Freiburg: Kore.

Wojak, I. (1998). Südafrika. In C. D. Krohn et al. (eds.), *Darmstadt Handbuch der Deutschsprachigen Emigration 1933–1945.* Darmstadt: Wissenschaftliche Buchgesellschaft, pp. 402–411.

KARL PELTZER
JOHANNES REICHMAYR

Aggression

In contrast to his libidinal instinct theory, Freud never fully developed his theory of aggression and its developmental vicissitudes. He eventually abandoned his early tentative position that cruelty and destructiveness arose from a mastery instinct which served an adaptive function, and was linked to self-assertion and motor activity. Turning away from clinical observation to biology, he sought to explain aggression as being solely self-destructive and in the service of returning the organism to its original state of nonbeing. From this point on, Freud abandoned his struggle for a clinically informed understanding of the puzzling phenomena of masochism, sadism, and the compulsion to repeat painful experiences. Gripped by the idea that the aim of instinctual life as a whole is to bring about death, for a time he even revised his view of the instincts of self-preservation, self-assertion, and of mastery: "They are component instincts whose function it is is to assure that the organism shall follow its own path to death" (1920, p. 39). Though he

later moved from this position to one that subsumed the self-preservation instincts under the sexual instinct, and in opposition to the death instinct, he never returned to a consideration of aggression as other than a destructive force.

Freud first wrote explicitly about aggression in *Three Essays on the Theory of Sexuality*, in the context of what he then termed the most common and significant of all the perversions—sadism and masochism (Parens, 1979, p. 44). In it he notes that the roots of sadism are easily found in normals, in that "the sexuality of most male human beings contains an element of aggressiveness—a desire to subjugate; the biological significance of it seems to lie in the need for overcoming the resistance of the sexual object by means other than the process of wooing. Thus sadism would correspond to an aggressive component of the sexual instinct which has become independent and exaggerated and, by displacement, has usurped the leading position" (1905, pp. 157–158) In a footnote later in the same work (p. 168), he again alludes to a separate instinct which is not sexual and which has its source in motor impulses.

In these early writings, Freud makes a connection between aggression and activity. He refers to an instinct for mastery and sees this as manifested in the activity of the somatic musculature. His reluctance to revise his first dual instinct theory is apparent in his disagreement with Alfred Adler in 1909: "I cannot bring myself to assume the existence of a special aggressive instinct alongside of the familiar instincts of self-preservation and sex, and on an equal footing to them" (1909, p. 140). He goes on to suggest that aggression is not a separate instinct but a universal and indispensable attribute of all instincts which accounts for their capacity to initiate movement. In a footnote to this work added in 1923, Freud admits that he had to acknowledge the existence of a separate aggressive instinct, but notes that it differs from Adler's concept of aggression as self-assertion. Freud called this aggressive instinct "the destructive or death instinct" (1909, p. 140).

Freud's views are explicated with greater assurance in *Civilization and Its Discontents*. He states unequivocally that "This aggressive instinct is the derivative and the main representative of the death instinct which we have found alongside of Eros and which shares world-dominion with it" (1930, p. 122).

Henceforth, Freud used the expressions "death instinct" and "destructive aggression" interchangeably.

A

In *The Ego and the Id* (1923), he posits that the death instinct expresses itself, at least in part, through the muscular apparatus as an instinct of destruction. Again in the *New Introductory Lectures on Psycho-Analysis* (1933), he offers his hypothesis that there are two different instincts—the sexual, which he calls "Eros," and the aggressive, whose aim is destruction. He returns to an examination of masochism and sadism, suggesting that the former is an expression of the destructive instinct and that sadism is the destructive instinct directed outward, "thus acquiring the characteristic of aggressiveness" (1933, p. 105).

Freud maintained his view of aggression as a manifestation of the death instinct even though, as he himself noted, it found little support at the time in psychoanalytic circles.

REFERENCES

Freud, S. (1905). *Three Essays on the Theory of Sexuality*. S.E. 7: 126–243.

————. (1909). Analysis of a phobia in a five-year-old boy. S.E. 10: 5–147.

————. (1920). *Beyond the Pleasure Principle*. S.E. 18: 7–64.

————. (1923). *The Ego and the Id*. S.E. 19: 12–59.

————. (1930). *Civilization and Its Discontents*. S.E. 21: 59–185.

————. (1933). *New Introductory Lectures on Psycho-analysis*. S.E. 22: 5–182.

Parens, H. (1979). *The Development of Aggression in Early Childhood*. New York: Jason Aronson.

                                        JENNIFER BONOVITZ

Aim See DRIVE THEORY.

Ambivalence

The term "ambivalence" connotes opposite feeling states toward a person or a thing. When mixed feelings of both love and hate exist, side by side, one experiences ambivalence. The use of the term in psychoanalytic writings, however, has undergone a refinement: a preambivalent state is distinguished from an ambivalent one. In a preambivalent state, there is alternation between a feeling and its opposite (i.e., a splitting apart of the two feelings); in an ambivalent state, there is a capacity to hold the opposite feelings simultaneously, in an integrated way.

Freud (1905, p. 199) acknowledged that he borrowed the "happily chosen" term "ambivalence" from Eugen Bleuler (1950), but his usage varied, and did not always correspond to Bleuler's. In *Three Essays on the Theory of Sexuality*, Freud uses the concept to refer to a form of sexual organization characterized by opposing pairs of instincts (1905, p. 199). In "Instincts and Their Vicissitudes," he characterizes the presence of an instinct and its passive opposite as "ambivalence."

In a 1912 paper, however, Freud speaks not of opposing instincts as ambivalence but of an "ambivalence of feeling." He points out that " . . . it [the negative transference] is found side by side with the affectionate transference, often directed simultaneously towards the same person" (1912, p. 106). In other writings, Freud uses the concept of ambivalence to refer to emotional impulses. In "The Devil as a Father-Substitute," he notes that an individual's relation to his father is ambivalent in that it contains two sets of emotional impulses: those of an affectionate and submissive nature, and hostile and defiant ones. He then applies the same idea to man's relation to God: "It is our view that the same ambivalence governs the relation of mankind to its deity" (1923 [1922], p. 85).

In post-Freudian writings, the term "ambivalence" is used in still other ways. Based on her observations of children in treatment, Melanie Klein (1940) postulated a specific developmental sequence in the infant's attitudes of love and hate. According to Kleinian theory, the infant perceives the world as split between all-good and all-bad experiences. The experience may be of a part of the maternal person, such as an experience of the mother's breast. The representing of the maternal part results in the perception of two separate mothers, one good and one bad. Similarly, the infant initially sees itself separately at times as all-good and and at other times as all-bad. As the child develops, it begins to see the mother as one person who has both good and bad qualities. At that stage, the child views itself as both good and bad. Thus, the child progresses from a split (preambivalent) phase to an integrated (ambivalent) phase.

Kernberg (1975) subsequently applied Klein's findings to adult patients with borderline pathology. He observed splitting being used as a defensive way of dealing with too much aggression. Patients with lower-level pathology tended to split apart positive and negative feelings. There might then exist a rapid alternation between love and hate toward the same person. Higher-level (less sick) patients were observed to be capable of integrating opposing feelings and simultaneously holding such feelings in awareness.

Preambivalence is characterized by splitting good and bad attitudes, or alternating from one to the other, occupying extreme all-or-none positions with the absence of gradations, an intolerance of ambiguity or mixed feelings. As a patient said, "If I felt two ways about something, I wouldn't know what I felt. I wouldn't know what I stood for. I wouldn't know who I was." Such are the characteristics of borderline and psychotic patients.

Ambivalence is characterized by the capacity to hold opposite attitudes concurrently, the ability to experience gradations of intensity of emotions, and the capacity to tolerate ambiguity. Ambivalence is a sign of a more healthy personality organization.

REFERENCES

Bleuler, E. (1950). *Dementia Praecox or the Group of Schizophrenias*. New York: International Universities Press.

Freud, S. (1905). *Three Essays on the Theory of Sexuality.* S.E. 7: 126–243.

———. (1909). Analysis of a phobia in a five-year-old boy. S.E. 10: 5–147.

———. (1912). The dynamics of transference. S. E. 12: 99–108.

———. (1923 [1922]). The devil as a father-substitute. S.E. 19: 83–92.

Kernberg, O. (1975). *Borderline Conditions and Pathological Narcissism*. New York: Jason Aronson.

Klein, M. (1940). Mourning and its relation to manic-depressive states. In her, *Love, Guilt and Reparation and Other Works: 1921–1945*, pp. 344–369. New York: The Free Press.

CLARENCE SCHULZ

Anaclitic Object

Freud used the term "anaclitic object" to denote an object choice made by a person on the basis of the instinct of self-preservation. The ensuing relationship is based on the model of the child-parent bond in that it guarantees the child nourishment, care, and protection.

The concept of anaclitic object was introduced by Freud in 1914, in an effort to distinguish between two kinds of object choice—the anaclitic and narcissistic. In fact, this idea grew out of his earlier theory of anaclasis, which designated the early relationship of the sexual instincts to the self-preservative instincts (Freud, 1905). The term "anaclitic" derives from the Greek meaning "to rest upon" or "to lean upon." Freud attempted to demonstrate the relationship between the sexual instinct and certain bodily functions. He felt that the infant's first sexual satisfaction arises out of the mechanisms neces-

sary for the preservation of life. This relationship is very evident in the oral activity of the infant at the breast: in the pleasure obtained from sucking, "the satisfaction of the erotogenic zone is associated, in the first instance, with the satisfaction of the need for nourishment" (1905, pp. 181–182). Hence, the breast primarily satisfies the hunger instinct but begins to become a source of sexual satisfaction as a bonus pleasure. Then the "need for repeating the sexual satisfaction . . . becomes detached from the need for taking nourishment" (p. 182). Thus, sexual instinct becomes independent at a later stage and functions in an autoerotic mode. Other erotogenic zones, labial and anal, are also suited to function as media through which sexuality may attach itself to other somatic functions.

Freud thus felt that "children learn to feel for other people who help them in their helplessness and satisfy their needs a love which is on the model of, and a continuation of, their relations as sucklings to their nursing mother" (pp. 222–223). Hence, according to the theory of anaclitic object choice, a man will love a woman who feeds him and a woman will love a man who protects her. The implication is that the man rediscovers a mother and the woman rediscovers a father. Hence, according to Freud's formulation, heterosexuality is anaclitic whereas homosexuality is narcissistic (a person chooses an object on the basis of some real or imagined similarity with himself). The anaclitic object provides psychic nourishment, and its loss can precipitate depression.

Many subsequent writers, such as Rene Spitz, Sidney Blatt, Robert Harmon, and Mary Ainsworth, have furthered our understanding of infant mental health in expanding upon the syndrome of "anaclitic depression." It is clinically important to recognize and understand this syndrome, to distinguish it from organic illness, and to treat it promptly. The term "anaclitic depression" was coined by Spitz in 1946, to denote a disturbance which resembles the clinical manifestations of adult depression but which develops by degrees in children who are deprived of their mother after having had a normal relationship with her during at least the first six months of life. It is characterized by weeping, wailing, weight loss, refusal of contact, lying prone in their cribs, motor retardation, and subsequent facial rigidity with physical illness. The syndrome progresses over three months, and the disturbance disappears with striking rapidity if the mother is restored to the baby or an acceptable substitute is found.

Anaclitic depression has been further distinguished from introjective depression. Anaclitic depression causes one to feel helpless, weak, depleted; to wish to be cared for, loved, fed, protected; and is accompanied by intense fears of abandonment, oral cravings, and an urgency to fill an inner emptiness. Introjective depression derives from a harsh, punitive conscience, resulting in feelings of inferiority, worthlessness, guilt, and a wish for atonement. The two syndromes can coexist in an individual.

While Freud used the concept of an anaclitic object to refer to a kind of choice, the expansion of the application of the concept in the clinical realm of infant mental health has been challenging, stimulating, and rewarding in the early detection and treatment of childhood disorders.

REFERENCES

Blatt, S. J. (1974). Levels of object representation in anaclitic and introjective depression. *Psychoanalytic Study of the Child*, 29: 107–158.

Freud, S. (1905). *Three Essays on the Theory of Sexuality*. S.E. 7: 125–243.

———. (1914). On narcissism: An introduction. S.E. 14: 73–102.

Spitz, R., and Wolf, K. (1946). Anaclitic depression, an inquiry into the genesis of psychiatric conditions in early childhood, II. *Psychoanalytic Study of the Child* 2: 313–342.

PURNIMA MEHTA

Anal Character

The anal stage, the second in Freud's chronology of the psychological and sexual development of the infant, lasts from one and a half years of age to about three. Unlike the oral stage, in which the child is expected to do little more than suck, feed, and sleep, and is reinforced for passivity and dependency, the anal stage is marked by parental (and societal) demands on the child to conform to local standards of neatness, cleanliness, and bodily control. Beginning with toilet training, children for the first time are indoctrinated to a lifetime need to conform to external demands in order to obtain love. Instead of releasing body waste products wherever and whenever they wish, children are asked to tolerate uncomfortable bodily tensions and to hold back the pleasure of relief until the right time and the right place. As was the case in the oral stage, some early theorists divided the anal stage into two phases—the anal retentive, or sadistic, and the anal erotic. Empirical research has failed to pro-

vide evidence for the utility of this distinction, and it has fallen into disuse.

As in the earlier oral stage, either indulgence of anal impulses or frustration of them is hypothesized to result in fixation. During this phase of life the child experiences both the pain from increased tension in bladder and bowel, and the pleasure that comes from discharging such tension. However easily this stage of development is resolved, remnants of the satisfactions and difficulties surrounding the process and control of defecation and urination, or more generally around the processes of refusing versus acceding to societal demands, can be found in adult behavior. Societies emphasizing cleanliness and obedience to parental demands, and depicting urine and feces as dirty and disgusting, can expect to experience greater struggles with the child over eliminatory processes than societies that are relatively relaxed about such activities. Sooner or later children become toilet trained, but the amount of effort put into this practice and the degree to which failures along the way are either ignored or criticized differ from family to family and group to group. The greater the insistence on toilet training, the greater the struggle between child and parent.

One obvious way children respond to adult pressures for toilet training is to refuse and disobey. The demand for toilet training is frequently transformed into a struggle for autonomy and independence—"you can't make me" is an easy solution to any adult request, whether for toilet training or not playing with food. Further, "you can't make me" is a sign that the child is different and separate from the parents, and signals the child's growing awareness of individuality and power.

Freud's clinical work with compulsive-obessive patients led him to observe that "the people I am about to describe are noteworthy for a regular combination of the three following characteristics. They are especially *orderly, parsimonious,* and *obstinate*" (1908, p. 169). These three traits, sometimes referred to as the three p's—pedantry, parsimony, and persistence—are all residues of the child's struggle to resolve competing needs—to enjoy immediate reduction of bodily tension or to please the parents by using the toilet appropriately. Obstinacy is left over from the "you can't make me" phase, when the child's easiest defense against parental demands is to refuse. A concern about being controlled and losing autonomy is easily manifested by refusal to be docile and compliant (or perhaps even being actively oppositional as well). The frugality that begins with the need to withhold pleasure and to save for a time one's bodily products may progress to a lifetime pattern of indiscriminate saving and indefinite withholding. Orderliness begins with the effort to avoid contact with feces or any form of dirt, and can escalate to more generalized patterns of ritual and phobic responses to disorganization.

Empirical research has generally supported these theoretical claims about the anal character type. All but one of about a dozen factor analytic studies have supported Freud's observation that the traits of parsimony, orderliness, and obstinacy form a cohesive cluster. People with one of these characteristics are quite likely to show the other two as well. Those with high scores on tests of anality learn more effectively for a reward of a penny than of a gum ball, and learn more quickly when criticized than when praised. Anal types in an experiment, particularly males, will attempt to disconfirm the experimenter's hypothesis, thus demonstrating the obstinacy Freud noted many years earlier. Research has also documented high anal scores in those with compulsive-obsessive characteristics. The exaggerated morality about dirt and waste products found in many anal personalities is also shown in their severely critical attitudes toward social problems. Highly anal people have been found to be as concerned with wasting time as they are with wasting money. Stamp collectors are more sensitive to anal stimuli than are control subjects.

Considerable ambiguity surrounds the circumstances that produce an anal personality. The simple assumption that time and intensity of toilet training lead to anal traits is not consistently supported by empirical evidence. It is more likely that parental attitudes about cleanliness, discipline, autonomy, and body parts are more important determiners of a child's anal orientation than the mechanical factor of the age at which toilet training is introduced.

Anality has been assessed using projective tests by Blum (1949) and Holt (1966). There are many objective tests assessing anal traits, including those by Lazare et al. (1966, 1970), Sandler and Hazari (1961), and Grygier (1961).

What evidence can be found in adults of the satisfactions and frustrations they experienced during the anal stage of toilet training? The derivatives of anal impulses can be seen in the triad of parsimony, cleanliness, and orderliness, and in all their vicissitudes—collecting objects of all varieties (stamps, coins, matchbooks, string, beer cans, etc.), hoarding, opposition for its own sake, rituals around cleaning, compulsive-obsessive traits, stringent, relatively inflexible attitudes about morality, and concerns about propriety all document the lingering effects of having to sublimate a basic bodily need.

REFERENCES
Blum, G. S. (1949). A study of the psychoanalytic theory of psychosexual development. *Genetic Psychology Monographs*, 39: 3–99.

Freud, S. (1908). Character and anal erotism. S.E. 9: 167–176.

Grygier, T. (1961). *The Dynamic Personality Inventory*. London: National Foundation for Educational Research.

Holt, R. R. (1966). Measuring libidinal and aggressive motives by means of the Rorschach test. In D. Levine (ed.), *Nebraska Symposium on Motivation*. Lincoln: University of Nebraska Press.

Lazare, A., Klerman, G. L., and Armor, D. J. (1966). Oral, obsessive and hysterical personality patterns. *Archives of General Psychiatry* 14: 624–630.

———. (1970). Oral, obsessive and hysterical personality patterns: Replication of factor analysis in an independent sample. *Journal of Psychiatric Research*, 7: 275–290.

Sandler, J., and Hazari, A. (1961). The "obsessional": On the psychological classification of obsessional character traits and symptoms. *British Journal of Medical Psychology*, 33: 113–121.

JOSEPH M. MASLING

Anal Eroticism See DEVELOPMENTAL THEORY.

Anal Stage See ANAL CHARACTER; DEVELOPMENTAL THEORY.

Analyzability

In "Freud's Psycho-analytic Procedure" (1904 [1903], p. 254), Freud stated some of the qualifications necessary for someone to be "beneficially affected by psychoanalysis." The patient "must be capable of a psychically normal condition," and "a certain measure of intelligence and ethical development" is also necessary. Freud also notes that "Deep-rooted malformations of character traits of an actually degenerate constitution" may lead to resistance that cannot be overcome in the analysis. He adds, "If the patient's age is in the neighborhood of the fifties, conditions for psycho-analysis become unfavorable." (p. 254).

A

In a later paper (1905 [1904], pp. 263-264), Freud delineates other necessary qualities. These include the possession of a reasonable degree of education and a reliable character structure. The patient also needs to be self-motivated, not being forced into treatment by the authority of relatives, and needs to be educable and in possession of a "normal mental condition" (p. 264). "Psychoses, states of confusion, and deeply-rooted . . . depression," Freud writes, "are therefore not suitable for psycho-analysis" (p. 264). He adds that the treatment should not be attempted when the speedy removal of dangerous symptoms is required: "as, for example, in the case of hysterical anorexia." He also states that "most valuable and most highly developed persons are best suited for this procedure" (p. 264).

Freud (1913, pp. 124–125) states that he takes a patient on provisionally for a period of one to two weeks. He feels this is useful, in that if one stops the treatment at this time, it spares the patient from being distressed by an impression of an attempted cure "having failed." He also sees diagnostic reasons for a trial treatment of one to two weeks, such as to identify dementia praecox (schizophrenia). Freud also indicates some of the situations that may make analytic treatment difficult or impossible: previous treatment by another method, previous acquaintance between the doctor and the patient, delaying treatment, and the existence of bonds of friendship or social ties between the analyst and his patient, or their families. In this trial period of analysis, Freud emphasizes the importance of the patient's free associations, for which "lengthy discussions and questions" are no substitute in determining the patient's suitability for analysis.

There have been a number of studies focusing on the issue of suitability for psychoanalysis. One is by Knapp, et al. (1960). Other studies were done by Klein and her group (1965) and by Erle and Goldberg (1984). Coltart (1992) wrote about diagnosis and assessment for suitability for psychoanalytic psychotherapy, and on assessing psychological-mindedness during the diagnostic interview (1988). Bachrach and Leaff (1978) undertook a systematic review of sixteen clinical and eight quantitative-predictive studies of analyzability. They concluded that good ego strength, intact reality testing, and capacity for sublimation are qualities found in individuals most suitable for psychoanalysis. Huxster et al. (1975, p. 100) state that "many developmental attributes (ego functions) must have been attained." These functions include capacities for object constancy, for differentiation of self, and for object representation, and also tolerance for anxiety, depression, and frustration. Huxster et al. (1975, p. 104) further stated "The presence of a capacity for meaningful conceptualization (not intellectualization) of human experiences and relationships" is important. This relates to the concept of psychological-mindedness. Significant also is a wish for growth and maturation (as differentiated from wishes for magic fantasy fulfillment) in the analysis. One looks for a pattern of relationships to significant people in the applicant's life; for achievements in everyday life, such as school and work, and marriage; for the capacity to "engage" with life, to withstand stress, disappointment, or misfortune; for depth and richness of his character; for flexibility; for the capacity for enjoyment; and for the capacity to persevere in the face of difficulties. These are all indicators of adequacy or inadequacy of many ego and personality attributes necessary to permit the analytic process to develop. The patient needs to have the capacity to form a stable therapeutic alliance and needs to be able not only to develop transference phenomena but also to be able to have sufficient observing ego to analyze these phenomena.

In addition to the patient's qualities, one has also to consider the importance of the match between the patient and the analyst. Kantrowitz (1995) studied this match. In addition, as Akhtar (1995) notes, there has been increasing understanding and research in child observation, and there are now multiple theoretical and clinical models. These new developments in psychoanalytic understanding and technique indicate that some individuals with more severe psychopathology, such as the personality disorders, may be analyzed successfully.

REFERENCES

Akhtar, S. (1995). *Quest for Answers. A Primer for Understanding and Treating Severe Personality Disorders.* Northvale, N.J., and London: Jason A.

Bachrach, H. M., and Leaff, L. A. (1978). Analysability: A systematic review of the clinical and quantitative literature. *Journal of the American Psychoanalytical Association*, 32: 881–919.

Coltart, N. (1988). The assessment of psychological-mindedness in the diagnostic interview. *British Journal of Psychiatry* 153: 819–829.

———. (1992). Diagnosis and assessment for suitability for psychoanalytic psychotherapy. In N. Coltart, *Slouching Towards Bethlehem.* New York: Guilford Press.

Erle, J. and Goldberg, D. (1984). Observations on the assessment of analyzability by experienced analysts. *Journal of the American Psychoanalytical Association*, 32: 715–737.

Freud, S. (1904 [1903]). Freud's psychoanalytic procedure. S.E. 7: 249–254.

———. (1905 [1904]). On psychotherapy. S.E. 7: 257–268.

———. (1913). On beginning the treatment. (Further recommendations on the technique of psychoanalysis I). S.E. 12: 123–144).

Huxster, H., Lower, R., and Escoll, P. (1975). Some pitfalls in the assessment of analyzability in a psychoanalytic clinic. *Journal of the American Psychoanalytical Association*, 23: 90–106.

Kantrowitz, J. (1995). The beneficial aspects of the patient-analyst match. *International Journal of Psycho-analysis*, 76: 299–313.

Klein, H. (1965). *Psychoanalysts in Training, Selection and Evaluation*. New York: Psychoanalytic Clinic for Training and Research, Department of Psychiatry, Columbia University College of Physicians and Surgeons.

Knapp, P., et al. (1960). Suitability for psychoanalysis: A review of one hundred supervised analytic cases. *Psychoanalytic Quarterly*, 4: 459–477.

PHILIP J. ESCOLL

Andreas-Salomé, Lou (1861–1937)

Lou Andreas-Salomé was an intellectual, a writer, and an analyst. She was a thinker concerned with questions basic to the human condition. Her intellectual gifts enabled her to establish contact with notable figures of her time with whom she could exchange ideas. In her circle of friends and acquaintances were some of the most interesting and influential members of the intellectual and cultural elite in the German-speaking countries. Friedrich Nietzsche's letters to her and her extensive correspondence with Rainer Maria Rilke, Sigmund Freud, and Anna Freud are part of the intellectual history of the period (1860–1940).

Salomé was the youngest child and only daughter of a German family living in St. Petersburg. Her father, Gustav von Salomé, was a general in the service of the czar, and the family lived in an apartment in the General Staff Building that stands opposite the Winter Palace. Growing up in a privileged family within an exclusive and cosmopolitan society in the capital of imperial Russia played its part in giving her the self-assurance that was an important trait in her personality. That self-assurance was also reflected in her bearing. Her intelligence, her vivid imagination, and her fierce determination to pursue her interests set her apart from other young girls of her time.

In 1880, accompanied by her mother, Salomé left St. Petersburg for Zurich in order to study philosophy and history of religion at one of the few universities that admitted women. She did not finish her studies. Plagued by recurring health problems, she was advised to seek a milder climate, and went to Italy. In 1882, in Rome, she met Paul Rée and, through him, Friedrich Nietzsche. Rée became her friend and later her housemate in Berlin. The friendship between Nietzsche and Salomé, important for both, was complicated by many factors and did not last long. Nevertheless, she was the first to write a book about him, *Nietzsche in Seinen Werken* (1894).

Probably to ensure that she would not have to return to her family in Russia, in 1887 Salomé entered into an unconventional marriage with Friedrich Karl Andreas, an orientologist who was fifteen years her senior. Living in Berlin, Salomé became part of the intellectual and literary avant-garde. She wrote articles and reviews for various journals including *Die Freie Bühne*, the official periodical of the German naturalist movement. She came to know actors, directors, and writers including Gerhart Hauptmann, the most important naturalist dramatist. Her involvement with the theater prompted her to write a study of Ibsen's female characters based on six of his dramas, one of the first books in Germany to deal with Ibsen.

Andreas-Salomé also wrote essays, novellas, and several novels. Perhaps her best-known novels are *Ruth* (1895), *Das Haus* (1919), and *Ródinka* (1923; dedicated to Anna Freud). Her collection of novellas *Im Zwischenland* (1902) concerns the emotions of adolescent girls. Her letters to a young boy in *Drei Briefe an Einen Knaben* (1917) attempt to explain sexuality to a boy at three different stages of his development. In her fiction, which often contained autobiographic components, Andreas-Salomé explored her ideas about women, femininity, and sexuality. She also dealt with women and sexuality in her 1899 essay "Der Mensch als Weib," which was later included in her book *Die Erotik* (1910). She wrote about issues of fundamental concern to the emerging women's movement in Germany. Some of her essays appeared in *Die Frau* and *Die Neue Generation*, two periodicals whose editors, Helene Lange and Helene Stöcker, were committed to the women's movement. She was also a friend of Ellen Key, a Swedish writer who fought for women's rights. Nevertheless, Andreas-Salomé did not consider herself a part of the women's movement, nor was she interested in promoting social reform.

She continued to write on philosophy and religion. Her 1896 essay "Jesus der Jude," which she considered

A

to be one of her best, brought her into contact with Rilke. Together they traveled to Russia in 1899 and in 1900. These trips had a profound effect on both of them and served as the inspiration for Rilke's *Book of Hours* as well for Andreas-Salomé's *Ródinka*. It also formed the basis of a lifelong bond between them, as their extensive correspondence illustrates. After Rilke's death Andreas-Salomé wrote her account of his life, *Rainer Maria Rilke* (1928). Her Russian experience became the impetus for her inward journey that ultimately led her to psychoanalysis.

In 1911, in the company of the Swedish physician Poul Bjerre, Andreas-Salomé attended the Third International Psychoanalytic Congress at Weimar. Subsequently she began an intense study of psychoanalytic texts. When she visited Karl Abraham in the spring of 1912, he was sufficiently impressed by her understanding of psychoanalysis that he wrote a letter of recommendation on her behalf to Sigmund Freud. Andreas-Salomé traveled to Vienna in 1912 in order to attend Freud's lectures. She kept a diary during her 1912–1913 stay in Vienna that was published posthumously as *In der Schule bei Freud* (1958). It contains not only an account of her activities, including contacts with Alfred Adler and Victor Tausk, but also her ideas and critical comments on topics covered in Freud's lectures and the discussions that took place during the Wednesday meetings of the Vienna Psychoanalytic Society.

Andreas-Salomé called her encounter with Freud and psychoanalysis "a turning point" in her life. She became a fiercely loyal supporter of Freud as well as a family friend. But she did not feel obliged to accept every aspect of Freud's theories, nor did Freud insist that she do so. In her essays "Zum Typus Weib" (1914), " 'Anal' und 'Sexual' " (1915/1916), and "Narzissmus als Doppelrichtung" (1921), published in the psychoanalytic journal *Imago*, she expresses opinions on female sexuality, narcissism, and the unconscious that are characteristically her own. She does not hesitate to point out these differences in her correspondence with Freud, which began in 1912 and ended at her death. Freud considered her ideas on anal eroticism to be important contributions to the understanding of the subject and referred to " 'Anal' und 'Sexual' " in his 1920 revision of *Three Essays on the Theory of Sexuality*.

Andreas-Salomé felt a deep gratitude to Freud that she mentioned many times in her letters to him as well as to Anna Freud. On the occasion of Freud's seventy-fifth birthday, she wrote a long essay in the form of an open letter, "Mein Dank an Freud" (1931). She insisted on that title although Freud objected to it, suggesting that she replace his name with "psychoanalysis." While expressing her thanks to Freud, she also used this letter to express her ideas on anal eroticism and sublimation.

In the fall of 1921, Andreas-Salomé returned to Vienna at the invitation of Freud. During that visit she was a guest at Freud's home at Berggasse 19 and came to know his daughter Anna. She became Anna's friend and confidante at a time when Anna was not sure about the direction of her personal or professional life. The yet unpublished correspondence between Anna Freud and Andreas-Salomé, begun after her 1921 visit to Vienna, shows that Andreas-Salomé played a crucial role in helping Anna Freud make important decisions in her life.

During Anna Freud's first visit in Göttingen, the two women worked together on a project that turned into "Beating Fantasies and Daydreams," Anna Freud's initial paper, which she presented to the Vienna Psychoanalytic Society on May 31, 1922. On the basis of that paper, both women became members of the society. They attended congresses together, exchanged ideas on psychoanalytic topics, and visited one another as frequently as they could. During the initial years of Freud's illness, their correspondence was a vital emotional link between them.

Anna Freud was very much aware how important "Lou," as she called her, was in her life. Time and again she wrote to Andreas-Salomé about issues that were of concern to her, and asked for her opinion and advice. In 1932 Anna Freud, by then an established analyst in her own right and her father's representative in the psychoanalytic community, wrote to Andreas-Salomé that she kept coming back to what Andreas-Salomé had once told her: it does not matter what one's fate is, as long as one lives it fully. This was Andreas-Salomé's adaptation of Nietzsche's "amor fati" (love of fate) from his *Ecce Homo*. She had turned it into an imperative that she also applied to herself.

From 1913 until about 1935, Andreas-Salomé was a lay analyst in Göttingen, where she and her husband had settled in 1903 after he obtained a position at the university. Göttingen was not very receptive to psychoanalysis, and it was difficult for her to get analysands who were willing to pay. Physically separated by distance, she felt isolated from the psychoanalytic community. She traveled, and corresponded with many analysts, including Freud, Sándor Ferenczi and Max Eitingon.

World War I and the 1917 revolution in Russia brought Andreas-Salomé the additional problem of divided loyalties, which she voiced in her letters to Rilke and Freud. She was living in Germany while her family was in Russia, on the side of the czarist regime. Financial problems brought about by the war and the subsequent inflation in Germany prompted Andreas-Salomé to go wherever her work took her. In 1922–1923 she spent several months in Berlin working at the Polyclinic while Eitingon's house guest. In 1923–1924 she went to Königsberg as a training analyst, only to find that what she had earned was wiped out by inflation. Freud and analysts from Berlin tried to help by sending referrals to her. Freud also gave her financial help. When he received the Goethe Prize in 1930, he sent her part of the prize money.

With the rise of National Socialism, Andreas-Salomé watched the emigration of her friends and colleagues in the psychoanalytic community. Health problems restricted her activities. Toward the end of her life she returned to writing, reworking old manuscripts and composing her reminiscences (*Lebensrückblick*, 1951). She died in Göttingen on February 5, 1937, shortly before her seventy-sixth birthday.

REFERENCES

For a comprehensive listing of Lou Andreas-Salomé's writings, see Binion; Livingstone; Welsch and Wiesner; Weber and Rempp (*Das "Zweideutige" Lächeln der Erotik*).

Andreas-Salomé, Lou. (1892). *Henrik Ibsens Frauengestalten. Nach seinen sechs Familiendramen: Ein Puppenheim/ Gespenster/Die Wildente/Rosmersholm/Die Frau vom Meere/Hedda Gabler.* Jena: 2nd ed., Berlin: 1906. Edited and translated by S. Mandel as *Ibsen's Heroines*. Redding Ridge, Conn.: Black Swan, 1985.

———. *Nietzsche in seinen Werken.* Vienna: Carl Konengen. 2nd ed., edited by E. Pfeiffer. Frankfurt: Insel Verlag, 1983. Edited and translated by S. Mandel as *Nietzsche*. Redding Ridge, Conn.: Black Swan, 1988.

———. (1895). *Ruth. Eine Erzählung.* Stuttgart: Cotta. 2nd ed., Stuttgart: Cotta, 1897.

———. (1896). Jesus der Jude. *Neue Deutsche Rundschau* 7: 342–351.

———. (1902). *Im Zwischenland. Fünf Geschichten aus dem Leben Halbwüchsiger Mädchen.* Stuttgart: Cotta.

———. (1914). Zum typus weib. *Imago* 3: 1–14. Reprinted in her *Das "zweideutige" Lächeln der Erotik*, edited by I. Weber and B. Rempp, pp. 87–103. Freiburg im Breisgau: Kore, 1990.

———. (1915/1916). "Anal" und "Sexual." *Imago* 4: 249–273. Reprinted in her *Das "Zweideutige" Lächeln der Erotik*, pp. 105–135.

———. (1917). *Drei Briefe an Einen Knaben.* Leipzig: Kurt Wolff Verlag. Reprinted in her *Das "Zweideutige" Lächeln der Erotik*, pp. 53–86.

———. (1919). *Das Haus. Eine Familiengeschichte vom Ende des Vorigen Jahrhunderts.* Berlin: 3rd ed., Berlin: Ullstein, 1987.

———. (1921). Narzissmus als doppelrichtung. *Imago* 7: 361–386. Reprinted in her *Das "Zweideutige" Lächeln der Erotik*, pp. 191–222.

———. (1923). *Ródinka. Eine russische Erinnerung.* Jena: Eugen Diederichs. 2nd ed., Berlin: Ullstein, 1985.

———. (1928). *Rainer Maria Rilke.* Leipzig: Insel. 2nd ed., Leipzig: Insel, 1928.

———. (1931). Mein dank an Freud. In *Offener Brief an Professor Sigmund Freud zu seinem 75. Geburtstag.* Vienna: Internationaler Psychoanalytischer Verlag. Reprinted in her *Das "Zweideutige" Lächeln der Erotik*, pp. 245–324.

———. (1951). *Lebensrückblick. Grundriss einer Lebenserinnerung.* Edited by E. Pfeiffer. Zurich: Max Niehans Verlag. 5th ed., Frankfurt: Insel Verlag, 1984. Translated by B. Mitchell and edited by E. Pfeiffer as *Looking Back: Memoirs of Lou Andreas-Salomé*. New York: Paragon House.

———. (1952). *Rainer Maria Rilke. Lou Andreas-Salomé: Briefwechsel.* Edited by E. Pfeiffer. Wiesbaden: Insel. 2nd ed., Frankfurt: Insel, 1975.

———. (1958). *In der Schule bei Freud. Tagebuch Eines Jahres.* Edited by E. Pfeiffer. Zurich: Max Niehans Verlag. 2nd ed., Berlin: Ullstein, 1983.

———. (1966). *Siegmund Freud. Lou Andreas-Salomé. Briefwechsel.* Edited by E. Pfeiffer. Frankfurt: S. Fischer Verlag. Translated by W. Robson-Scott and E. Robson-Scott, and edited by E. Pfeiffer as *Sigmund Freud and Lou Andreas-Salomé, Letters*. New York: Norton.

———. (1990). *Das "Zweideutige" Lächeln der Erotik.* Edited by I. Weber and B. Rempp. Freiburg im Breisgau: Kore.

Binion, R. (1968). *Frau Lou: Nietzsche's Wayward Disciple.* Princeton, N.J.: Princeton University Press.

Koepke, C. (1982). *Lou Andreas-Salomé: Ein Eigenwilliger Lebensweg.* Freiburg im Breisgau: Herder Verlag.

Livingstone, A. (1984). *Salomé: Her Life and Work.* Mount Kisco, N.Y.: Moyer Bell.

Martin, B. (1991). *Woman and Modernity: The (Life) Styles of Lou Andreas-Salomé.* Ithaca, N.Y.: Cornell University Press.

Michaud, S. (2000). *Lou Andreas-Salomé: L'Allie de la Vie.* Paris: Editions du Seuil.

Rothe, D. A. (1996). Letters of two remarkable women: The Anna Freud-Lou Andreas-Salomé correspondence. *International Forum for Psychoanalysis* 5: 233–245.

Welsch, U., and Wiesner, M. (1988). *Lou Andreas-Salomé: Vom "Lebensurgrund" zur Psychoanalyse.* Munich: Verlag Internationale Psychoanalyse.

DARIA ROTHE

A

Anna O. (1859–1936)

Anna O. (1859–1936), whose real name was Bertha Pappenheim, has a special place in the history of psychoanalysis. She was the first patient to be treated with a new form of psychotherapy which opened the way for psychoanalytic thinking.

In December 1880, Anna O., then twenty-one, developed a severe hysterical illness while caring for her father, Siegmund Pappenheim, a wealthy grain merchant who was slowly dying of a subpleural abscess. Josef Breuer, a prominent and much respected Viennese internist who was a mentor and friend of Sigmund Freud, became her physician. Anna's case is of great interest because of the complexity of her illness (Ernest Jones called it "a museum of symptoms") and because Breuer, quite serendipitously and guided by Anna herself, developed a new method of treatment. Breuer discovered that if he asked his patient, under light hypnosis, to tell him how particular symptoms had started, the symptoms disappeared or were temporarily attenuated. Instead of ordering the symptoms away, as in traditional hypnotic treatment, Breuer invited Anna to talk about them while he listened. The procedure, which involved a catharsis of the emotional material that had accumulated since the prior visit, was performed each day in the evening, and sometimes in the morning as well; it came to be known as "Breuer's method" or "the cathartic method." Anna herself called it "the talking cure." Prior to Breuer, probably no one had ever spent so much time listening to a psychiatric patient.

Freud was fascinated by the story he heard from Breuer, and was prompted to treat several other cases of hysteria by similar methods. The treatment of Anna O., however, had not gone well. In 1882, about a year after the death of her father, Anna had developed a pseudocyesis with the delusion that she was pregnant by Breuer. Breuer, unprotected by knowledge of the transference (which had not yet been discovered), was shaken by the experience and understandably reluctant to publish the case. Thirteen years elapsed. Finally, Freud was able to convince Breuer that the story of Anna O. was too important to be forgotten, and that they should collaborate on a book about their investigations, which would include also the case of Anna O. Titled *Studies on Hysteria*, (1895), the book remains a landmark contribution on hysteria and the origins of the psychoanalytic method.

Anna O.'s illness was not only difficult but prolonged, and required several hospitalizations, a fact which Breuer omitted from his 1895 report along with mention of her pseudocyesis. Her principal symptoms included intermittent psychosis; dissociative, conversion, and phobic manifestations; two personalities; an eating disorder; dramatic visual hallucinations; trigeminal neuralgia; and addiction to chloral hydrate and morphine which had been prescribed for sedation and analgesia. Breuer withdrew from the case in June 1882, when he referred Anna to the Sanatorium Bellevue in Kreuzlingen, Switzerland. In 1888 Anna O. finally recovered, moved permanently with her mother, Recha, to Frankfurt, Germany, where Mrs. Pappenheim had been born and where she still had many relatives. Anna's younger brother, Wilhelm, remained in Vienna, where he studied, and later practiced, law; Anna and Wilhelm were never close for reasons that are still unclear.

At this point the "second phase" of Anna's life began. A self-trained social worker, Anna founded and directed a home for orphaned Jewish girls. After the death of her mother in 1905, Anna lived alone and never married. Her illness did not return; she managed to achieve stability of a sort, based on a spartan lifestyle, unremitting hard work, and dedicated altruism. In addition to her work as director of the orphanage, she wrote plays, stories, and articles with a social background and a feminist orientation that dealt particularly with the relationship between the sexes. Typically, she saw women as victims and men as sexual predators. She became very occupied with the problem of prostitution—"white slavery," as it was called—and traveled far and wide, usually alone, from St. Petersburg to the Near East to New York City, inspecting brothels and the condition of Jewish prostitutes.

In 1935, for the first time since she had left Vienna in 1888, Anna returned for a final visit to her native city and to her brother Wilhelm; by then she was ill with cancer, and died a few months later. It is believed that during her stay in Vienna she may have destroyed letters and other documents pertaining to her youthful psychiatric illness. The Gestapo did not interfere with this frail and obviously ill woman. Afterward, however, they seized Hannah Karminski, Anna's friend and the assistant director of the orphanage; she disappeared in a concentration camp. Karminski had made plans to write a biography of Anna; a short biography of her was written much later by Dora Edinger, a distant relative. Anna never spoke of her youthful illness; she acknowledged it only once to Edinger, but gave no details.

There are many fascinating aspects to the story of Anna O. which have generated an extensive literature. These include the matter of her identity, various details of her illness which Breuer omitted for reasons of confidentiality, and her standing as a social activist and early feminist.

In his 1953 biography of Freud, Jones revealed Anna's real name because of her importance in the history of psychoanalysis. Her pseudocyesis came to light through disclosures by Freud: orally to Jones, Carl Jung, and his editor, James Strachey, as well as in several of his writings (e.g., in a letter of June 1932). The intriguing researches of Henri Ellenberger and Albrecht Hirschmüller have clarified Anna's illness and hospitalizations; Peter Swales has identified the place where Anna's father became ill. Ellenberger discovered from clues in a photograph of Anna that she had been hospitalized at the Sanatorium Bellevue; in the record room of the sanatorium he found Breuer's 1882 letter of referral, which is very similar to his 1895 case report but also differs in some important respects; he also found her discharge summary, written by a staff psychiatrist.

Anna O. remains, a century or so after her illness, a complex and strong-minded woman, idealistic and very much alive. In 1954 the German government issued a commemorative stamp with the portrait of a youthful Anna O. The legend reads, "Bertha Pappenheim Helfer der Menschheit" (helper of mankind).

REFERENCES

Breuer, J., and Freud, S. (1893–1895). *Studies on Hysteria.* S.E. 2.

Castelnuovo-Tedesco, P. (1994). On Re-reading the case of Anna O. More about questions that are unanswerable. *Journal of the American Academy of Psychoanalysis* 22: 57–71.

Edinger, D. (1963). *Bertha Pappenheim: Freud's Anna O.* Highland Park, Ill.: Congregation Solel.

Ellenberger, H. (1970). *The Discovery of the Unconscious.* New York: Basic Books.

———. (1972). The story of 'Anna O'. A critical review with new data. *Journal of the History of the Behavioral Sciences* 8: 267–279.

Freud, S. (1975). Letter to Stefan Zweig, dated June 2, 1932. In Ernst L. Freud (ed.), *Letters of Sigmund Freud,* pp. 412–413. New York: Basic Books.

Hirschmüller, A. (1989). *The Life and Work of Josef Breuer. Physiology and Psychoanalysis.* New York: New York University Press.

Jensen, E. (1970). Anna O. A study of her later life. *Psychoanalytic Quarterly* 39: 269–293.

Jones, E. (1953). *The Life and Work of Sigmund Freud.* Vol. 1. New York: Basic Books.

Swales, P. (1988). Anna O. in Ischl. *Werkblatt* 5: 57–64.

PIETRO CASTELNUOVO-TEDESCO

A

Anthropology, and Psychoanalysis

Anthropology was the first social science to utilize Freud's insights and findings to any degree. Though relatively few anthropologists have accepted and applied his psychological and cultural theories and methods wholesale, Freud and his followers have significantly influenced culture and personality studies and psychological anthropology (Bock, 1995; Heald and Deluz, 1994; La Barre, 1958; Le Vine, 1982; Wallace, 1983). A small but influential segment of cultural anthropologists have themselves been analyzed or received psychoanalytic training. Many more have collaborated closely with psychoanalytic psychiatrists and psychologists in the collection and interpretation of data (e.g., Ruth Benedict, Clyde Kluckhohn, Margaret Mead, Ralph Linton, Gregory Bateson, William Caudill, and Philip Bock). Journals such as *Ethos, Journal of Psychological Anthropology, Psychoanalytic Study of Society,* and *Journal of Psychoanalytic Anthropology* have remained important forums for such work.

Freud's anthropology and social thought generally are subject to a paradox. Ostensibly, his clinical and metapsychological writings are the meat of his corpus, whereas his sociocultural work is a late and (many feel) embarrassing development in the career of an otherwise brilliantly perspicacious psychologist. After all, his first major contribution to the topic (*Totem and Taboo*) did not appear until 1913, and others followed only sporadically: *Group Psychology and the Analysis of the Ego* (1921), *The Future of an Illusion* (1927), *Civilization and Its Discontents* (1930), and *Moses and Monotheism* (1939). Despite appearances, however, Freud's cultural concerns did not awaken until late in his career: "My interest," he wrote, "after making a long *detour* through the natural sciences, medicine and psychotherapy, returned to the cultural problems which had fascinated me long before, when I was a youth scarcely old enough for thinking" (1935, p. 72).

Second, Freud's anthropology was not isolated from the rest of his work. Nor were his anthropological writings merely an instance of "applied psychoanalysis." Rather, there was an intimate cross-fertilization between his anthropological reading and thinking, on the one hand, and his psychological reading, practice, and thinking, on the other. In fact, there is strong evidence for the influence of nineteenth-century cultural evolutionist writers (such as Herbert Spencer, Edward Tylor, and John Lubbock) on some of his most important psychological presuppositions and concepts—including projection, psychic causality, the omnipotence of thoughts, primary process thinking, neurosis as atavism, the Oedipus complex, the role of phylogeny in human psychology, and the psychic unity of mankind (Wallace, 1980, 1983).

Third, contrary to the impression conveyed by Ernest Jones (1953–1957), Freud was neither ignored by anthropologists nor given a wholly unfavorable reception by them. His impact on anthropology was definite and persistent. It began at least as early as 1920, when Alfred Kroeber published his review of *Totem and Taboo* in the *American Anthropologist*, and continued on through the work of such scholars as Charles Seligman, Edward Sapir, Bronislaw Malinowski, Melville Herskovits, Alfred Hallowell, Clyde Kluckhohn, and Margaret Mead. Generally, Freud's purely psychological writings were taken up more eagerly by anthropologists than his more specifically anthropological ones.

Freud read many of the writers who would influence his psychocultural thinking long before beginning work on *Totem and Taboo*. These included the philosophical and sociocultural reflections of David Hume, Ludwig Feuerbach, Friedrich Nietzsche, and Buckle; the biological and psychosocial writings of Darwin and Spencer; and a host of anthropologists, such as Tylor, Lubbock, Lewis Morgan, John F. McLennan, Johann Bachofen—and later James Frazer and Wilhelm Wundt. These philosophical and anthropological writers (read by Freud by 1900–1902) influenced his cultural and psychological ideas quite as much as did Darwin and the nineteenth-century biologists and sexologists emphasized by Sulloway (1979) (see Wallace, 1983).

While some of Freud's early letters, brief writings, and comments at the meetings of the Vienna Psychoanalytical Society reveal his cultural interests and insistence on parallels between the mental lives of "primitives" and neurotics, the earliest explicit psychoanalytic forays into anthropological, mythological, and artistic topics came from his disciples such as Otto Rank (1907, 1909, 1912), Alphonse Maeder (1908), and Karl Abraham (1908, 1912).

Stimulated partly by these colleagues and by the intensifying relationship with Carl Jung (who was writing his own psychocultural study, *Wandlungen und Symbole der Libido* [1912]), Freud began researching and writing *Totem and Taboo* in August 1911 (Wallace, 1983, pp. 59–64). From 1911 to 1913, Freud read a mass of ethnographic material—mostly by cultural evolutionists, who were themselves beginning to lose anthropological pride of place to the diffusionists and historical particularists ("Boasians"). Many anthropologists would criticize Freud's ready subscription to cultural evolutionist tenets such as psychic unity, the mental equivalence of adult contemporary "primitives" to prehistoric peoples and modern Western children, the notion of fixed and universal stages in cultural development, and the idea of psychic Lamarckianism and the biogenetic law.

Totem and Taboo appeared in 1913. Though it was never revised (unlike, for example, *The Interpretation of Dreams* and *Three Essays on the Theory of Sexuality*), many of its basic concepts reappeared in Freud's subsequent sociocultural works (1921, 1927, 1930, 1939), as well as in seminal psychological pieces such as "Mourning and Melancholia" (1917).

Totem and Taboo comprises four chapters. The first three deal with different aspects of the parallels between primitive and neurotic behavior. "The Horror of Incest" treats the sexual side of the Oedipus complex; "Taboo and Emotional Ambivalence" concentrates on the aggressive side; and "Animism, Magic, and the Omnipotence of Thoughts" expounds on the similarities in primitive and neurotic modes of thought. Finally, "The Return of Totemism in Childhood," which Freud considered the gem of the work, introduces the controversial theory of the primal horde and parricide, and proclaims the Oedipus complex the focal point of "the beginnings of religion, morals, society, and art" (1913, p. 156). Apart from Freud's attempt to demonstrate the primacy of projection, wishful thinking, and primary process modes of thought in magic and animism, this book proposes that cultural institutions (such as religion, totemism, exogamy rules, and the incest taboo) represent neurotic defenses and compromise formations (symptoms) at the group level. Totemism, which Freud saw as the precursor of religions such as Judaism and Christianity, was an ambivalent and guilt-laden attempt to come to terms with the sons' primordial oedipal aggression against the primal father. The Christian Eucharist, as well as certain Jewish rituals, continued the conflictual representation of the phylogenetically transmitted unconscious memory and remorse over the primal parricide. Exogamy rules and the incest taboo were further modes of atonement for this crime, as well as defenses against the sons' continued incestuous strings. *Moses and Monotheism* (1939) extended these themes to world historical religions such as Judaism and Christianity.

Despite some of the more fantastic theses in *Totem and Taboo*, many anthropologists have found considerable cogency in Freud's Oedipal (not phylogenetic) explanation of the incest taboo and exogamy rules (see, e.g., Stephens, 1962; D'Andrahl, 1961; Spiro, 1982). Similarly, Freud's idea that psychological conflicts, defenses, and compromise formations can become culturally institutionalized has borne important fruit (see Spiro, 1965; Le Vine, 1982).

Subsequent works, such as *Group Psychology and the Analysis of the Ego* (1921), placed more emphasis on personality and society/culture as an interactive process— for example, the individual's building of psychic structure through identification and through the internalization of social permissions and interdicts. And it was in this work that Freud wrote: "In the individual's mental life someone else is invariably involved, as a model, as an object, as a helper, as an opponent; and so from the very first individual psychology, in this extended but entirely justifiable sense of the words, is at the same time social psychology as well" (1921, p. 69).

Still, despite such insights, Freud's subsequent sociocultural work tended to explain culture and social institutions on the model of the individual neurotic writ large. It remained for post- or neo-Freudians such as Abram Kardiner (1939, 1945), Harry Stack Sullivan (1953), Erik Erikson (1950, 1962, 1970), and, much later, Robert Le Vine (1982) to develop more genuinely psychosocially interactive approaches. These writers also tended to emphasize, as did Frederic Bartlett (1939, p. 73), that it is not merely a question of conflicts between purely biological impulses and socially instituted inhibitions: "The driving forces are quite as much social [I would prefer to say "biosocial"] products as the social barriers which block them."

For example, in *The Future of an Illusion* (1927) Freud retained his 1907 diagnosis of religion as the "universal obsessional neurosis of humanity"—as he did that of philosophy as universal paranoia and art as universal hysteria. The upshot is clear: "If the development of civilization has such a far-reaching similarity to the development of the individual and if it employs the same methods," then we may be justified in diagnosing "some civilizations, or some epochs of civilization—*possibly the whole of mankind* [as] neurotic" (1927, p. 144; italics added). In *The Future of an Illusion*, we see the same emphasis on the crucial role of the leader (and the group members' internalization of his forceful precepts) in social cohesion as in *Group Psychology and the Analysis of the Ego*.

Civilization and Its Discontents (1930), Freud's most powerful social commentary, continues this emphasis on the ontogenetically and phylogenetically based internalization of the repressive dictates of the primal father. It is this internalized aggression (prompted by phylogenetic and ontogenetic remorse over the hostile component of the Oedipus complex) that establishes the superego, which is responsible for the self-restraint and social cohesion necessary for higher civilization. However, this internalization is also responsible for man's continued neurotic propensities and for the never optimum balance between the individual's demands for self-gratification and the inhibitory requirements for a civilized society. *Moses and Monotheism* (1939), Freud's last major sociocultural work, resurrects the primal parricide and inherited remorse of *Totem and Taboo*. Aptly subtitled *A Historical Novel*, it nonetheless furnished social scientists and historians with the hypothesis that whole nations or cultures can repress unpleasant or conflictual aspects of a history that may yet return to haunt them. Studies of the early post–World War II decades of Germany have examined this issue vis-à-vis the Holocaust.

In conclusion, Freud's thinking on cultural issues is far too complex to render adequately in a brief essay. By and large, anthropologists have not approached either Freud or psychoanalysis monolithically, but have discriminated among its tenets. While certain ideas—such as Freud's theory of totemism and the primal parricide— have tended to be overwhelmingly rejected, others have found a more favorable reception (the use of ambivalence to explain certain taboos and mourning behavior, of incestuous drives to explain incest taboos, of projection to explain animism, and of wish fulfillment and the omnipotence of thoughts to explain magic). But psychoanalysis, as Boyer (1978) points out, has not gone unaffected by its contact with anthropology—witness the neo-Freudian and dynamic culturalist schools, facets of ego and object relations psychology, and transcultural psychiatry. In short, Freud's impact on cultural

A

anthropology is far from dead. In many ways, he realized his lifelong dream of returning to the cultural issues that had gripped him since childhood.

REFERENCES

Abraham, K. (1908). Dreams and myths. *Journal of Nervous and Mental Disease* monograph no. 15, 1913.

———. (1912). Amenhotep IV (Echnaton): Psychoanalytische beiträge zum verstandis seinen personlichkeit und des monotheistische atonkultes. *Imago* 1: 334–360.

Bartlett, F. (1939). The limitations of Freud. *Science and Society* 3: 64–105.

Bock, P. (1995). *Rethinking Psychological Anthropology: Continuity and Change in the Study of Human Action.* Prospect Heights, Ill.: Waveland.

Boyer, B. (1978). The mutual influences between psychoanalysis and anthropology. *Journal of Psychological Anthropology* 1: 265–296.

D'Andrahl, R. (1961). Anthropological studies and dreams. In Francis Hsu (ed.), *Psychological Anthropology.* Homewood, Ill.: Dorsey.

Erikson, Eric. (1950). *Childhood and Society.* New York: Norton.

———. (1962). *Young Man Luther.* New York: Norton.

———. (1970). *Life History and the Historical Moment.* New York: Norton.

Freud, S. (1907). Obsessive actions and religious practice. S.E. 9: 117–127.

———. (1913). *Totem and Taboo.* S.E. 13: 1–161.

———. (1917). Mourning and melancholia. S.E. 14: 243–248.

———. (1921). Group psychology and the analysis of the ego. S.E. 18: 69–143.

———. (1927). *The Future of an Illusion.* S.E. 21: 5–56.

———. (1930). *Civilization and its Discontents.* S.E. 23: 7–137.

———. (1935). Postscript to an autobiographical study. S.E. 20: 71–74.

———. (1939). *Moses and Monotheism.* S.E. 23: 7–137.

Heald, S., and Deluz, A. (eds.). (1994). *Anthropology and Psychoanalysis: An Encounter Through Culture.* London: Routledge.

Jones, E. (1953–1957). *The Life and Work of Sigmund Freud.* 3 vols. New York: Basic Books.

Jung, C. (1912). *Wandlungen und Symbole der Libido.* Vienna: Deuticke.

Kardiner, A. (1939). *The Individual and His Society.* New York: Columbia University Press.

———. (1945). *The Psychological Frontiers of Society.* New York: Columbia University Press.

La Barre, W. (1958). The influence of Freud on anthropology. *American Imago* 14: 275–328.

Le Vine, R. (1982). *Culture, Behavior, and Personality* Rev. ed. Chicago: Aldine.

Maeder, A. (1908). Die symbolik in den legenden, marchen, gebrauchen, und traumen. *Psychiatrisch-Neurologische Wochenschrift* 10: 45–49.

Rank, O. (1907). *Der Kunstler.* Vienna: Heller.

———. (1909). *The Myth of the Birth of the Hero.* New York: Vintage, 1964.

———. (1912). *Das Inzestmotiv in Dichtung und Sage.* Vienna: Deuticke. Translated by Gregory Richter as *The Incest Theme in Literature and Legend.* Baltimore: Johns Hopkins University Press, 1992.

Spiro, M. (1965). Religious systems as culturally constituted defense mechanisms. In M. Spiro (ed.), *Context and Meaning in Cultural Anthropology*, pp. 100–113. New York: Free Press.

———. (1982). *Oedipus in the Trobriands.* Chicago: University of Chicago Press.

Stephens, W. (1962). *The Oedipus Complex Hypothesis: Cross-Cultural Evidence.* New York: Free Press.

Sullivan, H. S. (1953). *The Interpersonal Theory of Psychiatry.* New York: Norton.

Sulloway, F. (1979). *Freud: Biologist of the Mind.* New York: Basic Books.

Wallace, E. R. (1980). Freud and cultural evolutionism. In E. Wallace and L. Pressley (eds.), *Essays in the History of Psychiatry*, pp. 186–203. Columbia, S.C.: R. L. Bryan.

———. (1983). *Freud and Anthropology: A History and Reappraisal.* Madison, Conn.: International Universities Press.

                                   EDWIN R. WALLACE IV

Anxiety See ANXIETY AND DEFENSE; ANXIETY NEUROSIS.

Anxiety and Defense

Freud proposed one theory of anxiety and defense in the early years of his work, and a second theory from 1920 onward. The essential difference between the two is in the postulated causal relation between anxiety and defense. In the first theory, defense (repression, warding off) is a precondition of anxiety: after repression occurs, sexual striving (libido) and any affect can be expressed (discharged) in the form of anxiety. Repression causes anxiety. In the second theory, anxiety, or a signal thereof, causes defensive activity, a reversal of the previously postulated causal sequence. Furthermore, anxiety is no longer viewed as a "discharge process."

The second theory did not replace the first, but complemented it. For most clinical and developmental situations, anxiety as a signal instigating defense was said to be the relevant mechanism. In the explanation of certain other anxiety situations, however, the idea of anxiety as the discharge of transformed libido still prevailed.

1890–1900

In the early work, commencing in the 1890s, affect was seen by Freud as a "discharge process," meaning the discharge of energy, physiological or mental. In hysteria, for example, a trauma (an experience which evokes a distressing affect) is theorized to produce an increase in the sum of excitation in the nervous system, which must be discharged by a motor or verbal reaction (1893a), or divested by associative psychic activity (1893b). The process of "abreaction" (detaching an affect from the memory of a traumatic event) was conceptualized as a discharge of the excess excitation or affect.

In many of Freud's writings, the terms "affect" and "anxiety" are used interchangeably, as are the several terms for units of energy. There is, in addition, another ambiguity in his terminology. In *Project for a Scientific Psychology* (1895a) and in subsequent theoretical works, Freud tended to use the term "unpleasure" to designate anxiety, but he also used it to refer to other, perhaps less well delineated, affect states with an unpleasurable quality.

In his more clinical work, Freud usually used the term "anxiety" and, in this context, seemed to think first about somatic sexual factors. A major and permanent element in Freud's anxiety theory was his development of the concept of actual (*aktual*, or current) neuroses (1895b). These were conditions of altered excitation in the nervous system, not the product of mental conflict, and thus unlike the "neuropsychoses of defense" (1894a). The existence of these conditions, and the accompanying theory of anxiety, have been questioned by the great majority of other analysts ever since Freud introduced the ideas. Somatic and psychic sexual excitation are carefully differentiated in this period (see especially the sexual diagram, 1895c). In the theory of anxiety neurosis, one of the actual neuroses, anxiety is caused by undischarged somatic libido stemming from current (actual) sexual practices rather than from memories or traumatic experiences. In the neuropsychoses of defense, the excitation discharged as anxiety is said to arise from psychic libido. Once Freud discovered the roles of fantasy, infantile sexuality, and unconscious mentation, however, the distinction between somatic and psychic sexual excitation (libido) was no longer emphasized and, in fact, became deliberately blurred.

During this early period of work, Freud also introduced a relationship between anxiety and danger into the theory: a danger could arise from outside the organism, or from the accumulation of sexual excitation within the organism (1895b). He also related anxiety to breathing (1894b). It is important to keep in mind that in Freud's view, affects (i.e., anxiety) were discharge processes. There has to be a "something" to be discharged—some sort of energy—and energy must have a source.

1900-1920

After Freud proposed the topographic psychical systems (unconscious, preconscious, and consciousness), he saw the key to the "generation" of affects in the system unconscious: the entry of unconscious wishes into the preconscious may generate an unpleasure affect, that is, anxiety (1900). Two kinds of views of anxiety are now included in Freud's theory. One postulates a mechanism of anxiety production, either a response to external danger or the eruption of insufficiently disguised repressed wishes. The second view is concerned with energy sources: transformation of psychic libido, transformation of somatic libido, and cardiorespiratory or other somatic dysfunction. External stimuli can also be seen as an energy source. Structural relations (between the systems) and dynamic factors (mechanisms) have now been introduced into anxiety theory, in addition to energic considerations. The dynamic role of a signal of unpleasure (anxiety) was also introduced in the published work in 1900, but did not seem integral to the rest of the proposed sequences.

The period from 1902 to 1914 was one of expansion of clinical data for Freud. There were few major theoretical additions, relatively speaking, concerning anxiety. Anxiety remained an energic discharge of warded off libido, although "with the progress of repression . . . all affects are capable of being changed into anxiety" (1909, p. 35). The concept of a phylogenetic experience of birth was introduced to account for the particular quality of anxiety affect (1910), probably as a prototypic, universal experience of a disturbance of respiration.

Freud did not, however, allow his theory to interfere with the accumulation of observations that were not entirely convenient. In the report of the analysis of Little Hans (1909), he mentions that Hans's anxiety was related to longing for his mother; fear of punishment for hostile wishes against his sister; fear *of* his father because of his love for his mother; fear *for* his father because of his hostility toward his father; fear of repressed sadistic striving toward his mother; and distress about the small size of his penis. Neither the role of hostility nor the concern with penis size seems to fit readily into the libido *transformation theory.*

A

Significant consolidation occurred in Freud's anxiety theory during the period from 1914 to 1919. Anxiety remained, fundamentally, a discharge of libido. The theories of affects and energy remained largely indistinguishable. The relation between affect and buildup or discharge of excitation remained direct and explicit (1915a, 1915b, 1915c). The actual neuroses continued to be important in Freud's clinical scheme, although he mentioned that he no longer encountered such cases (1917, p. 386).

1920 Onward

In the years from 1920 until the end of his life, the changes Freud made in his theories of affects and energy were profound. In 1920, he altered an earlier fundamental hypothesis: he now said there is no simple relation between the quantity of excitation and the strength of feelings of pleasure and unpleasure (1920, pp. 7–8). This statement permits a distinction between the theory of affects and the theory of psychic energy: nondischarge affect states can now be described without doing violence to the theory of the pleasure principle. These steps are necessary precursors to altering the idea of anxiety as necessarily transformed libido. It is important to note, however, that Freud never discarded the idea that anxiety, at least in certain situations, is the product of the transformation of libido. He also began, explicitly, to differentiate anxiety and unpleasure (1926, p. 132): tension, pain, and mourning also have the quality of unpleasure.

From 1920 onward, Freud conceived of anxiety as an affective, unpleasurable state of expectation, of certain physiological accompaniments, and of perception of the physiological processes (1926, pp. 132–133, 161–165). He theorized that, in most situations, anxiety is an ego response to a dangerous situation, to be explained dynamically, genetically, structurally, and adaptively—but not as a discharge of energy.

Someone anticipating helplessness is in a "danger situation" (i.e., one perceived to be dangerous). The perceived threat may be external (physical helplessness) or instinctual (psychic helplessness). An experience of helplessness is a traumatic situation (1926, pp. 137, 166). Anxiety occurs in a particular (psychical) field: a situation perceived to be dangerous.

Once the ego-id-superego model of the mind was introduced (1923), conscious processes as well as regulatory functions were assigned to the ego. The ego then became "the actual seat of anxiety" (1923, p. 57); the ego alone could produce and feel anxiety (1926, p. 140; 1933, p. 85). From this (structural) viewpoint, there are three kinds of anxiety, depending on the source of the danger faced: neurotic (id danger), moral (superego threat), and real (external danger) (1923, p. 56). Anxiety is always a reaction to a dangerous situation; a drive is dangerous only if its satisfaction entails a real external danger (1926, pp. 126, 128).

States of helplessness are present from birth onward. The ability to anticipate helplessness does not, however, arise until later in development (1926, p. 136). Once that ability arises, the ego can produce an "anxiety signal," an anticipation of danger, which leads to a variety of responses, depending on the source of the danger and the level of development.

Early in life, before the anticipatory function develops, traumatic states occur as the result of energy disturbances produced by tension due to need, which echo the trauma of birth. After repeated experiences in which the infant's percept of the mother is associated with relief of growing tension due to need, the infant in that state of need takes the absence of the mother as the danger (1926, pp. 136–137). This is a change from an experience of trauma to a signal of anxiety (1926, p. 138). As development proceeds, a sequence of danger situations arises, each corresponding to a particular developmental phase (1926, p. 146): an experience of helplessness (trauma); absence of the object; loss of the object's love; castration; fear of the superego or the powers of fate (1926, pp. 139–143).

In Freud's later theory, there is no difference between anxiety and fear, except that for neurotic anxiety the source of the danger is unconscious (1926, pp. 108, 122, 126, 165). The affective reaction of anxiety is always a signal of a danger situation (1926, pp. 126, 128–129). Warding off of the drive derivative, the satisfaction of which is perceived as danger, is initiated by the anxiety signal: anxiety produces repression (defense) and not the other way around, as hypothesized earlier (1926, pp. 91–93, 108–109). "This causal sequence should not be explained from an economic point of view" (1926, p. 93)—that is, an energy source is not required as an integral part of the explanation.

There are exceptions to this formulation, however. Birth trauma is explained entirely in terms of energy discharge—a vast disturbance of the economy of narcissistic libido without psychic content (1926, pp. 135–136).

Growing tension due to need in early infancy, before development of the anticipatory function, results in a discharge of energy (1926, p. 137). Traumatic moments are not infrequent subsequently in infancy and childhood. In traumatic neuroses, the actual neuroses, and traumatic moments in adult life, anxiety is "involuntary, automatic and always justified on economic grounds . . ." (1926, p. 162).

Freud, in fact, consistently describes two types of anxiety from each of the metapsychological viewpoints. Economically, they are signal (nonenergic) anxiety and economic or generated anxiety. Structurally, anxiety may occur as a function of the ego organization or as a manifestation of the disruption of that organization (in a trauma). Developmentally, anxiety may occur as a response of the differentiated ego apparatus or as an experience of the undifferentiated apparatus. Dynamically, there may be a signal of impending helplessness or an experience of present helplessness. Adaptively, the anxiety response may be expedient or inexpedient.

Through most of the work reviewed here, Freud used the terms "repression" and "defense" synonymously. In some of the general, theoretical work and in the study of clinical entities, he sometimes specified a number of defenses, including repression (in a more limited sense), regression, reaction formation, undoing, identification, turning against the self, projection, and reversal (1915a, 1918, 1926). Defense, in Freud's work, was always a nuclear part of the ego concept (e.g., 1893a). Ego defenses, or self-preservative drives, ward off from consciousness certain drives or derivatives stemming from the unconscious or, later, the id. In the work prior to 1920, anxiety resulted from a failure of defense and an irruption of some unconscious content into the sphere of the ego with attendant discharge of libido. In the post-1920 work, anxiety occurred as a signal of danger aroused by activity of an id impulse or drive derivative. The signal caused defensive operations to occur. Defense, in Freud's work, was always directed against drive derivatives (1915c). In the early work, the presence of (neurotic) anxiety always indicated a failure of defense, manifested by the intrusion of an unacceptable drive derivative into consciousness.

REFERENCES

Freud, S. (1893a). On the psychical mechanism of hysterical phenomena: A lecture. S.E. 3: 27–39.

———. (1893b). Some points for a comparative study of organic and hysterical motor paralyses. S.E. 1: 157–172.

———. (1893c). Draft B. The aetiology of the neuroses. S.E. 1: 179–183.

———. (1894a). The neuro-psychoses of defense. S.E. 3: 45–61.

———. (1894b). Draft E: How anxiety originates. S.E. 1: 189–195.

———. (1895a). Project for a Scientific Psychology. S.E. 1: 281–397.

———. (1895b). On the grounds for detaching a particular syndrome from neurasthenia under the description "anxiety neurosis." S.E. 3: 90–117.

———. (1895c). Draft G. Melancholia. S.E. 1: 200–206.

———. (1900). The Interpretation of Dreams. S.E. 4 and 5.

———. (1909). Analysis of a phobia in a five-year-old boy. S.E. 10: 5–147.

———. (1910). A special type of choice of object made by men. S.E. 11: 165–175.

———. (1915a). Instincts and their vicissitudes. S.E. 14: 117–140.

———. (1915b). Repression. S.E. 14: 146–158.

———. (1915c). The unconscious. S.E. 14: 166–215.

———. (1917). Introductory Lectures on Psycho-Analysis. S.E. 15 and 16: 9–496.

———. (1918). From the history of an infantile neurosis. S.E. 17: 7–123.

———. (1920). Beyond the Pleasure Principle. S.E. 18: 7–64.

———. (1923). The Ego and the Id. S.E. 19: 12–59.

———. (1926). Inhibitions, Symptoms and Anxiety. S.E. 20: 87–172.

———. (1933). New Introductory Lectures on Psycho-analysis. S.E. 22: 5–185.

Stewart, W. (1967). Psychoanalysis: The First Ten Years. New York: Macmillan.

ALLAN COMPTON

Anxiety Neurosis

Anxiety neurosis is a condition in which neurotic solutions fail to deal effectively with inner conflicts, but the resulting anxiety is not attached to specific phobic objects or situations, so that the afflicted individual feels chronically or frequently anxious, in an unfocused, generalized, ill-defined manner.

In the course of his early clinical observations, Sigmund Freud, then a neuroanatomist and neurologist, became interested in a group of nervous patients who came with complaints of chronic, morbid anxiety associated with a variety of minor but troubling somatic disturbances. He separated off this group from those diagnosed as suffering from "neurasthenia," a term popularly used at that time to refer to patients complaining of nervousness, emotional and physical exhaustion, anhedonia, and a number of discomfiting somatic complaints, such as insomnia, shortness of breath, dyspepsia, flatulence, and headache. Neurasthenia seemed to occur in members of the more affluent, upper-middle and upper classes.

Freud connected neurasthenia with a lifestyle of self-centeredness and sybaritic self-indulgence, in which one prominent feature was solitary masturbation in the place of mature sexuality. The symptoms of the patients whom he separated off—those suffering from anxiety neurosis—seemed to him, on clinical grounds, to have a different etiology and significance than those of the neurasthenic patients.

The anxiety neurosis patients were tense, chronically anxious, and often hypochondriacal. They seemed to live in dread that something terrible was going to happen. They complained of periodic intense anxiety, associated with palpitations, shortness of breath, dizziness, paresthesia, and, at times, nausea, vomiting, and diarrhea. At first, Freud hypothesized that inadequate discharge of sexual excitement was at the basis of these patients' complaints. He observed that the condition occurred frequently in men with undischarged or inadequately discharged sexual excitement, because of sexual inhibition, coitus interruptus, or decreased sexual potency together with increasing libido during senescence. He also observed it in single women who were aroused sexually but lacked sexual outlets, in women who were anorgasmic or whose husbands were impotent or suffered from premature ejaculation, and in women who had lost their husbands and had no sexual outlets.

Freud constructed a working hypothesis that the anxiety experienced by these patients represented the transformation of their sexual tension, or "libido," into the affect of anxiety. He thought, in consonance with the mechanistic orientation prevalent in the medical community at that time, that dammed-up, inadequately discharged sexual excitation had somehow become transformed into nervous tension.

He soon realized, however, that it was not the state of arousal of feelings that was the problem; rather, there was inner awareness that disappointment, frustration, anger, vengefulness, temptation, and related feelings were impelling the individual toward actions that might very well lead to serious, untoward, even dangerous consequences. The person with anxiety neurosis felt helpless vis-à-vis the danger. He or she felt unable to cope with the situation, afraid of losing control, and thrust into a state of unrelieved nervousness, anxiety, and fear of something bad happening, but without knowing why this was happening. The cause of the anxiety was outside of awareness, because the individual was not able to face up to things consciously or to deal with them.

As time went on, and more and more clinical observations were accumulated, Freud and those who joined with him in carrying out psychoanalytic investigations came to recognize that anxiety is not just a passive experience. It is also actively generated within the psyche as a signal that a state of danger exists, in response to which some sort of effective action needs to be taken in order to deal with that danger. Effective action can consist of the employment of psychological mechanisms to deal with internally perceived danger and/or physical action to deal with an external situation. Patients with an anxiety neurosis are insufficiently able to do either of these things, so that the anxiety mounts and they feel overwhelmed, strained, stretched beyond their limits, unable to cope, and in need of help.

At first, Freud focused on sexual conflicts as being central to the neurosis, but it later became apparent that though these do play a prominent part in most, and perhaps even in all, neurotic constellations, for developmental reasons there are other, equally important factors that also are involved. These include conflicts over aggressive and destructive urges, conflicts involving self-esteem and self-image, moral issues, and other key aspects of personal and social functioning. The central dimension in anxiety neurosis is not so much what the person is struggling with psychologically as the person's inability to mobilize effective resources with which to deal with emotional stress and emotional conflict. Putting it in terms of Freud's heuristically valuable conceptualization of the structure of the mind, it is more a matter of ego vulnerability and weakness than it is of the strength of instinctual drives.

REFERENCES

Freud, S. (1895 [1894]). On the grounds for detaching a particular syndrome from neurasthenia under the description "*Anxiety Neurosis*." S.E. 3: 90–117.

———. (1926). *Inhibitions, Symptoms and Anxiety*. S.E. 20: 87–172.

———. (1933). *New Introductory Lectures on Psychoanalysis*. S.E. 22: 5–185.

MARTIN SILVERMAN

Aphasia

In his first book, *On Aphasia: A Critical Study* (1891), Freud conceives of the structure of the speech apparatus as the foundation of spontaneous speech. He was deeply impressed by Josef Breuer's description of Anna O., and dedicated the book to him: "... she [Anna O.] could be relieved ... if she was induced to express in words the affective phantasy by which she was at the moment dominated" (Freud, 1925, p. 20). Freud was fascinated, and concluded that "The state of things he [Breuer] had discovered seemed to me to be of so fundamental a nature that I could not believe it could fail to be present in any case of hysteria if it had been proved to occur in a single one" (p. 21). The power of the spoken word had taken over Freud's professional career, giving birth to psychoanalysis. He later acknowledged the debt: "The cathartic method was the immediate precursor of psychoanalysis; and, in spite of every modification of theory, is still contained within it as its nucleus" (1924, p. 194).

Two of Freud's patients, Frau Emmy von N. and Frau Caecilia M., continued to teach him about their need to say what they had to say, and the connection between words and bodily sensations (Rizzuto, 1989). Freud devoted most of his time at the end of the 1880s to reflecting about these patients, trying to understand what they were saying and what made it possible. The topic was scientifically important because the prominent neurologists of the time were creating models of the speech apparatus, with the goal of making intelligible the aphasias caused by neurological lesions.

Freud created his own model of the speech apparatus, intending to explain not only aphasias caused by lesions but also those due to a functional disconnection between a word and the thing it represented. His intent was to build a theoretical apparatus that could explain the "spontaneous speech" of his patients.

Freud's monograph is a masterpiece of tightly reasoned construction of a model based on published neurological cases as well as on his own observation. The model explains with sober elegance the clinical varieties of aphasia as well as the functional disturbances of speech due to "divided attention," intense emotions, or fatigue. Freud rejects any anatomical localization of speech functions, and describes the speech apparatus as a complex organization of associations from the periphery to the cortex that is at the service of the speech function.

The object associations forming the object representations appear as the cortically organized transformations of sensory perceptions and associations, particularly visual, tactile, and auditory sensations. They represent the body at the cortical level in a manner that is suitable for the speech function. We have no choice but to form mental representations of objects as long as we are capable of experiencing sensations in our bodies. To perceive is to associate (Rizzuto, 1993).

A word representation for an external object represented in the mind originates in the speaker's hearing the sound of the word as uttered by others; it completes its representational function with the kinesthetic image of its pronunciation, and the visual and motor images associated with writing. The meaning of the word emerges in the connections (*Verknüpfung*) between the object representation and the word representation. The most frequent link is between the visual components of the object representation and the sound image of the word used to refer to it.

Finally, Freud answered his own question about the need to speak by concluding that "All stimulations to speak spontaneously come from the region of object associations" (1953 [1891], p. 78). Therefore, "what stimulates us to speak willingly is a wish to express something related to memory images organized into visual object representations" (Rizzuto, 1993, p. 123).

Freud did not include his monograph on aphasia as part of his psychoanalytic writings. Despite his view, those who have studied it, such as Binswanger (1936), Bernfeld (1944), Stengel (1953, 1954), and Forrester (1980), consider it to be the foundation of psychoanalysis. Important psychoanalytic terms appear in it for the first time: associations, divided attention, cathexis, complex, connection, physiological correlate, impulse to speak, mnemic image, primary, representation, self-observation, spontaneous speech, and transference (Rizzuto, 1990). Their meaning evolved in Freud's later writings, but they have their earliest use in the monograph.

Freud's *The Unconscious* (1915) is so clearly related to *On Aphasia* that James Strachey, the editor of the *Standard Edition*, decided to add as Appendix C the portion of *On Aphasia* that deals with the function of speech. Freud's model of the speech apparatus, however, is tacitly present in all his works, both theoretical and technical.

REFERENCES

Bernfeld, S. (1944). Freud's earliest theories and the school of Helmholtz. *Psychoanalytic Quarterly* 13: 341–362.

Binswanger, L. (1936). Freud und die vervassung der klinischen psychiatrie. *Schweizer Archiv fur Neurologie und Psychiatrie* 37: 177–199.

Forrester, J. (1980). *Language and the Origins of Psychoanalysis*. New York: Columbia University Press.

Freud, S. (1924). *A Short Account of Psychoanalysis*. S.E. 19: 191–212.

———. (1925). *An Autobiographical Study*. S.E. 20: 1–74.

———. (1953 [1891]). *On Aphasia: A Critical Study*. New York: International Universities Press.

Rizzuto, A.-M. (1989). A hypothesis about Freud's motive for writing the monograph *On Aphasia*. *International Review of Psycho-analysis* 16: 111–117.

———. (1990). A proto-dictionary of psychoanalysis. *International Journal of Psycho-analysis* 71: 261–270.

———. (1993). Freud's speech apparatus and spontaneous speech. *International Journal of Psycho-analysis* 74: 113–127.

Stengel, E. (1953). *Introduction to Freud's Aphasia*. New York: International Universities Press.

———. (1954). A re-evaluation of Freud's book "On aphasia": Its significance for psychoanalysis. *International Journal of Psychoanalysis* 35: 85–89.

ANA-MARÍA RIZZUTO

Argentina, and Psychoanalysis

Toward the beginning of the 1930s, psychoanalysis entered medical practice in Buenos Aires: Celes Cárcamo came from a medical clinic; Arnaldo Rascovsky, from pediatrics; and Enrique Pichón Rivière from psychiatry. In 1936 Cárcamo, convinced of the need to complete psychoanalytic training, traveled to Europe and began studying at the Psychoanalytical Institute of Paris.

In 1938, Angel Garma arrived in Buenos Aires. He had completed his psychoanalytic training at the Psychoanalytical Institute of Berlin, where psychoanalysis had reached its maximum development. He was the foundation of the psychoanalytic movement in Argentina. In September 1939, Cárcamo ended his training in Paris and returned to Buenos Aires, where he met Garma, Rascovsky, and Pichón Rivère. In 1942, Maria Langer joined this group. In that same year, the Argentine Psychoanalytical Association (APA) was established and recognized as a component society of the International Psychoanalytical Association (IPA).

From the beginning, there was an active program of research, publication, and training, as attested by the *Magazine of Psychoanalysis*, the numerous books issued, and the reputation of the APA. The works published included *Psychoanalysis of Dreams*, by Angel Garma; *Fetal Psychism*, by A. Rascovsky; *Psychosis*, by E. Pichón Rivière and E. Rolla; *Communication*, by D. Liberman; *Psychoanalysis of Children*, by Arminda Aberastury, A. Garma, and S. Ferrer; *Psychoanalysis Technique*, by Enrique Racker; *Lethargy, Actual Neurosis and Somatic Manifestations*, by F. Cesio; *Counteridentification*, by L. Grinberg; *The Psychoanalysis of Becoming Ill*, by L. Chiozza; and *The Psychoanalytical Field*, by W. Baranger.

The work of Freud, the developments provided by Argentine pioneers, and the contributions of Melanie Klein are the foundation of the Argentine psychoanalytic movement.

On Garma's initiative in 1953, the annual symposia of the APA began; in 1956, the Latin American congresses that gave rise to the Psychoanalytical Federation of Latin America commenced; and in 1966, Garma and Rascovsky created the Pan-American congresses.

Psychoanalysis rapidly extended from Buenos Aires to the cities of the interior. Within a few years, psychoanalytic groups emerged in Mendoza, Bahía Blanca, Rosario, Tucumán, and Salta. Today, in each significant population center of the country, there is at least one group that studies and applies psychoanalytic theory and methods.

Horacio Etchegoyen created the group in Mendoza, which in 1973 was recognized by the IPA as a Study Group, in 1981 as a Provisional Society, and in 1983 as a Component Society.

In Córdoba, the group led by Beatriz Gallo, Enrique Torres, Marta Baistrocchi, and Diego Rapella was recognized by the IPA as a Study Group in 1981, a Provisional Society in 1991, and as a Component Society in 1993.

In 1992, the group in Rosario, led by Mario Bugacov, Juan Canale, and María Aidé Castellaro de Pozzi, was recognized by the IPA as a Study Group.

The pioneers of the APA helped to spread psychoanalysis to the Latin American countries. Medical doctors from those countries came to Buenos Aires to undergo psychoanalytical training; once it was completed, they returned to their home countries and formed psychoanalytic societies.

The E. Racker Investigation and Direction Center, created in 1961, is concerned with the treatment of institutional patients and the extension of psychoanalysis to hospitals and other institutions.

In 1974, the APA approved a program that established a system of credits awarded for scientific contributions, supervision, and teaching. It gives the vote to the adherent members, extends the didactic function to the full members who in fact exercise it, and grants curricular freedom. In 1977, as a result of their disagreement with this program, numerous members withdrew from the APA and entered the IPA as a Provisional Society. Two years later, that group was accepted as a Component Society, the Psychoanalytical Association of Buenos Aires. Among the founding members were analysts who had made a meaningful contribution to the development of the APA, such as David Liberman, León Grinberg, Horacio Etchegoyen, and Joel Zac.

In 1988, the First Argentine Congress of Psychoanalysis was held. At the second congress (1993), members of various societies recognized by the IPA attended.

Today, the Argentine psychoanalytical movement maintains the impetus given to it by its pioneers, which made the country, in particular the city of Buenos Aires, one of the most active psychoanalytical centers in the world. Its trunk, the APA, maintains the fundamental structure; it is the place where the movement's roots, its pioneers and its history, lie. The limbs, particularly Buenos Aires, Mendoza, Córdoba, and Rosario, have achieved a life of their own, and other groups continue their promising growth.

As of 2000, there were about two thousand members and candidates in the psychoanalytic societies belonging to the IPA, and even more belong to psychoanalytic centers detached from the IPA.

REFERENCES
Asociación Psicoanalítica Argentina. 1942–1982. (1982). Buenos Aires: A.P.A.
Cesio, F. (1981). Historia del movimiento psicoanalítico latinoamericano. *Revista de Psicoanálisis* 38: 695–713.
Cesio, F. (1991). Historia del movimiento psicoanalítico en la República Argentina. Paper presented at the 37th International Congress, Buenos Aires.
Cesio, F., Aberastury, A., and Aberastury, M. (1967). *Historia, Enseñanza y Ejercicio Legal del Psicoanálisis*. Buenos Aires: Bibliográfica Omeba.
Comunicaciones de Asociaciones Psicoanalisticas De (Communications of the Psychoanalytical Associations of) Buenos Aires, Mendoza, Córdoba, and Rosario.

FIDIAS CESIO

Art, and Psychoanalysis

See AESTHETICS, AND PSYCHOANALYSIS;
CINEMA, AND PSYCHOANALYSIS.

Association See FREE ASSOCIATION.   A

Australia, and Psychoanalysis

Although psychoanalytic practice in Australia did not commence until the early 1930s, the effects of the new and controversial discoveries of Freud were felt there twenty years earlier. Ernest Jones writes that in 1909, Freud reported having received a letter from Sydney telling him there was a group eagerly disseminating his works. Jones himself presented a paper to the 1914 Australian Medical Congress, "Some Practical Aspects of Psychoanalytical Treatment." In 1911, Freud, Carl Jung, and Havelock Ellis had been invited to read papers on psychoanalysis before the Australian Medical Congress in Sydney. None of them could attend, but Freud submitted a paper titled "On Psychoanalysis," which was read before the Congress and was printed, for the first time, in the October 1989 issue of *The Scientific Proceedings of the Australian Psychoanalytic Society*.

In the 1930s psychoanalytic ideas were considered revolutionary, and attitudes toward it, both in the medical profession and in the wider community, were polarized. Roy Winn was the first to practice psychoanalysis in Australia. As early as 1930 he was speaking, and writing in the *Medical Journal of Australia*, about the importance of psychoanalysis in medical practice. His papers provoked the most critical and scathing attacks by the then Professor of Medicine and from a number of other well-known psychiatrists. However, a minority of the medical fraternity was interested in and favorably disposed to psychoanalysis, and two prominent psychiatrists wrote to the editor of the *Medical Journal of Australia* supporting Winn's case, setting forth lengthy and detailed arguments in support of psychoanalysis and its practitioners.

In Melbourne, in the period before World War II, there was a growing interest in psychoanalysis by a vocal minority not only in psychiatry but also in the wider community. They had been intrigued by the promise and the challenge of the new "depth psychology." This group of enthusiasts worked to support the efforts of Ernest Jones and John Rickman to enable European psychoanalysts to migrate to Australia. As early as 1939, Jones had raised the possibility of six analysts from Europe migrating to Australia. As events transpired, permission was granted for only one, Dr. Clara Lazar-Geroe, to enter Australia. Although at that time there was one qualified training analyst in Sydney, Dr. Andrew Peto, Dr. Lazar-Geroe, because of the local support, settled in Melbourne.

The Melbourne Institute of Psychoanalysis was established shortly after she arrived, and for many years she alone dealt with the formidable task of establishing psychoanalysis and of training new analysts. Lazar-Geroe addressed the task of presenting psychoanalysis, and for many years, seminars were conducted for psychiatrists as well as for educators, parents, and teachers. She established the Melbourne Clinic, which provided psychoanalytic treatment as well as psychoanalytically oriented psychotherapy.

One of the arrangements made by those encouraging Lazar-Geroe's migration, notably Ernest Jones and Michael Balint, was that she be accredited as a training analyst of the British Psychoanalytical Society, and that the Melbourne Institute should act as the Australian branch of that society. From then on, psychoanalysis in Australia was closely tied to the British Society. It was not until after 1967, when the status of Australian analysis was questioned, that the International Psychoanalytic Association (IPA) established the Australian Study Group (1968) and the Australian Psychoanalytic Society (1971).

With the creation of the Australian Psychoanalytic Society (APS), attention was devoted to implementing a new system of training. Training had become such an issue that, for a while, very few other activities were undertaken. The climate at the time was full of uncertainty and insecurity. The almost exclusive concern with implementing the new training system inevitably involved confrontation with those who had grown up with and accepted the earlier system. This, together with rivalries between Adelaide, Melbourne, and Sydney; personal feelings; and theoretical differences, resulted in the IPA's appointing two site visiting committees. As a result, the structure of the APS was changed. Today it is governed by a nationally elected executive; it alone has ultimate authority to train and to qualify analysts; it is formally responsible for all national decisions concerning analysis, for holding regular scientific meetings, and for the publication of the *Scientific Proceedings*. Apart from the operation of the APS's executive and its various advisory bodies, there is very little in this "federation" that prevents the individual states from taking an independent approach to either training or public relations.

Great store is placed on the need to publicize psychoanalysis in the wider community and on forming links with other disciplines. Whereas previously many analysts had appointments to various hospitals and clinics, these were private arrangements. Today a great deal of psychoanalytic work, other than training, is being carried out by the institutes in Australia. This includes public lectures and workshops, seminars, and the provision of services such as supervision and clinical discussions for members of associated professions. In two of the institutes, the relationship of the literary arts to psychoanalysis has been seriously addressed, and a number of multidisciplinary conferences have been arranged, sometimes by the institute, and at other times in cooperation with other bodies.

Australia had one important feature which distinguished it from most other countries, and has played an important role in making psychoanalysis available to those who might otherwise be unable to pay. Until 1997, the Commonwealth Insurance Scheme, which was financed by the federal government, recognized patients who were in analysis with medical analysts as entitled to benefits under the scheme. The net result was that patients who were in analysis were entitled to medical benefits for the duration of their analysis; provided their analyst charged the "scheduled fee," the patients received their analysis free, apart from a nominal charge at the outset. The medical analysts, to ensure that their patients contributed financially to their analysis, in most cases charged a fee in excess of the benefit their patients received. This arrangement was altered in 1997 so that only patients suffering from a limited list of illnesses were entitled to 150 sessions a year; the bulk of patients were limited in their entitlement to fifty sessions per annum.

As of 2000, the membership of the APS is seventy-three, and twelve students are in training.

REGINALD T. MARTIN

Austria, and Psychoanalysis

See VIENNA, AND PSYCHOANALYSIS.

Autoerotism

"Autoerotism" is the term used to describe those forms of sexual activity that do not involve a sexual object.

The specifically psychoanalytic sense of "autoerotism" is distinct from its general sense as a synonym for masturbation, although this distinction is sometimes blurred by psychoanalytic writers. Freud's concept of autoerotism had important ramifications for several central components of psychoanalytic theory, including the problem of the choice of neurosis, psychosexual development, and the etiology of perversion. The thesis that infantile sexuality is predominantly autoerotic underwent a gradual attrition after its publication in 1905. The term "autoerotism" was introduced by the British sexologist Havelock Ellis (1898a), who used it to denote spontaneous, unprovoked episodes of sexual arousal. He published a second paper in 1898 linking the symptoms of hysteria to autoerotism, citing Freud and Josef Breuer (Ellis, 1898b), and sent an offprint to Freud.

Freud adopted the term a year later in a letter to Wilhelm Fliess in which he describes autoerotism as ". . . the lowest of the sexual strata . . . which dispenses with any psychosexual aim and seeks only locally gratifying sensations" (Masson, 1985, p. 390). Even at this point Freud defined the term differently than Ellis. As he later put it, ". . . the essential point is not the genesis of the excitation, but the question of its relation to an object" (1905, p. 181).

Freud made no published reference to autoerotism until the *Three Essays on the Theory of Sexuality* (1905), in which he cited Ellis's work and distinguished Ellis's views from his own. Freud distanced himself from Ellis's inclusion of "the whole of hysteria and all the manifestations of masturbation" (p. 181) under autoerotism. As he later made explicit, both hysterical symptoms and many examples of masturbation involve fantasied sexual objects, whereas autoerotism is not directed toward any object (1908).

Freud (1905, p. 207) believed the entire period of infantile sexuality to be "predominantly autoerotic, although not exclusively so, with object-choice prevailing only once puberty is reached," although over the next few years he began to qualify his emphasis on the autoerotic character of infantile sexuality (1907, 1909). Children initially stimulate their anal and genital zones to obtain pleasure without reference to a real or fantasied object (1909, 1910). Unlike early genital and anal impulses, the oral drive has an object from the beginning and only later becomes autoerotic (1905, 1910). Autoerotic activities become object-related by being brought into association with the psychological attitudes toward others (1907), or by the attachment of sexual instincts to vital, self-preservative activities requiring objects (1912).

During the autoerotic phase the components of the sexual drive behave autonomously, seeking gratification independently of one another: "each of them goes its own way to obtaining pleasure" (1916, p. 323). It is only at puberty that these drives are subordinated to the genital organization and to reproduction (1905). This feature of autoerotism, in conjunction with its objectlessness, determines the "perverse" character of infantile sexuality (1905).

In 1911, Freud introduced a modification into his developmental model of a stage of autoerotism giving way to object-related sexuality at puberty. He interposed a stage of narcissism (self-love) between autoerotic and mature sexuality. During the narcissistic stage the child takes himself as his first love object, and only later learns to love others. Freud thus distinguished between obtaining sexual pleasure *from* one's body without recourse to a real or imagined sexual object (autoerotism) and being sexually excited *by* one's body as a sexual object (narcissism), and went on to claim that paranoiacs are fixated in the stage of narcissism, whereas schizophrenics are fixated in the stage of autoerotism (1911). The unification of the sexual drive, which Freud had earlier claimed occurred only at puberty, is now described as a characteristic of the narcissistic stage (1911). The problem posed by Freud's 1911 thesis of the stages of autoerotism and narcissism as the respective fixation points for schizophrenia and paranoia was dealt with by abandoning the nosological distinction (Macmillan, 1991).

In "The Disposition to Obsessional Neurosis" (1913), Freud propounded the idea of a pregenital organization of the libido, the anal-sadistic stage, that follows the narcissistic stage. During this period "the component instincts have already come together for the choice of an object, and that object is already something extraneous . . ." (p. 321). Autoerotism was now implicitly confined only to the earliest phase of infancy.

In "On Narcissism: An Introduction" (1914), Freud altered his scheme by describing the original oral relation to the breast as an autoerotic sexual activity. "The first autoerotic sexual satisfactions," he wrote, "are experienced in connection with vital functions which serve the purpose of self-preservation" (1914, p. 87). The objectless oral sexual drive finds satisfaction through the necessarily object-directed self-preservative impulse to feed.

In "Instincts and Their Vicissitudes" (1915), the stage of autoerotism is abruptly dropped. Autoerotism becomes the characteristic mode of sexual activity during the narcissistic stage. Freud does not spell out the implications of this change for his earlier concept of the disunity of sexuality during the stage of autoerotism, and the view that autoerotism is a phenomenon of the narcissistic stage seems to preclude the existence of truly objectless sexuality. In the 1915 edition of the *Three Essays on the Theory of Sexuality* (1905), Freud emphasized that

> . . . the choice of an object, such as we have shown to be characteristic of the pubertal phase of development, has already been frequently or habitually effected during childhood: that is to say, the whole of the sexual currents have become directed towards a single person in relation to whom they seek to achieve their aims. (p. 199).

In the *Introductory Lectures on Psycho-analysis* (1916), Freud reverted to his earlier position on the primary object-directedness of the oral drive, a view that is reiterated in 1923. In the latter text, he also maintains the view that autoerotism is directed at the child's own body (i.e., that it is narcissistic).

> In the first instance the oral component instinct finds satisfaction by attaching itself to the sating of the desire for nourishment; and its object is the mother's breast. It then detaches itself, becomes independent and at the same time auto-erotic, that is it finds an object in the child's own body. (1923, p. 245)

Freud's last major statement concerning autoerotism is found in *An Autobiographical Study*. He returns to the notion of a "non-centralized" stage of autoerotism, but describes this as *preceding* the oral stage (1925, p. 35). This was the logical outcome of Freud's thesis of oral, anal, and phallic organizations of the libido (1925). His earlier concept of anarchic, unstructured sexual activity is not compatible with the concept of infantile sexual organizations unless it is taken to precede them. Freud regards it as likely that the infant does not distinguish the breast from its own body during the oral phase.

Freud's account of autoerotism became more and more contradictory and ambiguous during the course of his career. There is an ambiguity, for example, in his use of the term "object." Does it refer to a real object or a psychological object? This equivocation and confusion

have been discussed by several psychoanalytic commentators, notably Compton (1985, 1986) and Macmillan (1991).

REFERENCES

Compton, A. (1985). The development of the drive object concept in Freud's work: 1905–1915. *Journal of the American Psychoanalytic Association* 33: 93–115.

———. (1986). Freud: Objects and structure. *Journal of the American Psychoanalytic Association* 34: 561–590.

Ellis, H. (1898a). Autoerotism: A psychological study. *Alienist and Neurologist* 19: 260–299.

———. (1898b). Hysteria in relation to the sexual emotions. *Alienist and Neurologist* 19: 599–615.

Freud, S. (1905). *Three Essays on the Theory of Sexuality.* S.E. 7: 126–243.

———. (1907). The sexual enlightenment of children. S.E. 9: 131–139.

———. (1908). Hysterical phantasies and their relation to bisexuality. S.E. 9: 159–166.

———. (1909). Analysis of a phobia in a five-year-old boy. S.E. 10: 5–147.

———. (1910). Five lectures on psycho-analysis. S.E. 11: 9–55.

———. (1911). Psycho-analytic notes on an autobiographical account of a case of paranoia (dementia paranoides). S.E. 12: 9–79.

———. (1912). On the universal tendency to debasement in the sphere of love (contributions to the psychology of love II). S.E. 11: 179–190.

———. (1913). The disposition of obsessional neurosis. S.E. 13.

———. (1914a). On narcissism: An introduction. S.E. 14: 73–102.

———. (1915b). Instincts and their vicissitudes. S.E. 14: 117–140.

———. (1916). *Introductory Lectures on Psycho-analysis.* S.E. 15–16: 9–496.

———. (1923a). Two encyclopaedia articles. S.E. 18: 235–259.

———. (1923b). The infantile genital organization: An interpolation into the theory of sexuality. S.E. 19: 141–145.

———. (1925). *An Autobiographical Study.* S.E. 20: 7–74.

Macmillan, M. (1991). *Freud Evaluated: The Completed Arc.* Amsterdam: North Holland.

Masson, J. M. (1985). *The Complete Letters of Sigmund Freud to Wilhelm Fliess: 1887–1904.* Cambridge, Mass.: Harvard University Press.

DAVID LIVINGSTONE SMITH

Autonomy

In ordinary usage, the term "autonomy" refers to qualities of independence and self-direction. The term has also been used in a variety of ways in psychoanalytic theorizing.

Hartmann (1939) introduced the term into ego psychology, using it to refer to a relationship between the

A

ego and the id. He postulated that in adapting to reality, a person's ego has access to conflict-free functions which permit the autonomy of the ego from the id. Although this theory was first formulated by Hartmann, it had its roots in Freud's observation that the function of the ego is to reconcile the demands of the id, the superego, and reality (1923), and in Freud's description of the synthetic function of the ego (1926). Hartmann (1950) distinguished between ego apparatuses of what he termed "primary" and "secondary" autonomy. The former are theorized to be products of evolution which render the individual potentially adapted to reality at birth. They include perception, memory, language, and motility. The apparatuses of secondary autonomy initially arise from instinctual sources or defensive structures formed in response to instinctual pressures. In the course of development, they undergo a change of function, and secondarily become apparatuses serving adaptation to reality.

Erikson (1950), in his extension of the theory of reality relationships, outlined a sequence of phases of ego development, and theorized that social relationships influence the manner in which an individual deals with the tasks of each phase. He identified the task of the second phase as resolving tensions concerning autonomy, shame, and doubt. To develop autonomy, the child must feel that the trust in the self and the world established in the oral phase will not be jeopardized by the wish to make choices. The nature of the relationship between adult and child during the anal phase will influence the balance achieved between the child's cooperation and willfulness, and between self-expression and its suppression. Erikson described this process as follows: "From a sense of self-control without loss of self-esteem comes a lasting sense of autonomy and pride; from a sense of muscular and anal impotence, of loss of self-control, and of parental over control comes a lasting sense of doubt and shame" (Erikson, 1950, pp. 70–71). In Erikson's theory, a sense of personal autonomy is one criterion of mental health.

The relationship of autonomy to developmental processes, particularly those having to do with separation and individuation, has received further attention in the work of object relations theorists, self psychologists, and interpersonal psychologists (Mahler et al., 1975; Severino et al., 1987).

Object relations theorists postulated that successful "internalization" of the mother creates what is termed "object constancy," and is essential for creating an inter-

nal security that allows autonomous functioning in the world (Cashdan, 1988). Around the end of the first year of life, the infant is able to create mental representations of his or her caregiver. These representations serve many purposes, including initiating the development of autonomy. By using internalized representations as a self-reference, the infant is freed from the immediate influences of new encounters. Affect regulation can thus be internally regulated. This enhances autonomy while preserving the knowledge of interpersonal attunement.

Self psychologists (e.g., Kohut, 1971) and interpersonal relationships theorists (Emde, 1989; Stern, 1985, 1990) focus on the development of the infant's self in relation to caregivers (typically the mother). In the first year of life, the caregiver and infant are understood to interact in a symbiotic reciprocal reward system (Emde, 1989) which influences both the caregiver's and the infant's emotional experiences. This symbiosis occurs primarily through the visual process. When he or she is gazing at the infant, the caregiver's facial expressions stimulate and amplify the positive feelings of the infant. This positive affect, at times expanding to joy, is the product of mutual regulation of social exchanges by both caregivers and infants (Stern, 1990). Visual interaction is an intense form of interpersonal communication and sets the biological template for arousal, affect regulation, and a definition of self. The interpersonal fusion is the source of vitality (Stern, 1985), aliveness (Wright, 1991), and vigor (Izard, 1991) for the infant. Because the positive affect is enhanced by the sense of oneness with the other, the infant seeks the attention of the other to reactivate this pleasure. Under good enough circumstances, positive exchanges between caregiver and infant dominate the first year of life. The shared looking, smiling, and cooing create attachments, the natures of which are thought to be encoded in the orbitofrontal cortex and to influence all later socioemotional relationships (Schore, 1994).

REFERENCES

Cashdan, S. (1988). *Object Relations Theory*. Toronto: Penguin Books Canada.

Emde, R. D. (1989). Emotional availability: A reciprocal reward system for infants and parents with implications for prevention of psychosocial disorders. In P. M. Taylor (ed.), *Parent-Infant Relationships*, pp. 87-115. Orlando, Fla.: Grune and Stratton.

Erikson, E. H. (1950). Growth and crises of the healthy personality. In his *Identity and the Life Cycle*, pp. 51–107. New York: Norton.

Hartmann, H. (1939). *Ego Psychology and the Problem of Adaptation*. New York: International Universities Press, 1958.

———. (1950). Comments on the psychoanalytic theory of the ego. *Psychoanalytic Study of the Child* 5: 74–96.

Izard, C. E. (1991). *The Psychology of Emotions*. New York: Plenum Press.

Kohut H. (1971). *The Analysis of the Self: A Systematic Approach to the Psychoanalytic Treatment of Narcissistic Personality Disorders*. New York: International Universities Press.

Mahler, M., Pine, F., and Bergman, A. (1975). *The Psychological Birth of the Human Infant*. New York: Basic Books.

Schore, A. N. (1994). *Affect Regulation and the Origin of the Self: The Neurobiology of Emotional Development*. Hillsdale, N.J.: Lawrence Erlbaum.

Severino, S. K., McNutt, E. R., and Feder, S. L. (1987). Shame and the development of autonomy. *Journal of the American Academy of Psychoanalysis* 15, no. 1: 93–106.

Stern, D. N. (1985). *The Interpersonal World of the Infant*. New York: Basic Books.

———. (1990). Joy and satisfaction in infancy. In R. A. Glick and S. Bone (eds.), *Pleasure Beyond the Pleasure Principle*, pp. 13–25. New Haven, Conn.: Yale University Press.

Wright, K. (1991). *Vision and Separation: Between Mother and Baby*. Northvale, N.J.: Jason Aronson.

EDITH R. MCNUTT
NANCY K. MORRISON
SALLY K. SEVERINO

B

Baginsky, Adolf (1843–1918)

Adolf Baginsky was, for a very short period, an informal teacher of Sigmund Freud. This episode in Freud's career, ignored in his official biography, has only recently gained attention as a significant link between Freud's early work and the nineteenth-century history of the medicalization of infantile onanism (masturbation) and the use of castration as a medical procedure (Bonomi, 1994).

During Freud's 1885–1886 studies in Paris under Jean-Martin Charcot, Max Kassowitz offered him a post as neurologist in a polyclinic for ill children, a post Freud would hold from 1886 to 1896. Before accepting the post, Freud underwent neuropediatric training in March 1886 at a clinic for ill children run by Baginsky. Every afternoon for three weeks, Freud attended classes and demonstrations given by Baginsky. The courses were on the pathology and therapy of infantile illnesses, and on the dangers to which children were exposed in schools. Shortly after returning to Vienna, Freud began his private practice, in which he offered, among other services, the treatment of infantile nervous diseases. He also held classes on this topic at the Kassowitz Institute in Vienna (1887–1892).

Baginsky obtained a medical degree in 1866 and was appointed lecturer in children's medicine in 1882. In 1877, he published the work which created his professional reputation: the *Handbuch der Schul-Hygiene*, which went through a second edition in 1883. According to Baginsky, the community was the source of the most dangerous illnesses, the epidemics; moreover, he conceived masturbation in children as an "infection" which was dangerously spreading in the community. In his handbook the considerations about onanism were included in the chapter titled "Illnesses of the Nervous System." Baginsky stated that "masturbation appears in the earliest infancy . . . in babies" (1877, p. 465); he conceived of it as a contagious illness because "certain external stimuli are able to produce the evil and seduction [*Verführung*] plays . . . a very big role" (1877, p. 465). He stressed the great excitability of the nervous system in early infancy, and based his views mainly on the reflex neurosis theory. Because of the great excitability of the nervous system, he concluded that "insignificant stimulations coming from the periphery, which in adults pass without traces . . . are able to produce violent explosions by reflex. . . . With the advancement of the psychic development the excitability by reflex [*Reflexerregbarkeit*] becomes lower" (1877, p. 443).

Baginsky suggested that "sexual excesses of children" had to be taken into account as a direct causal element because of "the frequent excitation of the central nervous system" (1877, p. 451). He conceived masturbation mainly as a peripheral source of such excitation, and criticized the emerging tendency to reverse causes and effects, and to assume onanism as a mere consequence of the morbid state of the nervous system. According to Baginsky, onanistic children suffered underdevelopment of the musculature, appetite and sleep disturbances, rachitic changes, slow dentition, lowering of the forehead, and larger fontanels.

During his 1885–1886 study trip to Paris and Berlin, Freud became acquainted with contrasting views about the role of the genitals in hysteria. The peripheral conception held by Baginsky, which permitted him to stress the importance of "seduction" in the transmission of masturbation to young children, was at that time connected with the genital localization of the "evil" and its surgical removal. Charcot, in contrast, was moving toward a neuropsychic conception of hysteria, and was among the opponents of castration as treatment of hysteria. This opposition to castration was an important element of the young Freud's enthusiasm for Charcot. In his 1886 "Report on My Studies," Freud pointed out that the condition of hysterics was "under the odium of some very widespread prejudices," including "the supposed dependence of hysterical illness upon genital irritation." He praised Charcot for having attenuated "the connection of the neurosis with the genital system" (1886a, p. 11). He also referred to the crucial question of male hysteria precisely within this context (i.e., as a proof against the genital localization of the neuroses). A few months later, when he lectured on masculine hysteria at the Vienna Medical Society, on October 16, 1886, Freud again associated the two topics, claiming that Charcot had the merit of showing that hysteria did not result from a disease of the genital organs, and that male hysteria was much more frequent than generally admitted (Ellenberger, 1968, p. 124).

Similarly, Freud's early aversion to sexual etiology is well reflected in his 1886 article on hysteria, where it is stated that "the influence of abnormalities in the sexual sphere upon the development of hysteria" was, as a rule, overestimated (1886b, p. 51), and the assumption that "changes in the genital really constitute so often the sources of stimulus for hysterical symptoms" is qualified as "doubtful" (1886b, p. 56).

As becomes clear from his 1886 article on hysteria, Freud's original aversion to sexual etiology was directed only to the "strict sense" of the latter, which, being based on the anatomical explanation of the abnormalities of sexual life, was used to justify castration. More precisely, it was directed against the tendency to overestimate and exaggerate this kind of cause, to the contemporary tendency to find anatomical changes everywhere, which resulted in the mutilation or removal of healthy organs. Therefore, in this period, Freud embraced the strategy of reversing the cause-effect relationship between periphery and center, and explained hysteria as "a mere symptom of a deep-going degeneracy of the nervous system, which is manifested in permanent moral perversion" (1886b, p. 52). Significantly, he gave such an explanation while discussing the occurrence of hysteria in children.

In 1886, Charcot wrote a famous "lesson" on hysteria in boys ("A Fourteen-Year-Old Boy Accompanied by His Parents and His Doctor"), in which he claimed that hysteria is three-fourths psychic and that, therefore, it is necessary to treat it psychically. This lesson, which was translated into German and edited by Freud in 1892, is very important for the history of psychoanalysis, since it prompted in Freud the idea of "counter-will," his first model of the psychic mechanism of hysteria. The idea of a split within the will later grew into a more elaborate psychology, remaining a basic tenet of Freud's thought till the end of his life. Similarly and simultaneously, Freud moved away from Charcot, and turned again to sexual etiology, embracing the views he had earlier rejected and developing, between 1893 and 1896, an etiological speculation based on different types of sexual causes. Yet, his approach was new, at least with respect to the psychoneuroses, since it tried to combine the idea of a psychic mechanism of the neurosis with the idea of a sexual etiology. Precisely in this combination, we can recognize the search to overcome the split influence played by Charcot, on one side, and by Baginsky, on the other, during Freud's 1885–1886 study trip to Paris and Berlin.

Freud, however, denied such a combined influence. In the final chapter of the *Studies on Hysteria*, written in the spring of 1895, Freud wrote: "[initially] the expectation of a sexual neurosis being the basis of hysteria was fairly remote from my mind. I had come fresh from the school of Charcot, and I regarded the linking of hysteria with the topic of sexuality as a sort of insult" (Breuer and Freud, 1893, pp. 259–260). In this statement, Freud disavows the teaching of Baginsky, which was mainly based on "sexual neurosis," and utilizes the teaching of Charcot to conceal it. By presenting the theory of sexual etiology as a "sort of insult," Freud evokes the idea that the teaching of Baginsky had been an "insult" to him. This impression is further confirmed by the fact that Freud never mentioned Baginsky in any significant connection to his studies, and had a personal aversion toward him and his teaching. Yet, since being repelled by something is not less an influence than being attracted to it, it has been suggested that Baginsky's teaching on sexual etiology, though initially opposed and rejected, did indeed play an important and ignored role in shaping Freud's subsequent intellectual development.

REFERENCES

Baginsky, A. (1877). *Handbuch der Schul-hygiene*. Berlin: Denicke.

————. (1883). *Lehr der Kinderkrankheiten*, 3rd ed. Braunschweig: Verlag von Friedrich Wreden.

Bonomi, C. (1994). Why have we ignored Freud the paediatrician: The relevance of Freud's paediatric training for the origins of psychoanalysis. In A. Haynal and E. Falzeder (eds.), *100 Years of Psychoanalysis: Contributions to the History of Psychoanalysis*, pp. 55–99. Special issue of *Cahiers Psychiatriques Genevois*. London: Karnac.

————. (1997). Freud and the discovery of infantile sexuality: A reassessment. In T. Dufresne (ed.), *Freud Under Analysis: History, Theory, Practice. Essays in Honor of Paul Roazen*, pp. 37–57. Northvale, N.J., and London: Jason Aronson.

————. (1998). Sigmund Freud: Un neurologo tra sapere psichiatrico e sapere pediatrico del XIX secolo. *Psicoterapiae Scienze Umane* 32, no. 1: 51–91.

————. (1998b). Freud and castration: A new look into the origins of psychoanalysis. *Journal of the American Academy of Psychoanalysis* 26, no. 1: 29–49.

Breuer, J., and Freud, S. (1883–1893). *Studies on Hysteria*. S.E. 2: 19–305.

Ellenberger, H. F. (1968). Freud's lecture on masculine hysteria: A critical study. In M. S. Micale (ed.), *Essays of Henry Ellenberger in the History of Psychiatry*, pp. 119–135. Princeton, N.J.: Princeton University Press.

Fleischmann L. (1878). Über onanie und masturbation bei säugligen. *Wiener Medizinische Presse* 19: 8–10, 46–49.

Freud, S. (1886a). Report on my studies in Paris and Berlin. S.E. 1: 5–15.

————. (1886). Hysteria. S.E. 1: 41–57.

Schäfer, S. (1884). Über hysterie bei kindern. *Archiv für Kinderheilkunde* 5: 401–428.

CARLO BONOMI

Bauer, Ida See DORA.

Behaviorism, and Psychoanalysis

Conflicting approaches to the scientific study of behavior and its causes share several important similarities, as some behaviorists have noted. Although the behaviorist B. F. Skinner was skeptical about many of Freud's ideas, he also wrote: "Freud greatly reduced the sphere of accident and caprice in our considerations of human conduct" (1954, p. 300).

Both behaviorism and psychoanalysis presume a thoroughgoing causal determinism, focus on case histories of individual persons, often rely on explanation by reference to experienced associations between events, and assume that causes of behavior typically go unnoticed by the behaving person.

What, then, is the conflict? Behaviorism, immensely popular from about 1930 to 1960 in the Anglo-American psychological and philosophical community, is a surface psychology; psychoanalysis is a depth psychology. For behaviorism, behavior is a function of processes in the perceived environment of the behaving person—on the surface, as it were. These include processes of classical and operant conditioning, reinforcement, punishment, shaping, and extinction. For psychoanalysis, by contrast, behavior often is a function of forces beneath the conscious mind—in the depth, as it were. These forces include repression, reaction, sublimation, displacement, identification, and projection. In psychoanalysis, behavior expresses underlying mental activity; in behaviorism, behavior is produced by occurrences in the natural and social environment.

In its heyday, behaviorism offered two challenges to psychoanalysis. First, it insisted that theoretical terms which fail to refer to intersubjectively observable entities or events are scientifically illegitimate. "Repression," "sublimation," and various key descriptive and explanatory concepts of psychoanalysis fail to refer to observable entities or events. It follows that psychoanalysis is not proper science. Second, behaviorism insisted on experimental confirmation of hypotheses concerning the causes of behavior. Although Freud was not opposed to experimentation, he worried, in the words of Patricia Kitcher, that "experimental testing was relatively impractical for his theories" (1992, p. 190). Serious reservations about the accessibility of psychoanalytic theory to experimental confirmation (or falsification) led Skinner and other behaviorists to brand psychoanalysis ultimately as nonempirical speculation.

Striking parallels mark the histories of behaviorism and psychoanalysis. Each position was promoted by forceful personalities, foremost Skinner and Freud, respectively, who also were accomplished and prolific writers. Each tended to dismiss its critics as unenlightened and ill-informed. Each promoted itself as a welcome antidote to its challenger. Psychoanalysis dubbed behaviorism as mechanistic and dehumanizing, whereas behaviorism labeled psychoanalysis unscientific and obscurantist. Finally, each introduced and intellectually framed popular forms of therapy—behavior therapy, in the case of behaviorism—for emotional and behavioral disturbances.

Behavior therapy, unlike psychoanalytic therapy, stresses that behavior is under environmental control, even in cases of emotional disturbance. As in psychoanalytic therapy, individual case histories (in the language

B

of behaviorism, "learning histories") are required to support clinical treatment; in contrast to psychoanalytic therapy, patients typically need to be placed in controlled experimental settings (Rimm and Masters, 1974). For behavior therapists, psychoanalysis on a couch may produce beneficial side effects by providing emotional reinforcement and support, but actual environmental manipulation, not talk, constitutes the proper behavior therapeutic regimen.

Behaviorism has been severely criticized by Noam Chomsky (1959) and other cognitive scientists, in a manner at least loosely coincident with various commitments of psychoanalysis. Current consensus is that behaviorist insistence on an observational (sometimes also called "operational") definition of theoretic terms must be abandoned to permit reference to inner psychological causes (knowledge structures and information processing). Meanwhile, if experimentation is needed to vindicate scientific hypotheses, then accomplished sciences such as linguistics and astronomy fail as science. Thus, the demand for experimental confirmation is too severe and restrictive. Meanwhile, at least one doctrine common to both behaviorism and psychoanalysis has been modestly assimilated by contemporary cognitive science. This is the associationist notion that events frequently or otherwise saliently connected in experience sometimes therein control or contextually facilitate behavior (Fodor 1983, pp. 79–81). An employer's otherwise inexplicable anger at an employee may be a product of the employee's dress or physical appearance which the employer independently has had associated with aversive stimuli—perhaps having nothing at all to do with the employee himself. This is qualified associationism, to be sure, since contemporary cognitive science restricts the scope of associationist explanation to relatively unintelligent forms of behavior. However, both behaviorism and psychoanalysis, in distinctive and different ways, promoted association as an important variable in the production of human behavior. As Skinner remarked, "The Freudian argument that early emotional conditioning affects later personal adjustment presupposes such a process" (1953, p. 132).

REFERENCES

Chomsky, N. (1959). Review of *Verbal Behavior* by B. F. Skinner. *Language* 35: 26–58.

Fodor, J. (1983). *The Modularity of Mind: A Monograph on Faculty Psychology*. Cambridge, Mass.: MIT Press.

Kitcher, P. (1992). *Freud's Dream: A Complete Interdisciplinary Science of Mind*. Cambridge, Mass.: MIT Press.

Rimm, D., and Masters, J. (1974). *Behavior Therapy: Techniques and Empirical Findings*. New York: Academic Press.

Skinner, B. F. (1953). *Science and Human Behavior*. New York: Macmillan.

———. (1954). Critique of psychoanalytic concepts and theories. *Scientific Monthly* 79: 300–305.

GEORGE GRAHAM

Belgium, and Psychoanalysis

It is surprising that Belgium should have taken so long to become interested in Freudian ideas, especially since it is situated at a crossroads of many different cultures and languages. Indeed, it is because of this wide range of influences that Belgian universities have so much to offer.

At the end of the nineteenth-century and the beginning of the twentieth, medical training began to open up to certain Freudian ideas, though with some resistance among the older generation of teachers. Evidence of some interest in Freud's theories is found in one literary magazine and in the work of a small number of psychology teachers, but there is no sign that psychoanalysis was put into practice.

The one exception was Julien Varendonck (1879–1924), a teacher in Ghent who undertook a training analysis with Theodor Reik, following which he returned from Vienna to practice as an analyst in Ghent. In 1921, Freud wrote a preface to Varendonck's study "The Psychology of Daydreams," the first part of which was translated by Anna Freud. Varendonck became a member of the Dutch Psychoanalytical Society but died young, before training any pupils.

Shortly before World War II, Maurice Dugautiez (1893–1960) and Fernand Lechat (1895–1959), both interested in psychoanalysis, trained under a Viennese analyst who had settled in Antwerp to escape Nazi persecution. This was Dr. Ernst Hoffman, a follower of Freud and a brilliant student of Sándor Ferenczi. He was deported in 1942, and died in a concentration camp.

By then, the seed had been sown: since 1936, Dugautiez and Lechat had been practicing under the auspices of the Paris Society. In 1946 they were permitted to train analysts, and in 1947 the Association of Belgian Psychoanalysts was formed. Existing links with the Paris Society were never broken, as shown by the fact that Belgian analysts regularly and actively take part in the French-Language Congress for Romance Countries. Indeed, two members of the Association have written reports for this congress: Flagey (1972) on intellectual inhibition and Bauduin (1986) on the preconscious.

But French psychoanalysis has not been the only source of inspiration. Belgium's linguistic and cultural diversity has ensured a spirit of openness and an interest in all strands of contemporary psychoanalysis. One constant concern of the Association's membership is to remain close to clinical reality, and to evaluate any theory, however attractive, against that yardstick.

In 1960, the Belgian Association of Psychoanalysts became the Belgian Psychoanalytical Society. There followed a new generation of analysts, many of whom were trained by the founders, while others came in from abroad. Among them were Jacobs van Merlen, Bourdon, Flagey, Drapier, Vannypelseer, Pierloot, and Duyckaerts. Like any other society with a life of its own, the Belgian Psychoanalytical Society has undergone various reforms. Structures have been created to increase the involvement of the membership as a whole in issues such as the philosophy of analytic work, the organization of the Society, ethics, scientific thought, and publishing.

Belgium could not have remained unscathed by the dissent which occurred in France. Though the Belgian Psychoanalytical Society remained firmly outside the fray, a number of Belgian practitioners who returned home from abroad—several of them closely associated with the Catholic University of Louvain—decided not to join the Belgian Psychoanalytic Society, preferring to found the Belgian School of Psychoanalysis (1969). At that time, its theoretical approach closely followed the ideas of Jacques Lacan, though this influence is now less marked. When Lacan dissolved his Ecole Freudienne, various splits opened up, leading to the foundation of the Ecole de la Cause Freudienne, the Questionnement Psychanalytique, and the Association Freudienne de Belgique. These divisions clearly reflect the hazards of Lacanian succession.

To complete the picture, there is also the Belgian Society for Analytic Psychology, based on a Jungian approach, which was founded in 1975. The Belgian School of Jungian Psychoanalysis broke away from it in 1994.

Of these groups, only the Belgian Psychoanalytical Society is recognized by the International Psychoanalytical Association.

REFERENCES

Bauduin, A. (1987). Du préconscient. *Revue Française de Psychanalyse* 51: 449–538.

Berdondini, N. (1987). L'introduction de la psychanalyse en Belgique, 1900–1947: Examen critique des sources et des travaux. History thesis, Louvain-la-Neuve. (Revised in 1995.)

De Mijolla, A. (1993). Histoire comparé des débuts de la psychanalyse en Europe. *Revue Internationale de l'Histoire de la Psychanalyse* 6: 550–553.

———. (2000). *Dictionnaire de la Psychanalyse.* See entries Belgium (A. Alsteens), Dugautiez (D. Luminet), and Lechat (D. Luminet).

Flagey, D. (1972). Points de vue psychanalytiques sur l'inhibition intellectuelle. *Revue Française de Psychanalyse* 36: 717–798.

Freud, S. (1921). Introduction to Varendonck, *The Psychology of Day-Dreams.* S.E.18: 271.

Haber, M. (1992). Belgium. In P. Kutter (ed.), *Psychoanalysis International: A Guide to Psychoanalysis Throughout the World.* Vol. 1, *Europe.* Stuttgart: Frommann-Holzboog, pp. 25–33.

Labbee, P. (1955). Un psychanalyste belge peu connu, Julien Varendonck, 1879–1924. *Bulletin de l'Association des Psychanalystes de Belgique* 22.

Varendonck, J. (1921). *The Psychology of Day-Dreams.* London: Allen & Unwin.

ANDRÉ ALSTEENS

Binding

Many of Freud's psychoanalytic ideas were based on his speculative functional model of the central nervous system. "Binding" is one of these. Concepts of "free" and "bound" energy had been used in physics, notably by Hermann von Helmholz, prior to their incorporation by Freud into his neuropsychological theories (Holt, 1989).

Freud began his scientific career as a neurologist. In common with many neuroscientists of his day, he attempted to develop what are now called "functional" models of the way the brain instantiates mental processes. He represented the functional organization of the brain as an "apparatus" driven by "psychical energy."

Freud and Josef Breuer (1893) made use of a fundamental nineteenth-century neurophysiological principle in order to describe the way that psychical energy proliferated through the apparatus. Gustav Fechner, the father of the science of psychophysics, had claimed that the nervous system conforms to a "principle of stability" (Fechner, 1873). The brain is a self-regulating system which strives to keep its level of arousal at a constant level. When neural arousal exceeds the optimal threshold, the brain attempts to "discharge" the excess energy, thus restoring equilibrium. In accord with this, Freud and Breuer argued that beyond a certain threshold, psychic energy seeks discharge.

Drawing on a conventional neurophysiological distinction, Breuer believed that during waking life, neurons in the central nervous system maintain a constant, optimal level of excitation which facilitates the conduction of electrical impulses through the system. He called this *non-transmitted* charge "tonic excitation," If a neuron is already filled with energy, an additional excitation passed on to it by neighboring cells will immediately be discharged and transmitted to adjacent neurons. Freud (1900) used the term "binding" for Breuer's "tonic excitation."

According to Breuer's hypothesis, and that of the earlier work of Freud's friend Sigmund Exner (1894), energy proliferates most readily through those neurons that maintain a steady, tonic "bound" charge. Freud (1895) believed that when a neuron is tonically excited, it becomes more susceptible to further excitement because of a modification of its synaptic connection with adjacent neurons (a process now called "Hebbian learning"). The tonic excitation of neurons becomes fixed by processes of positive reinforcement. Networks of tonically excited neurons determine the channels (or what are now called "activation vectors") along which nerve signals will flow. Binding constrains neural (and therefore mental) activity. Freud used this principle to account for inhibition and defense. He had no concept of essentially inhibitory neurons, and postulated that assemblies of neurons carrying bound excitation can divert a mental process from its natural trajectory, and thus prevent its direct mental expression. He referred to the group of tonically excited neurons as "the ego."

The first and most elaborate published treatment of Freud's distinctive concept of binding is found in *The Interpretation of Dreams* (Freud, 1900). Unbound or "freely moving" (*frei bewegende*) energy proliferates in an unconstrained manner through the mind, one idea readily giving way to the next in the blind quest for discharge. This neurophysiological process underpins the "primary process," and is characteristic of unconscious mentation. It is only by means of binding that this gives way to the "secondary process," and therefore to rational, adaptive thinking (Freud, 1911).

It is clear that Freud often used the term "binding" in two distinct but closely related senses. He sometimes used it in a manner identical to Breuer's, to denote the hypothetical fixing of psychical energy in tonically excited neural groups. At other points in his writing, "binding" refers to the manner in which these neural groups constrain the trajectory of psychical energy through the mental apparatus. In his later work, Freud introduced a number of variations on these themes, such as the binding of anticathexes in states of mourning (Freud, 1917), the binding of anxiety (Freud, 1918), the use of binding to master energy breaking through the stimulus barrier (Freud, 1920), the use of binding to master trauma (Freud, 1920), the relationship between binding and mental pain (Freud, 1926), and the binding of the energy of the death instinct by the superego (Freud, 1933). A very detailed and comprehensive account of Freud's concept of binding can be found in Holt (1989).

Freud's basic theory of binding is strikingly reminiscent of contemporary "connectionist" models of mental functioning. Churchland, for example, asserts:

> The brain's global trajectory, through its own neuronal activation-space, follows the well-oiled prototypical pathways that prior learning has carved out in that space; and the brain's global trajectory shifts from one prototype to another as an appropriate function of the brain's changing perceptual inputs. (1995, pp. 171–172)

In schizophrenic thinking, which Freud regarded as conforming to the primary process, "the brain wanders uncertainly through its activation space, only loosely and fleetingly tied to its familiar causal prototypes" (Churchland, 1995, p. 172).

REFERENCES

Breuer, J., and Freud, S. (1893). *Studies on Hysteria.* S.E. 2.

Churchland, P. M. (1995). *The Engine of Reason, the Seat of the Soul: A Philosophical Journey into the Brain.* Cambridge, Mass.: Bradford/MIT Press.

Exner, S. (1894). *Entwurf zu Einer Physiologischen Erklarung der Psychischen Erscheinungen.* Vienna: Deutike.

Fechner, G. T. (1873). *Einige Ideen zur Schöpfungs- und Entwicklungsgeschichte zur Organismen.* Leipzig: Breitkopf und Hartel.

Freud, S. (1895). *Project for a Scientific Psychology.* S.E. 1: 283–397.

———. (1900). *The Interpretation of Dreams.* S.E. 4 and 5.

———. (1911). Formulations on the two principles of mental functioning. S.E. 12: 218–226.

———. (1917). Mourning and melancholia. S.E. 14: 243–260.

———. (1918). From the history of an infantile neurosis. S.E. 17: 7–123.

———. (1920). *Beyond the Pleasure Principle*. S.E. 18: 7–64.

———. (1926). *Inhibitions, Symptoms and Anxiety*. S.E. 20: 87–172.

———. (1933). *New Introductory Lectures on Psycho-analysis*. S.E. 22: 5–185.

Holt, R. R. (1989). *Freud Reappraised: A Fresh Look at Psychoanalytic Theory*. New York: Guilford.

DAVID LIVINGSTONE SMITH

Biography, and Psychoanalysis

Psychoanalysis began as a biographical enterprise. When Freud examined his patients' psychological problems, he could have remained strictly in the present (as certain later therapists have insisted on doing). However, he found it more productive to look at the analysand's entire life history. When Freud first pronounced that hysterics suffer from reminiscences, he was referring to their memories of significant life events, not to the processes of emotionally neutral short-term recall that experimental psychologists then and later studied. When he began to publish clinical case histories, he did not present merely a record of symptoms and treatments, as in other therapeutic areas; he wrote intimate biographies.

As Freud and his followers sought to apply psychoanalytic concepts beyond the consulting room, one of their first areas of application was biography: the lives of the famous and notorious. At early meetings of the Vienna Psychoanalytic Society, biographical studies were often presented, initially with Freud's encouragement. He expressed increasing dissatisfaction with these studies, however, objecting to their tendencies toward "pathography." When he proclaimed to Carl Jung in 1909 that it was time to "take hold of biography" (McGuire, 1974, p. 255), he had in mind much more than the identification of neurotic tendencies in well-known lives. He wanted to develop psychoanalysis into a general psychology, applicable to the full range of human experience.

Freud's first psychobiography was a brief book on Leonardo da Vinci (1910). Freud insisted on the book's first page that he intended to do more than "drag the sublime into the dust." Indeed, much of the book concerns Leonardo's creative efforts, seen by Freud as sublimations of sexual and aggressive urges. In discussing Leonardo's specific case, Freud pioneered most of the essential elements of subsequent psychobiographies. He applied a broad theoretical approach to his subject's personality, but modified its application to take account of Leonardo's unique personal history. Freud considered (at least briefly) Leonardo's cultural context, comparing him with other artists of the time to gain a sense of how idiosyncratic or culturally determined Leonardo's behavior might be. Freud closely examined the available information on Leonardo's life history, scrutinizing even the most trivial details in order to identify Leonardo's recurrent behavior patterns and unconscious conflicts.

However, Freud's scrutiny of Leonardo's life left much to be desired. Though he cautioned other biographers to avoid subjects that they might be inclined to idealize, Freud chose to write about Leonardo not only as someone he idealized but also as someone with whom he strongly identified. This identification led Freud to attribute features of personal history and personality to Leonardo that were more clearly attributable to Freud himself. Freud warned against resting any line of argument on a single biographical clue, but he did just that in an extensive interpretation of Leonardo's "memory" of a bird thrusting its tail into the infant Leonardo's mouth. Despite his own remonstrations against "pathographizing," Freud described Leonardo's alternation between art and science in terms that sound rather more pathographic than the evidence supports. In choosing Leonardo as a subject, Freud ignored his own warning against studying individuals about whom so little reliable biographical information exists that firm conclusions are impossible.

The Leonardo book remains, however, Freud's biographical masterwork. It offers valid insights into Leonardo's character at the same time that it illustrates important lessons (both positive and negative) for future biographers. Freud's further biographical efforts were more limited in scope, mainly repeating the Leonardo book's lessons through added examples. Freud's brief discussion of a childhood memory by Goethe (1917) notes the early importance of sibling rivalry without examining its role in any of Goethe's scientific or artistic creations. In the Goethe paper, Freud makes more explicit than in his Leonardo book the likelihood that prominent early memories are actually screen memories disguising important developmental dynamics. Freud's paper on Dostoyevsky (1928) is the most heavily pathographic of his biographical writings. Nonetheless, it adds to his previous work a more complex discussion of the role of the Oedipus complex in the male subject's attitudes toward father figures, especially in inducing appar-

B

ently groundless feelings of guilt and masochism. (A psychobiography of Woodrow Wilson, published as by Freud and William C. Bullitt [1967], appears to be largely if not entirely the work of Bullitt. In any case, it contributed nothing new either to Freud's biographical methods or to his theories.)

Moses and Monotheism, Freud's last contribution to biography, was also his final completed work (1939). The book's oddness and its shaky historical foundations were recognized by Freud, who originally planned to call it *The Man Moses: A Historical Novel*. Recent commentators have analyzed the book as a work of disguised autobiography, and to a considerable degree it is that. But at the same time, Freud (with great imaginative flair) posed two questions of interest well beyond his own autobiography: Why did the Egyptian-raised and perhaps Egyptian-born Moses want to lead the Jews, and why did the Jews want to be led by Moses? The raising of these questions, and the ways in which Freud sought to answer them, inspired subsequent psychobiographical studies of charismatic leaders by Erik Erikson (1958, 1969) and others, as well as broad analyses of charismatic leadership by such scholars as Saul Friedländer (1978).

Six decades after Freud's death, his direct and indirect influence on the writing of biography remains powerful, whatever the nature of the specific subject. Contemporary biographers may take their cue from such second-generation psychobiographers as Erikson and Leon Edel (1984); they may say little about Oedipal issues and id instincts; they may employ later expansions and modifications of psychoanalytic concepts by object relations theorists and self psychologists. But they are nonetheless likely to incorporate such distinctly Freudian features as (a) the shaping influence of the subject's early childhood; (b) the defensive distortion of the subject's memories and perceptions; (c) the symbolic significance of dreams, fantasies, and other imaginative products; and (d) most broadly, the role of unconscious motives and conflicts in the subject's adult behavior. Biographers have at times attempted to write psychological biographies that are totally non-Freudian, but with little success. Freudian concepts may have lost ground in other areas of intellectual enterprise, but in biography they continue to be useful, and therefore central.

REFERENCES

Edel, L. (1984). *Writing Lives: Principia Biographica*. New York: Norton.

Erikson, E. H. (1958). *Young Man Luther*. New York: Norton.

———. (1958). *Gandhi's Truth*. New York: Norton.

Freud, S. (1910). *Leonardo da Vinci and a Memory of his Childhood*. S.E. 11: 63-137.

———. (1917). A childhood recollection from "Dichtung und wahrheit." S.E. 17: 145-156.

———. (1928). Dostoevsky and parricide. S.E. 21: 175-198.

———. (1939). *Moses and Monotheism*. S.E. 23: 7-137.

Freud, S., and Bullitt, W. C. (1978). *Thomas Woodrow Wilson: A Psychological Study*. Boston: Houghton Mifflin.

Friedländer, S. (1978). *History and Psychoanalysis*. New York: Holmes and Meier.

McGuire, W. (ed.). (1974). *The Freud/Jung Letters*. Princeton, N.J.: Princeton University Press.

ALAN C. ELMS

Biology, and Psychoanalysis

Biological entities are inclined to cycle, and such is the case with psychoanalysis and its relationship with biology. Initiated by Freud, an experienced biologist, the explorations of the emotion-related mind began with his 1895 *Project for a Scientific Psychology*, an effort to model and establish a biological basis for the study of the mind. But in a short time, as he turned to clinical issues, Freud moved away from biology, setting a trend that was sustained for years. Psychoanalysis became a matter of psychological meaning and hermeneutics, and moved far from its biological roots.

Given that the human mind is part of living nature, arguments that psychoanalysis is not, or should not be, a biological science are highly suspect. The claim, for example, that every psychoanalytic treatment is a distinctive, nongeneralizable experience is a denial of science that would invalidate all of biology; it reflects a failure to appreciate that individuality always is constrained by and reflects core universals. Similarly, the contention that the mind is either unmeasurable or can be measured only through the highly unreliable process of introspection ignores the fact that communication through language is a mentally driven output that readily lends itself to quantitative, biological investigation.

All in all, there is no viable basis on which to exclude psychoanalysis from biology. Wilson (1998) has decried the isolation of the psychological sciences from the other sciences of nature, and has issued a call for the unification of the sciences—consilience, as he terms it—an effort that must begin by establishing a basic science in one's own field of endeavor. This pursuit, however, requires a deep appreciation for fundamental entities and an understanding of the powerful effects that formal science has on the theory and applications of any field of study to which it is applied.

Because psychoanalysis essentially has been a top-down, highly abstract, behavior-distant, impressionistic science, it has been difficult for psychoanalysts and others to appreciate the absolute need for a science of its own. It is only of late, perhaps since the 1990s, that this need has been seriously acknowledged and efforts have been made to bring psychoanalysis full circle, back into the biological fold. There is a growing consensus not only that the field needs to forge a basic science of its own, but also that it must pursue interdisciplinary collaborations with the other biological subsciences. These efforts promise to fortify the foundational base of psychoanalysis, promote the expansion and much-needed revision of its poorly substantiated theoretical precepts, enhance its clinical techniques, and solidify its position in the family of sciences. Efforts of this kind are now taking place on several fronts.

Evolutionary Biology

Evolutionary biology is the fundamental subscience of biology (Plotkin, 1994; Langs, 1996; Slavin and Kriegman, 1992). It has two components: evolution proper, which is the study of the long-term development of species—the distal causes of current behavior, broadly defined; and adaptation, which is the study of immediate means of coping, and thereby of the proximal causes of behavior. The focus in these investigations is on the universal attributes of a given species, around which individual differences are built. In order to fully understand an organism and its organ systems, it is essential to have knowledge of their evolutionary histories and present modes of adaptation.

The current theory of evolution proper is called the neo-Darwinian selfish gene theory (Dawkins, 1976). It views gene pools as the basic level of evolutionary activity. Essentially, the theory states that (the genes of) organisms within a species compete for survival and favored reproduction under prevailing environmental conditions. As they do so, a passive process of natural selection operates to favor the reproduction of those (genes of) organisms that are best suited to survive in the environment in which they live. In time, the environment of adaptation changes, new variants emerge to compete with existing organisms, and a new round of competition is initiated—and so on, ad infinitum.

Freud did not have an evolutionary or adaptive metapsychological position, so it is only in recent years that psychoanalysts have turned to evolutionary theory in an effort to understand psychoanalytic phenomena. Those who have done so, have explored the evolutionary roots and current adaptational roles of a variety of units of selection—particular mental entities and mechanisms that are subject to evolutionary forces. They have researched their chosen units, and have attempted to characterize their long-term development and their present adaptive functions.

Psychoanalysts have provided evolutionary scenarios for such entities as the Oedipus complex (as a means through which a child seeks to gain a larger than expected share of maternal or paternal care); the psychological defense of repression (as a descendant of deceptive practices among animals that, in humans, involves not knowing oneself so as to be able to deceive others and not give oneself away—and thereby gain a survival advantage); relationship structures (as a variety of means of gaining evolutionary advantages for one's genes); structures involved in affective responses—the so-called emotional mind (as an across-species means of rapidly activating survival-facilitating activities); and the structures involved in processing emotionally charged information and meaning—the so-called emotion-processing mind (as the means through which we adapt to emotion-related, animate and inanimate environmental events).

Evolutionary psychoanalysis is, today, an established interdisciplinary science. Its fundamental proposition is that the emotion-related human mind has evolved through the ages according to the same laws and regularities that apply to the physical body. It has offered perspectives on the emotion-related mind that are unavailable through other means.

To cite one such example, clinical study has shown that the emotion-processing mind is a mental module (a collection of functions organized around a particular set of adaptive tasks) that uses an inordinate amount of defensive denial in response to impacting, emotionally charged events and their most anxiety-provoking meanings. This is an unusual evolved attribute, in that natural selection almost always favors structures that increase an organism's knowledge of the environment, and denial involves a costly type of knowledge reduction.

Evolutionary study has clarified the preferred use of this mechanism by showing that the processing of emotionally charged meaning essentially is a language-based

B

function. This links the evolution of the emotion-processing mind to language acquisition, which occurred quite recently in terms of evolutionary time—about 200,000 years ago. Explorations of this momentous development have revealed that it provided *Homo sapiens* with enormous cognitive resources, and also led to the uniquely human development of a personal sense of identity and self, and the ability to anticipate the future.

These capabilities brought with them an awareness of human mortality and evoked powerful existential death anxieties. Given the ultimate helplessness of all humans in face of this inevitability, the pervasive use of denial mechanisms is readily understood, especially when it is realized that defenses directed against existential death anxieties have had very little evolutionary time in which to be selected. Trade-offs, such as anxiety reduction versus knowledge of one's living and nonliving environment and self, are common in evolutionary histories.

These are the special kinds of insights into distal causes that evolutionary theory offers to psychoanalysis. In so doing, evolutionary research has become a definitive means through which psychoanalytic phenomena have been afforded a biological cast.

Psychoneuroimmunology

Another relatively recent development that incorporates psychoanalysis into biology pertains to the new field of psychoneuroimmunology (Maier et al., 1994). This interdisciplinary science places the emotion-related mind in a biological matrix that includes the mind, the brain (especially the hypothalamus), the endocrine system, and the immune system. Much of this research is focused on the adaptive responses of this mind-body complex to a variety of stressors, with a growing consideration of psychodynamic factors.

Though blurred by many writers, this work calls for a clear distinction between the brain as a physical entity that is explored through a variety of anatomical, chemical, and electrical means, and the mind, which is an output and emergent property of the brain that is explored through other approaches, such as the study of behavior, communication, affects, and the like. The brain is the substrate and sponsor of the mind, but the mind has autonomous properties and capabilities of its own. There is also a circular, mutual feedback relationship between the mind and the brain. In this context, psychoanalysis can be understood to be the study of the

mental module responsible for adapting to emotionally charged events.

Clinically, the powerful interaction between the mind and the immune system is well established (Maier et al., 1994). There is a two-way flow of communication between the mind, the brain, and the immune system. Emotional experiences have been shown to have a variety of effects on brain and immune system activities, while changes in the immune system have been shown to have brain and mental consequences. The brain is capable of manufacturing immune system substances, and its autonomic system (a regulatory—sympathetic and parasympathetic—group of nerves) has nerve endings that reach immune system organs like the spleen and lymph nodes, and their lymphocytic cells. On the other side of this psychophysical partnership, the immune system is able to manufacture neurotransmitters and send chemical messengers to the mind via the brain.

Work also is being done to trace the pathways from the mind to the brain, and to the endocrine and immune systems, with an eye toward deepening our understanding of how humans respond to a wide range of stressful situations. Efforts are thereby being made to discover ways to enhance the adaptive capabilities of this crucial mind-body system.

A related line of study has been based on the proposition that the immune system shares the responsibility to protect humans from predatory threat with the previously mentioned emotion-processing mind—a mental module that is capable of both conscious and unconscious perception and processing of incoming information and meaning. The immune system deals with microscopic predators such as bacteria and viruses, while the emotion-processing mind deals with macroscopic, mainly conspecific (fellow human), predators.

Comparative study shows that these two systems have many features in common. They both are two-system entities, with B and T cells—lymphocytes—comprising the essence of the immune system, and conscious and deep unconscious processors making up the emotion-processing mind. Both the immune system and the emotion-processing mind also are capable of vigilance, memory, cloning successful adaptive responses, distinguishing self from non-self, self-monitoring, self-regulating, and communicating via encoded messages (chemically for the immune system, and through language-based messages for the emotion-processing mind). All in all, then, psychoneuroimmunology is a promising avenue for the biological investigation of the emotion-related mind and its adaptations.

A Formal Science of Psychoanalysis

There are four modes of science: qualitative (an impressionistic, unmeasured form that inevitably is rife with error); statistical (the use of measurement to facilitate the discovery of correlations without generating insight into underlying mechanisms); stochastic (a quantitative approach that requires time-series data and makes mathematically grounded postdictive or after-the-fact statements about hidden regularities); and formal (a quantitative approach to time-series data that allows for the discovery of predictive deep laws and regularities).

Freud viewed psychoanalysis as a science in the qualitative sense. In recent years, there have been many correlational studies related to psychoanalytic propositions like the Oedipus complex, repression, unconscious schema, psychological conflicts, and such. In general, the results of these studies have supported, but not significantly extended, present analytic thinking (Fisher and Greenberg, 1996).

Although it is essential that psychoanalysis become a full-fledged biological science, psychoanalysts have fashioned only a small number of stochastic and formal scientific investigations (Langs et al., 1996). There have, however, been some startling results.

Stochastic studies, for example, have shown several deep regularities for the speaker duration in psychotherapy sessions—the sequence of who speaks when and for how long. This work shows that therapy dialogues possess deep, stochastically defined stabilities, and that individual patients and therapists have mathematically definable, characteristic speaking and interrupting inclinations. It also has been found that the amount of time an individual spends speaking and not speaking in the course of therapy sessions produces curves that obey regularities characteristic of a pattern of phenomena, seen throughout biological nature, called Poisson processes.

There are as well formal science studies based on time series, quantitative measures of narrative and non-narrative forms of communication. Weighted scores were made for every ten seconds of analytic and therapeutic exchanges, for the newness of themes, the amount and power of storytelling versus intellectualizing, and the degree of positive and negative tone to the images. Using mathematical models borrowed from physics, a series of

psychobiological laws—mathematically predictable features—of human communication and the mind have been discovered.

There is, for example, a law of mental entropy or complexity that states that in the course of a therapy session, the complexity of the use of communicative vehicles (the above-mentioned four dimensions of expression) by any patient or therapist (and any couple engaged in an emotionally charged dialogue) grows as a logarithmic function of time. The same law has been found to govern the use of individual words.

This law indicates that in a mathematically definable manner, in the course of a therapy session, each party to therapy predictably makes use of many new communicative vehicles or words early in the hour, then invokes fewer and fewer new vehicles or words as the session goes on—but never stops turning to new forms. Further, each patient and therapist obeys this law in a personally characteristic manner—a clear example of a universal law, individually obeyed. In addition, there is evidence that the way in which an analyst adheres to these laws may offer a quantitative measure of countertransference. It was found, for example, that analysts who obtained higher total complexity scores than those of their patients showed other signs of emotional disturbance.

The discovery of formal laws of communication and the mind, and of measurable mental energy, establishes psychoanalysis as a unique and significant biological science.

Psychoanalytic Cognitive Neuroscience

Another group of psychoanalysts has been attempting to integrate psychoanalysis with both neuroscience and cognitive science. Efforts are being made to show the relevance to psychoanalysis of computer simulations of brain activities, of findings from direct studies of brain activity during aroused emotions and other emotion-related behaviors and communications, of explorations of brain development, of split brain studies, of research into the neurophysiology of psychological defenses and learning, and more.

On another front, findings from cognitive science research into memory, infant development and schema formation, consciousness, sensory reception, language development, and the like also are being integrated into psychoanalytic thinking.

We are, overall, rapidly moving toward a basic definition of psychoanalysis as the biological science of emotional adaptation, communication, development, and relating—a science that is certain to offer a sound foundation for its theoretical and clinical practices. The biological aspects of psychoanalysis hold the potential to revolutionize the field.

REFERENCES

Dawkins, R. (1976). *The Selfish Gene.* New York: Oxford University Press.

Fisher, S., and Greenberg, R. (1996). *Freud Scientifically Reappraised: Testing the Theories and Therapy.* New York: Wiley.

Freud, S. (1895). *Project for a Scientific Psychology.* S.E. 1: 281–397.

Langs, R. (1996). *The Evolution of the Emotion-Processing Mind, with an Introduction to Mental Darwinism.* London: Karnac Books.

———. (1996). *Psychotherapy and Science.* London: Sage.

Langs, R., Badalamenti, A., and Thomson, L. (1996). *The Cosmic Circle: The Unification of Mind, Matter and Energy.* Brooklyn, N.Y.: Alliance.

Maier, S., Watkins, L., and Fleshner, M. (1994). Psychoneuroimmunology: The interface between behavior, brain, and immunity. *American Psychologist* 49: 1004–1017.

Plotkin, H. (1994). *Darwin, Machines, and the Nature of Knowledge.* Cambridge, Mass.: Harvard University Press.

Slavin, M., and Kriegman, D. (1992). *The Adaptive Design of the Human Psyche.* New York: Guilford.

Wilson. E. (1998). *Consilience: The Unity of Knowledge.* New York: Knopf.

ROBERT LANGS

Bonaparte, Marie (1882–1962)

On the surface, Marie Bonaparte, the principal founder of the psychoanalytic movement in France, seems a most unlikely person to have become a practitioner of a predominantly Jewish, middle-class clinical specialty. A princess by birth, directly descended from the brother of Napoleon Bonaparte, she had every luxury and privilege available to a small child at the end of the nineteenth century. However, her mother died during her infancy, and this early loss may have stimulated her to find Sigmund Freud in the later years of her life. Bonaparte subsequently underwent an analysis with Freud, and she became one of his most loyal and cherished disciples, devoting her last decades to the perpetuation of Freud's work.

Born on July 2, 1882, in a château in Saint-Cloud, near Paris, Princess Marie Bonaparte, known affectionately as "Mimi," was the only child of Prince Roland Bonaparte, the grandnephew of Napoleon Bonaparte, and his wife, Princess Marie-Félix Bonaparte (née Blanc), the daughter of François Blanc, the founder of the Monte Carlo casino. Marie Bonaparte's mother died of an embolism less than one month after the child's birth, and the young princess spent a lonely and melancholic childhood in the care of her tyrannical grandmother, Princess Pierre Bonaparte. The small girl sought refuge in creative writing, and from a very early age began to record her dreams on slips of paper. In 1907 she traveled to Athens to marry Prince George of Greece, the son of King George I of the Hellenes and grandson of King Christian IX of Denmark. The marriage linked Bonaparte to the royal houses of France, Greece, and Denmark, an extraordinary combination of wealth and privilege which would later help her to rescue Freud and his family from the Nazis.

After a complicated extramarital tryst with the French politician Aristide Briand, and after the death of her father, Marie Bonaparte sought solace in the writings of Freud, having read the *Introductory Lectures on Psychoanalysis*, in French, at the bedside of the dying Prince Roland. Through a recommendation of René Laforgue, one of the earliest French psychoanalytic practitioners, Bonaparte met Freud, and she began her personal analysis with him in Vienna in 1925. Later, she returned to Paris, and in 1926 she became one of the prime instigators in the founding of the Société Psychanalytique de Paris, the first French psychoanalytic society. Thereafter, she assisted with the launching of the *Revue Française de Psychanalyse* in 1927, and of the Institut de Psychanalyse, the first formal French training institution, in 1934. She also translated some of Freud's writings from German into French, notably *Das Ich und das Es (The Ego and the Id)*.

Throughout her adult years, Bonaparte supported many psychoanalytic causes, rescuing the Internationaler Psychoanalytischer Verlag, the Viennese publishing firm, from bankruptcy, as well as helping to secure the safe passage of the Freud family from Nazi-governed Austria in 1938. She also financed some of the fieldwork of the pioneering psychoanalytic anthropologist Géza Róheim, so that he could travel to Australia, Somaliland, the United States, and elsewhere. After Freud's death in 1939, Bonaparte became one of the editors of the *Gesammelte Werke*, the eighteen-volume German edition of Freud's collected writings, published between 1940 and 1952, as well as an editor of Freud's correspondence with Wilhelm Fliess, which Bonaparte had purchased from a bookseller for safekeeping. Toward the end of her life, she became honorary president of the Société Psychanalytique de Paris, an honorary member of the American Psychoanalytic Association, and an honorary vice president of the International Psycho-Analytical Association.

Bonaparte wrote very little about the practice of psychoanalytic therapy, but she published a large number of clinical contributions, as well as books and articles on the application of psychoanalysis to works of literature. Her writings include psychoanalytic reflections on such diverse areas of inquiry as instinct theory, biology, anthropology, criminology, female sexuality (especially frigidity, passivity, and masochism), puberty, necrophilia, anti-Semitism, and the study of warfare. However, none of her works has exerted a truly lasting influence on the development of psychoanalytic theory or technique, though all of them display great sensitivity, creativity, and intelligence. They also demonstrate her tremendous allegiance to the work of Sigmund Freud, whom she esteemed above all other men.

In terms of her written work, Bonaparte will be best remembered for her ideas on female sexuality, which included not only an exploration of the factors preventing the fulfillment of full erotic functioning, but also the interconnection between frigidity and the fear of penetration. Bonaparte also provided a critique of Helene Deutsch's work on the passive, masochistic nature of certain components of female sexuality, as well as an attempt to classify female character into three types: feminine women, who derive primary pleasure from the vagina; bisexual women, who identify with men and obtain pleasure from the clitoris; and clitoral-vaginal women, who enjoy stimulation of both erotogenic zones.

Such a conceptualization of female sexuality would attract considerable suspicion from contemporary theorists of psychoanalysis and gender, but Bonaparte certainly helped to pave the way for contemporary discourse by being one of the first investigators, along with Helene Deutsch and Karen Horney, to explore the inner recesses of the sexual life of women. Students of applied psychoanalysis and psychoanalytic literary criticism appreciate Bonaparte's masterpiece on Edgar Allan Poe, in which she attempted to explain the American writer's obsession with death by linking his literary themes to events in his early childhood. Her study of Poe contains a particularly incisive analysis of the famous story "The Pit and the Pendulum," a tale of terrific anxiety, which Bonaparte regarded as indicative of our fear of being caught between the cutting pendulum (the father's penis) and the enveloping pit (the mother's vagina).

Bonaparte remained intellectually vigorous and industrious throughout her long life, and during her final years, she became a pioneer of psychoanalytic forensic psychology, exploring the psychodynamics of murder in particular. She became an increasingly outspoken critic of the death penalty, and she lobbied American government officials for the release of Caryl Chessman, a convicted killer awaiting execution in the California State Prison at San Quentin. Before her death, she had begun to prepare psychoanalytic studies of George Sand and Walt Whitman, and in the summer of 1961, at the age of seventy-nine, she even began to learn how to speak Russian, in anticipation of writing a study about Fyodor Dostoyevsky. After suffering from fibrillations of the heart, she developed leukemia, and she died on September 21, 1962, at a clinic in Saint-Tropez, France.

REFERENCES

Bertin, C. (1982). *La Dernière Bonaparte*. Paris: Librairie Académique Perrin.
Nacht, S. (1963). Marie Bonaparte: 1882–1962. *International Journal of Psycho-Analysis* 44: 516–517.
Schur, M. (1963). Marie Bonaparte: 1882–1962. *Psychoanalytic Quarterly* 32: 98–100.
Stein-Monod, C. (1966). Marie Bonaparte, 1882–1962: The problem of female sexuality. In F. Alexander, S. Eisenstein, and M. Grotjahn (eds.), *Psychoanalytic Pioneers.*, pp. 399–414. New York: Basic Books.

BRETT KAHR

Bound Energy See BINDING.

Brain Science, and Psychoanalysis

Many believe that mental life is dependent upon, and most likely originates in, the biological functions of brain/body. If this is so, it should be possible to reconcile a psychologically derived model of mind with a biologically derived model of brain. Freud understood and believed that. Yet he wisely abandoned his early attempt (1895) to reconcile his psychoanalytic (psychologically based) insights about mental function with the limited understanding of brain function available in his time. Instead he modeled his theory of mind exclusively upon his understanding of mental function, as he was able to observe it by using his special psychological method of inquiry (free association) into the mental life of his patients and of himself.

But much more is known about brain function now than was the case at the beginning of the twentieth century, surely enough to approach a more satisfactory reconciliation. But the reconciliation may never be complete unless or until a satisfactory solution is found to daunting procedural and conceptual problems that stand in the way.

The problem is that we have before us for consideration two different generic models or concepts of mind, different in that they derive from different domains:

1. That of mind and mental function.
2. That of brain and physiochemical physiological function.

There are, on the one hand, the subjectively based psychoanalytic models that have been derived primarily from the data of free association in clinical psychoanalytic process. On the other hand, there are the objectively based neurobiologic models that derive primarily from biologic study of the brain, including cognitive neuroscience and computer modeling of mental operations. The domain of mental science deals with meanings and motives of a psychological rather than material nature. Yet the domain of brain science deals with physiochemical phenomena, with matter and energy that are of a material nature. Furthermore, brain and mind sciences use different languages and different techniques, and their theories are framed at very different conceptual levels. Units are not interchangeable between domains, and covariance data cannot be sequentially or causally related. But emotion occupies both domains and may, when sufficiently understood, provide a key for understanding the mechanisms that link covariant mind and brain data. This is an exciting frontier for further research as new tools and techniques develop.

None of the models derived so far from one or the other domain alone is entirely satisfactory or complete. There are several possible ways to conceptualize the relationship (or lack thereof) between them:

Incompatible and Mutually Exclusive Models. The psychoanalytic and neurobiologic models are incompatible and mutually exclusive. Some brain scientists expect that the molecular biology of nerve cells will prove sufficient to provide full explanation of all mental phenomena. On the other hand, the hermeneutic school of psychoanalysis considers brain science to be irrelevant to psychologically derived understanding of the human mind.

Mutually Reducible or Translatable Models. Psychoanalytic and neurobiologic models will turn out to be mutually reducible or translatable one to the other, as Freud believed would ultimately be the case. But although information about the brain has accumulated exponentially in recent years, efforts to effect a diffuse global mapping of mind onto brain (which reflects this position) are less than fully satisfactory because of discrepancies in the nature of the data from the two domains. Development of new techniques, particularly noninvasive imaging techniques, have made it possible to study the brain during complex cognitive-emotional functions and behaviors, both in intact animals and in humans, and in experimentally lesioned animals as well as in patients with brain damage. Experimental cognitive-emotional neuroscience techniques have yielded much information about the relatively more superficial cognitive aspects of mental life. But much of psychoanalytic process and theory deals with content and mechanisms of "the dynamic unconscious" that have not (yet) been accessible to experimental investigation by those techniques. With notable recent exceptions (e.g., Shevrin et al., 1996; Solms, 1997), cognitive neuroscience has for the most part omitted consideration of the contents and mental mechanisms of the "dynamic unconscious," which is of such central interest in psychoanalysis.

This constitutes a major challenge for psychoanalysis! A leading scientific investigator of mind/brain, in discussing that patients with hippocampal damage who lack explicit memory are nevertheless capable of certain types of learning tasks that involve implicit memory, states:

> Here we have, for the first time, the neural basis for a set of unconscious mental processes. Yet this unconscious bears no resemblance to Freud's unconscious. . . . These sets of findings provide the first challenge to a psychoanalytically oriented neural science. Where, if it exists at all, is the other unconscious? What are its neurobiological properties? How do unconscious strivings become transformed to enter awareness as a result of analytic therapy? . . . At

its best, psychoanalysis could live up to its initial promise and help to revolutionize our understanding of mind and brain. (Kandel, 1998, p. 468)

Experimental Studies and Literature Searches. As a matter of fact, there are a number of promising empirically based ways of approaching the challenge of relating psychoanalysis to brain science. One is through experimental studies that combine the methods of psychoanalysis with those of brain science (Shevrin et al., 1996; Solms, 1997). Another is through literature searches in the two fields that aim to identify data that point to correspondences between psychoanalytically relevant mental functions and/or concepts, on the one hand, and independently derived data about brain structures and functions, on the other (Schore, 1997, pp. 807–840; Levin, 1991).

Still another way (a variant of the above) is for clinical psychoanalysis and experimental neuroscience to "collaborate" in a virtual dialogue in which the investigator compares data from the two fields that relate to specified mind/brain functions that are of common interest to both fields, and that are accessible to investigation by the methods of both. It is important for such studies to focus on function(s) about which the clinical psychoanalytic method can contribute data that are unique—unique in that they are not accessible by other methods. In contrast to a global mapping of mind onto brain, this approach aims to revise specific aspects of the separate psychoanalytic and neuroscience models of mind as data relevant to the same function(s) but obtained by the different methods converge. From this point of view, it seems more realistic at this stage of our knowledge to focus on specific functions and to aim at convergence rather than identity.

Such a dual-track converging process can be carried out in stages: retaining concepts from the two domains that are isomorphic with each other, modifying others to conform to each other as the data permit, and discarding or replacing outmoded concepts as new information accumulates. This can result in formulation of an intermediate (not final) composite model, identical with neither of the original models but taking into account key features of both. In the course of such a comparative process, findings in one realm may very well challenge concepts in the other and stimulate new research.

To illustrate, this article considers the convergence (developed by the use of such an approach) of psychoanalytic and neurobiologic concepts regarding perception, memory, dream process, and dream imagery.

Psychoanalytic Data and Concepts from the Mental Realm

The mental functions that engaged Freud's interest from the start included memory, perception, imagery, language, emotion, consciousness, the unconscious, and dreams. And he was concerned with understanding the functional interrelationships among them, formulating the concepts of repression, the dynamic unconscious, primary and secondary process, the reality and pleasure principles, transference, mental defense mechanisms, and his theory of dreaming. The first model of the mind that emerged was the topographic model (1900, pp. 536–541) that he formulated to account for the phenomena he had observed in his study of dreams. This hypothetical instrument contained three zones—conscious, preconscious, and unconscious—for processing, discharging, and/or storing stimuli that impinged upon it from the outside environment or from within the body (the internal environment). He postulated that this mental instrument would be stimulated to dream during sleep by a "wish." He defined a wish as the mental representation of an instinctual need, such as hunger, thirst, or sex, that arises from a somatic source in bodily processes. He eventually thought of the "wish" as the instigator of the dream in a special way, i.e., as the derivative of an instinct that is manifested in the mental realm as "a demand made upon the mind for work in consequence of its connection to the body" (1915, p. 122).

In his analysis of his "Dream of the Botanical Monograph" recounted in *The Interpretation of Dreams* (1900, p. 169), Freud observed that the ideas and memories represented in that dream were arranged in nodal networks. "Botanical" and "Monograph" were nodal points in that all ideas in the dream associations connected to one or the other of them. More recent clinical studies have led to the development of a central psychoanalytic concept of enduring nodal memory networks, in which memory traces are organized by affect—the principle of affective organization of memory (Reiser, 1990). It is summarized below.

Each of us carries within mind/brain an enduring network of stored memories encoded by images perceived during stressful life experiences. Such images and the memories they encode are associationally linked by shared potential to evoke identical or highly similar complexes of emotion. Such networks are organized around a core of perceptual images or part images encoding memories of early events experienced as highly stressful, even cataclysmic, by the child. As development proceeds, the networks branch out as later events evoke similar conflicts and emotional states. Encoded images that connect strongly and closely with several others in the network (and through them with still others) can be thought of as nodal points in the enduring memory networks of mind/brain, e.g., the dried plant "as if from an herbarium," in Freud's "Dream of the Botanical Monograph" (1900, p. 169). Here is a striking illustration of the idea noted earlier that emotion since it occupies both mental and biological domains may provide a *crucial key* for understanding the *linkage* between phenomena observed concurrently in the separate realms of *mind and body*.

From the Biological Realm

Beginning in the 1970s, experimental cognitive-emotional neuroscientific studies in animals including subhuman primates (Mishkin and Appenzeller, 1987, pp. 80–86; Squire, 1987) have led to development of the concept of neural memory networks. According to this concept, percepts encoding memories are inextricably linked by circuitry in cortical-limbic neural networks to the affects that accompanied their registration during meaningful life experiences. This concept is isomorphic (almost identical) with the psychoanalytically derived concept of enduring nodal memory networks that are organized by emotion. Studies of conditioned fear in rodents (LeDoux, 1996) have demonstrated that emotionally charged perceptual memories may be established via limbic pathways that bypass the cerebral cortex. This underlines the key role in memory of the neural circuits that mediate emotion.

Psychophysiologic studies of REM (dreaming) sleep (Hobson, 1988) indicate that mnemic perceptual images stored in the association cortex are activated during REM (dreaming) sleep by ascending excitatory (PGO) waves originating in the brain stem (pons). This activation is responsible for their appearance in the dream. The REM state itself is initiated by chemical changes in the pons.

Dialogue

Freud's concept of the wish as the instigator of the dream was not directly supported by these findings, and the psychoanalytic theory would have to be modified accordingly by distinguishing between the REM (dreaming) state as a physiological state of the brain during sleep and the subjective mental experience of the dream as recounted to the psychoanalyst or investigator. After all, a "wish" (mental realm) cannot instigate a dreaming state of the brain (biological realm); nor can a chemical change in the pons (biological realm) create a dream experience (mental realm).

Dream researchers (Hobson and McCarley, 1977, pp. 1335–1348) originally considered dream imagery to be randomly generated by the stimulating effect of the PGO waves on the cortex, and therefore devoid of primary meaning—only secondarily organized into narrative sequences that appear meaningful (similar to Freud's concept of secondary revision)—the *activation synthesis hypothesis*.

Meanwhile, clinical psychoanalytic studies indicated that current life conflicts, and conscious worries about them during the day, often find representation in the dream. It has been postulated that this occurs because current conflicts activate historically relevant memory traces and their associated affects, thus rendering the images that encode them more sensitive to stimulation by PGO waves during sleep (Reiser, 1990). Accordingly, the images appearing in dreams can be regarded as meaningfully related to both current and past conflicts. Furthermore, the activation-synthesis hypothesis could not account for repetitive dreams in which imagery appears repeatedly and without variation, and could hardly be regarded as randomly generated. Finally, recent PET imaging studies by Braun et al. (1998, pp. 91–95) demonstrate that the memory and emotional systems of the brain are active during REM sleep in human subjects. For these reasons the activation-synthesis must be modified to account for the meaningful content carried by dream imagery. All of this, considered together with psychophysiologic evidence of the memory-organizing function of dreaming sleep (Winson, 1985) led to a modified psychobiological definition of dream process:

> Dreaming in man can be defined as the subjective experience of vital memory and problem solving cognitive functions made possible by the special psychophysiological conditions that obtain in mind/brain-body during REM sleep. (Reiser, 1990, p. 200)

This is a contemporary psychobiologic definition of the dreaming process that conforms to both psychoanalytic and neuroscientific findings. Each separate theory had to be modified to achieve this new composite conceptualization, and each contributed unique material. It could not have been constructed from either side alone, illustrating how thoughtful dialogue between clinical psychoanalytic and cognitive neuroscience data and concepts can be reciprocally enriching and lead to appropriate modifications on both sides. This process then permitted construction of a composite psychobiologic formulation compatible with both clinical psychoanalytic and neurobiologic data, and useful to both disciplines. For clinical psychoanalysis it has important technical implications for working with dreams (Reiser, 1997).

Although this does not constitute a final or complete formulation and does not provide full understanding of dream process, it does represent progress. And it illustrates the promise of this approach for furthering understanding of the mind/brain problem. Space limitations do not permit review here of other promising investigative approaches (briefly mentioned earlier and reviewed elsewhere in this volume) that involve simultaneous and/or parallel investigations of mental functions by methods of both mind and brain science.

REFERENCES

Braun, A. R., Balkin, T. J., Wesensten, N. J., Gwadry, F., Carson, R. E., Varga, M., Baldwin, P., Belenky, G., and Herscovitch, P. (1988). Dissociated pattern of activity in visual cortices and their projections during human rapid eye movement sleep. *Science* 279: 91–95.

Freud, S. (1895). *Project for a Scientific Psychology.* S.E. 1: 283–297.

———. (1900). *The Interpretation of Dreams.* S.E. 4–5: 1–621.

———. (1915). Instincts and their vicissitudes. S.E. 14: 117–140.

Hobson, A. J. (1988). *The Dreaming Brain.* New York: Basic Books.

Hobson, A. J., and McCarley, R. W. (1977). The brain as a dream state generator. *American Journal of Psychiatry* 134: 1335–1348.

Kandel, E. R. (1998). A new intellectual foundation for psychiatry. *American Journal of Psychiatry* 155: 457–469.

LeDoux, J. (1996). *The Emotional Brain: The Mysterious Underpinnings of Emotional Life.* New York: Simon and Schuster.

Levin, F. M. (1991). *Mapping the Mind.* Hillsdale, N.J.: Analytic Press.

Mishkin, M., and Appenzeller, T. (1987). The anatomy of memory. *Scientific American* 256: 80–86.

Reiser, M. (1990). *Memory in Mind and Brain: What Dream Imagery Reveals.* New York: Basic Books. Paperbound ed., New Haven Conn.: 1994.

———. (1997). The art and science of dream interpretation: Isakower revisited. *Journal of the American Psychoanalytic Association* 45: 891–907.

Schore, A. M. (1997). A century after Freud's *Project*: Is a rapprochment between psychoanalysis and neurobiology at hand? *Journal of the American Psychoanalytic Association* 45: 807–840.

Shevrin, H., Bond, J. A., Brakel, L. A. W., Hertel, R. K., and Williams, W. J. (1996). *Conscious and Unconscious Processes: Psychodynamic, Cognitive, and Neurophysiological Convergences.* New York: Guilford Press.

Solms, M. (1997). *The Neuropsychology of Dreams: A Clinical Anatomical Study.* Institute for Research in Behavioral Neuroscience Monograph 7. Mahwah, N.J.: Erlbaum.

Squire, L. R. (1987). *Memory and Brain.* New York: Oxford University Press.

Winson, J. (1985). *Brain and Psyche: The Biology of the Unconscious.* New York: Doubleday/Anchor.

MORTON F. REISER

B

Brazil, and Psychoanalysis

An understanding of the relationships between psychoanalysis and Brazil requires a summary description of this extraordinary country with its unique culture.

The land area covered is of continental proportions. Brazil ranks among the ten greatest economic powers in the world. Its language, Portuguese, is the eighth most widely spoken language in the world, but its use renders Brazil culturally isolated from both the rest of Latin America and the Hispanic world, compounding the effects of its geographical isolation. The Portuguese colonization encountered a fragile indigenous culture that was easily crushed. After being colonized, Brazil received a large contingent of African slaves, who remained slaves until the end of the nineteenth century. In this same period, waves of European immigrants came—Italians, Germans, Polish—principally to the southern states. At the turn of the twenty-first century, Brazil has high-tech urban centers with all the sophisticated features found in the developed world, alongside poverty and illiteracy, and a serious national identity crisis. In short, it is a country of spectacular contradictions, many of which are revealed in its relationships with psychoanalysis.

Freud's ideas have penetrated Brazil since the late nineteenth century; references to them date back as early as 1899, at a conference held by Juliano Moreira, an erudite black professor of neuropsychiatry who is considered the founder of psychiatry in Brazil. In the 1910s, there is a record of conferences in Rio de Janeiro and São Paulo concerning psychoanalytical treatment, with descriptions of clinical experiences. The work of Freud was, step by step, being introduced and accepted by the Brazilian intellectuals. Not only did doctors and psychiatrists become interested in the new body of knowledge; so, too, did artists, anthropologists, and literary scholars. The relationships between the medical forerunners of psychoanalysis and the intellectuals were very close in this period. However, after the institutionalization of psychoanalysis, this relationship became more distant and problematic.

The first attempt to create a psychoanalytical institution in Brazil—at São Paulo in 1927—was made by two pioneering psychiatrists; Durval Marcondes and Franco da Rocha. They founded the short-lived Sociedade Brasileira de Psicanálise, which formed the basis for the later Sociedade Brasileira de Psicanálise de São Paulo. The latter is the largest Brazilian psychoanalytic association, boasting over 600 members (including associates and students). The founding of the Sociedade Brasileira was concomitant with the Semana de Arte Moderna (Modern Art Week), a project of intellectuals commemorating the centenary of Brazil's independence, during which poets, writers, and artists presented their works, inspired by European aesthetic movements but transformed by the influence of Brazilian culture. Also in the 1920s the Communist Party of Brazil was founded and the first labor syndicates were organized, reflecting the influence of the Italian anarchists.

The first visit by a didactic analyst recommended by the International Psychoanalytic Association (IPA) was in 1936, in São Paulo; the purpose was to commence the institutionalization of psychoanalysis in Brazil. The visitor was Adelheid Koch, trained in the Psychoanalytical Society of Berlin and analyzed by Otto Fenichel. The Sociedade Brasileira de Psicanálise de São Paulo was officially recognized by the IPA as a Society component in 1951.

The movement for the creation of psychoanalytical societies in Rio de Janeiro had characteristics different from those of São Paulo that were related to the postwar period. In the second half of the 1940s, through the IPA, Ernest Jones sent two European analysts to Rio. Mark Burke and Werner Kemper were refugees from the "German disaster"; the first was a Polish Jew, and the

second, a German member of the Goering Institute. At the same time, Brazilian doctors—Danielo and Marialzira Perestrello, Alcyon Bahia, and Walderêdo de Oliveira—went to Argentina for their training, and others went to London. Upon the return of these psychiatrists, and in conjunction with the training of those who had remained in Brazil, two societies were formed in Rio de Janeiro. The fact that these societies had been organized after World War II gave them particular characteristics, and affected the manner in which they have functioned in later crises involving the Rio societies and the IPA.

In Rio de Janeiro, in the 1950s, Iracy Doyle, a psychiatrist who had been trained in the United States, formed a psychoanalytical society that was not affiliated with the IPA, having a cultural orientation rather than a medical one.

In the 1940s, in Rio Grande do Sul state, in the city of Pôrto Alegre, the third focus of the diffusion of psychoanalysis occurred. Given the proximity of Argentina, then an important psychoanalytical center, the pioneers of psychoanalysis in this southern state underwent their training there. Mário and Zaira Martins, José Lemmertz, and Cyro Martins were members of this group, as was Celestino Prunes (coming from Rio de Janeiro). The society of Rio Grand do Sul was recognized officially by the IPA in the 1960s. Nevertheless, as in São Paulo and Rio de Janeiro, psychoanalysis in Rio Grande do Sul had been part of the psychiatric environment since the 1920s.

Psychoanalysis in Brazil has certain characteristics peculiar to the national culture and has been widely received, as is shown by the wide variety of schools. Its reception may be partly due to Brazil's being a young culture without great tradition and, consequently, without deeply rooted prejudice, as well as a greater acceptance of sexuality. However, psychoanalysis remained restricted to private practice and to the most economically privileged social classes, and, with regard to individual initiatives, was set apart from the university environment and social application. On the other hand, however, the media absorbed psychoanalytical ideas, often rendering them banal, making certain expressions popular—such as "Oedipus complex," "unconscious," and "repression"—but devoid of any more profound connotation. Despite the shallowness of many of the presentations, a venue was opened up, principally via television, for the majority of the population to discuss emotions, feelings, and conflicts outside the religious ambit or traditional morality.

The diffusion of psychoanalysis was strongest in the 1960s and 1970s. The therapeutic community and psychoanalytical group therapy were in their heyday. Some correlate this development with the repressive military regimes. In the same period Brazil, like other Latin American countries, was under military dictatorships. Psychoanalysis represented an "escape valve" for the feeling of impotence that dominated broad sectors of the middle class and the intellectual elite. This development was gradually restricted to psychoanalytical activity in consulting rooms, for the regime in power did not look favorably on the application of psychoanalysis to groups or to the treatment of large numbers of people. At the same time, there were frequent visits from foreign analysts, who, besides Argentines, included Wilfred Bion and Hans Thorner. They exerted a major influence on Brazilian psychoanalysis, then predominantly oriented to the views of Melanie Klein.

From the end of the 1970s into the 1980s, Lacanian psychoanalysis began to develop; it penetrated the universities, and today is a significant movement throughout Brazil. More recently, the influence of D. W. Winnicott and the French school, principally the thinking of André Green, has grown. These currents represent the second characteristic of psychoanalysis in Brazil: the sheer diversity of thought. The main scientific contributions come from research in mother-infant relationships, according to the Ester Bick method; six to eight decades of studying group analysis; a tradition of working with psychotic patients; and Bion's *Triology: Memoir of the Future.*

At the beginning of the 1980s, with the redemocratization of the country, two significant events occurred in Rio de Janeiro. The first was the restructuring of the Sociedade Brasileira de Psicanálise do Rio de Janeiro in a form that did not suit the IPA traditionalists (abolition of the category of associate member and of the prerogatives of didactic members; broad participation by students in the society's activities). The second was a discussion in the Sociedade Psicanalítica do Rio de Janeiro of the cover-up and bad handling by the psychoanalytical institutions, including the IPA, of the fact that one of their students had been a member of a torture group during the military regime. These events preceded the democratization and modernization of the IPA that began at the Congress of Rome (1989), and was strengthened in 1994 when the House of Delegates was made official. Both events in Rio de Janeiro resulted in interventions by the IPA.

Thus, another characteristic of psychoanalysis in Brazil is its questioning, polemical nature, raising issues that have remained unspoken in the international movement. The questioning with regard to the torturer/student had the effect of raising all the IPA's past relationships with Nazism. Likewise, the democratization of the institutions brought to the surface the dissatisfaction, principally of the Latin Americans, with the authoritarian manner in which the IPA had been treating the international psychoanalytical movement. It was not by chance that all of this coincided with the election of the first Latin American president of the IPA, Horácio Etchegoyen. He supported both further discussion of the institutional structure and the relationships between psychoanalysis and ethics.

As of 2000, the Brazilian societies affiliated with the IPA have 1,716 members (including associates and students), distributed among seven societies, four study groups, and eight nuclei; they are grouped under the Associação Brasileira de Psicanálise. There are over thirty Lacanian societies throughout the country.

REFERENCES

Anuário Brazileiro de Psicanálise no. 3 (1995).

Nosek, L., et al. (1994). *Album de Família: Imagens, Fontes e Idéias da Psicanálise em São Paulo.* São Paulo: Casa do Psicólogo.

Perestrello, M. (1988). Primeiros encontros com a psicanálise: Os precursores no Brasil (1899–1937). *Jornal Brasileiro de Psiquiatria, 35,* no. 4: 195.

———. (1987). *História da Sociedade Brasileira de Psicanálise no Rio de Janeiro: Origens e Fundação.* Rio de Janeiro: Imago.

Séreio, N. M. F. (1998). *Reconstruindo Farrapos. A Trajetória Histórica da SPRJ: Instituição e Poder.* Niterói: Centro de Estudos Gerais Graduação em História, Universidade Federal Fluminense.

NEY COUTO MARINHO

Brentano, Franz (1838–1917)

Franz Brentano was a German philosopher and psychologist whose early "intentionality thesis" is of significant interest to psychoanalysis, as well as being the foundation of Edmund Husserl's philosophical phenomenology. This thesis is elaborated in his text *Psychology from an Empirical Standpoint* (1874), in which he argues that every mental act has within it an object, although there are different ways in which thoughts may be direct-ed toward these "immanent" objects. This is the "mark of the mental," and defines the parameters within which the nascent science of psychology could be rigorously developed. The lineaments of Brentano's position are expressed most clearly as follows:

> Every mental phenomenon is characterized by what the Scholastics of the Middle Ages called the intentional (or mental) in-existence of an object, and what we might call, though not wholly unambiguously, reference to a content, direction towards an object (which is not to be understood here as meaning a thing), or imma-nent objectivity. Every mental phenomenon includes some thing as object within itself, although they do not all do so in the same way. In presentation something is presented, in judg-ment something is affirmed or denied, in love loved, in hate hated, in desire desired and so on. (Brentano, 1973 [1874], p. 88)

The distinction between "presentation" (*Vorstel-lung*), "judgment" (*Urteil*), and "love/hate," feeling or desire (*Gemütsbewegungen*) is central to Brentano's account of psychology. Each is an active mental process which refers to its object in a different way. A mental act may be directed toward any object, either physical or imaginary, or any mental act which is not identical with itself. Brentano regards presentations as the basic units of mental functioning; nothing can be desired or judged until it has first been presented to the mind. Each men-tal act contains the same object as the presentation to which it is connected; "nothing is an object of judgment which is not an object of presentation" (Brentano, 1973 [1874], p. 201). Furthermore, Brentano claims that every mental act is accompanied by the subject's awareness that he is involved in a cognitive process. In this sense, it is possible to question the truth or falsity of an object of thought, but not the fact that one is thinking.

Despite his own intellectual achievements, Brentano saw his primary role as that of teacher, and sought to be judged on the basis of his contribution to future gener-ations of thinkers. He achieved this aim through his stu-dents, including Alexix Meinong, Edmund Husserl, and Carl Stumpf. The influence of Brentano's teachings can also be found in the work of Sigmund Freud, who attended Brentano's philosophical lectures between the winter of 1874 and the summer of 1876. While a student at the University of Vienna, he was officially enrolled in the courses "Readings of Philosophical Writings," "Logic," and "The Philosophy of Aristotle." There is also evidence that Freud, like many students at the time, attended some of Brentano's lectures unofficially. This is most likely in the case of Brentano's ongoing course on psychology.

In his correspondence with his school friend Edward Silberstein, Freud frequently refers to Brentano. In a letter of March 7, 1875, he recounts his encounter with Brentano, whom he describes as a "remarkable man (a believer, a theologist (!) and a Darwinian and a damned clever fellow, a genius in fact), who is, in many respects, an ideal human being" (Boehlich, 1990, p. 95). Freud's devotion to Brentano and his philosophical ideas culminated in his decision to undertake a doctorate in philosophy and zoology under Brentano's supervision (Boehlich, 1990, p. 95). Although this intention was never realized, it indicates the seriousness with which Freud approached his philosophical studies.

Brentano's regard for his former student is marked by the fact that he recommended that Freud translate volume 12 of John Stuart Mill's *Collected Works*. Freud translated the four essays contained in this volume dur-ing his military service in the autumn and winter of 1879.

Brentano's contribution to Freud's development of psychoanalysis is apparent in several ways. First, Brentano considered himself to be a natural scientist, working objectively with experience as his guide. He insisted that "the true method of philosophy is none other than that of natural science": "*vera philosophia methodus nulla alia nisi scientia naturalis est.*" While drawing upon scientific methodology, Brentano sought to evolve beyond the scientific reliance upon empirical evidence gathered through external perception. He argued that philosophy, and the then emerging scientif-ic psychology, could attain a greater degree of certainty because they utilized both external perception and a form of introspection which he called "inner percep-tion" (*innere Wahrnemung*). Brentano believed that inner perception is a reflective process. In order to observe our own ideas or emotions, we must wait until they have passed. For example, "If someone is in a state in which he wants to observe his own anger raging within him, the anger must already be somewhat diminished and so his original object of observation would have disappeared" (Brentano, 1973, [1874], p. 30).

In Brentano's early philosophy, he was adamant that every mental act is based on a presentation: "We speak of a presentation whenever something appears to us. When we see something, a color is presented; when we hear something, a sound; when we imagine things, a fantasy image" (Brentano, 1872–1873, p. 198). Freud also considers every mental act to be based upon a presentation. In Brentano's terms, Freud's φ-system of the *Project for a Scientific Psychology* (Freud, 1895) would be equivalent to our initial perception of sensory information, before it becomes recognizable as a presentation. This division is apparent in Freud's letter to Wilhelm Fliess of June 12, 1896, in which he differentiates between "perception" and "perceptual signs," where perceptual signs are "the first registration of the perceptions" (Freud, 1950, p. 174). This is developed in *The Interpretation of Dreams* (Freud, 1900) and the short essay "A Note upon the 'Mystic Writing Pad'" (Freud, 1925). In these latter texts Freud explains that the first stage in memory, the Pcpt.-Cs system, ". . . receives perceptions but retains no permanent trace of them" (Freud, 1925, p. 230). The data merely pass through this part of the system without permanent record. It is at the next stage, where the perception is registered as a sign, that this presentation is coalesced with a wish (*Wunsch*). This is redolent of the intentional inexistence of the presented object in Brentano.

According to Brentano, we are performing two activities when we make a judgment. We judge that we are having an idea. This is the certain and indubitable aspect of any mental act. We also judge the truth or falsity of the object toward which that idea is directed. This distinction is also articulated by Freud, in particular in the *Project* and in his essay on "Negation" (Freud, 1925). Freud's concept of "reality-testing" also recognizes the difference between judgments which relate to the mental act and those which relate to the object of thought. This is further evidenced in his distinction between material reality and psychic reality; here the psychic reality of fantasy, it has been argued, enabled Freud to use a conceptual framework derived from Brentano to repudiate his seduction theory (Frampton, 1991).

Brentano's category of "love/hate" or desire (*Gemütsbewegungen*) also may have contributed to Freud's account of the "pleasure principle" as being responsible for guiding us toward acceptance of those objects which are good or pleasurable, and rejection of that which is bad or unpleasurable. Brentano taught that

"love/hate" is the instigator of our mental acts. He even suggests that the original motivating force of action may have been "lust and unlust" (Brentano, 1872–1873).

Thus Brentano's basic categories of presentation, judgment, and desire have a significant place in Freud's psychoanalytic thought, although the shift from a psychology of consciousness on Brentano's part, to Freud's analysis of unconscious mental processes, changes their conceptual import.

REFERENCES

Barclay, J. R. (1964). Franz Brentano and Sigmund Freud. *Journal of Existentialism* 5: 1–36.

Boehlich, W. (ed.). (1990). *The Letters of Sigmund Freud to Eduard Silberstein 1871–1881.* Translated by A. J. Pomerans. Cambridge Mass.: The Belknap Press of Harvard University Press.

Brentano, F. (1872–1873). Plan für das Psychologiekolleg. Unpublished manuscript, catalog number PS 62, in the possession of Dr. John C. M. Brentano, Highland Park; Ill.

———. (1973 [1874]). *Psychology from an Empirical Standpoint.* Translated by A. C. Rancurello, D. B. Terrell, and L. McAlister. New York: Humanities Press.

Frampton M. F. (1991). Considerations on the role of Brentano's concept of intentionality in Freud's repudiation of the seduction theory. *International Review of Psychoanalysis* 18: 27–36.

Freud, S. (1895). *Project for a Scientific Psychology.* S.E. 1: 283–397.

———. (1900). *The Interpretation of Dreams.* S.E. 4 and 5: 1–621.

———. (1925). A note on the "mystic writing-pad." S.E. 19: 227–232.

———. (1950). *The Origins of Psychoanalysis: Letters to Wilhelm Fliess, Drafts and Notes.* Edited by M. Bonaparte, A. Freud, and E. Kris. Translated by E. Mosbacher and J. Strachey. New York: Basic Books.

AVIVA COHEN

Breuer, Josef (1842-1925)

Josef Breuer, a Viennese internist who was Sigmund Freud's mentor, friend, and for a period, his collaborator, is remembered today mainly for the role he played in the prehistory of psychoanalysis. Breuer developed a form of psychotherapeutic treatment, the cathartic method, which depended on extended listening by the physician to the patient's verbalizations about her symptoms; Freud, in turn, elaborated and modified this method into a new system of therapy he called psychoanalysis. Yet this statement, though accurate, does not quite do justice to Breuer, who had other significant professional accomplishments that today they are largely forgotten and over-shadowed by his connection with psychoanalysis.

In his youth, Breuer had carried out research in physiology with substantial success. He first addressed the problem of fever—whether it had a neural or humoral origin—and succeeded in demonstrating by means of animal experiments that fever results when pyrogens are released into the bloodstream from the site of injury or inflammation. He then studied the mechanism controlling respiration. With his teacher, the physiologist Ewald Hering, Breuer clarified the role of inflation of the lungs as mediated by the vagus nerve. This became known as the Hering-Breuer reflex. Breuer's most ambitious experiments were those on the function of the semicircular canals of the ear; he concluded that they were not organs of hearing but part of the system controlling equilibrium.

Breuer also discovered that, despite the success of his research, his chances, as a Jew, of obtaining a full-time professorial appointment were slim. In 1871 he went into private practice, although for a number of years he continued to pursue his research on the semicircular canals, working at night in a small laboratory in his home.

Breuer became a foremost clinician and diagnostician, and was valued for his acumen, his dedication, and the thoughtful attention he gave his patients. He also had a warm and generous heart (when Freud was an impecunious student, Breuer loaned him money, and when, years later, Freud tried to repay it, Breuer would not accept it). Breuer came to be known as a doctor's doctor—perhaps the most genuine recognition the profession can bestow. Among his patients were members of the medical school faculty and their families, including Ernst Brücke, his teacher and professor of physiology; Theodor Billroth, professor of surgery; Rudolf Chrobak, professor of gynecology; and Moriz Kaposi, professor of dermatology. The philosopher Franz Brentano was one of his patients, as were others from the intelligentsia and upper bourgeoisie. He also became the physician of Anna O. (Bertha Pappenheim), the twenty-one-year-old hysteric with whose name Breuer's is firmly linked.

The story of Anna O. is told elsewhere in this work, but additional comments are relevant here. Anna's illness was very complex, and Breuer found himself involved in a therapeutic relationship that was much more intense than any he had experienced before. Relevant factors were the frequency of his visits and a special closeness that had developed between him and his patient. Probably of significance is that the patient's name (Bertha) was the same as that of Breuer's mother, who had died in childbirth when he was three. It was also the name of Breuer's eldest daughter, who was ten at the time of the treatment. Moreover, Anna O. was then approximately the age of Breuer's mother when she had died.

Breuer, unprotected by knowledge of the transference (which had not yet been discovered), was shaken and distressed when Anna developed a pseudocyesis and the delusional belief that she was pregnant by Breuer. Shortly afterward he withdrew from the case and referred Anna to the Sanatorium Bellevue in Switzerland.

The relationship between Breuer and Freud was in no small part connected to the case of Anna O. Breuer in his role as mentor told Freud, soon after his graduation from medical school, about this challenging case he was treating, and Freud never forgot it. Freud was convinced of the importance of the Anna O. case and eventually succeeded in persuading Breuer that it should be published (this was some thirteen years after Breuer had concluded his treatment of Anna). Breuer agreed to include the case in a book that he and Freud would co-author. Breuer also contributed a theoretical chapter on the psychopathology of hysteria and another chapter (in collaboration with Freud) on the mechanism of hysterical phenomena. Freud contributed four cases and a chapter on the psychotherapy of hysteria. Titled *Studies on Hysteria* and published in 1895, the book, according to Ernest Jones, was not particularly successful at first. Today, though, it is considered a landmark contribution on hysteria and the origins of the psychoanalytic method.

By the time the book appeared, Breuer's and Freud's views on the etiology of hysteria and, more generally, of the neuroses already were beginning to diverge. Freud was increasingly convinced that sexual traumata and a disturbance of the sexual function were fundamental, while Breuer grew more and more uncomfortable with this view and inclined not to accept it. They also differed in style and temperament; Freud was an audacious investigator of the mind and a theoretician, whereas Breuer was a highly accomplished but traditional physician. Their divergences increased. As Freud gradually became the recognized founder of the new discipline of psychoanalysis and an authority in his own right, the friendship between the two cooled, and finally they stopped seeing one another. Breuer was absorbed in his medical practice and did not pursue his investigations on hysteria.

There was no further scientific collaboration, but their personal relationship remained, at least outwardly, one of mutual consideration and respect. In his writings Freud repeatedly had occasion to praise Breuer for his contribution to the early development of psychoanalysis. When Breuer died, at eighty-three, Freud wrote one of the principal obituaries in which he conveyed his admiration and appreciation for Breuer. It may have been largely serendipity, but Breuer was the first to discover the therapeutic value of frequent visits, prolonged listening, and thoughtful attention to the patient's words, which later became central to psychoanalytic treatment.

REFERENCES:

Breuer, J., and Freud, S. (1895). *Studies on Hysteria.* S.E. 2, 19–305.

Castelnuovo-Tedesco, P. (1994). On re-reading the case of Anna O: More about questions that are unanswerable. *Journal of the American Acedmy of Psychoanalysis* 22, no. 1: 57–71.

Freud, S. (1925). *An Autobiographical Study.* S.E. 20: 3–74.

———. (1975). Letter to Stefan Zweig dated June 2, 1932. In Ernst L. Freud (ed.), *Letters of Sigmund Freud*, New York: Basic Books, pp. 412–413.

Ellenberger, H. (1970). *The Discovery of the Unconscious.* New York: Basic Books.

———. (1972). The story of "Anna O": A critical review with new data. *Journal of the History of the Behavioral Sciences* 8: 267–279.

Hirschmüller, A. (1989). *The Life and Work of Josef Breuer: Physiology and Psychoanalysis.* New York: New York University Press.

Jones, E. (1953). *The Life and Work of Sigmund Freud.* Vol. 1. New York: Basic Books.

PIETRO CASTELNUOVO-TEDESCO

B

C

Canada, and Psychoanalysis

In the early part of the twentieth century, psychoanalytic practice in Canada was minimal. D. Campbell Meyers and Ernest Jones (who lived in Toronto between 1908 and 1913) treated psychoneurotic patients in Canada. Jones and the Canadian John McCurdy were among the eight charter members of the American Psychoanalytic Association founded in 1911. These isolated activities, however, were insufficient to foster a psychoanalytic community at that time.

For the next three decades, individual Canadians trained abroad, mostly in the United States, where they stayed and contributed to their local societies. These included, in addition to McCurdy, who trained in New York, Hugh Carmichael, who trained in Chicago; Clifford Scott, in Britain; Douglas Noble, Washington, D.C.; and Grace Baker, Baltimore. Of this early group, only Scott returned to Canada, in 1954, the same year he became the president of the British Society.

The real history of psychoanalysis in Canada began in 1945 in Montreal, where Miguel Prados, a Spanish neuropathologist, started a study group with four residents. In 1946, the group was named the Montreal Psychoanalytic Club; by 1948 it had 40 members, some of whom went abroad to train. Several trained analysts moved to Montreal: Theodore Chentrier, a lay member from Paris (in 1948); Eric Wittkower and Alastair Macleod, both from London (in 1950); and George Zavitzianos, from the French Society (in 1951). With the return of Bruce Ruddick from New York, the group had five fully trained analysts as members, the number necessary to become an official study group of the International Psychoanalytic Association.

Conflict, however, surrounded the sponsorship of the application for full membership in the International Psychoanalytic Association. The original sponsor, the American Psychoanalytic Association, claimed suzerainty over psychoanalytic training in North America. Because it seemed to the Canadians that absorption by the American was its goal, the Canadian group applied for sponsorship by the British Society. In subsequent correspondence, the president of the American Psychoanalytic Association called the Canadian group "the Montreal toddlers."

By 1954, with the return of Scott from Britain, the recruitment of Johann and Gottfriede Aufreiter, and the return from London of the newly trained André Lussier to Montreal and Alan Parkin to Toronto, the membership in the Canadian group became twelve. Thus, on July 31, 1957, membership in the International Psychoanalytic Association was approved during its congress in Paris.

Further conflict about the control of the training program and the training of lay analysts occurred between the Canadian Society and the Department of Psychiatry at McGill University, the sponsor of several of the recruited analysts. Because of a very strong European influence, the Canadian Society had always supported training lay analysts. The medical emphasis in a department of psychiatry, as well as the fact that some analysts were not members of the faculty at the university, led to the establishment of an independent training program in psychoanalysis. In May 1959, the first training program under the auspices of the Canadian Society started in Montreal with ten candidates.

While these developments were taking place in Montreal, Toronto was in the process of establishing its own training programs. In 1956, a number of psychiatrists under the leadership of Alan Parkin formed the Toronto Psychoanalytic Study Circle. In 1960, this group became the Psychotherapy Section of the Ontario Psychiatric Association. Training in Toronto now became possible: candidates could have their analysis in Toronto and commute to Montreal for their courses and supervision. With the arrival of more American-trained analysts and the graduation of local candidates, a separate training program was started in Toronto in 1969.

In 1967, to accommodate the needs of French-speaking candidates, a French training program was initiated in Montreal. A short-lived fourth training program began in Ottawa in 1978. Only one class of candidates graduated from that program. Subsequent moves of training analysts from Ottawa closed down the program.

Currently, psychoanalysis thrives in Canada. Membership in the Canadian Psychoanalytic Society is approaching 350. Most Canadian analysts live in either Montreal or Toronto; however, there are medium-sized groups (10 to 20) in Ottawa and London, Ontario, and growing groups in Quebec City and western Canada, particularly in Vancouver, British Columbia, where training is possible through the cooperation of the Canadian Psychoanalytic Institute and the American Psychoanalytic Institute in Seattle. Training of Canadian psychoanalysts occurs under the auspices of the Canadian Psychoanalytic Institute in three training programs: two (one each in English and French) in Montreal and one in Toronto.

Like the Canadian Society, Canadian psychoanalysis reflects the confluence of North American and European, both English and French, influences. Consequently, in addition to what is often called mainstream North American psychoanalysis, the Canadian Psychoanalytic Society membership has a very active interest in and representation of self psychology, British object relations theories, Kleinian and post-Kleinian theories, French psychoanalysis, and Lacanian theories. The Canadian Psychoanalytic Society has been able to maintain its unity, despite major cultural and theoretical differences. At the beginning of the century, Canadian psychoanalysis is healthy but faces the challenges of psychoanalysis everywhere: problems with funding psychoanalytic treatment and the challenge of shorter and less intensive forms of treatment.

REFERENCES

Parkin, A. (1987). *A History of Psychoanalysis in Canada.* Toronto, Ontario: Toronto Psychoanalytic Society.

GEORGE A. AWAD

Castration Complex

The set of reactions, both mental and behavioral, to either the perceived fear of having one's penis cut off or the perception that one has already been castrated.

Freud's first published discussion of the castration complex appeared in his case history of Little Hans (1909), whose mother reportedly told him that if he continued to touch his penis, she would ask the doctor to cut it off (see "Little Hans," this volume). Freud realized, however, that overt, explicit threats of castrating children were not frequent enough to explain the prevalence, in fact the universality, of the castration complex. Rather male children more typically reacted to more subtle hints that castration was a realistic threat.

Both male and female children begin, at the age of three or earlier, by believing that everyone possesses a penis. If the male child sees a vagina by observing his sister or some other female, he initially disavows, Freud claims (1916–1917, p. 317), the evidence of his senses; for he cannot believe that any human creature would fail to possess a penis. That is his first reaction. Later, he becomes frightened that he too may have his penis removed. He thus "comes under the sway of the castration complex" (p. 317). The little boy experiences *castration anxiety*, anxiety about the possibility of his father castrating him as a result of his amorous advances toward his mother. How the male child reacts to this castration anxiety, Freud notes (p. 318), plays a key role in the construction of his character if he remains normal, and in his neurosis if he develops one; it also appears in his resistances if he should ever undergo analytic treatment.

The more immediate results of the threat of castration, Freud says (1940, p. 190), are "multifarious and incalculable." Rather than risk castration, the male child renounces the desire to sexually possess his mother. He continues to indulge in unconscious sexual fantasies involving his mother, but he ceases his overt sexual advances toward her. The whole experience, Freud says, is then subjected to a highly energetic repression. This repression of the child's wish to have sex with his mother generally leads to the termination of the Oedipal period.

Female children, quite obviously, are not likely to react in the way that boys do; they come to realize that they have no penis the loss of which can be threatened. Their reaction to this knowledge is to infer that they have already been castrated and to feel at a great disadvantage owing to their lack of a big, visible penis. As a consequence, they envy boys for possessing one, and this envy leads to their wish to become a man, a wish that reemerges later in any neurosis that may arise if they meet a mishap in playing a feminine role (1916–1917, p. 318). The female child also reacts by blaming her mother for lack of a penis. Because of her resentment, she gives up the mother as the object of her affection and substitutes the father (Freud, 1940: 193–194). She tries to take her mother's place with the father and begins to hate her mother, for two reasons: from jealousy and from mortification over being denied a penis. The little girl may at first wish to have her father's penis at her disposal, but eventually she wishes to have a baby from him. The wish for a baby thus takes the place of the wish for a penis, or at least has split off from it. The desire for a penis, however, is long lasting. If we ask an analyst, Freud writes, about what experience has shown to be the mental structures least susceptible to influence in his female patients, the answer will be: Her wish for a penis (Freud, 1940: 194).

The idea that females react to their anatomical discoveries by envying boys for possessing a penis has long been controversial, especially among Freud's feminist critics (see "Penis Envy," this volume). The idea that boys react to their observations of a female vagina or hints of the threat of castration by developing a castration complex has been much less disputed, even if this idea is also controversial. Some writers claim that analysts commonly encounter the castration complex in their analytic experience and suggest that the real problem is not to establish its existence, but to account for its all but universal presence in human beings when the threats from which it supposedly derives are far from being always evident (Laplanche and Pontalis, 1973: 57). However, it could reasonably be asked how contemporary analysts, or Freud himself, can know that what they are encountering in their clinical experience really is a castration complex. They cannot decide by asking the patient, for the constituent elements, including castration anxiety, are allegedly unconscious. Nor can they just ask small children about their fear of castration or the presence of other attitudes associated with the complex. Once again, the fear and additional attitudes are supposedly unconscious. Nor can the castration anxiety be directly observed.

Freud and many contemporary analysts would presumably reply that the presence of the castration complex is *inferred* from propositions about the observed behavior of both children and adult patients undergoing psychoanalysis. Still, a persistent critic will ask about the *basis* for that inference. At this point, one approaches

more general epistemological issues of the justification of psychoanalytic interpretations of clinical phenomena (see "Interpretation," this volume). Whatever one concludes about these issues, some have tried to avoid them by founding the castration complex on either anthropological or experimental evidence rather than the data from clinical case studies.

Whiting and Child (1953), for example, studied the antecedents of castration anxiety in seventy-two primitive societies. The antecedents included such items as overall severity of sex training and severity of punishment for disobedience. The authors do not establish empirically, however, that such items really are antecedents of castration anxiety. Without such evidence, the results do not support the existence, let alone the prevalence, of the castration complex.

In doing experimental studies of the castration complex, investigators face the same problem as those who rely on clinical observations: How do they detect the presence of the castration complex if it is unobservable? That problem need not be insuperable, but how is it to be overcome in any particular study? The standard solution has been to rely on projective tests. Friedman (1952), for example, used "castration fables" to measure castration anxiety; others have used the Blacky Test. The problem with such studies is obvious: How does one establish that the projective tests measure what they purport to measure? For arguments that some of these studies provide firm empirical support for at least the existence of castration anxiety, see Kline (1981 [1972]) and Fisher and Greenberg (1977); for dissenting arguments see Erwin (1996, pp. 155–158) and Eysenck and Wilson (1973).

REFERENCES

Erwin, E. (1996). *A Final Accounting: Philosophical and Empirical Issues in Freudian Psychology*. Cambridge, Mass.: MIT Press.

Eysenck, H. J., and Wilson, G. D. (1973). *The Experimental Study of Freudian Theories*. London: Methuen.

Fisher, S., and Greenberg, R. (1977). *The Scientific Credibility of Freud's Theories and Therapy*. New York: Basic Books.

Friedman, S. M. (1952). An empirical study of the castration and Oedipus complexes. *Genetic Psychology Monographs*, 46: 61–130.

Freud, S. (1909). Analysis of a phobia in a five-year old boy. S.E. 10: 55–149.

———. (1916–1917). *Introductory Lectures on Psycho-Analysis*. S.E. 15–16: 9–496.

———. (1940). *An Outline of Psycho-Analysis*. S.E. 23: 144–207.

Kline, P. (1981 [1972]). *Fact and Fantasy in Freudian Theory*, 2d ed. New York: Methuen.

Laplanche, J., and Pontalis, J. B. (1973). *The Language of Psychoanalysis*. Trans. D. Smith. New York: Norton; 1st ed., 1967: Presses Universitaires de France.

Whiting, J., and Child, I. (1953). *Child Training and Personality*. New Haven, Conn.: Yale University Press.

                                        EDWARD ERWIN

Catharsis

Cathartic therapies were widely used in the second half of the nineteenth century by Janet and Delboeuf (Macmillan, 1979); Binet, Bourru, and Burot (Jackson, 1994), Hoek (Van der Hart and Van der Velden, 1987), and others. Janet (1919/1925) employed "treatment by discharge" in which creative canalization of raw emotional energies raised the "psychological tension," or in Freud's terms, ego strength and enhanced personality integration. Fin de siècle conceptualizations such as these, however, were outstripped by those of Freud.

Freud's use of the concept of catharsis was influenced by his uncle Jacob Bernay's views on the Aristotelian idea of "purging" in theatrical tragedy and by the work of Josef Breuer. Drawing upon Breuer's treatment of Anna O (1893–1895), Freud conceptualized catharsis in terms of the emotional release of paralyzing affects associated with pathogenic traumatic memories. The term "catharsis" referred to the discharge of repressed quanta of emotional energy, theorized to be the precipitates of psychological trauma. The discharge was induced by the psychoanalytic technique of abreaction, first under hypnosis, and later by using the concentration technique.

Freud (1906) subsequently lost confidence in the therapeutic value of inducing catharsis. He came to regard it as a mere symptomatic treatment and as an obstacle to the analysis of resistance. To these objections, later Freudians added that catharsis could become a resistance in its own right (Greenson, 1967). Because of symptomatic overdetermination, cathartic treatment proved to be only partially effective, eventually leading to symptomatic recurrence and requiring further catharsis (Ferenczi, 1930). Ultimately it promoted passive dependence (Fenichel, 1945).

Freud subsequently subordinated the induction of catharsis to the promotion of conscious insight. Treatment by affective discharge ultimately gave way to the psychological analysis of resistance in the transference, and working through. But the idea of a modified catharsis continued to find a place in a number of psychodynamic approaches, particularly in the abreactive treatment of shell-shocked combatants in World War I and World War II (Brown, 1920).

Cathartic methods were taken up much more enthusiastically in the post–World War II years in the Human Potential movement in America. This development was spurred by wartime successes in inducing catharsis and by the contribution of émigré analytical psychotherapists to the United States. Most of their therapeutic formulations can be traced back to Reich's (1949) character analysis, in which emotional release is theorized to reverse chronically conditioned emotional inhibitions rather than reversing repression of prior traumas. Reich spoke of the release of "orgone energy" from intrapsychic and societal sexual repression, and of the undoing of what he called "somatic character armor." Other analysts, such as Perls (1951) and Moreno (1959), sought therapeutic liberation from unfinished emotional business through various forms of role play. Critics regarded these therapies as mere "ventilationist" approaches (Berkowitz, 1974), which were less emotionally liberating than their advocates claimed. More ominously, the use of such techniques risked the regressive destruction of necessary defenses (Lowy, 1970).

Nichols and Zax's (1977) watershed survey of the role of catharsis in psychotherapy covered accounts of catharsis in, among others, psychodynamic, behavioral implosion and Rogerian therapies, but cited only one empirical scientific study of catharsis (Nichols, 1974), and this study found only an equivocal curative effect. Further, when practiced alone, the inducement of catharsis risked stasis rather than emotional growth. Nichols and Zax (1977) nevertheless concluded that cathartic therapy had both central and adjunctive applications, but to be effective such therapy must release both cognitive and emotional components of repressed experience. Their most interesting conclusion, however, was that the inducement of catharsis is indicated for recent—rather than remote—emotional or traumatic distress.

Recently, cathartic methods have been recommended for the treatment of posttraumatic stress disorder (DSM-IV, 1994), generating some conceptual confusion. The conceptual issues, however, have been clarified by Van der Hart and Brown (1992). In essence, catharsis is one of three integral therapeutic processes: remembering, emotional release, and reintegration. The final treatment path is one of emphasis: humanistic therapies such as primal scream (Janov, 1970) emphasize emotional catharsis, while modern analytically oriented therapies and neo-Janetian approaches (Van der Hart, 1993) favor much more controlled cathartic release. The former combine remembering and controlled catharsis with the induction of insight, and the latter, neo-Janetian approaches, with memory and personality reintegration.

Some therapists warn of the risks associated with promotion of unrestrained reexperiencing of trauma emotions. Thus Silove (1992) writes of the potential for triple retraumatization: from the trauma itself, from symptomatic reexperiencing, and from therapeutic recovery. Hence most contemporary approaches encourage controlled emotional release rather than massive catharsis.

REFERENCES

Berkowitz, L. (1974). The case for bottling up rage. *Psychology Today,* 7:24–31.

Bibring, E. (1954). Psychoanalysis and the dynamic psychotherapies. *Journal of the American Psychoanalytic Association,* 2: 745–770.

Breuer, J. and Freud, S. (1893–1895). *Studies on Hysteria.* S.E. 2: 19–305.

Brown, W. (1920). The revival of emotional memories and its therapeutic value. *British Journal of Medical Psychology,* 1: 16–19.

DSM-IV (1994). *Diagnostic and Statistical Manual of Mental Disorders.* 4th ed., Washington D.C.: American Psychiatric Association.

Fenichel, O. (1945). *The Psychoanalytic Theory of Neurosis.* New York: Norton.

Ferenczi, S. (1930). The principal of relaxation and neocatharsis. *International Journal of Psychoanalysis,* 11: 428–443.

Freud, S. (1906). On psychotherapy. S.E. 7: 257–268.

Greenson, R. R. (1967). *The Technique and Practice of Psychoanalysis.* New York: International Universities Press.

Jackson, S. (1994). Catharsis and abreaction. *The History of Psychological Healing.* Psychiatric Clinics of North America, 3: 471–491.

Janet, P. (1919). *Les Médications Psychologiques.* Paris: Alcan. English Edition: *Psychological Healing.* (1925) E. Paul and C. Paul (translators). New York: Macmillan.

Janov, A. (1970). The primal scream. *Primal therapy: The Cure for Neurosis.* New York: Putnam.

Kernberg, O. (1984). *Severe Personality Disorders: Psychotherapeutic Strategies.* New Haven, Conn.: Yale University Press.

Lowy, F. H. (1970). The abuse of abreaction: An unhappy legacy of Freud's cathartic method. *Canadian Psychiatric Association Journal,* 15: 557–565.

Macmillan, M. (1979). Delboeuf and Janet as influences in Freud's treatment of Emmy Von N. *Journal of the History of the Behavioral Sciences,* 15: 299–309.

———. (1990). Freud and Janet on organic and hysterical paralyses: A mystery solved? *International Review of Psychoanalysis,* 17: 189–203.

Moreno, J. L. (1959). Psychodrama. In S. Arieti (ed.). *American Handbook of Psychiatry,* 2. New York: Basic Books, pp. 1375–1396.

Nichols, M. P. (1974). Outcome of brief cathartic psychotherapy. *Journal of Consulting and Clinical Psychology,* 42: 403–410.

Nichols, M. P., and Zax, M. (1977). *Catharsis in Psychotherapy.* New York: Gardner Press.

Perls, F., Hefferline, R. E., and Goodman, P. (1951). *Gestalt Therapy: Excitement and Growth in the Human Personality.* New York: Dell.

Reich, W. (1949). *Character Analysis.* New York: Orgone Institute Press.

Scheff, T. (1980). *Catharsis in Healing, Ritual and Drama.* Berkeley: University of California Press.

Silove, D. (1992). Psychotherapy and trauma. *Current Opinion in Psychiatry,* 5: 370–374.

Simmel, E. (1944). War neurosis. In S. Lorand (ed.). *Psychoanalysis Today.* New York: International Universities Press, pp. 227–248

Van der Hart, O., and Van der Velden, K. (1987). The hypnotherapy of Andries Hoek: Uncovering hypnotherapy before Janet, Breuer, and Freud. *American Journal of Clinical Hypnosis,* 29: 264–271.

Van der Hart, O. and Brown, P. (1992). Abreaction reevaluated. *Dissociation,* 5: 127–140.

Van der Hart, O., Steele, K., Boon, S., and Brown, P. (1993). The treatment of traumatic memories: Synthesis, realization, and integration. *Dissociation,* 6, 162–180.

Volkan, V. (1975). Regrief therapy. In B. Schoenberg et al. (eds.), *Bereavement: Its Psychosocial Aspects.* New York: Columbia University Press.

PAUL BROWN

Cathartic Method See CATHARSIS.

Cathexis

The term "cathexis" has been used by Freud and later analysts to express multiple concepts including the following: (especially) mental energy, a quantity of mental energy, charging with mental energy, emotional investment, and the focusing of interest.

The confusion surrounding the use of the term arises partly from Freud's usage, partly from the translation given by James Strachey, and partly from the variegated uses of later analysts.

Strachey's Translation

James Strachey, the best known of the many translators of Freud's works into English, accepted the authority of Ernest Jones (1953), who contended that psychoanalytic theory was, for the most part, unique. Although Jones was aware that Freud had used some previously known organizing metaphors at critical points, he believed that Freud's ideas had hardly been influenced by nineteenth-century neuroscience or philosophy (a view widely rejected today). Although Freud's sources remain unsettled, some version of his idea of psychological energy can be found in the works of his teachers and contemporaries as they try to picture a working model of the mind (Amacher, 1965).

Besides being influenced by Jones, Strachey also believed Freud's (1905) occasional claim that his "discoveries" were based altogether on his own observations. When translating Freud into English, Strachey thought that inventing some new technical terms to express psychoanalytic ideas might clarify differences between them and similar ideas from common sense psychology and from nonpsychoanalytic theories. A significant example is Strachey's coining of the term "cathexis."

Throughout his career, Freud used the concepts of "psychic energy" and "emotional investment," but used a single word to express both ideas: the German word *Besetzung*, a word he also used to express other ideas.

Strachey decided that the "right" (or, at least most useful) translation of *Betsetzung* was *cathexis*, a term he invented. He claimed to have based it on a classical Greek word *catechein*, which he said meant "to occupy." The difficulty, however, is that Freud used *Betsetzung* in multiple senses; so, "cathexis," rather than expressing a single, technical idea, took on all of the ambiguities of Freud's usage.

Strachey felt that the concepts Freud denoted by *Besetzungen* were widely misunderstood by Americans who:

> apparently had even less notion of the exact meaning of the word than I have myself. But they seemed to think that if they could be told the "right" translation the meaning would automatically be conveyed to them. I believe that if the "right" translation can be fixed upon as a word with no ostensible meaning at all, people may be induced to try and discover what the meaning really is. (Strachey in Ornston, 1985: 394).

Freud's Usage

Freud expressed unhappiness with Strachey's introduction of the term "cathexis" (Strachey, 1962) and generally continued to use instead the German term *Besetzung* even after the former term was introduced by Strachey in 1922 (an exception is Freud's use of "cathexis" in the original manuscript for his *Encyclopedia Britannica* article [1926, p. 266]).

The German word *Besetzung* is both ambiguous and protean. Used bluntly and by itself, its meaning is close to that of the English words "setting" or "putting." What Freud meant in using this term is generally clear enough in German; his intended sense can usually be determined by paying close attention to the context—in particular to his analogies or the specific problem he is addressing.

In one of his first papers about psychoanalysis, Freud (1894) said that among the psychic functions something can be distinguished that has all the qualities of a quantity although we have no way to measure it. This something may be enlarged, reduced, shifted, or discharged and spreads itself over the memory traces of ideas somewhat like the way an electrical charge spreads itself over the surface of the body. Although Freud did not use the term *Besetzung* to refer to this "something," Strachey took Freud's comment to be a definition of "cathexis."

In 1895, Freud extended and expanded his metaphor as he tried to put together an intricate psychoneurology of his own. He had hoped that this kind of fluid imagery about "excitation," or "activation," or "intensity" flowing through, occupying, and holding patterns of neurons might cut through the Gordian knot of neuropsychology—that is, explain the way mind interacts with matter. He postulated many distinct kinds of quantitative "energy" or "interest" that might mobilize and regulate the material of the mind. But his primary analogy was to electricity. When he realized that his model could not work, he repudiated these unfinished and untitled notes as some kind of "madness" (*Wahnwitz*). He was embarrassed when they turned up at the end of his life: he wanted them destroyed. Instead, his editors published the manuscript, calling it "The Project for a Scientific Psychology." Then "The Project" was used as a Rosetta stone in translating more obscure passages in Freud's later work. The value of "The Project" remains controversial.

Freud accumulated an untidy plethora of drives, energies, forces, conflicting intensities, and distinct kinds of activation, as well as "drive energies," "energy sources," "surges of need," "emerging excitations," "repressing interests," and many more such concepts. The referent of each was theorized to be a purposeful mental activity. Each was qualitatively different from all the others. Freud's translators' attempts to simplify by combining clusters of Freud's variations into single technical expressions such as "mobile cathexes" will not resolve the confusion afflicting any and every reader. For example, Freud used his own distinction between "bound" and "free" energy (or "cathexis") to elucidate at least a dozen different pairs of ideas (Holt, 1962). Some say these "economic" ideas are clinically useful, but many contemporary analysts disagree.

In common and everyday German usage, *Besetzung* is often used to designate something analogous to a military maneuver, such as occupying a post, or "taking over" or "holding" a position against attack. For decades, Freud's *Besetzung* was conventionally and correctly translated in this way—among others. In English, "occupation" resonates handily with "preoccupation." This may have become the most frequent translation of *Besetzung* because Freud's designated and prolific translator, Abraham Brill, preferred the idea of occupation, as did G. Stanley Hall. Other translations included "investing," "interest," "intensity," "excitation," "drive energies," "surges or quanta of energy," "nervous energy," and many more.

Freud translated his lectures into English for an American audience. His renderings of the various ideas that others translated by use of the single word "cathexis" were anything but technical. Some examples may help to understand what he had in mind and may be usefully compared to the translations given in *The Standard Edition*:

(1) Freud translates his German phrase *eines mit Affekt besetzten seelischen* as "a mental process which is emotionally colored . . ."

The *Standard Edition* has this as "an emotionally cathected mental process."

(2) *eine Gruppe von zusammengehoerigen, mit Affekt besetzten Vorstellungselementen* is translated by Freud as "a group of ideas which belong together and have a common emotive tone."

The *Standard Edition* puts this as "a group of interdependent ideational elements cathected with affect" (Ornston, 1992: 14–15).

In contrast to Strachey's views, (1) Freud never gave a definition of *Besetzung*; (2) he generally avoided the use of the technical term "cathexis"; and (3) he never said that this notion was fundamental, let alone "the most fundamental of his concepts" (Strachey, 1962). Freud also never published any direct discussion of his economics of nerve force (Laplanche and Pontalis, 1967; Holder, 1970).

On the other hand, Freud never gave up his analogy of a vague and immeasurable psychological "excitation," "activation," "force," or "stirring of a drive"—or some such quasi-quantitative conception as one way of portraying, if not explaining, unconscious life. He may not have understood that in mental life quantitative accounts are generally descriptive without being explanatory, can never describe more than rough estimates and often deflect attention from genuinely explanatory qualitative accounts. As Gill (1977, p. 594) notes: "Every time we accept or offer an explanation in terms of a shift in intensities, we are failing to see change in a qualitative pattern that would be a more specific and illuminating explanation."

In sum, there is no consensus among psychoanalysts about what "cathexis" means beyond the ancient and ambiguous, but at least candid, analogy of "mental energy."

REFERENCES

Amacher, P. (1965) Freud's neurological education and its influence on psychoanalytic theory. *Psychological Issues*, 4. Monograph 16. New York: International Universities Press.

Freud, S. (1894). The Neuro-psychoses of Defense. S.E. 3: 45–61.

———. (1905). *Fragment of an Analysis of a Case of Hysteria.* S.E. 7: 7–122.

———. (1916–1917). *Introductory Lectures on Psycho-Analysis.* S.E. 15–16: 9–496.

———. (1940). *An Outline of Psycho-analysis.* S.E. 23: 144–207.

Gill, M. (1977). Psychic Energy Reconsidered. *Journal of the American Psychoanalytical Association*, 25: 581–597.

Holder, A. (1970) Basic psychoanalytic concepts on metapsychology. In H. Nagera (ed.). *Conflicts, Anxiety, and Other Subjects.* The Hampstead Clinic Psychoanalytic Library, 4. London: H. Karnac Ltd.

Holt, R. (1962). A critical examination of Freud's concept of bound versus free cathexis. *Journal of the American Psychoanalytical Association*, 10: 474–525.

Jones, E. (1953). *The Life and Work of Sigmund Freud*, vol. 1. New York: Basic Books.

Laplanche, J., and Pontalis, J. B. (1973). *The Language of Psychoanalysis.* Translated by D. Nicholson-Smith. New York: Norton.

Ornston, D. G. (1985). The invention of "cathexis" and Strachey's strategy. *International Review of Psychoanalysis*, 12: 391–399.

———. (1992). *Translating Freud.* New Haven, Conn.: Yale University Press, 1992.

C

Strachey, J. (1962). *Editor's Appendix: The Emergence of Freud's Most Fundamental Hypotheses*. S.E. 3: 62–68

———. (1966). *Editor's General Preface, Dedication, and Notes on Some Technical Terms; Editor's Introduction, and Editor's Note*. SE 1: xiii–xxvi; 175–176; 283–293.

DARIUS ORNSTON

Character

"Character" refers in the broadest sense to those enduring traits, dispositions, attitudes, and behaviors that are typical of an individual. The concept of character received its first serious psychoanalytic consideration in Freud's classic essay "Character and Anal Erotism" (1908). Character traits, according to Freud's theory, are compromise formations resulting from the interplay of drives, defenses, the superego, and reality factors.

Character formation results from the interaction of many variables. Among the most important ones are constitutional factors that interact with the early instinctual drives. Defenses, too, play a role in determining the final shape of one's character. The process of character formation is also very dependent on the mechanism of identification. Initially, the child identifies with idealized images of the parents but later substitutes a more realistic assessment of the parent's qualities and attributes.

This change is in line with Freud's idea that "the character of the ego is a precipitate of abandoned object-cathexes and contains the history of those object choices" (Freud, 1917, p. 29).

From a developmental point of view, character does not emerge in its final form until after adolescence, although it is first solidified after the child passes through the Oedipal phase. The formation of character is a normal developmental step. Speaking of "character" implies by itself neither normality nor pathology, even though psychoanalysis is much more concerned with pathologic traits than with fundamentally adaptive character traits such as honesty, sense of humor, loyalty to one's friends, or reliability. The grouping of character traits into larger units constitutes the character "organization" (Baudry, 1989).

An individual does not generally complain about the nature of his or her character. Partly for this reason, character traits are said to be ego-syntonic in contrast to symptoms such as phobias or obsessions, which are ego alien. However, when an individual's character traits are sufficiently rigid and maladaptive, his or her overall functioning may be markedly impaired so as to constitute a character disorder. The psychoanalytic classification of character disorders is in a state of disarray. The classification is loosely based on a number of different organizing features such as neurosis (phobic, obsessional, or hysterical character), affective states (depressive character), or psychotic-like states (schizoid character). There are, in addition, a number of other conditions that do not fit in readily in any clear-cut schema. One example is "character neurosis," a phrase coined by Robert Waelder to refer to a character disorder that has a similar structure and function as a neurosis it has replaced.

Character problems were accorded their due in the theory of technique by Freud, Abraham, and most of all by Wilhelm Reich. The latter coined the term "character armor" to call attention to the narcissistic defensive function of character. Reich developed a technique of actively and aggressively tackling character defenses, but that technique has been largely discredited.

With the development of ego psychology, the renewed interest in the structuring effect of unconscious fantasy, and the importance of object relations, the concept of character has regained some of its popularity. In the light of these recent developments, it is possible to see character traits as the result of the influence of a number of key unconscious fantasies. The uncovering and working through of such fantasies is an important therapeutic task of analysis. Character can also be understood as resulting from the enactment of some crucial object relations scenarios that the individual replays time and time again. As many, if not most, of the patients now seen by analysts suffer from disorders of character, dealing with character in the analytic situation, particularly in the transference, has become particularly important.

The analysis of a patient's character is a complicated endeavor with few rules to decide when and how traits are to be confronted and analyzed. One generally accepted principle is that a trait cannot be successfully dealt with unless it is involved in some current conflictual situation. By its very nature, character tends to be viewed in moral terms; that is, most traits are seen as desirable or good, or undesirable and bad. Thinking of character traits in these terms raises a problem in clinical work. When analysts bring a particular trait to the patient's attention, most patients react as though their character is being criticized.

REFERENCES

Baudry, F. (1989). Character, character type and character organization. *Journal of the American Analytic Association* 37: 655–686.

Freud, S. (1908). *Character and Anal Erotism*. S.E. 9: 167–175.

———. (1917). *The Ego and the Id*. S.E.: 19–29.

FRANCIS D. BAUDRY

Character Neurosis

Freud said little about character neuroses, which he termed "character disorders." In the *New Introductory Lectures on Psycho-Analysis* (1933), Freud talks briefly about the treatment of character problems, but without providing any detailed analysis. After reiterating that the application of psychoanalysis is limited to the transference neuroses "phobias, hysteria, obsessional neurosis" (p. 155), he adds: "and further, abnormalities of character which have been developed in place of these illnesses" (p. 155).

Despite the paucity of Freud's writings on the subject, the distinction between neurotic symptom and character neurosis became important since it led to increased theoretical understanding of the neuroses and to improvements in therapeutic technique. Thus the discovery and recognition that psychic conflict may manifest itself via defensive character traits, or behavior patterns, or even as a pathological organization of the total personality structure, rather than merely by neurotic symptoms, widened the scope of psychoanalytic investigation. The fact that in character neurosis the pathology is "ego-syntonic" (i.e., in conformity with the ego) and that there are no "dystonic" (i.e., ego-alien) symptoms raised new questions as to the correct approach in dealing with resistance. A patient coming to psychoanalysis who was suffering from neurotic symptoms typically sought relief and to that extent, at least consciously, was eager for treatment. In most cases, the reverse was true for the character neurotic who had a narcissistic investment in his or her ego-syntonic traits. Though these traits were perceived by the analyst as neurotic, they were valued by the patient. Character-neurotic patients did not recognize that their modes of behavior led to recurrent and often permanent difficulties in their object relations and, consequently, generally did not seek treatment for them.

During the 1920s, analysts were occupied with the exploration of character, its origins, and development and especially with the impact of character on the analytic process. Finding appropriate methods of dealing with resistance in the treatment of the character neurotic posed a great challenge and led to theoretical differences and conflicts among analysts.

Wilhelm Reich (1949 [1933]) was foremost in the formulation of a theory and method of treatment for patients resistant to classical analysis. He envisioned the patient's character as an "armor" consisting of defensive attitudes that the patient utilized irrespective of verbalized content, and that were typical for the patient's object relations. According to Reich's findings, psychic predispositions were shaped by environmental forces. He maintained that "character armor" is the sum total of modes of reaction specific to a given personality. On the deepest level, Reich held, character formation was motivated by the unconscious anxiety caused by wishes for gratification of forbidden impulses. However, Reich recognized that though character is primarily a defensive reaction to keep anxiety unconscious, it also provides outlets for disguised instinctual gratification.

Reich (1949 [1933]) was the first to distinguish between transference resistance and character resistance. He also was the first to formulate a method for resistance analysis that he considered essential for the treatment of character neurosis. Since, according to Reich, character resistance did not manifest itself in the content of the material but only in the formal aspects of behavior, it is the latter that had to be the focus of the analytic thrust. Thus the patient's character resistance always remained the same, irrespective of the material against which it was directed. According to Reich, the consistent analysis of character resistance "provides an infallible and immediate avenue of approach to the central infantile conflict" (p. 93). He maintained that the negative transference is present in character neurotics from the beginning and has to be analyzed relentlessly. He considered an initial positive transference as merely a cover-up.

Reich stressed that in the process of analysis patients have to discover:

1. that they unconsciously defends themselves against something they consider dangerous;
2. what means they use for the purpose of defense;
3. against what this defense is directed.

Though Reich recognized that his method of analysis could be extremely painful to the patient and could even lead to a temporary "break down," he insisted that only a consistent, systematic, and historic approach would attain the desired analytic result.

Reich's method of character analysis evoked strong opposition among many analysts. One of these critics was Nunberg, 1928; another was Fenichel (1945, pp. 463–540), whose formulations of psychoanalytic characterology incorporate Freud's (1908; 1916; 1931) views and subsequent findings. Fenichel distinguished between sublimatory character traits present in healthy development and reactive character traits that are defensive and employ countercathexis to contain and repress forbidden instinctual forces.

In character neurosis, defensive character traits that are rigid and stereotyped predominate over sublimatory ones, leading to attitudes of avoidance (phobic reactions) and/or opposition (reaction formations). Flexible adaptability is lost. When reaction formation is used for the resolution of psychic conflict, the return of the repressed is precluded and therefore the need for subsequent secondary repression is avoided. Reaction formation is a "once and for all solution" that leads to definite personality changes. In such cases, the character appears as an essentially defensive formation designed to protect the individual against instinctual threat and outer danger (Fenichel, 1945).

Fenichel (1953 [1935]) formulated principles of technique for the treatment of character neurosis based on ego psychology. He stressed the significance of an optimal balance between interpretation of defense and interpretation of content. However, Fenichel did incorporate into his technique Reich's insistence that interpretation of defense always precedes interpretation of content. Fenichel recommended that the patient be helped to recognize that she is defensively resistive, how she does it, why she does it, and against which unconscious fantasies and/or conflicts the defense is directed. Fenichel (1945) maintained that in the treatment of character neurosis a "mobilization of conflicts" must take place that, when successful, changes the "character neurosis into a symptom neurosis, and character resistances into transference resistances" (p. 538).

To achieve these results is a difficult process. Schafer (1979) states that the self-confirming ego syntonicity present in character neurosis poses a great obstacle to treatment. Only when inconsistencies and experiential diversity can be pointed out to the patient is it possible to demonstrate contradictions and stimulate curiosity, which is necessary for undermining the pervasive characterological ego syntonicity. The exploration of contradictions (Kernberg, 1980, 1984; Schafer, 1982, 1983) is essential in making the patient aware of ego-dystonic elements, a process that, by undermining the pervasive ego syntonicity, leads to a disturbance in the neurotic equilibrium. Such changes are essential for making the patient accessible to analytic treatment.

Regardless of whether the analytic approach is confrontational (Kernberg, 1984) or tactful, nonadversarial, and even affirmative in some respects (Lax, 1988: 283–292; Schafer, 1982: 91–99), the analytic attention to incongruities and inconsistencies is experienced by the patient as an attack on his narcissistically invested character patterns that form his personality. It therefore is not surprising that the analytic exploration of character traits arouses the patient's anger and negative transference that she needs to express. The analyst's capacity to deal with this anger by analyzing his countertransference and own characterologic tendencies is essential to avoid entering into a power struggle with the patient. Persistence with the analytic investigation of the patient's contradictory wishes that lead to incongruous behavior patterns and nonadaptive, conflicted object relations increases the patient's awareness of dystonicity and thus facilitates the exploration of her unconscious conflicts.

The current position presented by Cooper (Panel, 1982) and adhered to by most analysts no longer considers the distinction between symptom analysis and character analysis as useful since from the dynamic, structural, genetic, and developmental vantage points, analysis of character is required in the psychoanalytic treatment of any type of neurosis. The concept of psychic structure tends to transcend the distinction between neurosis with symptoms and asymptomatic neurosis. Current emphasis is on the way impulse and defense are interactively organized in dealing with unconscious psychic conflict.

Though the outlook for a successful analysis of character that eventuates in meaningful structural change is guarded, such therapeutic change is possible. However, the attainment of this goal is long, arduous, and painful. Though most analysts agree that core character patterns do not change as a result of treatment, analysis that includes the exploration of psychic structures does contribute to modifications. Consequently, there is some alteration in, or resolution of, psychic conflict. When successful, analysis of character neurosis leads to greater flexibility and availability of energy for love and work.

REFERENCES

Bergmann, M. D., and Hartman, F. R. (1976). *The Evolution of Psychoanalytic Technique.* New York: Basic Books.

Fenichel, O. (1941). *Problems of Psychoanalytic Technique.* New York. *Psychoanalytic Quarterly.*

———. (1945). Character disorders. In O. Fenichel (author). *The Psychoanalytic Theory of Neurosis.* New York: Norton, pp. 463–540.

Freud, S. (1908). *Character and Anal Eroticism.* S.E. 9: 167–176.

———. (1916). *Some Character Types Met With in Psychoanalytic Work.* S.E. 14: 309–335.

———. (1923). *The Ego and the Id.* S.E. 19: 19–27.

———. (1926). *Inhibitions, Symptoms and Anxiety.* S.E. 20: 87–156.

———. (1931). *Libidinal Types.* S.E. 21: 215–222.

———. (1933). *New Introductory Lectures on Psycho-Analysis.* S.E. 22: 57–80.

Kernberg, O. F. (1980). *Internal World and External Reality.* New York: Jason Aronson.

———. (1984). *Severe Personality Disorders and Psychotherapeutic Strategies.* New Haven, Conn.: Yale University Press.

Lax, R. F. (1975). Some comments on the narcissistic aspects of self-righteousness: Defensive and structural considerations. *International Journal of Psychoanalysis,* 56: 283–292.

———. (1989). Comments on the narcissistic investment in pathological character traits and the narcissistic depression: Some implications for treatment. *International Journal of Psychoanalysis,* 70: 81–90.

Panel (1982). Problems of technique in character analysis. Discussion by A. M. Cooper. *Bulletin of the Association Psychoanalytic Medicine,* 21, no. 3: 110–118.

Reich, W. (1927). On the technique of interpretation and of resistance analysis. Chapt. 3 in W. Reich (author). *Character Analysis,* 3d enl. ed., pp. 20–38. Trans. P. Wolfe. New York: Orgone Institute Press, 1949. Reprint *Internationale Zeitschritt für Psychoanlyse.*

———. (1949 [1933]). *Character Analysis,* 3d enl. ed., Trans. P. Wolfe. New York: Orgone Institute Press.

Schafer, R. (1979). Character, ego-syntonicity, and character change. *Journal of the American Psychoanalytic Association,* 27: 867–890.

———. (1982). Problems of technique in character analysis. *Bulletin of the Association of Psychoanalytic Medicine,* 22: 91–99.

———. (1983). *The Analytic Attitude.* New York: Basic Books.

Sterba, R. R. (1953). Clinical and therapeutic aspects of character resistance. *Psychoanalytic Quarterly,* 22: 1–20.

RUTH F. LAX

Charcot, Jean-Martin (1825–1893)

Jean-Martin Charcot was born in Paris in 1825, the son of a carriage builder and decorator. Although it may not be true that he hesitated between a career as artist or physician, his medical work made much use of his artistic talents and interests. He entered medical school in 1843, serving internships in three of the main Paris Hospitals (Pitié, Charité, and Salpêtrière) before graduating in 1853. He published and lectured on a wide range of conditions but held no hospital post proper until 1852, when he transferred as Chéf de Clinique to the Salpêtrière as a junior consultant. In 1862 he was appointed Médicin de la Salpêtrière as chief of its medical services where, after conducting careful classificatory medical examinations with Claude Bernard Vulpain on the approximately five thousand mainly indigent patients there, he began investigating neurological diseases with Vulpain and Duchenne de Boulogne. He became Professor of Pathological Anatomy in 1872 and in 1882 was appointed to a Chair of Diseases of the Nervous System. It can almost be said that that appointment founded neurology as a medical specialty.

Charcot achieved an enormous national and international reputation. He founded or was an editorial adviser on a large number of the most important French medical journals, and was elected to the Académie Impériale de Médicine, the Académie des Sciences as well as numerous international medical societies, and his informal Tuesday lectures became important public events. Many of his patients were distinguished: Writers included Alphonse Daudet, Ivan Turgenev, and (possibly) Guy de Maupassant, and rulers and aristocrats included the queen of Spain, the emperor of Brazil, and the grand dukes Nicholas and Constantine of Russia. However, as a politically quiet republican he gave no preference to patients with high status. Charcot was named Commandeur, Légion d'Honneur, in 1892. Until that year he was active in French medical and artistic life (his *salons* were famous) but ill health, signaled by an attack of angina early in 1891, led to his death from pulmonary edema on August 16, 1893.

Charcot based his work on what he called the clinico-anatomical method. It required that what was revealed by the close analysis of symptoms be related to demonstrable lesions of the skeleto-muscular or nervous systems. He established the histopathology of many diseases, notably amyotrophic lateral sclerosis, tabes dorsalis and tabetic arthropathy, multiple sclerosis, which he differentiated from Parkinson's disease, and atrophic paralysis of childhood (now acute poliomyelitis). An early convert to the doctrine of cerebral localization, he conducted much valuable clinical work on it, taking a

C

position not unlike that of Hughlings Jackson, and not hesitating to disagree with authorities such as the great Paul Broca himself.

Charcot was a prodigious worker who wrote much, and what he wrote was and is much read. His completed works, comprising nine substantial volumes (and by no means complete), were published in five editions and translated, in whole or in part, into six languages. The New Sydenham Society (London) published a five-volume uniform edition of his clinical lectures, many of which have been reprinted, and other translations of them and of other works have been made. English reprints of all or some of these works appeared as recently as 1985 and 1991, and the records of his less formal Tuesday lectures, made by his students and published separately, were published in English in 1987. He promoted Désiré-Magloire Bourneville and Paul Regnard's use of photography at the Salpêtrière, and made detailed studies with Paul Richer of the appearance of the phenomena of physical and hysterical illnesses in art, the latter together with his works on possession and faith-cures, reflecting his muted anticlerical sentiments.

Late in his neurological career Charcot began the investigation of hysteria (1870) and hypnosis (1878), conditions that then had not much more than marginal medical status. His enormous reputation made hysteria and hypnosis legitimate areas of scientific investigation. He took his hysterical patients and hypnotized subjects seriously, bringing his clinico-anatomical method to bear on them in the hope of relating their phenomena to alterations in the nervous system. It is this aspect of his work that is most relevant to psychoanalysis.

Hysteria

In Charcot's day the term "hysteria" referred to a variety of conditions that resembled neurological disorders but in which pathological changes could not be demonstrated in the nervous system. Thus, one patient might be unable to see without there being anything wrong with the retina or visual pathways; another unable to walk with nothing wrong with the nerve supply to the muscles of the legs, and so on. Some symptoms were sensory, such as heightened or lost sensation (paraesthesias or anaesthesias); others were motor, among them paralyses, making it impossible for the patient to move a limb, contractures, which kept a hand or foot permanently contracted, and convulsions; and others were disturbances of consciousness and memory, including

hallucinations, mild *absences*, or complete losses of memory. The major alterations of personality known as multiple personality were included among the latter.

Hysterical symptoms were most often components of what Charcot called "major hysteria" a typical attack of which proceeded through four successive stages: the epileptoid or convulsive stage; the stage of clownism or major movements; *Attitudes passionelles* [hallucinatory stage]; and *decline terminal* [terminal confusion].

Frequently signaled by some unusual sensation or aura, such as a constriction in the throat, a throbbing in the temple, or a ringing in the ears, the attack would proceed with the tongue, mouth, and head being drawn to one side and the patient becoming unconscious. Convulsions proper began with the arms extending in a continuous or tonic contraction and the whole body turning to the side until it lay there completely. Clonic convulsions then replaced the tonic spasm and a momentary stage of complete relaxation followed the first stage. Large (major) movements of the body then began in which the bodily positions and the face often expressed emotions of exaltation, terror, or grief. The stage frequently ended with a convulsive arching of the back, the so-called *arc de circle* (the second stage). The patient then became delirious and had frightening hallucinations that seemed to be related to real events in the patient's past (third stage). The attack was terminated when the patient fell into a kind of sleep from which he or she woke confused and not knowing what had taken place (fourth stage).

Charcot differentiated "traumatic hysteria," in which the symptoms developed after the patient experienced a trauma. Generally the symptoms were alterations of function, like paralyses, contractures, and anaesthesias, or the sensory losses, rather than the more florid symptoms of major hysteria. Thus one of Charcot's patients had been knocked over by a horse-drawn van and fell, striking the back of his head on the roadside. After being unconscious for some days he woke complaining he could feel nothing in his legs and that the back of his head was hypersensitive. He frequently dreamed that the wheels of the van passed over his legs, and would call out and wake in a fright. In fact the van had not touched him and could not have been responsible for the loss of sensation. Nor was the loss of consciousness or the hyperaesthesia consistent with the injury to his head. Sigmund Freud and Josef Breuer adopted Charcot's traumatic hysteria as the model for all hysteria.

Differentiating Hysterical from Organic Symptoms

In one sense hysterical symptoms were readily distinguishable from their organically based counterparts. For example, the boundaries in hysterical anaesthesias did not match the pattern of innervation caused by nerve injury. Similarly the hysterical aphasias were usually less complete than the organic, were not accompanied by such signs of organic damage as those associated with cerebro-vascular accidents or strokes, and related functions like writing or second language use were not affected. Hysterical convulsions were not explicable by a neural discharge from some particular part of the brain.

Nevertheless, hysterics did not seem to produce their symptoms intentionally. Thus, Charcot's experiments seemed to show that when force was applied to an hysterical contracture of the thumb, the patient's breathing showed none of the signs of exertion typical of normal subjects. If hysterical symptoms did not seem to be intentional simulations of organic disorders what sort of nervous system lesion caused them? Clearly they had to be different from those known to cause organic symptoms but because the symptoms seemed so regular, law-like, and physiological, Charcot could attribute only a physiological basis to them. He called these lesions "dynamic" or "functional" but was never able to specify their nature.

Hypnosis

The word "hypnosis" seems to have been first used in France early in the nineteenth century, although the phenomenon itself had been known since ancient times. Hypnosis typically causes the hypnotized subject to behave toward things that have been suggested to him or her as if they were real. For example, a subject really looking at a piece of white card may report seeing a red after-image when the card is removed if it has been suggested that the white card is green. Similarly, a subject will neither report nor show signs of pain after a suggestion that no pain will be felt when an ordinarily painful electrical stimulus is applied.

Charcot's believed that there was a type of hypnosis, which he called "major" hypnosis, which consisted of three fundamental states. It was brought about or induced by prolonged visual fixation of an object. Some subjects then passed into a state that Charcot called *catalepsy* in which the limbs tended to remain for long periods in the positions the experimenter placed them.

Cataleptic subjects entered the state of *lethargy* when they closed their eyes. Muscles became flaccid, certain reflexes were altered, the pupils were contracted, and mechanical pressure on the nerves produced contractures of the kind caused by their electrical stimulation. In turn, pressure or light friction on the scalp during lethargy caused *artificial somnambulism*: The subject appeared to be asleep, the limbs resisted being moved, and sensory functions like hearing or touch were enhanced.

Charcot was convinced that each state was produced lawfully. First, all his hypnotic subjects passed into and through each state in almost exactly the same way. For example, lethargic subjects passed into artificial somnambulism with pressure on the top of the head. Second, his subjects showed essentially the same changes in nervous and muscular functioning. Thus, reflex changes in lethargy did not vary, or varied only slightly, among subjects. Third, what Charcot called changes in "neuro-muscular excitability" did not vary among subjects. All the changes or alterations in hypnosis seemed to be governed by physiological laws.

Charcot rejected the notions that hypnotic phenomena were due simply to the subject's increased suggestibility or that they were produced by unconscious suggestions from him. That could not explain the law-like nature of hypnosis. Were suggestion at work, each investigator would make slightly different suggestions and the phenomena would vary. Charcot made essentially the same points about hysteria. Its symptoms could not be produced by deliberate deception and were based on physiological alterations. Both hysteria and hypnosis obviously a physiological basis but Charcot could not specify exactly what it was.

"Realization" in Hysteria and Hypnosis

Charcot produced symptoms in hypnosis by "direct" and "indirect" suggestion that were the same as the hysterical. Thus, he would suggest directly to the subject that a function had been lost ("You no longer have any sensation/movement in your arm/leg" or "You can no longer see/hear"). Charcot gave "indirect" suggestions by suddenly striking his hypnotized subjects by, for example, hitting them sharply on the shoulder, and a short time later the arm would become anaesthetic or paralyzed. However produced, these experimental symptoms were absolute as well as restricted and the anaesthetic areas had the same well-marked boundaries as hysterical. None corresponded to anatomy or physiology.

Charcot began his explanation of paralyses with the then commonly accepted theory of ideo-motor action. According to it, in any action, like throwing a ball, the thrower had to have the idea of throwing in mind beforehand. Any movement was a "realization" of the idea of the movement in mind just before it was executed. Hypnosis was a state of "annihilation of the ego" in which the process normally transforming ideas into movement escaped the control of the conscious ego. The directly suggested idea of not being able to move had simply been transformed into a reality, or "realized," as a lack of movement. Similarly with the indirect suggestions: a blow to the shoulder necessarily called up sensations of a momentary numbness and a slight feeling of loss of movement and ideas of anaesthesia and paralysis. Ideas so suggested were also transformed into real symptoms. Charcot generalized this explanation to traumatic hysteria: the accident caused "an intense cerebral commotion" in which there was the same loss of ego-control as in hypnosis. Consequently, the sensations and ideas experienced during the accident were also realized as symptoms. Thus in a man who slightly injured his shoulder when he unexpectedly fell off a ladder, the sensations called up during his fright were later transformed into a real inability to move the arm.

There was another connection between hypnosis and hysteria. Charcot had observed that his best hypnotic subjects came from the ranks of hysterics, and having concluded that the fundamental cause of hysteria was an hereditary weakness, he went on to propose that the same weakness was present in the good hypnotic subject. In essence, hypnosis was an artificial hysteria.

Freud and Charcot

Freud went to Paris in November 1885 and spent four months at Charcot's clinic at the Salpêtrière. The primary purpose of his visit was to study its wealth of neurological cases, but he became very interested in Charcot's investigations of hysteria and hypnosis and persuaded by his explanations of them. In the same months that Freud was at the Salpêtrière, the Belgian psychologist J-R-L Delboeuf also visited but, unlike Freud, became convinced that all the hypnotic phenomena he saw there were due to Charcot's unconscious suggestions. Delboeuf experimentally trained previously naïve subjects to reproduce the Salpêtrière phenomena

and did so so convincingly that Alfred Binet, Charcot's co-worker and staunch defender, capitulated. Binet went on to say, in 1892, that all that had been written about the physiological basis of hypnosis seemed to be fanciful and that even unsatisfactory psychological hypotheses were to be preferred to false physiological ones.

At the time Freud was at the Salpêtrière, the apparently physiological basis of hysteria was as controversial as hypnosis; Charcot's four well-defined stages were observed practically nowhere other than the Salpêtrière. There is now no doubt that Charcot's patients learned from him and from other patients what an attack of major hysteria was supposed to be like. There were even visual guides. In André Brouillet's famous painting of Charcot demonstrating the phenomena of hysteria (*Une Leçon clinique à la Salpêtrière*), a large drawing by his artist-neurologist colleague Paul Richer hangs on the wall of the theater the patient is facing. It is of a second patient in the *arc-de-circle*, the very next substage into which the patient being demonstrated is about to pass.

Despite the critical evidence of Delboeuf and the criticisms of Charcot from outside the Salpêtrière, Freud adopted Charcot's defence against the charges of suggestion. Were the criticisms correct, said Freud, different symptoms would be produced by different experimenters, and it would never be known what alterations in excitability succeeded one another. All that could be learned were the intentions Charcot suggested unconsciously to his subjects, and that, he said, was entirely irrelevant to the understanding of hypnosis and hysteria.

Three other aspects of the influence of Charcot's conceptualizations on Freud are worth noting. First, despite his references to "lesions," Charcot also thought that hysterical symptoms had to explained by "unconscious or sub-conscious cerebration" (i.e., thinking) that had escaped the conscious ego. Freud's concepts of "unconscious mental processes" and "ego" were eventually very different from Charcot's but they owe their starting point to him. Second, Breuer's notion of the pathogenic effects of events taking place in an hypnoid state, with which he eventually explained Anna O.'s symptoms, is closely related to how Charcot thought of hypnosis. Third, Janet's explanation that the details Charcot had discerned in hysterical symptoms were determined by the popular idea of the functions affected, and the concepts of subconscious association and secondary consciousness that were partly formulated by him and Charcot's other colleagues, were used directly by Freud.

However, the most important influence of Charcot on Freud is almost always overlooked: the role of sensations in the trauma. Not only do the sensations call up the ideas realized in the symptoms, but exactly those sensations are present in the symptom itself. A sensation of slight loss of feeling or movement does not just call up any paralysis or anaesthesia; it calls up only the kind of paralysis or anaesthesia in the part of the body for which those sensations are appropriate. What Charcot demonstrated (but did not spell out explicitly) was that the sensory content of the trauma was represented or reflected in the sensory content of the symptom.

In investigating the psychoneuroses (hysteria and obsessional neuroses), Freud gave sensory content the highest place among his methods for identifying specific causal trauma. The trauma had to have the right "determining quality," and although Freud also did not define the concept explicitly, there is no doubt what he meant: The trauma had to have the same sensory content as the symptom, and that different neuroses had to be caused by different trauma.

By so relying on the lodestone of determining quality, Freud made two errors. He arrived at the ill-fated childhood seduction hypothesis in his search for the causes of the psychoneuroses by assembling his patients' (usually) fragmentary recollections into "memories" or "scenes" of perverse sexual experiences that had the same sensory content as the symptoms. Later it was the major influence on the way he conceptualized the childhood sexual drive. And, even before he investigated the psychoneuroses, the lodestone had led him to identify, quite erroneously, sexual factors as causes of the non-traumatic actual neuroses of neurasthenia and anxiety neurosis. There he also seemed to find that the same sensations as were contained in their apparently specific sexual causes were contained in their symptoms: Tiredness after early onset masturbation was reflected in the general weakness of neurasthenia, and the sensations of incomplete orgasm in the anxiety attack. In his later work, it provided the missing pieces of the puzzle through which the development of the neuroses could be reconstructed.

REFERENCES

Charcot, J. M. (1889). *Clinical Lectures on Diseases of the Nervous System.* (Trans. T. Savill). London: New Sydenham Society. (Original work published 1889.)

Ellenberger, H. (1970). *The Discovery of the Unconscious: The History and Evolution of Dynamic Psychiatry.* New York: Basic Books.

Guillain, G. (1959). *J. M. Charcot, 1835–1893: His Life, His Work.* Ed. and trans. P. Bailey. New York: Hoeber. (Original work published 1955.)

Goetz, C. G., Bonduelle, M., and Gelfand, T. (1995). *Charcot: Constructing Neurology.* New York: Oxford University Press.

Macmillan, M. (1997). *Freud Evaluated: The Completed Arc.* Cambridge, Mass.: MIT Press, especially chapters 2 and 3.

Owen, A. R. G. (1971). *Hysteria, Hypnosis and Healing: The Work of J. M. Charcot.* London: Dennis Dobson.

MALCOLM MACMILLAN

Child Abuse See SEDUCTION THEORY.

Child Psychoanalysis

Two fundamental presuppositions are as basic to child psychoanalysis as they are to adult psychoanalysis: psychic determinism and unconscious mental activity. It is assumed that one thought is connected to another but that the person may be unaware of the connections. Thus, in both adults and children, psychic activity deriving from earlier periods of life is assumed to have an impact on present unconscious conflicts. One aims to achieve the greatest degree of beneficial alteration of such conflicts, and, in the case of a child, to help the child resume a normal developmental path. There are additional similarities between child and adult psychoanalysis, but there are also important differences.

Motivation for Treatment and Parental Support

Adults who enter analysis need to be sufficiently motivated to benefit from treatment, but children usually do not have the same motivation or the same impetus to decide to enter treatment. Instead, their parents, who often suffer more from the children's symptoms than the children themselves, decide whether or not to initiate and maintain treatment. Another difference concerns fees and schedules. In adult cases, these are negotiated between analysand and analyst. Obviously, this is not the case with children. Thus, parents' emotional and realistic support are needed to sustain an analysis with a child.

In addition, throughout the analysis, the analyst may have to have regular ongoing contact with the parents to

C

allow the analysis to continue. The child psychoanalyst often obtains critical information from parents about events in the child's life that the child just may not reveal.

Method

Since in any individual, child or adult, only a finite number of dynamic mental structures are operative, an important hallmark of analytic work with children, as with adults, involves listening to and observing the repetitive ideas and themes that preoccupy the patient. As with adults, the child analyst attempts to establish an analytic process, utilizing defense interpretations as well as analysis of transference. However, with children, who do not, often cannot, free associate, the mental productions to which the analyst must attend include not only verbal utterances but also the child's actions and play.

Over time, the child communicates the essence of his or her dynamics in these various verbal and nonverbal activities. By virtue of carefully listening and observing the child's verbal associations as well as his or her play and other activities, the child analyst begins to make hypotheses about the significance of the verbal associations and nonverbal activities.

Since the child analyst interacts with the child, by playing with and conversing with him or her, the analyst has to be cognizant of his or her reactions to the child. As the child communicates the nature of his or her wishes and defenses, the child analyst gradually learns the child's language and metaphorical usages in order to communicate in a manner that the child understands. For example, children often understand the significance of the analyst's playful comments about "other children" and say, "I know you are talking about me."

In many respects, the furor and controversy surrounding the "real" relationship versus the transference relationship is puzzling. Child analysts, after all, always interact with their child analytic patients. It matters less exactly how one reacts, since one inevitably *does react* to children; what is central is trying to understand the *meaning* of the analyst's reaction to the child. However, child analysts often need to, and do, pay more attention to the therapeutic alliance than do adult analysts. Thus, although one has to work with the parents to foster the development of a therapeutic alliance with the child or adolescent, the child must feel that it is *his* or *her* treatment, *his* or *her* time, and *you* are *his* or *her* therapist (Byerly, 1993).

Indications for Treatment

Maturational and developmental forces in childhood lead to a great plasticity in the child's mental life. As a result, psychological dysfunction in children is usually manifested by a deviation in the child's developmental profile: disturbances appear in affect regulation, cognition, social relations, and ability to develop appropriate sublimations or interests. These disturbances can be severe or mild, thereby creating unclarity about deciding whether psychoanalysis is the best treatment for a child. In other words, when does a child have severe enough symptomatic and developmental disturbances to warrant treatment, yet also the psychological capacity to benefit from the psychoanalytic method? One cannot justifiably recommend analysis by simply looking at a group of symptoms and deciding that they are indicative of a childhood neurosis. An evaluation is needed.

During the evaluation, the child analyst has to assess whether the child has internalized neurotic conflicts that interfere with the child's expected development. Such a situation is a key indicator for child psychoanalysis. There are situations where psychoanalysis is contraindicated—in a child, for example, who is psychotic. Children who suffer from one or other variation of a severe pervasive developmental disorder need a great deal of cognitive support, but some of these children can very much benefit from intensive psychotherapy. Psychotherapeutic support can be very helpful: one can help them understand the circumstances under which they are provoked and become aggressive; one can help them master their anxieties and limit their aggressive outbursts; one can provide the child an object with whom to identify; and one can help the parents set appropriate limits for their child's behavior.

Interpretative work can be done with these more severely disturbed children but only in limited ways. In order for parents to agree to have their child in a psychoanalysis, they have to be in some way psychologically minded or at least accepting of the idea of an intensive treatment. In addition, psychoanalysis in children, as in adults, requires a certain degree of realistic stability. Thus, there are situations in which the family constellation may be a contraindication for psychoanalysis. If there is too great a degree of family disorganization and pathology, not only will the family not be able emotionally to support the analysis but the main work with the child may involve a lot of reality testing to help him or her interact more productively with the parents. If there is too much chaos in a family, other kinds of therapeutic interventions are necessary. Obviously, there are families whose psychopathology is not extreme but either for their own neurotic reasons or other reasons refuse to entertain the notion of analysis. In addition there are children who do not seem psychotic, retarded, or profoundly delayed, but who communicate an arid inner life. In such children, interpretative work does not lead to an elaboration of fantasies and there is no deepening of understanding.

Origins of Psychoanalysis

It is likely to be a surprise to readers of this encyclopedia that the first child psychoanalyst was not Anna Freud or Melanie Klein but Hermine Hug-Hellmuth, one of the first lay analysts and the first gentile and third woman member of the Vienna Psychoanalytic Society. Her work has been all but forgotten because of several tragedies in her life, including the notoriety of her "A Young Girl's Diary," claimed to be fraudulent, and her murder in 1924 by her nephew, Rolf. However, Hug-Hellmuth's original work as a child analyst well preceded that of Anna Freud and Melanie Klein.

She explicitly stated that her goal was to demonstrate the relevance to children of Freud's ideas and method. She clarified the differences between child analysis and adult analysis, and understood that no psychoanalytic treatment, in either adults or children, could occur without transference; she realized that the analyst represented both mother and father. She was extremely sensitive to children's feelings and stressed that the analyst needed to understand childhood narcissism and the effect on the child of blows to his narcissism. She cautioned analysts not to discuss positive transference feelings with children prematurely because children might experience a loyalty conflict and be forced to choose the parent over the analyst. At the same time, she understood the important concept that came to be known as "object removal" in puberty.

In the 1920s, Melanie Klein and Anna Freud disagreed in their approaches to children but both essentially ignored Hug-Hellmuth and her work. Anna Freud felt that one needed to include a preparatory phase in which the analyst essentially seduces the child into analysis by acting in powerful and protective ways, developing something like the "real relationship" or something akin to a holding environment. Klein, on the other hand, maintained that this phase interfered with the development of the transference. Another analyst, Berta Bornstein, was instrumental in the development of the technique of defense analysis with children, especially the interpretation of defenses against unwelcome intense affects. The introduction of understanding and interpreting the child's defenses against affects proved to be a nodal point in child analytic technique. With this understanding, it became unnecessary to try to seduce the child into developing a therapeutic alliance with the analyst, and the use of the preparatory phase became unnecessary. At the same time it became superfluous to introduce symbolic id-type interpretations early in the treatment. Instead the analyst observed the child's affects and defensive reactions to about-to-be-felt feelings. From the earliest points in the treatment, the analyst could interpret how the child, regardless of age or wish to communicate in words, coped with unpleasant feeling states. Armed with this understanding, the analyst could understand how the child managed his or her wishes.

Recent Developments

The most recent work in child analysis has included the critical research by Peter Fonagy and Mary Target of the Anna Freud Centre and the Menninger Clinic. Fonagy and Target have demonstrated that for children with anxiety and depressive disorders and for those with severe or multiple pathologies, intensive psychoanalytic treatment at four to five times per week is more efficacious than one to three times per week therapy, and treatment length is positively correlated with better outcome. Young children with the most severe emotional disorders respond best to psychoanalysis of six months or more. This intensive treatment has been shown to be more effective than shorter therapies or a combination of therapy and drugs. In addition, longer treatments were independently associated with greater improvement: 51 percent of the children studied improved if treated for one or two years, and 74 percent improved when treatment lasted at least three years. The study also found that more frequent treatment is the most effective therapy for older children and adolescents: 74 percent of preschool children significantly improved after long-term treatment, 67 percent of children six to twelve years old improved, and 58 percent of adolescents showed marked improvement with intensive psychoanalysis.

C

REFERENCES

Bornstein, B. (1945). Notes on child analysis. *Psychoanalytic Study of the Child*, 1: 151–165.

Byerly, L. (1993). The therapeutic alliance. In M. Hossein Etezady (ed.). *Treatment of Neurosis in the Young: A Psychoanalytic Perspective.* Northvale, N.J.: Jason Aronson.

Fonagy, P., and Target, M. (1996). Predictors of outcome in child psychoanalysis: A retrospective study of 763 cases at the Anna Freud Centre. *Journal of the American Psychoanalytic Association* 44: 27–77.

Freud, A. (1927). Four lectures on child analysis. In A. Freud (author). *The Writings of Anna Freud* 1, pp. 3–69. New York: International Universities Press, 1974.

Glenn, J. (1992). Indications and contraindications for child analysis. In J. Glenn (ed.). *Child Analysis and Therapy.* New York: Jason Aronson.

Hoffman, L. (1993). An introduction to child psychoanalysis. *Journal of Clinical Psychoanalysis*, 2(1): 5–26.

Grosskurth, P. (1986). *Melanie Klein: Her World and Her Work.* New York: Knopf.

Klein, M. (1975). The Psycho-Analysis of Children. (Translation by Alix Strachey). In M. Klein (author). *The Writings of Melanie Klein*, vol. 2. New York: Free Press.

MacLean, G., and Rappen, U. (1991). *Hermine Hug-Hellmuth: Her Life and Work.* New York: Routledge.

Sandler, J., Kennedy, H., and Tyson, R. L. (1980). *The Technique of Child Psychoanalysis: Discussions with Anna Freud.* Cambridge, Mass.: Harvard University Press.

Target, M., and Fonagy, P. (1994). Efficacy of psychoanalysis for children with emotional disorders. *American Academy of Child and Adolescent Psychiatry*, 33: 1134–1144.

Young-Bruehl, E. (1988). *Anna Freud: A Biography.* New York: Summit Books.

LEON HOFFMAN

Childhood Neurosis

Freud's conceptions of childhood (or "infantile") neurosis are set forth in two of his great case histories—"Little Hans" (1909) and "The Wolf-man" (1918). Each of these, concurrently and retrospectively, served to confirm and/or polemically defend his basic theories of infantile sexuality and its relations to psychopathology. Neuroses in children, like those in adults, are characterized by symptoms (phobias, obsessions/compulsions, hysterical phenomena) in the setting of an otherwise intact personality (not "degenerate" or psychotic). The symptoms must be distinguished, Freud emphasized, from functional inhibitions that represent ways of coping with the symptoms, though each has symbolic meaning (e.g., Little Hans's refusal to go out of doors was an inhibition; his fear of horses was a symptom).

In Freud's account, Little Hans's neurosis was precipitated by the birth of his sister when he was three. This event intensified his erotic longings for his mother; thus his unconscious Oedipal conflicts and associated fantasies (sexual possession of his mother, murderous wishes toward his father) led to fears of retaliatory castration from his father that were displaced onto horses. The resulting repression of his sexual wishes led to the damming up of his libido which was, somehow, transformed into anxiety. When, in "Inhibitions, Symptoms and Anxiety" (1926), Freud reformulated his anxiety theory, he reinterpreted Hans's neurosis in structural terms; the Oedipal conflict remained fundamental to its pathogenesis, but anxiety served the ego as a signal of danger (castration) that led to the repression of the Oedipal wishes and the definitive displacement to the now-feared extrafamilial object—the horse. Anxiety was now seen as the cause of repression rather than its consequence.

The basic pattern of Oedipal conflict, Freud maintained, was universal; thus some degree of "infantile neurosis" was an inevitable aspect of the human condition. Depending on the pattern of "resolution" of the Oedipus complex (1924), this normative psychological structure might be transitory or might evolve into a true childhood neurotic illness. In turn, this could be expected to form, as with the "Wolf-man," the nucleus of an adult neurosis. In other words, in Freud's view every adult neurosis would have its roots in an "infantile neurosis," but not every "infantile neurosis" need inevitably eventuate in an adult neurosis.

Freud's ideas about childhood neurosis have been extended and modified by many subsequent workers. A thorough review of recent psychoanalytic views from a variety of perspectives can be found in Etezady (1990).

REFERENCES

Etezady, M. H. (ed.) (1990). *The Neurotic Child and Adolescent.* Northvale, N.J.: Jason Aronson.

Freud, S. (1909). *Analysis of a Phobia in a Five-Year-Old Boy.* S.E. 10: 5–149.

———. (1924). *The Dissolution of the Oedipus Complex.* S.E. 19: 173–179.

———. (1918). *From the History of Infantile Neurosis.* S.E. 17: 7–123.

———. (1926). *Inhibitions, Symptoms and Anxiety.* S.E. 20: 87–172.

AARON H. ESMAN

Childhood Sexuality See INFANTILE SEXUALITY.

Chile, and Psychoanalysis

The history of psychoanalysis in Chile is well documented (Whiting, 1980; Nuñez, 1981; Florenzano, 1988; Arrué, 1988 and 1995; Oyarzún, 1990; Prat, 1990; Gomberoff, 1990).

It was Sigmund Freud himself who took note of the first psychoanalytic publication in Chile. In 1911 he reviewed "Sobre psicología y psicoterapia de ciertos estados angustiosos," by Germán Greve (1869–1954), a Chilean physician who did postgraduate studies in Germany (1893). This paper, which was presented at an international conference held in Buenos Aires in 1910, contains the first reference to psychoanalysis in Latin America. Freud considered it important enough to refer to it in his *On the History of the Psycho-analytic Movement* (1914).

Greve's experience with psychoanalysis, however, had no lasting effects. The diffusion of psychoanalysis in Chile began in 1925, when Fernando Allende Navarro (1890–1981) returned to Chile after completing his training in medicine, psychiatry, and psychoanalysis in Europe. In 1926, Allende Navarro validated his medical qualification with a dissertation on *El valor del Psicoanálisis en Policlínico: Contribución a la Psicología Chilena (The Value of Psychoanalysis in the Out-Patient Clinic: A Contribution to Chilean Psychology)*, which is probably the first paper by a Spanish-speaking psychoanalyst.

Allende Navarro did not associate himself with academic activities and restricted his work to the private practice of psychiatry and psychoanalysis. However, as a private practitioner, he achieved a significant degree of influence through personal psychoanalysis and the training of medical doctors who would become important names in Chilean psychiatry. The most outstanding of them were Carlos Nuñez Saavedra (1918–1981) and Ignacio Matte Blanco (1908–1995). The Jesuit priest Abdón Cifuentes (1878–1960), professor at the Faculty of Theology of the Catholic University, was another influential person to be trained by Allende Navarro. This fact is worth noting since it showed an unusual and still present receptivity toward psychoanalysis on the part of some sectors of the Catholic Church.

After specializing in psychiatry at Maudsley Hospital in London, Matte Blanco completed his psychoanalytic training at the Institute of the British Psycho-Analytical Society in the 1930s. On his return to Chile in 1943, he attracted an enthusiastic group of young psychiatrists with whom he formed a study group. On August 17, 1949, this group achieved recognition as a member of the International Psychoanalytical Association. The first president of the newly constituted Chilean Psychoanalytical Association was Allende Navarro. A few days before, on August 3, Matte Blanco, who had been previously short-listed for the post, was appointed to the chair of psychiatry at the Faculty of Medicine of the University of Chile.

The period between 1949 and 1960 can be considered as the golden age of psychoanalysis in Chile. Psychoanalysis during this period was closely associated with academia and with psychiatry. Several generations of psychiatrists, psychologists, and psychoanalysts received their training under the scientific leadership of Matte Blanco. The Psychiatric Clinic of the University of Chile, another initiative of its director, Matte Blanco, was the first to offer a dynamic orientation in psychiatry and psychology in the country. Among the psychiatrists and psychoanalysts trained in that period, Otto Kernberg ultimately achieved the greatest prominence. In the same period, Nuñez Saavedra was appointed professor of psychiatry at the Faculty of Medicine of the Catholic University, and the University of Chile and the Catholic University of Santiago created the first two schools of psychology in Chile, with a large number of psychoanalysts among their teaching staff.

In 1960, after the Third Latin American Congress of Psychoanalysis was held in Santiago, internal conflicts first emerged. These conflicts led to the massive resignation of psychoanalysts from the university, whose head of department was Matte Blanco, and to the creation of a Psychoanalytic Institute independent of the university. In 1961, Kernberg, the first of many analysts to emigrate in the 1960s, settled in the United States. In 1967, Matte Blanco and his family left for Rome, where he published his most important work. He was never to return to Chile. This state of affairs left the psychoanalytical institution bereft of its most active members, resulting in a period of stagnation lasting well into the 1980s. In a way, the Chilean Psychoanalytical Association underwent the same global crisis affecting the country from the 1960s to the late 1980s.

The liberalization of higher education in the last ten years has brought about a significant increase in the number of psychiatrists and psychologists seeking psychoanalytic training. These years have seen the birth of institutes of psychoanalytic psychotherapy, the creation of the Association of Psychoanalytical Psychotherapists, and the appearance of the Lacanian movement in the country.

For the first time, the provinces have been showing an interest in psychoanalysis. All this has represented new challenges for the Chilean Psychoanalytical Association. At the same time, within the Psychoanalytical Association there has been a strong movement of renovation and opening toward the community, which points to the end of the psychoanalytical doldrums. The association's constitution and bylaws are being revised to conform to more democratic conditions, and scientific activity has shown a steady growth. At present, the association has almost sixty members and there are no fewer than thirty candidates for membership. This makes it possible to forecast that the association will treble its membership in the next fifteen years. One-third of the members and candidates are university teachers, in the tradition of Matte Blanco. Also, the psychoanalytical group has been more closely involved with the artistic and cultural environments. In 1999, coinciding with the fiftieth anniversary of the recognition of the Chilean Psychoanalytical Association by the International Psychoanalytical Association, the forty-first International Psychoanalytical Congress was held in Santiago, bringing to Chile no fewer than 1,500 psychoanalysts from all over the world.

REFERENCES

Arrué, O. (1988). 40 años de Psicoanálisis en Chile. *Revista Chilena de Psicoanálisis*, 7: 3–5.

———. (1995). Chile. In P. Kutter (ed.), *Psychoanalysis International. A Guide to Psychoanalysis throughout the World.* Stuttgart-Bad Cannstatt: Fromman-Holzboog, pp. 74–92.

Florenzano, R. (1988). Estrategias de desarrollo y la Asociación Psicoanalítica Chilena, *Revista Chilena de Psicoanálisis*, 7: 20–28.

Gomberoff, M. (1990). Apuntes acerca de la historia del psicoanálisis en Chile. *Revista Chilena de Psiquiatría (Chile)*, 7: 379–389.

Nuñez, C. F. (1981). Allende Navarro. Editorial. *Revista Chilena de Psicoanálisis*, 3: 1–7.

Oyarzún, F. (1990). La significación del Profesor Ignacio Matte Blanco en la Psiquiatría Chilena. *Revista Chilena de Psiquiatría (Chile)*, 7: 375–378.

Prat, A. (1990). Historia de la Psiquiatría Dinámica en Chile. *Revista Chilena de Psicoanálisis*, 8: 5–8.

Whiting, C. (1980). Notas para la historia del psicoanálisis en Chile. *Revista Chilena de Psicoanálisis*, 2/1: 19–26.

JUAN PABLO JIMÉNEZ

China, and Psychoanalysis

Freud's ideas have had a limited and variable reception in China. A few articles appeared in the second decade of the twentieth century, and by the early eighties, fourteen of Freud's works had appeared in translation (Bauer and Wang, 1982). To date however, there has been no translation of Freud's complete works, though there have been numerous articles about his ideas. These were first taken seriously by intellectuals in the wake of the May Fourth Movement in 1919. This was a cultural development that sought to overthrow the feudal system and reevaluate traditional thinking. Freud's ideas were put to use at this time by social reformers. One of the earliest, Zhang Dongsun, wrote in 1929 that Freud's deterministic stance on slips and forgetting was "beyond the explanatory power of general psychology." While grudgingly acknowledging that much of Freud's theory was grounded in sexuality, it was his defense of sublimation that Zhang appealed to in corroborating a Buddhist saying, "the greatest wickedness is licentiousness" (*wan e yin wei shou*) by claiming Freud expounded "the elimination of human desires" (*jue ren yu*). In distorting Freud's meaning of the mechanisms of defense, he offers sublimation as a viable means of social reform (Zhang, 1989). All people should understand psychoanalysis, he argued, so that they could analyze their own thoughts and character, and improve themselves by removing their baser aspects through sublimation. Rather idealistically, he believed social problems would disappear. Nevertheless this line of argument could be addressed to parents and teachers since it stressed the importance of early development and children's special needs.

In spite of the intentions of social reformers, Freud's ideas had little impact on psychology in China in the thirties because of the dominance of behaviorism (Blowers, 1994). Also lessening the impact was the arbitrariness of the choice of Freud's works for translation, not to mention the whims of individual translators. Freud's name appears in ten different forms coming through transliterations of Japanese katakana—"furoito"—or of the mispronunciations of his name ("froit"). Many psychoanalytic terms were taken from Japanese, for which they already had other meanings in that language. For example, the "unconscious," rendered in Japanese (using Chinese characters) was *muisiki*, which in Chinese means "without consciousness." Translators debated whether to use this or coin a new term, and subsequently several variants were in use. It is now commonly expressed as *qian yi shi*, which means "hidden," "latent," or "submerged" consciousness. "Oedipus Complex" is usually translated as *lian mu qing jie*—the "romantic/sexual love of mother." Many early translations were creative revisions of the original text. The social reformer Zhang Shizhao, the only Chinese intellectual to correspond with Freud (Blowers, 1993), translated *Selbstarstellung* from German, producing a text heavy in classical Chinese allusion and in many places replacing clinical references with Chinese historical and cultural terms in keeping with Zhang's own partiality for ancient and Confucian teachings rather than new Western ideas.

By contrast, Gao Juefu, in his translations from English of the *Introductory* and *New Introductory Lectures* in the thirties, and again in the eighties, was scrupulous in avoiding vague and not widely understood terms. While admiring Freud's work, which he saw as liberating the modern world from the clutches of superstition, he was wary and critical of what he took to be Freud's pansexualist position and worried that in the hands of popularizers it could have a pernicious and corrupting effect on young people. Like many Chinese he expressed concern over a theory that seemed to grant primacy to a free-reigning sexuality, because it could be construed as a threat to the stability of family relations. His motive for translating Freud, he explains in one of his prefaces, was to alert readers to what a strange man Freud was (Blowers, 1995).

The Sino-Japanese War and the political upheaval that accompanied the Communist revolution gave intellectuals little time for further speculations on Freud. Following the formation of the People's Republic of China (PRC) in 1949 and the ushering in of a broad program of socialist reform, psychologists and psychiatrists, like other intellectuals, had to study Marxist philosophy and practice their disciplines according to two principles: that psychological phenomena are a product of the brain, and that mind is a reflection of outer reality. As Ding Zuan, the secretary of the Chinese Psychological Society in 1955 was to write, this left little room for Freud's "mysterious sexual drives." The ending of the twelve-year period known as the Cultural Revolution in 1978, during which virtually all intellectual development stopped, has seen a reemergence of interest in Freud's work. More translations have appeared and the debate about his ideas continues.

However, psychoanalysis as therapy had not until quite recently taken root in China. This is because, it has been argued, there has been no tradition of expressiveness in the doctor-patient relationship, and the doctor in a traditional Chinese setting adopts an authoritarian attitude toward patients. Before World War II there had been only one Chinese psychoanalyst, Bingham Dai, who trained under Harry Stack Sullivan and taught psychotherapy at Peking Municipal Psychopathic Hospital allied to the Peking Union Medical College from 1935 to 1939. While he was of the view that, but for the Japanese invasion, psychoanalysis might have taken root in China, he downplayed the theoretical importance Freud attached to the instinctual impulses, claiming that "the Chinese, by and large, have a rather natural attitude towards their biological needs" (Dai, 1987).

With the political upheavals in the early years of the PRC, there were no analysts. But there are recent signs of change. Since 1995, the International Psychoanalytical Association has begun reaching out to China, inviting professionals to its conferences and organizing a subcommittee for Asia. The Chinese-German Academy for Psychotherapy, comprising analysts interested in and familiar with Chinese culture, has initiated a wide range of training programs covering different behavioral, systemic, and psychoanalytic trends. Dynamic psychotherapy is being practiced in a variety of psychiatric settings in Beijing, Shanghai, and Wuhan, and a Chinese analyst trained in France recently founded a psychoanalytic center in Chengdu (Yuan, 2000). Freud's ideas have certainly contributed to this. However, the range and complexity of his ideas may not be fully appreciated unless and until a translation of more of his works is undertaken, clinical psychology gets more firmly established, and the therapeutic context is expanded to encompass through education a range of treatments and the possibilities of the individual psychotherapeutic scheme.

REFERENCES

Bauer, H. W. Von, and Hwang Shen-chang (1982). *German Impact on Modern Chinese Intellectual History. A Bibliography of Chinese Publications.* Wiesbaden: Franz Steiner Verlag.

Blowers, G. H. (1993). Freud's China connection. *Journal of Multicultural and Multilingual Development,* 14: 263–273.

———. (1994). Freud in China: the variable reception of psychoanalysis. In G. Davidson (ed.). *Applying Psychology: Lessons from Asia-Oceania.* Carlton, Victoria: Australian Psychological Society, pp. 35–49.

———. (1995). Gao Juefu: China's interpreter of western psychology. *World Psychology* 1(3): 107–121.

Dai, B. (1987). Psychoanalysis in China before the revolution. In R. Fine (ed.). *Psychoanalysis around the World.* New York: Howarth Press.

Yuan, T. S. (2000). China in the history of psychoanlysis: A possible fate for psychoanalysis at the dawn of the millennium.

Paper read at the *8th International Meeting of the International Association for the History of Psychoanalysis*. Versailles. July 20–22, 2000.

Zhang, Yingyuan (1989). *Sigmund Freud and Modern Chinese Literature*. Ph.D. diss., Cornell University. (University Microfilms).

GEOFFREY H. BLOWERS

Cinema, and Psychoanalysis

Freudian theories have played a prominent role in conceptualizing the nature of the motion picture experience and in analyzing films. Theorists who use Freud's ideas in the first way try to identify the ways in which motion pictures mobilize unconscious processes. A prime example is what has come to be known as the "Althusserean-Lacanian model."

This model combines political and psychoanalytic features. It is political in that it seeks to provide a conceptual map of the role that the experience of the motion picture plays in such political processes as reinforcing capitalism, maintaining patriarchy, and supporting racism. It is psychoanalytic in that it tries to explain in psychoanalytic terms why the motion picture experience has this effect. Louis Althusser provided the overtly political aspects of the model; Jacques Lacan provided a needed psychoanalytic aspect.

Althusser's Theory

Althusser (Althusser, 1971) asks the pointed question: given the social injustices that exist in society, why do not the people revolt against the existing power structure? His answer is that there are repressive and institutional state apparatuses that position citizens to believe in the efficacy of the existing power structures. The army, the police, and the courts are examples of repressive apparatuses. More subtle but just as effective are other institutional apparatuses such as the film industry. The experience of a motion picture in its typical mode (e.g., the classic Hollywood film, the most popular film form so far in the history of the medium) serves to "reproduce" capitalist subjects. By "reproduce," Althusser means that individuals leave an encounter with an institutional state apparatus continuing to believe in the capitalist system or to believe in the appropriateness of patriarchal organization in society; they are, moreover, reinforced in their tendencies to submit to the state's demands, and also to participate in its processes. The

Althusserean analysis, however, goes only so far. A question still remains: assuming that he is correct in his diagnosis, why do subjects encountering institutional state apparatuses such as the movies become "reproduced" as capitalist subjects or patriarchal subjects? The additional answer is supposedly provided by Jacques Lacan's radical transformation of orthodox Freudian theory and his analysis of the "mirror-stage."

Lacan's Theory

Unmodified Freudian theory has been thought less useful for the Althusserean-Lacanian radical political project because of a perceived gender bias in Freud's writings; i.e., it has been thought that Freud was overly focused on issues of male identity while being relatively inattentive to female identity. Lacan's interpretations of Freud, on the other hand, are thought to apply equally well to the experience of either gender. With the advent of feminism as a dominant force in later-twentieth-century film theory, a perceived gender bias is given great weight in deciding about fruitful directions in film theory, lending an attractiveness to Lacanian theory.

Of particular relevance to political-psychoanalytic theories of film experiences is Lacan's theory of the "mirror-stage." On his analysis, the process leading to being reproduced as a capitalist or patriarchal subject takes place on an unconscious level owing to what occurs in this stage of infantile development.

Lacan tells a story about an infant's first encounter with a mirror (Lacan, 1968). Film theorists have regarded this mirror-stage analysis as the needed psychoanalytic dimension of the political analysis. Lacan's view is that the individual becomes "constructed" during this very early period of psychosexual development. In a prenatal condition, the embryo has a sense of plenitude—a feeling of wholeness and completeness. Birth, however, severs the individual from the mother, creating a feeling of loss, alienating the individual and making its condition one dominated by a sense of lack. After birth, the infant feels dependent but wishes for wholeness. During this period, some time between six and eighteen months, the infant obtains its first sense of itself as individuated in its encounter with the mirror. In this moment, it recognizes (misrecognizes) itself. It sees itself but it sees itself wrongly. It sees what seems to be a whole being but what is really fragmented and dependent. Its feelings of fragmentation and dependency eventually give way. The infant obtains a sense of ideal unity and illusory autonomy in the mirror experience that triggers the creation of "the imaginary." The imaginary is a faculty something like the imagination in older theories of the mind. The infant is jubilant at the exercise of this illusion-making imaginary it has acquired. The imaginary stays with humans the rest of their lives, continuing to support their faith in a unified subjecthood. The imaginary, according to Lacan, functions in adult life to instill and support illusions of subject unity through pictorial representations and discourse, as in, for example, the experience of a motion picture. In watching a motion picture, adults are "positioned" like infants in their first encounter with a mirror. We think we see events and persons before us when we see only images that we merely construct under the sway of the imaginary. The illusions about the film interact with the illusions about the subject watching it, mutually reinforcing the illusion-making process. The belief in a unified, autonomous subject, created under the influence of the imaginary, is central to being reproduced as a capitalist or patriarchal subject since according to the political analysis in which the mirror-stage analysis fits, only an individual subject to the illusion of being a self can be influenced by an institutional state apparatus. Lacan's story about the mirror-stage and the imaginary is not based upon any empirical research, but since it supplies a needed psychoanalytic dimension to the political analysis that lies at the heart of late-twentieth-century film theory, it is widely accepted without confirmation.

Freudian Film Criticism

Psychoanalysis is at once a psychological theory, a therapy, and a critical discourse for analyzing art. It might seem that only the last aspect of Freud's work would come into play in Freudian theorizing about film, but that has proved to be not the case.

Psychoanalytic theory has been used to explain the behavior, relationships, actions, and motives of film characters. For example, it has been used in explaining abnormal behavior and dream content in Hitchcock's *Spellbound*. Psychoanalytic notions have been used to explain problematic aspects of films: the oral/narcissistic dilemma as a key to the meaning of Bergman's *Persona*; the Oedipus complex as central to Laurence Olivier's interpretation of *Hamlet*; the sense of the uncanny as described by Freud as underlying structure in Dreyer's *Vampyr*. Feminists have also analyzed the ways in which psychoanalysis as a discourse has been used to oppress women or to position them in stereo-

typical social roles. These applications involve psychoanalysis as both psychological theory and art critical tool. There are, however, some instances of film criticism and film theory that conflate psychoanalysis as therapeutic practice and psychoanalysis as art critical activity. Some critics do not distinguish between psychoanalysis as therapy for neurosis and psychoanalysis as a discourse used in critical analysis. The aims of the analyst in the therapeutic situation are nevertheless different from the aims of the film critic in interpreting the experience of a film. In the former case, the analyst, for instance, facilitates the dreamer in constructing a dream text partly via primary identification with the aim of understanding the individual's psychic life. By contrast, the appreciator and critic, in constructing interpretations of what they are experiencing in the motion picture, are involved only in secondary identification. To speak of transference in the context of a critical interpretation of a character in the same sense as referring to transference in the therapeutic situation blurs the distinction between psychoanalysis as therapeutic practice and as art critical discourse. There are those who strive to maintain the conceptual separation in critical practice among the three aspects of psychoanalysis, notably E. Ann Kaplan (Kaplan, 1990). It is through their guidance in conceptualizing psychoanalysis in relation to film criticism and film theory that critical work may find its most fruitful use of Freudian concepts in relation to film.

REFERENCES

Althusser, L. (1971). Ideology and ideological state apparatuses. *Lenin and Philosophy and Other Essays.* London: Monthly Review, pp. 127–186.

Kaplan, E. A. (1990). *From Plato's Cave to Freud's Screen. Psychoanalysis and Cinema.* New York: Routledge.

Lacan, J. (1968). The mirror-phase as formative of the function of the I. *New Left Review*, 51: 71–77.

ALLAN CASEBIER

Clinical Ethics See ETHIC, CLINICAL.

Clinical Theory

The Formation of the Primary Clinical Model

Freud's clinical theory logically takes as its starting point his study of hysterical symptoms. He had been exposed to hypnosis in the treatment of hysterical symptoms while studying with Jean-Martin Charcot at the Salpêtrière in

Paris during his fellowship there in 1885. Charcot, however, relied on hypnotic suggestion for symptomatic relief, providing an outcome that proved to be not only unreliable but without grounds for coherent explanation. That coherence began to appear in Freud's mind after he learned from Josef Breuer of the latter's treatment of Anna O. in the years 1880–1882 (Breuer and Freud, 1893–1895).

Anna O.'s symptoms were made up of motor paralysis, inhibitions, and disturbances of consciousness, originating during the period she nursed her sick father. At her request, Breuer set aside the suggestion technique employed at that time and listened to her describe how her symptoms began, allowing her to express freely her feelings and thoughts. Freud saw in this procedure something special. While under hypnosis, the patient spoke of memories associated with her father's illness. These memory reports were accompanied by expressions of painful feelings, at times of extraordinary intensity. Invariably, the hysterical symptoms disappeared as soon as the events that had given rise to them were reproduced in her hypnosis (1893–1895). For Freud, these observations contained the nucleus of all that was to follow.

An initial formulation emerged reflecting findings both in the case of Anna O. and subsequent studies of hysterical patients: (1) hysterical symptoms were associated with "dammed up" or undischarged affect, and (2) the affect was connected with memories that could not be admitted to consciousness because of the pain associated with them. In effect, symptoms were conceived of as a coherent expression of painful feelings and thus were meaningful.

The memories represented, in Freud's language, "pathogenic ideas," which were understood as the registrations of psychical trauma. Thus, his theory of hysteria began as a trauma theory. The affect associated with traumatic ideas could not be discharged along the normal emotional pathways but, becoming "strangulated," found expression in hysterical symptoms. Searching for the origin of the pathogenic images, a search that led ineluctably to the technique of free association and the fundamental rule, Freud was drawn into the patient's increasingly remote history. This history invariably revealed a sexual trauma. While the connection between hysterical symptoms and ordinary trauma was familiar to Freud, sexual trauma now replaced ordinary trauma, to which it was associatively or symbolically connected, in his thinking about hysterical neurosis. Investigating these

pathogenic sexual ideas, Freud inevitably came upon their elaboration in fantasy. A shift thereby occurred in his thinking away from the external world to the patient's inner world. His patients' reports of childhood seduction came to be seen not as accounts of actual seductions but as expressions of their inner life, having their origin in the patients' earliest years. This inner life, for Freud, involved the existence of sexual wishes.

Earlier, Freud had distinguished clinical entities that, according to the defenses they triggered, organized thinking and symptoms along the lines of hysterical or obsessive-compulsive neuroses. In each disorder, the unmastered sexual experience is both defended against and expressed. In hysteria, the defense displaces the experience to the area of the conversion symptom to which it is symbolically connected and through which it is symbolically experienced. The symptom is thus a compromise formation. Affect is discharged with the formation of the symptoms. In the obsessional neurosis, the traumatic sexual experience is first expressed actively via sexual sadistic acts that are then defended against by the operation of reaction formation, turning them into their opposites. These reaction formations result in patients reassuring themselves of the nature of their upstanding character against persistent doubt (associated with sadistic fantasies of which they are unaware). Once again, a compromise rendering of the trauma is achieved. This view of neurotic symptoms as a product of defense and discharge is an explicit theory of conflict.

Wishes and the Primary Model

It was primarily from the study of dreams (from his letters we know their prominence in his self-analysis) that Freud seems to have brought wishes to their central role in the inner life. For the mental apparatus to initiate work, he says in *The Interpretation of Dreams* (1900), there must be wishes. Thus, in his theory of dream formation, Freud found conflict to be in the central position, with the dream as the compromise through which wishes unacceptable to consciousness can be expressed in a disguised form. Freud assumed, furthermore, that the mechanisms governing dreams, as well as other normal phenomena such as slips, were the same as those underlying pathological phenomena such as obsessional ideas.

The Role of Sexuality

The prominence of sexual wishes in inner life led Freud to study the development of human sexuality. In describing that development he first placed sexuality in the context of the instincts. Sexuality was seen as omnipresent in infantile life. Freud noted its development from partial to complete instincts dominated by genital aims, and he described its clinical derivatives. The sources for the component instincts were the organs of the body, especially those that he called erogenous zones, but contributions to the libido were said to be made from every important functional process in the body.

Three stages of sexual development were described: oral, anal, and genital, each stage having its own particular wishes. The fulfillment of the wishes of each stage would occur in direct relation to its aim, which is always the satisfaction accompanying discharge. In seeking satisfaction, the wishes find which channels of discharge are in unconscious mental functioning, such as condensation and displacement. They appear in the external world in any derivatives from the pathological to the normal, in feelings, thought, and action.

The Role of the Oedipus Complex

Wishes appear whenever needs are unsatisfied. The earliest needs of the infant are provided for by the mother, the primary external object. The sexual instincts seek their gratification along the pathways established and provided for by the primary needs. As an example, oral satisfaction via biting, sucking, and the like is obtained along pathways already established for nourishment. Central is the position of the object world—the ministrations of the mother registered in the infant in terms of both their quantity and their quality. Thus the earliest wishes, the earliest pleasures, appear in concert with need satisfaction by the mother. These wishes, of oral (sexual) gratification, are associated with sensory impressions of the mother, the first object, and as the mental apparatus develops are elaborated in idiosyncratic fantasies.

The primary organizer of the wishes is the Oedipus complex. Freud felt there was a period of time, subsequent to the period of first object finding, a kind of latency during the unfolding of psychosexual development, in which the body and of course its mental representation was taken as the primary object. This he termed a period of "autoerotic stimulation," from the oral through the anal to the phallic phase, in which the child becomes, as it were, a pleasure machine. The central place of fantasy in the expression of wishes becomes manifest only at the time of genital primacy, when the Oedipus complex is in the foreground. Only at this time do the component

instincts seek once again an external object. It seemed particularly noteworthy to Freud that instincts belonging to the genital zone regularly passed through a period of intense autoerotic satisfaction: this seemed to prepare the way for the Oedipus complex. The child is now two to four years old, and the objects of this complex are his or her parents.

In Oedipal fantasies, the child seeks sole possession of the desired parent. Any person who has independent claims on that love object is regarded as a rival. Combinations are possible depending upon whether the subject is male or female, the love object mother or father. Opposite-sex attachments are labeled "positive," while the designation for same-sex attachments is "negative." Fantasy and its elaboration in the various designated sets are determined by genital wishes in combination with environmental impressions. Each Oedipal fantasy will favor one of the two parents, but both parents must occupy a place in the complete version of that fantasy. All Oedipal fantasies are rooted in an underlying bisexuality.

At the height of development of the fantasies driven by the wishes of the Oedipal phase, a period of latency ensues in which this excitement more or less dies down. Freud terms this a period of "retrogression" as, in his typical way, he contrasts the biology of human sexuality to its uninterrupted unfolding in other primates. During this period, the child's development provides the moral and intellectual apparatus that will be utilized in resolving Oedipal wishes. This concept of latency is analogous to what Freud describes as "deferred acts," a notion that appears in his earlier clinical formulation and reappears in different clinical contexts throughout his life. In that early model, the traumatic memories engender affect that could not be discharged by ordinary channels. Instead, it undergoes repression and there is a period of latency before that affect reappears in discharge in the form of an hysterical symptom. This term of latency was determined by the external world, for the symptoms were triggered by the appearance of some associated impression.

The Outbreak of Illness and the Compulsion to Repeat

The reappearance of the excitement engendered by Oedipal wishes occurs at puberty with its accompanying maturation of the sexual apparatus. Now the psyche will be challenged by its Oedipal wishes, the demands of which conflict with both reality and morality, or, as Freud writes "ethics and aesthetics." The results of this conflict have a far-reaching effect on the functioning of the ego and may ultimately result in the appearance of symptoms.

The second quantitative factor (after the effects of puberty), which can eventuate in a widening circle of defense and the appearance of symptoms, is the pressure of reality on the maturing adolescent. To the degree that the ego has already been constricted by the conflict over Oedipal wishes, it will find itself too crippled to deal with the demands of object choice and work.

It will be useful here to return to the state of the child's mental apparatus at the height of the Oedipus complex before the subsiding of sexual excitement at the beginning of latency. The experience of intense excitement in the first years of life—a product of external impressions and individual zonal and functional predispositions—will have determined the fixation points to which the child's fantasies will inevitably be attached in her striving to repeat these experiences. This led Freud to say that the neurosis may be regarded as a direct expression of a "fixation" to an early period of the child's life. We can conceive of these fixations, whether to the trauma or the pleasurable excitement, as the source of a compulsion to repeat. They determine the composition of the Oedipal wishes.

How do the conflicts of the Oedipal period arise? Freud thought that the child believed that his erotic and hostile wishes exposed him to a series of overwhelming dangers: of loss of love and fear of castration. These anticipated dangers evoke the defenses that mark the dangers that signal the resolution of the Oedipus complex. In certain individuals, the dangers are so threatening that a childhood neurosis ensues. These symptoms can divert the ego from its normal developmental course, but they rarely continue through latency.

Symptom Formation

The central factor in the character formation and neurosis of adolescence is quantitative—the degree of psychical intensity mobilized in the service of the compulsion. The repetition compulsion is expressed in what Freud characterizes as positive ways and negative ways. The positive expression of the fixation is manifested in character traits such as the type of object choice and the nature of relationships. In them, there is always an endeavor to revive the past, to remember the forgotten experiences, to return to the trauma or fixation by reexperiencing in the external world its underlying fantasy. These repetitive modes of discharge endow the ego with tendencies or character traits that may be looked upon

as normal or neurotic. Freud says that the negative reactions pursue the opposite aim: nothing is to be remembered or repeated of the conflicted wish. Instead, defensive reactions are evoked, such as avoidance or inhibition. These reactions, in the same way as the positive ones, enter into character formation reflecting once again the underlying fixations. Neurotic symptoms represent a compromise in which both the positive and the negative effects of the fixation enter, satisfying, via the compromise, the purposes of both discharge and defense.

Symptom Formation from the Point of View of Repression, Resistance, and the Return of the Repressed

Freud was referring to repression when he spoke of defense, the withdrawal by the ego from unacceptable impulses or memories so that these impressions or memories would not be available to the conscious mind and would not find access to motor discharge. These impressions and memories are incompatible with the ego's integrity and ethical standards; although repressed, they can be observed in therapy in the form of resistances, which by manifesting themselves betray their unconscious origin. Resistance in psychoanalysis is the particular way the ego's defense manifests itself in the psychoanalytic situation.

After the period of latency ends, the repression results in a buildup of sexual instincts, libido, in the unconscious, and inevitably their return to consciousness begins—the return of the repressed. For Freud, the symptom represents substitute sexual satisfaction. In hysteria, the mechanisms utilized by the return of the repressed are largely those of displacement and symbol formation, and in conversion hysteria, somatic compliances. In Freud's theory of obsessional neurosis, there is a stronger emphasis on the repressing factor than the wish-fulfilling impulses because of the presence of reaction formations that reassure against the sexual nature of the underlying wishes. Freud realized early on that the resistances were utilizing the transference to the analyst in both its positive and negative aspects. He saw that transference was used as a weapon by the resistance and that it was in transference that the resistances make their initial impression. It became clear that transference embodies in displacement the meaningful figures of the patient's past.

Dreams and Clinical Theory

To understand the causes of symptom formation, it is useful to return to the model that dominated Freud's clinical theorizing: his theory of dreams. On his theory, the dynamics of dream formation and symptom formation are the same, which means that the same causal factors operate in the normal as in the pathological. This insight led Freud to develop psychoanalysis into a depth psychology with relevance for religion, mythology, literature, and culture. The similarity is clear: what Freud calls the motor power in the formation of dreams are the unconscious impulses represented by the wishful life. Freud believed that these unconscious wishes combine with the latent dream thoughts stimulated by the residues of the preceding waking day to form a dream wish, which then is disguised by the mechanisms of the dream work—condensation, displacement, considerations of representability, and secondary revision. Thus the dream, no less than the hysterical symptom, represents a return of the repressed, made possible in this instance by the wish for sleep with the corresponding withdrawal of psychic investment from the external world. The dream represents wish fulfillment in compromise.

What draws our attention now is Freud's remark that the strangeness of the manifest dream is partly the effect of a restricting, critically disapproving agency of the mind, which he calls "dream censorship." This operation of conscience is present in symptom formation in the form of moral considerations that initiate defense and are represented in the compromise formation.

The Resolution of the Oedipus Complex and Its Effect on the Sexual Instincts

The overpowering fantasies of sole possession of the desired parent at the expense of the child's rival, which had been brought to a focus by the genital sexual organization, now undergo two extraordinary modifications. The parent represents all the dangers that the child fears from his external world: the loss of the love object, the withdrawal of love, and the threat of castration. Driven by another emotion, his love for the feared parent, as well as by his fears, the child internalizes parental prohibitions, thus providing the basis for the moral and ethical notions that will develop in latency. This identification with the parents' own consciences is the origin of a system of ideals, values, and standards that Freud termed the "superego." The dread of conscience now joins the series of dangers, the signals of which initiate the repression of the Oedipal fantasies.

The other fundamental modification, this at the expense of the sexual instincts themselves, is, in Freud's language, the aim inhibition of the drives. In the place of direct sexual satisfaction, satisfaction can now be attained by approximations. To this group of feelings belongs the affection between parents and children, the emotional ties in marriage, and feelings of friendship. Because their direct sexual aims, while held back from attainment, have not been abandoned, these affectionate feelings lead to especially strong and lasting attachments. This aim inhibition is the other sweeping consequence of repression during the resolution of the Oedipus complex.

Symptom Formation and Its Shaping by the Vicissitudes of the Instincts and the Strength of the Ego

We can now view symptom formation with a deeper understanding of the contending forces. First, let us outline the course taken by the Oedipal wishes. Under the sexual pressures of puberty, the Oedipal conflicts take on a renewed intensity. The aims of Oedipal fantasies have achieved some altered satisfaction via aim inhibition. Another, indeed the most important, instinctual satisfaction is obtained by sublimation in which both the aim and the object of the drives powering the wishes are changed. In place of the hostile and erotic wishes, satisfaction is found in achievements that Freud describes as of a higher social or ethical value. In place of the parental object, the objects become those of, for example, the larger artistic, scientific, or civic worlds. These sublimations have begun to take shape in latency, rising to a peak of intensity and focus in adolescence. In this setting, repression is attempting to withhold derivatives of the Oedipal wishes from consciousness and motor discharge. However, the intensity of the instinctual wishes under the compulsion to repeat becomes the determining factor. The instincts, becoming dammed up, regress to earlier developmental phases and correspondingly earlier attitudes toward objects. Reinforced by these fixation points, the instincts break through to consciousness and discharge as substitute sexual satisfaction (symptoms). In this process of regression to fixation points in order to achieve gratification, the instincts can replace one another, so that satisfaction of one can replace the satisfaction of another; they can combine with one another; they can change from activity to passivity; and the instinct's object can become the self.

C

Freud gives the example of a man who had repressed his all-consuming mother fixation from childhood; as an adult, he sought constantly for a woman to keep him. Here the Oedipal wish is realized in a type of object choice, which has been altered by regression and is in the symptomatic foreground as a neurotic character trait, constituting a major ego deformation.

The other side of the conflict arises from the ego. The Oedipal wishes, being incompatible with the integrity of the ego and with its ethical standards, are repressed. The series of dangers evoking catastrophic anxiety in the ego and a threat to its integrity have been noted above. All these dangers, no matter how early their origin, act as instigators or signals mobilizing defense, for the ego too has undergone regression to the fixation points of the childhood struggles over the Oedipal wishes. What defense then contributes is the modification of the wish expressed in symptoms, so that their sexual nature vanishes, and any satisfaction is unrecognizable. In this way, the symptom becomes a compromise formation in which the dangers to the ego that instigated defense are all represented.

The example of obsessional neurosis, with its reaction formation assuring the patient that her attitudes are the opposite of her unconscious sexual or hostile wishes, exhibits a symptom complex in which repression predominates. The danger conspicuously represented in the reaction formation is the voice of conscience. Freud gives another example of predominantly defensive reactions (mentioned above): those individuals whose character is marked by avoiding issues, people in whom inhibition and phobia tend to develop.

What about the strength of the ego? Freud conceived of the ego as the part of the psyche that carried out the biological functions of self-preservation. Thus all functions that carry out relations with the external world, that serve the most adequate adaptation to it, constitute the ego, such as logical thinking, reality testing, and the most effective use of one's mental and physical endowment. The strength of the ego enters from the outset of life into the potential for symptom formation. When we have spoken of the quantitative factor in symptom formation and of the propensity toward fixation, we have also been speaking of the ego's vulnerability to excitation. The psyche's capacity to hold excitation in check is the earliest measure of the ego's strength. Other important measures of ego strength are aim inhibition and, all important to Freud, the presence of a rich sub-

limatory endowment. The burdens imposed during adolescence reveal two different measures of the ego's strength. When symptoms appear, there has been a partial failure of the ego's defensive function, under the renewed pressure of the drives. (We should also mention another sort of pressure: that exerted by the conscience when its inflexibility overpowers the ego's defenses.) But there is still one more consequence of this defensive struggle, which occurs toward the end of adolescence: a weakening of the ego itself. As has been mentioned, character can be altered, albeit in disguised form, by the compulsions exerted by the demands of the hostile and erotic Oedipal wishes. Widespread avoidances and inhibitions may occur. Particular object choices and sexual attitudes that are all-encompassing and yet unpleasurable may develop. These compulsive patterns are independent of outer reality, of the demands of the real world, of reason. Although the ego attempts to organize its functioning in a self-preservative and adaptive way, it is markedly weakened by the compulsive psychical processes that Freud termed "a state within a state, useless for the commonweal." The demands of work and object choice, of what Freud calls "the problems of life," upon the ego that has been thus weakened are another cause of the outbreak of neurotic symptoms, with possibly devastating effects.

Clinical Theory and Narcissism

We have seen above that just as Freud's first clinical theory was conceived in the early efforts to treat hysteria, so later advances were each in turn intimately attached to a deepening understanding of the nature of psychoanalytic treatment. Freud's observations of resistance, and then of transference with its intense positive and negative aims, of fixation, repressed childhood sexual wishes and the Oedipus complex, the return of the repressed in symptom formation, and the symptom as compromise—each found its key place in clinical theory.

In contrast to his typically neurotic patients, Freud treated a class of patients in whom transferences never appeared. The feature common to these patients was the centering of the material of their associations on the self. Some of these patients, those suffering from severe depression, exhibited a relentless absorption with self-depreciation, self-reproaches, and delusion of inferiority and inadequacy. In another group, a paranoid quality was in the foreground. In some, delusions of observation were prominent, in others delusions of persecution. In still others, bodily and even mental preoccupations ranging from conviction of deficiency to delusions of damage and bizarre hypochondria were the essential feature.

Freud saw this unvarying investment of the self on the part of these patients as the determining feature in differentiating them from neurotic patients. He called their disorders the "narcissistic neuroses," in contrast to the transference neuroses. The onset of illness in these patients was marked by a withdrawal of libido from its investment in objects into any of various (distorted and fragmentary) aspects of the self-image. (Freud felt that this occurs under pressure of the drive toward discharge of the infantile wishes. In these narcissistic patients, the investment of the love object has collapsed under that pressure.) In severe depression, the withdrawal of libido is precipitated by an emotional or actual loss of the loved one. The regressive effort to retain investment of the object, to save it, results in an (orally determined) identification with it. The cruel self-depreciation, self-criticism, and self-reproaches are transformed into unconscious attacks on the disappointing object. These attacks on the ego by its self-critical function result from the ego's having retained its forbidden love object. In delusions of observation, the withdrawal of the libido results in the disintegration of the superego.

With the understanding gained from his study of the narcissistic neuroses, Freud's view of libidinal development became more global. He saw the primary libidinal investment as being of the ego. The state of primary narcissism is interrupted by the infant's periods of wakefulness. All subsequent interruptions of the primary state by differentiations of the psyche are marked by libidinal investments. In this way Freud revised his theory of the ego. The primary identification with the parent, who is the small child's model and whose place he wishes to take, is the first appearance of the ego ideal invested with narcissistic libido. Subsequently, as the parents become the objects of the Oedipal wishes, narcissistic libido has become object libido. Accompanying this crucial change in the distribution of the libido is the expansion of the ego ideal into the superego, so that it becomes the carrier of conscience and the instigator of repressing forces. In Freud's words, "the ego ideal has become the heir of the original narcissism." For Freud the self-preservative instincts, too, turn out to be a function of narcissistic aims. Thus any privation such as hunger, cold, or pain is at the same time a narcissistic frustration and occasions a libidinal investment—in this case, of the sensory images

of the primary object, the mother, who restores the state of satiety. As development proceeds, because of the increasing limitations on the child's self-sufficiency and the difficulties in meeting the demands of her environment, she must search increasingly for her narcissistic satisfaction in her acceptance and realization of the standards and values of her ego ideal. The repressing forces in neurotic conflict are now seen by Freud as the narcissistically charged wishes of the ego ideal: the repressed forces, the unconscious Oedipal wishes.

Clinical Theory and Aggression

Transference had one more significant contribution to make to theory: a recognition and deeper understanding of the omnipresence of sadism and masochism. Freud found that there was a class of patients who gave paradoxical responses to his interpretations. Usually, a patient would respond to a piece of insight, or indeed to any intervention regarded as an indicator of progress, by displaying symptom relief or some sign of improvement. But in this particular group of patients, there was invariably a worsening of their illness. Freud termed this response a "negative therapeutic reaction." In his words, "recovery . . . is dreaded as if it were a danger." Among the different resistances to recovery, he considered this one the most powerful. Its prominent feature is a need for punishment, a need invariably satisfied, at the least, by the suffering imposed by the neurotic illness. The need for punishment arises from a sense of guilt of which the patient is unconscious. Freud observed this phenomenon in extreme instances, such as moral masochism, but also felt that the severity of any neurosis varied directly with the severity of the superego and the consequent degree of the need for suffering.

In his studies of obsessional neurosis and melancholia, Freud remarked on the special intensity in them of the sense of guilt. In the obsessional neurosis, the outcome is a ceaseless tormenting criticism of the (unconscious) aggressive impulses on the one hand and on the other a torturing of the object to the degree that defense permits it. In melancholia, there is an unchecked violent attitude of the superego directed against the ego.

The sweep of these clinical considerations, taken together with other investigations that do not belong here, led Freud to revise his theory so that sadism and masochism would occupy a fundamental place. From the clinical side, it took this form. The aggressive instinct appears in development in two ways. On the one hand, it will be directed toward the outer world and is served by the muscular apparatus. On the other hand, aggression is more or less fused with the sexual drive whether oral, anal, or genital. Thus sadism and masochism manifest themselves in each libidinal phase. For example, the wish to devour and the fear of being eaten are characteristic of the oral phase.

Degrees of fusion of aggression with libido may also be observed in the instinctual vicissitudes. When the superego arises out of parental identifications, in each of these identifications a desexualization (in the form of aim inhibition) takes place with the consequent liberation of a quantity of the aggression with which the sexual aim had been fused. This diffusion results in a particular harshness of conscience, via its self-critical and self-punitive functions. In pathology, for example, in which the reaction formation of the obsessional turns the aggression toward the object into its opposite, the patient's superego becomes the vehicle of this aggression directed as unrelenting criticism against the ego. The superego's harshness has taken on sadistic coloring independently of instinctual regression. In melancholia, the identification with the object results in abolishing the externalization of aggression, and the individual's sadism is directed completely internally, against the self, by the superego. In patients suffering from moral masochism, a different vicissitude of aggression is in the foreground. These patients need suffering and seek punishment from the external world, which is their surrogate for parental powers or the superego. In the misfortunes they undergo, they seem victims of fate. Freud points out that the suffering at the behest of external powers (at bottom a beating fantasy) is tantamount to a (regressed) resexualization of the superego and satisfies unconscious negative Oedipal wishes. To this degree, it exemplifies a fusion of aggression and libido and achieves a sexual satisfaction.

Conclusion

To Freud, all human life is marked by its vulnerability to unhappiness. From the outset, falling like a shadow over every child's life is the significance of early injuries to the self in determining later neurotic conflict. Even under the most optimal circumstances, the inevitable feelings of failure, and loss of love in connection with Oedipal disappointments and jealousies, will leave a permanent injury to self-regard, a kind of narcissistic scar that then must burden the child's later development.

The advances in clinical theory have been made through addressing the problem of neurotic suffering. Where were the resistances? Why was it so difficult for the patient to relinquish the painful experience of the past and of the present? Freud summed up the discoveries through which neurosis could be understood: "the foundation . . . is the assumption that there are unconscious mental processes, the recognition of the theory of resistance and repression, the appreciation of the importance of sexuality and of the Oedipus complex" (1923 [1922]), p. 247).

REFERENCES
Breuer, J., and Freud, S. (1893–1895). *Studies on Hysteria*. S.E. 2: 1–310.
Freud, S. (1900). *The Interpretation of Dreams*. S.E. 4–5: 1–621.
———. (1923 [1922]). *Two Encyclopaedia Articles*. S.E. 18: 235–259.

GEORGE E. GROSS
ISAIAH A. RUBIN

Cognition See COGNITIVE PSYCHOLOGY; AND PSYCHOANALYSIS; PRECONSCIOUS UNCONSCIOUS.

Cognitive Psychology, and Psychoanalysis

Many of Freud's methodological assumptions occupy a central place in contemporary cognitive psychology, and many of his distinctive topics are reemerging as important areas of study for cognitive psychologists. Freud and contemporary cognitive psychologists agree that, contrary to the approach of behaviorism, any adequate explanation of human behavior must appeal to mental events, and any adequate explanation of human mentality must move beyond the surface phenomena of behavior to underlying psychical and neurophysiological mechanisms that bring it about.

Methodological Assumptions

Most contemporary cognitive psychologists are similar to Freud in their commitment to physicalism, nonreductionism, and a thoroughly interdisciplinary approach.

a. Physicalism: Cognitive psychologists agree with Freud's view that the brain and central nervous system constitute the organs of thought. Like Freud, they also tend to accept physicalism, the thesis that thinking and all other mental states and events are physical. Besides the many paradoxes produced by mind-body dualism, one attraction of physicalism is the discipline that it brings to psychological theorizing. Cognitive psychologists believe, as Freud did, that a touchstone for the truth of any psychological theory is that it be compatible with known properties of the central nervous system. Although some theorists raise the possibility of "emergent" properties, these properties are thought to emerge from the complex interaction of physical substances.

b. Antireductionism: Despite their acceptance of physicalism, most cognitive psychologists, like Freud, reject the reductionist thesis that ultimately psychological explanations will be replaced by neurophysiological ones. While Freud recognized that some psychotic conditions were the result of relatively simple chemical imbalances in the nervous system, a view that is widely accepted today, he never accepted the idea that psychoanalytic or other psychological categories could be given up in favor of purely neurological descriptions. To understand the rich texture of human mentality, he assumed that it would be necessary to consider general features of development, as well as individual psychological histories.

The "reductionist" label has seemed applicable to Freud, in part, because of his interests in other sciences, particularly neurophysiology and evolutionary biology. In much the fashion of current interdisciplinary cognitive science, Freud's intention was not, however, to reduce psychology to a more basic science, but to draw on other sciences for inspiration and constraints for his psychological models.

Possibly through the common influence of the philosopher Franz Brentano (1838–1917), both Freud and contemporary cognitive psychologists regard the brain as having ideas or representations, which (a) represent various aspects of the external world, (b) are manipulated by various processes, (c) are causally efficacious in bringing about behavior, and (d) may be inaccessible to conscious awareness. The psychologist George Mandler identifies the commitment to a representation/process model of the mind as the central tendency of contemporary work in cognitive psychology. Freud's frequent and cogent defenses of the need for unconscious ideas very probably made the adoption of this model easier than it otherwise would have been, but cognitive psychologists would be right to note a salient difference. In cognitive psychology, representations are regarded as unconscious by virtue of the large amount of information that needs to be processed and the seemingly limited resources of consciousness, and not because they are kept out of consciousness by some special psychic force, such as repression.

Common Topics

a. Consciousness: To some degree, the commonality of topics between psychoanalysis and contemporary work in cognitive psychology is a reflection of a common freedom from behaviorist strictures against any appeal to mentalistic causation. This freedom is most evident in the current resurgence of interest in *consciousness*. Cognitive psychologists would like to understand the properties, function, and cerebral location of conscious thought. Although psychoanalysis focused on the other half of the dichotomy, the unconscious, Freud also attempted to characterize conscious phenomena along these three dimensions. Oddly, contemporary attempts to make sense of the "qualitative" character of conscious phenomena often pursue the same line that Freud took in the *Project*, and assume that qualitative differences noted in conscious phenomena must ultimately be explained in terms of quantitative features of neural action. Because Freud differed from cognitive psychologists in his explanation of the unconscious status of many ideas, he had a much easier time in providing a function for consciousness. Since unconscious ideas were kept apart from sensory evidence and rational thought processes, the function of consciousness was, in a very real sense, liberation. By making unconscious ideas conscious, agents could bring the ideas that led them to act under rational control. Given the utility and sophistication of unconscious mental processes, cognitive psychologists have been at a loss to determine what additional benefits consciousness could confer, and there is little agreement on this issue.

b. Development: Although he recognized the importance of neural functioning, Freud's theories of the mind were largely developmental. This emphasis was a reflection of nineteenth-century views that complex phenomena could be understood only by tracing their development. Largely through the influence of Jean Piaget (1896–1980), this tradition is strongly represented in contemporary *developmental psychology*. As had Freud, Piaget proposed a fairly rigid sequence of developmental states leading to full adult competencies. Recent work has questioned a number of Piaget's claims about the age and order of various cognitive achievements, and

C

current researchers have been much more willing to allow greater influence from innate developmental patterns in addition to learning. Although topics are beginning to change, the focus of much work has been the development of cognitive—as opposed to emotional—capacities.

c. Personality Types: Freud's heirs offered theories of personality types and, after a number of years of eclipse, this topic is beginning to be addressed again. Some recent work has achieved interesting results by combining the notion of enduring personality traits with process models of mental functioning. The hypothesis is that what is stable in individuals are ways of dealing with certain kinds of situations, even though there may be considerable variation in their behavior across situations. Other research has suggested that personality characteristics that are detectable quite early in life have a lasting, recognizable influence on later behavioral tendencies. Although these research programs are relatively new and limited, they may indicate future trends, since cognitive psychology is currently committed to both processing models and work in development.

d. Emotions: As the name suggests, "cognitive" psychology recognizes an important distinction between cognitive processes and the emotions. Ulrich Neisser's seminal text, *Cognitive Psychology,* included no chapters on the emotional side of mental life. By contrast, Freud had a thoroughly cognitive theory of emotions, with emotions having both an affective and an ideational component. Some recent work indicates that the foundational distinction between cognitive processes and others may be breaking down. In a widely reported case of frontal lobe damage (EVR), Antonio Damasio has suggested that although the patient's cognitive capacities, such as IQ, remain intact, emotional deficits create difficulties for his ability to engage in rational planning. From the other side, a number of psychologists have argued that there is an important cognitive component in the emotions. As with recent trends in personality theory, it remains to be seen whether this work will lead to a more central place for the study of emotions in cognitive psychology.

e. Memory: Memory has been an active area of research in cognitive psychology for many years, with different theorists positing a variety of possible memory systems, including short-term and long-term memory, semantic (for words and facts) versus episodic memory, declarative memory versus memory for skills,

and sensory memory "buffers." The focus on the mechanisms of memory has generally led researchers to slight such important questions as the mechanisms of forgetting and the nature of the material that is remembered. Recent empirical work and the methodological assumption that cognition is "constructed" have opened up some new directions that are closer to the traditional concerns of psychoanalysis. The work of Elizabeth Loftus and her colleagues, for example, strongly suggests that memories are nothing like photographic images of past events, but are constructed and reconstructed through time on the basis of various sources of information, including the event itself, later inferences, and the ways in which questions about the event are framed.

f. Self-knowledge: Memory is an important source of self-knowledge, and the view that memories are constructed fits naturally with the resurgence of interest in self-knowledge. Within the behaviorist framework, self-knowledge had no sources of evidence, since both introspection and complex mental processing were ruled out as potential sources. In recent years, however, there has been increasing interest in questions about "metacognition"—our understanding thought processes themselves. One active area of research concerns the so-called theory of mind that children are thought to develop (or have innately) that enables them to understand the actions of others. Another investigates the relation between self-understanding and self-control. In particular, Albert Bandura and his colleagues have argued at length about the importance of the perception of self-efficacy in the performance of different tasks.

g. Dreams: Oddly, considering the blistering criticisms directed at Freud's theory of dreams, a few contemporary scholars have returned to the problem of trying to understand the significance of dreams. In keeping with the computer model of the mind, Crick and Mitchison have suggested that the function of dreaming is to make the brain more efficient, by enabling it to eliminate unwanted information and possibly unwanted neural oscillations. J. Allan Hobson has hypothesized that dreaming is the result of periodic self-stimulation of the brain that leads to a great deal of mental activity, which the synthetic-interpretive processes of the brain try to put in some order, with the result that dreams are partially coherent and partially bizarre. Although Hobson is highly critical of Freud, his attempts at dream interpretation invoke a number of similar ideas, including the classification of dreams into different forms, attempts to understand different types of dream processes, issues of temporality and logic, day residues, and association.

Differences

There are a number of similarities between the overall shape of Freud's project, and the topics that were crucial to it, and contemporary work in cognitive psychology, but there are also striking differences. Nothing in current cognitive psychology echoes Freud's joint emphases on the problems of sexuality and the psychical mechanisms of repression. Even where there are interesting convergences, as in the study of consciousness, the degree of influence is not clear. Freud's diminished reputation in the scientific community is not likely to encourage individuals to claim psychoanalysis as a forebear. If some recent trends in research in personality theory, the relation between emotions and cognition, the construction of memory, and the role of self-knowledge continue, however, and cognitive psychologists try to understand some of the same important, complex, and difficult phenomena that Freud did, they may become more patient with his errors and more interested in his speculations.

REFERENCES

Bandura, A. (1986). *Social Foundations of Thought and Action.* Englewood Cliffs, N.J.: Prentice-Hall.

Crick, F., and Mitchison, G. (1983). The function of dream sleep, *Nature*, 304: 111–114.

Damasio, A. (1994). *Descartes' Error.* New York: Putnam.

Hobson, J. (1988). *The Dreaming Brain.* New York: Basic Books.

Kagan, J. (1994). *Galen's Prophecy: Temperament in Human Nature.* New York: Basic Books.

Leslie, A. (1994). Pretending and believing: Issues in the theory of ToMM. *Cognition*, 50: 211–238.

Loftus, E., and Palmer, J. (1974). Reconstruction of automobile destruction: An example of the interaction between language and memory. *Journal of Verbal Learning and Verbal Behavior*, 13: 585–589.

Mandler, G. (1985). *Cognitive Psychology: An Essay in Cognitive Science.* Hillsdale, N.J.: Lawrence Earlbaum Associates.

Mischel, W., and Shoda, Y. (1995). A cognitive-affective system theory of personality: Reconceptualizing situations, dispositions, dynamics, and invariance in personal structure. *Psychological Review*, 102: 246–268.

Neisser, U. (1967). *Cognitive Psychology.* Englewood Cliffs, N.J.: Prentice-Hall.

PATRICIA KITCHER

Committee, The Secret

C

From the "Protocols of the Vienna Psychoanalytical Society" (Nunberg and Federn, 1962–1975) and other sources, it is known that psychoanalysis as a movement started as early as 1902. The decisive step came with the Second International Psychoanalytical Congress, held in Nuremberg in 1910, where the movement laid down its first formal structures—its articles of association.

In his *An Autobiographical Study*, Freud (1925) noted this important administrative step and indicated the motivation for setting up such an association: "The result of the official Anathema against psycho-analysis was that the analysts began to come closer together. At the second Congress, held in Nuremberg 1910, they formed themselves, on the proposal of Ferenczi, into an 'International Psycho-Analytical Association,' divided into a number of local societies but under a common President. The Association survived the Great War and still exists, consisting today of branch societies in Austria, Germany, Hungary, Switzerland, Great Britain, Holland, Russia, and India, as well as two in the United States" (1925: 50).

According to Ernest Jones: "In these years was launched what was called the 'Psycho-Analytical Movement'—not a very happy phrase, but one employed by friends and foes alike" (Jones, 1955:74). Freud employed this expression for the first time in a letter to Jung, dated February 18, 1908.

An important development within the psychoanalytic movement was the formation of the "Secret Committee," the name Freud gave to a small circle of his colleagues and pupils. Hanns Sachs, in his memoirs *Freud, Master and Friend*, writes for the first time of the existence of this committee: "In these days it was a limited small group of intimates who received this distinction, consisting of Abraham, Eitingon, Ferenczi, Jones, Rank and myself. The devotion to psychoanalysis, as our predominating common interest, the frequent exchange of opinion and ideas, and the cooperation in building up an organized psychoanalytic movement had already done a great deal to bring us closer together" (Sachs, 1944: 153).

The fact that Freud attached much importance to the formation of the Secret Committee and everybody's struggle for the common cause is shown in the symbolic meaning of the ring carrying a Greek gem that he gave to his fellows to express his respect and as an intimate gesture of appreciation. Those honored in such a way wore the ring as a sign of solidarity. Sachs further reports: "The gift of the rings had a certain symbolical significance; it reminded us that our mutual relations had the same center of gravity. It made us feel that we belonged to a group within the group although without any formal ties or the attempt to become a separate organization. Freud changed this state of things during the Convention (Congress) at the Hague, Holland, in 1920" (Sachs, 1944: 153–154). The Secret Committee soon became the leading organ of the psychoanalytic movement because of the introduction of the "circular letter" correspondence.

Freud himself proposed that the committee members exchange circular letters on a regular basis. At weekly intervals, each member was to write a letter on the same day about personal matters, the state of the various psychoanalytic societies, or scientific issues (Grosskurth, 1991). The letters were sent to each member of the Secret Committee but not to other members of the International Association.

Since Hanns Sachs himself was a member of this "mysterious" group of colleagues, contributing decisively toward the scientific and organizational structure and improvement of the psychoanalytic movement, his memories have to be judged critically in regard to the image of Freud as a hero. His information on the conception of the group members, however, still attests to the significance of this institution for the psychoanalytic movement and the administration of psychoanalysis. The history of the Secret Committee's formation and its effects on the psychoanalytic movement have been reconstructed several times, each time with a different emphasis (Grosskurth, 1991; Schröter, 1995; Wittenberger, 1995).

With the first "Statutes of the International Psychoanalytic Association" worked out by Ferenczi together with Freud, an important goal was reached. With the formation of the Secret Committee, an apparent counterprocess of the organizational development took place in 1912. As an informal institution within the association, it originated in response to the tension between Freud and his Swiss "crown prince," C. G. Jung. Jung increasingly disagreed with Freud, and the resulting tension culminated in his rejecting clinical psychoanalysis and breaking off personal correspondence and professional relations with Freud in the years 1910 to 1912.

The history of the Secret Committee can be divided into three phases:

1912–1920: The members of the Secret Committee correspond with each other without any binding rules.

1920–1927: The Secret Committee introduces the circular letter correspondence on certain weekdays.

1927–1936: The Secret Committee forms the board of the International Psychoanalytic Association and continues the circular letter correspondence (Wittenberger and Tögel, 1999).

From the first working period—the period from the formation of the committee in the summer of 1912 to The Hague Congress in 1920—we know from five committee letters so far that the early letters do not have the character of the circular letters. Nevertheless, it can be noted from these early letters that the members of the committee arranged and agreed upon their proper policy together even in its early phase (Wittenberger, 1996). The middle phase, 1920–1927, encompasses the true history of the institution of the Secret Committee. During this period—from September 1920 to March 1926—an extensive correspondence of around 400 letters was maintained.

Because of his leading role in the international psychoanalytic movement at its peak, the departure of Otto Rank from the Secret Committee (at the end of 1924/beginning of 1925) was the most important event leading to its destabilization and final breakup (Lieberman, 1985). Other significant factors in the breakup were Freud's cancer (spring 1923) and the death of Abraham (December 1925). The reasons for the breakup pertained to both the group dynamics of the "study group" and the specific dynamic in Otto Rank's relationship to Sigmund Freud on the one hand and to his colleagues—rivals who all had hopes of succeeding the "master"—on the other.

A gap of around two years exists (from April 1924 to November 1926) between the gradual termination of the circular letter correspondence and its official renewal. The committee members compensated for this communication gap by intensifying their private correspondence with Freud. Only after the sending of the Vienna circular letter, dated November 23, 1926, and written by Anna Freud from Freud's dictation, was a new agreement on reintroducing the circular letter correspondence made possible, and finally achieved.

Thus, the third working phase (1927–1936) of the former Secret Committee began, as the committee was transformed into a board of the International Psychoanalytic Association. As Jones notes: "After the Innsbruck Congress we changed the structure of the Committee by converting it into a group, no longer private, of the officials of the International Association. They were Eitingon, the President; Ferenczi and myself, Vice-Presidents; Anna Freud, Secretary, and van Ophuijsen, Treasurer" (Jones, 1957: 143–144.) During this period, Hanns Sachs left the committee.

The board later renewed the tradition of the committee again and continued the circular letter correspondence. Known to us so far are 83 circular letters from this last period before World War II; they provide only a small insight into the efforts and difficulties of those forced to emigrate because of the seizure of power by the Fascists.

REFERENCES

Freud, S. (1925). *An Autobiographical Study.* S.E. 20: 7–70.

Grosskurth, P. (1991). *The Secret Ring. Freud's Inner Circle and the Politics of Psychoanalysis.* Reading, Mass.: Addison-Wesley.

Jones, E. (1955). *Life and Work of Sigmund Freud, vol. 2: Years of Maturity, 1901–1919.* London: Hogarth Press.

———. (1957). *Life and Work of Sigmund Freud, vol. 3: The Last Phase, 1919–1939.* London: Hogarth Press.

Lieberman, E. J. (1985). *Acts of Will. The Life and Work of Otto Rank.* New York: Free Press.

Nunberg, H., and Federn, E. (eds.) (1962–1975). *The Minutes of the Vienna Psychoanalytic Society, 1906–1918.* 4 vols. New York: International University Press.

Sachs, H. (1944). *Freud—Master and Friend.* Cambridge, Mass.: Harvard University Press.

Schröter, M. (1995). Freuds' Komitee 1912–1914. Ein Beitrag zum Verständnis psychoanalytischer Gruppenbildung. *Psyche,* 49: 513–563.

Wittenberger, G. (1995). *Das "Geheime Komitee" Sigmund Freuds. Institutionalisierungsprozesse in der Psychoanalytischen Bewegung zwischen 1912 und 1927.* Tübingen: Edition Diskord.

———. (1996). The Circular Letters (Rundbriefe) as a means of communication of the "Secret Committee" of Sigmund Freud. *International Forum of Psychoanalysis,* 5: 111–121.

Wittenberger, G., and C. Tögel (1999). *Die Rundbriefe des "Geheimen Komitee," Band 1: 1913–1920.* Tübingen: Edition Diskord.

GERHARD WITTENBERGER

Compulsion and Obsession

Freud described many of the key elements of obsessional neurosis in his early psychoanalytic writings. In 1894 he noted that those people who lack the hysteric's "aptitude" for the use of conversion to manage an incompatible (unacceptable) idea must instead hold in their minds the affect associated with this idea, but separate it from its ideational content. This separated, "free" affect, he wrote, "attaches itself to other ideas which are not in themselves incompatible; and thanks to this 'false connection', those ideas turn into obsessional ideas" (p. 52). Two years later (1896), Freud expanded this view, saying that obsessional neurosis is triggered by "*return of the repressed memories*" (p. 169), which, however, do not return in their original form. Rather, by combining with their associated "self-reproaches," obsessional ideas and affects are created that are "structures in the nature of a *compromise* between the repressed ideas and the repressing ones" (p. 170). At this early point, Freud also distinguished obsessional ideas resulting from the substitution of something current for the repressed content, from obsessions that represent principally transformation of the repressed self-reproach. In the latter case, he found the basis for many instances of obsessional shame, hypochondriacal worry, social anxiety, and depression (melancholia). Finally, he explained many complex obsessional rituals as the result of transferring energy from simply defending against the original forbidden thought to secondary "protective measures" also designed to ward off awareness, but whose connections to the underlying forbidden thought are initially obscure. For instance, he analyzed complex bedtime rituals showing their symbolic protection against actual or fantasied sexual seduction.

Freud's next major advance with respect to obsessionality was to define the basic tenets of obsessional character, namely, orderliness, parsimoniousness, and obstinacy (1908). He related these characteristics to sublimation of, or reaction formation to, underlying anal erotism (the theory of which he had introduced three years before in the *Three Essays on Sexuality* [1906]). Later, he introduced the concept of the anal-sadistic stage, the first of the pregenital stages of development defined by a component instinct, which gave a locus for fixation, or a locus to which the psyche could regress, in obsessional neurosis (1913). Regression to the anal-sadistic phase became from that point forward a central element in the understanding of obsessional neurosis.

In his analysis of the Rat Man, Freud gave his most comprehensive description of the pathology and technique of treatment with an obsessional patient (1909, S.E. 10: 153–318). The case illustrates the complex, condensed nature of apparently illogical symptomatology and many of the characteristic defenses of obsessional neurosis:

doing and undoing, isolation of affect, reaction formation, displacement and generalization, obsessive doubt, corruption of the intellect for defensive purposes ("the capacity for being illogical" [p. 208]), and ambivalence. Seventeen years later, in *Inhibitions, Symptoms and Anxiety* (1926), Freud could add to this list the tendency of obsessionals to suffer with a severe superego.

Since Freud, there has been surprisingly little psychoanalytic focus on obsessional neurosis, with the exception of the 1965 international congress that was devoted to this topic. There, Sandler and Joffe (1965) described the basis for the use in obsessional neurosis of ego functions that develop during the anal phase as arising owing to ego, not only drive, regression. They also described an ego style linked with fixation at the anal phase that is distinct from anal character—a style that involves delay and control in thinking, speaking, and acting. Post-Freudian analytic literature also has reexamined the specific case of the Rat Man (Zetzel, 1966; Lipton, 1977; Muslin, 1979; Blacker and Abraham, 1982–1983) and the relationship of obsessionality to the psychiatric diagnosis of obsessive-compulsive disorder (Esman, 1989).

Shengold (1967, 1971, 1982, 1985) has written of the continued importance in psychoanalytic thinking of drive theory, particularly of anality. He describes the narrowing, in people with defensive anality and anal narcissism, of one's world view to create a controlled anal world in which objects and feelings are rendered devalued and the same—fecalized, and in which the individual is king. He describes this restriction of experience as like the function of the anal sphincter: fulfilling an essential task of being able to close off, to create a boundary, between oneself and the world in order to have a sense of self, while also maintaining a limited form of object relationship. People who have suffered early traumatic experience may have had to defensively create such a closed system that is lacking in flexibility and the capacity to fully value others as people. Shengold's work has added to our understanding of the experience and defensive structure of many obsessional patients.

Dodes (1996) suggests a redefinition of "compulsion" in the light of his work on addiction. His formulation of addictive behavior as an unconscious effort to restore a sense of narcissistic potency against traumatically perceived helplessness—an effort driven by narcissistic rage at helplessness—applies also to a great many compulsions. He suggests that addictions can be under-

stood to be a subset of compulsions, while many compulsions can be more deeply understood with this formulation to be true addictions. Although addiction and compulsion clearly have in common a quality of "compulsiveness," this was the first attempt to demonstrate their psychodynamic unity.

REFERENCES

Blacker, K. H., and Abraham, R. (1982–83). The rat man revisited: Comments on maternal influences. *International Journal of Psychoanalysis and Psychotherapy*, 9: 705–727.

Dodes, L. (1996). Compulsion and addiction. *Journal of the American Psychoanalytic Association*, 44: 815–835.

Esman, A. (1989). Psychoanalysis and general psychiatry: Obsessive-compulsive disorder as paradigm. *Journal of the American Psychoanalytic Association*, 37: 319–336.

Lipton, S. D. (1977). The advantages of Freud's technique as shown in his analysis of the rat man. *International Institute of Psychoanalysis*, 58: 255–273.

Muslin, H. L. (1979). Transference in the rat man case: The transference in transition. *International American Psychoanalytic Association*, 27: 561–579.

Sandler, J., and Joffe, W. G. (1965). Notes on obsessional manifestations of children. *Psychoanalytic Study Child*, 20: 425–438.

Shengold, L. (1967). The effects of overstimulation: Rat people. *International Journal of Psychoanalysis*, 48: 403–415.

———. (1971). More about rats and rat people. *International Journal of Psychoanalysis*, 52: 277–288.

———. (1982). Anal erogeneity: The goose and the rat. *International Journal of Psychoanalysis*, 63: 331–345.

———. (1985). Defensive anality and anal narcissism. *International Journal of Psychoanalysis*, 66: 27–73.

Zetzel, E. R. (1966). Additional notes upon a case of obsessional neurosis: Freud 1909. *International Journal of Psychoanalysis*, 47: 123–129.

LANCE DODES

Compulsion to Repeat

See REPETITION COMPULSION.

Confidentiality

The principle that certain types of information learned in a professional relationship will remain private.

The need for absolute confidentiality, however, varies. The accountant-client relationship is a confidential one, but by agreement its results are reported to government taxing agencies. The clergyman-penitent relationship is granted unique status in some jurisdictions; in California the legal privilege (see below) of confidentiality may be asserted by the clergyman as well as the penitent, contrary to the legal rights of any other professional. The confidentiality of the Catholic confessional is considered by the church to be inviolate.

In recent years, the psychoanalytic requirement of total confidentiality has been asserted to be equal to that of the penitential relationship. That is so because, unlike all other confidential situations, the patient reveals to the analyst not just conscious information, but in the course of the analytic process, information heretofore unconscious to the patient himself. Free association, the core technique of the psychoanalytic process, maximizes the emergence of unconscious contents.

The term "psychotherapy" needs careful definition. In its broadest meaning, it includes psychoanalysis proper. Other therapies that work by the same core principles but are typically of a shorter duration may called "psychoanalytically oriented psychotherapy," or just "psychoanalytic psychotherapy."

At the other end of the so-called therapy spectrum are professional services that are more aptly called guidance, counseling, educational counseling, social welfare, or, as has recently been proposed by Bollas and Sundelson (1995), "social counseling." The provision of these services should be distinguished from psychoanalysis and psychoanalytic psychotherapy, even if performed by a psychoanalyst. In counseling, unconscious contents are not sought by the psychoanalytic technique of free association. The need for confidentiality in this kind of counseling is not as essential as it is in psychoanalysis and psychoanalytic psychotherapy.

In the legal process, evidence is needed to support the two sides in each case, and citizens are required to give sworn testimony supplying that evidence. The law provides certain exceptions to that requirement, stating that certain information is "privileged." The concept of privilege needs definition because of its close association with confidentiality.

"Privilege" means that some evidence otherwise open to litigating parties may be kept from them by some holders of evidence under certain circumstances. For example, the client's communications with his lawyer are held to be confidential, protected by a legal privilege. If a client is asked, "What did you tell your attorney?", he may say, "I assert my client-attorney privilege to not reveal that information." The client holds the privilege, not the attorney. The attorney *must* assert it if the client is silent. The client, however, has the right to *waive* his privilege, break the confidentiality, and give the information. The professional party may not.

As stated above, in some jurisdictions the clergyman has a unique privilege, independent of the penitent, which he may assert. California is one such jurisdiction.

In *In re: Lifschutz* (1970), the California Supreme Court did not sustain Dr. Joseph Lifschutz in his contention that the psychoanalytic psychotherapist merited the same independent privilege granted in California to the clergyman. Otherwise, this opinion strongly supported the general need for psychotherapist-patient privacy.

The importance of that opinion of the California Supreme Court arises from the fact that it was the first psychotherapeutic confidentiality case, federal or state, determined by an appellate court opinion.

In July 1976, the California Supreme Court rendered an opinion in the case of *Tarasoff v. the Regents of the University of California* that has had far-ranging legal effects in all jurisdictions in the United States. Tatania Tarasoff, a student at the University of California at Berkeley, was murdered there. Her assailant had been in psychotherapy at the University Student Health Service. The court held that it was the duty of the psychotherapist to *warn* and *protect* the victim of a potentially violent patient, that confidentiality was superseded in such circumstances. This so-called Tarasoff rule to warn and protect is frequently quoted.

In July 1977, Dr. George Caesar of Marin County, California, spent three days incarcerated by a Superior court judge for refusing to testify about a patient, a litigant in a civil suit. His argument was that if he testified publicly, he was very likely to cause his patient great mental and emotional distress, and that he would thereby be violating that part of his Hippocratic oath that says "primum non nocere" (first do no harm). Caesar's case had been appealed to the United States Ninth Circuit Court of Appeals (*Caesar v. Montanos*), which ruled against Caesar. An extensive minority opinion was written, supporting Caesar and the fundamental right of psychotherapeutic confidentiality.

A number of other cases have occurred since then in various jurisdictions in the United States, none of which have prevented the gradual and by now extreme erosion of psychotherapeutic privacy, especially after 1985. This has been dramatically documented by Bollas and Sundelson in *The New Informants: The Betrayal of Confidentiality in Psychoanalysis and Psychotherapy* (1995). The insurance industry today takes for granted that detailed information about patients in psychoanalysis and psychotherapy must be available to them to permit

C

insurance support of the treatment. These issues are dealt with in detail by Bollas and Sundelson, who decry the passivity and inaction of all the therapy professional associations in the face of this undermining of a central psychotherapeutic requirement.

In the United States, there were, until recently, no formal rules and regulations relating to privilege and confidentiality under federal law. This situation changed as a result of the case of *Jaffe v. Redmond*. In June 1991, an Illinois police officer, Mary Lu Redmond, shot and killed Ricky Allen Sr. in the line of duty. After the shooting, Officer Redmond sought counseling (or therapy?) from a licensed clinical social worker. Allen's family sought damages for his death, and subpoenaed the social worker and her records. She refused to give up her records, and after much legal maneuvering, the trial judge instructed the jury "that it could draw an adverse inference from the defendant's [Redmond's] failure to produce the social worker's notes." The jury voted in favor of the plaintiff's (Allen's) family. Upon appeal to the United States Court of Appeals, Seventh Circuit, the court reversed the ruling and asserted: "[r]eason and experience compel the recognition of a psychotherapist/patient privilege." The Seventh Circuit Court referred to *In re: Lifschutz* (quoting *Griswold v. Connecticut*): "We believe that a patient's interest in keeping such confidential revelations from public purview, in retaining this substantial privacy, has deeper roots than the [state] statute and draws sustenance from our constitutional heritage. . . . [T]he United States Supreme Court declared that 'Various guarantees [of the Bill of Rights] create zones of privacy,' and we believe that the confidentiality of the psychotherapeutic session falls within one such zone."

After the ruling of the Appeals Court, several professional psychotherapy organizations wrote amicus curiae briefs to the United States Supreme Court urging concurrence with the opinion of the Seventh Circuit Court of Appeals in *Jaffee v. Redmond*. In 1996, the United States Supreme Court affirmed the judgment of the Court of Appeals, holding that federal law recognizes privilege protecting confidential communication between a psychotherapist and her patient.

REFERENCES

Bollas, C., and Sundelson, D. (1995). *The New Informants: The Betrayal of Confidentiality in Psychoanalysis and Psychotherapy*. Northvale, N.J.: Jason Aronson.

Caesar v. Montanos. (1976). 542 F.2nd 1064 (9th Cir.).

Griswold v. Connecticut. (1965). 381 U.S. 479 85 S.Ct. 1678.

In re: Lifschutz. (1970). 2 Cal 3rd 415.

Jaffee v. Redmond. (1996). U.S. Supreme Court Case #95-266.

Tarasoff v. Regents of the University of California. 17 Cal. 3rd 425, 131 Cal Rptr. 14.

JOSEPH E. LIFSCHUTZ

Conflicts, Theory of

The concept of conflict was at the center of Freud's understanding of the mind's functioning in everyday life and in all forms of psychopathology. The pleasure principle, which Freud believed motivates human beings, creates ubiquitous social conflicts and, eventually, internal conflicts, as aspects of social convention and prohibition are encoded within each individual. Freud developed the analytic process to facilitate the working through and resolution of these internal, unconscious conflicts.

Freud's Evolving Theory of Conflict

In Freud's early work with Breuer (Breuer and Freud, 1893–1895), conflict was theorized to revolve around the moral prohibitions and injunctions of society and the buried, undifferentiated, often primitive affects associated with traumatic events. Freud introduced the concept of conflict when he encountered what he termed "resistance" in his patients, once he gave up use of the technique of hypnosis. In asking patients to say as much as possible of what came to mind (free association), he noted that all patients resisted. The resistance was explained in terms of patient conflicts.

Freud (1900; 1905) later began to think of ways in which conflict involved internal forces and not exclusively actual traumatic events. He also began to think about instincts more than affects as internal sources of conflict.

In Freud's original theory of conflict, aggressive drives were not featured. Instead, conflicts were between sexual and ego self-preservative instincts (Freud, 1910; 1914). Freud later (1920) introduced aggressive drives; conflicts were now theorized to be between instinctual drives and defense mechanisms employed to prevent their emergence into the individual's awareness. On this view, the death (or destructive) instinct manifests itself in various forms in human life, including the pervasiveness of an unconscious feeling of guilt. The aggressive drives are also manifested in the resistance against the uncovering of defense, and in the unanalyzable residue

C

of masochism. Finally, Freud (1937) described the need for suffering and a propensity for inner conflict. He viewed inner conflict as the result of the turning inward of our aggressiveness (1937). This would have happened "in the course of man's development from a primitive state to a civilized one. If so, his internal conflicts would certainly be the proper equivalent for the external struggles that have then ceased" (1937, p. 244).

Conflict and Defense

While Freud's theory of defenses went through several stages of development, the concept of defense was always important in his theory of conflict. Freud's paper on *The Neuro-psychoses of Defense* (1894) spelled out a view of cathexis and countercathexis that involved both his early theory of conflict and defense. In this paper, he postulates a force (cathexis) spread out like an electric charge that meets up with a counterforce (or countercathexis) to impede its emergence into consciousness. Thus, there was from the outset a postulated conflict between opposing forces.

In Freud's paper on the neuropsychoses of defense (1894), defense is conceptualized in terms of repression and repressing forces. In his early view of defense contained in the topographic model (1901), there are essentially two parts of a conflict: the unconscious (id) and censorship (defense). In his theory of dreams, for example, repression is said to undergo a relaxation of censorship through a kind of compromise formation in which the individual's wish is expressed in a disguised form in accordance with certain censorship demands.

With the introduction of the structural model (Freud, 1923) and the theory of signal anxiety (Freud, 1926), defenses were associated with the ego and were more sharply defined in terms of function and motive. They functioned to keep forbidden, instinctual impulses unconscious. Symptoms were seen as a kind of compromise formation between instincts and defense. Anxiety was viewed now as the motive for defense. Long after Freud's contributions, the importance of defenses continued to be intrinsic to the study of conflict in the work of such writers as Gill (1963), Schafer (1968), and Brenner (1975; 1982).

Thus psychoanalytic theory has, from the beginning, understood the organization of the psychic apparatus in terms of defense and conflict. Freud understood the relationship between the individual and the environment as basically antagonistic. He assumed that an environmen-

tal stimulus is something hostile to the individual and to the nervous system. Ultimately, instinct is understood as a need or compulsion to abolish stimuli. Any stimulus represents a threat. Freud concludes that "at the very beginning it seems the external world, objects, and what is hated are identical" (1915, p. 136).

Conflict and the Structural Theory

In *Beyond the Pleasure Principle* (Freud, 1920) and *The Ego and the Id* (Freud, 1923), Freud changed his views about the nature of neurotic conflict. In moving to a structural view, Freud no longer viewed conflict as between conscious and unconscious ideas or wishes. Now, he viewed conflict as existing between the coherent ego and the repressed. In his new formulation, what causes conflict is not the fact that what is repressed is unconscious (which it is by definition). Instead, it is that this repressed content is split off from the coherent ego. Within the structural model, neurotic symptom formation was largely understandable in terms of conflict among the different psychic structures.

In Freud's structural theory, conflict occurs among the id, the ego, and the superego. The id is the source of impulses derived from drive tensions. The superego consists of internalized images of parental figures derived from instinctual tensions. The ego tries to negotiate between the demands and requirements of the outside world, the id's demand for impulse gratification, and the superego's prohibitions. Except for its role as mediator, the ego is said to have no clearly defined interests of its own other than the completion of these negotiations with the least anxiety possible. This view of the ego contrasts with that of ego psychology, a post-Freudian theory developed largely in the United States, which characterizes the ego as having dynamic qualities in its own right, not simply as a mediator of internal conflicts.

Brenner (1975) suggests that although the concept of psychic conflict occupied an important position in psychoanalytic theory from the start, it was not truly central to Freud's theory of neurosis prior to 1926. Before this time, Freud viewed anxiety as a consequence of the failure of repression rather than the motive for repression, but in a 1926 paper, he gave conflict and anxiety central roles in the formation of neurosis. Specifically, he identified several "danger" situations associated with childhood instinctual life, engendering anxiety and conflict throughout the life of the individual. The danger situations, or "calamities of childhood," that Freud identified were object loss, loss of love, and castration. According to Freud, these situations are the ideational content of anxiety aroused by drive derivatives.

Conflict and the Compulsion to Repeat

An important aspect of conflict is how it relates to repetition and the repetition compulsion. Freud emphasized psychosexual development and its importance in the formation of neurosis. Conflicts are repeated throughout development. For example, in puberty there is the danger that sexuality will be drawn into the process of repression, as was infantile sexuality during earlier development. In puberty, the Oedipal situation is often repeated; Freud emphasized that the danger is that in its repetition, the individual will not be able to avail him- or herself of the augmented ego development occurring during latency and early adolescence. Instead, repression of Oedipal conflict occurs more in the context of infantile prototypes. During analysis, the conflict is made to be repeated or reactivated through interpretation. Through the process of interpretation, the ego is called upon for its observational capacities during the reactivation of the conflict. This process is what allows repeating to include remembering and the transformation of infantile repressed conflicts into novel configurations.

The compulsion to repeat unconscious conflicts and wishes more passively is due to their not having been exposed to the influence of the organizing activity of the ego. In other words, conflicts are likely to be repeated because they have remained under the influence of repression. This was one of Freud's major discoveries concerning psychic determinism. In developing the concept of psychic determinism, Freud suggested that behaviors were partly determined by unconscious memories and conflicts. The notion that so much of our behavior was determined by psychic conflict made it possible to develop a treatment technique organized around the modification and reorganization of psychic conflict.

The patient is compelled to repeat, in the transference, unconscious infantile experience and conflict. The analyst, by bringing these experiences into consciousness, is moving toward mitigating the compulsive component of the behavior through the broadening of the ego's observing capacity. What is being observed are the affective components of conflict attached to infantile fantasies and experience. As these conflicts are observed,

the patient can remember and integrate affects surrounding the conflicts in a new way. Transference is often the medium through which the patient learns that certain kinds of psychic experiences involving wishes and conflict have been automatic or reflexive. As Loewald (1980, p. 92) put it: "The analyst, in other words, tends to evoke in the patient a sense of personal psychic involvement as compared with purely unconscious automatic process. We try to make the patient see, or rather feel, that he as an actor is or can be involved, that he was compelled by his unconscious because it had been automatic and autonomous."

Post-Freudian Conceptualizations of Conflict

One issue that arose in post-Freudian theorizing concerns the infant's interest in external reality. For Freud, such interest develops only as a result of conflicts arising from the failure to gratify instinctual needs. This idea was first challenged by Hartmann (1939; 1950; 1958; 1964), who introduced the concept of "autonomous ego function" and a conflict-free sphere, suggesting that the infant can become interested in reality independently of the frustration of instinctual needs. The concept of a conflict-free area further suggested a functional area in ego development that is, in the main, neither complicated nor stimulated by conflict.

Freud's thesis about the infant's interest in reality was also challenged from a very different perspective than Hartmann's. Freud's belief in the reality principle suggests that the only way to be directed toward the external world through perception and memory is through conflict. From the perspective of British object relations theory, Fairbairn (1952) argued, in contrast to Freud's view, that there is a drive that is inherently interested in and directed toward objects existing in reality.

Another issue addressed by Fairbairn (1952) concerns motivation and conflict. For Freud, the central conflict within an individual arises from clashes of instinctual aims, social demands, and external reality. For Fairbairn, the central conflict involves maintaining the wholeness of experiences of the self in relation to other people.

Kernberg (1975) built on the contributions of both Fairbairn's object relations theory and Hartmann's ego psychology in spelling out his view of conflict, particularly for severe character pathology. According to Kernberg's development of Fairbairn's psychology, unconscious intrapsychic conflicts are not simply conflicts between impulse and defense. These conflicts include two opposing units or sets of internalized object relations. Each of these units involves a self and an object representation under the impact of a drive derivative (clinically, an "affect disposition"). Both impulse and defense are expressed through an internalized object relation that has been imbued with a particular affect disposition.

Rejecting much of Fairbairn's metapsychology, a great deal of relationally oriented theory in the United States during the last twenty years (e.g., Mitchell, 1988; 1997) has tried to redefine conflict in terms of internalized relational configurations. In American relational theory, conflict relates to varying affects, but affects are always tied inextricably to objects. For example, Loewald, as early as 1960, suggested that all drives and objects are integrated from the outset of development.

Much of the post-Freudian development of conflict theory has been concerned with the nature of defensive functioning and the Freudian emphasis on drives as instinctually based phenomena. Gill's (1963) main emphasis was on what he called "hierarchical layering" of the defensive and conflict apparatus. Gill was interested in defenses as behaviors, affects, and ideas that can be either conscious or unconscious, that can serve simultaneously as drives that are more primitive, and that are more socially acceptable. Gill (p. 123) states that "any behavior simultaneously has impulse and defense aspects. . . . What is defense in one layer is impulse in relation to another layer. . . . In general, a behavior is a defense in relation to a drive more primitive than itself, and a drive in relation to a defense more advanced that itself." Defenses are also for Gill a form of compromise formation in that the same mechanism can serve both defense and impulse-expression purposes.

Schafer (1968) was also interested in the layering of conflict and defense, and particularly in the notion of defense as compromise formation. He argues that Freud's theory of conflict and defense ignored a theoretical problem about the unconscious status of defenses themselves. In conceptualizing ego defenses in the structural model as being organized against id impulses, Freud minimized the issue of why defenses are by definition unconscious in nature. Schafer (1968) holds that it is more accurate to think of the ego's mechanisms of defense as themselves having a dynamic nature consisting of ego wishes as a part of defensive activity. In a sense, Schafer is arguing that conflict is even more ubiq-

uitous than Freud suggested in his structural model. In Schafer's view, each of the agencies is riddled with conflict including wishes, demands, and prohibitions.

Charles Brenner (1975) has been one of the most active and prolific writer about conflict theory. He claims that the unpleasurable affects that trigger psychic conflict are of two kinds, anxiety and depressive affect (p. 55). For Freud, conflict occurs whenever gratification of a drive derivative is associated with a sufficiently intense, unpleasurable affect. This includes, for example, superego demands and prohibitions that arouse anxiety or depressive affect of varying levels of intensity. Both depressive affect and anxiety are unpleasurable and differ only in their ideational content. They are both based on the calamities of childhood that Freud (1926) identified as the typical dangers of childhood psychic life. According to Brenner, anxiety and depressive affect differ along the lines of a temporal component. An experience of unpleasure and the idea that one or more calamities has happened is what leads to or constitutes depressive affect. In contrast, an experience of unpleasure and the idea that one or more calamity *will* occur is what constitutes anxiety.

This change by Brenner also led him to revise his theory of defense, again in a manner importantly related to his concept of conflict. He suggests that there are no special mechanisms of defense: "Whatever ensues in mental life which results in a diminution of anxiety or depressive affect—ideally in their disappearance—belongs under the heading of defense (1975, p. 72). Unlike Schafer (1968), Brenner does not see defenses as a form of compromise formation, or "double agents" in Schafer's terminology. Instead, a defense "is an aspect of mental functioning which is definable only in terms of its consequence: the reduction of anxiety and/or depressive affect associated with a drive derivative or with superego functioning" (p. 72).

Another issue in post-Freudian theorizing about conflict concerns the role of the self. George Klein (1976) tried to reformulate psychoanalytic theory as a theory of the self and to alter the Freudian account of the essential nature of conflict. If at the heart of Freud's perspective lie the individual's attempts at "constant resolution of incompatible aims and tendencies," then Klein suggested that the resolution of these incompatibilities was motivated by the need for an integrated and coherent self. For Klein, conflict does not occur between forces but in relation to self-experience and self-conception.

C

This implies that repression relates to "lived meanings," which are in some way dissociated or separated from the self, in contrast to the notion that repression occurs as a defense against unconscious content.

A. Kris (1982) differentiated between two kinds of conflict encountered through the process of free association. He refers to the "conflicts of defense" as the resistance or reluctance that is encountered in the patient's attempt to free-associate. This is one of Freud's earliest and most important discoveries and gave rise to what later became known as "defense analysis." Kris notes that the second broad group of conflicts centers around what he refers to as "conflicts of ambivalence." Freud thought of ambivalence as simultaneous feelings of love and hate or arising between active and passive libidinal aims; Kris, in contrast, argues that conflicts of ambivalence are manifested in many ways during the process of free associating. For example, they may appear in the context of what Kris (1977) refers to as "either-or" attitudes. This sort of attitude creates a sense in the patient of having insoluble problems because of the unconscious threat of loss. Other manifestations of conflicts of ambivalence involve self-critical attitudes in which an injunction is experienced that the individual should give up one side of a conflict.

A major issue related to conflict theory throughout the history of post-Freudian psychoanalysis has hinged on the question of whether conflict is at the center of all forms of psychopathology. There has been a repeated argument that some forms of psychopathology have included certain kinds of deficits, or what has been termed "developmental arrest." Patients exhibiting such pathologies are viewed as not having reached a developmental stage in which conflict and problems of ambivalence are prominently featured. Kohut (1971) suggests a dichotomy between developmental self-defects and intrapsychic conflict. On his view, patients with narcissistic personality disorders in particular are less likely to experience Oedipal conflicts than more primary self-defects. Many psychoanalysts have debated the merits of viewing psychopathology in bifurcated terms or, instead, as seeing conflict as a ubiquitous part of experience at all levels of psychopathology.

Conflict remains a linchpin concept in the psychoanalytic vision of human functioning, even though the basis for conflict and its referent points has been broadened. In fact, the diversification of perspectives about the nature and basis of conflict is probably, at the core, the most significant part of a vastly diversified theoretical body within contemporary psychoanalysis.

REFERENCES

Brenner, C. (1975). Affects and psychic conflict. *Psychoanalytic Quarterly*, 44: 5–28.

———. (1982). *The Mind in Conflict*. New York: International Universities Press.

Breuer, J. and Freud, S. (1893–1895). *Studies on Hysteria*. S.E. 2: 19–305.

Fairbairn, R. (1952). *An Object Relations Theory of the Personality*. New York: Basic Books.

Freud, S. (1894). *The Neuro-Psychoses of Defense*. S.E. 3: 43–61.

———. (1900). *The Interpretation of Dreams*. S.E. 4–5: 1–621.

———. (1901). *On Dreams*. S.E. 5: 633–686.

———. (1905). *Three Essays on Sexuality*. S.E. 7: 130–243.

———. (1910). *Five Lectures on Psycho-Analysis*. S.E. 12: 1–82.

———. (1914). *On Narcissism: An Introduction*. S.E. 14: 67–72.

———. (1915). *Instincts and Their Vicissitudes*. S.E. 14: 117–140.

———. (1920). *Beyond the Pleasure Principle*. S.E. 18: 3–64.

———. (1923). *The Ego and the Id*. S.E. 19: 1–66.

———. (1926). *Inhibitions, Symptoms and Anxiety*. S.E. 20: 75–175.

———. (1937). *Analysis Terminable and Interminable*. S.E. 23: 209–253.

Gill, M. (1963). *Topography and Systems in Psychoanalytic Theory*. New York: International Universities Press.

Hartmann, H. (1939). *Ego Psychology and the Problem of Adaptation*. New York: International Universities Press.

———. (1950). Psychoanalysis and developmental psychology. *Essays on Ego Psychology*. New York: International Universities Press, 1964.

———. (1958). Comments on scientific aspects of psychoanalysis. *Essays on Ego Psychology*. New York: International Universities Press, 1964.

———. (1964). *Ego Psychology and the Problem of Adaptation*. New York: International Universities Press.

Kernberg, O. (1975). *Borderline Conditions and Pathological Narcissism*. New York: Jason Aronson.

Klein, G. (1976). *Psychoanalytic Theory: An Exploration of Essentials*. New York: International Universities Press.

Kohut, H. (1971). *The Analysis of the Self*. New York: International Universities Press.

Kris, A. (1977). Either-or dilemmas. *Psychoanalytic Study of the Child*, 32: 91–117.

———. (1982). *Free Association*. New Haven, Conn.: Yale University Press.

Loewald, H. (1980). *Papers on Psychoanalysis*. New Haven, Conn.: Yale University Press.

Mitchell, S. (1988). *Relational Concepts in Psychoanalysis*. Cambridge, Mass.: Harvard University Press.

Schafer, R. (1968). The mechanisms of defense. *International Journal of Psycho-analysis*, 49: 49–65.

STEVEN H. COOPER

Conscience See SUPEREGO.

Consciousness

Freud's views about consciousness evolved in line with advances in his general psychoanalytic theory. In early writings on pathological defense (1894), Freud equated consciousness with the ego, or, more accurately, he assumed that any ideas attributed to the self were conscious ideas. Consequently, in discussing hysteria, where repressed ideas give rise to somatic sensations, he refers to this phenomenon as a "splitting of consciousness"; the unwanted ideas become dissociated from the other ideas that form the content of the normal ego's consciousness and form a secondary consciousness. In speaking of ideas that make up the content of consciousness, Freud was apparently acquiescing to the Cartesian tradition in which "idea" could refer indiscriminately to sensations, images, concepts, propositions, or thoughts.

In 1896, Freud abandoned the split-consciousness theory in favor of a theory of unconscious ideas. Thereafter, he insisted that a theory of unconscious ideas was preferable to the notion of a secondary consciousness of which its owner was unaware. Consciousness was thus bound up with awareness, and the repressed became the prototype of unconscious mentality. But this division of the psychic apparatus into conscious and unconscious called for a further elaboration of consciousness; for if psychoanalysis was to be given a firm theoretical basis, Freud needed to show how his conscious-unconscious distinction could provide an explanation of how repression occurs and how it can be removed. This need was satisfied in his topographical model of the mind that appeared in the *Interpretation of Dreams* (1900).

The topographical model offers a functional account of the mental apparatus—a flowchart of inputs and outputs—with no further attempt to localize these functions neurologically, though Freud apparently continued to hold that these functions were carried out somewhere in the central nervous system. The model is constructed on the basis of a reflex arc, beginning with a perceptual system (*Pcpt.*) and ending with a preconscious system (*Pcs.*) that precedes motor activity. The function of the apparatus is to maintain a homeostatic balance by discharging excess excitations. Following and dependent upon the perceptual system is a secondary one in which a series of memory traces are laid down (*Mnem.*). Closest to the motor end of the apparatus, the *Pcs.* system serves to explain both the occurrence of dreams and the phenomenon of repression.

The processes of the *Pcs.* can enter actual consciousness without hindrance if certain other conditions are fulfilled, such as either reaching a degree of intensity or being subject to attention. Behind the preconscious system is that of the unconscious (*Ucs.*), whose processes can enter consciousness only after being filtered through the *Pcs.* and modified accordingly. Dreams are a result of this filtering process, being symbolic translations of uncensored material, whereas unconscious processes blocked by the *Pcs.* are said to be repressed and must remain unconscious. In this scheme, the *Ucs.* is restricted to the repressed, whereas what belongs to the *Pcs.*, although not conscious in actuality, is accorded a place in the system of the conscious (*Cs.*) by virtue of its capacity for becoming conscious.

The model explains mental events by charting their psychical topography. For instance, if a wish appears as a neurotic symptom instead of as part of a train of rational thought, then this is due to an abnormal translation across the barrier from *Ucs.* to *Pcs./Cs.* In this scheme, consciousness seems to arise only toward the motor end of the apparatus, after the *Pcpt.* system transmits its impulses to deeper within the apparatus. By 1917, however, Freud came to regard consciousness and perception as belonging to the same system (*Cs./Pcpt.*); this subsequently allowed him to distinguish between a primitive perceptual consciousness and a more advanced and "secondary" thought-consciousness.

By 1920, Freud had abandoned his topographical theory because of the phenomenon of "unconscious ego resistance." Resistance of the patient to the therapist's suggestions during treatment showed Freud that he could no longer distinguish sharply between the systems *Ucs.* and *Pcs./Cs.*, since the resistance to treatment could only be said to flow not from what was repressed in the *Ucs.* but from those higher-level systems (*Pcs./Cs.*) that originally carried out the repression. Yet the motives for these resistances and the resistances themselves could be unconscious only at the beginning of treatment. Thus, the three systems of the topographical model (*Cs., Pcs.,* and *Ucs.*) came to be replaced by an explanatory model of structural agencies: ego, id, and superego. Though everything in the id remained unconscious, parts of the ego and superego had to be unconscious as well. Thus Freud despaired of being able to show any precise parallel between the structural agencies and the psychical

C

"qualities" of consciousness and unconsciousness, and this led to his pessimism about the systematic importance of the psychical qualities themselves. The distinction between these qualities now seemed to tell us little or nothing about the functioning of the mind.

Despite Freud's pessimism, however, the concepts of consciousness and unconsciousness continued to have significance for his later theory, especially since the goal of psychoanalysis was to effect a cure by helping the patient overcome resistances and facilitate the bringing to consciousness of that which had been hidden from it.

The account of Freud's theorizing thus far has been concerned with the explanatory role of consciousness, not with its nature. But the nature of consciousness becomes important in explaining how to replace what is unconscious in a patient with what is conscious. This cannot be done, according to Freud, simply by the therapist's communicating the content of some unconscious memory to the patient, for this just amounts to another idea in the patient's consciousness alongside the unconscious one. Instead, the unconscious memory can become conscious and the repression lifted only when the unconscious memory trace has itself been made conscious. But to understand how one and the same idea can first be unconscious and then later conscious requires saying more about what Freud took the nature of consciousness to be.

Freud had outlined an ambitious neurological theory that touched on the nature of consciousness in his *Project for a Scientific Psychology*, written in 1895. In this posthumously published work, he set out to make psychology into a natural science by reducing all psychical processes to quantitatively determinate states of "neurones," the basic material units of the central nervous system. The neurones tend to divest themselves of quantities of energy (Q) according to a "principle of inertia" (homeostasis); yet one system of neurones discharges Q more readily than a second system, which is capable of a retention (cathexis) of Q. The first system is responsible for perception, whereas the second accounts for memory and learning.

Freud also insisted that his quantitative theory find a place for the content of consciousness, or the "quality" of sensations. This led him to posit a third system of neurones "whose states of excitation give rise to the various qualities—that is to say, are—*conscious sensations*" (1895:309). But this statement seems ambiguous between a dualistic account of consciousness in terms of psychi-

cal qualities *caused* by neuronal excitation, and a materialistic account in which the states of excitation are identical with consciousness. The fact that he did not publish the *Project*, and even tried to destroy it, offers some reason for thinking that he resolved the ambiguity by denying the identity between neurological and psychological processes, instead adopting a metaphysical dualism of the mental and physical. Further evidence for this view resides in the fact that Freud made no reference to this third system of neurones in his later writings regarding consciousness.

Despite this evidence, it is more likely, however, that Freud discarded the neurological model only because it failed to explain psychological functions, and not because that he came to believe that some psychical processes were nonphysical. The fact that he abandoned his attempts to localize psychical processes in specific parts of the central nervous system shows only that he disavowed any specific identity between psychological and physical properties. But this is consistent with saying that each psychological process is some (unknown) process in the central nervous system.

The account Freud apparently adopted, however, was not a straightforwardly materialistic one in which the property of being conscious was some unknown physical property. Even though every conscious process was some physical process or other, Freud seemed to think that certain perceiver-dependent properties of mental processes called "qualities" were not themselves reducible to any neurological properties. Instead, by attaching themselves to certain neurological processes such as sensations, these qualities thereby serve to render these sensations conscious. Thus, Freud seems to adopt a "double-attribute" theory of conscious processes, each of which has both neurological attributes and also a "subjective side": the qualitative attributes that constitute the immediate objects of our awareness.

The double-attribute view can be employed to resolve a tension in Freud's thought about the function of consciousness. On the one hand, he wanted consciousness to play a regulative role in mental functioning—by expediently directing the discharge of retained energy throughout the psychical system. On the other hand, his structural-agency view of mental functioning (id, ego, superego) seemed to relegate consciousness to being a "mere quality"—or an epiphenomenal reflection of such functioning. Distinguishing between conscious processes and their dual properties allows him to address both these points. The double-attribute view gives a causal role to conscious processes solely in virtue of their neurological properties, whereas any "quality" of consciousness serves no other purpose than that of making such processes perceptible. Thus Freud can plausibly be seen as trying to steer a middle course between materialism and dualism with regard to consciousness.

The double-attribute view also seems presupposed in Freud's explanation of how unconscious ideas can become conscious: they do so by becoming invested with qualities that enable them to be perceived as belonging to oneself. How these perceptual qualities manage to emerge and attach themselves to quantitative neurological items is problematic, but Freud thought the manner in which they did so was similar to the way in which perceptual qualities arise from the transaction between our sense organs and the external world. Here he adopts a representative theory of perception: a world of matter in motion affects our material sense organs and gives rise to a representation—describable either as an idea or as a brain process—that is invested with perceptual quality. Simply to have one's representation bear this perceptual quality is to be perceptually conscious. But Freud also held (from 1917 on) that perceptual quality was present in all forms of consciousness—either of the world, in dreams, in hallucinations, or of our own thoughts and feelings. Dream consciousness is a form of hallucination; perceptual quality is present but it is not an "indication of reality," since the latter requires an external source.

What first distinguishes thought-consciousness from mere perceptual consciousness is the twofold way in which the psychical function of attention is manifested. Perceptual consciousness (awareness of perceptual quality) automatically attracts the attention of the ego as being a possible "indication of reality." Perceptual consciousness is thus prior to such attention. Thought-consciousness, on the other hand, is not generated spontaneously, since memory traces do not automatically give rise to perceptual quality. Instead, such quality must be aroused internally by a contribution of energy from the ego; that is, it must first be generated by the ego's attention. Such attention consists of the ego's linking of memory traces with the words describing them (or with the impulses to speak about them). These reactivated impulses to speak possess perceptual quality sufficient once more to attract the ego's attention, resulting in consciousness of thought. Unconscious ideas thus become conscious when translated by the subject into words that properly describe them, and it is by this means that the therapist seeks to counteract repression.

From the foregoing, it can be seen that perceptual consciousness, as awareness of perceptual quality, can be present with or without attention. Without attention, it is mere qualitative content, or sensory stimulation, without associative links to other ideas (or brain processes) constituting the ego. With attention, perceptual qualities can be related first to the self and then to the world; one becomes aware of oneself as being presented with qualities that arise spontaneously, and one is able to infer the world as their source. Freud thus borrows Leibniz's (and Kant's) distinction between perception and apperception to distinguish mere awareness of content from ego-based awareness.

Mental processes are in themselves unconscious, and perception of them is analogous to perception of the external world by means of the sense organs. Just as perception of an external world (as opposed to the mere presence of qualitative content) requires an apperceptive awareness, Freud also conceived thought-consciousness apperceptively, as being more than a mere "indication of quality." Unconscious ideas might be the bearers of perceptual qualities, as in dreams and symptoms, but such ideas are not made conscious if they lack the required associative links connecting them to the self. To make an unconscious idea conscious, one must be able to describe it in a way that embeds it in the network of coherent ideas that constitute the ego. Only on the basis of qualities that prompt such apperceptive awareness can a healthy self-consciousness be achieved.

REFERENCES

Freud, S. (1894). *The Neuro-psychoses of Defense.* S.E. 3: 45–61.

———. (1895). *Project for a Scientific Psychology.* S.E. 1: 283–397.

———. (1900). *The Interpretation of Dreams.* S.E. 4–5: 1–621.

L. S. CARRIER

Conversion

In a paper on the defense neuropsychoses, Freud (1894) introduced the term "conversion" to designate an unconscious psychic process that renders an unbearable idea innocuous "by the quantity of excitation attached to it being transmuted into some bodily form of expression."

In his joint study with Breuer (1895), and in his "Fragment of an Analysis of a Case of Hysteria" (1905), Freud later showed that conversion in hysteria proceeds along the line of motor and/or sensory innervations that are more or less intimately related to a psychically traumatic experience. This relationship is symbolic, representing a compromise among leading mental conflicts. Sometimes, as when conversion follows a physical injury, the effects of the injury are exaggerated or prolonged, and then become a form of symbolic expression. For in the bodily symptoms of conversion, there is an expressive function in which previously repressed instinctual impulses, and defenses against them, are symbolized.

The conversion symptoms, then, result from an attempt at expression that is in the direction of discharging the tension associated with intrapsychic conflict. Drive and defense are simultaneously symbolically expressed in "body language," short-circuiting conscious perception of the conflict originating from the early family drama experienced by the afflicted patient. The expression of the ego-alien symptoms, resulting in the reduction of inner tension, is the so-called primary gain of the bodily impairment. The "secondary gain" consists in the subsequent utilization by the ego of the perceived bodily distress to communicate to others, usually in a more or less transparent attempt at manipulation of them, but also in an attempt to provide a rationalization for the self. Such maneuvers, based much more on misinterpretation of the meaning of the experienced symptoms than on sound interpretation of them, may be elaborated in speech as part of an effort to manipulate other people, and through them, a current frustrating life situation. The attention-attracting function of the symptoms, be they gross paralysis, spasmodic or convulsive motor disturbances, exaggeration, diminution or perversion of sensation, or dumbness, deafness or blindness, may be emphasized by associated nonverbal behavior as well as verbal communication. Similarly, the sympathy, dominance, and compensation-gaining functions of the symptoms may be elevated into the foreground, and may be justified both nonverbally and verbally. The fact that this secondary gain from somatoform disorder is accomplished through more secondary process-associated ego activity does not necessarily indicate that such gain is a matter of secondary importance to the patient emotionally. In the complex stratification of the psychic life, these strivings are derivatives of frustrated oral-dependency needs, and of anal-manipulative needs for mastery. The importance of secondary gain in the psychic economy of the patient is maximal in instances in which there is heavy quantitative loading of pregenital fixation. While in conversion hysteria, genital wishes and fantasies from the realm of the Oedipus complex find a distorted expression in the symptoms of somatic disorder; in some instances pregenital fixation may actually determine the selection of the organ involved in disordered function (Abse, 1987). Moreover, there are pregenital conversions where the unconscious impulses expressed symbolically in the symptoms are predominantly pregenital. As Marmor (1953) has emphasized, in many cases of hysteria, fixations in the Oedipal phase of development are themselves the outgrowth of pre-Oedipal fixations, chiefly of an oral nature.

In his early papers on the defense neuropsychoses, Freud (1894; 1896) discussed conversion with reference to traumatic sexual experiences. Ferenczi (1919) similarly indicated in his paper on materialization that repressed libidinal drives find expression in an alteration of physical functioning, the involved organ representing the genitals—a form of archaic symbolism. Later, it became clearer that repressed hostility and the turning of the aggression against the self are also important elements in the conversion process. This is starkly evident in convulsive forms of hysteria, when aroused hostility, often generated by frustration of genital libidinal trends, finds release in seizures (Abse, 1987).

The essential messages in a conversion reaction are thus embodied cryptically in the somatic symptoms. Word language is reduced and compressed in inaudible symbols of primitive character, and in such a way that the subject is unaware of their essential meaning. In conversion, there are six interrelated communicative aspects of motor and sensory phenomena as enumerated below:

(1) Sexual symbolic references couched in cryptophoric symbolism.
(2) Distorted affect expressions, e.g., of appeal, of resentment, of weeping, of joy, and so on.
(3) Condensation of identifications.
(4) Associated connotations relating to conflicting fantasies—both wish-fulfilling and punitive.
(5) Denotational propositional pantomimic movements—often truncated, or with reversals in sequence, or other disguises.
(6) Metaphorical embodiments.

These aspects of the communicative disorder that is the essence of conversion are illustrated in a plethora of psychoanalytic case studies. They show that the conversion process is a regressive defense that alters the patient's body image as a substitute for a more realistic adaptation that the patient feels helpless to achieve. The highly condensed symbolic process encountered in conversion phenomena is of a different order from the symbolic process in waking thought and language. Freud was impressed by parallels between the nature of the conversion process and dreaming. As he notes (1909), not only are the forces producing the distortion of the expression of wishes the same as those in dreams, but the technique of the distortion is also similar. In particular, the type of symbolism employed in a conversion resembles that of the manifest dream.

While not all conversion symptoms are readily translatable into easily recognizable metaphors of speech such as "a pain in the neck" or "seeing red," sometimes a preliminary retranslation of part of the meaning of somatic symptoms to metaphorically embellished language facilitates access to the emotions of the patient (Abse, 1971).

These emotions, when released in treatment, reveal fantasies associated with repressed drive derivatives. They are defended against because they conflict with the patient's beliefs about how he or she ought to feel and act. In employing unconscious defenses, the patient loses effective communication with his or her self. Both self-related means of expression and communication with others become progressively more distorted—beneath a shell of rationalization that, together with the conversion symptoms, are eventually proffered to the physician, to whom he or she turns for help.

REFERENCES

Abse, D. W. (1959). Hysteria. In S. Arieti (ed.). *American Handbook of Psychiatry*. New York: Basic Books, vol. 1, pp. 272–292.

———. (1971). *Speech and Reason. Language Disorder in Mental Disease and a Translation of the Life of Speech*, Philip Wegene. Charlottesville, Va.: University Press of Virginia.

———. (1987). *Hysteria and Related Mental Disorders*. Bristol, England: John Wright.

Breuer, J., and Freud, S. (1895). *Studies on Hysteria*. S.E. 2: 19–305.

Ferenczi, S. (1919). The phenomena of hysterical materialization. In *Further Contributions to the Theory and Technique of Psycho-Analysis*. London: Hogarth Press, 1926.

Freud, S. (1894). The neuro-psychoses of defence. S.E. 3: 43–61.

———. (1908). *Some General Remarks on Hysterical Attacks*. S.E. 9: 227–234.

———. (1920). *Beyond the Pleasure Principle*. S.E. 18: 7–64.

———. (1952). Further remarks on the neuropsychoses of defence. Part I: The specific etiology of hysteria. S.E. 3: 162–168.

———. (1953). Fragment of an analysis of a case of hysteria. S.E. 7: 3–122.

Marmor, J. (1953). Oratory in the hysterical personality. *Journal of the American Psychoanalytic Association*, I: 656–71.

Krohn, A. (1978). *Hysteria: The Elusive Neurosis*. New York: International Universities Press.

Noble, D. (1951). Hysterical manifestations in schizophrenic illness. *Psychiatry*, 14: 153–160.

Rangell, L. (1959). The nature of conversion. *Journal of the American Psychoanalytic Association*, 7: 632–662.

D. WILFRED ABSE

C

Counter-Transference See TRANSFERENCE.

Creativity

Freud's attitude toward creativity is best characterized as acutely ambivalent. He never presented a systematic analysis of the subject, and his many writings reflect inconsistent and, at times, contradictory opinions. Nevertheless, Freud's interest in art lasted throughout his lifetime, and he did not heed his own "hands off" policy warning: "Before the problem of the creative artist analysis must, alas, lay down its arms" (1928, S.E. 21: 177). He argued, on the other hand, that artists and their works are not beyond psychological comprehension, "like any other fact of human life" (1914: 212).

For the most part, Freud spoke of artists with an enormous amount of respect and regard; he claimed that artists "are far in advance of us everyday people," and their knowledge has always served as a precursor of scientific discoveries (1907/6: 8). Freud believed artists possessed special qualities, such as "a certain flexibility [*Lockerheit*] of regression," which enabled them to tap into and use experiences from childhood (1917: 376). This insight provided the foundation for Kris's (1952) concept, "regression in the service of the ego."

Freud initially applied psychoanalytic methods, derived from his study of neurotics, to the understanding of artists and their works. In his earliest speculations, he believed that the artist's highly private and unacceptable unconscious fantasies and built-up tensions do not find gratification in the real world and are therefore released in disguised form onto an audience as a way of relieving internal pressure and obtaining pleasure. The artwork resembles a symptom in that it is essentially a safety valve that helps bind the artist's repressions. Freud therefore wrote that "the mechanism of poetry [creative writing] is the same as that of hysterical phantasies" (1897: 256). Although he believed the artist to be "not far removed from neurosis" (1917: 376), Freud nevertheless tried to distinguish the two. Sublimation, the transformation of instinctual energies into "higher ones of art or culture," functions as a cultural outlet for powerful sexual excitations, thereby resulting in an "increase in psychical efficiency" (1905: 238). In his *Introductory Lectures*, Freud further asserted that the artist succeeds in finding his or her way back to reality while the neurotic does not. According to Freud, this is accomplished by the artist's molding his fantasies (e.g., the winning of "honour, power and the love of women") into truths that are appreciated by others as reflections of reality (i.e., the artistic illusion) (1917: 376–377).

Freud pointed out that the artist's alterations in the external world are made possible only because others deal with similar conflicts and dissatisfactions, and therefore unconsciously identify with artworks while escaping their own censorship (1908, p. 153). Indeed, he considered the process of identification to be at the root of aesthetic experience. For instance, he explained the appreciation of Shakespeare's Hamlet as deriving from the idea that "Each member of the audience was once, in germ and in phantasy, just such an Oedipus" (1897: 265).

Freud's view of the artist's instinctual conflicts and their resolution through sublimation led him to analyze art as he would a dream; that is, by primarily deciphering the symbolic content to arrive at an understanding of the artist's unconscious motives. As a matter of fact, he placed little emphasis on the formal aspects of artworks, just as he left unattended aspects of the manifest dream. Freud admitted his one-sided approach to art when he confessed: "the subject-matter of works of art has a stronger attraction for me than their formal and technical qualities" (1914: 211). His emphasis on the content of art resulted in his failure to explain the difference between great art and mediocre or bad art. Indeed, his detailed analyses of distinguished works, like Leonardo da Vinci's *Virgin and St. Anne with the Infant Jesus* (1910) and Michelangelo's *Moses* (1914) differ little from his analysis of a lesser work of literature, Jensen's *Gradiva* (1907/6).

Psychoanalytic theorists on creativity, from Rank (1932) to Gilbert Rose (1980), have attempted to amend Freud's neglect of form. These theoreticians claim that the meaning of a work of art is to be found in the form no less than, and perhaps more than, in the content. However, it is not entirely accurate to state that Freud did not address the formal aspects of art altogether. Freud recognized the aesthetic value of artistic form when he designated it as a "bribing fore-pleasure," a facade that distracts our attention while simultaneously allowing for the discharge of otherwise inhibited cathexes (1905: 152). Under the mask of form, Freud claimed, "the artist softens the character of his egoistic daydreams by altering and disguising it, and he bribes us by the purely formal—that is, aesthetic—yield of pleasure which he offers us in the presentation of his phantasies" (1908: 153).

In his book on jokes, Freud paid the most attention to formal aspects of creative works, such as rhyme and rhythm. Unlike dreams, unconsciously motivated and geared toward avoiding displeasure, both jokes and art represent social phenomena aimed at obtaining pleasure. Freud's attention to the aesthetic and playful aspects of jokes led him to draw a direct comparison between creative writing and children's play: "Every child behaves like a creative writer, in that he creates a world of his own, or, rather, re-arranges the things of his world in a new way which pleases him" (1908: 143–144). Freud traced a direct line from the child's imaginative play through daydreaming and fantasy, to the creative work of the artist, particularly the writer. His attention to child's play as a serious activity comparable to the creative process influenced later writers on psychoanalysis and art, like Winnicott (1971) and Ehrenzweig (1967), to elaborate on the childhood origins of the creative process.

In 1920, Freud once more drew a comparison between child and artist, explaining how both repeat painful experiences as a way of gaining mastery over them. Art does not "spare the spectators (for instance, in tragedy) the most painful experiences and can yet be felt by them as highly enjoyable (1920: 17). In contradistinction to his earlier writings, which view the artist primarily as a person saved from neurosis by sublimation, his later work considers the artist as someone who gains mastery over his impulses and who, through the use of formal techniques, enjoys the act of doing so. This sense of mastery applies not only to the artist's experiences during the creative process but also to the manner in which the artist is able to control the audience's reactions: "the storyteller has a peculiarly directive influence over us; by means of the moods he can put us into, he is able to guide the current of our emotions, to dam it up in one direction and make it flow in another" (1920: 251).

REFERENCES

Ehrenzweig, A. (1967). *The Hidden Order of Art*. Berkeley: University of California Press.

Freud, S. (1897). *Letter to Fleiss*. S.E. 1: 256.

———. (1897). *Letter to Fleiss*. S.E. 1: 265.

———. (1905). *Jokes and Their Relation to the Unconscious*. S.E. 8.

———. (1905). *Three Essays on the Theory of Sexuality*. S.E. 7: 130–243.

———. (1907/6). *Delusions and Dreams in Jensen's Gradiva*. S.E. 9: 7–95.

———. (1908). *Creative Writers and Daydreaming*. S.E. 9: 141–153.

———. (1910). *Leonardo da Vinci and a Memory of his Childhood*. S.E. 11: 59–138.

———. (1914). *The Moses of Michelangelo*. S.E. 13: 211–236.

———. (1917). *A General Introduction to Psychoanalysis*. S.E. 16: 370–371.

———. (1920). *Beyond the Pleasure Principle*. S.E. 18: 3–64.

———. (1928). *Dostoevsky and Parricide*. S.E. 21: 175–196.

Kris, E. (1952). *Psychoanalytic Explorations in Art*. New York: International Universities Press.

Rank, O. (1932). *Art and Artist*. New York: Agathon Press.

Rose, G. (1980). *The Power of Form*. New York: International Universities Press.

Winnicott, D. W. (1971). Creativity and its origins. In *Playing and Reality*. London: Tavistock, pp. 65–85.

DANIELLE KNAFO

Criminality, and Psychoanalysis

There are intriguing paradoxes in the interrelation of Freud and concepts of criminality. He was not experienced with criminals; he was pessimistic about the contribution of psychoanalysis in the treatment of the criminal; he concerned himself little with criminality—writing only a few papers specifically on the subject—yet his views continue to influence profoundly psychodynamic thinking within the forensic field. Freud's "material" upon which he based his hypotheses concerning criminality came partly from his analytic work with his private patients, partly from his knowledge and occasional comments on real-life crime from information in the public domain, but predominantly from his reading and interpretations of the great literary texts.

Oedipal Themes and Criminality

In thinking about crime, one of Freud's preoccupations was with Oedipal themes and the crimes of parricide and incest. Thus he writes, "It can scarcely be owing to chance that three of the masterpieces of the literature of all time—the 'Oedipus Rex' of Sophocles, Shakespeare's 'Hamlet', and Dostoevsky's 'The Brothers Karamazov'—should all deal with the same subject, parricide. In all three, moreover, the motive for the deed, sexual rivalry for a woman, is laid bare" (Freud, 1916: 188).

This essentially Oedipal theme had formed the basis of the now classic short paper, "Criminals From a Sense of Guilt" (Freud, 1916: 333), in which Freud writes: "mankind's sense of guilt in general . . . [is] derived from the Oedipus complex and was a reaction to the two great criminal intentions of killing the father and having sexual relations with the mother." He continues: "We must in this connection remember that parricide and incest with the mother are the two great human crimes, the only ones which, as such, are pursued and abhorred in primitive communities." Freud acknowledges that the role of "the essential characteristics"—universality, content, and fate (of the Oedipus complex)—were recognized long before the days of psychoanalysis, by that "acute thinker Diderot in 'Le neveu de Rameau'" (Freud, 1931 [1930], p. 251). Freud quotes Diderot, in Goethe's translation, "If the little savage were left to himself, preserving all his feebleness and adding to the small sense of a child in the cradle, the violent passions of a man of thirty, he would strangle his father and lie with his mother" (Freud, 1931 [1930] ibid.).

In opposition to Freud's view, Fonagy and Target (1996) write: "In his paper on character types encountered in the course of psychoanalytic work (Freud, 1916, p. 333) he [Freud] traces all crimes to either incest or parricide. His argument for this is less than compelling and has largely been abandoned by later writers." It is true that a theory of such universal (unconscious) fantasy tells us nothing about the specific factors that cause, rather rare, acts of parricide or mother incest (or their displacement equivalents). Freud, however, was aware of the problem; he writes in the "Halsmann Case": "Precisely because it is always present, the Oedipus complex is not suited to provide a decision on the question of guilt . . . it is a far cry from there to the causation of such a deed" (Freud, 1931 [1930]: 252).

On the Education of Juvenile Delinquents

Freud also applied his theories to juvenile crime, although he doubted that child offenders possessed the characteristics necessary to benefit from standard psychoanalytic treatment. Thus, he writes in his Preface to (August) Aichorn's *Wayward Youth* (Freud, 1925)—which deals specifically with the place of psychoanalytic thought in the education of juvenile delinquents—"The possibility of analytic influence (generally) rests on quite definite preconditions which can be summed up under the term 'analytic situation'; it requires the development of certain psychical structures and a particular attitude to the analyst. Where these are lacking—as in the case of children, of juvenile delinquents, and, as a rule, of impulsive criminals—something other than analysis must be employed, though something that will be at one with analysis in its *purpose*" (Freud, 1925: 274). It is here, too, that Freud makes his well-known recommendation that all those involved in the education of children (including delinquent children) "should receive a psychoanalytic training . . . since without it the object of (his) endeavours must remain an inaccessible problem (to him). A training of this kind is best carried out if such a person himself undergoes an analysis and experiences it on himself: theoretical instruction in analysis fails to penetrate deep enough and carries no conviction" (Freud, 1925: 274).

Aggression, Psychopathy, and Crime

Freud was slow to develop a theory of aggression and destructiveness, and indeed said so—"why have we ourselves needed such a long time before we decided to recognise an aggressive instinct? Why did we hesitate to make use, on behalf of our theory, of facts which were obvious and familiar to everyone?" However, there is reference in many of Freud's early papers to aggression and destructiveness, specifically to "untamed aggression," for example, and of aggression in personality disorder—especially narcissistic personality disorder, and an explicit link is made between narcissistic personality and psychopathy (1914).

In a 1916 paper (1916: 332–333), Freud also described the psychopath as one "who develops no moral inhibitions" that inhibit his potential for criminal activity. This is in line with later classical, phenomenological descriptions of the psychopath as in Cleckley (1941), and the "primary psychopath" as in Hare and Cox (1987). However, later psychoanalytic theorists have regarded the superego functions of many criminals as typically excessively harsh. They describe a vicious cycle of defensive projective identification, of persecutory superego internal objects, which then are experienced as externally persecutory, and therefore need further violent projection psychologically or, in some cases, physically. This was first adumbrated by Greenacre (1945) and is central to all Kleinian writing on this subject now.

When Freud did develop a theory of aggression, he immediately linked it up to the (much disputed) "Death Instinct" and so-called internalized aggression—which may then be projected outward as "normal" or pathological aggression (Freud, 1921). These concepts provided fertile theoretical ground for later authors, in particular Melanie Klein, who identified "primary envy" as a manifestation of the death instinct. In the view of many writers, however, including this one, it is unfortunate that other theories of aggression (and the "component" affects, e.g., destructiveness and hostility) had to wait the attention of later object relations theorists, for example, Fairbairn, Winnicott, Bowlby, and others who saw the need to postulate neither a death instinct nor a so-called aggressive instinct. Aggression was seen by these authors as more a secondary phenomenon in reaction to frustration and perceived deprivation.

An excellent discussion of early views of aggression, and of the theoretical revisions of the 1920s, is given in Waelder (1960). Later developments of the evolution of conceptualizations of sadism, hatred, and destructiveness are well reviewed by Thomä and Kächele (1994). These authors, too, dispense with the arguments for an aggressive instinct.

Guilt, Envy, and Crime

Freud lists as his central *specific* contribution to the theory of criminality the idea of unconscious guilt as an important causal factor in the commision of crimes. He writes in *The Ego and the Id* (1923): "In many criminals, especially youthful ones, it is possible to detect a very powerful sense of guilt which existed before the crime, and is therefore not its result but its motive. It is as if it was a relief to be able to fasten this unconscious sense of guilt on to something real and immediate" (Freud, 1923, p. 52).

Freud explores, too, in *Group Psychology and the Analysis of the Ego* (1921) the destructiveness of envy—for example, in his interpretation of the motives of the women in the Judgement of Solomon. Most significantly, Freud opposes Trotter's theory of the "herd instinct," and of human beings as primarily social animals. None of this, he says, is evident in young children. Only in the face of rivalry and envy for parental love, he notes, is the child forced to identify with other children, and is thus compelled (secondarily, as it were) into communal and group feeling. Put another way, "The first demand made by this reaction-formation is for justice [and] for equal treatment for all. The core of this argument is founded upon the transformation of envy; . . . without envy, not only would there be no need for a judicial apparatus, there would not even be a desire for justice" (Forrester, 1996, p. 132). In this argument, the psychological basis of justice and our system of justice—and its transgression by criminals—is explained as being rooted in envy and destructiveness.

Far more significant than Freud's specific contributions to theories of crime and criminality are the conceptual tools he developed for understanding states of mind and motivation. The core psychoanalytic concepts of the unconscious; the defense mechanisms—including the now contentious concepts of the different forms of repression and the vicissitudes of memories of trauma, actual or in fantasy, and of remembering and repeating, if not worked through; the basic writings on psychosis (especially on Schreber, 1911); the developmental theory of infantile, adolescent, and adult sexuality (1905); the core paradigm of conflict within the self and theories of "splitting" of the object and the ego; and the concept of acting out—all these have provided the essential groundwork for later psychoanalytic views about criminality.

Post-Freudian Psychoanalytic Views on Crime

Anna Freud described a developmental theory of psychopathology with evolution through stages, and specifically included the harnessing of aggression and component affects. She also provided a developmental model of antisocial and narcissistic personality disorder (1949), which focused upon early failures by an absent, neglectful, or ambivalent primary object. This influence was continued, especially by the psychoanalyst Edward Glover, whose specifically criminal psychology writings are collected in *The Roots of Crime* (1960).

Separately, powerful clinical and theoretical developments within the diversely represented object relations school were to change the way that, on the one hand, severe borderline, narcissistic, and psychotic patients, and, on the other, criminality and criminal acts, were conceptualized and understood. For Fairbairn (1940), the schizoid personality originates from early infantile trauma, with infantile anxiety concerning maternal destructiveness (by lack or withdrawal of love) leading to narcissistic withdrawal. Fairbairn also elaborated a theory of the "functional self" and its response to early trauma by developing multiple self-representations. This is similar to the "false self" theory of Winnicott, and has some affinity with a Dissociative Identity Disorder as formulated in DSM(IV).

In parallel, Melanie Klein laid the way for further understanding of psychotic processes and defenses, first with her accounts of the use of toys in play with very young children; the later descriptions of different psychic "positions"—the "depressive" and "paranoid schizoid"; the formation of the persecutory superego; and of primitive defenses of splitting and of projective and introjective identification. These ideas have become highly influential in British practice, and in some areas of Europe, in the understanding and treatment of patients with psychotic structures, or actual psychotic illness, and also in criminality. While Fairbairn had not written directly on criminality, Klein had written two early papers on the "criminal" fantasies and play of the children whom she analyzed (1927, 1934).

Other object relations contributions came from Winnicott, who make use of his concepts of the transitional object, the false self, and the ability of the child to "use" that object. His paper, "The Antisocial Tendency" (1956), has achieved classic status. No less significant is the work of Bowlby on "Attachment and Loss" (Bowlby, 1988), with its now specific and empirical applications to research in delinquency and criminality (Fonagy et al., 1997). Bowlby's early empirical study of 44 juvenile thieves (Bowlby, 1944) remains an exemplary use of psychoanalytical hypotheses to explain the acts of youngsters caught in a stage of what he called "affectionless psychopathy." Both Winnicott and Bowlby specifically addressed what today we think of as the "acquisitive" offender, redressing the common emphasis—which continues—on the violent, possibly sexual, severely personality disordered patient.

C

Later influential writers in Britain have included Glasser (1979) in the Freudian tradition, and Hyatt-Williams (1982) and Gallwey (1996) in the Kleinian tradition.

The development of self-psychology sets its stall, too, within the area of object seeking and the finding of an adequate "self object" (Kohut, 1977) as an essential foundation for a viable sense of self, i.e., a stable identity. It, therefore, lends itself to the interpersonal, and by extension, to wider application within groups and society—within which context the psychodynamics of the criminal and his act are located. However, for the British analyst, the practices of self-psychology emphasize insufficiently the "negative transference" that is so crucial in the practice of the talking therapies with the criminal patient.

Finally, Kernberg (1992) has attempted to bring together ego psychological and Kleinian object relations conceptualizations, based upon his extensive experience with severely personality disordered patients. His work with such patients concentrates predominantly on the here and now, eschewing attempts at reconstruction, and avoiding issues of distinction between Oedipal and pre-Oedipal pathology. These clinical and theoretical accounts have yet to be applied directly in the forensic sphere but do address the common elements in the psychopathology of many criminal offenders.

REFERENCES

Bowlby, J. (1944). Forty-four juvenile thieves: Their character and home life. *International Journal of Psychoanalysis*, 25: 1–57, 207–228.

———. (1988). *A Secure Base: Clinical Application of Attachment Theory*. London: Routledge.

Carveth, D. L. (1996). Psychoanalytic conceptions of passions. In J. O'Neill (ed.). *Freud and the Passions*. University Park: Pennsylvania State University Press.

Cleckley, H. (1941). *The Mask of Sanity*. St Louis: Mosley.

Erikson, E. H. (1963). *Childhood and Society*. 2d ed. New York: Norton.

Fairbairn, W. R. D. (1940). Schizoid factors in the personality. In W. R. D. Fairbairn (author). *An Object-relations Theory of the Personality*. New York: Basic Books.

Fonagy, P., and Target, M. (1996). Personality and sexual development. In C. Cordess and M. Cox (eds.). *Forensic Psychotherapy. Crime, Psychodynamics and the Offender Patient*. London: Jessica Kingsley.

Fonagy, P., Target, M., Steele, H., Steele, M., Leight, T., Levinson, A., and Kennedy, R. (1997). Morality, disruptive behaviour, borderline personality disorder, crime and their relationship to security of attachment, In L. Atkinson and K. Zucker (eds.). *Attachment and Psychopathology*. New York: Guildford Press.

Forrester, J. (1996). Psychoanalysis and the history of the passions: The strange destiny of envy. In J. O'Neill (ed.). *Freud and the Passions*. University Park: Pennsylvania State University Press, pp. 127–149.

Freud, A. (1949). Certain types and stages of social maladjustment. In K. R. Eissler (ed.). *Searchlights on Delinquency*. New York: New International Press.

Freud, S. (1905). *Three Essays on the Theory of Sexuality*. S.E. 7: 130–243.

———. (1911). *Psychoanalytic Notes on an Autobiographical Account of a Case of Paranoia* S.E. 12: 9–82.

———. (1914). *On Narcissism: An Introduction*. S.E. 14: 73–102.

———. (1916). *Criminals From a Sense of Guilt*. S.E. 14: 332–333.

———. (1918). *Beyond the Pleasure Principle*. S.E. 18: 7–64.

———. (1921). *Group Psychology and the Analysis of the Ego*. S.E. 18: 65–143.

———. (1923). *The Ego and the Id*. S.E. 19: 2–66.

———. (1925). Preface to Aichhorn's *Wayward Youth*. S.E. 19: 273–275.

———. (1928). *Dostoevsky and Parricide*. S.E. 21: 177–196.

———. (1931). *The Expert Opinion in the Halsmann Case* [1930], S.E. 21: 251–253.

———. (1933). *New Introductory Lectures on Psychoanalysis* [1932], S.E. 22: 5–185.

Friedlander, K. (1945). Formation of the antisocial character. *Psychoanalytic Study of the Child*, 1: 189–203.

Gallwey, P. (1966). Psychotic and borderline processes. In C. Cordess and M. Cox (eds.). *Crime, Psychodynamics and the Offender Patient*. London: Jessica Kingsley, pp. 153–174.

Glasser, M. (1979). Some aspects of the role of aggression in the perversions. In I. Rosen (ed.). *Sexual Deviation*. Oxford: Oxford University Press.

Glover, E. (1960). *The Roots of Crime: Selected Papers on Psychoanalysis*. vol. 2. New York: International Universities Press.

Greenacre, P. (1945). Conscience in the psychopath. *American Journal of Orthopsychiatry*, 15: 495–509.

Hare, R. D., and Cox, D. N. (1987). Clinical and empirical conceptions of psychopathy, and the selection of subjects for research. In R. D. Hare and D. Schalling (eds.). *Psychopathic Behaviour: Approaches to Research*. Toronto, Ontario: Wiley.

Holmes, J. (1998). Psychodynamics, narrative and "intentional causality." Editorial. *British Journal of Psychiatry*, 173: 279–280.

Hyatt-Williams, A. (1982). Adolescence, violence and crime. *Journal of Adolescence*, 5: 125–134.

Jacobson, E. (1964). *The Self and the Object Word*. New York: International Universities Press.

Jaspers, K. (1923). *General Psychopathology*. Translated from the German by J. Hoenig and Max Hamilton. Manchester, England: Manchester University Press, 1963.

Kernberg, O. F. (1992). *Aggression in Personality Disorders and Perversions*. New Haven, Conn.: Yale University Press.

Klein, M. (1927). Criminal tendencies in normal children. In M. Klein (author). *The Writings of Melanie Klein*. vol. 1. London: Hogarth Press.

———. (1934). On criminality. In M. Klein (author). *The Writings of Melanie Klein.* vol. 1. London: Hogarth Press.

Kohut, H. (1977). *The Restoration of the Self.* New York: International Universities Press.

Thomä, H., and Kächele, H. (1994). *Psychoanalytic Practice Principles.* vol. 1. Northvale, N.J.: Jason Aronson.

Waelder, R. (1960). *Basic Theory of Psycho-Analysis.* New York: International Universities Press.

Winnicott, D. W. (1956). The antisocial tendency. In D. W. Winnicott (author). *Collected Papers: Through Paediatrics to Psychoanalysis.* London: Tavistock, 1958.

CHRISTOPHER CORDESS

Criticisms of Psychoanalysis

See CRITIQUE OF PSYCHOANALYSIS; EXPERIMENTAL EVIDENCE, FREUDIAN; PSEUDOSCIENCE, AND PSYCHOANALYSIS.

Critique of Psychoanalysis

Introduction

The most basic ideas of psychoanalytic theory were initially enunciated in Josef Breuer and Sigmund Freud's "Preliminary Communication" of 1893, which introduced their *Studies on Hysteria.* But the first published use of the word "psychoanalysis" occurred in Freud's 1896 French paper on "Heredity and the Aetiology of the Neuroses" (1896, p. 151). Therein Freud designated Breuer's method of clinical investigation as "a new method of psycho-analysis." Breuer used hypnosis to revive and articulate a patient's unhappy memory of a supposedly *repressed* traumatic experience. The *repression* of that painful experience had occasioned the first appearance of a particular hysterical symptom, such as a phobic aversion to drinking water. Thus, Freud's mentor also induced the release of the suppressed emotional distress originally felt from the trauma. Thereby Breuer's method provided a catharsis for the patient.

The cathartic *lifting* of the repression yielded relief from the particular hysterical symptom. Breuer and Freud believed that they could therefore hypothesize that the *repression*, coupled with affective suppression, was the crucial cause for the development of the patient's psychoneurosis (1893, pp. 6–7; 1893–1895, pp. 29–30).

Having reasoned in this way, they concluded in Freud's words:

Thus one and the same procedure served simultaneously the purposes of [causally] investigating and of getting rid of the ailment; and this unusual conjunction was later retained in psychoanalysis. (1924, p. 194)

In a 1924 historical retrospect (1924, p. 194), Freud acknowledged the pioneering role of Breuer's cathartic method:

The cathartic method was the immediate precursor of psychoanalysis; and, in spite of every extension of experience and of every modification of theory, is still contained within it as its nucleus.

Yet Freud was careful to highlight the contribution he made himself after the termination of his collaboration with Breuer. Referring to himself in the third person, he tells us:

Freud devoted himself to the further perfection of the instrument left over to him by his elder collaborator. The technical novelties which he introduced and the discoveries he made changed the cathartic method into psycho-analysis. (1924, p. 195)

These extensive elaborations have earned Freud the mantle of being the *father* of psychoanalysis.

By now, the psychoanalytic enterprise has completed its first century. Thus, the time has come to take thorough *critical* stock of its past performance qua theory of human nature and therapy, as well as to have a look at its prospects. Here I can do so only in broad strokes.

It is important to distinguish between the validity of Freud's work qua *psychoanalytic* theoretician, and the merits of his earlier work, which would have done someone else proud as the achievement of a lifetime. Currently, Mark Solms, working at the Unit of Neuro-surgery of the Royal London Hospital (Whitechapel) in England, is preparing a five-volume edition of *Freud's Collected Neuroscientific Writings* for publication in all the major European languages. One focus of these writings is the neurological representation of mental functioning; another is Freud's discovery of the essential morphological and physiological unity of the nerve cell and fiber. They also contain contributions to basic neuroscience such as the histology of the nerve cell, neuronal function, and neurophysiology. As a clinical neurologist, Freud

C

wrote a major monograph on aphasia (Solms and Saling, 1990). As Solms points out in his preview *An Introduction to the Neuro-Scientific Works of Sigmund Freud* (unpublished), Freud wrote major papers on cerebral palsy that earned him the status of a world authority. More generally, he was a distinguished pediatric neurologist in the field of the movement disorders of childhood. Furthermore, Freud was one of the founders of neuropsychopharmacology. For instance, he did scientific work on the properties of cocaine that benefited perhaps from his own use of that drug. Alas, that intake may well also account for some of the abandon featured by the more bizarre and grandiose of his psychoanalytic forays.

As Solms has remarked (private conversation), it is an irony of history that Freud, the psychoanalyst who postulated the ubiquity of bisexuality in humans, started out by deeming himself a *failure* for having had to conclude that eels are indeed bisexual. In a quest to learn how they reproduce, one of Freud's teachers of histology and anatomy assigned him the task of finding the hitherto elusive testicles of the eel as early as 1877, when he was twenty-one years old. After having dissected a lobular organ in about four hundred specimens in Trieste, Freud found that this organ apparently had the properties of an ovary no less than those of a testicle. Being unable to decide whether he had found the ever elusive testicles, Freud inferred that he had failed, as he reported in a rueful 1877 paper.

In 1880, he published a (free) translation of some of J. S. Mill's philosophical writings (Stephan, 1989: 85–86). Yet he was often disdainful of philosophy (Assoun, 1995), despite clearly being indebted to the Viennese philosopher Franz Brentano, from whom he had taken several courses: The marks of Brentano's (1995) quondam representationalist and intentionalist account of the mental are clearly discernible in Freud's conception of ideation (see "Brentano, Franz," this volume). And the arguments for the existence of God championed by the quondam Roman Catholic priest Brentano further solidified the thoroughgoing atheism of Freud, the "godless Jew" (Gay, 1987: 3–4).

History and Logical Relations of the "Dynamic" and "Cognitive" Species of the Unconscious. Freud was the creator of the full-blown theory of psychoanalysis, but even well-educated people often don't know that he was certainly *not at all* the first to postulate the existence of *some kinds*

or other of unconscious mental processes. A number of thinkers did so earlier to explain conscious thought and overt behavior for which they could find no other explanation (1915a, p. 166). As we recall from Plato's dialogue *The Meno*, that philosopher was concerned to understand how an ignorant slave boy could have arrived at geometric truths under mere questioning by an interlocutor with reference to a diagram. And Plato argued that the slave boy had not acquired such geometric knowledge during his life. Instead, he explained, the boy was tapping prenatal but *unconsciously stored* knowledge, and restoring it to his conscious memory.

At the turn of the eighteenth century, Leibniz gave psychological arguments for the occurrence of *subthreshold* sensory perceptions, and for the existence of unconscious mental contents or motives that manifest themselves in our behavior (Ellenberger, 1970: 312). Moreover, Leibniz (1981, p. 107) pointed out that when the contents of some forgotten experiences subsequently emerge in our consciousness, we may *misidentify* them as *new* experiences, rather than recognize them as having been unconsciously stored in our memory. As Leibniz put it (1981, p. 107):

> It once happened that a man thought that he had written original verses, and was then found to have read them word for word, long before, in some ancient poet. . . . I think that dreams often revive former thoughts for us in this way. As Rosemarie Sand has pointed out (private communication), Leibniz's notion anticipates, to some extent, Freud's dictum that "*The interpretation of dreams is the royal road to a knowledge of the unconscious activities of the mind,*" (1900, p. 608)

Before Freud was born, Hermann von Helmholtz discovered the phenomenon of "unconscious inference" as being present in sensory perception (Ellenberger, 1970: 313). For example, we often unconsciously infer the *constancy* of the *physical* size of nearby objects that move away from us, when we have *other* distance cues, although their *visual* images decrease in size. Similarly, there can be unconsciously inferred constancy of brightness and color under changing conditions of illumination, when the light source remains visible. Such unconscious *inferential compensation* for visual discrepancies also occurs when we transform our *non*-Euclidean (hyper-

C

bolic) binocular *visual* space into the "seen" Euclidean physical space (Grünbaum, 1973: 154–157).

Historically, it is more significant that Freud also had other precursors who anticipated some of his key ideas with impressive *specificity*. As he himself acknowledged (1914, pp. 15–16), Arthur Schopenhauer and Friedrich Nietzsche had speculatively propounded major psychoanalytic doctrines that he himself reportedly developed independently from his clinical observations only thereafter. Indeed, a new German book by the Swiss psychologist Marcel Zentner (1995) traces the foundations of psychoanalysis to the philosophy of Schopenhauer.

Preparatory to my critical assessment of the psychoanalytic enterprise, let me emphasize the existence of major differences between the unconscious processes hypothesized by current cognitive psychology, on the one hand, and the unconscious contents of the mind claimed by psychoanalytic psychology, on the other (Eagle, 1987). These differences will show that the existence of the *cognitive* unconscious clearly fails to support, or even may cast doubt on, the existence of Freud's *psychoanalytic* unconscious. His so-called *dynamic* unconscious is the supposed repository of repressed forbidden wishes of a sexual or aggressive nature, whose reentry or initial entry into consciousness is prevented by the defensive operations of the ego. Though socially unacceptable, these instinctual desires are so imperious and peremptory that they recklessly seek immediate gratification, independently of the constraints of external reality.

Indeed, according to Freud (1900, pp. 566–567), we would not even have developed the skills needed to engage in cognitive activities if it had been possible to gratify our instinctual needs without reliance on these cognitive skills. Thus, as Eagle (1987, p. 162) has pointed out:

> Freud did not seem to take seriously the possibility that cognition and thought could be inherently programmed to reflect reality and could have their own structure and development—an assumption basic to cognitive psychology. After World War II, the psychoanalyst Heinz Hartmann was driven, by facts of biological maturation discovered *non*-psychoanalytically, to acknowledge in his so-called "ego psychology" that such functions as cognition, memory and thinking can develop autonomously by *innate genetic programming*, and independently of instinctual drive gratification. (Eagle, 1993: 374–376).

In the cognitive unconscious, there is great rationality in the ubiquitous computational and associative problem-solving processes required by memory, perception, judgment, and attention. By contrast, as Freud emphasized, the wish content of the dynamic unconscious makes it operate in a highly illogical way.

There is a further major difference between the two species of unconscious (Eagle, 1987: 161–165): The dynamic unconscious acquires its content largely from the unwitting repression of ideas in the form they originally had in consciousness. By contrast, in the generation of the processes in the cognitive unconscious, neither the expulsion of ideas and memories from consciousness nor the censorious denial of entry to them plays any role at all. Having populated the dynamic unconscious by means of repressions, Freud reasoned that the use of his new technique of free association could *lift* these repressions of instinctual wishes, and could thereby bring the repressed ideas back to consciousness *unchanged*. But in the case of the cognitive unconscious, we typically cannot bring to phenomenal consciousness the intellectual processes presumed to occur in it, although we can describe them theoretically.

For example, even if my life depended on it, I simply could not bring into my phenomenal conscious experience the elaborate scanning or search process by which I rapidly come up with the name of the Russian czarina's confidante Rasputin when I am asked for it. Helmholtz's various processes of "unconscious inference" illustrate the same point. By glossing over the stated major differences between the two species of unconscious, some psychoanalysts have claimed their compatibility within the same genus without ado (Shevrin et al., 1992: 340–341). But Eagle (1987, pp. 166–186) has articulated the extensive modifications required in the Freudian notion of the dynamic unconscious, if it is to be made compatible with the cognitive one.

More important, some Freudian apologists have overlooked that even after the two different species of the genus "unconscious" are thus made logically *compatible*, the dynamic unconscious as such cannot derive any *credibility* from the presumed existence of the cognitive unconscious. Nonetheless, faced with mounting attacks on their theory and therapy, some psychoanalysts have made just that fallacious claim. Thus, the Chicago analyst Michael Franz Basch (1994, p. 1) reasoned in vain that since neurophysiological evidence supports the hypothesis of a *generic* unconscious, "psychoanalytic theory has passed the [epistemological] test with flying colors." On the contrary, we must bear in mind that evidence for the cognitive unconscious does not, as such, also furnish support for the dynamic unconscious as such.

Has Psychoanalytic Theory Become a Staple of Western Culture?

In appraising psychoanalysis, we must also beware of yet another logical blunder that has recently become fashionable: The bizarre argument recently given by a number of American philosophers (e.g., Nagel, 1994) that the supposed pervasive influence of Freudian ideas in Western culture vouches for the validity of the psychoanalytic enterprise. But this argument is demonstrably untenable (Grünbaum, 1994).

Even its premise that Freudian theory has become part of the intellectual ethos and folklore of Western culture cannot be taken at face value. As the great Swiss scholar Henri Ellenberger (1970, pp. 547–549) has stressed in his monumental historical work, *The Discovery of the Unconscious*, the prevalence of vulgarized *pseudo*-Freudian concepts makes it very difficult to determine reliably the extent to which *genuine* psychoanalytic hypotheses have actually become influential in our culture at large. For example, *any* slip of the tongue or other bungled action (parapraxis) is typically yet incorrectly called a "Freudian slip."

But Freud himself has called attention to the existence of a very large class of lapses or slips whose psychological motivation is simply *transparent* to the person who commits them or to others (1916, p. 40). And he added commendably that neither he nor his followers deserve any credit for the motivational explanations of such perspicuous slips (1916, p. 47). In this vein, a psychoanalyst friend of mine provided me with the following example of a *pseudo*-Freudian slip that would, however, be wrongly yet widely called "Freudian": A man who is at a crowded party in a stiflingly hot room starts to go outdoors to cool off but is confronted by the exciting view of a woman's *décolleté* bosom and says to her: "Excuse me, I have to get a *breast* of *flesh* air." Many otherwise educated people would erroneously classify this slip as Freudian for two *wrong* reasons: First, *merely* because it is motivated, rather than a purely mechanical *lapsus linguae*, and, furthermore, because its theme is sexual.

Yet what is required for a slip or so-called parapraxis to qualify as *freudian* is that it be motivationally *opaque* rather than transparent, precisely because its psycho-

logical motive is repressed (1916, p. 41). As the father of psychoanalysis declared unambiguously (1901, p. 239): If psychoanalysis is to provide an explanation of a parapraxis, "we must not be aware in ourselves of any motive for it. We must rather be tempted to explain it by 'inattentiveness', or to put it down to 'chance'." And Freud characterized the pertinent explanatory unconscious causes of slips as "motives of unpleasure." Thus, when a young man forgot the Latin word "*aliquis*" in a quotation from Virgil, Freud diagnosed its interfering cause as the man's distressing unconscious fear that his girlfriend had become pregnant by him (1901, p. 9). *If* that latent fear was actually the motive of the slip, it was surely *not apparent* to anyone.

Once it is clear what is *meant* by a *bona fide* Freudian slip, we need to ask whether there *actually exist* any such slips at all, that is, slips that *appear* to be psychologically *unmotivated* but are actually caused by repressed, unpleasant ideas. It is very important to appreciate how difficult it is to provide cogent evidence for such causation. K. Schüttauf et al. (forthcoming) claim to have produced just such evidence. They note that, according to psychoanalytic etiologic theory, obsessive-compulsive neurosis is attributable to an unconscious conflict whose repressed component features anal-erotic and sadistic wishes, which are presumably activated by regression. Then they reason that when such conflict-laden material is to be verbalized by obsessive-compulsive neurotics, Freudian theory expects a higher incidence of misspeakings (slips of the tongue) among them than among normal subjects. And these researchers report that all their findings bore out that expectation.

This investigation by Schüttauf et al. differs from Bröder's (1995) strategy, which was designed to inquire into "the possible influence of unconscious information-processing on the frequency of specific speech-errors in an experimental setting." Thus, Bröder and Bredenkamp (1996, Abstract) claim to have produced experimental support for the "weaker Freudian thesis" of verbal slip-generation by unconscious, rather than repressed, thoughts: "Priming words that remain unconscious induce misspeaking errors with higher probability than consciously registered ones."

As for the soundness of the design of Schüttauf et al., Hans Eysenck (private communication to Rosemarie Sand, March 1, 1996; cited by permission to her) has raised several objections: (1) "as the author [Schüttauf] himself acknowledges, this is not an experiment, as ordinarily understood; it is a simple correlational study . . . correlation cannot be interpreted as causation, which he unfortunately attempts to do." (2) The members of the experimental group were severely neurotic, while the control group were normals. But "the proper control group would have been severely [disturbed] neurotics suffering from a different form of neurosis than that of obsessive compulsive behaviour." (3) "Freudian theory posits a causal relationship between the anal stage of development and obsessive compulsive neurosis; the author does not even try to document this hypothetical relationship." (4) "[O]bsessive-compulsive neurotics suffer from fear of dirt and contamination, so that on those grounds alone they would be likely to react differentially to stimuli suggesting such contamination. . . . It is truly commonsensical to say that people whose neurosis consists of feelings of dirt will react differentially to verbal presentations of words related to dirt."

Naturally, I sympathize with Schüttauf and his coworkers in their avowed effort (Section 4) to escape my criticism (Grünbaum, 1984: 202–205) of an earlier purported experimental confirmation of Freud's theory of slips by M. T. Motley (1980). I had complained that the independent variable Motley manipulated in his speech-error experiments did *not* involve *unconscious* antecedents— only conscious ones. As Schüttauf et al. tell us, precisely to escape my criticism of Motley, they relied on Freud's etiology of obsessive-compulsive neurosis to infer that subjects who exhibit the symptoms of that neurosis fulfill the requirement of harboring repressions of anal-sadistic wishes. Thus, *only* on that etiologic assumption does their use of compulsive subjects *and* their manipulation of words pertaining to anal-sadistic themata warrant their expectation of a higher incidence of verbal slips in this group than among normals.

Surely one could not reasonably expect the authors themselves to have carried out empirical tests of the etiology on which their entire investigation is *crucially predicated*. But nonetheless Eysenck's demand for such evidence is entirely appropriate: Without independent *supporting* evidence for that etiology, their test is definitely not a test of Freud's theory of slips of the tongue, let alone—as they conclude—a confirmation of it.

Thus, as long as good empirical support for the Freudian scenario is unavailable, we actually don't know whether any *bona fide* Freudian slips exist at all. Just this lack of evidence serves to undermine Nagel's thesis that cultural influence is a criterion of validity. After all, if we

have no cogent evidence for the existence of genuinely Freudian slips, then Freud's theory of bungled actions ("parapraxes") might well be false. And if so, it would not contribute one iota to its validity, even if our entire culture unanimously believed in it and made extensive explanatory use of it: When an ill-supported theory is used to provide explanations, they run the grave risk of being bogus, and its purported insights may well be *pseudo*-insights.

A second example supporting my rejection of Nagel's cultural criterion is furnished by the work of the celebrated art historian Meyer Schapiro of Columbia University. Schapiro saw himself as greatly influenced by Freud in his accounts of the work of such painters as Paul Cézanne, who died in 1906 (Solomon, 1994). Of course, Schapiro never actually put Cézanne on the psychoanalytic couch. But he subjected artists indirectly "to his own [brand of speculative] couch treatment" (Solomon, 1994). In his best-known essay, Schapiro "turns the Frenchman into a case history." Indeed, a recent tribute to Schapiro's transformation of scholarship in art history (Solomon, 1994) says that his "accomplishment was to shake off the dust and open the field to a style of speculation and intellectual bravura that drew . . . most notably [on] psychoanalysis" (Solomon, 1994: 24). Reportedly, "his insights into . . . the apples of Cézanne" (Solomon, 1994: 24) make the point that Cézanne's "depictions of apples contain [in Schapiro's words] 'a latent erotic sense'."

But if apples are held to symbolize sex unconsciously for Cézanne or anyone else, why doesn't *anything else* that resembles apples in some respect (e.g., being quasi-spherical) do likewise? Yet we learn that Schapiro's 1968 publication "The Apples of Cézanne" is "His best known essay" (p. 25). Alas, if Schapiro's claim that Cézanne was "unwillingly chaste" is to be a psychoanalytic insight gleaned from his art, rather than a documented biographical fact, Schapiro's psychodiagnosis is an instance of what Freud himself deplored as "'Wild' Psycho-Analysis" (1910, pp. 221–227). In any case, *pace* Nagel, such art-historical invocation of Freud, however influential, does nothing, I claim, to enhance the *credibility* of psychoanalysis.

For centuries, even as far back as in New Testament narratives, both physical disease and insanity have been attributed to demonic possession in Christendom, no less than among primitive peoples. That demon theory has been used, for example, to explain deafness, blindness, and fever as well as such psychopathological conditions as epilepsy, somnambulism, and hysteria. Our contemporary medical term "epilepsy" comes from the Greek word *"epilepsis"* (*seizure*) and reflects etymologically the notion of being seized by a demon. Since exorcism is designed to drive out the devil, it is the supposed *therapy* for demonic possession. In the Roman Catholic exorcist ritual, which has been endorsed by the present pope and by the late John Cardinal O'Connor of New York, the existence of death is blamed on Satan. And that ritual also survives in baptism as well as in blessing persons or consecrating houses.

How does the strength of the cultural influence of such religious beliefs and practices compare to that of Freud's teachings? Though Freud characterized his type of psychotherapy as *"primus inter pares"* (1933, p. 157), he conceded sorrowfully: "I do not think our [psychoanalytic] cures can compete with those of Lourdes. There are so many more people who believe in the miracles of the Blessed Virgin than in the existence of the unconscious" (1933, p. 152). Clearly, the psychoanalytic and theological notions of etiology and of therapy clash, and their comparative cultural influence cannot cogently decide between them. But if it *could*, psychoanalysis would be the loser! This alone, I claim, is a reductio ad absurdum of the thesis that the validity of the psychoanalytic enterprise is assured by its wide cultural influence.

Nor can Nagel buttress that thesis by the dubious, vague declaration that psychoanalysis is an "extension" of common sense. As I have shown elsewhere (Grünbaum, forthcoming), the term "extension" is hopelessly unable to bear the weight required by his thesis, if actual psychoanalytic theory is to square with it. What, for example, is *commonsensical* about the standard psychoanalytic etiologic explanation of male diffidence and social anxiety by repressed adult "*castration* anxiety" (Fenichel, 1945: 520), or of a like explanation of a male driver's stopping at a *green* traffic light as if it were red (Brenner, 1982: 182–183)? Common sense rightly treats such explanations incredulously as bizarre, and rightly so: As I have shown (Grünbaum, 1997), these etiologic explanations rest on quicksand, even if we were to grant Freud's Oedipal scenario that all adult males unconsciously dread castration by their fathers for having lusted after their mothers.

Critique of Freudian and Post-Freudian Psychoanalysis

Let me now turn to my critique of the core of Freud's original psychoanalytic theory and to a verdict on its fun-

damental modifications by two major post-Freudian sets of hypotheses called "self-psychology" and "object relations theory."

The pillars of the avowed "cornerstone" of Freud's theoretical edifice comprise several major theses: (1) Distressing mental states induce the operation of a psychic mechanism of repression, which consists in the banishment from consciousness of *unpleasurable* psychic states (1915b, p. 147). (2) Once repression is operative (more or less fully), it not only banishes such negatively charged ideas from consciousness, but plays a *further* crucial multiple causal role: It is *causally necessary* for the pathogens of neuroses, the production of our dreams, and the generation of our various sorts of slips (bungled actions). (3) The "method of free association" can identify and lift (undo) the patient's repressions; by doing so, it can identify the pathogens of the neuroses and the generators of our dreams, as well as the causes of our motivationally opaque slips; moreover, by lifting the pathogenic repressions, free association functions therapeutically, rather than only investigatively.

Freud provided two sorts of arguments for his cardinal etiologic doctrine that repressions are the pathogens of the neuroses: His earlier one, which goes back to his original collaboration with Josef Breuer, relies on purported *therapeutic successes* from lifting repressions; the later one, designed to show that the pathogenic repressions are sexual, is drawn from presumed reenactments ("transferences") of infantile episodes in the adult patient's interactions with the analyst during psychoanalytic treatment.

It will be expositorily expeditious to deal with Freud's earlier etiologic argument below, and to appraise the subsequent one, which goes back to his "Dora" case history of 1905, after that. But also for expository reasons, it behooves us to devote an introduction section to his account of the actuation of the hypothesized mechanism of repression by "motives of unpleasure."

Negative Affect and Forgetting. As Freud told us, "The theory of repression is the cornerstone on which the whole structure of psycho-analysis rests. It is the most essential part of it" (1914, p. 16). The *process* of repression, which consists in the banishment of ideas from consciousness or in denying them entry into it, is itself presumed to be unconscious (1915b, p. 147). In Freud's view, our neurotic symptoms, the manifest contents of our dreams, and the slips we commit are each constructed as "compromises between the demands of a repressed impulse and the resistances of a censoring force in the ego" (1925, p. 45; 1917, p. 301). By being only such compromises, rather than fulfillments of the instinctual impulses, these products of the unconscious afford only *substitutive* gratifications or outlets. For brevity, one can say, therefore, that Freud has offered a unifying "compromise model" of neuroses, dreams, and parapraxes.

But what, in the first place, is the *motive* or cause that initiates and sustains the operation of the unconscious mechanism of repression *before* it produces its own later effects? Apparently, Freud assumes *axiomatically* that distressing mental states, such as forbidden wishes, trauma, disgust, anxiety, anger, shame, hate, guilt, and sadness—all of which are *unpleasurable*—almost always actuate, and then fuel, *forgetting* to the point of repression. Thus, repression regulates pleasure and unpleasure by defending our consciousness against various sorts of *negative affect*. Indeed, Freud claimed perennially that repression is the paragon among our *defense* mechanisms (Thomä and Kächele, 1987: vol. 1, 107–111). As Freud put it dogmatically: "The tendency to forget what is disagreeable seems to me to be a quite universal one" (1901, p. 144), and "the recollection of distressing impressions and the occurrence of distressing thoughts are opposed by a resistance" (1901, p. 146).

Freud tries to disarm an important objection to his thesis that "distressing memories succumb especially easily to motivated forgetting" (1901, p. 147). He says:

> The assumption that a defensive trend of this kind exists cannot be objected to on the ground that one often enough finds it impossible, on the contrary, to get rid of distressing memories that pursue one, and to banish distressing affective impulses like remorse and the pangs of conscience. For we are not asserting that this defensive trend is able to put itself into effect *in every case* . . . (p. 147, italics *added*)

He acknowledges as "also a true fact" that "distressing things are particularly hard to forget" (1916, pp. 76–77).

For instance, we know from Charles Darwin's autobiography that his father had developed a remarkably retentive memory for painful experiences (cited in Grünbaum, 1994), and that a half century after Giuseppe Verdi was humiliatingly denied admission to the Milan

Music Conservatory, he recalled it indignantly (Walker, 1962: 8–9). Freud himself told us as an adult (1900, p. 216) that he "can remember very clearly," from age seven or eight, how his father rebuked him for having relieved himself in the presence of his parents in their bedroom. In a frightful blow to Freud's ego, his father said: "The boy will come to nothing."

But Freud's attempt here to uphold his thesis of motivated forgetting is *evasive* and *unavailing*: Since some painful mental states are vividly remembered while others are forgotten or even repressed, I claim that *factors different from their painfulness determine whether they are remembered or forgotten*. For example, personality dispositions or situational variables may in fact be causally relevant. To the great detriment of his theory, Freud never came to grips with the *unfavorable* bearing of this key fact about the mnemic effects of painfulness on the tenability of the following pillar of his theory of repression: When painful or forbidden experiences are forgotten, the forgetting is tantamount to their repression *owing to their negative affect*, and thereby produces neurotic symptoms or other compromise formations. Thomas Gilovich, a professor of psychology at Cornell University, has done valuable work on the conditions under which painful experiences are *remembered*, and on those *other* conditions under which they are forgotten.

The numerous and familiar occurrences of vivid and even obsessive recall of negative experiences pose a fundamental *statistical* and explanatory challenge to Freud that neither he nor his followers have ever met. We must ask (Grünbaum, 1994): Just what is the *ratio* of the forgetting of distressing experiences to their recall, and what *other* factors determine that ratio? Freud gave no statistical evidence for assuming that forgetting them is the *rule*, while remembering them is the exception. Yet as we can see, his theory of repression is devastatingly undermined from the outset if forgettings of negative experiences do not greatly outnumber rememberings statistically. After all, if forgetting is not the rule, then what *other* reason does Freud offer for supposing that when distressing experiences are actually forgotten, these forgettings are instances of genuine repression due to affective displeasure? And if he has no such other reason, then, a fortiori, he has no basis at all for his pivotal etiologic scenario that forbidden or aversive states of mind are usually repressed and thereby cause compromise formations.

Astonishingly, Freud thinks he can parry this basic statistical and explanatory challenge by an evasive dictum

C

as follows: "mental life is the arena and battle-ground for mutually opposing purposes [of forgetting and remembering] (1916, p. 76) . . .; there is room for both. It is only a question . . . of what effects are produced by the one and the other" (p. 77). Just that question cries out for an answer from Freud, if he is to make his case. Instead, he cavalierly left it to dangle epistemologically in limbo.

The Epistemological Liabilities of the Psychoanalytic Method of Free Association. Another basic difficulty, which besets all three major branches of the theory of repression alike, lies in the epistemological defects of Freud's so-called fundamental rule of free association, the supposed microscope and X-ray tomograph of the human mind. This rule enjoins the patient to tell the analyst without reservation whatever comes to mind. Thus it serves as the fundamental method of clinical investigation. We are told that by using this technique to unlock the floodgates of the unconscious, Freud was able to show that neuroses, dreams, and slips are caused by repressed motives. Just as in Breuer's cathartic use of hypnosis, it is a cardinal thesis of Freud's entire psychoanalytic enterprise that his method of free association has a twofold major capability, which is both investigative and therapeutic: (1) It can *identify* the unconscious causes of human thoughts and behavior, both abnormal and normal, and (2) by overcoming resistances and lifting repressions, it can remove the unconscious pathogens of neuroses, and thus provide therapy for an important class of mental disorders.

But on what grounds did Freud assert that free association has the stunning investigative capability to be *causally probative* for etiologic research in psychopathology? Is it not too good to be true that one can put a psychologically disturbed person on the couch and fathom the etiology of her or his affliction by free association? As compared to fathoming the causation of major somatic diseases, that seems almost miraculous, *if at all true*. Freud tells us very clearly (1900, p. 528) that his argument for his investigative tribute to free association as a means of uncovering the causation of neuroses is, at bottom, a *therapeutic* one going back to the cathartic method of treating hysteria. Let me state and articulate his argument.

One of Freud's justifications for the use of free association as a *causally probative* method of dream investigation leading to the identification of the repressed dream thoughts, he tells us (1900, p. 528), is that it "is

identical with the procedure [of free association] by which we resolve hysterical symptoms; and there the correctness of our method [of free association] is warranted by the coincident emergence and disappearance of the symptoms." But as I have pointed out elsewhere (Grünbaum, 1993: 25–26), his original German text here contains a confusing slip of the pen. As we know, the patient's symptoms hardly first emerge simultaneously with their therapeutic dissipation. Yet Strachey translated Freud correctly as having spoken of "the coincident emergence and disappearance of the symptoms." It would seem that Freud means to speak of the *resolution* (German: *Auflösung*), rather than of the emergence (*Auftauchen*), of the symptoms as coinciding with their therapeutic dissipation. Now, for Freud, the "resolution of a symptom," in turn, consists of using free association to uncover the repressed pathogen that enters into the compromise formation that is held to constitute the symptom. This much, then, is the statement of Freud's appeal to therapeutic success to vouch for the "correctness of our method" of free association as causally probative for etiologic research in psychopathology.

To articulate the argument adequately, however, we must still clarify Freud's original basis for claiming that (unsuccessful) repression is indeed the pathogen of neurosis. Only then will he have made his case for claiming that free association is etiologically probative, because it is uniquely capable of uncovering repressions. The pertinent argument is offered in Breuer and Freud's "Preliminary Communication" (1893, pp. 6–7). There they wrote (p. 6, italics in original):

For we found, to our great surprise at first, that *each individual hysterical symptom immediately and permanently disappeared when we had succeeded in bringing clearly to light the memory of the event by which it was provoked and in arousing its accompanying affect, and when the patient had described that event in the greatest possible detail and had put the affect into words.* Recollection without affect almost invariably produces no result. The psychical process which originally took place must be repeated as vividly as possible; it must be brought back to its *status nascendi* and then given verbal utterance.

Breuer and Freud make an important comment on their construal of this therapeutic finding:

It is plausible to suppose that it is a question here of unconscious suggestion: the patient expects to be relieved of his sufferings by this procedure, and it is this expectation, and not the verbal utterance, which is the operative factor. This, however, is not so. (p. 7)

And their avowed reason is that, in 1881, i.e., in the "'pre-suggestion' era," the cathartic method was used to remove *separately* distinct symptoms, "which sprang from separate causes" such that any one symptom disappeared only after the cathartic ("abreactive") lifting of a *particular* repression. But Breuer and Freud do not tell us why the likelihood of placebo effect should be deemed to be lower when several symptoms are wiped out *seriatim* than in the case of getting rid of only one symptom. Thus, as I have pointed out elsewhere (Grünbaum, 1993: 238), to discredit the hypothesis of placebo effect, it would have been essential to have comparisons with treatment outcome from a suitable control group whose repressions are *not* lifted. If that control group were to fare equally well, treatment gains from psychoanalysis would then be placebo effects after all.

In sum, Breuer and Freud inferred that the therapeutic removal of neurotic symptoms was produced by the cathartic lifting of the patient's previously ongoing repression of the pertinent traumatic memory, not by the therapist's suggestion or some other placebo factor (See Grünbaum, 1993: chap. 3 for a very detailed analysis of the placebo concept). We can codify this claim as follows:

T. Therapeutic Hypothesis: Lifting repressions of traumatic memories cathartically is *causally relevant* to the disappearance of neuroses.

As we saw, Breuer and Freud (p. 6) reported the immediate and permanent disappearance of each hysterical symptom after they cathartically lifted the repression of the memory of the trauma that occasioned the given symptom. They adduce this "evidence" to draw an epoch-making inductive *etiologic* inference (p. 6), which postulates "a causal relation between the determining [repression of the memory of the] psychical trauma and the hysterical phenomenon." Citing the old scholastic dictum *"Cessante causa cessat effectus"* (When the cause ceases, its effect ceases), they invoke its contrapositive (p. 7), which states that as long as the effect (symptom) persists, so does its cause (the repressed memory of the psy-

chical trauma). And they declare just that to be the pattern of the pathogenic action of the repressed psychical trauma. This trauma, we learn, is *not* a mere *precipitating* cause. Such a mere *"agent provocateur"* just releases the symptom, "which thereafter leads an independent existence." Instead, "the [repressed] memory of the trauma . . . acts like a foreign body which long after its entry must continue to be regarded as an agent that is still at work" (p. 6).

The upshot of their account is that their observations of positive therapeutic outcome upon the abreactive lifting of repressions, which they interpret in the sense of their therapeutic hypothesis, spelled a paramount etiologic moral as follows:

E. Etiologic Hypothesis: An ongoing repression accompanied by affective suppression is causally necessary for the initial pathogenesis *and* persistence of a neurosis.

(This formulation of the foundational etiology of psychoanalysis supersedes the one I gave at the hands of a suggestion by Carl Hempel and Morris Eagle [in Grünbaum, 1984: 181, last paragraph]. The revised formulation here is faithful to Breuer and Freud's reference to "accompanying affect" [p. 6] apropos of the traumatic events whose repression occasioned the symptoms.)

Clearly, this etiologic hypothesis *E* permits the *valid deduction* of the therapeutic finding reported by Breuer and Freud as codified in their therapeutic hypothesis *T*: The cathartic lifting of the repressions of traumatic memories of events that occasion symptoms engendered the disappearance of the symptoms. And as they told us explicitly (p. 6), this therapeutic finding is their "evidence" for their cardinal etiologic hypothesis *E*.

But I maintain that this inductive argument is vitiated by what I like to call the *"fallacy of crude hypothetico-deductive ("H-D") pseudo-confirmation."* Thus note that the remedial action of aspirin consumption for tension headaches does not lend H-D support to the outlandish etiologic hypothesis that a hematolytic aspirin *deficiency* is a causal *sine qua non* for having tension headaches, although such remedial action is validly deducible from that bizarre hypothesis. Twenty-five years ago, Wesley Salmon called attention to the fallacy of inductive causal inference from mere valid H-D deducibility by giving an example in which a deductively valid pseudoexplanation of a man's avoiding pregnancy can readily give rise

C

to an H-D pseudoconfirmation of the addle-brained attribution of his nonpregnancy to his consumption of birth-control pills. Salmon (1971, p. 34) states the fatuous pseudoexplanation:

> John Jones avoided becoming pregnant during the past year, for he had taken his wife's birth control pills regularly, and every man who regularly takes birth control pills avoids pregnancy.

Plainly, this deducibility of John Jones's recent failure to become pregnant from the stated premises does not lend any credence at all to the zany hypothesis that this absence of pregnancy is *causally attributable* to his consumption of birth-control pills. Yet it is even true that any men who consume such pills *in fact* never do become pregnant. Patently, as Salmon notes, the fly in the ointment is that men just do not become pregnant, whether they take birth-control pills or not.

His example shows that neither the empirical truth of the deductively inferred conclusion and of the pertinent initial condition concerning Jones nor the deductive validity of the inference can provide bona fide confirmation of the causal hypothesis that male consumption of birth-control pills prevents male pregnancy: That hypothesis would first have to meet other epistemic requirements, which it manifestly cannot do.

Crude H-D confirmationism is a paradise of spurious causal inferences, as illustrated by Breuer and Freud's unsound etiologic inference. Thus, psychoanalytic narratives are replete with the belief that a hypothesized etiologic scenario embedded in a psychoanalytic narrative of an analysand's affliction is *made credible* merely because the postulated etiology then permits the logical deduction or probabilistic inference of the neurotic symptoms to be explained.

Yet some apologists offer a facile excuse for the fallacious H-D confirmation of a causal hypothesis. We are told that the hypothesis is warranted by an "inference to the best explanation" (Harman, 1965). But in a careful new study, Salmon (2001) has argued that "the characterization of nondemonstrative inference as inference to the best explanation serves to muddy the waters . . . by fostering confusion" between two sorts of why-questions that Hempel had distinguished: *Explanation*-seeking questions as to why something is the case, and *confirmation*-seeking why-questions as to why a hypothesis is *credible*. Thus, a hypothesis that is pseudoconfirmed by some data

cannot be warranted qua being "the only [explanatory] game in town." Alas, "best explanation"–sanction was claimed for psychoanalytic etiologies to explain and treat the destructive behavior of sociopaths *to no avail* for years (cf. Cleckley, 1988, Section Four, esp. pp. 238–239 and 438–439).

I can now demonstrate the multiple failure of Freud's therapeutic argument for the etiologic probativeness of free association in psychopathology, no matter how revealing the associative contents may otherwise be in regard to the patient's psychological preoccupations and personality dispositions. Let us take our bearings and first encapsulate the structure of his therapeutic argument.

First, Freud inferred that the therapeutic disappearance of the neurotic symptoms is *causally attributable* to the cathartic lifting of repressions *by means of the method free associations*. Relying on this key therapeutic hypothesis, he then drew two further major theoretical inferences: (1) The seeming removal of the neurosis by means of cathartically *lifting* repressions is good inductive evidence for postulating that repressions accompanied by affective suppression are themselves *causally necessary* for the very existence of a neurosis (1893, pp. 6–7), and (2) granted that such repressions are thus the essential causes of neurosis, *and* that the method of free association is uniquely capable of uncovering these repressions, this method is uniquely competent *to identify the causes* or pathogens of the neuroses. (Having convinced himself of the causal probativeness of the method of free associations on therapeutic grounds in the case of those neuroses he believed to be successfully treatable, Freud also felt justified in deeming the method reliable as a means of unearthing the etiologies of those other neuroses—the so-called narcissistic ones, such as paranoia—that he considered psychoanalytically *untreatable*.)

But the argument fails for the following several reasons: In the first place, the durable therapeutic success on which it was predicated did not materialize (Borch-Jacobsen, 1996), as Freud was driven to admit both early and very late in his career (1925, p. 27; 1937, pp. 23, 216–253). But even insofar as there was transitory therapeutic gain, we saw that Freud *failed* to rule out a rival hypothesis that undermines his attribution of such gain to the lifting of repressions by free association: The ominous hypothesis of placebo effect, which asserts that treatment ingredients *other than* insight into the patient's repressions—such as the mobilization of the patient's hope by the therapist—are responsible for any resulting improvement (Grünbaum, 1993: chap. 3). Nor have other analysts ruled out the placebo hypothesis during the past century. A case in point is a forty-five–page study "On the Efficacy of Psychoanalysis" (Bachrach et al., 1991), published in the official *Journal of the American Psychoanalytic Association*. Another is the account of analytic treatment process by Vaughan and Roose (1995).

Last, but not least, the repression etiology is evidentially ill founded, as we saw earlier and will see further in the next section. It is unavailing to the purported *etiologic* probativeness of free associations that they may lift repressions, since Freud failed to show that the latter are pathogenic. In sum, Freud's argument has forfeited its premises.

Freud's Etiologic Transference Argument.
Now let us consider Freud's argument for his cardinal thesis that *sexual* repressions in particular are the pathogens of all neuroses, an argument he deemed "decisive." Drawing on my earlier writings (1990, pp. 565–567; 1993, pp. 152–158), we shall now find that this argument is without merit.

According to Freud's theory of transference, the patient *transfers* onto his or her psychoanalyst feelings and thoughts that originally pertained to important figures in his or her earlier life. In this important sense, the fantasies woven around the psychoanalyst by the analysand, and quite generally the latter's conduct toward his or her doctor, are hypothesized to be *thematically recapitulatory* of childhood episodes. And by thus being recapitulatory, the patient's behavior during treatment can be said to exhibit a thematic kinship to such very early episodes. Therefore, when the analyst interprets these supposed reenactments, the ensuing interpretations are called "transference interpretations."

Freud and his followers have traditionally drawn the following highly questionable causal inference: Precisely in virtue of being thematically recapitulated in the patient-doctor interaction, the hypothesized earlier scenario in the patient's life can cogently be held to have originally been a *pathogenic* factor in the patient's affliction. For example, in his case history of the "Rat-Man," Freud (1909) infers that a certain emotional conflict had originally been the precipitating cause of the patient's inability to work, merely because this conflict had been thematically reenacted in a fantasy the "Rat-Man" had woven around Freud during treatment.

Thus, in the context of Freud's transference interpretations, the thematic reenactment is claimed to show that the early scenario had originally been *pathogenic*. According to this etiologic conclusion, the patient's thematic reenactment in the treatment setting is also asserted to be *pathogenically* recapitulatory by being pathogenic in the adult patient's here and now, rather than only thematically recapitulatory. Freud (1914, p. 12) extols this dubious etiologic transference argument in his *History of the Psycho-Analytic Movement*, claiming that it furnishes the most unshakable proof for his sexual etiology of all the neuroses:

> The fact of the emergence of the transference in its crudely sexual form, whether affectionate or hostile, in every treatment of a neurosis, although this is neither desired nor induced by either doctor or patient, has always seemed to me the most irrefragable proof [original German: "unerschütterlichste Beweis"] that the source of the driving forces of neurosis lies in sexual life [sexual repressions]. This argument has never received anything approaching the degree of attention that it merits, for if it had, investigations in this field would leave no other conclusion open. As far as I am concerned, this argument has remained the decisive one, over and above the more specific findings of analytic work.

On the contrary, the patient's thematically recapitulatory behavior toward his doctor *does not show* that it is also *pathogenically* recapitulatory. How, for example, does the reenactment, during treatment, of a patient's early conflict show at all that the original conflict had been pathogenic in the first place? Quite generally, how do transference phenomena focusing on the analyst show that a presumed current replica of a past event is *pathogenic* in the here and now?

Therefore, I submit, the purportedly "irrefragable proof" of which Freud spoke deserves more attention *not* because its appreciation "would leave no other conclusion open," as he would have it; instead, I contend that the "Rat-Man" case and other such case histories show how baffling it is that Freud deemed the etiologic transference argument cogent *at all*, let alone unshakably so.

Marshall Edelson (1984, p. 150) has offered a rebuttal to my denial of the cogency of the etiologic transference argument:

C

. . . . in fact, in psychoanalysis the pathogen is not merely a remote event, or a series of such events, the effect of which lives on. The pathogen reappears in all its virulence, with increasing frankness and explicitness, in the transference—in a new edition, a new version, a reemergence, a repetition of the past pathogenic events or factors.

And Edelson elaborates (p. 151):

The pathogen together with its pathological effects are [sic], therefore, under the investigator's eye, so to speak, in the psychoanalytic situation, and demonstrating the causal relation between them in that situation, by experimental or quasi-experimental methods, surely provides support, even if indirect, for the hypothesis that in the past the same kind of pathogenic factors were necessary to bring about the same kind of effects.

But how does the psychoanalyst demonstrate, within the confines of his or her clinical setting, that the supposed current replica of the remote, early event is presently the virulent cause of the patient's neurosis, let alone that the original pathogen is replicated at all in the transference? Having fallaciously identified a conflict as a pathogen because it reappears in the transference, many Freudians conclude that pathogens must reappear in the transference. And in this way, they beg the key question I have just asked. How, for example, did Freud show that the "Rat-Man"'s marriage conflict depicted in that patient's transference fantasy was the current cause of his ongoing death obsessions? Neither Edelson's book nor his (1986) paper offers a better answer. Thus, in the latter paper, he declares: "The psychoanalyst claims that current mental representations of particular past events or fantasies are constitutive (i.e., current operative) causes of current behavior, and then goes on to claim that therefore past actual events or fantasies are etiological causes of the analysand's symptoms." And Edelson concludes: "Transference phenomena are . . . nonquestion-begging evidence for . . . inferences about causally efficacious psychological entities existing or occurring in the here and now" (p. 110).

In sum, despite Edelson's best efforts, the etiologic transference argument on which both Freud and he rely is illfounded: (1) They employ epistemically circular reasoning when inferring the occurrence of infantile episodes from the adult patient's reports, and then claiming that these early episodes are thematically recapitulated in the adult analysand's conduct toward the analyst; (2) they beg the etiologic question by inferring that, qua being thematically recapitulated, the infantile episodes had been pathogenic at the outset; (3) they reason that the adult patient's thematic reenactment is pathogenically recapitulatory such that the current replica of the infantile episodes is pathogenic in the here and now.

Freud went on to build on the quicksand of his etiologic transference argument. It inspired two of his further fundamental tenets: first, the investigative thesis that the psychoanalytic dissection of the patient's behavior toward the analyst can reliably identify the original pathogens of his or her long-term neurosis; second, the cardinal therapeutic doctrine that the working through of the analysand's so-called "transference neurosis" is the key to overcoming his or her perennial problems.

Free Association as a Method of Dream Interpretation. Yet as we learn from Freud's opening pages on his method of dream interpretation, he extrapolated the presumed causally probative role of free associations from being only a method of etiologic inquiry aimed at therapy, to serving likewise as an avenue for finding the purported unconscious causes of dreams (1900, pp. 100–101; see also p. 528). And in the same breath, he reports that when patients told him about their dreams while associating freely to their symptoms, he extrapolated his compromise model from neurotic symptoms to manifest dream contents. A year later, he carried out the same twofold extrapolation to include slips or bungled actions.

But what do free associations tell us about our dreams? Whatever the manifest content of dreams, they are purportedly wish-fulfilling in at least two logically distinct specific ways, as follows: For every dream D, there exists at least one normally unconscious infantile wish W such that (1) W is the motivational cause of D, and (2) the manifest content of D graphically displays, more or less disguisedly, the state of affairs desired by W. As Freud opined (1925, p. 44): "When the latent dream-thoughts that are revealed by the analysis [via free association] of a dream are examined, one of them is found to stand out from among the rest . . . the isolated thought is found to be a wishful impulse." But Freud manipulated the free associations to yield a distinguished wish motive (Glymour, 1983).

Quite independently of Freud's abortive therapeutic argument for the causal probativeness of free association, he offered his analysis of his 1895 "Specimen Irma Dream" as a *non*therapeutic argument for the method of free association as a cogent means of identifying hypothesized hidden, forbidden wishes as the motives of our dreams. But in my detailed critique of that unjustly celebrated analysis (Grünbaum, 1984: chap. 5), I have argued that Freud's account is, alas, no more than a piece of false advertising: (1) It does not deliver at all the promised vindication of the probativeness of free association, (2) it does nothing toward warranting his foolhardy dogma that *all* dreams are wish-fulfilling in his stated sense, (3) it does not even pretend that his alleged "Specimen Dream" is evidence for his compromise model of manifest-dream content, and (4) the inveterate and continuing celebration of Freud's analysis of his Irma Dream in the psychoanalytic literature as the paragon of dream interpretation is completely unwarranted, because it is mere salesmanship.

Alas, Freud's 1895 neurobiological wish-fulfillment theory of dreaming was irremediably flawed from the outset (Grünbaum, forthcoming). Furthermore, he astonishingly did not heed a patent epistemological consequence of having abandoned his 1895 *Project's* neurological energy model of *wish-driven* dreaming: By precisely that abandonment, he himself had *forfeited* his initial biological *rationale* for claiming that at least all "normal" dreams are wish fulfilling. *A fortiori*, this forfeiture left him without any kind of energy-based warrant for then *universalizing* the doctrine of wish fulfillment on the psychological level to extend to *any* sort of dream. Yet, unencumbered by the total absence of any such warrant, the *universalized* doctrine, now formulated in psychological terms, rose like a Phoenix from the ashes of Freud's defunct energy model.

Once he had clearly *chained* himself gratuitously to the universal wish monopoly of dream generation, his interpretations of dreams were constrained to reconcile *wish-contravening* dreams with the decreed universality of wish fulfillment. Such reconciliation demanded imperiously that all other parts and details of his dream theory be obligingly *tailored* to the governing wish dogma so as to sustain it. Yet Freud artfully obscured this *dynamic* of theorizing, while begging the methodological question (1900, p. 135). Wish-contravening dreams include anxiety dreams, nightmares, and the so-called "counter-wish dreams" (1900, p. 157). As an example of

the latter, Freud reports a trial attorney's dream that he had lost all his court cases (1900, p. 152).

Freud's initial 1900 statement of his dual wish fulfillment in dreams had been: "*Thus its content was the fulfilment of a wish and its motive was a wish*" (1900, p. 119). But the sense in which dreams are wish fulfilling *overall* is purportedly *threefold* rather than only two fold: One motivating cause is the universal *preconscious* wish to sleep, which purportedly provides a generic causal explanation of dreaming *as such* and, in turn, makes dreaming the guardian of sleep (1900, pp. 234, 680); another is the individualized *repressed* infantile wish, which is activated by the day's residue and explains the *particular* manifest *content* of a given dream; furthermore, as already noted, that manifest content of the dream graphically displays, more or less disguisedly, the state of affairs desired by the unconscious wish. The disguise is supposedly effected by the defensive operation of the "dream-*distortion*" of the content of forbidden unconscious wishes.

But this theorized distortion of the hypothesized latent content must not be identified with the very familiar *phenomenological bizarreness* of the manifest dream content! That bizarreness stands in contrast to the stable configurations of ordinary waking experiences. By achieving a compromise with the *repressed* wishes, the postulated distortion makes "plausible that even dreams with a distressing content are to be construed as wish fulfillments" (1900, p. 159). Accordingly, Freud concedes: "The fact that dreams really have a secret meaning which represents the fulfillment of a wish must be proved afresh in each particular case by analysis" (1900, p. 146).

But in a 1993 book (Grünbaum, 1993, chap. 10; and in Grünbaum, forthcoming), I have argued that this dream theory of universal wish fulfillment should be presumed to be false at its core rather than just ill founded.

More conservatively, the psychoanalysts Jacob Arlow and Charles Brenner (1964) had claimed, for reasons of their own, that "A dream is not simply the visually or auditorily hallucinated fulfillment of a childhood wish" (Arlow and Brenner, 1988: 7). And they countenanced a range of dream motives *other than* wishes, such as anxiety, though ultimately still rooted in childhood (p. 8).

But this modification did not remedy the fundamental epistemological defect in the claim that the method of free association can reliably identify dream motives. Undaunted, Arlow and Brenner declare (1988,

p. 8): "The theory and technique of dream analysis [by free association] in no way differs from the way one would analyze . . . a neurotic symptom, . . . a parapraxis, . . . or any other object of [psycho]analytic scrutiny." By the same token, these analysts insouciantly announce: "Dreams are, in fact, compromise-formations like any others" (pp. 7–8). Yet this ontological conclusion is predicated on the ill-founded epistemological thesis that free associations reliably identify repressions to be the causes of symptoms, dreams, and slips.

Careful studies have shown that the so-called free associations are not free but are strongly influenced by the psychoanalyst's subtle promptings to the patient (Grünbaum, 1984: 211–212). And recent memory research has shown further how patients and others can be induced to generate *pseudo*-memories, which are false but deemed veridical by the patients themselves (Goleman, 1994).

As a corollary of the latter epistemological defects of the method of free association, it appears that such associations *cannot* reliably vouch for the *contents* of presumed past repressions that are lifted by them. Thus, the products of such associations cannot justify the following repeated claim of the later (post–1923) Freud: The mere painfulness or unpleasurableness of an experience is *not itself* the prime motive for its repression; instead, its negativity must involve the conscious emergence of an instinctual desire recognized by the superego as illicit or dangerous (1940, pp. 184–187; 1933, pp. 57, 89, 91, 94; 1937, p. 227).

But since Freud had also stressed the well-nigh universal tendency to *forget* negative experiences *per se*, his later view of the dynamics of repression disappointingly leaves dangling theoretically (1) the relation of forgetting to repression, and (2) why some forgettings, no less than repressions, supposedly cannot be undone without the use of the controlled method of free association. In James Strachey's *Standard Edition*, (1901, p. 301), the general index lists two subcategories, among others, under "Forgetting": (1) "motivated by avoidance of unpleasure," and (2) "motivated by repression." But alas, Freud himself leaves us in a total quandary whether these two categories of Strachey's represent a distinction without a difference.

The Explanatory *Pseudo*-Unification Generated by Freud's Compromise Model of Neuroses, Dreams, and Slips. My indictment of the compromise model, if correct, spells an important

lesson, I claim, for both philosophical ontology and the theory of scientific explanation. Advocates of psychoanalysis have proclaimed it to be an explanatory virtue of their theory that its compromise model gives a *unifying* account of such *prima facie* disparate domains of phenomena as neuroses, dreams, and slips, and indeed that the theory of repression also illuminates infantile sexuality and the four stages hypothesized in Freud's theory of psychosexual development. In fact, some philosophers of science, such as Michael Friedman, have hailed explanatory unification as one of the great achievements and desiderata of the scientific enterprise. Thus, one need only think of the beautiful way in which Newton's theory of mechanics and gravitation served all at once to explain the motions of a pendulum on earth and of binary stars above by putting both terrestrial and celestial mechanics under a single theoretical umbrella.

Yet, in other contexts, unification can be a vice rather than a virtue. Thales of Miletus, though rightly seeking a rationalistic, rather than mythopoeic, picture of the world, taught that everything is made of water. And other philosophical monists have enunciated their own unifying ontologies. But the Russian chemist Dmitry Mendeleyev might have said to Thales across the millennia in the words of Hamlet: "There are more things in heaven and earth, Horatio, than are dreamt of in your philosophy" (Shakespeare, *Hamlet*, Act I, Scene V).

As I have argued, the same moral applies to Freud: By invoking the alleged causal cogency of the method of free association as a warrant for his compromise model, he generated a *pseudo*-unification of neurotic behavior with dreaming and the bungling of actions. This dubious unification was effected by conceiving of the normal activities of dreaming and occasionally bungling actions as *mini*-neurotic symptoms, of a piece with *abnormal* mentation in neuroses and even psychoses. To emphasize this monistic psychopathologizing of normalcy, Freud pointedly entitled his magnum opus on slips *The Psychopathology of Everyday Life* (1901). To this I can only say in metaphorical theological language: "Let no man put together what God has kept asunder," a gibe that was used by Wolfgang Pauli, I believe, against Einstein's unified field theory.

The "Hermeneutic" Reconstruction of Psychoanalysis. The French philosopher Paul Ricoeur (1970, p. 358), faced with quite different criticisms of psychoanalysis from philosophers of science during the 1950s and 1960s (von Eckardt, 1985: 356–364),

hailed the *failure* of Freud's theory to qualify as an empirical science by the received standards as the basis for "a counter-attack" against those who deplore this failure. In concert with the other so-called hermeneutic German philosophers Karl Jaspers and Jürgen Habermas, Ricoeur believed that victory can be snatched from the jaws of the *scientific failings* of Freud's theory by abjuring his scientific aspirations as misguided. Claiming that Freud himself had "scientistically" misunderstood his own theoretical achievement, some hermeneuts misconstrue it as a semantic accomplishment by trading on the multiply ambiguous word "meaning" (Grünbaum, 1984: Introduction, Sections 3 and 4; 1990; 1993, chap. 4). In Freud's theory, an overt symptom manifests one or more underlying unconscious causes and gives evidence for its cause(s), so that the "sense" or "meaning" of the symptom is constituted by its latent motivational cause(s). But this notion of "meaning" is different from the one appropriate to the context of *communication*, in which *linguistic* symbols *acquire semantic* meaning by being used deliberately to designate their referents. Clearly, the relation of being a manifestation, which the symptom bears to its cause, differs from the semantic relation of designation, which a linguistic symbol bears to its object.

The well-known academic psychoanalyst Marshall Edelson (1988: chap. 11, "Meaning", pp. 246–249) is in full agreement with this account and elaborates it lucidly:

> For psychoanalysis, the *meaning* of a mental phenomenon is a set of unconscious psychological or intentional states (specific wishes or impulses, specific fears aroused by these wishes, and thoughts or images which might remind the subject of these wishes and fears). The mental phenomenon substitutes for this set of states. That is, these states would have been present in consciousness, instead of the mental phenomenon requiring interpretation, had they not encountered, at the time of origin of the mental phenomenon or repeatedly since then, obstacles to their access to consciousness. If the mental phenomenon has been a relatively enduring structure, and these obstacles to consciousness are removed, the mental phenomenon disappears as these previously unconscious states achieve access to consciousness.

That the mental phenomenon substitutes for these states is a manifestation of a causal sequence. (pp. 247–248) And drawing on Freud's compromise model of symptoms in which symptoms are held to provide *substitutive* outlets or gratifications, Edelson continues:

> Suppose the question is: "Why does the analysand fear the snake so?" Suppose the answer to that questions is: "A snake stands for or symbolizes, a penis." It is easy to see that by itself this is no answer at all; for one thing, it leads immediately to the question: "Why does the analysand fear a penis so?" The question is about an inexplicable [unexplained] mental phenomenon (i.e., "fearing the snake so") and its answer depends on an entire causal explanation. . . . "A snake stands for, or symbolizes, a penis" makes sense as an answer only if it is understood as shorthand for a causal explanation. . . . Correspondingly, "the child stands for, or symbolizes, the boss" is not a satisfactory answer (it does not even sound right) to the question, "Why does this father beat his child?"

For my part, in this context I would wish to forestall a semantic misconstrual of the perniciously ambiguous term "symbol" by saying: In virtue of the similarity of shape, the snake *causally* evokes the unconscious image of a feared penis; thereby the snake itself becomes a dreaded object.

Speaking of Freud's writings, Edelson (1988, p. 247) says illuminatingly:

> Certain passages (occasional rather than preponderant) allude, often metaphorically, to symbolizing activities in human life. I think it could be argued that these indicate an effort on Freud's part to clarify by analogy aspects of the subject matter he is studying, including in some instances aspects of the clinical activity of the psychoanalyst—while at the same time perhaps he paid too little attention to disanalogies—rather than indicate any abandonment on his part of the [*causally*] explanatory objectives he so clearly pursues. There is no more reason to suppose that just because Freud refers to language, symbols, representations, and symbolic activity (part of his subject matter), he has

rejected, or should have rejected, canons of scientific method and reasoning, than to suppose
that just because Chomsky studies language (his
subject matter), his theory of linguistics cannot
be a theory belonging to natural science and
that he cannot be seeking causal explanations in
formulating it.

The "hermeneutic" reconstruction of psychoanalysis slides illicitly from one of two familiar senses of
"meaning" encountered in ordinary discourse to another.
When a pediatrician says that a child's spots on the skin
"*mean* measles," the "meaning" of the symptom is constituted by one of its *causes*, much as in the Freudian
case. Yet, the analyst Anthony Storr (1986, p. 260), when
speaking of Freud's "making sense" of a patient's symptoms, conflates the fathoming of the *etiologic* "sense" or
"meaning" of a symptom with the activity of making
semantic sense of a text (Grünbaum, 1986: 280), declaring astonishingly: "Freud was a man of genius whose
expertise lay in semantics." And Ricoeur erroneously
credits Freud's theory of repression with having provided,
malgré lui, a veritable "semantics of desire."

In a book that appeared before (Grünbaum, 1990;
1993, chap. 4), Achim Stephan (1989, Section 6.7,
"Adolf Grünbaum," pp. 144–149) takes issue with some
of my views. (Quotations from Stephan below are my
English translations of his German text.) He does not
endorse Ricoeur's "semantics of desire" (p. 123). But he
objects (p. 146, item [3]) to my claim that "In Freud's
theory, an overt symptom manifests one or more underlying unconscious causes and gives evidence for its
cause(s), so that the 'sense' or 'meaning' of the symptom
is constituted by its latent motivational cause(s)."

As Stephan recognizes (p. 27), Freud (1913, pp.
176–178) avowedly "overstepped" common usage when
he generalized the term "language" to designate not only
the verbal expression of thought but also gestures "and
every other method . . . by which mental activity can be
expressed" (p. 176). And Freud declared that "the interpretation of dreams [as a cognitive activity] is completely
analogous to the decipherment of an ancient picto-
graphic script such as Egyptian hieroglyphs" (p. 177).
But surely this common challenge of *problem solving*
does not license the assimilation of the *psychoanalytic*
meaning of manifest dream content to the *semantic*
meaning of spoken or written language (Grünbaum,
1993: 115).

Stephan does countenance (p. 148) my emphasis on
the distinction between the relation of manifestation, which
the symptom bears to its cause, and the semantic relation
of designation, which a linguistic symbol bears to its object.
Yet his principal objection to my view of the psychoanalytic "sense" of symptoms as being causal manifestations
of unconscious ideation is that I assign "exclusively non-
semantic significance" to them by *denying* that they also
have "semiotic" significance like linguistic symbols (pp.
148–149). He grants that Freud did not construe the sense
or meaning of symptoms as one of semantic reference to
their causes. Yet according to Stephan's own reconstruction of Freud's conception, "he did assume that the manifest phenomena [symptoms] semantically stand for the
same thing as the (repressed) ideas for which they substitute," i.e., "they stand semantically for what the repressed
(verbal) ideas stand (or rather would stand, if they were
expressed verbally)" (p. 149).

Searle (1990, pp. 161–167) has noted illuminatingly
(p. 175) that, unlike many mental states, language is *not
intrinsically* "intentional" in Brentano's directed sense;
instead, the intentionality (aboutness) of language is
extrinsically imposed on it by deliberately "decreeing" it
to function referentially. Searle (pp. 5, 160, and 177)
points out that the mental states of some animals and of
"pre-linguistic" very young children do have intrinsic
intentionality but *no* linguistic referentiality.

I maintain that Stephan's fundamental hermeneuticist error was to slide illicitly from the *intrinsic, nonse-
mantic* intentionality of (many, but *not* all) mental states
to the *imposed*, semantic sort possessed by language.
Moreover, *some* of the neurotic symptoms of concern to
psychoanalysts, such as diffuse depression and manic,
undirected elation even *lack* Brentano intentionality.

Finally, the aboutness (contents) of Freud's repressed
conative states is avowedly different from the intentionality (contents) of their psychic manifestations in symptoms. But Stephan erroneously insists that they are the
same.

Yet some version of a hermeneutic reconstruction of
the psychoanalytic enterprise has been embraced with
alacrity by a considerable number of analysts no less than
by professors in humanities departments of universities.
Its psychoanalytic adherents see it as buying absolution
for their theory and therapy from the criteria of validation mandatory for causal hypotheses in the empirical
sciences, although psychoanalysis is replete with just
such hypotheses. This form of escape from accountabil-

ity also augurs ill for the future of psychoanalysis, because the methods of the hermeneuts have not spawned a single new important hypothesis. Instead, their reconstruction is a negativistic ideological battle cry whose disavowal of Freud's scientific aspirations presages the death of his legacy from sheer sterility, at least among those who demand the validation of theories by cogent evidence.

Post-Freudian Psychoanalysis. But what have been the contemporary *post*-Freudian developments insofar as they still qualify as psychoanalytic in content rather than only in name? And have they advanced the debate by being on firmer epistemological ground than Freud's original major hypotheses (Grünbaum, 1984: chap. 7)? Most recently, the noted clinical psychologist and philosopher of psychology Morris Eagle (1993) has given a comprehensive and insightful answer to this question on which we can draw.

Eagle (1993, p. 374) begins with a caveat: "It is not at all clear that there is a uniform body of thought analogous to the main corpus of Freudian theory that can be called contemporary psychoanalytic theory. In the last forty or fifty years there have been three major theoretical developments in psychoanalysis: ego psychology, object relations theory, and self-psychology. If contemporary psychoanalytic theory is anything, it is one of these three or some combination, integrative or otherwise, of the three." Eagle makes no mention of Lacan's version of psychoanalysis, presumably because he does not take it seriously, since Lacanians have avowedly forsaken the need to validate their doctrines by familiar canons of evidence, not to mention Lacan's willful, irresponsible obscurity and notorious cruelty to patients (Green, 1995/1996).

Previously we had occasion to note that Heinz Hartmann's ego psychology departed from Freud's instinctual anchorage of the cognitive functions. But more important, both Heinz Kohut's self-psychology and the object relations theory of Otto Kernberg and the British school more fundamentally reject Freud's compromise model of psychopathology. Indeed, self-psychology has repudiated virtually every one of Freud's major tenets (Eagle, 1993: 388). Thus, Kohut supplants Freud's conflict model of psychopathology, which is based on the repression of internal sexual and aggressive wishes, by a psychology of self-defects and faulty function caused by hypothesized *environmental events* going back to the first two years of infancy. Relatedly, Kohut denies, contra Freud, that

insight is curative, designating instead the analyst's empathic understanding as the operative therapeutic agent (Kohut, 1984). Again, the object relations theorists deny that the etiology of pathology lies in Freudian (Oedipal) conflicts and traumas involving sex and aggression, claiming instead that the quality of maternal caring is the crucial factor.

Yet these two post-Freudian schools not only diverge from Freud but also disagree with each other. Thus, the orthodox psychoanalysts Arlow and Brenner speak ruefully of "the differences among all these theories, so apparent to every observer" (1964, p. 9), hoping wistfully that refined honing of the psychoanalytic method of free association will yield a common body of data, which "would in the end resolve the conflict among competing theories" (p. 11). But their hope is utopian, if only because of the severe probative limitations of the method of free association. How, for example, could a method of putting adults on the couch possibly have the epistemological resources to resolve the three-way clash among the Freudian and two post-Freudian schools in regard to the *infantile* etiologies of psychopathology? Otto Kernberg's (1993) account of the "Convergences and Divergences in Contemporary Psychoanalytic Technique" does not solve that problem. And as other psychoanalysts themselves have documented, there are several clear signs that the future of the sundry clinical and theoretical enterprises that label themselves "psychoanalytic" is now increasingly in jeopardy. For example, the pool of patients seeking (full-term) psychoanalytic treatment in the United States has been steadily shrinking, and academic psychoanalysts are becoming an endangered species in American medical schools (Reiser, 1989). No wonder that the subtitle of the 1988 book *Psychoanalysis* by the well-known analyst Marshall Edelson is "*A Theory in Crisis*" (Edelson, 1988).

But what about the evidential merits of the two post-Freudian developments usually designated as "*contemporary* psychoanalysis"? Do they constitute an *advance* over Freud? The answer turns largely, though not entirely, on whether there is *better evidential support* for them than for Freud's classical edifice. But Eagle (1993, p. 404) argues that the verdict is clearly negative: "the different variants of so-called contemporary psychoanalytic theory . . . are on no firmer epistemological ground than the central formulations and claims of Freudian theory. . . . There is no evidence that contemporary psychoanalytic theories have remedied the epistemological and

C

methodological difficulties that are associated with Freudian theory."

What Are the Future Prospects of Psychoanalysis? Finally, what are the prospects for the future of psychoanalysis in the twenty-first century? In their 1988 paper on that topic, the psychoanalysts Arlow and Brenner (1988, p. 13) reached the following sanguine conclusion about both its past and its future:

> Of some things about the future of psychoanalysis we can be certain. Fortunately, they are the most important issues as well. Psychoanalysis will continue to furnish the most comprehensive and illuminating insight into the human psyche. It will continue to stimulate research and understanding in many areas of human endeavor. In addition to being the best kind of treatment for many cases, it will remain, as it has been, the fundamental base for almost all methods that try to alleviate human mental suffering by psychological means.

By contrast, a dismal verdict is offered by the distinguished American psychologist and psychoanalyst Paul E. Meehl (1995, p. 1021). Since one of my main arguments figures in it, let me mention that apropos of my critiques of Freud's theories of transference and of obsessional neurosis ("Rat-Man"), I had demonstrated the *fallaciousness* of inferring a *causal* connection between mental states from a mere "meaning" or thematic connection between them. Meehl refers to the latter kind of shared thematic content as "the existence of a theme":

> His [Grünbaum's] core objection, the epistemological difficulty of inferring a causal influence from the existence of a theme (assuming the latter can be statistically demonstrated), is the biggest single methodological problem that we [psychoanalysts] face. If that problem cannot be solved, we will have another century in which psychoanalysis can be accepted or rejected, mostly as a matter of personal taste. Should that happen, I predict it will be slowly but surely abandoned, both as a mode of helping and as a theory of the mind [reference omitted].

Returning to Arlow and Brenner, I hope I have shown that, in regard to the last hundred years, their rosy partisan account is very largely ill founded, if only because the lauded comprehensiveness of the core theory of repression is only a *pseudo*-unification, as I have argued. Among Arlow and Brenner's glowingly optimistic statements about the future, just one is plausible: The expectation of a continuing heuristic role for psychoanalysis. Such a function does *not* require the correctness of its current theories at all. As an example of the heuristic role, one need only think of the issues I raised apropos of Freud's dubious account of the relation of affect to forgetting and remembering. These issues range well beyond the concerns of psychoanalysis. As the Harvard psychoanalyst and schizophrenia researcher Philip Holzman sees it (Holzman, 1994: 190): "This view of the heuristic role of psychoanalysis, even in the face of its poor science, is beginning to be appreciated only now." Holzman (private communication) mentions three areas of inquiry as illustrations: (1) The plasticity and reconstructive role of memory as against photographic reproducibility of the past, (2) the general role of affect in cognition, and (3) the relevance of temperament (e.g., shyness) in character development, as currently investigated by Jerome Kagan at Harvard.

REFERENCES

Arlow, J., and Brenner, C. (1964). *Psychoanalytic Concepts and the Structural Theory.* New York: International Universities Press.

———. (1988). The future of psychoanalysis. *Psychoanalytic Quarterly,* 57: 1–14.

Assoun, P. (1995). *Freud, la Philosophie, et les Philosophes.* Paris: Presses Universitaires de France.

Bachrach, H., et al. (1991). On the efficacy of psychoanalysis. *Journal of the American Psychoanalytic Association,* 39: 871–916.

Basch, M. (1994). Psychoanalysis, science and epistemology. *Bulletin of the [Chicago] Institute for Psychoanalysis,* 4, no. 2: 1; 8–9.

Borch-Jacobsen, M. (1996). *Remembering Anna O.: 100 Years of Psychoanalytic Mystification.* New York: Routledge.

Brenner, C. (1982). *The Mind in Conflict.* New York: International Universities Press.

Brentano, B. (1995). *Psychology from an Empirical Standpoint.* New York: Routledge & Kegan Paul, Ltd.

Breuer, J., and Freud, S. (1893). On the psychical mechanism of hysterical phenomena: Preliminary communication. S.E. 2: 1–17.

Bröder, A. (1995). *Unbewusstes semantisches Priming laborinduzierter Sprechfehler.* Bonn: University of Bonn. *"Diplomarbeit"* in psychology.

Bröder, A., and Bredenkamp, J. (1996). SLIP-Technik, Prozessdissoziationsmodell und multinomiale Modellierrung: Neue

C

Werkzeuge zum experimentellen Nachweis "Freudscher versprecher"? *Zeitschrift für experimentelle Psychologie*, 43: 175–202.

Carrier, M., and Mittelstrass, J. (1991). *Mind, Brain, Behavior: The Mind-Body Problem and the Philosophy of Psychology.* New York: Walter de Gruyter.

Cleckley, H. (1988). *The Mask of Sanity*, 5th ed. Augusta, Ga.: Emily S. Cleckley.

Eagle, M. (1987). The psychoanalytic and the cognitive unconscious. In R. Stern (ed.). *Theories of the Unconscious and Theories of the Self.* Hillsdale, N.J.: Analytic Press, pp. 155–189.

———. (1993). The dynamics of theory change in psychoanalysis. In J. Earman, A. Janis, G. Massey, and N. Rescher (eds.). *Philosophical Problems of the Internal and External Worlds: Essays on the Philosophy of Adolf Grünbaum.* Pittsburgh: University of Pittsburgh Press, Chapter 15.

Edelson, M. (1984). *Hypothesis and Evidence in Psychoanalysis.* Chicago: University of Chicago Press.

———. (1986). Causal explanation in science and in psychoanalysis. *Psychoanalytic Study of the Child*, 41: 89–127.

———. (1988). *Psychoanalysis: A Theory in Crisis.* Chicago: University of Chicago Press.

Ellenberger, H. (1970). *The Discovery of the Unconscious.* New York: Basic Books.

Fenichel, O. (1945). *The Psychoanalytic Theory of Neurosis.* New York: Norton.

Freud, S. (1893). *On the Psychical Mechanism of Hysterical Phenomena.* S.E. 3: 27–39.

———. (1896). *Heredity and the Aetiology of the Neuroses.* S.E. 3: 143–156.

———. (1900). *The Interpretation of Dreams.* S.E. 4–5: 1–621.

———. (1901). *The Psychopathology of Everyday Life.* S.E. 6: 1–279.

———. (1905). *Fragment of an Analysis of a Case of Hysteria.* S.E. 7: 249–254.

———. (1909). *Notes Upon a Case of Obsessional Neurosis.* S.E. 10: 155–318.

———. (1910). *'Wild' Psycho-Analysis.* S.E. 11: 219–230.

———. (1913). *The Claims of Psycho-Analysis to Scientific Interest.* S.E. 13: 165–190.

———. (1914). *On the History of the Psycho-Analytic Movement.* S.E. 14: 7–66.

———. (1915a). *The Unconscious.* S.E. 14: 166–215.

———. (1915b). *Repression.* S.E. 14: 146–158.

———. (1916–1917). *Introductory Lectures on Psycho-analysis.* S.E. 15–16: 9–496.

———. (1924). *A Short Account of Psychoanalysis.* S.E. 19: 191–209.

———. (1925). *An Autobiographical Study.* S.E. 20: 7–74.

———. (1933). *New Introductory Lectures on Psychoanalysis.* S.E. 22: 5–185.

———. (1937). *Analysis Terminable and Interminable.* S.E. 23: 209–253.

———. (1940). *An Outline of Psycho-Analysis.* S.E. 23: 139–207.

Gay, P. (1987). *A Godless Jew: Freud, Atheism, and the Making of Psychoanalysis.* New Haven, Conn.: Yale University Press.

Glymour, C. (1983). The theory of your dreams. In R. S. Cohen and L. Laudan (eds.). *Physics, Philosophy, and Psychoanalysis: Essays in Honor of Adolf Grünbaum.* Dordrecht: Reidel, pp. 57–71.

Goleman, D. (1994), "Miscoding Is Seen as the Root of False Memories," *New York Times* (May 31): C1 and C8.

Green, A. (1995–1996). Against Lacanism. *Journal of European Psychoanalysis*, 2: 169–185.

Grünbaum, A. (1973). *Philosophical Problems of Space and Time*, 2d ed. Dordrecht: Reidel.

———. (1984). *The Foundations of Psychoanalysis: A Philosophical Critique.* Berkeley: University of California Press. Translations are available in German, Italian, Japanese, and French.

———. (1986). Is Freud's theory well-founded?. *Behavioral and Brain Sciences*, 9: 266–281.

———. (1990). "Meaning" connections and causal connections in the human sciences: The poverty of hermeneutic philosophy. *Journal of the American Psychoanalytic Association*, 38: 559–577.

———. (1993). *Validation in the Clinical Theory of Psychoanalysis: A Study in the Philosophy of Psychoanalysis.* Madison, Conn.: International Universities Press.

———. (1994). Letter to the Editor, *New York Review of Books*, 41, no. 14 (August 11): 54–55. Contra Thomas Nagel's "Freud's Permanent Revolution."

———. (1997). Is the concept of "Psychic Reality" a theoretical advance? *Psychoanalysis and Contemporary Thought*, 20, no. 2: 83–105.

———. (Forthcoming). Critique of Freud's neurobiological and psychoanalytic dream theories. To appear in A. Grünbaum, *Philosophy of Science in Action*, vol. 2, Part 2. New York: Oxford University Press.

Harman, G. (1965). Inference to the best explanation. *Philosophical Review*, 74: 88–95.

Holzman, P. (1994). Hilgard on psychoanalysis as science. *Psychological Science*, 5, no. 4 (July): 190–191.

Kernberg, O. (1993). Convergences and divergences in contemporary psychoanalytic technique. *International Journal of Psychoanalysis*, 74: 659–673.

Kohut, H. (1984). *How Does Analysis Cure?* Chicago: University of Chicago Press.

Leibniz, G. (1981). *New Essays on Human Understanding.* Trans. P. Remnant and J. Bennett. Cambridge University Press. The original publication date was circa 1705.

Meehl, P. (1995). Commentary: Psychoanalysis as science. *Journal of the American Psychoanalytic Association*, 43, no. 4: 1015–1021.

Motley, M. (1980). Verification of "Freudian Slips" and semantic prearticulatory editing via laboratory-induced spoonerisms. In V. Fromkin (ed.). *Errors in Linguistic Performance: Slips of the Tongue, Ear, Pen, and Hand.* New York: Academic Press, pp. 133–147.

Nagel, T. (1994). Freud's permanent revolution. *New York Review of Books*, 41, no. 9 (May 12): 34–38.

Reiser, M. (1989). The future of psychoanalysis in academic psychiatry: Plain talk. *Psychoanalytic Quarterly*, 58: 158–209.

Ricoeur, P. (1970). *Freud and Philosophy*. New Haven, Conn.: Yale University Press.

Salmon, W. (1971). *Statistical Explanation and Statistical Relevance*. Pittsburgh: University of Pittsburgh Press.

———. (2001). Explanation and confirmation: A Bayesian critique of inference to the best explanation. In G. Hon and S. S. Rackover (eds.). *Explanation: Theoretical Approaches and Applications*. Dordrecht: Kluwer.

Schapiro, M. (1968). The apples of Cézanne. *Art News Annual*, 34: 34–53.

Schüttauf, K., et al. (forthcoming). Induzierte "Freudsche Versprecher" und zwangsneurotischer Konflikt. To appear in the journal *Sprache und Kognition*.

Searle, J. (1990). *Intentionality*. New York: Cambridge University Press.

Shevrin, H., et al. (1992). Event-related potential indicators of the dynamic unconscious. *Consciousness and Cognition*, 1: 340–366.

Solms, M., and Saling, M. (Trans. and eds) (1990). *A Moment of Transition: Two Neuroscientific Articles by Sigmund Freud*. New York: Karnac Books.

Solomon, D. (1994). Meyer Schapiro. *New York Times Magazine* (August 14): 22–25.

Stephan, A. (1989). *Sinn als Bedeutung: Bedeutungstheoretische Untersuchungen zur Psychoanalyse Sigmund Freuds*. Berlin: Walter de Gruyter.

Storr, A. (1986). Human understanding and scientific validation. *Behavioral and Brain Sciences*, 9: 259–260.

Thomä, H., and Kächele, H. (1987). *Psychoanalytic Practice*. Berlin: Springer-Verlag.

Vaughan, S., and Roose, S. (1995). The analytic process: Clinical and research definitions. *International Journal of Psycho-Analysis*, 76: 343–356.

von Eckardt, B. (1985). Adolf Grünbaum and psychoanalytic epistemology. In J. Reppen (ed.). *Beyond Freud: A Study of Modern Psychoanalytic Theorists*. Hillsdale, N.J.: Analytic Press, pp. 353–403.

Walker, F. (1962). *The Man Verdi*. New York: Knopf.

Zentner, M. (1995). *Die Flucht ins Vergessen: Die Anfänge der Psychoanalyse Freuds bei Schopenhauer*. Darmstadt, Germany: Wissenschaftliche Buchgessellschaft.

ADOLF GRÜNBAUM

Czech Republic, and Psychoanalysis

"[F]or me, an old man, it will be quite a satisfaction that despite the well known proverb I might be able to make myself useful in my fatherland," writes Sigmund Freud in the preface to the first Czech edition of "Lectures on the Introduction to Psychoanalysis," dated April 4, 1935. However, to fulfill his words required much effort and unfortunately also blood. Psychoanalysis in the Czech lands thrived and lan- guished depending on the fortunes or misfortunes of the time.

A circle interested in psychoanalysis formed around J. Stuchlik (1890–1967) in Kosice in the 1920s. Among others, Emanuel Windholz, Sandor Lorand, and Jan Frank were members of this group. At the same time, Nikolai Jefgrafovic Osipov (born in Moscow in 1877) translated Freud into Czech and lectured at the university level. In 1931, Stuchlik and Osipov initiated an effort to unveil a memorial plaque on the house in Pribor where S. Freud was born. Eitington, Federn, and Anna Freud took part in the ceremony, at which Anna Freud read a letter of her father's.

In the early 1930s, Emanuel Windholz returned to Prague having studied at the Berlin Institute of Psychoanalysis, and in 1932 he edited *Compendium of Papers in Psychoanalysis*. A study group was established from previously existing cells, and at the request of the International Psychoanalytic Association (IPA), Otto Fenichel was sent to Prague by the Vienna Psychoanalysis Association as a professional training analyst. As of 1935, he was expected to develop the field in collaboration with Anna Reich and Steffi Bornstein. In 1936, with the support of the Vienna Psychoanalytic Association, the Czech association became a member of the IPA at the 14th International Congress of Psychoanalysis in Mariánské Lázné (Marienbad). E. Windholz became its first president, with R. Karpe, M. Karpe, O. Brief, M. Brief, T. Bondy, B. Dosuzkov, J. Frank, and others as its members. Given the growing pressure of the fascist terror in Germany, Prague became a transit stop for a number of German and Austrian analysts. Having stayed for three years in Prague, Fenichel left for the United States, where he then organized a group of analysts in Los Angeles. His future wife, H. Heilbron, left with him. Karpe and his wife, J. Loewenfeld, A. Reich, K. Olden, and Otto Friedman also emigrated.

The Czech association ceased to exist in the dark year of 1939. Those who stayed soon perished, Otto Brief in 1943 in Buchenwald concentration camp, his wife in 1944 in Auschwitz, Theresa Bondy in 1941 in Auschwitz; in addition, Steffi Bornstein-Windholz died suddenly in 1939. Only Theodor Dosuzkov continued to work. He organized anew a small group of psychoanalysts during World War II.

After the war, Dosuzkov renewed contact with Fenichel, and as a member of the IPA, he was confirmed as a training analyst. In 1947 and 1948, he edited The

C

second and third *Yearbook of Psychoanalysis*. Dosuzkov continued to write and was preparing to establish an institute when the Communist takeover in 1948 again forced psychoanalysis to its knees. Some professionals left the field. Other future members of the IPA remained, namely Otokar Kucera (1906–1981) and Marie Benova (1908–1987), as did Ladislav Haas, who emigrated in 1966 and died in England in 1984. Dosuzkov attempted a synthesis of the research of I. P. Pavlov, Freud, and his own psychoanalytical understanding of psychopathology. His innovative approach to scoptophobia (fear of looking) as the fourth transference neurosis is an insufficiently recognized part of subsequent interest in narcissist structure.

Signs of progress were trampled by the Soviet-led Warsaw Pact invasion in 1968. The period of repression that followed forced psychoanalysis into the scientific underground. Surprisingly, the training of several professionals was completed: Bohumila Vackova and Miroslav Borecky by Dosuzkov; Václav Mikota, Jiří Kocourek, Petr Prihoda, and Vera Fischelova by Kucera; Hana Junova by Benova; Michael Sebek by Tautermann and others. After Kucera and Dosuzkov died, this psychoanalytical generation finally created a full organizational structure according to IPA rules and established the Psychoanalytical Institute. Even though they worked in the scientific underground, for a number of reasons they did not experience much interference (see M. Borecky, "What is the Prague psychoanalyst afraid of in post-totalitarian society?" *Zeitschrift für Psychoanalytische Theorie and Praxis*, Sonderheft 1992). Some Western literature was received. There was, however, a lack of personal contacts and experience.

During the 1980s, a number of professionals underwent psychoanalytical training. A significant amount of literature was translated and published in samizdat form. It was not until the late 1980s that the Prague association was visited and motivated by H. Luidpold Loewenthal, the Sandlers, Rolf Klüwer, and J. Groen-Prakken.

In 1989, the 36th International Psychoanalytical Congress in Rome accepted five Czech analysts as direct associate members of the IPA, and in that same year, prior to the revolution, the Czech Psychoanalysis Association was finally accepted into the prestigious Purkyne's Medical Society as the Working Group for the Study of Psychoanalysis. The independent Czech Psychoanalysis Association was officially established at the beginning of 1990.

At the end of the 1980s and in the early 1990s, the active interest of the IPA and the European Psychoanalysis Federation (EPF) was expressed by dispatching a number of supervising professionals to Czechoslovakia: R. Klüwer, N. Treurniet, and A. Vatillon. Also, the Frankfurt Psychoanalysis Association (FPV) and the Sigmund Freud Institute in Frankfurt provided significant support. It was there that the Czech analysts Eugenia Dosuzkov-Fischer, Rene Fischer, and Mr. and Mrs. Erdely had worked since the late 1960s.

At the 38th Congress of the IPA in Amsterdam in July 1993, the Czech Psychoanalysis Association was reinstated in the IPA as "a research group." Thus, the work of generations of Czech psychoanalysts, who, except in a few short periods, were a clandestine society, was de facto recognized. Furthermore, the continuity of psychoanalytical training in Prague from the prewar years to the present time was confirmed.

IPA representatives Fridrich Wilhelm Eickhof, Heyde Faimberg, and Ralf Moses, who are members of the IPA sponsoring committee, are presently participating in the further development of Czech psychoanalysis.

The transition of psychoanalysis from dissent to official recognition created a number of problems for Czech psychoanalysts. In the past the existence of a common enemy enhanced the cohesion of the group. However, professional quality was threatened and there was the danger of amateurism. It appears that these risks were confined within reasonable limits. In the new democratic environment, it will be necessary to reformulate the identity of psychoanalysis and face the loss of an alibi that frequently presented itself under totalitarian pressure.

At the end of 1997, the Czech Psychoanalysis Association (the IPA Study Group) had twelve full members and ten contributing members. Of these, nine are full IPA members and twelve are associate members. The Prague Institute of Psychoanalysis has seven training analysts (Miroslav Borecky, Vera Fischelova, Jiří Kocourek, Václav Mikota, Michael Sebek, Zdenek Sikl, Bohumila Vackova). Martin Mahler was its president. Kocourek's Psychoanalytical Publishing House is gradually publishing Freud's works. Approximately thirty candidates are in training. Conceivably, Freud's wish will finally be realized in the Czech lands.

REFERENCES

Borecky, M. (1992). Die Befürchtungen eines tschechischen Psychoanalytikers in der posttotalitären Gesellschaft. Zeitschr. f. psychoanal. *Theorie und Praxis*, Sonderheft, s. 45–51.

————. (1996). Die Konkurrenz und die Identität in verwechselten sozialpsychologischen Bedingungen der Tschechische Republik, Zeitschfr. f. psychoanal. *Theorie und Praxis*, 6, 4: 401–409.

Fischer, R. (1975). Zur Geschichte der Psychoanalytischen Bewegung in der Tschechoslowakei. *Psyche*, 29: 1126–1131

Kocourek, J. (1992). *Horizonty psychoanalyzy*, pp. 101–114. Prague.

Sebek, M. (1992). Lorsqu'une psychanalyse est clandestine: quelques problemes de transfert et de contre-transfert. *Revue Française Psychoanal*, 2: 413–421

Sebek, M. (1992). La psychanalyse, les psychanalystes et la periode staliniennne de l'après-guerre. La situation tchécoslovaque. *Revue internationale d'historie de la psychoanalyse*, 5: 553–568.

MIROSLAV BORECKY

D

Defense Mechanisms

In *The Ego and the Id*, Freud (1923) postulated that the neurotic conflict took place between the ego, which is the center of consciousness, and the id, the unconscious province of the mind wherein lie instinctual drives. The ego seeks to bar entry into consciousness of certain instinctual impulses and other painful feelings by employing the defense mechanisms. These defense mechanisms, it is important to note, are unconscious. They give rise to behavior, therefore, of which the purpose and motives are hidden from the subject. Thus they are of crucial importance to the understanding and the study of human psychology, because if it can be established that defense mechanisms are, indeed, operating, then many current procedures in social science research, notably questionnaires and interviews, are rendered of little value.

The defense mechanisms have been carefully described in classical psychoanalytic texts, notably Fenichel's *The Psychoanalytic Theory of Neurosis* (1945) and Anna Freud's *The Ego and the Mechanisms of Defence* (1946), and the definitions in this article are based upon them. First, a general point should be noted. It is customary to classify defenses as successful or unsuccessful. Successful defenses allow the expression of the instinctual drive; these are known as sublimations. Unsuccessful defenses simply block the drive and thus have to be in operation all the time.

Sublimation

The most usual concept of sublimation involves the deflection of aims. Among childless persons, maternal love can he sublimated into a love of others' children or even pets. Pottery, in which clay is handled, is regarded as the sublimation of the repressed desire to handle feces. In Freudian theory, this is known as anal erotism. Sadism can be sublimated into masochism in which the sadism is turned onto self, a defense sometimes referred to as "turning round" on subject.

As stated above, most defenses are unsuccessful and these will now be described.

Repression

The essence of repression is rejecting and keeping something out of consciousness (Freud, 1915). In fact, there are two types of repression: primal repression and repression proper. Because the whole notion of repression has been the subject of so much recent discussion and debate, it will be considered in some detail.

Primal repression is the denial of entry into consciousness of the mental presentation of the instinct. However, this is accompanied by fixation in which this mental presentation remains unaltered, and the instinct remains attached to it. In repression proper, the mental derivatives and associations of the repressed presentation are also barred entry into consciousness, and repression proper is sometimes referred to as "after expulsion." The mental energy, which is part of repressed instincts, is transformed into affects—especially anxiety. Thus repression is a pathogenic defense. From this description, it is clear that repression is a fundamental concept in psychoanalysis, and the unblocking of repression is a critical aspect of psychoanalytic therapy.

Denial

When the ego has to ward off some painful aspect of the external world, the perceptions that bring this to knowledge are denied. Freud has a classic example of this defense. A patient answering the question as to who an individual was in a dream claims that it was not his mother. Freud amends this accordingly in the light of denial: so it was his mother.

Reaction-formation

Reaction-formations create conscious attitudes and feelings opposite to those in the unconscious. The most usual example is the disgust that most individuals feel concerning feces. This is regarded in psychoanalytic theory as a reaction formation against the pleasure in handling feces and in anal erotism generally (Freud, 1908).

Undoing

This is regarded in psychoanalysis as a kind of negative magic that does away with the consequences of some event, and even the event itself, usually by motor symbolism. It is, therefore, typical of obsessional neurosis (Freud, 1909), where patients often feel compelled to make special ritual gestures before they can proceed with their normal daily tasks. Acts of expiation can be seen as forms of undoing.

Projection

Projection is the attribution of one's own unacceptable impulses onto others. Freud (1911) characterized this as the mechanism, together with reaction formation (against homosexuality), that created the persecutor's delusions of paranoia. "I love him" becomes "I hate him," which, in turn, becomes "He hates me."

The meaning of "projection" in the term "projective tests" is quite different from its use in referring to a defense mechanism. In interpreting these tests, it is assumed that subjects project aspects of their personality onto the test stimuli; it is not assumed that they are attributing their own characteristics to other people.

Isolation

In isolation, experiences are separated from their feelings and emotions. Commonly, at least at the turn of the nineteenth century, isolation could be observed in those men who separated the tender components of sexuality from the sensual (Freud, 1910). These individuals can have satisfying sexual relations only with women whom they despise. In some men, this isolation is so complete that sexuality is isolated from the rest of life, and such individuals can express their sexual drives without guilt.

Regression

In regression, individuals resort to thinking and behavior typical of much earlier phases of development. This is common in the early stages of development in children but Freud (1925) argues that it can also have a defensive purpose.

Such are, in psychoanalytic theory, the defense mechanisms, all unconscious ego processes, aimed at barring the emergence into consciousness of instinctual impulses or unacceptable thoughts. In addition, however, there are defenses against affect. The main defense against affect is *displacement*. Freud has many well-known examples of displacement, of which the most famous is Little Hans (Freud, 1905). Here, fear of the father was displaced to fear of horses. Sometimes displacement of affect is accompanied by postponement, when the pain is felt some time after the event.

Finally, mention should be made of a defense that Anna Freud (1946) described and of which much use is made in more recent psychoanalysis. This is *identification with the aggressor*. This mechanism is employed as a defense against anxiety. A well-known phenomenon said to exemplify this defense is the anti-Semitism of certain Jews.

In discussing the main defense mechanisms, certain points are critical. First, these are unconscious processes. This is important because suppression, which is a conscious decision not to talk about some sensitive matter, is confused with repression. Furthermore, in recent research into personality conducted by psychologists, the term "defense mechanism" is often used. However, examination of this work indicates that this has become an umbrella term incorporating genuinely psychoanalytic mechanisms and other methods of dealing with emotional problems that are conscious and can even include having a cup of tea. A full discussion of all this work can be found in Hentschel, Smith, Elhers, and Draguns (1993).

There is a logical objection to the notion of denial, which to some extent applies to all defenses. It runs as follows. How can a threat be denied if it has not been perceived? If it has been perceived, as it apparently must have been, there is no function served by the denial. However, this objection can be refuted. It has been shown experimentally that subjects can reliably utilize the semantic and structural aspects of stimuli with no awareness of the presence of that stimulus, a phenomenon not unlike the blindsight of certain patients with cortical blindness who nevertheless can pick their way through obstacles. Whatever the relation of these studies of the cognitive unconscious to the psychodynamic, Freudian unconscious remains contentious (but see Hentschel, Smith, Elhers, and Draguns, 1993). What is not contentious, however, is the importance of these defense mechanisms in understanding human behavior and motives. For example, all studies of racism that ignore the defense of projection are likely to be doomed to failure. In this connection, the descriptions of despised races or outgroups are often remarkably similar, and in the case of Jews contradictory, suggesting their unconscious, nonrational basis.

Indeed, it can be argued that in all matters that are of real emotional and psychological importance to human beings, defense mechanisms are bound to be brought into play because of the affect and instinctual behavior involved. Hence, discussion of all such human affairs, without recourse to defenses, is bound to end in failure. Experience of attempts to end wars and conflicts all over the globe, to establish justice and the rule of law, even to regulate such matters as the treatment of children, birth control, torture, and the role of women surely bear out this point.

In conclusion, it seems clear that psychoanalytic defense mechanisms deserve to be studied in all their aspects, and it is to be hoped that such research will be conducted both by analysts and by psychologists who by use of the appropriate scientific methods can hone down the brilliant Freudian insights into an accurate and sober account that cannot be rejected by those who regard only scientifically verifiable knowledge as useful. Fortunately, such work has now begun and is fully discussed in Hentschel, Smith, Elhers, and Draguns (1993).

REFERENCES

Fenichel, O. (1945). *The Psychoanalytic Theory of Neurosis.* New York: Norton.

Freud, A. (1946). *The Ego and the Mechanisms of Defence.* London: Hogarth Press and the Institute of Psychoanalysis.

Freud, S. (1905). Fragment of an analysis of a case of hysteria. S.E. 7: 7–122.

———. (1908). Character and anal erotism. S.E. 9: 169–175.

———. (1909). Notes upon a case of obsessional neurosis. S.E. 10: 155–310.

———. (1910). A Special Type of Choice of Object Made by Men (Contributions to the Psychology of Love I). S.E. 11: 165–175.

———. (1911). Psycho-analytic notes on an autobiographical account of a case of paranoia. S.E. 12: 9–82.

———. (1915). Repression. S.E. 14: 146–158. S.E. 14: 143).

———. (1923). *The Ego and the Id.* S.E. 19: 12–59.

———. (1925). *Inhibitions, Symptoms and Anxiety.* S.E. 20: 87–172.

Hentschel, U., Smith, G. J. W., Ehlers, W., and Draguns, J. G. (eds.). (1993). *The Concept of Defence Mechanisms in Contemporary Psychology.* New York: Springer-Verlag.

PAUL KLINE

D

Delusions

Delusions are strongly believed ideas that are false. Freud saw delusions as existing on a continuum from the "psychopathology of everyday life" to severe manifestations of psychopathology in hysteria, paranoia, and schizophrenia, in which a return of the repressed makes unwavering demands on the ego, which then must adapt itself to them.

There are two basic processes in delusion formation: (1) a turning away from reality; and (2) the influence exerted by wish fulfillment on the content of the delusion. But these processes, Freud argues, may be linked in that the repressed, in its drive toward consciousness, exploits the ego's turning away from reality. But then, the resistances stirred up by the emergence of the repressed lead to distortion and displacement, much as they do in dream formation. Many other mechanisms of dream formation apply to delusions as well. In both dreams and in delusions, for example, absurdity can express ridicule and derision.

Freud discusses delusions in his paper on Schreber (Freud, 1911). Daniel Paul Schreber was a German judge of high cultivation and professional accomplishment who nevertheless had severe delusions revolving around the idea that "after all it really must be very nice to be a woman submitting to the act of copulation." Schreber published his *Memoirs of a Nerve Patient*, in which he described his system of delusions, involving hypochondriacal ideas and methods of uncanny influence between himself, his physicians, and God. Freud, analyzing Schreber's memoirs, concluded that the driving force behind the delusions was an unacceptable homosexual impulse. He proposed that such an impulse might be the unconscious force behind all paranoia, although the methods of defense against such impulses might result in different pathological manifestations.

Psychotic delusions may include fragments of historical truth; delusions attain their force precisely because of their being rooted in actual early experience. This viewpoint was greatly reinforced after Freud's death, when close examination of the books of Schreber's father on child rearing revealed a striking similarity between his mechanical devices to insure proper posture and the contents of Schreber's delusions. The Schreber findings did, however, undermine somewhat Freud's view of the exclusively sexual etiology of paranoid delusions. It is possible that the great power of homosexual ideation to carry feelings of ignominy in our culture may be at the root of their connection with paranoia, and that in other cultures where homosexuality is less stigmatized, other factors may become the central force behind paranoid delusions. Weinstein (1962), for example, found that none of the paranoid schizophrenic patients he studied in the Caribbean island of St. Thomas had delusions concerning homosexuality, but rather formed delusions around issues of fertility.

From a therapeutic standpoint, it is futile to try to talk a patient out of his or her delusions. Freud found that clinical progress depends on the recognition of the "kernel of truth" on which the delusion is based. This is the fundamental principle of post-Freudian psychotherapeutic developments dealing with analysis of delusions, as illustrated in the work of Sullivan, Fromm-Reichmann, Searles, and Selzer.

Freud noted the frequent appearance of projection in the development of delusions, and referred to a planned work on projection that was either not written or lost. Nevertheless, he noted how many irrational delusions can be better understood as projections of one's internal state. For example, delusions of the approach of the end of the world may be a projection of a sensed internal catastrophe. In addition, Freud noted that delusions, despite their grossly pathological appearance, may have a constructive value. In the face of psychotic withdrawal from the world, delusions may be seen as an attempt at recovery and reconstruction, an attempt to recapture relations with people even if those relations are manifestly destructive.

Delusions, like hallucinations, can represent a form of "endopsychic perception," in which the delusion expresses an insight into the structure of the mind. Thus, Paul Schreber's belief that the world must come to an end because his ego was attracting all the rays of God to itself represents the withdrawal of object libido into narcissism in certain clinical states and in sleep.

Freud saw delusions as appearing on a continuum that included both psychotic and neurotic manifestations. In both, the psychic bases of the delusion are analyzable. For example, ideas of reference may appear in everyday life, such as in the misreading of words as if they are one's own name. Freud cites Bleuler, who kept misreading the word "Blutkörperchen" (blood corpuscles) as his own name and, upon analysis, realized that the entire passage in which the word occurred was about bad style in scientific writing, of which Bleuler felt guilty.

Another common manifestation of delusions is in certain religious systems, where mythic beliefs are accepted as real. Such delusions have the advantage over psychotic delusions in that they are shared and can forestall certain neurotic difficulties. Like all delusions, religious beliefs can reflect the unconscious needs of the believer, needs that may apply to the majority of humankind, such as the experience of a needed but feared protector, transposed from father to God (hence, "God the father").

REFERENCES

Freud, S. (1911). Psycho-analytic notes on an autobiographical account of a case of paranoia (dementia paranoides). S.E. 12: 9–79.

Weinstein, E. A. (1962). *Cultural Aspects of Delusions*. New York: Free Press.

MARK J. BLECHNER

Denial

One of the least complex mechanisms of defense. Freud (1911, 1923, 1924) originally conceptualized denial as acting to ward off perceptions of external reality that would be upsetting. In such a case, the person would not perceive external stimuli that were apparent to others. Subsequently, the concept of denial was expanded (Freud, 1925; Fenichel, 1945; Jacobson, 1957) to include a failure to perceive certain internal stimuli, including thoughts, feelings, and wishes that, if acknowledged, would bring about psychological distress.

To accomplish this "warding off," or failure to perceive external or internal stimuli, several mental operations may be used. At first, Freud explained the "failure to see" in terms of the individual withdrawing attention from the stimulus; unless some attention is deployed to the stimulus, it will not be perceived. Subsequently, other mental operations were added to attention withdrawal as means for carrying out denial. For example, a person may perceive the stimulus but ignore it (Freud, 1940). Alternatively, the stimulus may be *mis*perceived and turned into something more desirable. These manifestations of denial are all closely tied to the perceptual system.

Denial may take other forms as well. The development of language provides the individual with the possibility of disavowing an experience ("It did not happen that way"). Or the anxiety-arousing experience may be minimized, or ridiculed, or otherwise distorted so that the arousal of negative affect is diminished. Denial may also be carried out through "enacted daydreams" (A. Freud, 1936), in which a person superimposes his or her own personally satisfying fantasy onto a situation that, if perceived accurately, would be a source of psychological distress. In turn, this fantasy may result in an attitude of unfounded optimism, sometimes referred to as "Pollyannaish denial."

Denial is generally considered to be an immature defense; in its simplest, prototypical form, it requires only attaching a negative marker, or minus sign, to the perception. Because of its simplicity, it is easily seen through, once an individual's cognitive development has matured somewhat. However, for young children, denial is an age-appropriate defense. For an infant, toddler, or preschooler, who may have little capacity to change a distressing reality situation, denial may be an effective mechanism for protection from what would otherwise be overwhelming anxiety. In fact, research studies show that denial is a frequently used defense among children below the age of five. After that time, children begin to be able to "see through" the defense, and so it is no longer effective in warding off anxiety. (For a summary of this research, see Cramer, 1991; also, Cramer, 1997; Smith and Danielsson, 1982).

The use of denial by adults, if it takes the form of perceptual malfunction—not seeing what is there, or misperceiving what is there—is often taken as evidence of psychosis. However, there are circumstances in which even this extreme form of denial may be adaptive, and not evidence of pathology. For situations in which external reality is overwhelmingly painful and immutable—extreme natural disasters, horrors of wartime, terminal illness—when the adult, like the young child, has no way to modify reality, then "denial in the service of the need to survive" (Geleerd, 1965) should not be considered to be psychotic.

Adults may also use denial in its cognitive form by imposing a personal fantasy onto an otherwise stressful situation, as occurs with individuals who suffer from a personality disorder (Vaillant, 1992, 1994). These individuals do not misperceive physical reality, but they fail to comprehend the psychological implications of what they perceive; instead, they impose their own wished-for fantasy onto the situation. In general, in the absence of overwhelming external conditions over which an individual has no control or hope of changing, the extensive use of denial by an adult is indicative of psychopathology. There is recent empirical research evidence that this pathology has its origins in the early years of the individual's development (Cramer and Block, 1998).

REFERENCES

Breznitz, S. (1983). The seven kinds of denial. In S. Breznitz (ed.). *The Denial of Stress*. New York: International Universities Press, pp. 257–280.

Cramer, P. (1991). *The Development of Defense Mechanisms*. New York: Springer-Verlag.

———. (1997). Evidence for change in children's use of defense mechanisms. *Journal of Personality*, 65: 233–247.

Cramer, P., and Block, J. (1998). Preschool antecedents of defense mechanism use in young adults. *Journal of Personality and Social Psychology*, 74: 159–169.

Fenichel, O. (1945). *The Psychoanalytic Theory of Neurosis*. New York: Norton.

Freud, A. (1936). *The Ego and the Mechanisms of Defense*. New York: International Universities Press.

Freud, S. (1911). Formulations on the two principles of mental functioning. S.E. 12: 218–226.

———. (1923). *The Ego and the Id*. S.E. 19: 12–59.

———. (1924). The loss of reality in neurosis and psychosis. S.E. 19: 183–190.

———. (1925). Negation. S.E. 19: 235–239.

———. (1940). Splitting of the ego in the process of defence. S.E. 23: 271–278.

Geleerd, E. R. (1965). Two kinds of denial: Neurotic denial and denial in the service of the need to survive. In R. Loewenstein (ed.). *Drives, Affects and Behavior*, vol. 2. New York: International Universities Press, pp. 118–127.

Jacobson, E. (1957). Denial and repression. *Journal of the American Psychoanalytic Association*, 5: 61–92.

Smith, G. J. W., and Danielsson, A. (1982). *Anxiety and Defense Strategies in Childhood and Adolescence*. New York: International Universities Press.

Vaillant, G. E. (1992). *Ego Mechanisms of Defense: A Guide for Clinicians and Researchers*. Washington, D.C.: American Psychiatric Press.

———. (1994). Ego mechanisms of defense and personality psychopathology. *Journal of Abnormal Psychology*, 103: 44–50.

PHEBE CRAMER

Denmark, and Psychoanalysis

As in all parts of the Western world, psychoanalysis in Denmark has had a profound impact on fields such as culture, art, pedagogy, and the like, as well as a major, though indirect, influence on psychiatry and psychology.

When in the 1920s Freud's thoughts reached Denmark, they were seized with enthusiasm by artists, intellectuals, and in particular a group of so-called cultural radicals with liberal sexual political views, whereas the psychiatric establishment and academic psychology repudiated psychoanalysis, comparing it to superstition. Wilhelm Reich's short visit to Copenhagen in 1933 did not improve the situation (Jensen and Paikin, 1980: 103–116). When the attempts to establish contact with the International Psychoanalytic Association in the 1930s proved futile, it was left in the hands of self-taught individuals from the above group to represent psychoanalysis to the public, which made things very easy for the critics. However, that was not the worst part of it; these "wild" analysts practiced what they called psychoanalysis to the detriment of their patients as well as the reputation of psychoanalysis. Thus, in all conceivable ways, clinical psychoanalysis had a very unfortunate beginning in Denmark, and only gradually are we beginning to overcome these difficulties. The repercussions of the "wild" analysis are still highly visible, because some of the societies established in the 1920s and 1930s continued to train "analysts," some of whom are still practicing in the pervasive gray-black psychotherapeutic supermarket.

The Danish Psychoanalytic Society became a component Society of the International Psychoanalytic Association (IPA) in 1957 after having been a Study Group under Swedish sponsorship for four years (see Jensen and Paikin, 1980: 103–116). The core of the newly founded society was an IPA-approved Swedish training analyst and two Danish psychiatrists, who returned from training in New York and Vienna, respectively. The society got off to a flying start through the successful arrangement of the international congress in 1959 in Copenhagen.

Nevertheless the society stagnated shortly after its start. One reason—of many, presumably—was that the society led a highly restrictive policy for the acceptance of new candidates, and when this became known, many interested psychiatrists and psychologists gave up in advance. Another contributing factor might have been that—inspired by the practice of analysis in the United States—it attempted to integrate psychoanalysis into psychiatry. Thus the only two psychiatric professors in Denmark at the time were formal members of a selection committee who were to assess applicants for the psychoanalytic training. This did not, of course, change the fact that psychiatry in Denmark has always been predominantly biologically/genetically oriented.

Whatever the explanation, the fact remains that for a substantial period during the 1960s and 1970s, only two candidates completed the training. Of the original group of fifteen trained analysts, all but a few ceased to practice as analysts. In this way, the society lost one or maybe even two generations of analysts. One of the training analysts, who was among the founders, lost interest in psychoanalysis and left the society. The other, active as a training analyst, fell ill and died in 1972 (Paikin, 1992: 50–53).

In 1975, the society began training candidates from southern Sweden. Although psychoanalysis thrived in Sweden, it was only in Stockholm—about six hundred kilometers from southern Sweden—that psychoanalytic training was available. The intake of Swedish candidates into training analysis and to the seminars was a much welcomed stimulus for the Danish society.

Since then, the society has regularly arranged theoretical and clinical training programs of three—recently four—years' duration for classes of five to ten candidates. The increasing intake of candidates obliged the society to start new classes every second year.

Because of this increase, the society today (1998) has thirty-six members (including six associate members) and twenty-four candidates. About 50 percent of the members live and work in southern Sweden, and approximately 30 percent are Swedish. In 1996, the Swedish members also obtained membership in the Swedish Psychoanalytic Society, so that now most of them have double membership.

Conditions for psychoanalytic practice in Denmark have never been favorable, partly because neither psychoanalytic treatment nor training has been subsidized, in spite of Denmark's being a welfare society, where all medical and social support is at the public expense—paid for by a high personal income tax. This means that only very few people can afford a psychoanalysis. The advantage until now is that psychoanalysis has been able to avoid interference from the authorities.

During the last ten to fifteen years, the Danish society has experienced considerable progress. As mentioned above, the society has increased and the majority of the members now practice psychoanalysis to a greater or lesser degree. This progress is mostly due to the assistance and contributions of a number of outstanding analysts from abroad (Ronald Baker, London; Janice de Saussure, Geneva; Michael Feldman, London; Martin Miller, London) who have been supervisors for members and candidates and advisers for the society on a regular basis since 1987. At the occasion of the society's fortieth anniversary, they were all elected honorary members of the Danish society.

Because of its smallness and for fear of being identified with the "wild" analysts, the society has until recently been reluctant to become more visible to the public. With the recent positive development, however, the society has gained the strength and courage to change these policies. It has produced an informative brochure as well as a public relations organ, "Psychoanalytic Debate," which sets up public meetings where its members or prominent analysts from abroad present papers on psychoanalytic topics. This activity has brought clinical psychoanalysis to the fore.

Paradoxically, clinical psychoanalysis has been almost unknown even to professionals, whereas at the same time there has been a keen interest in psychoanalytic theory (and in Freud as a person) among academics. In particular, within the field of literary research, psychoanalytic viewpoints have been applied, e.g., in literary interpretation. And the translation into Danish of some of Freud's works has been done by highly proficient men of letters without any psychoanalytic training whatsoever.

Although the psychiatric establishment in Denmark has been ambivalent toward psychoanalysis, psychoanalytic ideas have, at least in some places, had a marked indirect influence in the form of the so-called psychoanalytically oriented psychotherapy. The psychological faculties of the Danish universities have been equally ambivalent; there have been lectures in psychoanalytic theory, but there has never been a chair in psychoanalysis, nor has clinical psychoanalysis had any support (Paikin, 1992: 50–53). However, several psychoanalytic dissertations by the members of the society have been accepted by the psychological and medical faculties of the Danish universities.

For the small Danish society, it has been of immeasurable value to be part of IPA and the European Psychoanalytic Federation (EPF). The cooperation with the Nordic societies has been of equally great importance. The evolution of the society has made it possible to host Nordic and EPF conferences and the Second Joint Clinical Meeting of the EPF and the American Psychoanalytic Association in 1992.

The head office of the *Scandinavian Psychoanalytic Review*, an English-language journal published jointly by the four Nordic societies, was situated in Denmark from its very beginning in 1978 and remained there until 1988. During this period the journal succeeded in attracting international recognition (Lind, 1989: 3–4). A steadily increasing number of Danish analysts now write articles for the journal.

REFERENCES

Jensen, R., and Paikin, H. (1980). On psychoanalysis in Denmark. *Scandinavian Psychoanalytic Review*, 3: 103–116.

Lind, L. (1989). Editorial. *Scandinavian Psychoanalytic Review*, 12: 3–4.

Paikin, H. (1992). Denmark. In P. Kutter (ed.). *Psychoanalysis International*. Stuttgart–Bad Cannstadt: Frommann-Holzboog, pp. 50–53.

HENNING PAIKIN

Depression

The first contribution to the psychoanalytic understanding of depression was made by Karl Abraham (1911). He posited that the origins of the illness lay in significant experiences of disappointment and frustration, related to the infant's failing to have his or her needs gratified. Occurring early in life, these events are associated with profound feelings of despair and being unloved.

In a further contribution, Abraham (1924) elaborated on the earlier theory, specifically linking the unfulfilled gratification to intense, constitutional oral needs. He believed that such susceptible infants inevitably experienced frustration and disappointment in their first love relationships, resulting in a fixation at the oral level of development. In adult life, similar disappointments may lead to a regression to the infantile oral phase, with the accompanying affect.

Freud (1917), like Abraham, was struck by the similarities between depression ("melancholia") and mourning. He observed that the critical difference lay in the self-reproaches, diminished self-esteem, and expectation of punishment experienced by the depressed individual. In contrast, he noted, "Mourning is regularly the reaction to the loss of a loved person, or to the loss of some abstraction which has taken the place of one, such as one's country, liberty, an ideal, and so on" (p. 243).

Accordingly, whereas the bereaved individual experiences the world as "poor and empty," the depressed person feels himself or herself to be "poor and empty."

Freud observed that depression, in the adult, is initiated by a significant disappointment with a loved person from whom one's love has become "detached." Instead of that love being displaced onto another person, the disappointment is brought into the individual's psyche, where it forms the nucleus of an identification with the lost object. The now devalued external object becomes part of the self, the source of devaluation of the self, and of feelings of impoverishment.

The two major preconditions for the foregoing process, Freud noted, are that the depressed person shall have a significant emotional investment in the beloved object, and that the original investment shall have been importantly colored by fragile, narcissistic, self-serving needs, creating a strongly ambivalent relationship. In addition to the powerful influence of life experiences, Freud did not dismiss the role of constitutional factors.

Later analysts added to and emended these views. Melanie Klein (1935) hypothesized that at around six months of age, the infant "introjects" good and bad aspects of the mother, which come to represent good and bad impulses in the infant. At some point, the infant becomes aware of his or her destructive impulses toward the mother and is afraid that they may lead to losing her. This "depressive position" can, under appropriate circumstances, be reactivated in adult life.

Starting from an ego-psychological perspective, Bibring (1953) regarded depression as an affective state of helplessness and hopelessness resulting from an inability to have responded to a situation of danger. This state is associated with feelings of not being lovable, not being able to love, and being incompetent. The precursor to depression, Bibring said, lies in an overwhelming, shock-like state of hopelessness and helplessness that can occur in any phase of childhood. Adult experiences that resonate with the earlier affect would initiate depression.

Bibring's views were echoed by Zetzel (1965), who described a "depressive character structure" that, in addition to its chronicity, is characterized by the inability of such individuals to "bear depression"; consequently, they more readily succumb to depressive illness.

Jacobson (1971) drew attention to what she saw as a central aspect of depression, that it is "the outcome of an aggressive conflict, caused by a lack of understanding and acceptance by the mother that reduces the child's self-esteem" (p. 180).

Also from an ego-psychological perspective, Brenner (1991) stressed that depression is an affect and not an illness per se. In contrast to anxiety, which represents the fear of an anticipated occurrence, depressive affect results from the actual occurrence of the event. The major calamities, he stated, are loss of the love of the object, loss of the object, and castration and punishment. Brenner also believes that depression may accompany any psychic conflict; what varies is its role in the resulting "compromise formation."

Another schema of depression was developed by Kohut (1977), based on a self-psychology perspective. Similarly to the previous authors, Kohut implicated early life experiences in the later onset of depression. Kohut observed that as children, depressed adults had experienced the unavailability of a "mirroring and idealizing self-object." From this point of view, depression does not involve guilt or a punitive superego but arises from profound feelings of mortification and failure. Accordingly, suicide represents a "remedial act," seeking to erase the pain of such unbearable emotions.

In summary, most psychoanalytic authors assume that there is a constitutional susceptibility to depression; that early childhood experiences may create a vulnerability to depression; and that the occurrence of events in adult life that resonate with the affective and or cognitive nature of the childhood events may lead to depressive illness.

REFERENCES

Abraham, K. (1911–1968). *Selected Papers*. London: Hogarth Press, pp. 137–156, 418–501.

Bibring, E. (1953). The Mechanism of Depression. In P. Greenacre (ed.). *Affective Disorders*. New York: International Universities Press, pp. 13–47.

Brenner, C. (1991). A psychoanalytic perspective on depression. *Journal of the American Psychoanalytic Association*, 39: 25–43.

Freud, S. (1917). *Mourning and Melancholia*. S.E. 17: 239–258.

Jacobson, E. (ed.) (1971). *Depression: Studies of Normal, Neurotic and Psychotic Conditions*. New York: International Universities Press.

Klein, M. (1921–1945). *Contributions to Psycho-Analysis*. London: Hogarth Press, 1948, pp. 282–310.

Kohut, H. (1977). *The Restoration of the Self*. New York: International Universities Press.

Zetzel, E. (1965). *The Capacity for Emotional Growth*. New York: International Universities Press, 1970, pp. 82–114.

DAVID S. WERMAN

Deutsch, Helene (1884–1982)

The first leading woman member of Freud's Vienna Psychoanalytic Society, Helene Deutsch is best known for developing and influencing his ideas about women's psychology and for her theory of the "as if" personality. Born Helene Rosenberg on October 9, 1884, in Przemysl, Galicia (present-day Poland), she claimed in old age that she had always hated her housewife mother and idealized her lawyer father. In her teens she ran away from home and in 1907 became one of the first women to study medicine at the University of Vienna, where she first learned about psychoanalysis through reading Wilhelm Jensen's novella, *Gradiva*, and Freud's analysis of it.

Seeking to free herself from an affair, beginning when she was sixteen, with a married man—the prominent socialist leader and lawyer Herman Lieberman—Helene briefly left Vienna for a year's study in Munich in 1910. In 1912, she married Felix Deutsch, later known for his psychoanalytic work in psychosomatic medicine.

After qualifying as a doctor, Helene worked in pediatrics and then in psychiatry. She gave birth to her and Felix's only child, Martin, in 1917. The next year she went into analysis with Freud; took on her first psychoanalytic patient, Victor Tausk, in 1919; and gave her first Psychoanalytic Congress paper (about Martin) in The Hague in 1920.

Three years later, in 1923, she went into analysis with Karl Abraham in Berlin. From there she gave a talk at the 1924 Salzburg Psychoanalytic Congress. It formed the basis of her 1925 monograph, *The Psychology of Women's Sexual Functions*. Drawing on several years' work with women, it was the first book devoted by a psychoanalyst to women's psychology. Ridiculed at the time by Karen Horney for characterizing childbirth as "an orgy of masochistic pleasure" (Deutsch, 1950: 172) and lambasted subsequently by feminists for reiterating Freud's seeming equation of women with masochism, Deutsch's work has subsequently been welcomed by some feminists (notably by Barbara Webster, 1985) for attending, unlike Freud, to the problems posed for women by identifying with their mothers in being female like them.

Deutsch's work on women's psychology continued through the 1920s on her return from Berlin to Vienna. In 1925, she became the first president, for the next decade, of Vienna's Psychoanalytic Training Institute, which she helped inaugurate after being involved in the training established at the Berlin Psychoanalytic Institute, founded in 1920. Her case history accounts of women's psychology—including linking women's suicidal, phobic, agoraphobic, obsessional, and depressive symptoms to ambivalent identification with their mothers—provided the material for much of her next book, *Psychoanalysis of the Neuroses*, published in 1930. She followed this with a 1931 essay, recently approved of by feminists Noreen O'Connor and Joanna Ryan (1993) for its sympathetic analysis of lesbianism in contrast to the prevailing pathologizing of homosexuality by Freud's followers today.

As for Deutsch, she increasingly turned her attention through the 1930s from the specifics of women's psychology to what has become her most enduring contribution to psychoanalysis, her theory, first formulated in 1934, of "as if" identification of men, as well as women, with those they happen to meet as adults in place of secure childhood identification with their parents. This theory was subsequently incorporated into US ego and self psychology, to which Deutsch contributed both with her 1934 paper and with the papers and books she wrote following her move, with Martin and Felix, from Vienna to Boston in 1935. Here she worked with social work and other cases in the psychiatric unit established in 1934 by Stanley Cobb in Boston's Massachusetts General Hospital.

Deutsch included descriptions of many of these cases in her two-volume book, *The Psychology of Women*, published in 1944 and 1945. Following the war, however, she turned increasingly from women's to men's psychology. She continued to develop her theory of "as if" identification, illustrating it with examples from fiction (e.g., Thomas Mann's *Felix Krull*) and from her clinical work. These and her other post-1930 papers, together with the English translation of *Psychoanalysis of the Neuroses*, constituted her 1965 book, *Neuroses and Character Types*.

Next, returning to the subject of adolescence, with which she began *The Psychology of Women*, and drawing on her experience as grandmother to Martin's college student sons and on interviews with Harvard students, she wrote two final books about psychoanalysis—*Selected Problems of Adolescence* and *A Psychoanalytic Study of the Myth of Dionysius and Apollo*. They were published in 1967 and 1969, respectively, over a decade before her death, at age ninety-seven, in 1982.

D

Accounts of her life and work can be found in her 1973 autobiography, *Confrontations with Myself*; in Paul Roazen's biography, articles about, and introductions to translations of her work into English; and in my 1991 book, *Mothers of Psychoanalysis*.

REFERENCES

Deutsch, H. (1950). The psychology of women in relation to the functions of reproduction. In R. Fliess (ed.). *The Psycho-Analytic Reader*. London: Hogarth Press, pp. 165–179.

O'Connor, N., and Ryan, J. (1993). *Wild Desires and Mistaken Identities*. London: Virago.

Roazen, P. (1985). *Helene Deutsch*. New York: Meridian.

Sayers, J. (1991). *Mothers of Psychoanalysis: Helene Deutsch, Karen Horney, Anna Freud, Melanie Klein*. New York: Norton.

Webster, B. (1985). Helene Deutsch. *Signs*, 10: 553–571.

JANET SAYERS

Developmental Theory

Freudian theory has been characterized by developmental propositions from its inception. In *Studies on Hysteria*, Freud (1893–1899) sought to establish the origins of hysteria in early sexual seductions. Although he did not report any such seduction in the years below eight, he did establish the core idea that there can be no adult neurosis without a childhood or infantile neurosis. When Freud shifted to the postulation of fantasied rather than actual seduction in childhood, he did not abandon the idea of real "out of phase" sexual experience but rather gave up the idea of early sexual seduction of the child as the core of neuroses. He did, however, introduce the premise of polymorphous infantile sexuality (many forms of sexual arousal without copulation) as the basis of drive representation in infancy.

On this new theory, infantile sexuality culminates in the Oedipus constellation, following which the full, mature mental apparatus is established with id, ego, and superego in place. The proposal for many forms of sexual experience in infancy led to the introduction of narcissistic, oral, anal, and phallic stages of development, which Erickson referred to as the tragedies and comedies that occur around the orifices of the body. However, these stages, or "way stations," were meant as designations of the themes found in fantasy life, and were not considered to be ego developmental milestones. Hartmann posited that the stages were *maturational*, implying that they were features of an emergent focus on body ego to be expressed in accord with an invariant course only to lead to interaction with experience by chance. The word "development" was reserved for the full range of biological and experiential contributions, and included biological maturation.

Together, these way stations were called "libido theory." This theory offered a wide-ranging, all-encompassing attempt to explain symptom formation, character, and perversions in a single parsimonious developmental model. While the source of the drives in the body could not be explored by the psychoanalytic method, the aims and objects of a person's desire could be studied psychoanalytically by examining the derivatives of the combinations and permutations of active and passive libidinal and aggressive wishes that were attached to "objects" (mental representations of early figures in an infant's life) culminating in the attachments and conflicts that inevitably cluster around the triadic Oedipal configuration. In this earliest of Freud's genetic models, symptom specificity was thought to derive from the level of fantasy (oral, anal, phallic, Oedipal). Indeed, if the person had a fixation at the anal level, the resulting perversion would contain elements of pleasurable anal activity. If a constellation of neurotic symptoms ensued from the same level, a regressive constellation of compromise formation would lead to an obsessive-compulsive neurosis, and if an ego-syntonic character structure were to emerge, the traits of orderliness, stinginess, and punctiliousness would be prominent. As can be seen, the theory was based upon retrospective genetic propositions that constituted a significant commitment to prospective developmental principles that were thought to be at work throughout the life cycle.

In 1926, Freud reexamined his somewhat rigid biopsychological model and determined that a revision in the theory of anxiety was necessary. He moved from a hydraulic proposal that dammed libido was expressed as anxiety to a psychological theory that anxiety was the result of the ego's response to a sequence of dangers, each of which belonged to a specific stage of development. The earliest danger is helplessness, the next separation, and then castration. Once the tripartite structure of the mind was in place, superego anxiety ensued, with the ego recoiling from infantile wishes that were not acceptable in response to the demands of the superego, i.e., conscience.

All of the foregoing was part of Freud's retrospective reconstructive psychology that was to be designated as "genetic theory" by Rapaport. Prospective developmental theory, by contrast, grew out of the propositions outlined. However, this time, empirical investigators and clinicians observed children and infants directly to determine the path of becoming a fully functioning member of the species and also to determine which, if any, of the retrospective propositions could be verified. The remainder of the history of psychoanalytic developmental theory can be found in many of the empirical and clinical observations of the twentieth century. Some psychoanalyst-researchers should also be acknowledged as pioneers in forming and re-forming psychoanalytic developmental psychology. But before we enter that arena, we should note that the emergence of ego psychology changed the orientation of this early view from a depth psychology by adding the surface experiences of the relationship of fantasy to reality. Freud's programmatic look at the role of the pleasure and reality principles in development gave rise to Ferenczi's attempt to map the stages in the appreciation of reality that became a precursor to our current perspective on the role of the ego in development and adaptation.

On the clinical side, we cannot ignore the work of Melanie Klein, Anna Freud, and D.W. Winnicott, all of whom changed Freud's initial views. Klein exploited the newly introduced play therapy as a means of understanding the child's inner world. She posited a highly truncated developmental progression from an initial need for attachment through the inability to fuse early experience of pleasure and pain with an initial mental designation of a good and bad breast and mother. The bad and unpleasant interactions were externalized and thus experienced as paranoid persecutory objects, and then with increasing mental development, the depressive position was adopted with the persecutor within. Defenses such as splitting and projective identification are seen to derive from these early primitive experiences.

Anna Freud also used play therapy but focused on the adaptive ego, offering the proposal that psychoanalysts study the repercussion of events on the mind and not the events alone. Moreover, we can follow developmental lines as the best means of grasping the significance of symptoms. She also disavowed infantile psychologizing (especially during the first year), modeling her ideas on her father's work. She designated the first six months of life as the period of the *need satisfying object*, rejecting Klein's idea of an infant under one year of age having structured mental contents. Rather than making diagnoses, Anna Freud saw symptoms as

indicators of arrest or regressive adaptation in developmental lines ranging from the following sorts of progression: from egocentricity to companionship, from soiling and wetting to bodily control, and so on.

Winnicott, on the other hand, stated, as did Klein, that infants were object seeking, and that attachment took place on a "built-in" need for mothering, in contrast to the Freudian notion of its anaclitic origins, where the attachment leaned against physiologic needs. It was Winnicott who coined the phrase "good enough mothering," and who said, "there is no such thing as a baby." The latter was invoked to remind the observer that human infancy is a dependent existence—more precisely, an interdependent state of being with fuzzy self-other boundaries. Winnicott also introduced the term "transitional object" to designate that hypothetical space that is not I or you during the predifferentiated stage in infancy and that becomes the anlage for creative imagination. The objects that infants cling to during this period have been called "transitional objects" because they mediate tolerance for separation in fantasy.

Although Freud, as well as his early followers, placed much weight on the first five years of life, he also designated the period following the resolution of the Oedipus complex as a latency period, which then gave way to adolescence following puberty. Latency was seen as the result of the suppression of infantile sexuality that follows the response to castration anxiety at the close of the Oedipal stage. The Oedipal boy's wish for his mother was seen in the child's mind as forbidden by the father, generating castration anxiety; the resolution of this conflict would constitute the various constellations of male-female relationships in later life. Similarly, the girl child being disappointed by her mother, who was seen as figuratively castrated, would turn to her father with the hope of bodily restitution or its substitute, a baby.

These early Freudian formulations of unconscious fantasies have been revised under the influence of later clinical and feminist critiques, with the most prominent one being the feminine genital castration complex taking the form of fear of damage to the genitals. The penis envy proposal is given second place in this formulation as it is activated in a male-dominated social milieu. Regardless of which position has been espoused, most psychoanalytic thinkers do believe that a change occurs following the resolution of the Oedipus complex, ushering in the latency period during which drive derivatives of early sexuality are suppressed. Shapiro and Perry

D

(1976) also argued for the discontinuity in development called "latency," but not on grounds of suppressed sexuality alone. Rather, by age six or seven, a child's thinking and neurodevelopmental course changes, facilitating learning and the industry that Erickson claims for the period.

Adolescence is the next major developmental step that includes the psychological changes that ensue following the effects of puberty and the new social demands on the sexually competent preadult. There is a revival of Oedipal struggles and a need for removal from the incestuous objects of earlier years, as well as a significant struggle to integrate one's newly configured body into a new body image. The capacity of being fully sexual and able to procreate creates new burdens, and the fantasies employed for arousal in masturbation must finally be harnessed in object finding and new linkages as social opportunities arise. The central conflicts during adolescence develop around the issues of dependency and autonomy, and drive satisfaction and restraint. Studies of adolescents have helped to define adolescence better and will be described below following a review of empirical studies in earlier infancy.

In the United States, prospective empirical studies stimulated by psychoanalytic theory became prominent, and baby watching took on new meanings. The movement was spearheaded by Rene Spitz and Margaret Mahler, both practicing medical psychoanalysts. Spitz pioneered work on early caretaking and its significance for depression, and is responsible for the elaboration of an ego psychological scheme that defined the emergence of a competent child. He called his theory a genetic field theory of development based on an embryological model of three maturational landmarks to be traversed, which can be designated as organizers. The landmarks are empirically observed and derived, and refer to significant achievements in coming to grips with the external world. The first achievement is the social smile that regularly can be observed at six weeks, marking the appreciation of the human facial configuration as a signal for pleasure and contact. The second landmark is represented in the six-month stranger response that is presumed to represent the initial attachment to the mother, and the third, the establishment of a meaningful use of the word "no," signifying separateness at two to three years.

Mahler in turn revised developmental ego psychology without discarding earlier libido theory but enriched and embellished it in accord with the observations made of mothers and infants and toddlers in interaction. She elaborated Freud's ideas about development in her separation individuation theory, which takes the infant from the earliest *autistic* phase through psychological hatching and the capacity to maintain a mental image of the mother that is stable and sustaining in her absence. The *symbiotic* phase follows on the heels of the *autistic* phase, and gives way to the *separation individuation process* and its subphases. The first subphase is called the *practicing period*, in which the toddler's newfound locomotion and growing capacity for language are expressed in what has been called a love affair with the world with high spirits and reckless abandon. The *rapprochement subphase* that follows is more low-keyed, finding a more solemn and fretful toddler who has learned that the world as experienced is not as joyful and is less dependable on wishes, and more arbitrary. Mother leaves, her whereabouts are not known; the child must check on her frequently and "refuel" until she can achieve the next phase of confident expectation that memory sustains, allowing the child to trust that there are reliable caretakers who return and sometimes even gratify wishes. The establishment of a stable representation of the primary caretaker is termed "object constancy."

Following empirical studies of the devastating effects of the Second World War on separated children and the distressing outcome of delinquency derived from deprivation, John Bowlby, a psychoanalyst nurtured in London in the intellectual ferment of the Kleinian and Freudian theoretical frames, developed a unique theory of attachment that has given rise to an enormous volume of empirical and theoretical investigation. His contribution has dominated psychoanalytic and academic developmental laboratories. The theory is derived from an amalgam of clinical and nonclinical observations, psychoanalytic theory, and ethological modeling. Bowlby has fused theories and has transcended some of the parochialism of clinical psychoanalysis. He used the observations of the regularly appearing constellation of protest, despair, and detachment seen in separated children to develop a model of attachment that is the backdrop against which these responses occur. Each response is related sequentially to a mental mechanism with separation anxiety first, grieving second, and denial last. These mechanisms are set into motion following the establishment of attachment that is the process guaranteeing adaptive survival for the human infant. Bowlby utilizes the construct of an inborn response system (IRS) as an ethological trigger to these dangers to attachment. Attachment in turn is considered not as an anaclitic process but as a built-in tendency of human biopsychology. Thus, Freud's partial instinct theory was revived by Bowlby to explain the attachment bond in a number of inborn infantile reflexes such as clinging, sucking, and following, and two responses that "bring the mother halfway," smiling and crying.

Ainsworth and others, working from Bowlby's attachment model, have devised a test of attachment to be used during the second year of life that permits children to be classified as to attachment type. This strange situation paradigm has been shown to be predictive of healthy and maladaptive outcomes that are empirically founded. The developmental implications of this paradigm have also been carried into adulthood by Mary Main in the adult attachment interview (AAI). The parent's attachment status as determined by a semistructured interview offers insight into the conservative transmission of secure attachment versus insecure attachment, and most strikingly has been shown to predict the nature of the mother's attachment in the next generation to the newborn child. These are powerful tools for prospective prediction in a system that derives from psychoanalytic theory.

Other areas of observational research that derive from psychoanalytic models and that have influenced developmental theory come from the work of Roiphe and Galenson, Stern, and Emde. Roiphe and Galenson described an early genital phase that precedes the phallic Oedipal awareness in children. They relate the preoccupations that derive from that period to perceptual experiences that direct body focusing and that may be accentuated by inadvertent body trauma. The stronger focus may lead to fixations and distortion in genital body image. The data are largely anecdotal but are clinically relevant.

Stern has used dyadic film and video to explicate early infantile attunement between mother and infant and later codetermination of dialogues that aid in the emerging competence of the self. His data have been used by those representing the school of Kohut in regard to their view of empathy and the narcissistic line of development. In a self-psychological model for the development of self-esteem, the infant must initially mirror and then seek a coherent self amid the emerging threats to self-cohesion. The extravagant demands of the line of development of narcissism have been built from the early data on the empathic interactions of the early dyad.

Emde has provided an array of new information concerning the early role of social referencing as a sign of approaching separation and the need for maternal affirmation. He also has demonstrated the early roots of constraint and moral internalization in three year olds even prior to the resolution of the Oedipus complex. These are but a few of the forays into the development of the mental life of children as they relate to basic psychoanalytic theory. Each new finding has been used to direct our attention to the understanding of the evolution of the developmental process in an individual regardless of culture. Each new finding has also permitted revision of theory to fit the new data and to direct clinical progress.

Perhaps most striking in this arena is the new information about adolescence. The earliest view of adolescence as a time of instinctual drive increase and maximum turmoil has been revised. There is need to integrate new body experiences and new functions and appearances in a new body image. Moreover, new social opportunities and object removal remain prominent themes. Procreative readiness, as noted earlier, offers new challenges to these young adults within a context of changing social mores. The psychological integration of all these momentous events is no easy task, and "romantic crushes," as well as falls from idealized grace and dependency struggles with parents, are prominent. Nevertheless, most current observers of adolescents have described a smoother path, with fewer bumps for most, than the initial psychoanalytic observers suggested. A significant number of adolescents, however, become depressed or fall prey to drugs and alcohol, or become psychotic or borderline as new challenges arise.

The psychoanalytic theorists have invoked the challenge of a new version of the Oedipal struggles with strong issues related to negative Oedipal mastery and object removal as paramount conflicts. Erickson introduced the concept of struggle for identity, both sexual and role identity, as well as the establishment of life goals as keys to understanding this period. The persistence of identity diffusion was seen as a maladaptive outcome in this struggle. The rising rates of depression as adolescence proceeds may be relevant to the struggle in a world that seems to hold less promise than in prior generations in our culture. Whatever the reason, psychoanalytic adolescent developmentalists continue to be most insistent on studying the interplay of culture and fantasy as a means of grasping the compromises and adaptive outcomes in adolescence.

D

In psychoanalytic theory, there is no terminus to development. It may be studied throughout the life cycle as Erickson has suggested, but at all points a psychoanalytic view includes the interplay of fantasy and reality in relation to adaptation. There is also no way to continue to add to our knowledge without some cross-fertilization of knowledge gained from Freud's psychoanalytic method in combination with empirical research.

REFERENCES
Ainsworth, M. D. S., Blehar, M. D., Waters, E., et al. (1978). *Patterns of Attachment: A Psychological Study of the Strange Situation*. Hillsdale, N.J.: Erlbaum.

Bowlby, J. (1969). *Attachment and Loss*, vol. 1. New York: Basic Books.

Buchsbaum, H. K., and Emde, R. N. (1990). Play narrations in 36-month-old children: Early moral development and family relationships. *Psychoanalytic Study of the Child*, 40: 129–155.

Emde, R. N. (1992). Social referencing research: Uncertainty, self, and the search for meaning. In S. Feinman (ed.). *Social Referencing and the Social Construction of Reality in Infancy*. New York: Plenum Press.

Fonagy, P., Steele, H., and Steele, M. (1991). Maternal representations of attachment during pregnancy predict the organization of infant-mother attachment at one year of age. *Child Development*, 62: 891–905.

Freud, A. (1974). A psychoanalytic view of developmental psychopathology. *Journal of the Philadelphia Association for Psychoanalysis*, 1: 7–17.

Freud, S. (1926). *Inhibitions, Symptoms, and Anxiety*. S.E. 20: 75–175.

Mahler, M. S. (1975). *The Psychological Birth of the Human Infant: Symbiosis and Individuation*. New York: Basic Books.

Roiphe, H., and Galenson, E. (1980). The pre-oedipal development of the boy. *Journal of the American Psychoanalytic Association*, 28: 805–827.

Shapiro, T., and Hertzig, M. (1995). Normal child and adolescent development. In J. Talbott (ed.). *Textbook of Psychiatry*. Washington, D.C.: American Psychiatric Press.

Shapiro, T., and Perry, R. (1976). Latency revisited: The age 7 plus or minus 1. *Psychoanalytic Study of the Child*, 31: 79–105.

Stern, D. N. (1985). *The Interpersonal World of the Infant: A View from Psychoanalysis and Developmental Psychology*. New York: Basic Books.

THEODORE SHAPIRO

Displacement

Displacement has a special position among the defense mechanisms. It belongs to those few defenses that have been described as "archaic," and it also leads to a resolution different from the others.

Freud mentions displacement in his *Interpretation of Dreams* (1900), assuming that dream formation uses displacement under the influence of censorship as an endopsychic defense. As such, he considers displacement to be an archaic mode of thinking that leads to a change from the latent to the manifest dream content.

During this early time it was thought that displacement changes the intensity of an idea to an associated "place," one that is more acceptable to the ego. In Anna Freud's "The Ego and the Mechanisms of Defense" (1936), she lists ten defense mechanisms but does not include displacement. She may have failed to mention it because she understood it to express primary process functioning, or as Freud stated, that it is archaic in nature. She does not believe that repression, as one example, can occur before there is a division between conscious and unconscious ego, or between ego and id (A. Freud and Sandler, 1985).

As development proceeds, a progressive differentiation between ego and id occurs, and displacement thus takes on a changing role in defending the ego from unacceptable influences. Anna Freud, though omitting displacement from her list, includes it in her discussion of the case of Little Hans and his animal phobia, as she explores the defense against his aggression, against his father, and against Little Hans's fear of retaliation by his use of displacement to avoid these threatening consequences (A. Freud, 1966: 71).

When a child attacks or destroys the enemy when playing with toys, or adults attack their boss instead of their father, they use a defense different from that of, say, repression or denial. These latter defenses eliminate the threat to the ego, restraining the drive derivative, whereas displacement places them where the ego has a chance to achieve mastery over them. By placing apparently unresolvable conflicts from the primary relationship into a new situation, the ego allows the pursuit of solutions. The shift of the primary conflict in transference—and transference neurosis—is an example of displacement's use in this context.

Beyond the archaic nature of the earliest function of displacement, Anna Freud elaborates on the developmental role of this defense mechanism during puberty: "Prohibited forms of gratification are exchanged for other modes of enjoyment through a process of displacement and reaction formation." She then states that during adolescence, "instead of compromise formations and the usual processes of displacement, regression . . . we find . . . a swing over from asceticism to instinctual excess" (A. Freud, 1966: 155–156). Developmental organization and reorganization changes the employment of displacement as a defense mechanism.

Finally, in defense mechanisms such as repression and denial, the ego eliminates conflict from its domain, whereas in displacement the ego is allowed to seek new solutions. This consideration has implications for therapeutic intervention (Neubauer, 1994). In the play of children, for instance, displacement should be studied to observe how and to what degree the child's ego searches for and achieves a resolution of conflicts. A premature interruption of play by the therapist, by placing the conflicts into the primary relationship, may circumvent the positive function of displacement. The therapist should observe whether the play reaches conflict resolution or at what point further intervention will be required. The counterpart of play in adult life will demand similar technical consideration.

REFERENCES

Freud, A. (1966). The ego and the mechanisms of defense. In A. Freud (author). *The Writings of Anna Freud*. rev. ed. New York: International Universities Press, pp. 42–53.

———. (1966). Analysis of a phobia in a five-year-old boy. In A. Freud (author). *The Writings of Anna Freud*, vol. 2. rev. ed. New York: International Universities Press, pp. 71–74.

Freud A., and Sandler, J. (1985). *The Analysis of Defense: The Ego and the Mechanisms of Defense Revisited*. Madison, Conn.: International Universities Press.

Freud, S. (1900). *The Interpretation of Dreams*. S.E. 4–5: 1–621

Neubauer, P. B. (1994). The role of displacement in psychoanalysis. In A. J. Solnit, P. B. Neubauer, S. Abrams, and A. S. Dowling (eds.). *The Psychoanalytic Study of the Child*. New Haven, Conn.: Yale University Press, pp. 107–118.

PETER B. NEUBAUER

Dissociation

Dissociation—a symptom characterized by "a disruption in the usually integrated functions of consciousness, memory, identity, or perception of the environment" (American Psychiatric Association, 1994, p. 231). Originally termed by Janet as "disaggregation," dissociation was thought to be a passive disintegration or splitting up of the mind owing to psychic trauma in those who were organically predisposed. Freud, too, studied this phenomenon, observing that this "splitting of the mind is the consummation of hysteria . . . one part of the patient's mind is in the hypnoid state permanently but with a varying degree of vividness in its ideas and is always prepared whenever there is a lapse in waking thought to assume control over the whole person" (Breuer and Freud, 1893–1895: 249–250). In contrast to Janet, however, he thought that this condition was due to repression, which was an active mental process, and concluded that "Janet's opinion that mental weakness is in any way at the root of hysteria or splitting of the mind is untenable" (Breuer and Freud, 1893–1895: 233).

Repression, not dissociation, was responsible for the organization of the mind into Consciousness and the Unconscious, according to Freud's topographic model of the psyche. Because this model could not explain certain complexities, such as unconscious guilt, Freud sought a more sophisticated theory, eventually revolutionizing psychology with his structural theory or tripartite model of the mind. Subsequently, his writing on dissociation and hypnosis declined and mainstream psychoanalysis followed. Freud, however, continued to wrestle with Janet's notion of a split in the psyche, and this theme is still very much with us.

Interestingly, the term "dissociation," despite its "checquered history," did not completely leave the analytic literature, although it was used more descriptively than scientifically. A number of writers did continue to study the essence of it, describing such related phenomena as psychological sleep, hypnoid states, déjà vu, depersonalization, and autohypnotic defenses.

With the renewed interest, over the last fifteen years, in the condition known as "multiple personality," an abundance of data has been collected, linking this and other so-called dissociative disorders with severe, early childhood trauma. As a result of the importance of this rediscovery, the great debate between Freud and Janet, i.e., repression versus dissociation, has been revived and continues a century later. However, this matter is not easily resolved because the evolution of analytic theory led to ego psychology, self-psychology, and object relations theory, theories that have pursued a related but different defensive operation, that of splitting. At the same time, the direction of American psychiatry has been to stay on the surface, to emphasize phenomenology and categorization. What has resulted, therefore, is a void in our deeper understanding of these very perplexing and not so rare dissociative conditions. Although they have been identified and are being extensively studied, they have not been thoroughly reexamined through the psychoanalytic lens. Mistakenly thought by some to be outside the perimeter of Freudian thought, the application of psychoanalytic principles to the understanding and treatment of these entities is essential.

One recent effort to bridge the ever widening chasm between Freud's ideas and general psychiatry redefines dissociation as a defensive operation that, like other defenses, reduces anxiety. In this theory, dissociation, through the use of autohypnotic altered states, augments repression or primitive splitting of ego, depending on the level of integration of the psyche. These autohypnotic states originate in response to externally derived trauma, but through a change of function get reactivated in the service of warding off the anxiety of here and now intrapsychic conflict. They may also achieve a degree of secondary autonomy, which could explain why they may be accessed through hypnosis.

In those individuals for whom dissociation is the predominant defensive operation, it may become a central feature of their personalities. These people might be considered to have a "dissociative character," which could span a broad range of psychopathology depending on the level of integration of aggressively and libidinally derived self and object representations. For example, it is hypothesized that "multiple personality" (D.I.D., or dissociative identity disorder) is at the severe end of such a continuum, a lower-level dissociative character, in which the encapsulation of profound amounts of aggression is the central task of the developing ego. Other emerging theories overlap this model, and more research is needed to help determine which blueprints are the most useful for the psychoanalytically informed, contemporary approach to dissociation.

REFERENCES

American Psychiatric Association (1994). *Diagnostic Criteria from D.S.M. IV.* Washington, D.C.: American Psychiatric Association.

Brenner, I. (1994). The dissociative character: A reconsideration of 'multiple personality.' *Journal of the American Psychoanalytic Association*, 42: 819–846.

———. (1996). The characterological basis of multiple personality. *American Journal of Psychotherapy*, 50: 154–166.

———. (2001). *Dissociation of Trauma: Theory, Phenomenology, and Technique.* Madison, Conn.: International Universities Press.

Breuer, J., and Freud, S. (1893–1895). *Studies on Hysteria.* S.E. 2: 19–305.

Freud, S. (1923). *The Ego and the Id.* S.E. 19: 12–59.

Janet, P. (1889). *L'Automatisme Psychologique.* Paris: Bailliere.

Kluft, R. F. (1984). Treatment of multiple personality: A study of 33 cases. *Psychiatric Clinics of North America*, 7: 9–29.

IRA BRENNER

Dora

"Dora" was the pseudonym given by Freud to his patient Ida Bauer, whom he treated between October and December 1900. He wrote his account of that brief analysis shortly after it ended, but it was published only in 1905, entitled "Fragment of an analysis of a case of hysteria" (Freud, 1905). In recent years, the case of Dora has become the most intensely debated of Freud's case studies.

Ida Bauer was born November 1, 1882, in Vienna (at Berggasse 32, a few buildings from where Freud saw her). Her parents were Phillip Bauer, a Jewish industrialist (who suffered from tuberculosis, a detached retina, and syphilis, and was often nursed by his daughter), and Katharina Bauer, described by Freud as a housewife tormented by a cleaning compulsion. Ida's brother, Otto Bauer (1881–1938), became a leader of the Austrian Socialist Party and Austria's foreign minister in 1918–1919 (Rogow, 1979). An important part in the family drama was played by their friends, Hans Zallenka and his wife Peppina, (called by Freud "Herr and Frau K."). Hans referred Phillip to Freud as a physician for his syphilitic symptoms. Later on, when Phillip brought his daughter Ida to Freud, following her suicide threats, her analysis was colored by her awareness of the love affair that had developed between her father and Peppina, and by her intense reactions to Hans's repeated attempts to seduce her, which her parents dismissed as her fantasy. Ida told Freud "she had been handed over to Herr K. as a price for his tolerating the relations between her father and his wife" (Freud, 1905: 34).

Ida terminated her analysis abruptly and one-sidedly, and when she asked Freud to accept her back, in 1902, he turned her down, doubting her motives. She married Ernst Adler, a Jewish engineer and an unsuccessful composer, in 1903; their son Kurt later became a prominent musician and conductor. Following his birth, Ida and Ernst converted to Christianity. In 1922, Ida consulted analyst Felix Deutch about her nervousness, anxiety, and somatic symptoms; his harsh judgment of her character (Deutch, 1957) may have been colored by his wish to support Freud's pessimistic view of her. Later on she became a teacher of bridge, collaborating with Peppina Zallenka, who also helped her escape the Nazis after the *Anschluss*. In 1939, Ida, who was widowed, emigrated to the United States, and then died in New York City in 1945 (Decker, 1991; Mahony, 1996).

Numerous sources have been offered to explain Freud's choice to call Ida "Dora": the name Freud's sister gave a nursemaid in her house whose actual name was identical to her own (Freud, 1901: 241); the related associations Freud may have had to the seductive caretaker who played a major role in his childhood (Glenn, 1986); the childish wife of David Copperfield, Freud's beloved protagonist (Marcus, 1975); Dora Breuer, the same-aged daughter of Freud's alienated friend (Decker, 1991); the vengeful protagonist of a play that had impressed Freud, Theodora (Decker, 1991); and Pandora, representing dangerous femininity in Greek mythology (Malcolm, in Bernheimer and Kahane, 1990).

Freud, in his brief work with "Dora" (the name that will be used from here on), was strongly motivated by his wish to substantiate his theoretical models regarding the formation of hysterical symptoms and regarding his technique of dream interpretation (his initial title was "Dreams and hysteria"). These goals are clearly stated in his Prefatory Remarks, which are characterized by an apologetic and defensive style, mobilizing the reader as an ally in an attack on all potential critics (Mahony, 1996). Freud's view of hysteria dominates the subsequent chapter, "The Clinical Picture," in which he discusses incoherent narration as an indication of neurosis, describes Dora and her milieu, and attempts to develop a full explanatory hypothesis for each of Dora's symptoms—nervous cough, hoarseness, avoidance of passionate couples, aphonia, and the like.

Freud judgmentally portrays Dora's negative reaction to Herr K.'s first attempted seduction, in his store, as a major indication of her hysteria, and interprets her subsequent disgust as a displacement from her genital excitation. (He says Dora was fourteen at the time, but she was actually thirteen and a half). The case can be seen as standing halfway between Freud's earlier seduction hypothesis and his full Oedipal model (Blass, 1992), and the focus is on Dora's repressed attraction toward Herr K., while the attraction to her father is portrayed as secondary and defensive.

The next two chapters are organized around two central dreams explored in the analysis: the dream of escaping from a house on fire, and the dream of wandering in an unknown town and hearing of her father's death. Both dreams are related to a second major seduction attempt, by the lake, when Dora was fifteen and a half. Dora's and Freud's associations are discussed extensively, and Freud demonstrates how he reaches his interpretations regarding Dora's underlying unconscious wishes, about which she usually remains skeptical. The second dream actually ushers in her decision to leave analysis, which takes Freud by surprise and disappoints him (his subsequent refusal to accept her again may point to his vindictiveness). He realizes she may have stayed had he shown a warm personal interest in her, but rejects this option, calling it "acting a part."

In the Postscript, probably written closer to the time of publication, Freud argues for sexuality as providing the motive power for every single symptom. He also discusses his realization that he had not paid sufficient attention to Dora's transferences toward him, and to her homosexual attraction to Frau K.

While some critical reviews by nonanalysts (Kiell, 1988) raise as early as 1905–1906 concerns about Freud's view of Dora's seduction, the Dora case was unanimously revered by early generations of psychoanalysts as a source of major theoretical insights about the dynamics of neurosis. Lacan's (1952) analysis of the dialectical turnabouts in the case first points to Freud's prejudices and blind spots as blocking its resolution: Freud puts himself too much in the place of Herr K., and fails to understand Dora's problem in accepting herself as an object of desire for the man. Wolstein (1954) is the first to discuss Freud's lack of attention to Dora's loveless relationship with her mother. The turning point in the literature on Dora appears, however, to be Erikson's (1962) critique. Erikson suggests that Freud failed to appreciate adolescent Dora's crucial developmental need to get straight her historical past and to call infidelities by their name, as a stage in forming her own identity.

Subsequently, numerous papers (see Jennings, 1986) explore the relevance of the growing understanding of adolescence to the case. There is also much attention to problems in Freud's technique, especially his suggestive pressure on Dora to accept his interpretations, which often block her own free associations; his disregard of her difficulty with his blunt sexual communications; and his blindness to the impact of his prior ties with Dora's father and with Herr K., which unavoidably strengthen her justified suspiciousness as to whose agent her therapist is (a major issue in the treatment of adolescents). Freud's own unhappiness with his "interpret at all costs" technique with Dora may have contributed to his later realization that an emotional attachment of the patient to the analyst is a crucial precondition for interpretations to be effective, and that premature interpretations may arouse animosity (Freud, 1910). This realization may be seen as a first stepping-stone toward analytic models, from Ferenczi on, that turn the analytic relationship itself into a central curative factor.

Starting with Lacan (1952), many authors identify in the text indications of Freud's countertransferential identification with Dora's father and with Herr K., and some suggest that like these two, Freud tried to make Dora fulfill his own needs—in his case, confirm his interpretations, supplying evidence for his new controversial theories. This agenda may have distanced Freud from an empathic listening to Dora's deep vulnerability, related by Ornstein (1993) to her growing up with an unempathic mother, incapable of mirroring, and to the collapse of her idealizations of her father and of Herr and Frau K., whose functioning as her newly found self-objects was short-lived, soon destroyed by their exploitative and dishonest behavior. This left her with a desperate need for a self-object (a need that, in another paradigm, may be called a need for holding), but Freud's unempathic interpretations, critical judgments, and eventual rejection totally frustrated this need.

Marcus (1975) and Hertz (in Bernheimer and Kahane, 1990) express the recent trend to treat Freud's cases (and at times theoretical papers too) as works of fiction, a strategy consistent with hermeneutic and narrative models within psychoanalysis. They compare Freud to modern novelists such as Proust or James, and utilize literary analysis to pinpoint the text's subtleties and paradoxes, including Freud's presence as an unreliable narrator, his constant struggle with his own feminine identifications, and the ways Freud and Dora mirror each other. Decker (1991) supplies a rich historical context to the encounter between Freud and Dora, emphasizing their similar Jewish identity and destiny on the background of Austro-Hungarian discrimination and anti-Semitism. She also underlines Dora's fate as a woman in an authoritarian, patriarchal social structure, which viewed "hysterical" women with suspicion and animosity, promoted treatment methods for them that bordered on torture, and allowed Dora's brother many more outlets for ambition and for protest than she could ever find.

The extensive feminist critique of the case (see Bernheimer and Kahane, 1990), often drawing upon Lacan's work but criticizing him too, points to Freud's collusion in sexist societal norms, identifying femininity with servitude, failing to see how both the masculine and the feminine roles are cultural rather than natural and are affected by symbolic castration, and refusing to consider female sexuality as an active, independent drive. Dora is portrayed by some feminist critics as a defeated victim of exploitation, and by others as a core example of the protesting force of women, of their struggle to become subjects and not merely objects of desire or of study. Moi (in Bernheimer and Kahane, 1990) analyzes Freud's phallocentric epistemology in treating Dora and discussing her: the male as the bearer of knowledge, having alone the power to penetrate woman, and to penetrate the text.

A contemporary reading, no longer bound by "the myth of the analytic situation" (Racker, 1968) as involving an insightful analyst objectively deciphering the inner life of a distortion-prone, sick patient, may instead portray Dora and Freud as partners in a complex, intersubjective encounter in which Freud's countertransference is omnipresent (Berman, 1993).

This countertransference, in the broadest sense of the term, includes sociocultural aspects, such as conventional views of femininity typical of the period, and uniquely individual aspects, such as the impact of Freud's childhood relationships with his mother and his nursemaid. It also includes conscious levels, such as Freud's ambition to find support for his theoretical views, and unconscious levels, such as his struggle with feminine identifications and homosexual urges; permanent character traits, such as his tendency for authoritative conclusions (described by Marcus, 1975, as hubris or chutzpah), and specific reactions, such as his anger at Dora for depriving him of a full success. Finally, the countertransference includes as well "concordant" identifications (Racker, 1968) of Freud with his patient, which lead to some of the more empathic interpretations, and "complementary" identifications with figures in Dora's life such as Herr K., which eventually appear to have the upper hand; affective manifestations, such as open annoyance at her for turning Herr K. down, and cognitive manifestations, including Freud's consistent errors regarding the time of the analysis (reported as 1899—deeper into Freud's friendship with Fliess, marred by his jealous wife, Ida) and regarding Dora's age (turning her older, which makes the sexual abuse appear slighter); direct countertransference to young and attractive Dora, and "indirect" countertransference (Racker, 1968) influenced by Freud's relationships with Breuer or Fliess.

While many authors describe the analysis as a total failure, Decker (1991) reminds us that Freud listened to Dora more than any prior physician did, and was the first person to believe her stories, although he remained unempathic to her plight. Though truncated and faulty, the brief analysis helped her confront Herr and Frau K. with the truth, and subsequently separate from her parents, get married, and become a mother.

Moreover, while Freud presents Dora through his own prism, he appears to allow her personality and voice enough presence—as a subtext (Mahony, 1996)—to enable contemporary readers to form an identification with her, formulate their own original interpretations, and script alternative ways of treating her, thus fulfilling the powerful rescue fantasies her drama appears to arouse.

REFERENCES

Berman, E. (ed.) (1993). *Freud and Dora*. Tel Aviv: Am Oved (Hebrew).

Bernheimer, C., and Kahane, C. (eds.) (1990). In Dora's case: Freud-Hysteria-Feminism. 2d ed. New York: Columbia University Press.

Blass, R. (1992). Did Dora have an Oedipus complex? *Psychoanalytic Study of the Child*, 47: 159–187.

Decker, H. (1991). *Freud, Dora and Vienna 1900*. New York: Free Press.

Deutch, F. (1957). A footnote to Freud's "Fragment of an analysis of a case of hysteria." *Psychoanalytic Quarterly*, 26: 159–167.

Erikson, E. H. (1962). Reality and actuality: An address. *Journal of the American Psychoanalytic Association*, 10: 451–474.

Freud, S. (1901). *The Psychopathology of Everyday Life*. S.E. 6: 1–279.

———. (1905). Fragment of an analysis of a case of hysteria. S.E. 7: 7–122.

———. (1910). "Wild" psychoanalysis. S.E. 11: 221–227.

Glenn, J. (1986). Freud, Dora and the maid: A study of countertransference. *Journal of the American Psychoanalytic Association*, 34: 591–606.

Jennings, J. (1986). The revival of "Dora": Advances in psychoanalytic theory and technique. *Journal of the American Psychoanalytic Association*, 34: 607–635.

Kiell, N. (ed.) (1988). *Freud without Hindsight: Reviews of His Work, 1893–1939*. Madison, Conn.: International Universities Press.

Lacan, J. (1952). Intervention on transference. In J. Mitchell and J. Rose (eds.). *Feminine Sexuality*. New York: Norton, pp. 61–74.

Mahony, P. J. (1996). *Freud's Dora*. New Haven, Conn.: Yale University Press.

Marcus, S. (1975). Freud and Dora: Story, history, case history. In *Representations*. New York: Random House.

Ornstein, P. H. (1993). Did Freud understand Dora? In Barry Magid (ed.). *Freud's Case Studies: Self-Psychological Perspectives*. Hillsdale, N.J.: Analytic Press.

Racker, H. (1968). *Transference and Countertransference*. London: Maresfield.

Rogow, A. (1979). Dora's brother. *International Review of Psycho-Analysis*, 6: 389–411.

Wolstein, B. (1954). *Transference: Its Meaning and Formation in Psychoanalytic Therapy*. New York: Grune and Stratton.

EMANUEL BERMAN

Dreams, Theory of

Freud always considered *Die Traumdeutung* (*The Interpretation of Dreams*, 1900) to be his masterwork, and for good reason. It demonstrated how unconscious forces shape our mental and emotional lives, surely his most important discovery. His clinical method of interpretation, still the most effective tool of the psychoanalyst, was described and convincingly illustrated in the dream book. Whatever criticism of Freud's theories that can be made today or substantiated in the future, his reputation as one of the world's most original and influential thinkers rests on the pioneering work of this volume.

Freud made a number of original and remarkable observations about dreams and dreaming. With respect to dreams themselves, *The Interpretation of Dreams* showed that they were meaningful expressions of the dreamer's experience and fantasy life, not random neurological accidents as some researchers still claim. Freud saw that dreaming is both meaningful and motivated, that dream images are motivated by the biological and emotional needs of the dreamer, by his or her most vital concerns and conflicts.

Dreams depict events and situations desired or feared by the dreamer. The struggle between the expressive and defensive forces at work in the dream is an example of unconscious intrapsychic conflict. Here again the dream is paradigmatic of a more general feature of unconscious mental activity. Biological and emotional needs are often conflicting, especially when the need for action opposes the need for safety and security. Since action in the dreamer's external world must be unified and coordinated, these conflicts have to be kept out of consciousness for long stretches of time.

During the Rapid Eye Movement (REM) phase of sleep, when most dreams occur, the dreamer's body is disabled for action. The skeletal muscles are in a state of inhibition. This allows the conflicting forces in the dreamer's psyche to be represented in the dreams without the danger of disrupting his or her actions in the surrounding world. However, the dream censorship reacts to *representations* of anxiety-laden events as if they were actions in the real world. Although Freud was unaware of the REM state, he realized that dreaming was a safer alternative to impulsive action. Dreaming was a situation in which unconscious conflict could be observed and understood.

Freud showed how this could be true even when the superficial content of the dream appears to be either trivial or fantastic. He made this discovery by noticing that much of the material on display in the imagery of a dream is ordinarily inaccessible to the dreamer's waking consciousness. He observed that much of this dream imagery is linked associatively with thoughts and feelings not represented directly, yet capable of explaining the otherwise mysterious activity displayed in a dream.

He concluded that this material was originally part of the process of dream construction but was excluded from the dream imagery by a mechanism he called "the dream censorship." This insight allowed him to distinguish between the "manifest dream," the dream as reported by the dreamer, and the "latent dream," the dream that would have emerged if the censorship had not intervened.

He recognized two distinct classes of dream imagery, one derived from the current life situation of the dreamer, which he called "the day's residues," and the other from the remote past, called "the repressed infantile wishes." He realized that every dream contained imagery from both these sources, from both the past and the present.

By exploring the dreamer's associations to individual items in the manifest dream, Freud discovered that the psychoanalyst could often recover the latent dream material denied expression by the censorship. The censorship mechanism interfered with the direct expression of anxiety-laden memories. It substituted related but less objectionable ideas and events for those it excluded from the manifest dream content. He recognized that the dream censorship is part of the larger system of psychological defenses that constantly monitor the mental life of every person. Because dreams are so visible, the dream censorship has come to be the paradigm for the defense mechanisms in general.

Freud's discovery that material apparently excluded from the dream imagery could be recovered by his method of free association stimulated him to develop a theory of dream construction that would account for the censorship of this "objectionable" unconscious material. This theory was based largely on the biology and physics of Freud's time.

With some modifications, Freud's method for recovering the unconscious material excluded from the dream imagery, his method of interpretation, has stood the test of time. When the analyst helps the patient reconstruct the meaningful links that connect a reported dream to the associations it evokes, useful analytic work is accomplished. Although we now understand more fully how the method works, Freud's clinical discovery is still the cornerstone of the psychoanalytic process. His theory of dream construction, on the other hand, has lost its credibility as our scientific knowledge of the sleeping brain continues to increase.

Freud's theory of dream construction, based on nineteenth-century science, has not been able to explain the new observations about dreaming made in the twentieth. It now appears both inconsistent and inaccurate. Unfortunately, many psychoanalysts still believe that Freud's method of interpretation is dependent on his theory of dream construction. They imagine that to give up the theory would be to invalidate the method of interpretation. Even worse, some analysts have devalued dream interpretation because the theory of dream construction no longer makes sense to them.

The remainder of the article will explain how Freud's theory of dream construction can be modified to bring it up to date. Making his dream theory compatible with contemporary science actually provides a much greater degree of support for Freud's method of interpretation than his own out-of-date assumptions (Palombo, 1978, 1992).

First of all, REM sleep studies have shown that dreaming is not an ad hoc process as Freud supposed. Dreaming takes place in regular ninety-minute intervals during the course of a night. Periods of dreaming last ten to twenty minutes, growing somewhat in length as sleep continues. Deprivation of REM sleep in animals and narcoleptic patients impairs their ability to consolidate the memory of recently learned tasks. Deprivation of REM sleep in humans causes a number of unpleasant psychological symptoms including disorientation and sometimes hallucinations.

These new data show that dreaming is part of the normal information-processing activity of the brain. Dreaming has an adaptive as well as a defensive function. It is not initiated by the content of particular impulses striving for expression, as Freud believed. Freud's idea that dreaming occurs spontaneously to preserve sleep by neutralizing objectionable impulses has to be modified. Dreaming cannot be, as Freud put it, "the guardian of sleep."

The fact that dreaming has an adaptive function indicates that the dream censorship need not be active continuously throughout every dream. Dreams occur whether or not the censorship is active. A close study of dreams shows that the dream censorship does intervene spontaneously in dreams in response to anxiety-provoking content. Thus the dream censorship is the guardian of the adaptive process that takes place when an ongoing dream is threatening. This is the more precise formulation that Freud's proposal anticipated.

Dreaming is a critical step in the transfer of representations of current events into long-term memory. Because long-term memory is episodic and associative, new information can be introduced into suitable locations only by matching it with items stored there previously. Dream imagery is a composite of superimposed representations of present and past experiences. As in the case of Galton's superimposed photographs (mentioned by Freud in the *traumdeutung* and *On Dreams* [1901] on four different occasions), the common features reinforce one another while the different ones cancel one another out. If the superimposition is coherent, with reinforcing imagery predominating, then a new association is formed between the two in long-term memory.

Freud was alert to these two sources of dream material, as illustrated in this passage from *On Dreams*:

From every element in a dreams's content associative threads branch out in two or more directions; every situation in a dream seems to be put together out of two or more impressions or experiences. For instance, I once had a dream of a sort of swimming-pool, in which the bathers were scattered in all directions; at one point on the edge of the pool someone was standing and bending towards one of the people bathing, as though to help her out of the water. The situation was put together from a memory of an experience I had had at puberty and from two paintings, one of which I had seen shortly before the dream. (p. 648)

The superimposition of images from present and past is what Freud referred to as *condensation*. Freud believed that condensation is a mechanism of the dream censorship, like *displacement*, although in his *Introductory Lectures* (1917), he acknowledged that condensation is part of the basic mechanism of dreaming while displacement is a purely defensive operation. One can now say simply that while displacement is the modus operandi of the dream censorship, condensation is an adaptive mechanism.

This was difficult for Freud to see for two reasons, one having to do with his own ideological bias, the other with the dynamics of dream construction. Freud was committed to the idea that dreaming is an eruption of unconscious impulses without adaptive significance. This conviction was very likely due to Freud's fear that his discovery of the power of unconscious and irrational forces would not be adequately understood or appreciated.

Second, it is easy for any observer to miss the adaptive function of condensation, because the images being condensed are themselves often the result of displacement by the censorship from emotionally powerful but "objectionable" experiences. This is the case with day residues as well as with repressed infantile experiences. The "trivial" day residue, "without associative valence," as Freud put it, is itself a displacement from more troublesome experiences of the day. It is these more troublesome experiences that act as "instigators" of individual dreams (but not of the dreaming state itself).

The dream images associated with "repressed infantile wishes" are also subject to displacement *prior to* the superimposition that forms the composite dream structure. In many dreams, the image derived from childhood experience is a displaced substitute for a more frightening memory. Freud postulated that the day residue was "trivial" in order to explain the frequent affective neutralization of the childhood memory present in the dream. A close examination of dream imagery reveals that the repressed childhood wish is usually represented by a "trivial" substitute drawn from long-term memory. Both the day residue and the repressed childhood memory superimposed in the dream are displacements produced by the censorship.

Freud's idea that the trivial day residue becomes the disguise for the repressed childhood wish seemed at the time to solve the problem he created by his denial of an adaptive function of dreams. Without an information-processing function that brought the representations of current and past experience together for an adaptive purpose, one would have to wonder why the two are superimposed in the dream. Freud ingeniously brought them together by short-circuiting the work of the dream censorship. Freud's intuition in filling the gaps in the scientific knowledge of his time was brilliant, so brilliant that one has trouble even today in realizing how much he was forced to leave out. But one now has the luxury of new science that shows how close Freud came to fore-seeing the actual mechanisms of dream construction.

This new knowledge can also be helpful in clinical practice. Dreams are still one of the analyst's major points of access to a patient's unconscious wishes and fantasies. Freud's view of the dream censorship is still valid, although it works a little differently from the way he imagined. The analyst can expect to find evidence of repressed childhood wishes in the patient's association to the content of a dream. These wishes are attached to the memories of events in which they were expressed in the past, events from all stages of the patient's emotion-al development. Experiences from the more recent past are often substituted for childhood experience, in the dream censorship's effort to reduce the anxiety that often attends the construction of a dream.

Childhood memories can be retrieved from dream associations more often than one may have realized. Even if they do not come up in the patient's spontaneous asso-ciations to the dream, they can often be evoked by a question from the analyst. All the analyst needs to say is something like, "Does anything in the dream imagery remind you of an actual event in the past?" More often than not, the appropriate memory rises to consciousness.

The frequent recovery from the patient's associa-tions of a significant day residue not represented in the dream (often with transference implications) is no acci-dent. The censorship regularly substitutes for such events during the process of dream construction. The analyst should be as alert to this source of instinctual material as he or she is to the patient's childhood memories.

These suggestions extend the analyst's usual atten-tion to the hidden instinctual content of a dream. How-ever, there is another useful source of information in the dream that analysts have not sufficiently exploited. This source is the adaptive function that links the day residues with childhood memories.

When a day residue and a childhood memory are superimposed in a dream image, one can assume that the mechanism of dream construction has already recog-nized some resemblance between them. This resem-blance may not hold up, if the composite formed by the superimposition turns out not to be self-reinforcing. But it indicates that the patient's unconscious has already taken the first step in assimilating the new experience to the content of long-term memory.

This step often reveals a bias of the patient's uncon-scious that leads it to misinterpret new experience as if it were no more than a repetition of what has happened before. By monitoring the combinations of day residue and childhood memory that occur in patients' dreams, the analyst can trace the neurotic mechanisms that dis-tort patients' understanding of themselves and their emo-tional world. Because of this, the process of dream interpretation is a microcosm of the analysis as a whole. This was clearly Freud's understanding, although his denial of the adaptive function of dreams made it diffi-cult for him to formulate this insight as forcefully as he might have.

Condensation, or superimposition, creates a com-parison, like Galton's method of superimposing photo-graphs. Freud's explanation for condensation finessed the question of the resemblance between the day residue and the childhood memory. The implication, however, was that the day residue had to be enough like the child-hood memory to be useful as a disguise for it, but not enough like it to give away the connection between them. Only a very sophisticated information-processing mech-anism could make such an assessment, but Freud thought it could be done with nothing but the brute force of the unconscious impulse.

The mechanism of condensation actually is a sophis-ticated information-processing mechanism, as befits the adaptive process that sorts and stores new experience in long-term memory. Analysts can avail themselves of its sophistication by noticing that the connections it makes are meaningful in themselves, not only as the by-products of the censorship process.

Freud's belief that a dream originated with the break-out of an unconscious impulse made him suspicious of any continuity between dreams, or between dreams and the events of analysis. He warned that "corroboration dreams," dreams that seem to corroborate the analyst's interpretations, cannot be trusted. He thought they were most likely the product of the patient's wish to please the analyst. But sleep laboratory studies indicate the wish to please the analyst has little influence over the content of dreams, which have their own adaptive purposes.

Corroboration dreams are more likely to be a sign that an analysis is working effectively than an obstacle thrown up by the patient. When continuity of theme between dreams and the events of analysis is observed, it shows that the analytic work is being successfully incorporated into the patient's long-term memory, where it acts to counteract the effects of earlier repression.

The adaptive function of dreams makes what Freud called "the royal road to knowledge of unconscious mental activity" into a two-way street. Dreaming works both to reveal the contents of the unconscious *and* to expand and modify it. Through dreams, the connections made by the analyst between events defensively isolated within the patient's mind become new connections in the patient's long-term memory. The adaptive function of dreaming is at the core of the adaptive purpose of the analytic process.

Freud's theory of dream construction was certainly a start in the right direction. One does not have to choose between taking it whole, just as he left it, or discarding it altogether. The findings of the laboratory, if we read them correctly, have shown us what needed to be changed. They have shown us, for example, that the dreaming state is not initiated by the content of individual dreams (or impulses coming directly from the unconscious) but by the physiological process that supports the adaptive information-processing function of dreaming. They have not shown, however, that the content of individual dreams is the product of random stimulation of the cerebral cortex.

Pathways leading from the brain stem to the cortex are involved in the onset of dreaming. Unfortunately, this finding has been widely misunderstood to mean that individual dreams are unmotivated and meaningless. There is *no* evidence, however, that the content of individual dreams is determined or even influenced by those pathways. The brain stem connections have to do with the initiation of the REM state as such, not with the initiation of individual dreams that take place during the REM state. Their job is to prepare the sensory projection areas of the cortex for whatever content is displayed when current and past experience are matched in a dream.

Of course, Freud did not have all the answers about dreaming. But he asked most of the right questions. When he was mistaken, it was hardly ever because the question was inappropriate. There is still much to be learned by going back to his questions and trying to answer them with contemporary knowledge.

There was a great deal that Freud did not know in 1900 about the circumstances in which dreaming occurs. In many cases, his personal and ideological biases prevented him from taking his theory of dream construction further. Yet, he was able to make dream interpretation a fundamental and integral part of psychoanalytic thought and practice, and the paradigm for the interpretation of unconscious material from every source.

REFERENCES

Freud, S. (1900). *The Interpretation of Dreams.* S.E. 4 and 5: 1–627.

———. (1901). *On Dreams.* S.E. 5: 631–686.

Palombo, S. R. (1978). *Dreaming and Memory: A New Information-Processing Model.* New York: Basic Books.

———. (1992). The Eros of dreaming. *International Journal of Psychoanalysis,* 73: 637–648.

STANLEY R. PALOMBO

Drive Theory

The term "drive" (*Trieb*) first appeared in Freud's writings in 1905. His use of drivelike constructs began at least a decade earlier, however, when Breuer and Freud (1895) reported that the emergence into consciousness of traumatic memories resulted in the alleviation of hysterical symptoms.

Early Stirrings

To account for these findings, they built upon the then prevailing view that hysterical symptoms were related to nervous system excitation. They assumed that when the nervous system is exposed to high levels of excitation, it tries to divest itself of some of it. Such excitation may originate externally or internally. If the source is external, it is usually possible to lessen excitation by simply leaving the scene. But if the source of excitation is internal, there is no escape. Wherever the person goes, he or she carries the excitation with him or her.

Applying this model to their findings, Breuer and Freud (1895) argued that traumatic memories tend to be kept out of consciousness because they clash with the moral standards of society. The affect accompanying these memories is thereby prevented from being expressed or discharged. Instead, it is dammed up and adds to nervous system excitation. In order to divest itself of some of this excess internal excitation, the affect is displaced onto some environmental object or converted into some sort of somatic complaint, or a combination of the two. It thereby finds expression or is discharged in the form of a hysterical symptom (cf. Rapaport, 1960). Bringing the memory to consciousness allows for more direct and complete expression of the affect and the symptom subsequently disappears. In this early model, sexuality, which was to become central to Freudian drive theory, was seen as just another source of internal excitation.

From Memories to Wishes

By 1900, Freud had come to a radical conclusion that moved him further toward a true theory of drives. He now believed that what emerged into consciousness in his patients were not memories at all. They were instead fantasies expressing the patient's unconscious and repressed wishes. These same wishes underlay the content of dreams (Freud, 1900). He now wrote of a conflict between wishful impulses and an internal censor attempting to prevent expression of these wishes. The result of this conflict was a compromise between the wish and the repressing censor. This compromise found form in symptoms and anxiety. Traumatic experiences were no longer necessary to account for the production of neurosis. Symptomatology and anxiety were natural outgrowths of endogenous processes shaped to some degree by experience. Freud's model had become universal; it now applied to all of humankind and could explain normal phenomena like dreams.

The Beginnings of a Real Drive Theory

Freud's efforts to understand the endogenous wishful impulses he described in 1900 led him to propose a bona fide drive theory by 1905. In *Three Essays on the Theory of Sexuality* (Freud, 1905), Freud introduced the term *Trieb*. This term refers to a dynamic process consisting of an irresistible pressure or push to expression. It captured the peremptory quality of the unconscious wishes that impressed Freud so greatly in 1900. *Trieb* referred to a general orientation rather than a precise goal, thereby allowing for the variety of expression he found.

Freud concentrated his attention on sexuality because it was the drive that most allowed for variety of

expression and had the most far-ranging effects. It also appeared to account for the wishes he was uncovering in his patients. So for Freud, the sexual drive consists of a general peremptory pressure toward some vaguely defined sexual satisfaction. Freud (1905) now believed that the sexual drive is present at birth and is the major source of the endogenous nervous system excitation he wrote about earlier. He called upon the sexual drive to explain all of his previous findings regarding symptomatology and the wishes underlying symptoms and dreams. Freud connected the unconscious fantasies and dream wishes he had uncovered earlier with the actions of sexual perversions (cf. Compton, 1981a). In the case of the perversions, the development of this drive is seen as having gone awry. Its influence is present in all of us, however, as evidenced by universal unconscious wishes that mirror the perversions.

The sexual drive passes through several developmental stages from infancy through adolescence; that is, sexuality is expressed through different parts of the body, termed erotogenic zones, as the person develops. At first, sexual satisfaction is concentrated around the mouth; this is termed the oral stage. Next, at around age two, satisfaction can be obtained through the anal area; this is the anal stage. When the child is about four or so, sexual satisfaction is focused on the genital area; this is termed the phallic stage. A diminution of sexual activity occurs at about this time and lasts until adolescence; this is termed latency. And finally, in adolescence, sexuality reaches procreative maturity in the genital stage. These erotogenic zones serve as way stations in the development of the sexual drive. They are points of application or expression of the drive. They are not sources of separate drives. There is a single central sexual drive whose main focus moves from zone to zone (Rapaport, 1960). This part of Freudian drive theory remained unchanged.

The 1905 paper also presaged later developments in Freudian drive theory. Although he implied it in his 1905 book, Freud did not directly write of other drives opposing the sexual drive. In 1910, however, he made explicit the conflict between self-preservation drives, or ego instincts, and the sexual drive. The self-preservation drives represent needs associated with bodily functions necessary for personal survival, like hunger. Freud elaborated on this theme in 1911 and 1914 when he referred to conflict between libidinal (sexual) and ego instincts. He argued that the sexual instinct becomes repressed through the defensive motive of self-preservation (cf. Brunswick, 1954). Symptoms and psychopathology emerge from this conflict. This gave substance to the workings of the internal censor Freud referred to in 1900. The energy for the internal censor, as well as the person's reality orientation, stemmed from these ego instincts. This view was to change as Freud proposed different sets of conflicts in his later writings.

Another concept Freud referred to in his 1905 paper was "libido." He had used this term before but it had no consistent meaning across his writings. Freud began using the term clearly and more consistently as he related it to the concept of narcissism (Freud, 1914). (See Compton, 1981c, for a more complete discussion of this.) "Libido" was defined as the energy underlying the sexual drive. It is initially unfocused but is then directed toward the infant's own body. Freud termed this ego or narcissistic libido. In its later development, it can be expressed through external objects (object libido) or back to the self (ego libido). Finally, Freud first introduced the notions of source, aim, and object of drives in 1905. They helped explain the particulars of drive functioning. A more detailed and complete exposition appeared in his 1915 paper *Instincts and Their Vicissitudes*. This latter version endured in all of his subsequent writings on this topic.

Drive Theory Takes Center Stage

A landmark year for Freudian drive theory was 1915. Freud wrote three papers that systematically presented his views on drives that year: *Instincts and Their Vicissitudes, The Unconscious*, and *Repression*. The most complete and systematic presentation is contained in *Instincts and Their Vicissitudes*. In this paper, Freud offered his most complete exposition of the pressure, source, object, and aim of drives. First, Freud (1915b) defined a drive or instinct as "a concept on the frontier between the mental and the somatic, as the psychic representative of the stimuli originating from within the organism and reaching the mind, as a measure of the demand made upon the mind for work in consequence of its connection with the body" (pp. 121–122). The source of a drive is, therefore, a physiological process. The drive itself is a mental representation of that physical phenomenon. Freud called it a sort of delegate sent into the psyche by the soma. Thus, drive is a demarcatory concept between psyche and soma (Vermorel, 1990). The actual physiological process or

processes involved lie outside the realm of psychology, and Freud did not concern himself with them.

Freud averred that there are two major classes of drives or instincts relevant to psychology. These are the sexual and the self-preservation, or ego, drives. All of drive psychology can be understood in terms of the interplay of these two drives (Compton, 1981b). The sexual drive is the more interesting because it allows for avenues of expression.

The concept of pressure is represented by "the demand made upon the mind for work" (Freud, 1915: 122). This pressure manifests itself as a kind of uncomfortable mental tension, varying in degree, depending upon the momentary demand of the drive. Pressure therefore represents a quantitative, economic factor of mental functioning (Lampl-de Groot, 1956).

The aim of the drive is satisfaction. In line with Freud's previous theorizing, this entails discharge or expression of nervous system excitation. Since Freud now focused largely on the sexual drive, satisfaction consists of relief from sexual tension. So the aim of the sexual drive is expression of sexuality. Such expression results in a feeling of satisfaction. Failure to express these needs results in feelings of chronic dissatisfaction. The combination of pressure and aim explains the peremptoriness of the drive. When expression is delayed or prevented, the person is in psychic discomfort because the pressure is unrelenting. When the drive is expressed (which is its aim), he or she experiences satisfaction. This is also an example of the operation of the pleasure principle.

Expression of the sexual drive was not limited to genital satisfaction. Instead, Freud saw the possibilities for satisfaction as being enormously varied. This notion was contained in his conception of the object of the drive. The object is the thing or person in regard to or through which the drive can achieve its aim or expression. Objects can and do change in the course of life experience and because of developmental changes. In the best-case scenario, the drive passes through the developmental stages described in Freud (1905) and culminates in the aim of mature genital union, consistent with reproduction. Similarly, the ultimate object choice would be a partner suitable for reproductive activity. Perversions result from developmental arrests in the aim and/or object sequence. Symptomatology results from displacement and/or conversion of the energy (libido) of the sexual drive. Aberrations in either object or aim result in psychopathology. The concepts of pressure, source, aim, and object, as

D

described above, remained consistent in all further developments of Freudian drive theory.

The Emergence of Aggression in Drive Theory

The next change in drive theory came about as a result of Freud's efforts to understand aggression. In 1915 (Freud, 1915a), he argued that frustration led to aggression. More specifically, thwarted self-preservation drives in conflict with sexual drives led to angry outbursts and destructive inclinations. But this formulation soon seemed inadequate. It could not account for masochism, chronic hostility evidenced in many long-term relationships, or the apparent need to reenact unpleasant experiences in the psychoanalytic relationship (cf. Compton, 1981d). These considerations led Freud (1920) to invoke a death instinct in *Beyond the Pleasure Principle*. He now subsumed the self-preservation drives under the sexual drives and referred to this combination as the life instincts, or Eros. The life instincts strive to bind together and to preserve. They are unifying and constructive (Lampl-de Groot, 1956). The aim of the newly proposed death instincts or drives is to return to a nonliving, inorganic state. More abstractly, they seek an absolute equalization of energy or tension. They are a biological form of entropy. The conflict was now between the life and death instincts and their opposing aims. But these drives not only oppose one another, they can also combine, as they do in eating where the destructive actions of chewing and cutting lead to the life-giving effects of nutrition. Moreover, the aggressive drive passes through the same developmental sequence as the sexual drive. Thus, biting represents the aggressive drive in the oral stage just as sucking represents the sexual drive in the oral stage (Brenner, 1955).

Drives and the Structural Model of the Mind

Freud's final position on drive theory was presented in 1923 with the publication of *The Ego and the Id*. In this book, he proposed his famous tripartite structure of the mind. The life and death instincts now existed side by side in one of these structures, the id. Their conflict was no longer stressed. Instead both were said to strive constantly for expression with no regard for one another. The ego, the mental structure charged with responsibility for reality and survival, tries to defend against potential dangerous consequences of unbridled expression of the id drives by holding off, delaying, or altering such expression. Its mechanisms for doing so were termed "defenses." The representative of moral injunctions, the superego, may try to oppose drive expression outright if it deems them wrong. Psychopathology was understood as maladaptive compromise among id drives, ego defenses, and superego moral injunctions. The conflict was now between mental structures and not between types of drives. But the drives were still critical. They set the whole mental apparatus in motion. This position never changed and can be seen in all of Freud's subsequent works. Freud used these concepts to explain an amazing range of human behavior and cultural phenomena.

An Ahistorical Summary of Freudian Drive Theory

We have traced the historical development of Freudian drive theory. We would now like to describe it in its final form, independent of historical considerations. For a more complete treatment, see Rapaport (1960).

The Freudian concept of drives was designed to explain the variability of behavior under identical stimulus conditions as well as the relative constancy of behavior under changing stimulus conditions. The concept of displacement of drive energy (libido) so that its expression could be almost infinitely variable was the major conceptual tool employed to account for these phenomena.

Drives are defined as appetitive internal forces. Their internal loci differentiates them from external sources of influence. They are mental representations of unspecified nervous system excitation related in some way to sexual and aggressive urges. Their appetitive nature makes them motivational constructs, thereby differentiating them from other internal influences on behavior and thought.

The appetitive nature of drives is manifested in their peremptory, cyclic, and displaceable features. "Peremptoriness" refers to the irresistible and relatively inescapable pressure to express the drive. Successful expression of a drive leads to a temporary lowering of its peremptoriness. Gradually, however, the pressure builds anew. Thus, there is a cyclic rise and fall to the pressure of a drive. The means of expression or object of a drive is variable. If one object is unavailable, another will be chosen. Similarly, if there is resistance to one form of expression, another will be found. This quality of displacement is a major innovation and contribution of Freudian drive theory.

The defining characteristics of drives are their source, pressure, aim, and object. The sources of the drives are the aforementioned nervous system excitations having to do with urges of binding together (Eros) and pulling apart (aggressive or death instinct). It is beyond the scope of psychology to investigate the physiological underpinnings of these drives. Psychology deals with the psychic representations and effects of these physiological urges.

"Pressure" refers to how demanding or peremptory a drive is. This can be determined by how many mental and emotional resources it demands. This is a critical part of the appetitive nature of drives, described above. The aim of the drive is always to be expressed so as to relieve the aforementioned pressure. This is experienced as satisfaction if it occurs in behavior and as wish fulfillment if it occurs cognitively (e.g., through fantasy, dreams, and/or delusions). When satisfaction is only partial or is chronically blocked, the person experiences psychic discomfort. These processes underlie the pleasure principle. Symptoms reflect unsatisfactory partial expression of drives.

The object of the drive is the thing or person through which the drive achieves its aim of being expressed. This is the most variable aspect of the drive. No object is automatically connected to a drive but comes to be associated with it if it allows for satisfaction of drive expression. Possible objects are not infinitely variable, however. They must allow for expression of drives and so have some limitations. The object can be a part of the person's own body (e.g., erotogenic zone) or external to the person (e.g., a loved one). The object may be and is changed any number of times through development. The normal development of the sexual drive from oral to anal to phallic to genital illustrates such change. It can and does also change on the basis of experience. This means that learning plays a large role in object choice so that people's object choices will vary greatly depending on their personal histories. Changes in object choice are termed displacements and allow for great variety in human functioning. In fact, objects and their potential displacements give Freudian drive theory a flexibility enjoyed by few other theories of motivation.

The drives are housed in the id, where they constantly apply pressure as they strive for expression. The drives motivate most behavior; they supply the energy to get the mental apparatus running. The ego is charged with keeping the drives under control by providing realistic and safe avenues for their expression. The superego condemns and tries to block drives it believes will be frowned upon by society. The interactions and conflicts of these three agencies account for all of mental life.

REFERENCES

Brenner, C. (1955). *An Elementary Textbook of Psychoanalysis*. New York: International Universities Press.

Breuer, J., and Freud, S. (1895). *Studies on Hysteria*. S.E. 2: 19–305.

Brunswick, D. (1954). A revision of the classification of instincts or drives. *International Journal of Psychoanalysis*, 35(2): 224–228.

Compton, A. (1981a). On the psychoanalytic inquiry of instinctual drives. II: The sexual drives and the ego drives. *Psychoanalytic Quarterly*, 50(2): 219–237.

———. (1981b). On the psychoanalytic theory of instinctual drives. III: The complications of libido and narcissism. *Psychoanalytic Quarterly*, 50(2): 345–362.

———. (1981c). On the psychoanalytic theory of instinctual drives. IV: Instinctual drives and the ego-id-superego model. *Psychoanalytic Quarterly*, 50(2): 363–392.

———. (1983). The current status of the psychoanalytic theory of instinctual drives. I: Drive concept, classification, and development. *Psychoanalytic Quarterly*, 52(3): 364–401.

Freud, S. (1900). *The Interpretation of Dreams*. S.E. 4 and 5: 1–621.

———. (1905). *Three Essays on the Theory of Sexuality*. S.E. 7: 130–243.

———. (1910). Five lectures on psycho-analysis. S.E. 11: 9–55.

———. (1911). Formulations on the two principles of mental functioning. S.E. 12: 218–226.

———. (1914). On narcissism: An introduction. S.E. 14: 73–102.

———. (1915a). *Instincts and their Vicissitudes*. S.E. 14: 117–140.

———. (1915b). Repression. S.E. 14: 146–158.

———. (1915c). The Unconscious. S.E. 14: 166–215.

———. (1920). *Beyond the Pleasure Principle*. S.E. 18: 7–64.

———. (1923). *The Ego and the Id*. S.E. 19: 12–59.

Lampl-de Groot, J. (1956). The theory of instinctual drives. *International Journal of Psychoanalysis*, 37(4): 354–359.

Rapaport, D. (1960). On the psychoanalytic theory of motivation. In M. Jones (ed.). *Nebraska Symposium on Motivation*. Lincoln: University of Nebraska Press.

Vermorel, M. (1990). The drive (Trieb) from Goethe to Freud. *International Review of Psychoanalysis*, 17(2): 249–256.

JOEL WEINBERGER
JEFFREY STEIN

D

E

Education, and Analysts

Education for the practice of psychoanalysis is post-graduate and consists of three interrelated elements: personal analysis, supervision, and formal courses. Standards defining these elements vary widely among disparate psychoanalytic groups. The oldest credentialing body is the International Psychoanalytical Association, founded in 1908 by Sigmund Freud and his associates. It continues to actively monitor psychoanalytic education around the world.

The formal education of analysts begins with a prior training in psychology, social work, or psychiatry. In addition, analytic training is sometimes available to educators, social scientists, or those engaged in the humanities. Personal suitability for formal analytic education is more salient in the selection of students than is prior professional background.

Psychoanalytic training institutes vary not only in professed orientation—the degree to which Freudian emphases predominate, the admixture of Kleinian views, the contributions of the interpersonal school, and quite a number of other vantage points as well—but also in the relative stress on formal requirements, ranging from prescribed curricula to informal training arrangements.

The more formal Freudian tradition flows from the overarching International Psychoanalytical Association and its member societies, each of which separately trains candidates interested in practicing psychoanalysis. In the United States, most of these societies are part of the American Psychoanalytic Association. In addition, there are four so-called independent societies, independent in the sense of not being part of the American Psychoanalytic Association, although part of the International Psychoanalytical Association. Outside these established domains, there are quite a number of other organizations that educate following different traditions.

The centerpiece of a psychoanalyst's education is her or his own personal analysis. Within the Freudian tradition, this consists of analysis on the couch four or five times a week, which is necessary to achieve a thorough understanding of one's own inner mental workings—to properly prepare for the analyzing of others. Some other orientations require fewer than four sessions a week, following different rationales.

A second element in the education of analysts is the supervised treatment of patients. Students in training meet with supervisors on a weekly basis and discuss in detail their analytic sessions with their own patients. In the Freudian tradition, two or three cases of the student are each supervised intensively by two or three supervisors. These arrangements, too, may vary with the orientation and educational aims.

Courses and seminars complete the picture of analytic training. The formal Freudian institutes ordinarily prescribe a four-year sequence of classes in current Freudian theory and practice. These courses are generally given at night once or twice a week through the academic year. Naturally, the content of the courses and seminars varies with the theoretical orientation, although the night school atmosphere is endemic across other differences.

Ongoing monitoring of a student's progression through the training program, including presentation of case material for examination, typically takes place under many different formats and orientations. The degree of structured evaluations likewise varies among institutes—Freudian and others. Some institutes provide a formal graduation procedure as well as a procedure for inclusion into the ranks of psychoanalysts.

MOSS L. RAWN

Ego

The ego is usually considered to be the executive organ of the mind. It negotiates the demands of the outside world; it negotiates demands from the other mental agencies (the id and the superego); it negotiates resolutions of the conflicts that arise from competing demands; it orders the contents of the mind; and it is crucial to adaptation.

As a structure of the mind, the ego can share some of its contents and functions with the other psychic structures. For example, both the ego and the id attempt to satisfy the pleasure principle, but their methods of going about it are radically different: the id insists on immediate gratification without regard to the consequences or steps necessary to achieve it, whereas the ego's task is to factor in those very issues about how to make the original wish or a substitute gratification (or a delay in gratification) possible. Similarly, the superego insists on total and immediate compliance with its (usually moral) demands, and it does so without regard to any mitigating circumstances and without concern about the costs or the consequences of its requirements; the ego facilitates, transforms, or deflects those demands. It does so by taking into account the very factors that the superego ignores. What differentiates the psychic structures, then, is not so much their specific contents and functions (since many of these features are so often shared) but the overarching organization of how those contents and functions are employed and implemented in the mind.

The ego (as an organized psychic structure) is presumed to emerge from situations in which some mental conflict needs to be resolved, and it is assumed that it grows stronger and more articulated every time the management of a conflict has been successful. A structured ego is not presumed to exist at birth (at least not in mainstream analytic thinking: the Kleinians, as one example, would disagree); however, the capacity to develop as a potential structure, as well as some of its contents and functions, are assumed to be present at birth. Babies, for example, have certain perceptual abilities and sensational capacities. They are born with the ability to reduce tension through bodily movement (motility), and they have the potential to acquire memory engrams and traces, however primitive or transient they may be at first. These are the basic materials out of which the ego will be built.

Partly because of its bodily origins, particularly perception, Freud described the nascent ego as the "ego-percept." Viewing it as the mental organ that makes an interchange possible between inner and outer demands and realities, he likened it to an orange, the meat of the orange corresponding to inner (psychological) life, and the ego-percept represented by the rind (which is in continuous contact with both the inside and the outside at all times). Since Freud's time, analysts have thought of the early stages of the ego-in-formation as being first and foremost a "body-ego" (illustrating yet another way that the ego and the id can share certain contents and functions while, at the same time, having distinct characters of their own).

The management of conflict and its ability to work toward adaptation are the ego's most characteristic operations: it balances and counterbalances the drives using sublimation, neutralization and drive-fusion; it sets up defensive systems designed to ameliorate or to avoid entirely dysphoric affect states; it is the home of secondary process mental functioning (bringing into the mind such things as a relation to reality, the measurement of time, the ability to link cause and effect as well as other kinds of logical operations, and the capacity to symbolize experience, among other things). The ego operates in both consciousness and unconsciousness; it is the reservoir of both object relations and identifications (at least until the superego develops its own unique variety of aim-inhibited identifications); it is the agent of narcissistic regulatory processes; and it facilitates the wishes of both id and superego (as well as its own wishes) in the sense that these structures each provide an impetus for mental action. The ego transforms those pressures into the action itself (for example, the superego demands punishment and the ego responds with the production of guilt); and its most psychologically sophisticated activity is its synthetic function, which operates entirely in unconsciousness and without volitional control. Even in the realm of psychopathology the ego's influence is brought to bear on the development of symptom formation in such a way that the compromise-formations underlying a complex of symptoms both defend against and gratify unacceptable wishes at one and the same time.

In the clinical setting, many factors (the innate ego-strength of the patient, the potential safety of the analytic setting, identifications with the "analytic" ego and superego of the analyst, among others) influence what makes the usefulness of interpretation (as a therapeutic tool) possible for a patient. However, the specific purpose of interpretation itself is to give the mature ego material to grapple with, in the patient's attempt to sort out his or her problems and difficulties. The alliance that makes an analysis possible is, in large part, based directly on the relationship formed between the egos of the patient and the analyst (although other factors are at work as well). In psychoanalytic treatment, as contrasted with psychotherapy, the aim is not to ameliorate symptoms but to better organize the psychic structures (one result of which is the amelioration of symptoms). The therapeutic goal—achieving a higher degree of psychic structuralization—is directly dependent on the degree to which more autonomous ego functioning (that is, a relative independence from the drives, from the other psychic structures, from "outside" influences, and from the total, concrete, absoluteness of reality) is made possible by the analysis.

RICHARD LASKY

Ego Psychology

Freud uses the concept of the ego throughout his studies of the mind and the mental apparatus (Hartmann, 1946; Schur, 1966). In fact, the term "ego" (or rather, its German equivalent, "*Das Ich*") is among the most commonly used terms in Freud's corpus, but it is used in two distinct senses. As pointed out by his editor, James Strachey, in his Introduction to *The Ego and the Id* (Freud, 1923), Freud sometimes uses "ego" to refer to a person's self as a whole (the self concept) and sometimes to a particular part of the mind characterized by special attributes and functions (the agency concept). The self concept is germane to Erikson's ideas about identity and Kohut's work on self psychology, but it is the agency concept of the ego that is central to ego psychology (see Hartmann, 1964: 114).

The ego was first seen as a variable positioned between inside and outside, allowing one to distinguish between memory and perception (Freud, 1895). As Freud developed his theory, the concept of ego was broadened in scope. In the topographical model, the ego

appeared as a set of functions interposed between consciousness and unconsciousness. In the structural model, Freud's ego concept evolved further; the ego was theorized to be an active, intervening agency.

The Pre-Topographical Status of the Ego

To understand the significance of the topic, it is important to review Freud's steps in building his model of the mind and how the ego concept became a part of it. Apparently, the first use of the term "ego" occurred in an 1892–1893 paper on hypnotism in which its use was ambiguous but related to the self concept. In 1894, however, the agency functions of the ego are clearly illustrated by Freud's suggestions that it fends off intolerable ideas by a flight into psychosis, which "eludes the subject's self-perception" (p. 59). This is perhaps the first mention of the ego's defensive properties. In Freud's first trauma model of neurosis, the mind was assumed to be reflexively neurotogenic. However, Freud soon introduced an intervening variable—memory—noting that hysterics suffered "*mainly from reminiscences*" (Breuer and Freud, 1893–1895: 7). Trauma was neurotogenic but, more important, so was its recall (Freud, 1896). In Freud's *Project for a Scientific Psychology* (1895), the ideas of reality testing, perception, memory, thinking, and judgment were already included in his ego concept, in addition to defense (Hartmann, 1964). The ego was described in the *Project* as a set of stable, intercollated functions mediating interference and inhibition between memory and perception, making it possible to understand how the mind distinguishes between perception and memory: "*inhibition by the ego . . . makes possible a criterion for distinguishing between perception and memory*" (1895, p. 326). Furthermore, Freud suggested that the ego might be both investigative and purposive (1895, p. 374), or even "tendentious" in its substitution of one version of history for another (1899).

In his paper on "screen memories" (1899), such memories are theorized to be not substitutes for earlier ones but rather are falsifications—memory-fantasy complexes—developed under the influence of ego operations. Freud noted that such ego activity was a product of motivated "conflict, repression [and] substitution involving a compromise" (1899, p. 308) and that "These falsifications of memory are tendentious—that is they serve the purposes of repression and replacement of objectionable or disagreeable impressions" (1899, p. 322).

E

In a systematic, functional sense, the ego was referred to as "acting," "recollecting," and "working over" impressions from experience (p. 321).

The Ego in the Topographical Model

In Freud's first major model of the mind, the "topographical" model, the mind is divided into conscious, preconscious, and unconscious sectors. Since the task of psychoanalysis was to remove barriers to consciousness, making the unconscious conscious, ego functions were largely conceived of as defensively maintaining the unconsciousness of wishes and impulses. As Rapaport conceptualized the "first phase" of ego psychology, the major concept was defense, the operation of which forestalled "the experience of an unacceptable and thus painful affect," prevented "recall and re-encounter of a reality experience," and circumvented memories "incompatible with . . . [the] dominant mass of ideas" (Rapaport, 1958b: 746).

The exploration of instinctual drives dominated the second phase of ego psychology (Freud, 1911; Rapaport, 1958b: 747), owing, in part, to Freud's adherence to his "libido theory." Freud explained the intricate relationship between id and ego functions as follows: "the id sends part of this libido out into erotic object cathexes," to which the ego responds by mediating, even mastering that function (Freud, 1923: 46). Because a drive-dominated ego could scarcely be considered autonomous, the view of a basically passive psychic apparatus was retained (Holt, 1965: 106). The ego continued to be viewed by Freud as largely oppositional, and for some time its functions were described in a form "limited to that of mechanisms of defense at its disposal" (Hartmann and Kris, 1945: 24). In fact, the ego and its defenses were themselves treated as instinctual vicissitudes (Rapaport, 1958b: 747).

Nonetheless, the evidence for a more sophisticated ego continued to accumulate. In *The Interpretation of Dreams* (1900), for example, the ego was assigned the roles of dream censorship and secondary revision, the nuclei of the synthetic function (Hartmann, 1946). Interestingly, the development of agency and self aspects of the ego concept intersected in "On narcissism" (1914). Although the term "ego" in this work is used primarily in its "self" sense and is considered central to the development of self psychology, "agency" ego elements were also suggested. For example, decision functions mediating between anaclitic or narcissistic object choices (p. 87) were attributed to the ego. Ego ideal and con-

science concepts were also present in rudimentary form, concepts later to be crucial in Freud's elaboration of the structural ego.

The Structural Ego

According to Rapaport (1958b), the third stage of ego psychology began with the formulation of the structural model in Freud's *The Ego and the Id* (1923), with the ego being considered one of the three major psychic structures (or agencies). In this tripartite model, Freud delineates the three mental agencies in the following order: id, the primary agency, which is unconscious; ego, the secondary agency, considered to be both conscious and unconscious; and the superego, the tertiary agency, seen as largely unconscious (Boesky, 1995).

The ego of the structural model is seen as mediating among the id's instincts and drives, the superego's idealizations and prohibitions, and the external world's adaptive necessities. It is described as having a set of powerful tools to aid it in its tasks: perception, memory, will, defense, synthetic ability, and motility, among others. As Freud (1923) described the ego, there is a "coherent organization of mental processes; and we call this the *ego* . . . it is the mental agency which supervises all its own constituent processes" (p. 17).

The ego, as conceptualized in the structural model, was theorized to be a relatively weak system caught between the powerful id and superego, retaining some of the character of a passive reflex apparatus (Holt, 1965: 104). However, with the formulation of Freud's second theory of anxiety, in *Inhibitions, Symptoms, and Anxiety* (1926), the ego was conceptualized as having the capacity to initiate defense autonomously, turning passive reflexivity into active anticipation (Freud, 1926: 92–93). Among other far-reaching changes, the ego was conceptualized as the source of repression (p. 91), as having extensive influence over processes in the id (p. 92), as organizing symptoms and adapting to them until the symptom "gradually comes to be the representative of important interests" (pp. 98–99), and as being "characterized by a very remarkable trend towards unification, towards synthesis" (1926, p. 196). By 1926, the ego was clearly viewed as structuring internal and external reality into derivative form (Rapaport, 1958b: 794).

Later Developments in Ego Psychology

Although Freud introduced the concept of the ego and gave it a prominent place in his theory of mental functioning, he did not fully develop the theory of the ego, nor did he elaborate its clinical applications. These tasks were taken up by authors who came later.

In Rapaport's view (1958b, p. 750), Anna Freud's (1946 [1936]) work on the ego and its defense mechanisms ended the third phase of ego psychology; the fourth began with Hartmann's (1958 [1939]) work on adaptation, a major ego function. While Anna Freud's focus had been on the clinical situation, Hartmann and his colleagues were more concerned with formulating a general theory of psychology based on a psychoanalytic foundation, a theory that was to be compatible with findings in other branches of science.

Rapaport saw a major theoretical challenge lying in "conspicuous gaps" in theory regarding reality and object relations and their psychosocial implications (1958b, p. 750). In his view, Hartmann's work on adaptation and Erikson's development of his psychosocial theories began the process of bridging those gaps. Their work "showed a clear awareness of the foundations which existed in psychoanalysis for a theory of reality relationships in general, and interpersonal (psychosocial) relationships in particular" (Rapaport, 1958b: 750).

Modern ego psychology views the ego as a strategically placed agency with a set of important functions. As such, the ego is one part of the structural model, whose components are "structures" in the sense that they are postulated to possess related clusters of more or less observable, durable functions and operations (Hartmann et al., 1946; Rapaport, 1960; Beres, 1965; Meyer, 1988b). Although the ego is only part of the structural model, its functions are of the greatest importance and have been progressively emphasized, leading Schur to complain that the ego was "crowding out the other two structures, especially the id" (1966, p. 23). Its self-observational and interactional functions are sufficiently impressive to take seriously the possibility that everything we know about the patient on a firsthand basis comes to us through observing operations of the ego.

Current ego psychology favors a view in which the past is represented in the structural, symbolic, screen, representational, and synthetic functions of ongoing ego activities. This view subsumes rather than excludes the functions of recall, repression, and opposition to recall that were more prominent in Freud's topographical model.

Ego psychology is sometimes said to have reached its high-water mark prior to 1980 and then receded, but that is true only of discussions of the ego in the context of Freud's metapsychology. In fact, ego psychology is evolving vigorously, and its advances are being incorporated into technique.

REFERENCES

Beres, D. (1965). Structure and function in psychoanalysis. *International Journal of Psychoanalysis*, 46: 55–63.

Boesky, D. (1995). Structural theory. In B. Moore and B. Fine (eds.). *Psychoanalysis: The Major Concepts*. New Haven, Conn.: Yale University Press, pp. 494–507.

Freud, A. (1946 [1936]). *The Ego and the Mechanisms of Defense*. New York: International Universities Press.

Freud, S. (1892–1893). A case of successful treatment by hypnotism. S.E. 1: 117–128.

———. (1894). The neuro-psychoses of defense. S.E. 3: 41–61.

———. (1950 [1895]). Project for a Scientific Psychology. S.E. 1: 281–397.

———. (1896). The aetiology of hysteria. S.E. 3: 187–221.

———. (1899). Screen memories. S.E. 3: 301–322.

———. (1900). *The Interpretation of Dreams*. S.E. 5: 339–627.

———. (1911). Formulations on the two principles of mental functioning. S.E. 12: 213–226.

———. (1914). Remembering, repeating, and working through. S.E. 12: 145–156.

———. (1923). *The Ego and the Id*. S.E. 19: 12–59.

———. (1926). *Inhibitions, Symptoms, and Anxiety*. S.E. 20: 77–174.

Hartmann, H. (1958 [1939]). *Ego Psychology and the Problem of Adaptation*. New York: International Universities Press.

———. (1964). *Essays on Ego Psychology: Selected Problems in Psychoanalytic Theory*. New York: International Universities Press.

Hartmann, H., and Kris, E. (1945). The genetic approach in psychoanalysis. *Psychoanalytic Study of the Child*, 1: 11–30.

Hartmann, H., Kris, E., and Loewenstein, R. (1946). Comments on the formation of psychic structure. *Psychoanalytic Study of the Child*, 2: 11–38.

Holt, R. (1965). A review of some of Freud's biological assumptions and their influence on his theories. In N. Greenfield and W. Lewis (eds.). *Psychoanalysis and Current Biological Thought*. Madison: University of Wisconsin Press, pp. 93–124.

Meyer, J. (1988). The concept of adult psychic structure. *Journal of the American Psychoanalytic Association*, 36: 319–346.

Rapaport, D. (1958b). A historical survey of psychoanalytic ego psychology. In M. Gill (ed.). *The Collected Papers of David Rapaport*. New York: Basic Books, 1967, pp. 745–757.

———. (1960). The structure of psychoanalytic theory. *Psychological Issues*, 2, no. 2, Monogr. 6. New York: International Universities Press.

Rapaport, D., and Gill, M. (1959). The points of view and assumptions of metapsychology. *International Journal of Psychoanalysis*, 40: 153–162.

Schur, M. (1966). *The Id and the Regulatory Principles of Mental Functioning*. New York: International Universities Press.

JON K. MEYER
BRENDA BAUER

E

Eissler, Kurt (1908–1999)

Kurt Eissler was born in Vienna in 1908. He earned the Ph.D. in psychology in 1934 at the University of Vienna. His Ph.D. thesis under Professor Karl Bühler concerned the constancy of visual configurations in the variation of objects and their representation. In 1937, Eissler was awarded the M.D. degree, also by the University of Vienna. He was trained in psychoanalysis at the Vienna Psychoanalytic Institute. One of his principal teachers was August Aichhorn, to whom Eissler served as an assistant at the institute's consultation service. Eissler became a member of the Vienna Psychoanalytic Society in 1938. In the same year, he started to practice psychoanalysis but left when Germany annexed Austria.

Eissler emigrated to the United States, settled in Chicago, and became a diplomate of the American Board of Psychiatry. He again began to practice psychoanalysis but in 1943 volunteered for service in the U.S. Army. As a captain of the medical corps, he directed a consultation service in a training camp of the U.S. ground forces. He described his army experiences in a lengthy unpublished manuscript, as well as in articles on malingering and on the efficient soldier. After the war he moved to New York, where he remained in psychoanalytic practice until his death in 1999.

Among books Eissler published are a work on *The Psychiatrist and the Dying Patient* (1955); a study of Hamlet; an examination of medical orthodoxy and the future of psychoanalysis; a two-volume investigation of Goethe's first ten years in Weimar; and a study of the enigma of Leonardo da Vinci's art. Taking a polemical stance, in *Talent and Genius* Eissler corrected misstatements by Paul Roazen, and in *Tausk's Suicide* documented the causes of Tausk's self-destruction. Other books dealt with Freud as an expert witness at the trial of Julius Wagner-Jauregg after the First World War, and with Freud and the University of Vienna. Eissler wrote papers on delinquency, schizophrenia, and metapsychology, as well as on survivors of concentration camps and on parents who saw their children killed.

In 1952, Eissler was among the group of psychoanalysts who founded the Freud archives, at which he accepted the position of secretary. The purpose of the archives was to collect letters by and to Freud, and interviews with persons who knew him, and to deposit these documents in the U.S. Library of Congress. Subsequently, Eissler also was instrumental in establishing the Anna Freud Foundation and the Freud Literary Heritage Foundation.

One of the few who admired Freud's works to such an extent that he only rarely found anything to criticize, Eissler is known for what many persons consider his dogmatic insistence that Freud's basic theories are correct. He documented his position in a comprehensive manuscript, "Freud and the Seduction Theory: A Brief Love Affair."

Eissler's parents were Jewish. Eissler himself was an atheist who never participated in a religious ritual.

EDITH KURZWEIL

Eitingon, Max (1881–1943)

Although he made very few contributions to the development of psychoanalysis as either a body of theory or as a clinical technique, Max Eitingon, one of the early members of Sigmund Freud's inner circle, will remain an important figure in its history in view of his tireless dedication to the development of psychoanalytical causes, first in Germany, where he helped to create the Berlin Psycho-Analytical Society, and later in Palestine, where he established the Chewra Psychoanalytith b'Erez Israel, the forerunner of the Israeli psychoanalytical movement, thus promulgating psychoanalytical ideas on at least two continents. Plagued by a slight speech defect, Eitingon maintained a quiet but nevertheless committed position in the psychoanalytical movement.

Born on June 26, 1881, in Mogilev, in the Galician region of Russia, to a family of wealthy, Orthodox Jewish furriers, Eitingon grew up to become one of the few colleagues to whom Freud could entrust the perpetuation of his work. At the age of twelve, Eitingon moved to Leipzig, where he spent his adolescence and, subsequently, undertook university studies in history, literature, and philosophy. Eitingon commenced medical studies at the University of Marburg, then journeyed to Zürich to continue his education. In 1907, he became a voluntary assistant (*Volontär*) at the famous Burghölzli psychiatric clinic, studying with Professor Eugen Bleuler; while at the Burghölzli, Carl Gustav Jung introduced him to psychoanalytic concepts. On January 23 of that same year, Eitingon visited Freud in Vienna, the first person from a country outside of Austria to attend a meeting of the Vienna Psycho-Analytical Society, whereupon he became increasingly preoccupied with psychoanalytical ideas. Freud analyzed Eitingon on long walks through the park. Eitingon finally received his medical degree in 1909, but although he possessed the M.D. qualification, he failed to take an important entry examination; thus, he never possessed a legal license to practice medicine. Sensitive to this matter, he later became one of the few medically qualified champions of "lay analysis." He thereupon moved to Berlin, and with the cooperation of Karl Abraham, Freud's first serious German disciple, he helped to establish the Berlin Psycho-Analytical Society in 1910, eventually becoming its secretary. Eitingon worked doggedly to develop a psychoanalytic culture in Germany and, with the assistance of Abraham and colleagues, created a climate in which psychoanalytic theory could begin to take root.

During World War I, Eitingon served as a captain in the Austrian Medical Corps and ran a hospital in Miskolc, Hungary, specializing in the treatment of the war neuroses. He also used some of his private funds to obtain cigars for Freud, which proved difficult to purchase during the war years. Afterwards, in 1919, Freud had invited Eitingon to become a member of his secret committee of loyal followers. In the following year, Eitingon instigated the founding of the famous Poliklinik für Psychoanalytische Behandlung Nervöser Krankheiten, the well-known free mental health clinic for the indigent of Berlin, which would also train psychoanalysts, ably aided by both Karl Abraham and Ernst Simmel.

In 1924, the Poliklinik changed its name to the Berlin Psycho-Analytical Institute, thus becoming the first formal training body for psychoanalytic candidates in the world. For many years, Eitingon devoted the bulk of his energy, as well as a large part of his private fortune (through an anonymous donation), to the development of the training institute in Berlin, overseeing everything from the chairmanship of the Training Committee, the development of a library, the statistical tabulation of the results of treatment, and the editing of the annual reports, to the hanging of a picture and the choice of letterheads. Eitingon's report on the clinical activities of the Poliklinik may well be the first piece of formal psychotherapy outcome research. The Berlin training institute served as the model for all future psychoanalytic institutions around the world, incorporating the components of a training analysis, clinical supervision or "control analysis," and classroom seminars. In 1925, Eitingon proposed that the Berlin system should become standardized throughout the world as the model for psy-

choanalytic training, and this proposal became formally adopted at the International Psycho-Analytical Congress in Bad Homburg, with Eitingon serving as president of the International Training Commission, a post that he held until his death almost two decades later.

In 1926, Eitingon was elected president of the International Psycho-Analytical Society, following the death of his colleague Karl Abraham, having previously served as Abraham's secretary. Being able to read English, French, German, Hebrew, Polish, and Russian, Eitingon participated in the development of psychoanalytic groups in both Paris and Moscow. His colleagues reelected him for another term as president in 1929. He also became a director of the Internationaler Psychoanalytischer Verlag, the Vienna-based publishing house, and he contributed financial support to the activities of Freud's press.

His published contributions to the literature include papers on lay analysis, genius and talent, misreadings, and Friedrich Nietzsche. He also scripted many congress reports and miscellaneous documents; but on the whole, he confined his energies to clinical pursuits, teaching, and organizational activities, rather than to scientific writing.

In 1928, Eitingon suffered a serious financial reversal, and in 1932 he succumbed to a mild cerebral thrombosis with paresis of the left arm. By 1934, with the advent of Nazism, Eitingon moved to Jerusalem with his wife, Mira. Eitingon's father had bought land in Palestine many years previously, and after Eitingon arrived, he created the first psychoanalytic institution in Palestine, serving as the inaugural president of the Chewra Psychoanalytith b'Erez Israel. With the help of Moshe Wulff, a psychoanalyst who had emigrated from Russia, Eitingon set up small study groups in Haifa and Tel Aviv, as well as in Jerusalem. He also became a benefactor of the Hebrew University of Jerusalem, one of his many philanthropic activities, attempting to establish a medical chair for psychoanalysis in the university, albeit unsuccessfully, and a lecture series on "Psychoanalysis for Physicians and Educators." An ardent Zionist who had long dreamed of dying in Jerusalem, Eitingon lived out the remainder of his days there. He died on July 30, 1943, at the age of sixty-two, after enduring a painful cardiac illness of coronary thrombosis with angina pectoris. His remains were interred on Mount Scopus, in Jordan.

REFERENCES

Brill, A. (1943). Max Eitingon. *Psychoanalytic Quarterly*, 12: 456–457.

E

Jones, E. (1943). Max Eitingon. *International Journal of Psycho-Analysis*, 24: 190–192.

Pomer, S. (1966). Max Eitingon. 1881–1943: The organization of psychoanalytic training. In F. Alexander, S. Eisenstein, and M. Grotjahn (eds.). *Psychoanalytic Pioneers*. New York: Basic Books, pp. 51–62.

Rosenbaum, M. (1954). Freud-Eitingon-Magnes correspondence: Psychoanalysis at the Hebrew University. *Journal of the American Psychoanalytic Association*, 2: 311–317.

Sachs, H. (1943). Max Eitingon: 1880–1943. *Psychoanalytic Quarterly*, 12: 453–456.

                                                    BRETT KAHR

Electra Complex

Carl Jung used the term "Electra Complex" to describe the feminine Oedipus complex in order to demonstrate the parallel attitude of the children of both sexes toward the parents.

It seems to be a widely held impression that a girl's psychosexual development was originally labeled the "Electra Complex" by Freud. Contrary to this popular belief, it was in fact Jung who introduced the expression in his *Theory of Psychoanalysis* (Jung, 1915). In Freud's writings, there are three references to the Electra Complex, either in a footnote or parentheses, all declaring that he was unable to see the usefulness of such a term. This may have been a result of his conflicts with Jung at the time. Freud states in his essay on "Female Sexuality" that "Oedipus Complex applies with complete strictness to the male child only and that we are right in rejecting the term 'Electra Complex' which seeks to emphasize the analogy between the attitude of the two sexes" (Freud, 1931: 229). He further asserts: "It is only in the male child that we find the fateful combination of love for the one parent and simultaneous hatred for the other as a rival" (p. 229). In fact, Freud actively recommends disuse of the term. He states: "I do not see any advance or gain in the introduction of the term 'Electra Complex' and do not advocate its use" (p. 155). Although he strongly disagreed with Jung, Freud is also known to have claimed, both in his professional writings and in personal correspondence, not to have understood female sexuality. Hence, although Freud dismissed the use of the Electra myth, it seems relevant to consider its use for attempting to understand female development.

In the Greek myth, Electra is the daughter of Agamemnon and Clytemnestra. Agamemnon is the general-in-chief of the Greeks and during his absence, his wife betrays him by bringing home her lover, Aegisthus. Electra is enraged at her mother for her betrayal of her father and awaits her father's return. Unfortunately, her father is murdered by her mother and Electra's rage escalates. Electra, overcome with grief at the loss of her father, plans to murder her mother, not directly but by encouraging her brother Orestes to fulfill his duty of avenging his father's death, and he ultimately does so. Finally, Electra is left without both parents, immobilized and mourning.

This story reveals the triangular love relationship, the longings and rivalry of every child, but it is different from the Oedipal myth. While Oedipus consummates incest with Jocasta, is the actual murderer of Laius (his father), and ends up assuming all guilt, with subsequent punishment by blindness and exile, Electra has no incest with her father, does not murder her mother, and makes a murderer out of her brother. She is seen as longing and waiting for each parent to provide comfort and gratification. In fact, the Greek word *Electra* means "the unmarried."

Bernstein (1993) describes these affects and attitudes to be central to the girl's development. She feels that the "Electra myth" describes a point in female development when the girl must integrate her sexuality into her self-image, achieving a childhood identity synthesis. This must contain a stable, individuated self-image with sexuality integrated into her core-gender identity. To achieve this, satisfying relationships and identifications with *both* parents are critical (Bernstein, 1993: 116–117).

Electra, however, remains paralyzed and helpless, isolated in erotic mourning, awaiting her father's rescue but left disappointed. This contrasts with the boy's development in the Oedipal theme where Oedipus achieves mastery by taking his fate in his own hands. In fact, the psychic state of Electra can allow one to speculate the themes of masochism and longing so well depicted by writers and poets in themes of women, both loved and betrayed. Although Freud dismissed the Electra myth, presumably linked to his own rivalry with Jung, Electra "waits" around to be rediscovered by contemporary analysts to help throw light on the "dark continent" that Freud felt women were.

REFERENCES

Bernstein, D. (1993). *Female Identity Conflict in Clinical Practice*. New York: Jason Aronson.

Freud, S. (1920). The psychogenesis of a case of homosexualilty in a woman. S.E. 28: 147–172.

———. (1931). Female sexuality. S.E. 21: 225–243.

Holme, B. (1993). *Bulfinch's Mythology: The Greek and Roman Fables Illustrated*. New York: Viking.

Jung, C. G. (1915). *The Theory of Psychoanalysis*. New York: Journal of Nervous and Mental Disease Publishing Company.

PURNIMA MEHTA

Elizabeth von R.

Elizabeth von R. is the subject of one of Freud's most detailed case presentations in *Studies on Hysteria* (Breuer and Freud, 1895), designated by him as "the first full length analysis of a hysteria" (p. 139). Freud saw this twenty-four-year-old woman from the fall of 1892 to the summer of 1893. Her main symptoms were pains in her legs, difficulties in walking, and fatigue. These symptoms had been present with varying degrees of intensity for about two years. Because of the indefinite nature of her symptoms, her relative indifference to them, and her expression of pleasure when the painful areas of her legs were stimulated (including by electric shocks, which Freud, in keeping with standard methods at the time, initially administered), Freud decided that he was dealing with a case of hysteria.

Freud made a point of stressing that Elizabeth was an intelligent, capable, and lively woman, without any of the signs of intellectual and/or moral weakness that, at the time, were generally considered characteristic of hysterics. The story that she told Freud was an unhappy one, filled with losses and misfortunes. The youngest of three daughters, she had been her father's favorite. Her father had died two years earlier after a long illness during which Elizabeth was his primary nurse and caretaker. Then her mother had become ill, and Elizabeth nursed her also, the mother remaining a chronic invalid in Elizabeth's care. The older of her sisters had married and moved away from the family. The middle sister, to whom Elizabeth was very close, had also married but died suddenly during her second pregnancy. Freud decided that this "unhappy story," while worthy of "deep human sympathy" (p. 144), did not provide a specific explanation of her symptoms: "I firmly expected that deeper levels of her consciousness would yield an understanding both of the causes and the specific determinants of the hysterical symptoms" (p. 145). Freud compared his goal of clearing away pathogenic psychical material, layer by layer, to that of excavating a buried city—a comparison he was to use frequently in his later writings.

His attempts to use hypnosis with Elizabeth failed, so Freud used a modified new technique, the "pressure technique." Freud would apply pressure with his hand to the patient's forehead while instructing her "to report to me faithfully whatever appeared before her inner eye or passed through her memory at the moment of the pressure" (p. 145). If nothing occurred to the patient, Freud insisted that there must be something that she was deliberately or unwittingly concealing (p. 153f). This technique thus used physical pressure and suggestion to overcome resistance. Freud seems to have used this pressure technique with a few patients at the time but to have abandoned it around 1895 (for reasons he never spelled out). Historically, the pressure technique can be seen as a transition from the use of hypnosis and direct suggestion to the final technique of the "basic rule," urging the patient to free-associate without withholding anything that comes to mind. This technique may also be seen as the enactment of a fantasy (a kind of conversion in reverse, from the physical to the mental) by Freud, as if hidden repressed thoughts could be somehow squeezed out of the head by physical pressure.

On the basis of progressively recovered memories, Freud concluded that Elizabeth's physical symptoms were mostly the expression of conflicts around erotic feelings and fantasies. More specifically, Freud concluded that Elizabeth had been secretly in love with her brother-in-law, but finding such feelings completely unacceptable to her moral principles, she had completely repressed her love. She remembered having had the momentary intrusive thought at her sister's deathbed, "Now he is free again and I can be his wife" (p. 156). "She repressed her erotic idea from consciousness," Freud writes (p. 164), "and transformed the amount of its affect into physical sensations of pain." While admitting that he did not know how such a conversion comes about, Freud maintained his overall formulation that repressed traumatic memories (usually acting in a cumulative way) get transformed into symptoms. In this case of Elizabeth, the trauma theory had already become a *conflict* theory. External events are traumatic to the extent that they create or exacerbate an inner conflict.

Elizabeth's choice of symptoms was overdetermined. Some organic predisposition such as rheumatism is likely to have contributed to her symptoms. This is an early example of what Freud later (1905) called somatic convergence (*entgegenkommen*, commonly mistranslated as somatic "compliance"). Also, much of her pain was especially sharp in an area of her thigh that had come in contact with her father's swollen leg, while she daily changed his bandages. Here we have association by contiguity (and maybe an indication of what would later be interpreted as an expression of Oedipal conflicts). Furthermore, her symptoms, Freud tells us, may also have had a "symbolic" meaning, as a concretized metaphor or body language. Freud stated that "by means of symbolization . . . she had found . . . a somatic expression for her lack of an independent position and her inability to make any alteration in her circumstances, and that such phrases as 'not being able to take a single step forward', 'not having anything to lean upon', served as a bridge for this fresh act of conversion" (p. 176). This implied that linguistic usage plays a significant role in the choice of symptoms (an assumption central to the theories of Jacques Lacan). But Freud believed that verbal metaphors are themselves originally derived from somatic expressions of affect: "both hysteria and linguistic usage alike draw their material from a common source" (p. 181).

The case of Elizabeth is of great value for those interested in the historical development of Freud's clinical theory and technique. It illustrates and clarifies the increasing role of inner conflict over external trauma, and shows aspects of the transition from hypnosis to free associations. In 1895, Freud's focus was still very much on the explanation and cure of specific symptoms rather than with lasting character issues, and on the exploration of the recent past, rather than the reconstruction of early childhood.

The case is presented in an open-minded, lively, and exploratory manner. Freud apologized for its reading like a short story rather than a scientific presentation, which contrasts with the more self-assured (authoritative), predictable, and theory-dominated style of his later, more famous case presentations.

REFERENCES

Breuer, J., and Freud, S. (1895). *Studies on Hysteria*. S.E. 2: 19–305.
Freud, S. (1905). Fragment of an analysis of a case of hysteria. S.E. 7: 7–122.

JEAN G. SCHIMEK

Ellis, Havelock (1859–1939)

Havelock Ellis's remarkable life and career run in almost perfect synchroneity with those of Freud. Both men died in 1939, with Freud being the older by three years. Their earliest explorations of sexual themes are almost simultaneous, and it seems clear that neither borrowed from the other during those pre-1900 years, though each was well aware of the other. Their forays into medical school were not pleasurable. A career in psychiatry (Freud) or even that of a writer on sexology (Ellis) was not possible, absent a medical degree. Each man knew this at an early age and each attended medical school mainly as a rite of passage.

Ellis was eventually to be completely overshadowed by the great Viennese psychoanalyst, but the Englishman's prominence was extraordinary in the period 1897–1910 when his six-volume *Studies in the Psychology of Sex* appeared. These volumes, startlingly bold for late Victorian times, were soon banished from England. The themes with which Ellis was concerned had already been dealt with by others, most notably by Krafft-Ebing, but the latter's approach was more conventional, more conservative, more in keeping with sexual propriety. Ellis broke with Victorian mores by defending the so-called sexual aberrations (i.e., perversions) as extensions of normal sexuality that, taken all by themselves, had no pathological tendencies.

The first of his volumes, *Sexual Inversion*, dealt with what we now call homosexuality. Krafft-Ebing regarded it as "degenerate," an acquired disease probably caused by masturbation, itself a pathology in his view. Freud, too, was later to pronounce homosexuality as an illness originating in the unsuccessful resolution of the Oedipus complex. In a more modern spirit, Ellis insisted that anything to be classified as illness had to be some sort of dysfunctionality. He denied that homosexuality was usually accompanied by any particular dysfunctionality and thought the problems of homosexuals stemmed from the manner in which they were treated and regarded by others. Ellis ridiculed the idea, once Freud put it forward, that homosexuality could be cured via talk therapy. Indeed, he thought there was nothing to be cured, and his book is largely taken up with case studies of gifted, famous men who were homosexual. The studies even suggest that homosexuality is curiously well suited to help develop the talents for which these men were celebrated. Ellis was convinced that homosexuality was congenital, probably genetic in origin, making the notion of change via talk seem preposterous.

Ellis's second volume, *Auto-erotism*, defends masturbation as harmless. Ellis certainly had his work cut out for him when we consider that masturbation criticism, or at least its residue, still finds expression one hundred years later. *Auto-erotism* was written in reaction to the very influential *Functions and Disorders of the Reproductive Organs* by William Acton, which appeared in 1857. Acton's view that excessive masturbation leads to insanity was echoed just a couple of decades later by Krafft-Ebing. These men, typical of their era, also found masturbation to be revolting, independent of any harmful consequences to which it allegedly led. Acton and his followers thought masturbation to be a gender-based activity, and Ellis, by claiming it was even more common among women, the so-called genteel sex, managed in that way to rob masturbation of its viciousness. In his enthusiasm for masturbation, Ellis proclaimed the view, adopted by Kinsey a half-century later and then by Masters and Johnson, that masturbation, rather than interfering with the ability to perform interpersonally, improves sexual capacity.

In his third volume, *The Analysis of The Sexual Impulse, Love and Pain, The Sexual Impulse in Women*, Ellis analyzed sadism and masochism and insightfully pointed out that an interest in pain, not in cruelty, motivated the sadistic impulse. Moreover, sadism and masochism were not exclusive character traits but were to be found in one and the same person at different moments. Freud accepted this analysis wholeheartedly in his *Three Essays on the Theory of Sexuality* (1905). Indeed, rather than give illustrative examples, Freud contented himself with the remark that a citation from Havelock Ellis will do nicely. (The citation is from Ellis's *The Second Impulse*, published in 1903.) Of course, in the matter of the etiology of sadism and masochism, Freud went his own way and examined them far more deeply than Ellis was inclined to. It is a hallmark of Ellis's work that he preferred painting large scenes and never plumbed the depths of any topic to the extent that Freud did.

In his fourth volume, *Sexual Selection in Man* on sexual selection, Ellis anticipated a currently commonly held view that smells, touch, and hearing are as powerful as vision in driving people to select mates. Ellis's fifth volume, *Erotic Symbolism, the Mechanism of Detumescence, the Psychic State of Pregnancy*, is a curious redefining of tumescence. Ordinarily understood as the purely physical phase of erection, Ellis saw some virtue in identifying it with the whole process of arousal during courtship. Nothing much can be said about this reconceptualizing, and nothing much has come of this useless but harmless notion. Volume six is something of a prototype of a modern how-to sex manual, with little significance for Freudian theory.

Not well known at all is the fact that Ellis and Freud maintained a correspondence from the late 1890s up to the year in which they both died. At times, the correspondence was a lively exchange of ideas from which they both benefited, but more usually it consisted of criticisms that Ellis leveled at Freud and Freud's defenses of himself. For Freud, these defenses grew tiresome, and long periods would elapse between responses. In private conversation with Ernest Jones, Freud said, "It's not so much Ellis' ignorance that matters; it's his knowing so many things that are not so." Still, Freud admired Ellis so much as a man that he kept a photo of him in his study.

Fundamentally, although he conceded major contributions to Freud, Ellis was skeptical about the whole psychoanalytic enterprise. He maintained that neither Freud nor Breuer can be given credit for innovativeness. In his *History of the Psychoanalytic Movement*, written some time after January 1915, Ellis insisted that Schopenhauer anticipated the most important aspects of the unconscious, claimed that Freud's doctrines concerning autoerotism, particularly as expressed in *Three Essays on the Theory of Sexuality*, were derived from him, and that the idea that dreams were always symbolic came from Albert Scherner and J. Popper. In "Unlocking the Heart of Genius" (*The Nation*, 1919), Ellis stated that even the psychoanalytically oriented Albert Mordell admitted that, so far as dream theory is concerned, Hazlitt "gave almost complete expression to the views of Freud." Unquestionably, this is not true, but it gives us a good sense of how reluctant Ellis was to regard Freud as the more significant psychologist. In this same article, Ellis pointed to Bagehot as having psychoanalyzed Shakespeare well before Freud came on the scene. In his "Open Letter to Biographers," Ellis stated that psychology became a science under Wundt and that he, Ellis, learned to obtain by "exact methods a true insight into the processes of the average human mind" from Stanley Hall, Jastrow, and Munsterberg. There is no mention of Freud.

More intriguing than his theoretical doubts were Ellis's occasional attitudes of outright contempt and hostility. Again, in "Unlocking the Heart of Genius," Ellis described psychoanalytic writings as "random and unsupported," adding that there is "something unpleas-

E

ant in the theories of psychoanalysis, even when applied to the ordinary population, and it is natural they should seem more offensive when applied to genius." In a middle-period article entitled "The New Psychology" (*Forum*, 1926), Ellis wrote that Freud was "head of a sect on the model of those religious sects to which the Jewish mind has a ready tendency to lend itself, as the whole Christian world exists to bear evidence." He tacked on the little taunt that this does "not lend itself to scientific ends." This rather out-of-character insult caused a rift between the two men but for a surprisingly short time.

Despite his remark that Ellis knows so many things that are not so, Freud was always pleased to have Ellis on his side. In "Transformations of Puberty," Freud (1905) used the ad hominem that Ellis agrees with him that there is no wickedness in the fondling, kissing, and sexual excitement a mother derives from her child. In his autobiography, Freud generously admitted that he learned from Ellis that Plato is the originator of the idea that hysteria and sexuality are connected. Freud was also instrumental in correcting an error of attribution concerning Ellis's work. It was he who pointed out that Ellis, not Nocke, deserved credit for introducing the term "narcissism."

So much of early anti-Freudianism (the writings of Jung, Adler, etc.) strikes the casual observer as internecine warfare, since all parties seemed committed to some version of psychoanalysis, broadly conceived, but Ellis was the most prominent critic from outside the psychiatric circle, certainly at least in England. Ellis mocked the idea of infantile sexuality and rejected entirely the notion of an Oedipus complex. He held that the experience of sexuality had no place in children's experience in any genuine sense. A mother may derive sexual pleasure from fondling her child, but this appeared to Ellis to be a one-way street. Nor did Ellis see a need for complex explanations for incest taboos. For him, familiarity blunts sexual attraction. Appealingly facile, this view unfortunately fails to account for the existence of legal prohibitions. Why make illegal that which people have no inclination to do?

Ellis conceded that dreams have an importance of some sort, that they "reveal to us an archaic world of vast emotions," but said that this has been known for thousands of years. Still, he underestimated the Freudian contribution, for whether the Freudian account is correct or not, it added so much rich content concerning symbolic meanings and images that allegedly universally represent objects that prior notions about dreams pale in comparison. Freudian theory, correct or not, extends to dreams a power and significance not anticipated by Freudian predecessors.

In his *History of the Psychoanalytic Movement*, Ellis wrote that the doctrine of suppression and resistance "is the foundation stone on which the edifice of psychoanalysis rests." This is not quite true, of course, and perhaps helps explain why Ellis, believing suppression to be an old doctrine, is reluctant to ascribe innovativeness to Freud. Nevertheless, Ellis granted that even the field of criminology (one of his areas of expertise) owed a great deal to Freud. Ellis claimed that at least 7 percent of criminals, and probably a much higher percentage, are criminals because of inner conflicts that are mostly sexual.

Ellis was a remarkable man of letters whose humanistic range was far broader than Freud's. He wrote on every humanistic subject imaginable and was personally acquainted with the literary giants of his time. Perhaps this renaissance-like thirst contributed to his being a bit superficial, especially when compared with Freud. Still, Ellis remains the father of modern sexology, the first great revolutionary against Victorian prudery, and his graceful style makes him worth reading even today. As an antidote to Freudian excesses, however, Ellis's essays have seen their best day, and skeptical readers must turn to more recent critiques.

REFERENCES

Ellis, H. (1890). *The Criminal*. London: W. Scott, Ltd.
———. (1926a). *Affirmations*. London: Constable, 1st ed., 1898.
———. (1926b). *Man and Woman: A Study of Secondary Sexual Characteristics*. London: A.C. Black, 6th ed.
———. (1936). *Studies in the Psychology of Sex*. New York: Random House.
———. (1939). *My Life: Autobiography of Havelock Ellis*. Boston: Houghton Mifflin.
Freud, S. (1905). *Three Essays on the Theory of Sexuality*. S.E. 7: 126–243.

SIDNEY GENDIN

Envy

Freud emphasized the importance of envy and other emotions for the understanding of human functioning but never developed a consistent theory about envy in particular. Rather, his views about this emotion can be found scattered in different writings about, for example, female development and social psychology. Of special interest are his theory of "penis envy" and his views of the functions of envy in a social group, as dealt with in *Group Psychology and the Analysis of the Ego* (1921).

The Cognitive Comparison Model

Freud's views on envy may be usefully compared with a more current, general theory of the development, phenomenology, and function of envy and other emotions. This model integrates current theoretical considerations and empirical findings from research on the emotions (cf., Bänninger-Huber and Widmer, 1996).

In terms of this model, emotions can be understood as consequences of cognitive evaluations of specific situations (Scherer, 1984). Envy, in particular, develops when a person becomes aware of an advantage enjoyed by another, and desires to possess the same advantage. In this sense, envy is the result of a comparison that takes place in a real or imagined social context. The relevant emotional wish is aimed not at the other person (as, e.g., in the case of love or jealousy) but at the other person's envied possession. For Freud, too, processes of comparison are essential for the elicitation of envy, at least in the case of a little girl's penis envy: "She has seen it and knows that she is without it and wants to have it" (1925, p. 252).

If such comparisons lead to the conclusion that there is a significant difference (between one person and another in respect to a desired possession or attribute), the cause of this difference can be seen by the subject as "internal"—caused by him or her—or "external"—caused by something outside the subject (Weiner, 1985). In his reflections on penis envy, Freud also describes possible internal and external attributions with respect to envy. While at first, a girl interprets her failure to possess a penis as a punishment for wrongdoing (1925, p. 253), she later holds her mother responsible (1925, p. 254).

The Objects of Envy

What we envy can vary, depending on time and culture. It is specific to envy, however, that the "wished for" object belongs to someone else and has great personal or social relevance (Salovey, 1991). The relevant attributes that are envied are often associated by the subject with well-being, success, happiness, or prestige. With regard to Freud's idea of penis envy, it has long been disputed whether the envied object is the anatomical difference per se or rather the social privileges associated with the male gender.

Envy occurs in the context of real or fantasized *object relations* in which the subject can compare him- or herself with the object of envy. The more similar the object is to oneself, the more the perceived differences are experienced as unfair and hurtful. The subjective experience of envy is less intensive, however, when the other person is viewed as completely different. Freud (1925, p. 121) points out, for example, that a leader's privileges are generally not envied by the members of a group, as long as all members are treated as equals.

Aspects of Envy

A single *emotional experience* specific to envy does not seem to exist. Envy, rather, seems to be a complex emotion consisting of different experiences (or emotional episodes). These include the experiencing of the wish to possess what the other has, aggressive feelings, negative self-feelings such as feelings of inferiority, and hurt feelings or irritation. Freud (1925, p. 253) describes the following psychic consequences of envy for the penis: "After a woman has become aware of the wound to her narcissism, she develops, like a scar, a sense of inferiority."

With respect to *motivational aspects* of envy, we can differentiate between *intrapsychic, interactive*, and *behavioral* features. Being envious, I may wish my rival bad luck; or I may devalue the envied person or advantage; or I may destroy his or her possession. According to Freud, an important (intrapsychic) strategy for coping with envy is *reaction-formation*. He illustrates this phenomenon by using the example of the initial envy displayed by the elder child toward the younger sibling. Because the parents love the younger child as much as the older one, the latter's hostile reaction cannot be prolonged without damaging him- or herself. Therefore, the elder child is forced into identifying with the younger sibling or other children (1921, p. 120). The result is a communal or group feeling among the children that may further be developed during latency.

Which strategies are mentioned by Freud to cope with penis envy? According to his theory, the envied difference is an unchangeable, anatomical fact. This fact—of a perceived lack and not merely a "neutral" difference—has to be accepted by the envious female. Only when a girl replaces her wish for a penis with a wish for a child, taking her father as a love-object, can her penis envy be overcome. Dealing with this Oedipal wish finally leads to the formation of the superego (Bänninger-Huber and Widmer, 1996). The alleged anatomical basis of penis envy, however, has been severely criticized for a long time (see, e.g., Horney, 1923). In Freud's theory, any female wish to participate in male privileges would be interpreted as a sublimation of the anatomically determined disadvantage.

In our culture, envy is usually condemned. In our view, however, a difference that is envied may provide a person with the necessary motivational power for change.

REFERENCES

Bänninger-Huber, E., and Widmer, C. (1996). A new model of the elicitation, phenomenology and function of emotions in psychotherapy. In N. H. Frijda (ed.), *Proceedings of the IXth Conference of the International Society for Research on Emotions*. Toronto, pp. 251–255.

Freud, S. (1921). *Group Psychology and the Analysis of the Ego*. S.E. 18: 67–143.

———. (1925). Some psychical consequences of the anatomical distinction between the sexes. S.E. 19: 248–258.

Horney, K. (1923). Zur Genese des weiblichen Kastrationskomplexes. *Internationale Zeitschrift für Psychoanalyse*, 9: 12–26.

Salovey, P. (1991). *The Psychology of Jealousy and Envy*. New York: Guilford Press.

Scherer, K. R. (1984). On the nature and function of emotion: A component process approach. In K. R. Scherer and P. Ekmans (eds), *Approaches to Emotion*. Hillsdale, N.J.: Lawrence Erlbaum Associates.

Weiner, B. (1985). An attributional theory of achievement, motivation and emotion. *Psychological Review*, 92: 548–573.

EVA BÄNNINGER-HUBER
CHRISTINE WIDMER

Ethics, Clinical

The term *clinical ethics* refers to the normative standards and virtues governing a clinical practice, such as psychoanalysis. That psychoanalysis as a practice is inevitably bound up with certain moral values has been questioned on the grounds that it is allegedly a value-free inquiry. For example, the influential psychoanalytic ego psychologist Heinz Hartmann (1960) contends that psychoanalysts study values and other contents of mental life as facts. The analyst describes, classifies, and explains mental phenomena, without passing judgment as to what is good or bad, Hartmann (1960) writes.

Warrant in Freud's writings for treating psychoanalysis as value-free is sometimes found in occasional statements about the scientific credentials of psychoanalysis, but it is doubtful that Freud imagined the sciences to be entirely value-free. He wrote frequently of the scientist's commitment to the intrinsic value of truth, with which he allied psychoanalysis (see, e.g., Freud, 1933: 158–159). And he was not embarrassed to write that the psychoanalyst has a "*duty* . . . to carry on . . . research without consideration of any immediate beneficial effect" (1916–1917, p. 255) and that "psychoanalysis is committed to the same moral goals as religion: namely the love of man and the decrease of suffering" (1927, p. 53).

Philip Rieff (1961) has argued that Freud's devotion to truth was contentless and that he pursued truth at the expense of the patient values commonly associated with health care, such as respect for patient autonomy, relief of suffering, beneficence, and altruism. But the dichotomy Rieff draws between truth and health values is false. Freud viewed the pursuit of the deep, hidden truths about patients and their behavior as contributing to the relief of suffering and the realization of such values for the patient as freedom and happiness. His writings are full of references to the value of relieving suffering and to the selflessness of the physician committed to ferreting out truths that heal. He says of psychoanalysis that "knowledge . . . [and] therapeutic success" are inseparable; it is "impossible to gain fresh insight without perceiving its beneficent results" (1926, p. 256).

Freud is famous for urging psychoanalysts to practice their craft "coolly," that is, with the personal detachment of a surgeon or the impersonality of a mirror. But Freud did not believe analysis could occur without "sympathy and respect" (1893, pp. 282–283; 1905, p. 16; 1915a, p. 165). He criticized some of his early disciples for taking his recommendations about analytic neutrality "literally or exaggerat[ing] them" (Meng and Freud, 1963: 113). The attitude Freud appears to have had in mind is what is now called, following Greenson (1958) and Stone (1961), "benevolent" or "compassionate" neutrality—that is, a warmly tolerant, nonjudgmental approach. The analyst creates a benignly supportive environment, in part by refraining from giving voice to customary forms of moral censure and didactic instruction, not because the analyst is neutral about values but because beneficence dictates that in the analytic setting the best therapeutic method is to concentrate on clarifying and interpreting nonjudgmentally. "The analyst inhibits the wish to heal now, adopting a stance of temporary goallessness, for the sake of the long-range goal of analysis—namely, to heal as effectively as possible" (Wallwork, 1991: 212).

The practice of psychoanalysis is marked by a particularly high regard for the patient's autonomy. The analyst avoids suggestions and advice not only because interpretation is ultimately more beneficial, but also because it is to respect the patient. Indeed, one of the prime goals of analysis is to augment the patient's independence and autonomy, for example, by enabling the patient to employ self-analytic tools in improved decision making. As Freud puts it, "analysis . . . set[s] out . . . to give the patient's ego *freedom [Freiheit]*" (1923, p. 50n.1). In contrast to therapies that try to convert the patient to the therapist's personal values or world view, as Freud suspected Jung and Putnam of doing, Freud says regarding the value of autonomy to psychoanalytic treatment: "The analyst respects the patient's individuality and does not seek to remold him [or her] in accordance with his [or her] own—that is, according to the physician's—personal ideals; he [or she] is glad to avoid giving advice and instead to arouse the patient's power of initiative" (1923, p. 127; see also 1919, pp. 164–165; Wallwork, 1991: 213). Respect for the patient's autonomy also means that the analyst has a duty to provide the patient with the information necessary for an informed choice prior to treatment and to respect the patient's right "to break off [treatment] whenever he [or she] likes," even when the analyst believes this will be harmful (1913, p. 129). In this situation, the analyst has a moral responsibility to share his or her concerns about the probable consequences of early termination, but the decision is finally the patient's (1913, pp. 129–30).

Promise keeping and truthfulness are central moral dimensions of what Freud calls the "pact" that the patient and analyst make at the outset of treatment. The patient promises to practice "the fundamental rule" of free association, which entails the most complete candor and truthfulness possible (1940, p. 173). Such truthfulness goes beyond ordinary truth telling, because the patient is encouraged to tell not only whatever he or she thinks consciously, but also whatever he or she has difficulty knowing because it is too shameful or awful to admit to oneself, much less to someone else (1926, p. 188; 1940, pp. 172–174). The analysand promises, Freud writes, "to tell us not only what he can say intentionally and willingly, what will give him relief like a confession, but everything else as well that his self-observation yields

him, everything that comes into his head, even if it is *disagreeable* for him to say it, even if it seems to him *unimportant* or actually *nonsensical*" (1926, p. 207). The analyst has a correlative responsibility to eschew customary moral reactions to even the most distasteful communications, including those that hurt the analyst. The analyst especially avoids retaliating, injuring, exploiting, or otherwise harming the patient, who, by virtue of the transference, is peculiarly vulnerable. This abstinence includes, of course, sexual responses to the temptations aroused by the eroticization of the transference. In Freud's unambiguous words, "to yield to the demands of the transference, to fulfil the patient's wishes for affectionate and sensual satisfaction, is . . . justly forbidden by moral considerations" (1926, p. 227).

Psychoanalytic ethics particularly stresses confidentiality—namely, the therapist's duty not to betray the patient's privacy by revealing what is communicated in the therapeutic relationship to persons outside it. The analyst's commitment to confidentiality needs to be steadfast for the analysand to develop the kind of archaic trust necessary to share what is ordinarily not allowed to enter consciousness. Of course, analysts needs to discuss patients with colleagues for the advancement of the mental health field and for educational purposes. For such communication to occur ethically, Freud realized, the case material must be disguised so as to prevent identification of the particular patient, or the patient's informed consent must be obtained. Freud initially thought the analyst's responsibilities to science and to "the many other patients who are suffering or will some day suffer from the same disorder" meant that case material could be shared with colleagues as long as it was well disguised. He wrote in the prefatory remarks to the "Dora" case that he had taken "every precaution to prevent my patient from suffering any . . . injury [from being identified]" (1905, p. 8). However, Freud worried, as psychoanalysts continue to do today, that his disguises might alter facts that would end up misleading colleagues. "One can never tell what aspect of a case may be picked out by a reader of independent judgment, and one runs the risk of leading him [sic] astray," Freud wrote in 1915b (p. 263). But we know now that Freud's disguises were not thick enough. All but one of the patients in his published cases have been identified. In his later writings, Freud sometimes recommended that the analyst obtain the patient's consent, as Little Hans's father consented to publication of his son's case history. However, the problem of how truly informed consent can be obtained within the context of the transference continues to plague psychoanalysts who worry about the voluntariness of permission under these special circumstances and about patients being inadvertently harmed in ways they failed to anticipate when consenting to disclosures that ended up compromising their privacy (see Stoller, 1988).

Psychoanalysis is not value-free, then, at least not in the sense of "anything goes." Rather, psychoanalytic treatment is predicated on the establishment of a nonjudgmental milieu, a "holding environment" to use Winnicott's felicitous term (1965), in which the patient develops sufficient trust in the analyst to say whatever comes to mind, including the most despicable, shameful things. The clinical ethics that govern psychoanalytic treatment gives pride of place to respect for autonomy, nonmaleficence, truthfulness, promise keeping, and confidentiality. The analyst's unusual tolerance of beliefs, values, and actions that violate the analyst's own values are based on a moral stance that combines the values of truthfulness and respect for autonomy with the belief that a nonjudgmental approach is most beneficial to the patient in the therapeutic relationship.

REFERENCES

Breuer, J., and Freud, S. (1893–1895). *Studies on Hysteria*. S.E. 2: 19–305.
Freud, S. (1905). Fragment of an analysis of a case of hysteria. S.E. 7: 7–122.
———. (1913). On beginning the treatment. S.E. 12: 123–144.
———. (1915a). Observations on transference love. S.E. 12: 159–171.
———. (1915b). A case of paranoia running counter to the psycho-analytic theory of the disease. S.E. 14: 263–272.
———. (1919). *Lines of Advance in Psycho-analytic Therapy*. S.E. 17: 159–168.
———. (1923). Two encyclopaedia articles. S.E. 18: 235–259.
———. (1926). *Inhibitions, Symptoms and Anxiety*. S.E. 20: 77–172.
———. (1926). *The Question of Lay Analysis*. S.E. 20: 183–258.
———. (1927). *The Future of an Illusion*. S.E. 21: 5–56.
———. (1933). *The New Introductory Lectures on Psychoanalysis*. S.E. 22: 5–182.
———. (1940). *An Outline of Psycho-Analysis*. S.E. 23: 144–207.
Greenson, R. (1958). Variations in classical psychoanalytic technique: Introduction. *International Journal of Psychoanalysis*, 39: 200–201.
Hartmann, H. (1960). *Psychoanalysis and Moral Values*. New York: International Universities Press.
Meng, H., and Freud, E. (eds.) (1963). *Psychoanalysis and Faith: The Letters of Sigmund Freud and Oskar Pfister*. New York: Basic Books.
Rieff, P. (1961). *Freud: Mind of the Moralist*. Garden City, N.Y.: Doubleday, Anchor Books.
Stoller, R. (1988). Patients' responses to their own case reports. *Journal of the American Psychoanalytic Association*, 36: 371–391.
Stone, L. (1961). *The Psychoanalytic Situation*. New York: International Universities Press.
Wallwork, E. (1991). *Psychoanalysis and Ethics*. New Haven, Conn.: Yale University Press.
Winnicott, D. W. (1965). *The Maturational Processes and the Facilitating Environment*. New York: International Universities Press.

ERNEST WALLWORK

Existentialism

Existentialism is a philosophical movement initiated by the German philosopher Martin Heidegger (1889–1976), which grew out of a fusion of Edmund Husserl's phenomenology and the writings of Kierkegaard and Nietzsche.

Freud had a certain amount of intellectual contact with precursors of existentialism. Both he and Husserl were students of the philosopher Franz Brentano at the University of Vienna. Freud was also influenced by the early phenomenologist Theodor Lipps, and admired Nietzsche. Among the psychoanalysts, Freud's friend and colleague Ludwig Binswanger (1881–1966) and, later, Medard Boss (1903–1990) attempted to reformulate psychoanalysis on the basis of Heidegger's philosophy. Boss collaborated with Heidegger to this end. However, most of the contemporary literature on the relationship between existentialism and psychoanalysis deals not with Heidegger's work but rather with Jean-Paul Sartre's (1943) criticism of Freud's theory of unconscious mental states.

Freud had no direct contact with existentialism and would have been uncomfortable with its central doctrines of radical human freedom, the primacy of consciousness, and its antireductionism. As a philosophical materialist and scientific naturalist, Freud ascribed to the metaphysical theory of "psychic determinism": the view that mental events are subject to the same causal laws as all other events in the material universe. The doctrine of psychic determinism does not deny that human beings make choices, but it does deny that these choices are themselves uncaused. The existentialist doctrine of the primacy of consciousness and the rejection of the hypothesis of radically unconscious mental states are part of the Cartesian philosophical tradition that Freud was anxious to refute. Finally, Freudian theory rested on the belief that at bottom all mental states supervene upon the material processes of the central nervous system and are *in principle* explicable in neurophysiological terms, a position antagonistic to the existentialist rejection of any program for scientifically explaining human existence.

There has been speculation that Nietzsche's work exercised considerable influence on Freud's developing theories, and that Freud failed to give the philosopher credit for this (Ellenberger, 1970; Sulloway, 1979; Esterson, 1993). Although Freud purchased a set of Nietzsche's *Collected Works* in 1900, there is no evidence that he studied these, and Freud repeatedly asserted up until 1925 that he had never studied Nietzsche, and remarked at several points up until 1925 that he had never read Nietzsche (Freud in Nunberg and Federn, 1962; Freud 1925). Freud's close colleague Otto Rank (1884–1939), who *did* study Nietzsche and who gave Freud another set of Nietzsche's *Collected Works* on his seventieth birthday, corroborated Freud's claims in a letter stating that Freud read Nietzsche "only in his later years" (Rank, cited in Kaufmann, 1980: 269) but stressed that Nietzsche's ideas permeated the intellectual atmosphere during Freud's formative period.

REFERENCES

Ellenberger, H. (1970). *The Discovery of the Unconscious: The History and Evolution of Dynamic Psychiatry*. New York: Basic Books.

Esterson, A. (1993). *Seductive Mirage*. Chicago: Open Court.

Freud, S. (1925). *An Autobiographical Study*. S.E. 20: 7–74.

Kaufmann, W. (1980). *Discovering the Mind, vol. 3: Freud Versus Adler and Jung*. New York: McGraw-Hill.

Nunberg, H., and Federn, E. (eds.) (1962). *Minutes of the Vienna Psychoanalytic Society*. New York: International Universities Press.

Sartre, J. P. (1943). *Being and Nothingness: An Essay on Phenomenological Ontology*. Trans. H. E. Barnes. New York: Philosophical Library, 1957.

Sulloway, F. (1979). *Freud: Biologist of the Mind: Beyond the Psychoanalytic Legend*. New York: Basic Books.

DAVID LIVINGSTONE SMITH

Experimental Evidence, Freudian

Freud relied very heavily on evidence from clinical case studies to support his theoretical hypotheses, although he also appealed to other sorts of data, such as facts about the psychopathology of every day life, myths, and literature. He did not, however, see the need for *experimental* studies to confirm his theories. He published only one experimental study, and that was on the effects of cocaine, not on psychoanalysis (1885).

Whether Freud's opinion about experimental evidence is correct has been central to disagreements about the existing empirical support for his theories. He, and many who came after him, provided numerous methodological arguments to show that support for his theories does not generally require experimental confirmation. Other Freudian arguments are not directly concerned with epistemology or methodology; they bear directly on the truth of Freudian theory. Nevertheless, they have methodological import; if some of them are cogent, then Freud's opinion about not needing experimental evidence has been vindicated.

Assessing all of these arguments is a complex endeavor requiring attention to the relevant empirical details, issues about meaning and the interpretation of Freudian theory (see "Meaning, and Psychoanalysis"; "Hermeneutics, and Psychoanalysis," this volume), the vexed issue of suggestion, and many other matters (on Freud's arguments, see "Critique of Psychoanalysis," this volume). There is one issue, however, that has stood in the way of resolving some of these other issues: What are the correct standards for evaluating the Freudian evidence? Answering this question cannot by itself settle issues about the truth or falsity of Freudian theory, but it is important given that much of the disagreement is about standards. The same issue obviously bears on the evaluation of the Freudian experimental evidence.

Conceptual Standards

Issues about Freudian standards can be divided into conceptual and epistemological questions. An obvious conceptual question is: For what theory is the evidence being assessed? There are now various kinds of psychoanalytic theories besides Freud's and some of the recent experimental studies are relevant to psychoanalysis but not necessarily to Freud's. If we confine ourselves to the Freudian experimental evidence, questions often arise about the *distinctiveness* of the Freudian hypothesis. For example, some scholars (Levy, 1996) take the existence of the unconscious to be one of the most important issues dividing Freudians and non-Freudians. If that is the issue, then one is free to appeal to semantic priming experiments and other experiments concerning the cognitive unconscious. However, given that virtually no recent critic of Freud, excluding certain behaviorists, has denied the existence of unconscious events, this is really a nonissue. Both sides agree about the existence of the unconscious; there is disagreement, however, about Freud's specific theory of the dynamic unconscious.

There are many other instances where the experimental evidence may well support Freud's views, but the views are those shared by his critics as well. For example, if an experiment provides evidence of the existence of dream symbols, that supports an implication of Freud's dream theory, but the existence of dream symbols is accepted by many rival theories of dreams as well as commonsense psychology. Some scholars deal with this problem of competing theories having some of the same logical implications by distinguishing between hypotheses that are *distinctively* Freudian and those that are not (Kline, 1981). This suggests an initial conceptual standard: If Freudian experimental evidence is to be relevant to the confirmation or disconfirmation of Freudian theory, the hypothesis being assessed must be distinctively Freudian (i.e., peculiar to his theories).

A second conceptual standard concerns centrality. Some experimental investigators try to study hypotheses that are "closer to the observations." For example, Luborsky et al. (1985) claim to have verified experimentally what they term Freud's "grandest hypothesis": the transference. However, an examination of their results shows that their evidence does not support what is central to Freud's theory of the transference: the emergence in psychoanalytic sessions of infantile prototypes. At most, what they confirm are propositions rather peri phial to Freud's theory (Erwin, 1996: 287; Eagle, 1986). To take another example, Fisher and Greenberg (1977) cite experimental evidence in support of three propositions constituting Freud's Oedipal theory. Two of these propositions, that males and females are closer to their mother than their father in the pre-Oedipal period and that, later, each sex identifes more with the same-sex parent than with the opposite sex parent, are implications of the Oedipal theory (at least when it is combined with other reasonable assumptions). Neither proposition, however, is central to the theory; they could both be true and yet it could be false that males generally want to have sex with their mothers during the Oedipal period or that they suffer from castration anxiety.

The above examples suggest a second conceptual standard: that the hypothesis being assessed is central (to some degree) to Freudian theory. There is a connection between the two standards: If one confirms an implica-

tion of Freudian theory that is not central, then the hypothesis will often not be distinctively Freudian either. However, some hypotheses might meet the first standard but still not be central to any Freudian theory.

Both of the above standards are somewhat vague; so, it cannot be discerned in every single case whether or not they have been met. More importantly, neither of these conceptual standards need be met in order for Freudian experimental evidence to have value. What is important is what question is being addressed. If the question is merely whether one of Freud's claims is supported—e.g., if one is asking whether there are unconscious mental events of some sort or other, not whether there exists a dynamic unconscious; or, whether some slips are motivated, not whether they are motivated by repressed wishes; or, whether childhood events sometimes contribute to the development of adult neuroses, not whether the causes are of a sexual nature—then one need not be concerned about whether the hypothesis is distinctively Freudian or not. Likewise, if the issue is merely whether an implication of Freudian theory is true or false, then the issue of centrality need not arise. However, the cost of not adhering to both of these conceptual standards or something like them is that the conclusion that is reached will be irrelevant to any live debate about Freudian theory.

Epistemic Standards

There has been much disagreement about the basic epistemic standards appropriate for judging the Freudian evidence. A recent trend among psychoanalytic theorists is the denial of *objective* epistemic standards for judging any psychological theory and a commitment to some form of postmodernism. If this position is correct, then ultimately issues about the status of the Freudian evidence, experimental and non-experimental, may be subjective (for a critique of postmodernist epistomologies, see Erwin, 1996, chapter 3). A related strategy is to adopt some form of relativism. In a report on psychoanalytic therapy by A Subcommittee on Efficacy Research of the Committee on Scientific Activities of the American Psychoanalytic Association, the authors cite the work of Thomas Kuhn to justify epistemic standards peculiar to a psychoanalytic paradigm, standards that do not require evidence from controlled experiments (Bachrach et al., 1991; for a critique of their view, see Erwin, 1996, chapter 6).

Assuming that there are at least some objective epistemic standards—the correctness of which does not depend on what anyone believes—there is still much room for disagreement. In some of his writings, Freud worried about the need to rule out a constant threat to his clinical arguments: that his data could be equally well explained by appealing to unwitting suggestion instead of psychonanalytic hypotheses. There is an empirical issue here concerning the details of these suggestion hypotheses, but suppose in a given experimental study, a solid case is made that a suggestion (or placebo) hypothesis is at least as credible as the psychoanalytic hypothesis being tested. Does that mean that there is no confirmation of the psychoanalytic hypothesis? Some scholars would say that depends; the ruling out of credible hypotheses is not necessary for confirmation (Fine and Forbes, 1986; Wilkes, 1988). Some psychoanalytic investigators implicitly commit as well to denial of the need to rule out credible alternatives when they claim that if a prediction is derived from a Freudian hypothesis, and the prediction is experimentally confirmed, then that is always sufficient for confirmation—regardless of whether credible rivals are ruled out (Hall, 1963). For an argument that there is no confirmation of an hypothesis at all if there is a failure to rule out even one credible rival, see Erwin, 1996: 44–54; Erwin and Siegel, 1989.

Another disputed issue concerns the appeal to inference to the best explanation. Freud sometimes took the position that the fact that his theory would, if true, explain certain facts provided some grounds for thinking that his explanation is correct. This view has been expressed as a rule of inference by some philosophers: If H explains certain facts (i.e. it would explain the facts if it were true), and no available competing hypothesis explains the facts as well, then one can infer that there is some empirical evidence for H. Without being formally stated, this rule is often relied on in the Freudian experimental literature (for arguments that it is incorrect, see Erwin, 1996: 62–73).

There are other standards in dispute in the Freudian experimental literature, concerning, for example, the role of simplicity and systematicity, and standards for assessing causal relevance (see Erwin, 1996, chapter 2). Enough has been said, however, to suggest that there is much room for reasonable disagreement in assessing the Freudian experimental literature. Given that there are over 1,500 Freudian experimental studies to evaluate, the task of reaching a reasoned, defensible overall assessment is difficult. However, that task has been made easier by the valuable work of Kline (1981) and Fisher and Greenberg (1985) who sift the experimental record and try to distinguish the sound studies from the unsound. As these scholars argue, there are many Freudian experimental studies that fail to meet reasonable evidential standards. Apart from individual design flaws, in many cases, there are one or two experimental studies with a positive outcome, but the absence of any sustained efforts to replicate the studies. This failure is doubly important: Without multiple replications reasonable alternative explanations of the original data are often left undiscovered and there is the additional problem of generalizing the results to larger populations.

Despite the problems, both Kline (1981) and Fisher and Greenberg (1985) reach a favorable verdict about some of the studies. As Kline puts it, his review of the Freudian experimental literature shows that not all of Freud's theory is supported but that "much of it has been confirmed" (p. 441) (see as well, "Scientific Tests of Freud's Theories and Therapy"; and "Research on Psychoanalysis," this volume). Erwin (1996) reviews the same experimental studies as these other scholars, plus some more recent studies, and concludes that virtually no distinctively Freudian theoretical hypothesis is well supported by the experimental evidence.

Whatever verdict is the correct one, it is subject to modification if new Freudian experimental studies warrant a different assessment. There is also an important point to consider made by Eagle (2000, p. 167): "In my view, as one increasingly attempts a systematic empirical, but ecologically valid, investigation of psychoanalytic ideas, propositions, and concepts, they will not necessarily survive in their original and unaltered form." Eagle gives as an example recent empirical work on repressive style, the concept of which is both similar to but also different from Freud's concept of repression (see Eagle, 2000, and "Repression," this volume).

One could be interested in the Freudian experimental literature for multiple reasons. Some scholars are primarily interested in making sense of *Freud's* overall contribution, to sift the true from the false in his work; for them, the issue of whether experimentally tested propositions are distinctively Freudian is important. Some philosophers, however, are primarily interested in the epistemological issues raised by Freud's arguments; many of these issues could just as well be raised about non-Freudian psychoanalytic theories, as well as certain cognitive and behavioral theories. For someone interested primarily in the epistemology, the question of whether certain tested propositions are distinctively

E

Freudian or merely resemble Freudian concepts may be only marginally important. One could also be primarily interested in certain psychological ideas whether they are genuinely Freudian or merely suggested by things that Freud wrote. From the latter point of view, insisting that the hypotheses being evaluated be distinctively Freudian is to adopt the wrong standard.

REFERENCES

Bachrach, H., Galatzer-Levy, Skolnikoff, A., and Waldron, S. (1991). On the efficacy of psychoanalysis. *Journal of the American Pschoanalytic Association*, 39: 871–916.

Eagle, M. (1986). Critical Notice: A. Grünbaum's The Foundations of Psychoanalysis: A Philosophical Critique. *Philosophy of Science*, 53: 65–88.

———. (2000). Repression Part II of II. *The Psychoanalytic Review*, 87 (2): 161–187.

Erwin, E. (1996). *A Final Accounting: Philosophical and Empirical Issues in Freudian Psychology*. Cambridge, Mass.: MIT Press.

———. (1997). *Philosophy and Psychotherapy: Razing the Troubles of the Brain*. London: Sage.

Erwin, E., and Siegel, H. (1988). Is confirmation differential? *British Journal for the Philosophy of Science*, 40: 105–119.

Eysenck, H. J., and Wilson, G. D. (1973). *The Experimental Study of Freudian Theories*. London: Methuen.

Fine, A., and Forbes, M. (1986). Grünbaum on Freud: Three grounds for dissent. *The Behavioral and Brain Sciences*, 9: 237–238.

Fisher, S., and Greenberg, R. (1977). *The Scientific Credibility of Freud's Theories and Therapy*. New York: Basic Books.

———. (1996). *Freud Scientifically Appraised: Testing the Theories and Therapy*. New York: Wiley.

Freud, S. (1885). Contribution to the knowledge of the effect of cocaine. In R. Byck (ed.). *Cocaine Papers: Sigmund Freud*. New York: New American Library.

Grünbaum, A. (1984). *The Foundation of Psychoanalysis: A Philosophical Critique*. Berkeley, Calif.: University of California Press.

———. (1993). *Validation in the Clinical Theory of Psychoanalysis*. Madison, Conn.: International Universities Press.

Hall, G. S. (1963). Strangers in dreams: An experimental confimation of the Oedipus complex. *Journal of Personality*, 3: 336–345.

Kline, P. (1981). *Fact and Fantasy in Freudian Theory*, 1st ed., 1972. London: Methuen.

Levy, D. (1996). *Freud Among the Philosophers*. New Haven, Conn.: Yale University Press.

Luborsky, L., Mellon, J., van Ravenswaay, P., Childress, A., Cohen, K., Hole, A., Ming, S., Crits-Christoph, P., Levine, F., and Alexander, K. (1985). A verification of Freud's grandest clinical hypothesis: The transference. *Clinical Psychology Review*, 5: 231–246.

Wilkes, K. (1990). Analyzing Freud. *Philosophical Quarterly*, 40: 241–254.

EDWARD ERWIN

F

Family Romance

At Christmastime in 1908, Sigmund Freud wrote a few short pages about a concept that has come to be called the "family romance," which Otto Rank inserted into his own book on *Der Mythus von der Geburt des Helden (The Myth of the Birth of the Hero)*, published in 1909. The full article by Freud, *Der Familienroman der Neurotiker (Family Romances)*, did not appear as a separate published contribution until 1931 in a German-language volume of Freud's technical papers; and a proper English translation did not become available until 1950. Nevertheless, the concept of the family romance has remained very important in work with both adult patients and child patients.

A family romance may be defined as a deep-seated wish, which begins in early childhood, to become a member of a highly idealized family, such as a royal family, in preference to being a member of one's own biological family. As childhood unfolds, young boys and girls discover many different mechanisms, both creative and defensive, to avoid psychic pain, and the use of the family romance idea becomes one way of dealing with some of the unhappiness in one's own family home. By becoming the long lost son or daughter of a rich, famous, loving king or queen, one can temporarily escape from the unpleasantness or drudgery of one's actual mother and father.

Freud has suggested that this family romance may be regarded as a universal feature of psychic life, and that everyone will have indulged in one or more variants of a particular family romance throughout childhood, although such fantasies often become forgotten in later life. Freud did, however, posit that family romance fantasies may be recovered at some future date during the course of psychoanalytic treatment.

Freud has noted that envy of other peoples' parents can often fuel the development of a family romance—thus anticipating some of the ideas of Melanie Klein developed years later. In the more neurotic individuals, often punished in childhood for "sexual naughtiness" (Freud, 1909: 240), the mental strategy of replacing one's own parents with more ennobled ones gratifies the "motive of revenge and retaliation" (p. 239), thereby suggesting that the family romance contains a sadistic component. But Freud also recognized that the family romance can help young children to begin to separate from their actual parents, thereby anticipating the work of Margaret Mahler, Donald Winnicott, and other developmental psychologists. Such fantasies also assist in the growth of the child's imagination.

Freud identified a variation of the family romance wherein the child becomes chosen as the favorite by the parents, while all the brothers and sisters become bastardized. One can find this theme in the biblical story of Joseph and his brothers, one that held a special attraction for Freud, who had seven younger siblings with whom he had to contend. Freud also noted that family romance fantasies can help the child to bypass the danger of the incest taboo. If a little boy decides that he really is the son of the lord and lady of the manor, to use one of Freud's examples, then he need not worry about his incestuous feelings toward his actual mother or sister.

Very little secondary literature has developed around the concept of the family romance, although many clinicians still find it a useful idea in work with patients of all ages. Donald Winnicott, the British psychoanalyst, draws upon this implicitly in his work on transitional objects, namely, objects or fantasies that help a child to separate both physically and psychologically from the influence of the parents.

REFERENCES

Freud, S. (1909). *Family Romances*. S.E. 9: 237–241.

Winnicott, D. W. (1953). Transitional objects and transitional phenomena: A study of the first not-me possession. *International Journal of Psychoanalysis*, 34: 89–97.

———. (1971). *Playing and Reality*. London: Tavistock Publications.

                                                        BRETT KAHR

Fantasy (Phantasy)

In the first volume of the *Standard Edition of the Complete Psychological Works of Sigmund Freud*, the editor, James Strachey, notes that the word "phantasy" (imagination, visionary notion) conveys the sense of the original German "Phantasie" more accurately than "fantasy" (caprice, whim, fanciful invention). This convention, used throughout the Hogarth Press *Standard Edition*, will be adhered to in the following discussion.

The concept of *phantasy* plays a fundamental role in Freud's theoretical expositions and is one of the basic concepts of psychoanalysis. It generally denotes an unconscious psychical structure underlying (and generating) neurotic behavioral traits or symptoms, though Freud occasionally used it in the everyday sense of an imaginative narrative or scenario experienced consciously, as in a daydream.

The psychoanalytic theory of unconscious phantasies has its origins in speculative notions Freud employed in 1897 in the course of his investigations into the etiology of hysteria and obsessional neurosis (Masson, 1985: 239, 240–242, 246–248). At that time, he had postulated that repressed memories of sexual traumas in early childhood were the cause of his patients' symptoms, and had utilized his newly developed psychoanalytic technique as a means of revealing the unconscious memories. When he came to doubt that the "sexual scenes" that his clinical procedure had purportedly revealed represented genuine experiences in the infancies of his patients, he posited that they were mostly unconscious phantasies rather than repressed memories. The uncovering of the contents of his patients' unconscious phantasies became central to his therapeutic procedure, and played a major role in the first published psychoanalytic case history, the analysis of the patient known as "Dora," who was treated in 1900 (Freud, 1905). It was with his description of this case (*Fragment of an Analysis of a Case of Hysteria*, written in 1901) that the psychoanalytic technique was first given a detailed public presentation, though the basic elements of the methodology were implicit in *The Interpretation of Dreams* (1900).

The importance of the concept under discussion may be perceived from the fact that psychoanalysis may be regarded, in practical terms, as essentially a procedure by means of which unconscious ideas, or phantasies, may be divined. In Freud's words: "We have discovered technical methods of filling up the gaps in the phenomena of our consciousness. . . . In this manner we infer a number of processes which are in themselves 'unknowable' and interpolate them in those that are conscious to us" (1940, pp. 196–197). The "unknowable" processes are associated with unconscious phantasies that, unbeknown to the individual, influence much of human behavior; a major part of Freud's analyses was devoted to the uncovering of the postulated phantasies.

In an early exposition on the subject of "hysterical phantasies," Freud maintained that "[t]he motive forces of phantasies are unsatisfied wishes, and every single phantasy is the fulfilment of a wish, a correction of unsatisfying reality" (1908a, p. 146). Such wishes are almost invariably of a sexual nature and ultimately derive from infantile experiences (p. 147). The parallel between these notions and Freud's theory of dreams implies that the latter should also be viewed as phantasies; for instance, both are wish fulfillments and both are based to a great extent on impressions of infantile experiences (1900, p. 492).

Freud was professionally concerned with psychoneurotics, whose symptoms he posited to be the result of the conversion of unconscious phantasies into corresponding somatic manifestations or behavioral traits. Implicit in his theory is the notion that in the process of the formation of phantasies, disturbing thoughts or instinctual sexual impulses are repressed from consciousness; indeed, the motivation for the generation of phantasies is precisely the banishment from consciousness of unacceptable ideas (Masson, 1985: 240). The phantasy incorporates elements based on the repressed material (in disguised form), together with items derived from genuine (though usually innocuous) childhood experiences. In one of his earliest formulations, Freud postulated that "hysterical symptoms" are a consequence of phantasies "mostly produced during the years of puberty, which on the one side were built up out of and over the [repressed] childhood memories and on the other side were transformed directly into the symptoms" (1906, p. 274). Typically such childhood memories might relate to infantile autoerotic activities, or to infantile sexual impulses arising from the Oedipus complex. Freud maintained that the technique of psychoanalytic reconstruction, utilizing the interpretation of free associations and dreams, as well as of the somatic symptoms and neurotic behavioral traits themselves, enabled him to ascertain both the contents of the underlying unconscious phantasies and the infantile experiences or impulses that were the ultimate source of the phantasies.

In his paper *Hysterical Phantasies and Their Relation to Bisexuality*, Freud (1908b) provides a description that exemplifies his view of the origins and function of unconscious phantasies. The context is a discussion of the conscious daydreams (almost invariably of an erotic nature) of young men and women. Unconscious phantasies may be the derivatives of such daydreams that have been repressed, or they may have been unconscious all along. Either way, the phantasies derive from a previous period of masturbatory activity, during which the masturbatory act (in the widest sense of the word) was compounded of two parts. One was the evocation of a phantasy and the other some active behavior for obtaining self-gratification at the height of the phantasy. This in turn can be traced back to an infantile autoerotic practice for the purpose of obtaining pleasure from some particular part of the body, which subsequently became merged with a wishful idea from the sphere of object love. When, in adulthood, masturbatory satisfaction is renounced, the phantasy becomes entirely unconscious. In the absence of other modes of sexual satisfaction, if the subject does not succeed in sublimating his or her libido—that is, deflecting the sexual excitation to higher aims—the condition is fulfilled for the unconscious phantasy to generate pathological symptoms (1908b, pp. 159–161).

This exposition illustrates the indispensable role that the concept of unconscious phantasies plays in Freud's theory of neuroses. The ultimate cause of the neurotic symptom is a repressed memory of infantile sexual activity. The adult manifestation of the neurosis is a somatic (or behavioral) symptom. The unconscious phantasy provides the link between these two phenomena, without which an explanation of the symptom in terms of

Freud's theory of infantile sexuality would be incoherent. Seen in terms of his basic notions of psychical processes, the energy associated with the original childhood experience is held, or bound, in the unconscious phantasy before its eventual discharge in the form of a somatic symptom in the event of a sufficiently powerful conflict with the ego (1916–1917, pp. 373–375).

In psychoanalytic terms, phantasies may thus be considered as a neurotic substitute for sexual satisfaction. From a therapeutic viewpoint, their elucidation constitutes the first stage in uncovering the infantile experiences and impulses that lie at the root of neurotic symptoms. In Freud's words: "The technique of psychoanalysis enables us in the first place to infer from the symptoms what those unconscious phantasies are and then to make them conscious to the patient" (1908b, p. 162). But the interpretive process is actually two stage. For, as he observed in relation to "seduction phantasies," Freud had "learned to explain [these phantasies] as attempts at fending off memories of the subject's own sexual activity (infantile masturbation)" (1906, p. 274). In other words, both the unconscious phantasies underlying neurotic symptoms and the infantile impulses and experiences that were the prime source of the phantasies were inferred by Freud by means of the psychoanalytic reconstructive technique.

Clinical examples

To understand fully these notions, it is helpful to examine specific examples of their application. A clear exposition of the kinds of processes involved in the formation of phantasies and their manifestation in symptoms is to be found in Freud's analysis of what he called "hysterical attacks," that is, epileptic attacks that he believed to be of psychogenic origin. The basic premise is that as an infant the patient had engaged in autoerotic activity, without ideational content. The same satisfaction is then connected with an associated phantasy, which later replaces the original activity. The essential components comprising the subsequent neurosis are the *repressed memory* of the infantile sexual activity, the *phantasy* generated at a later date (usually around puberty) in which the repressed memory plays a disguised role (enabling the subject to still obtain sexual satisfaction), and the *neurotic symptom*, resulting from repression of the phantasy (1909, pp. 232–233).

In the "Dora" case history, Freud made implicit use of these notions in his analysis of the patient's asthmatic attacks, which he regarded as hysterical and originating from childhood masturbation: "Hysterical symptoms hardly ever appear so long as children are masturbating, but only afterwards, when a period of abstinence has set in; they form a substitute for masturbatory satisfaction, the desire for which continues to persist in the unconscious until another and more normal kind of satisfaction appears—where that is still attainable." The precipitating factor in Dora's case, which "replaced her inclination to masturbation by an inclination to anxiety," was identified as her overhearing sexual intercourse taking place between her parents. A short time after this experience, when her father was away and the child was wishing him back, she reproduced in the form of an attack of asthma the impression she had received. She had preserved in her memory (in symbolic form) the event that occasioned the first onset of the symptom (1905, pp. 79–80). The process, then, can be seen to be essentially the same as that described above: childhood masturbatory activity was repressed, and in its place there occurred an unconscious phantasy with a sexual content. The asthma attacks were a consequence of the conversion of the psychical energy associated with the unconscious phantasy into somatic symptoms.

The same process was thought by Freud to underlie obsessional behavior. In his chapter on "The Sense of Symptoms" in *Introductory Lectures on Psycho-analysis* (1916–1917), he described the role of unconscious phantasy in the case of a young woman who felt compelled to perform a sleep ceremony each night before retiring to bed. Among other rituals, the large pillow at the top end of her bed had not to touch the wooden back of the bedstead, and a small top pillow had to lie precisely on the large pillow so as to form a diamond shape. Her head had then to lie exactly along the long diameter of the diamond. Finally, the eiderdown had to be shaken in such a way that the bottom end became very thick, and this accumulation of feathers was then evened out. The unconscious phantasy underlying these actions was uncovered on the basis of proposed interpretations and the analysis of associations. The patient regarded the large pillow as representing a woman, and the upright wooden back of the bed a man: thus she had devised a magical way of keeping the man and woman apart—that is, to prevent her father and mother from having sexual intercourse. In Freud's interpretation, the shaking down of the eiderdown until all the feathers were at the bottom end represented making a woman pregnant: the

smoothing out procedure was to ensure that she was not presented with a competing sibling. Finally, the big pillow being a woman, it followed that the small top pillow stood for the daughter. The diamond shape represented the open female genitals. Thus when she placed her head in position she was herself playing the man and replacing the male organ with her head. Linking this analysis of the patient's sleep ceremonial with her other symptoms, Freud concluded that at a deeper level the girl was exhibiting an erotic attachment to her father, the origins of which went back to early childhood (1916–1917, pp. 264–269). In other words, the obsessional behavior was the acting out of unconscious phantasy, the contents of which could be traced to repressed memories of infantile (Oedipal) impulses. As is the case with other neurotic symptoms, obsessional behavior derives from sexual impulses in early childhood that have been repressed and find expression in unconscious phantasy.

Critical Appraisal

For the critic of psychoanalysis, Freud's theory of unconscious phantasies is problematic because of its heavy reliance on analytic assumptions. In Freud's schema, as we have seen, such phantasies have their origins ultimately in infantile sexual impulses, notably autoerotic behavior or Oedipal wishes. The contents both of the phantasies and of their purported infantile origins are arrived at by analytic inference. But the above examples, which are entirely characteristic, indicate that the latter depends heavily on preconceived notions that largely, if not wholly, determine the direction of the analysis. As Freud himself observed, the crucial infantile experiences were not obtainable any longer as such (i.e., as memories) but had to be determined by interpretation of transferences and dreams (1900, p. 184). In other words, as he explained in an article on his psychoanalytic procedure, the unconscious material (both the inferred phantasy and the infantile impulse or experience from which it derives) had to be reconstructed by the analyst from patients' associations (1904, p. 252). The building blocks of such reconstructions, whether of the phantasies underlying symptoms or of the infantile experiences that determine the contents of the phantasies, were Freud's own hypothetical conceptions. The critic of psychoanalysis may conclude, with some justification, that this procedure is essentially circular, and that clinical findings based on such an approach are generated not so much by the patients' productions as by the input of the analyst. The findings claimed to have been obtained by such a procedure are therefore questionable.

Nevertheless, whatever the shortcomings of Freud's specific notions, a more flexible concept of unconscious phantasies has remained influential in psychoanalytic theory and practice, both in regard to the analysis of neurotic symptoms and in relation to theories of child development. (At one extreme, in the work of Melanie Klein and her followers, the latter application has been extended to an analysis of the earliest months of childhood.) In its more generalized form, the notion of unconscious phantasies refers to internalized psychical structures that govern a person's more or less irrational assumptions and responses in relation to events and to individuals. Life experiences and relationships with individuals may then be endowed with a significance determined by unconscious phantasy rather than by reality, resulting in inappropriate behavior on the part of the person concerned. In psychoanalytic theory, if a person undergoes a psychoanalysis, the transference relationship with the analyst will inevitably be colored by the patient's unconscious phantasies, so that neurotic relationships will be reenacted in the therapeutic setting, and hence will be amenable to modification once the source of the inappropriate behavior has been brought to consciousness. The detecting and uncovering of these phantasies is thus a central concern of the analyst, and largely determines the direction of the analysis.

Freud expressed these latter notions in the following terms: "The patient . . . directs towards the physician a degree of affectionate feeling (mingled, often enough, with hostility) which is based on no real relation between them and which . . . can only be traced back to old wishful phantasies of the patient's which have become unconscious. Thus the part of the patient's emotional life which he can no longer recall to memory is re-experienced by him in his relation to the physician; and it is only his re-experiencing in the 'transference' that convinces him of the existence and of the power of these unconscious sexual impulses" (1910, p. 51). The therapeutic process requires the physician to convince the patient that "his feelings do not arise from the present situation and do not apply to the person of the doctor, but that they are repeating something that happened to him earlier. In this way we oblige him to transform his repetition into a memory. By that means the transference . . . becomes [the treatment's] best tool, by whose help the most secret compartments of mental life can be opened" (1916–1917, pp. 443–444).

As George Klein writes, "[t]he principle of the motivational activity of repressed schemata has been an enormously generative one in psychoanalytic thought and has led to a number of vital analytic propositions; e.g., the notion of an inner reality of unconscious fantasy in which introjected relationships hemmed in by contradictory affects and conflicts are nonetheless active in producing and responding to replicas of such relationships in interpersonal encounters" (Klein, 1976: 255). Marshall Edelson describes such schemata as "master stories," generally concerned with the fulfillment of a childhood sexual or hostile wish, and asserts as an empirical claim of psychoanalysis that stories told by an analysand in the therapeutic context are unwitting "derivatives" of such unconscious master stories. In the course of therapy, "[t]he psychoanalyst repeatedly intervenes in ways that are designed to make fully accessible to consciousness what the analysand struggles to keep unconscious— namely, an unconscious fantasy and also that fantasy's immediate particular links to external reality" (Edelson, 1992: 104–107, 113).

These modern formulations, while perhaps persuasive in abstract terms, are less so in practice. The observation that the determining of the contents of the unconscious phantasies is overdependent on the preconceptions of the analyst remains apposite. That the patient's own perceptions, and even memories, of his or her past may be contaminated by preconceived notions conveyed by the analyst has been amply demonstrated (Grünbaum, 1984: 208–215, 241–245; Erwin, 1996: 98–106). The compliance of patients toward interpretations proposed by analysts cannot necessarily be taken as an indication of the truth of the interpretations, however broadly one defines the notion of "truth" (Macmillan, 1991: 562 [1997: 575–576]). Nor does there seem to be any way to validate specific interpretations. Reputable analysts may detect unconscious phantasies of a character that eludes the investigations of other eminent analysts. This is especially so in regard to the findings claimed by different schools of psychoanalysis (pp. 572–575 [1997, pp. 585–589]).

In an historically based appraisal of the analytic interpretive process, Donald Spence writes that, for the psychoanalyst, "[t]he world of natural objects has become, once again, a world of hidden and not-so-hidden meanings, opaque to the naïve but transparent to the initiated who can see below the surface into the depths of being. . . . The analyst scans the world (and the patients' free-associations) for resemblances that will tell the analyst what latent content lies beneath the surface appearance." But in adopting this approach, Spence argues, the analyst is not only using an outmoded form of reasoning, based on the natural, but often fallacious, tendency to look on similar patterns as somehow related, he or she also tends to listen to the clinical material with a favorite set of theoretical predispositions. Moreover, the belief that a well-crafted interpretation can bring about a significant clinical effect is one that has never been validated (Spence, 1992: 561–563).

The concept of unconscious phantasy nevertheless remains a potent force within psychoanalytic theory and practice. On the assumption that early experiences color our emotional and psychological responses in later life, it encapsulates a way of envisaging the psychological processes involved. This view has been succinctly expressed by Ilham Dilman in terms that do not necessarily presuppose invariable features of early childhood experiences, and are thus without the problematic elements of more specifically psychoanalytic formulations: "What thus 'migrates' into a person's later relationships, his interests and preoccupations, are constellations of feeling, the contents of which are rudimentary thoughts and expectations which originally found expression in his emotional reactions as a child" (Dilman, 1984: 36). If one does not presume that such constellations of feelings are necessarily fixations, unmodified by subsequent experiences, it is in such terms that the concept of unconscious phantasy may best be understood in its least controversial form.

REFERENCES

Dilman, I. (1984). *Freud and the Mind*. Oxford: Basil Blackwell.

Edelson, Marshall. (1992). Telling and enacting stories in psychoanalysis. J. Barron, M. Eagle, and D. Wolitzky (eds.). In *Interface of Psychoanalysis and Psychology*. Washington, D.C.: American Psychological Association, pp. 99–124.

Ellenberger, H. F. *Beyond the Unconscious: Essays of Henri F. Ellenberger in the History of Psychiatry*. Introduced and edited by M. S. Micale, Translated by F. Dubor and M. S. Micale. Princeton, N.J.: Princeton University Press.

Erwin, E. (1996). *A Final Accounting: Philosophical and Empirical Issues in Freudian Psychology*. Cambridge, Mass.: MIT Press.

Freud, S. (1900). *The Interpretation of Dreams*. S.E. 4–5: 1–621.

———. (1904). Freud's psycho-analytic procedure. S.E. 7: 249–254.

———. (1905). Fragment of an analysis of a case of hysteria. S.E. 7: 7–122.

———. (1906). My views on the part played by sexuality in the aetiology of the neuroses. S.E. 9: 271–279.

———. (1908a). Creative writers and day-dreaming. S.E. 9: 143–153.

———. (1908b). Hysterical phantasies and their relation to bisexuality. S.E. 9: 159–166.

———. (1909). Some general remarks on hysterical attacks. S.E. 9: 229–234.

———. (1910). Five lectures on psycho-analysis. S.E. 11: 7–55.

———. (1916–1917). *Introductory Lectures on Psycho-analysis*. S.E. 15–16: 9–496.

———. (1940). *An Outline of Psycho-analysis*. S.E. 23: 144–207.

Grünbaum, A. (1984). *The Foundations of Psychoanalysis: A Philosophical Critique*. Berkeley: University of California Press.

Klein, G. S. (1976). *Psychoanalytic Theory: An Exploration of Essentials*. New York: International Universities Press.

Macmillan, M. (1991). *Freud Evaluated: The Completed Arc*. Amsterdam: Elsevier North-Holland; Rev. ed., Cambridge, Mass.: MIT Press, 1997.

Masson, J. M. (translator and editor). (1985). *The Complete Letters of Sigmund Freud to Wilhelm Fliess 1887–1904*. Cambridge, Mass.: Harvard University Press.

Spence, D. P. (1992). Interpretation: A critical perspective. In J. W. Barron, M. N. Eagle, and D. L. Wolitzky (eds.). *Interface of Psychoanalysis and Psychology*. Washington, D.C.: American Psychological Association, pp. 558–572.

ALLEN ESTERSON

Fechner, Gustav Theodor (1801–1887)

Myths cloak this founder of experimental psychology in the robes of a bizarre panpsychic mystic with an oriental strain. Yet, his famous *Elemente der Psychophysik* (1860) created the field of experimental psychology and is regarded as the major work on experimental design before the 1935 appearance of Sir R. A. Fisher's *Design of Experiments*. *Elemente* also developed many ideas about mind that caused Freud to regard Fechner's work with undisguised enthusiasm, referring to "the great Fechner" and to Fechner's works in such books as *The Interpretation of Dreams*, *Beyond the Pleasure Principle*, and *The Wit and the Unconscious*. Freud declared: "I have followed that thinker upon many important points" (Freud, 1925: 59; Sulloway, 1979).

Born in 1801 in the village of Gross-Särchen near Muskau, Niederlausitz, Gustav Theodor Fechner was son and grandson of Presbyterian ministers. His father died when the son was five years old, but not before

Fechner learned to speak with him in Latin as well as German. During the next nine years Fechner and his brother lived with an uncle, also a minister. At age sixteen, Fechner matriculated at Leipzig University as a medical student. He studied under Ernst Heinrich Weber, the anatomist-physiologist and, in 1823, passed the Magisterexamen (Rigorosum), which included the degree of doctor of philosophy. His humorous side appeared in his first publication, a piece written under his lifelong nom de plume "Dr. Mises," satirizing the popular use of iodine as a panacea ("Proof that the moon is made of Iodine," 1821).

Although his interest in physiological processes never waned, he soon began studies of physics and the experiments on Ohm's law that made him famous. His slim means required that he support his scientific work by applying his skill at languages. During the next ten years he translated to German from French some four volumes of Biot's *Experimental Physics* and seven volumes of Thénard's *Textbook of Theoretical and Practical Chemistry*—a total of nearly eight thousand pages—and edited the pharmaceutical journal *Pharmaceutisches Centralblatt*.

His own writings were equally voluminous: *A Catechism or Examination of Human Physiology, A Catechism on Logic or the Laws of Thought,* and many smaller works. In 1830, he published *An Elementary Textbook on Electromagnetism* and in 1831 received the title extraordinary professor of philosophy at Leipzig University. His three-volume *Repertory of Experimental Physics* appeared in 1832. He also edited, and wrote in large part, the eight-volume *Hauslexicon* of nearly nine hundred pages per volume. By age thirty-two, Fechner was well known for his physics experiments and translations, and was acquainted with the greatest modern physicists in Germany and France. In 1834, he became professor in ordinary at Leipzig University. He founded and directed Leipzig's first Institute of Physics, and remained part of Leipzig and the intellectual community of the *deutscher Gelehrter* until his death in 1887.

Fechner's ideas about the mind developed in the intense intellectual climate of nineteenth-century Germany. The air was alive with speculation about the mind, or soul, owing in part to Herbart's famous *Psychologie als Wissenschaft* (1824–1825). E. H. Weber, wondering how the mind creates the concept of external space, explored the question through experimentation. His renowned physiopsychological studies of touch in rela-

tion to the concept of space appeared in Leipzig in 1834 (*De Tactu*). Stimulated by Weber, Fechner's first semi-psychological papers on subjective complementary colors appeared in 1838. Important work on afterimages surfaced in 1840. The speculative philosopher in Fechner wondered about the relationship between the external world and the soul, between physical processes and the mind. The physicist in Fechner wondered how aspects of the mind, such as Herbart's threshold of consciousness or Weber's threshold of sensation, might be measured.

In 1839, following a decade of strenuous work and disastrous retinal damage created during his introspective studies of visual afterimages, he collapsed into what William James later diagnosed as a "habit neurosis." Henri Ellenberger described Fechner's illness as a severe neurotic depression with hypochondriacal symptoms, if not "sublime hypochondriasis, a creative illness from which a person emerges with a new philosophical insight and a transformation in their personality" (1970, p. 216). Fechner himself describes in detail the suffering and uncontrolled thoughts experienced during this difficult time.

The three-year illness did not escape later attention from psychoanalysts interested in Fechner's life work. Imre Hermann's *A Psychoanalytical Study of Individual Personality as the Basis for the Development of Scientific Ideas* (1926) describes Fechner's secluded life in a darkened room as a womblike existence, during which both his mother and his wife read to him, and from which Fechner was reborn. The rebirth melded together the religious heritage of a son of the manse with the intellectual rigor of a seasoned scientist.

After nearly three years, Fechner miraculously recovered and entered a phase of elation that culminated in the discovery of his first law of the mind, "das Lust-princip des Handelns" (the pleasure principle of action). *On the Highest Good (Über das höchste Gut)*, a study of the *Lustprincip*, appeared in 1846. Fechner argued that the search for pleasure and the avoidance of unpleasure were forces driving human conduct.

In 1848, in his famous *Nanna, oder über das Seelenleben der Pflanzen* (of the soul-life of plants), he conjectured: "and now one can ask whether such a life [of animate creatures] pertains also to the plants, whether they too are animate individuals for themselves, combining in themselves impulses and sensations, or maybe more psychic experiences. If this were so, then the plants along with men and animals would constitute a common contrast to stones and all the things we call dead" (Lowrie, 1946: 164).

Fechner's 1851 rendering of *Zend-Avesta, Über die Dinge des Himmels und des Jenseits : vom Standpunkt der Naturbetrachtung* (about heavenly things and the hereafter from the standpoint of contemplating nature) established the idea that all life forms were self-aware, conscious. Even more, that consciousness pervaded all things, was in all and through all. Earth itself was conscious. Fechner did not choose the title by whim. *Zend-Avesta*, the sacred book of Zoroastrianism, contains the teachings of their prophet Zoroaster.

Fechner's *Zend-Avesta* describes the moment on October 22, 1850, when he awoke with an answer to his question about the relation between mind and body. He suddenly saw a new interpretation of Weber's discovery that a just noticeable difference (*jnd*) in sensation is felt when a new stimulus increases by a fixed constant proportion beyond the magnitude of the stimulus against which it is judged. This law of increased sensation established the *jnd* as a unit of psychological experience, as important to psychology as the mole is to chemistry or the quantum to physics. The *jnd* allowed Fechner to create his second law—a formula describing the relation between physical magnitudes and sensation magnitude. The formula set Fechner on the course of scientific experimentation that marks the origin of experimental psychology.

The experimentation culminated in the two-volume 907-page *Elemente der Psychophysik* (1860). In this breathtaking work, Fechner creates another pillar for his foundation for the scientific study of the mind—the theory of mental discrimination. Fechner proposed that the senses act as a measuring device for the mind. However, the measuring device is not perfect. The sensory measurements are disturbed by the same form of intrinsic measurement error previously proposed by Gauss in the *Theory of Celestial Motions* (1809).

Given that sense-error clouds our perceptions, how does the mind distinguish so accurately between two quite similar stimuli? The theory, presented early in *Elemente*, vol. 1 (pp. 85–91), generates the first experimental tests of invisible actions of the mind. Today the theory is called statistical decision theory and, specifically in engineering and psychology, ideal observer theory.

In the last two hundred pages of *Elemente*, vol. 2, Fechner defines "inner psychophysics," the study of the mind without regard to its sensory connections. Here he discusses mental energy, the structure of the mental landscape, the use of dreams for investigating the workings of the mind, the nature of consciousness and subconsciousness, memory, hallucinations, and illusions and psychophysical continuity and discontinuity. Many of these ideas formed the foundation for generations of psychological research and theorizing.

The last twenty-seven years of his life saw an astonishing number of publications that expanded his ideas about the mind and consciousness. In 1861, he published *Über die Seelenfrage : ein Gang durch die sichtbare Welt, um die unsichtbare zu finden* (*Concerning the Soul*), and in 1863, *Die Drei Motive und Gründe des Glaubens* (*The Three Motives and Grounds of Faith*). His 1866 publication *Das Associationprincip in der Aesthetik* foreshadowed the founding of the field of experimental aesthetics. In 1871, the path was set with *Zur experimentellen Aesthetik*. The two-volume *Vorschule der Aesthetik* (1876) established the field. Returning to psychophysics in 1877, he published *In Sachen der Psychophysik*, in 1882 *Revision der Hauptpunkte der Psychophysik* and in 1884 the extensive, 310-page theoretical and experimental study, *On the Method of Right and Wrong Cases*.

Throughout his long career as student-physician, physiologist, physicist, chemist, psychophysicist, aestheticist, philosopher, professor, poet, and satirist, Fechner called upon the world to recognize the fundamental unity of mind and physical reality. To prove his point, he created a theory of mind and a scientific method to investigate it—a theory that remains as vital today as it was astonishing in 1850.

REFERENCES

Altmann, I. (1995). *Bibliographie Gustav Theodor Fechner.* Leipzig: Verlag im Wissenschaftszentrum Leipzig.

Ellenberger, H. F. (1956). Fechner and Freud. *Bulletin of the Menninger Clinic*, 20: 201–214.

———. (1970) *The Discovery of the Unconscious: The History and Evolution of Dynamic Psychiatry.* New York: Basic Books.

Fechner, G. T. (1860). *Elemente der Psychophysic.* Leipzig: Breitkopf and Härtel.

Freud, S. (1925). *An Autobiographical Study.* S.E. 20: 7–74.

Hermann, I. (1926). *Gustav Theodor Fechner, eine Psychoanalytische Studie über individuelle Bedingtheiten Wissenschaftlicher Ideen.* Leipzig: Internationaler Psychoanalytischer Verlag.

Lowrie, W. (1946). *Fechner, Religion of a Scientist.* New York: Pantheon.

Marks, L. E. (1992). Freud and Fechner, desire and energy, hermeneutics and psychophysics. In H. G. Geissler, S. W. Link, and J. T. Townsend (eds.) *Cognition, Information Processing and Psychophysics: Basic Issues.* Hillsdale, N.J.: Lawrence Erlbaum Publishers.

Sulloway, F. J. (1979). *Freud, Biologist of the Mind: Beyond the Psychoanalytic Legend.* New York: Basic Books.

Villa, G. (1903). *Contemporary Psychology.* New York: Macmillan.

STEPHEN W. LINK

Feminism, and Psychoanalysis

The early relationship between the feminist movement to improve women's condition in society and the theories and practices of Freud and his followers was markedly antagonistic. Beginning in the 1970s, however, some feminists defended psychoanalysis as necessary for understanding, and so for transforming, the unconscious ways people internalize the rules and values of male-dominated cultures where women take care of children. In recent decades, academic feminists have extended psychoanalytic approaches to literature and culture, while practicing therapists have assimilated many feminist views.

Freud's View of Feminism

Freud disparaged the nineteenth- and early-twentieth-century European and American feminists who sought social equality and the vote; post–World War II feminists, in turn, condemned Freud and his theories on the grounds that psychoanalysis devalued women and encouraged conformity to unjust societies.

Although Freud's opinions about women and femininity were complex, he was consistently antagonistic to feminism. He first developed his theories in clinical work with troubled women. Sometimes he saw women as similar but inferior to men; sometimes he stressed women's different nature; sometimes he assumed an original bisexuality; often he ignored gender differences. Yet throughout his life, he ridiculed feminist insistence on women's equality with men, which he interpreted as the false claim that women were identical to men in function and value.

When courting Martha Bernays, Freud wrote her criticizing John Stuart Mill's vision of women as potential competitors rather than as charming helpmates: "women are different beings—we will not say lesser, rather the opposite—from men" (Jones, 1953: 176). During the suffrage campaigns, he claimed that only a few women benefited from the women's movement. In this period, he believed that boys and girls began their development in parallel, that the sexual drive in both sexes was masculine, that women's anatomy prefigured their lesser destiny, but that women's intellectual inferiority might be attributed to the stricter morality imposed on them by society.

In the 1920s and 1930s, Freud changed his views on women in response to other analysts, particularly Karen Horney and Ernest Jones. He professed ignorance of the "dark continent" of women's sexuality (1926, p. 212) but still judged women to be morally weaker than men, a view he defended against "the denials of the feminists, who are anxious to force us to regard the two sexes as completely equal in position and worth": "the feminist demand for equal rights for the sexes does not take us far," he pronounced, because "Anatomy is Destiny" (1924, p. 178).

Feminist Responses to Freud

As Freudian psychology gained ascendancy after Freud's death, especially in the United States, the influence of feminism waned, ushering in a postwar period of conformity, family values, and misogyny that the revivers of feminism later attributed, in part, to popularized psychoanalysis. In *The Second Sex* (1949), Simone de Beauvoir developed a feminist critique of psychoanalysis that was repeated for decades. She charged that Freud saw only men as fully human, regarding women as mutilated men, relegating them to the position of the Other with respect to the male self. Moreover, de Beauvoir claimed, Freud slighted women in his studies and falsely credited anatomy for male supremacy in culture and public life. She argued, instead, that social factors explained the observable characteristics and relationships of the sexes. Like many of Freud's early feminist critics, she found the concept of women's penis envy particularly galling, interpreting it as evidence of displaced male penis pride. She claimed that the phallus in Freud's and Jacques Lacan's thought symbolized male social dominance but could not explain it, adding that the concept of the unconscious undermined the moral responsibility necessary for women as well as men to choose transcendence. Unfortunately, according to de Beauvoir, psychoanalysis tied individuals to a determined childhood past rather than inspiring them to find future freedom.

F

In the United States, Betty Friedan's *The Feminine Mystique* (1963) inaugurated the women's liberation movement by calling attention to "the problem without a name," the unhappiness of educated, middle-class suburban women. Friedan saw Freud as a prisoner of his Victorian culture who wanted to adapt people to society rather than fight social injustice, and she accused him of sexual solipsism. In Friedan's view, however, the popularizers who made psychoanalysis an American religion were worse than Freud. They preached sexual activity as the road to happiness and derided feminists for their neurotic failure to be real women. In contrast, Friedan argued that wives and mothers were unhappy not because they were neurotic, but because their justified yearnings for equal opportunity were stifled.

Many feminists agreed that Freud was limited by the sexist ideas of his culture; they saw psychoanalysis as a conformist force that demeaned women and sought to confine them to limited roles within the family. They repeatedly attacked Freud's belief in female inferiority and his narcissism in assuming a male norm for humanity. The French psychoanalyst Luce Irigiray, like Horney earlier, compared Freud's views on sexual differences to childish prejudices. Irigiray concluded that psychoanalysis understood only the male sex and defined women as castrated men. Even more reprehensible to many feminists was Freud's conclusion that women were morally inferior to men and less able to reason abstractly because they lacked castration anxiety as an incentive for identification with civilized law. These feminists charged psychoanalysis with placing women in a double bind: the normal woman was passive, masochistic, narcissistic, and morally inferior, but the woman who lacked these traits was masculine, abnormal, developmentally arrested, and neurotic. Popular psychoanalysis defined female activity outside the home through such negative characterizations as "masculine protest" and "the masculinity complex," and it stigmatized lesbians as neurotic and perverse.

Feminists also objected to Freud's view that the Oedipal stage of child development was the necessary gateway to normal gender development, heterosexuality, and civilization. They felt that Freud justified paternal power and slighted mothers; they especially objected to the "mother blaming" of popularized Freudianism, including the anti-Mommism of the 1950s and the postulation in the 1960s of the so-called schizophrenogenic mother. Doris Lessing's influential novel *The Golden Notebook*, for example, portrayed infantile men who quote analysts against mothers, wives, and mistresses. The radical feminist Mary Daly charged that psychoanalysis blamed both female patients and their mothers for the unhappiness, injury, and abuse inflicted on women by men—variations of the practice of blaming the victim.

Fundamental to these objections is the feminist belief that psychoanalysis diverts attention from real social problems by pathologizing women's misery and attributing it to their unconscious desires; for example, feminists thought that depression in middle-aged women was caused by their overinvestment in feminine roles, so that selfless mothers were left desolate when children outgrew the nest. Some feminists questioned the existence of the unconscious altogether.

As psychoanalytic practice spread in the United States, feminists condemned it as another instance of men's manipulation of women for their own benefit. Daly defined "therapist" as "the/rapist," and claimed that psychoanalysts colonized women's bodies and controlled their minds. Other feminists were suspicious of the intimacy of transference, particularly between male analyst and female patient, and charged some analysts with seducing their patients, taking sexual and financial advantage of their vulnerability and so impeding a genuine cure. The most extreme critics today charge that Freud's texts encourage criminal violence against women. For example, Andrea Dworkin calls Freud a philosopher of sex and death whose devaluation of women's genitals contributes to their rape and murder.

Among the most controversial recent attacks on psychoanalysis is the contention that it protects incest and child abuse by attributing such allegations to the victim's fantasies rather than to repressed and then recalled memories of real events. Former members of the analytic community, such as Jeffrey Moussaieff Masson, join radical feminists in thinking that Freud's earliest views on the origins of neurosis in sexual abuse were correct and that he only disavowed them due to professional ambition, cowardice, or identification with the male perpetrators. They support victims who confront their attackers and institute criminal proceedings. Other feminists acknowledge that crimes against women and children are widespread and underreported, yet they fault poorly trained therapists for implanting false memories in women's minds; some question the concept of repression; others criticize notions of women's and children's purity that ignore unconscious fantasy and the malleability of memory.

Feminist Defenses of Psychoanalysis

Despite the hostile relationship between Freud and feminism, early psychoanalysis depended on women as patients, patrons, and practitioners. Breuer's patient Bertha Pappenheim, or "Anna O.," invented the talking cure and pioneered social work, and Fliess's patient Emma Eckstein was the first analyst Freud trained. Freud defended women's rights to become analysts, even as he praised his female acolytes for their masculine minds; in his final years, his daughter Anna often publicly presented his views. Psychoanalysis remained much more inclusive of women than did traditional medicine, especially in those communities that did not require analysts to be physicians. Anna Freud and Melanie Klein were leading figures in British psychoanalysis, while many European female analysts emigrated to the United States and Latin American after World War II.

In addition to the important role played by women in the psychoanalytic movement, some psychoanalytic feminists have recently defended Freud. Some dispute feminist critiques of Freud on the grounds that they are based on a misreading of Freud or on an erroneous blaming of psychoanalysis for the mistakes of its popularizers. The first specifically feminist defense of psychoanalysis was Juliet Mitchell's *Psychoanalysis and Feminism* (1974; reprinted as Mitchell, 2000). A British socialist influenced by Lacan, Mitchell argued that psychoanalysis was a liberating theory of creative human nature that feminists neglected at great risk to their cause. Although she conceded Freud's sexism, she claimed that psychoanalysis could be purged of its misogyny by stricter adherence to its own scientific methods. Psychoanalysis described social reality but did not prescribe it, and only psychoanalysis could adequately explain how masculinity, femininity, heterosexuality, and the social organization of gender are reproduced deep in each person's psyche and hence why patriarchy is so resistant to change. According to Mitchell, psychoanalytic theory describes not actual women but Woman as an oppressive idea within patriarchal cultures and a defensive system of male dominance built on men's insecurities. Thus psychoanalysis proves traditional gender arrangements are not natural but cultural, and it exposes their instabilities to the possibility of revolutionary change.

In recent decades, feminists of many sorts have assimilated Freud's ideas, methods, and techniques. All feminists believe that women's secondary status is unjust and must be changed. However, opinions differ regarding the causes and cures for women's subordination. Liberal feminists, such as Friedan, fight discrimination against women and seek to make their legal and economic positions equal to men's. Currently, they are more likely to fight over access to professional training or specific diagnostic categories applied to women, such as post-traumatic stress disorder, than to attack psychoanalysis as a whole. Radical feminists, who see women as united under patriarchal oppression, have most consistently opposed psychoanalysis as its agent. They see its sexism contributing to violence against women, and they prefer women-centered therapies that promise women empowerment. In contrast, cultural feminists emphasize the positive aspects of women's traditional roles, such as nurturance and empathy, while postmodernist feminists question all identities, including the very category of "women."

Those feminists who defend psychoanalysis and adapt its methods to feminist goals are sometimes grouped together under the rubric of "psychoanalytic feminism," although they divide into the allies, respectively, of cultural and postmodern feminisms.

In the United States, the most important use of psychoanalysis for feminism has been through feminist object relations theory, which focuses on the pre-Oedipal development of gender characteristics. Like cultural feminism, it is especially attentive to the bonds between women, especially between mothers and daughters. The other dominant mode within psychoanalytic feminism is Lacanian, sometimes called "French feminism," as represented by Hélène Cixous, Irigiray, and Julia Kristeva. This form of postmodernism emphasizes the contradictory, discursive construction of subjectivity, gender, desire, and sexuality. In addition, feminists use many other psychoanalytic theories, so that, for example, feminist Jungians and self-psychologists analyze gender in relation to concepts from archetypes to narcissism.

American feminist object relations theorists cite the role of the English School of psychoanalysis, especially the work of Melanie Klein and D. W. Winnicott, in developing areas neglected by Freud, particularly the pre-Oedipal psychology of infants in relation to their mothers.

Dorothy Dinnerstein proposed that mother-dominated child rearing in all known cultures caused both boys and girls to fear unconsciously an overwhelming maternal power capable of giving or withholding life and so to fear

F

female autonomy; the result has been the toleration of a sexual double standard and the perpetuation of dangerous military and environmental policies.

Nancy Chodorow has also addressed the psychic consequences of mother-dominated child rearing, especially in isolated middle-class families. She focused on the asymmetrical personality structures developed by girls and boys. She proposed that because of their early, intense identification with their mothers, girls' sense of self typically remains relational and fluid, and girls develop capacities and desires for maternal nurturance and empathy that lead them to reproduce the psychology of mothering in the next generation. Boys, in contrast, individuate themselves against their mothers and so become more autonomous and emotionally constrained.

Carol Gilligan extended this hypothesis about women's relational character to moral development, and so reassessed Freud's notorious judgments. Gilligan proposed that female moral development was not inferior but complementary to men's: women typically think of moral choices in terms of individual cases rather than abstract rules; and women are more likely than men to achieve moral maturity through a path of interdependence as they moderate both infantile selfishness and socially sanctioned female self-abnegation, thus balancing the claims of self and other.

The psychoanalytic feminists who use object relations theories are sometimes referred to as "mothering theorists." They criticize Freud for neglecting maternal subjectivity in his case studies and theories, and for endorsing the child's view that the mother exists solely for the child. Debunking fantasies of perfect mothers, they instead give mothers a voice.

Their critics charge these mothering theorists with sentimentalizing certain traits, such as empathy, which spring from women's subordinate status; with falsely attributing these traits to a fixed female nature; and with inverting, rather than displacing, traditional gender stereotypes. They also complain of an unwarranted extrapolation of the characteristics of privileged women, although since the 1980s the mothering theorists have become more attentive to class, racial, sexual, and individual differences among women.

Because they believe that the unconscious is structured like a language, Lacanian and other postmodernist feminists have been prominent in the analysis of literature and culture. They often put Freud and feminism in dialogue, reinterpreting Freud's texts for feminist ends.

For example, Cixous has written a play that dramatizes the conflicting interests in Dora's case, including Freud's. Irigiray and others subject Freud's and Lacan's works to close readings regarding slips, jokes, repetitions, and omissions. Feminist film critics analyze the content and apparatus of cinema, which took shape in the same era as psychoanalysis, as in Laura Mulvey's influential thesis that the camera in classic Hollywood movies gazes at the female star as a male voyeur would.

One consequence of the pre-Oedipal emphasis in psychoanalytic feminism is a debate about the necessity of a passage through the Oedipus stage for entry into sanity, gender development, heterosexuality, and civilization. Some feminists deny that a paternal threat of castration is necessary to disrupt the allegedly symbiotic relationship between mother and child, a premise disputed by developmental psychologists. These feminists believe that the child's loss of fantasied union with the mother or with its own body is sufficient to begin the work of mourning, guilt, or reparation that matures the psyche.

Although Freud insisted on the "psychological consequences of the anatomical distinction between the sexes," he thought, even in his most biologistic musings, that gender identity and the formation of sexual desire were not the inevitable results of nature but rather were complex and difficult formations with many possible outcomes. He typically viewed homosexual or lesbian object choice as immature and perverse, but not as either immoral or qualitatively different from heterosexual choices. Although orthodox American psychoanalysis originally barred homosexuals from analytic training, it wrote little about them. Now some lesbian and queer theorists enlist Freud as an ally against biologistic essentialism and conservative moralism, and for the fluidity and variability of all sexual desires and gender identities. In addition, psychoanalytic feminists examine the unconscious repercussions of other social categories such as race, class, and age in relation to gender. For example, Freud assumed that women atrophied psychologically in middle age, whereas feminist theorists are rethinking female maturity and are analyzing projections onto elderly women of cultural fears about embodiment, dependence, and death.

In practice, many psychoanalysts currently combine drug and insight therapies to treat the depressions and compulsions from which many women suffer. Popular psychology continues to borrow psychoanalytic approaches to disorders that are considered women's diseases, such as anorexia and bulimia. Feminist therapy centers and training institutes now treat women and train mental health professionals. They modify psychoanalytic technique, adding feminist commitments to an egalitarian process, women's empowerment, and sometimes mutual self-disclosure. Some feminists claim that psychoanalytic methods are intrinsically feminist because they resemble the consciousness raising practiced in the women's liberation movement. According to this view, psychoanalysis, like consciousness-raising, is a transformative process through which women articulate their dissatisfactions with society and achieve self-actualization through empathy and insight. From this utopian perspective the psychoanalytic transference is seen as a relationship of mutual emotional and intellectual engagement.

The relationship between psychoanalysis and feminism is no longer exclusively antagonistic, but rather interactive and complex. Psychoanalysis maintains a strong position within contemporary feminist theories and therapies. Conversely, it is likely that mainstream psychoanalysis will continue to respond to feminist analyses of gender and society.

REFERENCES

Barrett, M., and Gardiner, J. K. (1992). Psychoanalysis and feminism: Current controversies. *Signs*, 17: 435–66.

de Beauvoir, S. (1949). *The Second Sex*. Paris: Librairie Gallimard. Trans. H. M. Parshley (ed.). New York: Knopf, 1952.

Buhle, M.J. (1998). *Feminism and Its Discontents: A Century of Struggle with Psychoanalysis*. Cambridge, Mass.: Harvard University Press.

Chodorow, N. (1999). *The Reproduction of Mothering: Psychoanalysis and the Sociology of Gender*. Berkeley: University of California Press, 1st ed., 1978.

Dinnerstein, D. (1976). *The Mermaid and the Minotaur: Sexual Arrangements and Human Malaise*. New York: Harper and Row.

Feldstein, R., and Roof, J. (eds.) (1989). *Feminism and Psychoanalysis*. Ithaca, N.Y.: Cornell University Press.

Freud, S. (1924). *The Dissolution of the Oedipus Complex*. S.E. 19: 173–187.

———. (1926). *The Question of Lay Analysis: Conversations With an Impartial Person*. S.E. 20: 183–258.

Friedan, B. (1963). *The Feminine Mystique*. New York: Dell.

Gilligan, C. (1982). *In a Different Voice: Psychological Theory and Women's Development*. Cambridge, Mass.: Harvard University Press.

Irigiray, L. (1974). *Speculum: Of the Other Woman*. Paris: Minuit. Trans. Gillian Gill. Ithaca, N.Y.: Cornell University Press, 1985.

Jones, E. (1953). *The Life and Work of Sigmund Freud*. vol. 1. New York: Basic Books.

Mitchell, J. (2000). *Psychoanalysis and Feminism: A Radical Reassessment of Freudian Psychoanalysis*. New York: Random House.

Wright, E. (ed.) (1992). *Feminism and Psychoanalysis: A Critical Dictionary*. Oxford: Blackwell.

JUDITH KEGAN GARDINER

Fenichel, Otto (1897–1946)

Otto Fenichel was born in Vienna on December 2, 1897, to a bourgeois Jewish family. His father, Leo Fenichel, a court attorney, was originally from Galicia.

Fenichel finished his high school studies at the Vienna Akademisches Gymnasium in 1915 and enrolled at the Vienna Medical School in the fall of that year. Active in the Vienna youth movement around Siegfried Bernfeld, Fenichel belonged to the "left wing," which championed sexual, cultural, and educational reforms. Siegfried Bernfeld, an important leader of the youth movement before World War I and a mentor of the scholarly analytic research on youth after the war, cited Fenichel, at the time only nineteen years old, in his study "Die Psychoanalyse in der Jugendbewegung" (Psychoanalysis in the Youth Movement), in which he claimed that psychoanalysis contributes to clarifying the sexual revolt of youth.

Some of Fenichel's longtime friendships were based on common experiences in the youth movement. Fenichel was exempted from war service, and from 1915 onward he attended Sigmund Freud's lectures at the University of Vienna. As part of his medical studies, Fenichel moved for a semester to Berlin but graduated at the Vienna University in 1921. In February 1919, Fenichel had founded the Wiener Seminar für Sexuologie (Vienna Seminar for Sexology) at the university as a protest against the deficit in the school of medicine. The orientation of the seminar had been under the sway of psychoanalysis since the beginning, and Fenichel had attended the meetings of the Vienna Psychoanalytic Society since January 1918. In April 1918, he gave his first lecture; two years later, after he presented "Über Sexualfragen in der Jugendbewegung" (On Sexual Issues in the Youth Movement), he was elected a member of the Vienna Society. He began analysis with Paul Federn and continued it, after relocating to Berlin in 1922, with Sándor Radó at the Berlin Psychoanalytic Institute.

F

Fenichel became a member of the teaching staff of the Berlin Institute and transfered his membership to the German Psychoanalytic Society. In 1924, he organized a seminar for younger colleagues, the so-called Kinderseminar (Children's Seminar), an open discussion group on psychoanalytic issues apart from the meetings of the institute, which he led until his emigration in 1933.

In 1931, Fenichel was in charge of editing the *Internationale Zeitschrift für Psychoanalyse* in Berlin, following Radó in this position when the latter moved to the United States. In 1932, the publication of the journal was again transferred to Vienna and Fenichel lost the job. He organized private meetings for Marxist political discussions with a small group of the Kinderseminar including, besides himself, Edith Jacobson, Annie and Wilhelm Reich, Erich Fromm, and George Gerö among its members. Fenichel sympathized with the views of Marxism and, like Wilhelm Reich, who had joined the Communist Party, undertook "field trips" to the Soviet Union. Because of theoretical, personal, and political differences between Fenichel and Reich, the two distanced themselves from each other.

In 1933, after Hitler's rise to power in Germany, Fenichel emigrated to Oslo, Norway, and became secretary of the Danish-Norwegian Psychoanalytic Society. In 1934, after the Berlin analysts had become dispersed through their expulsion by the Nazis, Fenichel began work on his secret *Rundbriefe*, a continuation in written form of the discussion group in Berlin. He wrote a total of 119 circular letters, which spanned a period of more than eleven years.

In 1935, Fenichel moved to Prague and took over the Psychoanalytic Study Group, succeeding Frances Deri in this position. The group was affiliated with the Vienna Psychoanalytic Society, and Fenichel once again became a member of the Vienna Society. After the *Anschluss* and the occupation of Austria by German troops, the Vienna Psychoanalytic Society was dissolved and, with it, the Study Group in Prague. Fenichel emigrated to the United States in the spring of 1938 and settled in Los Angeles. He became a member of the Los Angeles Psychoanalytic Study Group and was elected a training analyst. In 1939, he became one of the editors of *Psychoanalytic Quarterly*. He was the head of the translation committee for Freud's collected works. In 1940, Fenichel separated from his first wife, Claire Nathanson, and married his colleague from Berlin and Prague, Hanna Heilborn. In 1942, he was one of the

founding members of the San Francisco Psychoanalytic Society and, in 1944, elected vice president.

In Los Angeles, Fenichel published his *Psychoanalytic Theory of Neurosis* (1945) and received the reputation of being the "encyclopedia of psychoanalysis" (Greenson, 1966). His book is still viewed as one of the most important and influential reference works for psychoanalytic doctrine and training. Fenichel's organization of the *Rundbriefe*, which—because of its vastness—is as long as all his prior publications together, was finished six months before his death in Los Angeles on January 22, 1946.

Fenichel's priority was the establishment of the requirements and the fundamentals for the "correct application of psychoanalysis" (Fenichel, 1998), which were based on scientific Freudian psychoanalysis. In addition to his reputation as the encyclopedia of psychoanalysis, he can be seen as an historiographer and as the first author of a consistent social history of the psychoanalytic movement.

REFERENCES

Fenichel, O. (1998). 119 Rundbriefe (1934–1945). vol. 1, *Europa* (1934–1938). J. Reichmayr and E. Mühlleitner (eds.). vol. 2, *Amerika* (1938–1945). E. Mühlleitner and J. Reichmayr (eds.). Frankfurt am Main: Stroemfeld Verlag.

Greenson, R. (1966). Otto Fenichel 1898–1946. The Encyclopedia of Psychoanalysis. In F. Alexander et al. (eds.) *Psychoanalytic Pioneers*. New York: Basic Books, pp. 439–449.

Jacoby, R. (1983). *The Repression of Psychoanalysis. Otto Fenichel and the Political Freudians*. New York: Basic Books.

Mühlleitner, E., and Reichmayr, J. (1998). Otto Fenichel—historian of the psychoanalytic movement. *Psychohistory Review, Studies of Motivation in History and Culture*, 26: 159–174.

ELKE MÜHLLEITNER

Ferenczi, Sándor (1873-1933)

Sándor Ferenczi was not only a pioneer in psychoanalytic technique but also held a special place in Freud's affection. Born in Miskolc, Hungary, Alexander Fränkel was the son of the booksellers Baruch and Rosa (Eibenschütz) Fränkel, who Magyarized the family name to Ferenczi in 1879. Ferenczi received his medical degree from the University of Vienna in 1896. Fascinated by Freud's *Interpretation of Dreams*, which he read in 1907, he met Carl Gustav Jung, whose association experiments were also of great interest to him. Ferenczi was first introduced to Freud in 1908, and joined him (and Jung) on the well-known 1909 visit to Clark University in Worcester, Massachusetts. Thus began an intimate, sometimes stormy, twenty-five-year relationship as disciple, analysand, and colleague ending with Ferenczi's death from pernicious anemia in 1933. Many details of their relationship are preserved in their letters, which number more than 1,200.

Ferenczi is a complex, often contradictory, important personality in the history of psychoanalysis. Brilliant, passionate, charming, creative, and initially totally devoted to Freud, Ferenczi was especially close to Freud during the dark years of World War 1. Freud wrote to Ferenczi on July 31, 1915: "You are the only one who still works beside me." A leitmotiv in their relationship was Ferenczi's frustrated wish to engage Freud, the father of psychoanalysis and seventeen years his senior, in an equal, open, mutual relationship. Sensitive to issues of power, abuse, and trauma, Ferenczi emphasized the therapeutic importance of a holding environment, tenderness, and nurturance. Some authors refer to him as the nurturing "mother" of psychoanalysis, in contrast to Freud, the frustrating and depriving "father." Toward the end of Ferenczi's life, intense disagreements about analytic technique and the nature of the analytic relationship threatened—but did not destroy—their relationship.

Ferenczi's Relationship and Analysis with Freud

After many years, Ferenczi finally persuaded a reluctant Freud to analyze him. Freud's reluctance was based on his "dearth of inclination to expose one of my indispensable helpers to the danger of personal estrangement brought about by the analysis" (May 4, 1913). Freud "analyzed" Ferenczi in three brief periods of analysis— one in 1914 and two in 1916—each lasting only about three weeks, with one consisting of two sessions per day. Central to the analysis was Ferenczi's ambivalence about whom he wanted to marry—his mistress, Gizella, eight years his senior, or her daughter, Elma. Freud, abandoning neutrality, consistently interpreted Ferenczi's reluctance to marry Gizella as a resistance to allowing himself to achieve the forbidden Oedipal goal of marrying the symbolic mother. Partly complying with Freud, partly following his own wishes, he finally married Gizella in 1919. Subsequently, Ferenczi never forgave Freud for influencing him to marry Gizella, regretting the decision not to marry Elma, who offered him sensuality and the prospect of fatherhood.

Through Groddeck's 1917 correspondence with Freud, Ferenczi first learned of Georg Groddeck, the author of *The Book of the It (Das Buch vom Es)* and recognized as one of the fathers of psychosomatic medicine. Ferenczi was initially disparaging of Groddeck's mystical predilections. However, after meeting him in 1920 at the International Psycho-Analytical Association Congress in The Hague, the Netherlands, Ferenczi was quite taken with Groddeck's way of bringing together psychosomatics and psychoanalysis. He and his wife went to Groddeck's sanatorium in Baden-Baden, Germany, for the first time in 1921. Soon they became very close friends and engaged in a kind of informal mutual analysis. Ferenczi confided in Groddeck the negative side of his ambivalence toward Freud and how intimidated he was by him. "He was too much the father for me," Ferenczi averred.

In their later correspondence, Ferenczi reproached Freud directly for not having analyzed his negative transference. Freud responded in a 1937 paper ("Analysis Terminable and Interminable," p. 221) with the assertion that when negative transference does not appear spontaneously in the analysis, analytic technique does not justify provoking the patient's hostility.

Ferenczi's Psychoanalytic Contributions

Today the best known of Ferenczi's earlier psychoanalytic contributions include "Introjection and Transference" (1909), "Stages in the Development of the Sense of Reality" (1913a), and "A Little Chanticleer" (Ein kleiner Hahnemann) (1913b). A little-known paper, "The Effect on Women of Pre-mature Ejaculation in Men" (1908), is significant because it exemplifies Ferenczi's sensitivity to gender inequality, a position highly unusual for an Austro-Hungarian man of that era. Indeed, the fact that Ferenczi sometimes advocated feminist points of view contributes to his contemporary appeal. From time to time, he engaged Freud in speculations about telepathic communication that he approached with great interest, still tempered by skepticism. Both Freud and Ferenczi were fascinated by the work of the pre-Darwinian Jean-Baptiste Lamarck, who believed in the inheritance of acquired characteristics. Although their oft-discussed joint work on Lamarck never materialized, they took pleasure in "indulging themselves" in metabiological speculations. Their speculations led to Freud's postulating the inheritance of prehistoric traumatic memories as a "phylogenetic factor" in the etiology

F

of neuroses and to Ferenczi's monograph, *Thalassa (Versuch einer Genitaltheorie, 1924)*. Ferenczi's work on neuroses resulting from wartime experiences ("Two Types of War Neuroses" 1916–1917) along with that of Abraham, Jones, and Simmel contributed to the growing popularity of psychoanalysis during World War I and in the postwar period.

At the Budapest Congress in 1918, Freud (1919) introduced the technique of "activity" that extended the analyst's role beyond passively responding to the analysand's free associations with evenly suspended attention and interpretations of the unconscious. Freud proposed this new "activity" for those patients who avoided confronting their fears. Initially, the term referred to the analyst's active encouragement of phobic patients to confront their phobias. Subsequently, he advocated the setting of a termination date for obsessives who endlessly prolonged their treatment by turning the analysis itself into a compulsion (see Freud's case of the "Wolf Man" [1918]). After 1918, Freud encouraged Ferenczi to develop the active technique on his own. Ferenczi took Freud's notion of activity to an extreme as he tried to promote progress with "stalemated" analyses. He coined the term "masturbatory equivalent" and urged patients to refrain from any motion on the couch that might deflect libidinal energy from the analytic process. His technique involved imposing prohibitions alternating with demands on his patients to bring hitherto hidden energies, feelings, and conflicts into the transference and into the "psychical field" of verbal associations. Indeed, by the early 1920s, Ferenczi was best known for his "active technique" of psychoanalysis.

In 1924, Ferenczi, with Otto Rank, published an important monograph, *The Development of Psychoanalysis (Entwicklungsziele der Psychoanalyse)*, which advocated the analyst's use of activity, time limits, and consistent transference interpretation, particularly of the negative transference, to bring the patient's "unwinding libido" more fully into the transference relationship. By attributing the chief role in analytic technique "to repetition instead of remembering," they challenged Freud's earlier emphasis "on remembering in the psychical field." The concession notwithstanding that "in the end, remembering remains the final factor in healing," their challenge had far-reaching consequences. This work can be viewed retrospectively as a watershed in the history of psychoanalysis because of its "modern" emphasis on analytic process, enactment, and subjectivity in the here-

now experience (*Erlebnis*) over intellectual insight (*Einsicht*). Herein are to be found the seeds of rebellion against the assumption of the analyst's objectivity and detached authority, and the germination of contemporary perspectives on countertransference and analysis as a two-person process.

Then, in 1925, Ferenczi reversed himself on some of his views on activity in his paper "Contraindications to the 'active' technique." This reversal heralded his far-reaching discovery of the potential for unrecognized traumatic repetitions of deprivation and harsh parental abuse inherent in a repressive, authoritarian analytic relationship. This discovery formed the basis of his revolutionary views of the analytic relationship, countertransference, enactments, trauma, technique, and therapeutic action. First came a series of technical papers that, while initially complementary to Freud's technical recommendations, ultimately opposed them. These papers began with: "The Elasticity of Psychoanalytic Technique" (1928) and included "The Principles of Relaxation and Neocatharsis" (1930) and "Child Analysis in the Analysis of Adults" (1931). In bending over backward to undo the traumas he believed he had re-created using his active technique, Ferenczi advocated tempering Freud's techniques of abstinence and frustration with those of gratification, indulgence, and relaxation. He viewed the analysand as a traumatized child who needed to be held by the sensitive analyst's tact and empathy (Einfühlung) to reexperience safely the childhood traumas and recover from them. As he worked with patients considered to be "hopeless cases," he became known as "the analyst of last resort." Tolerating severe regressions and emphasizing the holding, containing, corrective parental function of the analyst, Ferenczi witnessed and described primitive defense mechanisms in the service of psychic survival. These included dissociative states, identification with the aggressor, splitting, and fragmentation.

By the late 1920s and early 1930s, Ferenczi and Freud were at loggerheads about the role of actual trauma, infantile sexuality, technique, enactments, countertransference, and countertransference enactments. In his efforts to provide what his pupil Franz Alexander later termed "a corrective emotional experience" in the analysis for the traumatized child within the adult, Ferenczi participated in enactments that Freud critically regarded as his "kissing technique." He went on to accuse Ferenczi of "playing mother to your fantasy children." In his clinical diary of 1932, Ferenczi, wounded by these criticisms, accused Freud of "loving his theories more than his patients." (Freud may have seen the diary but not during Ferenczi's lifetime.) It was characteristic of Ferenczi to explicitly (and not infrequently through self-revelation) blame therapeutic failures not on the patient but on the analyst's hypocrisy, resistance, and other personal or technical shortcomings. Freud made it known that he believed Ferenczi suffered from a *furor sanandi*, excessive therapeutic ambition.

The nadir of their relationship was reached in September 1932 immediately before the Wiesbaden Congress. Ferenczi, now ill with undiagnosed pernicious anemia, visited Freud and insisted on reading him his paper "Confusion of Tongues between Adults and the Child: The Language of Tenderness and of Passion." Freud was displeased. He saw in it a regressive return to his abandoned seduction theory of neurosogenesis and a disavowal of the centrality of infantile sexuality, unconscious fantasy, and the Oedipus complex. More important, Freud objected to Ferenczi's efforts to cure patients by providing them with the love for which he himself longed. Freud was deeply concerned that Ferenczi's blurring of patient-analyst boundaries (now termed boundary crossings and violations) was dangerous to his own reputation and the future of the psychoanalytic cause. Ernest Jones allowed Ferenczi to present that paper at the Wiesbaden International Psychoanalytic Congress over the objections of Freud and Eitingon, but subsequently reneged on his promise to him to publish it in English. It was not until 1949 that Michael Balint, Ferenczi's student, analysand, and champion, finally succeeded in overcoming Jones's refusal to publish the "Confusion of Tongues" paper in English. Jones, who had been Ferenczi's analysand, stated in his Freud biography (vol. 3, p. 149) that Ferenczi had "violent paranoic and even homicidal outbursts." There is evidence that he did suffer from a brief, acute, and self-limited organic psychosis in March 1933 brought on by neurological complications of pernicious anemia. However, there is no convincing evidence to support Jones's suggestion that he was suffering from a progressive paranoia over the six years during which he wrote his controversial technical papers. The Freud-Ferenczi controversy continues even to this day, unfortunately at times in a polemical spirit, with the suggestion of one camp that Ferenczi's alleged psychosis is reason to ignore his clinical and theoretical contributions. The Ferenczi camp views such claims as false and politically motivated.

In the end, Ferenczi became a dissident, not a defector. He was viewed by some Freudians as an enfant terrible of psychoanalysis. His radical experiments in analytic technique culminated in trying out "mutual analysis" (1932–1933) with one patient (referred to as "RN" in his clinical diary) and possibly with one or two others. In that experimental technique, Ferenczi reversed roles and allowed himself to be analyzed temporarily by these patients in an effort to overcome impasses in treatment. He soon stopped his experiments with mutual analyses, for practical, not theoretical, considerations related to the confidentiality of other patients. His rebellion notwithstanding, Ferenczi never fully broke with Freud to start a new school of psychoanalysis. Indeed, Freud eulogized Ferenczi in his obituary, observing that his works have "made all analysts into his pupils."

Organizational Contributions to Psychoanalysis

At the Second International Psycho-Analytical Congress in Nuremberg in 1910, Ferenczi, in accordance with Freud's wishes, publicly proposed the founding of the International Psychoanalytic Association with Jung as the first president. In 1912, Ferenczi and Jones, before the imminent break with Jung, who was still president of the IPA, formed the idea of a "secret committee" to keep psychoanalysis "pure" and to protect Freud from having to engage in political matters. Ferenczi strongly advocated affectively deep—not pedagogical—analyses of future analysts, announcing the analyst's analysis as the "second fundamental rule" of psychoanalysis. (Free association was the first fundamental rule.) He expressed a wishful fantasy that members of the International Psychoanalytic Association, comprised of well-analyzed analysts, would pursue analytic knowledge and reach agreements unimpeded by petty jealousies or political rivalries.

In 1913, Ferenczi founded the Budapest Psychoanalytic Society. Five years later, a few weeks before the end of World War I, he was elected president of the International Psycho-Analytical Association at the Budapest Congress at a time when Budapest was being considered as the possible new center of psychoanalysis. Hungarian right-wing anti-Semitic and antipsychoanalytic politics prevented that development, virtually cutting off Hungary from international communication. For these reasons, Ferenczi himself had to resign as president a year later in favor of Jones in England. In 1926–1927, Ferenczi

F

traveled to America and taught at the New School for Social Research in New York City, where he lectured widely and maintained a busy psychoanalytic practice. He also visited the Washington, D.C. area, by invitation of William Alanson White (St. Elizabeth's Hospital), where he met the interpersonalist Harry Stack Sullivan and visited Chestnut Lodge, a well-known private mental hospital in Maryland. In 1932, Freud was eager for Ferenczi to accept the presidency of the International Psychoanalytic Association in an effort to bring him back from his isolation into the psychoanalytic mainstream. Ferenczi declined because he felt his ideas were not compatible with the role of president; he also wanted to allow himself time "to pursue his technical research."

Analysands, Followers, and Legacy

Ferenczi analyzed, among others, Michael Balint, Izette de Forest, Ernest Jones, Melanie Klein, Vilma Kovács, Sándor Lorand, John Rickman, Géza Róheim, Elizabeth Severn, Eugénie Sokolnicka, and Clara Thompson. His influence was spread internationally by his analysands and pupils: in Hungary, by Imre Hermann and Vilma Kovács; in England by Balint, Jones, Klein, and Rickman; in France, Eugénie Sokolnicka helped found the Société Psychanalytique de Paris; in America, Franz Alexander founded the Chicago School; in New York, Sándor Rádo helped found the Columbia University Psychoanalytic Clinic in 1946; Géza Róheim directed research at the New York Institute, and Clara Thompson with Erich Fromm, Karen Horney, and Harry Stack Sullivan helped found the Association for the Advancement of Psychoanalysis in 1941. Robert Bak, Theresa Benedek, and Margaret Mahler were also Ferenczi's pupils and influential in their own right.

The suppression of Ferenczi's innovations in the English-speaking countries began to lift, as noted, in 1949 when Balint prevailed upon Jones to publish "Confusion of Tongues between Adults and the Child" in English in the *International Journal of Psycho-Analysis*. But only in recent years has there been a resurgence of interest in Ferenczi's contributions. His emphasis on interaction, egalitarianism, countertransference, subjectivity, and his self-revealing candor occupies center stage in some countries in this postmodern era. Ferenczi is now heralded by many as the originator of the currently popular relational, constructivist, intersubjective, and interpersonal approaches. As analysis has widened its scope to include more disturbed patients, often victims

of incest or other severe traumas, Ferenczi's therapeutic ambition, activity, and understanding of defenses serving psychic survival have become increasingly relevant. An historical time line of Ferenczi's relational emphasis can be traced from Balint through Winnicott to Kohut and Modell. Indeed, Kohut's interest in narcissism and disturbances of the self lies very close to the problems that Ferenczi elucidated. Ferenczi is now slowly reclaiming the prominent position he held in the early 1920s when he was recognized, with Freud, as one of the two giants of psychoanalytic technique.

REFERENCES

PAPERS

Ferenczi, S. (1908). The effect on women of premature ejaculation in men. In M. Balint (ed.). *Final Contributions to the Problems and Methods of Psycho-Analysis*. Trans. E. Mosbacher et al. London: Karnac, 1980, pp. 291–294.

———. (1909). Introjection and transference. In M. Balint (ed.). *First Contributions to the Problems and Methods of Psycho-Analysis*. Trans. E. Mosbacher et al. London: Karnac, 1980, pp. 35–93.

———. (1913a). Stages in the development of the sense of reality. Ibid., pp. 213–239.

———. (1913b). A little chanticleer. Ibid., pp. 240–252.

———. (1921). The further development of the active therapy in psychoanalysis. In J. Rickman (ed.). *Further Contributions to the Problems and Methods of Psychoanalysis*. Trans. J. Suttie. London: Karnac, 1980, pp. 198–217.

———. (1926). Contraindications to the active psychoanalytical technique. Ibid., pp. 217–230.

———. (1928). The elasticity of psychoanalytic technique. In M. Balint (ed.). *Final Contributions to the Problems and Methods of Psycho-Analysis*. Trans. E. Mosbacher et al. London: Hogarth Press, 1955, pp. 87–101.

———. (1930). The principles of relaxation and neocatharsis. Ibid., pp. 108–125.

———. (1931). Child-analysis in the analysis of adults. Ibid., pp. 126–142.

———. (1933). Confusion of tongues between adults and the child: The language of tenderness and passion. Ibid., pp. 156–167.

Freud, S. (1919). *Lines of Advance in Psychoanalytic Therapy*. S.E. 17: 157–168.

BOOKS

Aron, L., and Harris, A. (1993). *The Legacy of Sándor Ferenczi*. Hillsdale, N.J.: Analytic Press.

Barande, I. (1972). *Sándor Ferenczi*. Paris: Payot.

Bokanowski, T. (1997). *Sándor Ferenczi*. Paris: P.U.F.

Brabant, Falzeder, et al. (1993), vol. 1; Falzeder and Brabant (1996), vol. 2; Falzeder and Brabant (2000), vol. 3, *The Correspondence of Sigmund Freud and Sándor Ferenczi*. Trans. P. Hoffer. Intro: A. Haynal, (vol. 1); A. Hoffer, (vol.

2); J. Dupont, (vol. 3). Cambridge, Mass.: Harvard University Press.

de Forest, I. (1954). *The Leaven of Love*. New York: Harper and Brothers.

Dupont, J. (1932) [1988]. *The Clinical Diary of Sándor Ferenczi*. Trans. M. Balint and N. Jackson. Cambridge, Mass.: Harvard University Press.

Falzeder, E. (1986). *Michael Balints über Entstehung und Auswirken früher Objektbeziehungen*. Salzburg: Salzburger Sozialisationsstudien Nr. 10.

Ferenczi, S. (1938). *Thalassa: A Theory of Genitality*. New York: Psychoanalytic Quarterly.

Ferenczi, S., and Rank, O. (1925). *The Development of Psychoanalysis*. New York: Nervous and Mental Disease Publishing Co.

Haynal, A. (1988). *The Technique at Issue*. London: Karnac.

Rachmann, A. (1955). *Sándor Ferenczi the Psychotherapist of Tenderness and Passion*. Northvale, N.J.: Aronson.

Rudnytsky, P. L., et al. (1996). *Ferenczi's Turn in Psychoanalysis*. Rudnytsky, P. L., Giampieri-Deutsch, P., Bókay, A. (eds.). New York: New York University Press.

Sabourin, P. (1985). *Ferenczi, Paladin et Grand Vizir Secret*. Paris: Éditions Universitaires.

Stanton, M. (1991). *Sándor Ferenczi—Reconsidering Active Intervention*. Northvale, N.J.: Aronson.

AXEL HOFFER

Fetishism See PERVERSIONS.

Finland, and Psychoanalysis

Psychoanalysis became rather slowly known in Finland. Sigmund Freud's name was mentioned for the first time in 1894, in a Finnish medical journal, for his cocaine experiments. As early as 1905, G. Mattson, a writer, wrote an article for a larger audience on Freud's book *Jokes and Their Relationship to the Unconscious*. In academic and literary circles, psychoanalysis was discussed in the period between 1910 and 1940. Philosophers, psychiatrists, psychologists, and artists were the most interested in it.

Among them was also Yrjö Kulovesi (1887–1943), who paid his first visit to Freud in 1924 and underwent two separate analyses (with Edward Hitschmann and Paul Federn). Kulovesi was a friend of Frans Emil Sillanpää, who was awarded the Nobel Prize in literature in 1939, shortly before the Soviet Union attacked Finland, and who helped him publish in 1933 the first introductory book on psychoanalysis in Finnish with Finnish terminology. Kulovesi was elected a full member of the Viennese Psychoanalytical society in 1931 and became a training analyst in 1936. His publications, totaling over thirty articles, displayed a wide range of subjects. Otto Fenichel mentioned three of his papers in his book *The Psychoanalytic Theory of Neurosis* (1945). Together with the Swedish-born Alfhild Tamm (1876–1959), he founded the Finnish-Swedish Psychoanalytical Society in 1934 in Stockholm under the auspices of the International Psychoanalytical Association (IPA).

After World War II, there was another Finnish physician, Benjamin Rubinstein (1905–1989), who had been in analysis in the late 1930s in London. He introduced psychoanalytic ideas to his Finnish colleagues in Helsinki in the 1940s. David Rapaport invited him to the United States in 1948, and in 1954 he became a member of the New York Psychoanalytic Association.

In postwar Finland, an increasing interest in psychoanalysis developed among young colleagues. The general atmosphere in Finland was favorable for psychoanalysis, and there were no strong prejudices against it at that time. A society was founded to promote the cause of psychoanalysis in 1952. But those who wanted psychoanalytic training had to study abroad.

Stig Björk was the first who went to Stockholm in 1948, and was succeeded by Pentti Ikonen, Carl Lesche, Tapio Nousiainen, and Veikko Tähkä. All of them became members of the Swedish Psychoanalytical Society in the middle fifties. More followed in their footsteps to Sweden (Eero Rechardt, Gunvor Vuoristo, Reijo Holmström, Mikael Enckell, Matti Tuovinen). Three of them (Henrik Carpelan, Lars-Johan Schalin, and Leena-Maija Jokipaltio) went to Switzerland for training and became members of the Swiss Psychoanalytical Society in the 1960s.

The origins of organized psychoanalysis in Finland date back to 1964, when the Finnish analysts had returned to Finland and were granted the status of a study group by the Executive Council of the IPA. Tähkä was elected chairman and Carpelan secretary. The president of the IPA elected the sponsoring committee under the chairmanship of Donald Winnicott, its secretary being Pearl King. In Copenhagen in 1967, the Finnish study group was elevated to the status of a provisional society. The society was accepted two years later as a component society of the IPA in Rome. From 1964 to 1980, the membership of the society grew from 11 to 56, with 34 candidates in training. In the year 2000, the number of members was 176, including 16 child analysts and 25 training analysts, with 31 candidates in training.

Finland plays a prominent part in the Nordic psychoanalytic publication *Scandinavian Psychoanalytic*

Review, founded in 1978. Nordic orientation played a highly important part in the work of the society. Many of its members have published books about psychoanalysis and related topics. The society has published a series of books of its own as well. The thirty-second International Psychoanalytic Congress of the IPA was held in Helsinki in 1981 at Finlandia House, designed by Alvar Aalto. Eero Rechardt was the host and the chairman of the Finnish organizing committee, and was elected vice president of the IPA for 1981–1983. The fifth Scientific Symposium of the European Psychoanalytical Federation was held in 1992 in Helsinki.

For more than thirty years, there have been over 500 scientific meetings of the society. Many well-known foreign analysts have visited the society. A more or less classical Freudian orientation characterizes Finnish psychoanalysis, but recent developments are well known in the society. Training closely resembles that of other psychoanalytic societies. The organized training began in 1965. The first training course in child analysis, with Leena-Maija Jokipaltio as teacher and supervisor, was established in 1978. In 1990, five Lithuanians began their psychoanalytic training in Helsinki and were graduated in 1996. Also two Estonians were in training as of 2001.

Psychoanalysis in Finland found a relatively favorable response in the medical faculties in the 1970s, although the state of affairs has recently changed in favor of biological psychiatry. Still, one can say that psychoanalysis has been able to arouse continued interest among physicians and psychologists.

REFERENCES

Kulovesi, Y. (1927). Der Raumfaktor in der Traumdeutung. *internationale Zeitschritz für Psychoanalyse* 13, 56–58.

Laine, A., Parland, H., and Roos, E. (1997). *Psykoanalyysin uranuurtajat Suomessa (The Pioneers of Psychoanalysis in Finland)*. Kemijärvi, LPT.

Roos, E. (1992). Psychoanalysis in Finland. In P. Kutter (ed.), *Psychoanalysis International*, vol. 1. Stuttgart: Fromman Verlag, pp. 55–67.

ESA ROOS

Fliess, Wilhelm (1858-1928)

Fliess was a German physician with a practice in Berlin who treated patients with ear and nose problems, but he also did research and developed original theories about the nasal reflex neurosis, bisexuality, and so-called "periodic phenomena." He is primarily known today because of his strange theories and his relationship with Sigmund Freud.

In 1887, Fliess, at the suggestion of Breuer, met Freud and discussed some of his ideas with him. Later, they had periodic meetings in Berlin, Vienna, Salzburg, Dresden, Nuremberg, Breslau, and Innsbruck, and carried on a regular correspondence from 1887 to 1904. Ernest Kris, in his introduction to the first publication of the letters written by Freud to Fliess, reports that Fliess was Freud's closest friend; Kris also expresses a largely favorable opinion of Fliess, based on a reading of his writings and from questioning those who knew him: "All who knew him emphasize his wealth of biological knowledge, his imaginative grasp of medicine, his fondness for far-reaching speculation and his impressive appearance; they also emphasize his tendency to cling dogmatically to a once-formed opinion" (Kris, 1954: 4).

One of Fliess's first speculative theories concerned the role of the nose in producing certain somatic complaints. However, unlike some of his other theories, this one was not entirely speculative, at least not initially, but rather was based on his clinical findings from his own practice. He found that some of his patients exhibited a consistent set of symptoms, including headaches, pains in the arm, stomach, and spleen, and disturbances in the respiratory system, the heart, and the digestive system. Despite the very large—and varied—set of symptoms, Fliess was convinced that he had discovered a clinical syndrome: the nasal reflex neurosis. He also concluded that the symptoms resulted from a disturbance in the nose. He apparently reached this conclusion when he discovered that he could eliminate the symptoms, at least temporarily, by anaesthetizing with cocaine the responsible area in the nose.

Fliess allowed for the possibility that the nasal reflex neurosis could result from infections, but he also held that it could result from a functional disturbance. The postulation of the latter cause would explain why, Fliess notes, "neurasthenic complaints, in other words the neuroses with a sexual aetiology, so frequently assume the form of the nasal reflex neurosis" (Fliess, quoted by Kris, p. 5). To explain this correlation between a disorder with a sexual etiology and the nasal reflex neurosis, Fliess postulated that there is a special connection between the nose and the genitals. Part of his evidence for this connection was the finding that women sometimes had nose bleeds in place of menstruation and experienced miscarriages resulting from administering cocaine to the nose.

The cocaine treatment apparently brought only temporary relief to those suffering from the nasal reflex neurosis. Fliess concluded that a permanent cure for at least some of the symptoms was an operation on the nose to remove the nasal disturbance. His embracing this theory led to his operation on Emma Eckstein.

Eckstein was Freud's patient; she suffered from, among other things, stomach and menstrual pains. Because Freud apparently believed that her problems had a sexual etiology, and because of the nature of the symptoms, he invited Fliess to treat her. Fliess responded in February of 1895 by operating on Emma's nose, removing part of the bone. Fliess, however, placed a large piece of gauze in the woman's nose and forgot to take it out. The result was that Eckstein later began hemorrhaging and almost bled to death. The attractive young woman was also permanently disfigured (Macmillan, 1991: 226; Sulloway, 1979).

Fliess's next theory was more speculative than the first. He theorized that all human beings are bisexual and that this physiological fact was of fundamental importance for understanding neuroses (Sulloway, 1998: 64). Fliess apparently communicated his theory to Freud as early as 1897 at one of their "congresses" (Freud's term for their meetings). Freud took note of Fliess's bisexuality theory in his *Three Essays on the Theory of Sexuality* (1905). In writing of the implications of Fliess's theory for the understanding of psychoanalysis, Freud speaks of bisexuality as "the decisive factor" and adds that "without taking bisexuality into account I think it would scarcely be possible to arrive at an understanding of the sexual manifestations that are actually to be observed in men and women" (quoted in Sulloway, 1998: 66).

Fliess considered his theory of bisexuality to be extremely important, and after ending his close friendship with Freud, his letters show a deep annoyance at Freud because of his alleged role in the "theft" of the bisexuality theory by Otto Weininger. Weininger published a book in 1903 making use of Fliess's ideas but without crediting Fliess; shortly after the publication of his book, Weininger committed suicide. In his letter to Freud dated July 20, 1894, Fliess complains that Weininger obtained knowledge of his ideas about bisexuality from Freud (through the intermediary of Freud's patient, the philosopher Swoboda) and demands a "frank reply" (Freud, 1895: 463). Freud replied on July 23, 1904, saying "I too believe that the late Weininger was a burglar with a key he picked up" (Freud, 1985: 464).

Freud, however, downplayed his role in the affair and even suggested that the criminal Weininger could have gotten the idea from other sources given that the idea of bisexuality had figured in the literature for some time—thus suggesting a lack of originality on Fliess's part. Fliess was not satisfied and in a later letter queried Freud about this literature allegedly discussing bisexuality. By the time of these exchanges of letters, however, the Freud-Fliess friendship was virtually ended. The decisive point was their last meeting, which took place at Anchensee in the summer of 1900; a hostile encounter in which Fliess's most speculative theory, his theory of periodicity, was partly the cause of the disagreement.

According to a monograph Fliess published in 1897, all human beings are subject to two periodic cycles: in the male, a 23-day cycle and in the female, a 28-day cycle. These exact cycles were causally connected, in Fliess's view, to all sorts of things, including the development of tissues, the appearance of teeth, first attempts at walking and speaking, etc. (Sulloway, 1998: 57). The theory in fact purports to explain a great deal more: As Fliess notes, "Consideration of these two groups of periodic phenomena points to the conclusion that they have a solid connection with both sexes. . . . Recognition of these things led to the further insight that the development of our organism takes place by fits and starts in these sexual periods, and that the day of our death is determined by them as much as is the day of our birth. The disturbances of illness are subject to the same periodic laws as are these periodic phenomena themselves" (Fliess, quoted by Kris, 1954: 7).

The illnesses to which Fliess applied his theory were not just organic; they were psychic as well. At first, the application to psychic problems enabled Fliess to come to Freud's defense. Later, it led to conflict with Freud.

In 1895, Ludwig Löwenfeld published a criticism of Freud's early theory of anxiety neurosis and Freud replied in his 1895 paper. Fliess also replied, defending Freud's theory. As Kris points out (1954, p. 37), Fliess's defense of Freud's theory of anxiety neurosis laid the groundwork for a subsequent disagreement between the two men. Fliess argued that the appearance of anxiety attacks was bound up with certain periodic dates. On certain dates, he theorized, a substance is secreted in the body which affects the nervous system and results in feelings of anxiety, but only on definite days, a fact that Löwenfeld's criticisms of Freud's theory ignores.

F

In the summer of 1900, Freud and Fliess had one of their "congresses," in Achensee. It proved to be their last. Fliess raised several objections to Freud's theories. One was that periodic processes had an effect on the psychopathic phenomena that Freud was trying to explain. Hence, Fliess reasoned, neither sudden deteriorations nor sudden improvements in Freud's patients were to be attributed to the psychoanalysis and its influence alone. Fliess also accused Freud of projecting his own ideas into the minds of his patients (Freud, 1954: 324, footnote 1).

Fliess's periodic theory was quite speculative, if not an outright piece of quackery. By 1900, Freud probably did not give it much credence, at least insofar as it rivaled his own theory. The idea, however, that he projected his theoretical views into the minds of his patients presented a more serious challenge. He addresses the challenge—that his theories and clinical results are due to his suggestions—in his Little Hans paper (1905) and more thoroughly in his *Introductory Lectures on Psycho-Analysis* (1916–1917).

Most of the letters that Fliess wrote to Freud have not survived, but we do have a record of Fliess's reaction to the Anchensee meeting. According to Fliess, after he presented his objections to Freud's claims, Freud "showed a violence" toward him. During the rest of the meeting, Fliess continues, he detected a personal animosity against him on Freud's part that sprang from envy. The result of the situation at Achensee, Fliess writes, is that he "quietly withdrew from Freud and dropped our regular correspondence" (Fliess in Freud, 1954: 324).

REFERENCES

Freud, S. (1895). A reply to criticisms of my paper on anxiety neurosis. S.E. 3: 123–139.

———. (1909). Analysis of a phobia in a five-year-old boy. S.E. 10: 5–149.

———. (1916–1917). *Introductory Lectures on Psycho-Analysis.* S.E. 15–16: 9–496.

———. (1954). *The Origins of Psycho-Analysis: Letters to Wilhelm Fliess, Drafts and Notes: 1887–1902.* New York: Basic Books

Kris, E. (1954). Introduction. In M. Bonaparte, A. Freud, and S. Kris (eds.). *The Origins of Psycho-Analysis: Letters to Wilhelm Fliess, Drafts and Notes: 1887–1902.* New York: Basic Books, pp. 3–47.

Macmillan, M. (1991). *Freud Evaluated: The Completed Arc.* New York: North Holland. 2d ed., 1997. Cambridge, Mass.: MIT Press.

Sulloway, F. J. (1979). *Freud: Biologist of the Mind.* New York: Basic Books.

———. (1998). The rhythm method. In F. Crews (ed.). *Unauthorized Freud: Doubters Confront a Legend.* New York: Viking, pp. 54–68.

EDWARD ERWIN

France, and Psychoanalysis

In France, as everywhere else, the psychoanalytic community is going through a difficult time. This situation arises out of the general crisis affecting advanced industrial societies afflicted with high unemployment, reduced incomes, lack of job security, and deteriorating working conditions—contributing to a sense of hopelessness, disillusion, and a questioning of democratic values. Besides these economic and social factors, which vary from country to country, the rise of cognitive and behavioral therapies and pharmacological treatments, quicker and cheaper than psychoanalysis, have also contributed to a loss of confidence in the methods introduced by Freud.

The present crisis, like that of the 1930s, has seen a great expansion in the far right—which is fascist, populist, racist, and anti-Semitic, and which has managed to make large inroads into social constituencies formerly dominated by the left, whether centrist, socialist, or communist. It was in these constituencies that Freudianism succeeded in establishing itself in France after the end of the Second World War, largely through such major republican institutions as schools of higher education, universities, and centers concerned with mental health (psychiatric hospitals, medicopsychological clinics, etc.). So the undermining of these constituencies is one of the dangers that practitioners of psychoanalysis have to face. Moreover, at the same time as on the administrative side they are subjected to economic imperatives incompatible with the requirements of long-term Freudian treatment, they also have to contend in the field not only with authoritarian dictates excluding any spirit of tolerance or humanism, but also with extreme situations of violence and delinquency.

Thus up to a point Jacques Derrida was right when in a recent text he compared contemporary psychoanalysis to an out-of-date medicine relegated to the back of the pharmacy: "It may come in useful in an emergency or a shortage, but we've done better since." Neglect of the valuable doctrine born in Vienna at the end of the nineteenth century has been accompanied by the revival of a purely organicist and mechanistic explanation of psychological phenomena.

But the French psychoanalytical community is still strong, even though the situation outlined above makes it more fragile than it was twenty years ago. There are five thousand psychoanalysts in France, divided among twenty or so different associations; i.e., eighty-six psychoanalysts for every million inhabitants. This is the highest ratio in the world—higher than in Argentina or Switzerland. Out of this total, between about eight and nine hundred French psychoanalysts (the figure includes their trainees) are members of the two associations—the Société Psychanalytique de Paris (SPP) and the Association Psychanalytique de France (APF)—that belong to the International Psychoanalytic Association (IPA). Most of the others belong to groups and associations deriving from the former École Freudienne de Paris (EFP), founded by Jacques Lacan in 1964 and dissolved in 1980, while he was still alive.

Historians of the psychoanalytic movement have got into the habit of dividing into generations the groups and individuals that make up the Freudian saga. The evolution of the movement is presented as a kind of family tree tracing the genealogy of Sigmund Freud's various disciples and showing the connections between different interpretations of the founder's original work, the way different schools succeeded one another, and the dialectic through which clinical and political conflicts led to schisms. There are two ways of looking at this evolution. First, on an international scale covering all members of the psychoanalytical diaspora throughout the world; and second, at a national level, showing the transference relationships between individual psychoanalysts (who analyzed whom), starting from a pioneer group (which in some countries consists of only one person) regarded as having introduced the doctrine and practice of psychoanalysis into a particular country.

In France, there have been three generations. The first was that of the pioneers who founded the SPP in 1926. Three people played a fundamental role here: Marie Bonaparte, René Laforgue, and Rudolph Loewenstein. Bonaparte, through her friendship with Freud, her celebrity, and her permanent activity as a translator and a militant devoted to the cause, was the chief organizer of the movement. Laforgue and Loewenstein became the SPP's two main teachers, and in the period between the two world wars they trained the second generation of French psychoanalysts, among them those who were

to be the "leaders" of the movement after 1945: Daniel Lagache, Jacques Lacan, Françoise Dolto, Sacha Nacht, and Maurice Bouvet.

Then came the third generation, born between 1920 and 1930, and taught by the second generation. They were confronted by two schisms, the first in 1953, arising out of the question of lay analysis, and the second ten years later (1963), when Lacan was denied admission to the IPA as a teacher because of his refusal to submit to the current rules about training analyses and the length of sessions. Lacan proposed several modifications of established clinical practice. He rejected the idea of a fixed fifty-five-minute session and suggested it be interrupted not in obedience to preestablished standards but according to the content of the patient's discourse. In his view a "punctuation" or interruption was necessary at especially significant moments in the treatment if the analytical interpretation was to be effective. Lacan also disagreed with the idea that an analysis should end with the dissolution of the transfer. He thought an analysis depended on a transference relationship that never ended. Lastly, he rejected the idea that there was a fundamental difference between a so-called training analysis and a so-called therapeutic or personal one. He also believed a candidate for training should be free to chose his or her analyst without having to select one from a list of authorized senior practitioners.

The second schism, which was far more serious than the first, was dramatic both for Lacan himself, who had never contemplated abandoning the official Freudian tradition, and for the third generation of French psychoanalysts. The most brilliant members of that generation had been analyzed by Lacan, and suddenly he and they found themselves on different sides. In one camp were the members of the APF, affiliated with the IPA in 1965. In the other were the members of the EFP, who, though definitively disowned by the official institutions of Freudianism, considered themselves much more Freudian in reality than their counterparts and rivals in the IPA.

Unlike their American and British colleagues, those members of the third generation of French psychoanalysts who belonged to the IPA never formed a homogeneous school. That is why the main currents of international Freudianism—these included Ego Psychology, Kleinianism, "Annafreudianism," the Self-Psychology of Heinz Kohut, and the post-Kleinian theories of Wilfred Ruprecht Bion—never became established in France.

F

It is Lacanianism alone that for more than thirty years has polarized the field of French psychoanalysis. On one side are the non-Lacanians (also called "orthodox Freudians"), and on the other the Lacanians. Both sides, of course, see themselves as "Freudians." This polarization was emphasized by the presence of Françoise Dolto in the ranks of the EFP. Dolto, who possessed an extraordinary clinical genius, was the founder of child psychoanalysis in France and occupied a position parallel to that of Melanie Klein vis-à-vis the British school, though her ideas were closer to those of Anna Freud. But in 1953 Dolto too was refused admittance to the IPA, though the reasons given in her case were quite different from those invoked against Lacan. Dolto was criticized not for "short sessions" (hers obeyed the rules) but for being too charismatic as a training analyst to conform with traditional standards. In reality, Dolto inherited some of the IPA leadership's hostility toward her own analyst, René Laforgue, whose technique and practice they regarded as "deviant" (i.e., too close to those of people like Ferenczi and Rank). So by 1964, the teaching of both Dolto and Lacan, the two great French masters of psychoanalysis, was being delivered outside the IPA. This was a bizarre situation.

The conflicts that divided the third generation of French psychoanalysts had important repercussions for the next two generations, born between 1935 and 1950. For fifteen years, they had to endure the narcissistic and damaging quarrels of their brilliant elders. They admired their seniors for their work and for their competence as teachers but had to look on as they tore one another to pieces around one omnipresent master—Lacan. While the two French IPA societies (especially the SPP) condemned his practice, underrated his teaching, and demonized his person, in his own school Lacan was now idolized to the point of absurdity.

So in both camps the two newest generations (the fourth and fifth) inherited a Manichaean idea of reality handed down to them both by Lacan's fellow travelers, who often imitated the style of the master, and by Lacan's adversaries, who hated and caricatured him. While the two IPA societies denounced the Lacanians as non-Freudians or even charlatans, the Lacanians regarded their IPA colleagues as bureaucrats who had betrayed psychoanalysis and turned it into an adaptive psychology in the service of triumphant capitalism. In short, the IPA party saw the Lacanians as irresponsible sorcerer's apprentices who indulged in "five-minute" sessions and were inca-

pable of producing a serious structure, technique, or theory based on transference, while the Lacanians regarded the IPA party as deintellectualized stick-in-the-muds who had bowed the knee to "American" psychoanalysis (a description intended as a supreme insult).

An attempt to break down this compartmentalization was made in the late 1970s when René Major, a teacher who belonged to the SPP but appreciated Lacan's culture and clinical practice, and Serge Leclaire, a loyal Lacanian but also an advocate of a Freudian republic, joined together to try to allow clinicians of the younger generations to come together at last outside their respective associations, the legitimacy of which they were beginning to question. This period of "confrontation" made it possible for practitioners of all parties to criticize the ossification of their institutions and exchange points of view about how psychoanalysis could best be practiced. While the two IPA societies were riven by conflicts about training, the EFP was also going through a serious crisis arising out of the failure of the experiment of the "passe" (pass).

The name of this procedure derives from the French verb *passer*, meaning "to pass" in general; but there is a particular sense in which a *passeur* is a ferryman or someone who helps fugitives across frontiers, as during the 1939–1945 war. The passe was invented by Lacan in 1967 and introduced into his school in 1969. An analysand or "passant" who aimed at becoming a training psychoanalyst him- or herself had to outline his or her life-history and the analysis previously undergone to some of his or her senior colleagues (passeurs), and explain how these experiences had made him or her want to be an analyst. The passeurs reported on the passant's motivation to a jury of training analysts, then the panel decided whether or not to admit the candidate. The objective of the procedure was to replace the traditional system for training analysts, now considered inadequate to the task of evaluating a candidate's real abilities, by a genuine examination of a training analyst's status. Hence the famous formula that caused so much ink to flow: "Psychoanalysis is authorized only by itself."

Lacan wanted to emphasize that the transition to being an analyst was a subjective test linked to the transference, in which both the candidate and the training analyst experienced a state of loss, castration, and perhaps even melancholy.

The idea of studying the true function of the initiatory passage or transition was interesting in itself, but the institutional realization of the passe fell short of expectations. It led the EFP first to breakdown then to dissolution, after a third schism, in 1989, brought about the departure of several clinicians, including François Perrier and Piera Aulagnier. They founded a fourth analytical group—the Organisation Psychanalytique de Langue Française (Organization for French-Speaking Psychoanalysis, or OPLF).

The two most recent generations of French psychoanalysts were then obliged to plan their future in terms of the past history of those who had been their analysts. The Lacanians' situation has proved to be different, however, from that of analysts with IPA training. Generally speaking the younger generation of Lacanians feel freer vis-à-vis the people who taught and trained them. As a result of the dissolution of the EFP and the breaking down of Lacanianism into various different trends (post- or neo-Lacanian), they have been able to create their own groups and associations and thereby achieved both political and psychoanalytical maturity. They have freed themselves from subservience toward the masters of the third generation and rid themselves of any idea of an ideal institution. They no longer dream of the type of school once envisaged by Lacan.

The younger generations of analysts in the SPP and the APF are more affected by the quarrels and disappointments of their elders. They are more deeply committed transferentially to their training analysts, who remain unchallenged leaders, very attached to their rights and privileges. So the younger SPP and APF members are more likely to be upset whenever some conflict breaks out. Hence the great but often hidden institutional violence permeating the two IPA societies. The APF is seriously afflicted by gerontocracy, with the age of its full members averaging seventy and that of its associate members sixty. As for the "pupils," their average age is fifty and they have little hope of rising in the hierarchy. Their frustration is reflected in scorn for any kind of institutional authority.

The Lacanians, scattered among fifteen or so associations, are now divided among themselves both on practice and on training. While most of their groups have retained the procedure of the passe, they have changed it into a more or less ordinary rite of passage. As for the length of sessions, almost all the Lacanians have definitely adopted the idea of "punctuation" (interruption of the therapy session). They have also retained the principle by which the analysand is free to choose his or her analyst.

But none of them has reduced the length of the sessions to five minutes, still less to just one minute. This practice, adopted by Lacan in the last five years of his life, is now imitated by only a handful of practitioners, and they must be described as charlatans pure and simple. And as such they are marginalized by the Lacanian community as a whole. But they do exist, behaving as pathological tyrants and presenting a disastrous public image of psychoanalysis, which the media and the anti-Lacanians exploit every so often to discredit Freudianism itself or deny Lacan's contribution to Freudian thought.

The Lacanians themselves give sessions that vary in length between half an hour and forty minutes—longer (about an hour) when the patient attends once a week. Some—especially in the École de la Cause Freudienne (ECF), founded by Jacques-Alain Miller—have reduced the length of their sessions to twenty or even fifteen minutes. But this practice is criticized by most other Lacanians.

There is a great difference between the clinical practice of the Lacanian Freudians and that of the Freudians who are members of the IPA. In the two IPA societies the length of the session is fixed (in theory), and each one lasts about forty-five or fifty minutes. Though their hierarchies and training programs conform to international standards, there are certain differences here between the two IPA societies.

In all the psychoanalytical groups there are good and bad practitioners. No one psychoanalytical society—and this is a new phenomenon—now has the monopoly of either good or bad clinical practice. All are weakened by schisms, conflicts, and institutional sclerosis, and their prestige has fallen so low that many practitioners no longer bother to apply to join them. Some analysts even belong to two groups simultaneously.

The crisis and dislocation to be observed among the psychoanalysts is reflected in those who consult them. The patients of the early 2000s are quite different from those of earlier days. They mostly present narcissistic or depressive symptoms, and suffer from loneliness, instability, and loss of identity. They no longer wish to undergo long courses of treatment, and refuse to see their analyst regularly enough for the treatment to be useful. Either they skip sessions or they will agree to attend only once or twice a week. As soon as they see an improvement in their condition they break off the treatment, invoking a kind of ego-omnipotence. When new symptoms appear they go back to their analyst. In short, they treat analy-

F

sis as a kind of medicine. The classic or traditional analytical situation is rare. So the "armchair-and-couch" model (involving exploration of the unconscious, interpretation of dreams, and a strong transference relationship) is becoming extinct or limited to special cases. For most young therapists, psychoanalysis is no longer a full-time occupation: it has been supplemented or replaced by varieties of verbal psychotherapy.

But if the patients are no longer the same, the younger generations of psychoanalysts too are quite unlike their elders. There is scarcely any difference now between Lacanians and non-Lacanians. Today's psychoanalysts have nearly all had a similar training in psychology, and all practice another profession as well as that of psychoanalysis. Whatever school they belong to they have few private patients (between four and ten on average). They work mostly in various institutions, where they employ other techniques such as psychodrama and group and family therapy. All spend some of their time in services catering for drug addicts, prostitutes, delinquents, and so on.

Access to the profession is now much more often through psychology than through medical or literary studies. The intellectual level of the average psychoanalyst is lower than it used to be. One often comes across young therapists who know no more of Freud, Klein, or Winnicott than what they have read in collections of extracts. This means they are in danger of adopting all kinds of clinical approaches that have little to do with Freudianism.

But despite all these problems, the psychoanalysts of today do represent a revival of Freudianism. They are nearer than their predecessors to the social deprivation they have to confront in their work. They are more pragmatic, simpler, more humanistic, and more alive to all forms of mental suffering, even if they are sometimes less cultured than earlier generations of psychoanalysts. Finally, they are more unprejudiced about all forms of therapy, as if declining to be imprisoned in dogma or sectarianism.

The danger in this broadening process is that it may lead to a lessening of theoretical rigor and even to the abandoning of all reference to a coherent and universalist system of Freudian thought.

REFERENCES

Derrida, J. (1996). *Résistances de la psychanalyse.* Paris: Galilée.

Roudinesco, É. (1994). *Histoire de la psychanalyse en France,* vol. 1 (1982), vol. 2 (1986). Paris: Fayard. Trans. In English by Jeffrey Mehlman as *Jacques Lacan and Co. A History of Psychoanalysis in France 1925–1985.* Chicago: University of Chicago Press, 1990.

———. (1993). *Jacques Lacan. Esquisse d'une vie, histoire d'un système de pensée.* Paris: Fayard. Trans. In English by Barbara Bray as *Jacques Lacan.* New York: Columbia University Press, 1997.

Roudinesco, É., and Plon, Michel (1997). *Dictionnaire de la psychanalyse.* Paris: Fayard. Trans. from the French by Barbara Bray.

ÉLISABETH ROUDINESCO

Free Association

Free association is the term used to describe the patient's uninhibited, stream-of-consciousness verbalization during a psychoanalytic session. Free association has remained one of the cornerstones of psychoanalytic therapy for nearly a century, primarily because the fundamental aim of free association is in many ways similar to the fundamental aim of psychoanalysis itself: It is intended to make unconscious material conscious, and bring it under the control of the ego, where it can be dealt with by the patient in a more modulated, realistic, and rational manner. Freud (1900) provided a succinct summary of his views regarding the purpose of free association and its importance for the psychoanalytic process, when he argued that "psychotherapy can pursue no other course than to bring the unconscious under the domination of the [conscious]" (p. 578).

When psychoanalytic patients are asked to engage in free association, they are given a set of instructions that seem, on the surface, quite simple: They are asked to say anything that comes to mind, no matter how silly, nonsensical, illogical, or embarrassing it may appear. They are told to be as uninhibited as possible—to censor nothing as they verbalize every thought, feeling, wish, idea, and fantasy that enters into consciousness. This lowering of inhibitions and removal of normal everyday censorship activities is sometimes referred to as the "basic rule" of free association; it helps create the mind-set and attitude that set in motion the associative process.

The analyst's role during free association is straightforward. The analyst listens for hidden meaning in the patient's associations, for patterns of thought and emotion that the patient cannot recognize. In particular, the analyst is trained to listen for remnants of unconscious material slipping unobtrusively into consciousness during the free association process. By providing periodic feedback to the patient in the form of psychoanalytic interpretations, the analyst can help the patient gain a better understanding of thoughts, feelings, and motives lying outside of consciousness that previously had affected behavior. In this way, free association leads to insight and enhanced self-awareness.

Engaging in free association would seem an easy task, but it is in fact exceedingly difficult for many people. As Korchin (1976, p. 327) noted, "One cannot readily wipe away years of commitment to logical thought nor easily bypass the conventions and inhibitions which guide ordinary social intercourse. Even with the best intentions, we are loathe to speak about things that seem trivial, illogical, embarrassing, or irrelevant." Although psychoanalysts have used a variety of means to encourage patients to free-associate (e.g., having the patient lie on a couch, minimizing distracting materials within the therapy room, deliberately sitting outside the patient's view), it remains a challenging task for most patients.

Anecdotal accounts confirm Korchin's speculation that many psychoanalytic patients are in fact unable to free-associate productively during the course of psychodynamic therapy. Such patients are said to be resistant to insight and therapeutic change. Resistance may be conscious and deliberate, or unconscious and unintentional, but regardless of its source, it is almost always an obstacle to successful treatment. In extreme cases, strong and insurmountable resistance may render free association impossible and preclude psychoanalytic treatment entirely.

Free association has come to be intimately connected with Freud's psychotherapeutic technique in the minds of most mental health professionals, but the free association method did not emerge full-blown at the birth of psychoanalysis more than a century ago. Instead, Freud's early efforts at recovering unconscious material employed variants of the therapeutic approaches that were in vogue during the latter part of the nineteenth century, namely, hypnosis, massage, water immersion, electrotherapy, and the now famous "pressure technique," wherein Freud placed his hand upon the patient's forehead in an effort to stimulate recall of repressed memories.

Over time, Freud found that the pressure technique—like hypnosis and other memory-enhancement strategies used by nineteenth-century therapists—produced modest and inconsistent results at best. Conse-

quently, he discarded all these earlier approaches in favor of free association. Freud came to believe that patients were better able to verbalize psychodynamically relevant information when (paradoxically) they relaxed their efforts to recall unconscious material directly, and simply spoke about whatever thoughts, feelings, or ideas happened to enter their mind at the moment.

In replacing the pressure technique with free association, Freud introduced a fundamental shift in the nature of psychoanalytic therapy—and in the epistemological underpinnings of psychoanalytic theory as well. Simply put, Freud stopped trying to gain *direct* access to unconscious memories and instead decided to take a more *indirect* route, circumventing the patient's resistance via free association rather than confronting this resistance directly via increased (and apparently fruitless) efforts to bring repressed material into consciousness through sheer force of will. Erdelyi (1985, p. 36) summarized nicely this evolution in psychoanalytic technique, noting that "Freud shifted from an overbearingly pushy cognitive approach for recovering lost memories to a totally permissive one. . . . Free associating is a cognitive form of 'doing without doing.' The patient lies back passively and tries not to force past structures or constraints upon his thinking and verbalizations. Ultimately, however, in Freud's estimate, it is a far more potent device for consciousness-raising than either hypnosis or pressure, for with free association the patient gains access not only to lost memories (hypermnesia) but to inaccessible meanings as well (insight)."

Freud's belief that indirect approaches to recovering unconscious material were more useful than the earlier direct approaches ultimately led to the development of several important therapeutic strategies, including dream interpretation and analysis of parapraxes (i.e., slips of the tongue). In a sense, dream interpretation and parapraxis analysis are both variants of Freud's basic free association technique: In both dreams and parapraxes, unconscious material is presumed to be revealed indirectly, and the patient (and analyst) can gain insight into the meaning of a dream or parapraxis only through free association.

Empirical research on the recovery of unconscious memories via free association began shortly after Freud's initial writings on the topic, and was initiated by Otto Poetzl's classic experiments demonstrating that aspects of a briefly presented image that participants could not describe directly emerged indirectly in subsequent dream imagery. This finding—which came to be known as the

F

Poetzl Phenomenon—was subsequently replicated and extended by Charles Fisher in an influential series of studies conducted during the 1950s and 1960s. Ultimately, Matthew Erdelyi and his colleagues followed up on the earlier work of Poetzl and Fisher, using improved methodologies and experimental procedures. In a series of experiments conducted during the 1970s and early 1980s, Erdelyi tested directly Freud's hypothesis that free association is a particularly powerful method for recovering inaccessible memories.

Erdelyi's investigations produced mixed results with respect to Freud's hypothesis. On the one hand, these studies demonstrated that individuals who are asked to free-associate following exposure to a series of verbal or pictorial stimuli do in fact show enhanced recall for the stimuli relative to individuals who are not asked to free-associate following stimulus exposures. However, Erdelyi and his colleagues found that this "hypermnesia effect" was stronger for pictorial than for verbal stimuli. Moreover, additional experiments indicated that other activities (e.g., silent concentration) could produce hypermnesia for previously inaccessible memories comparable to that obtained when free association was used to enhance recall. In the end, cognitive and psychodynamic researchers concluded that free association is only one of several strategies that may be used to gain access to unconscious memories.

Erdelyi's studies marked a turning point in the psychoanalytic conceptualization of free association. Following his seminal investigations, clinicians introduced other, more structured and directive approaches for eliciting psychodynamically relevant material during therapy, and researchers began to explore alternative ways of recovering inaccessible memories in the laboratory. By the late 1980s, comparatively little was being written on the topic of free association in psychoanalysis.

The 1990s witnessed a revival of interest in the free association method, for several reasons. First, clinicians have revised their understanding of the value of free association within the psychoanalytic session. It now appears that while free association is not a uniquely powerful tool for recovering unconscious memories, it is a useful method for encouraging patients to generate a large amount of material during the analytic session (Bornstein, 1993: 337–344). To the extent that a psychoanalytic patient is encouraged to produce a large quantity of verbal material, psychodynamically relevant content is more likely to emerge.

In addition, recent writings on clinical technique have offered alternative approaches to utilizing free association productively during psychodynamic therapy. For example, in lieu of focusing primarily on unconscious content and hidden meaning in a patient's free associations, some psychoanalysts now advocate interpreting the patient's stream-of-consciousness verbalizations from an ego psychological perspective (Busch, 1997: 407–423). In this approach, the analyst uses associative material to better understand the means through which patients shape their internal and external reality. The analyst also uses this associative material to better understand the role of the ego in structuring the patient's conscious and unconscious experience, to gain insight into the representational world of the patient, and to obtain information regarding the ego defenses used most (and least) frequently by the patient.

With these latest innovations, an updated and refined conceptualization of free association has emerged, helping to revitalize psychoanalytic practice and move it closer to theories and findings in other areas of psychology, psychiatry, and cognitive science. As clinicians and researchers learn more about the value and limits of the free association method, it is likely that additional connections will emerge between this important psychoanalytic concept and related constructs in other areas of inquiry.

REFERENCES

Bornstein, R. F. (1993). Implicit perception, implicit memory, and the recovery of unconscious material in psychotherapy. *Journal of Nervous and Mental Disease*, 181: 37–344.

Busch, F. (1997). Understanding the patient's use of the method of free association: An ego psychological approach. *Journal of the American Psychoanalytic Association*, 45: 407–423.

Erdelyi, M. H. (1985). *Psychoanalysis: Freud's Cognitive Psychology*. New York: W. H. Freeman.

Freud, S. (1900). *The Interpretation of Dreams*. S.E. 4 and 5: 1–621.

Korchin, S. J. (1976). *Modern Clinical Psychology*. New York: Basic Books.

ROBERT F. BORNSTEIN

Free Will

Freud's Rejection of Free Will

Freud gave an unequivocal verdict on the traditional philosophical question of freedom of the will: There is no such thing. Our belief in free will is deeply rooted, but is nonetheless illusory.

In his *Introductory Lectures* (1916–1917), Freud writes: "You nourish the illusion of there being such a thing as psychical freedom, and you will not give it up. I am sorry to say I disagree with you categorically over this" (p. 49). Later in the same work, he refers to a faith in undetermined psychical events and freedom of the will as "unscientific": "Once before [p. 49] I ventured to tell you that you nourish a deeply rooted faith in undetermined psychical events and in free will, but that this is quite unscientific and must yield to the demand of a determinism whose rule extends over mental life" (p. 106).

Freud (1901, pp. 253–254) also gives a partial explanation of why most of us tend to believe in free will. When we make important decisions, there is a feeling of psychic compulsion, but in making unimportant, indifferent decisions, there is an appearance of a causal "gap"; there is nothing, as far we can tell, that caused us to decide. In making the unimportant decisions, there is a sense that ". . . we have acted of our free—and unmotivated—will" (p. 254). This gap, however, disappears once we postulate unconscious causes: "If the distinction between conscious and unconscious motivation is taken into account, our feeling of conviction informs us that conscious motivation does not extend to all our motor decisions. . . . But what is thus left free by the one side receives its motivation from the other side, from the unconscious; and in this way determination in the psychical sphere is still carried out without any gap" (p. 254).

In his paper "The 'Uncanny'" (1919), Freud cites our belief in future possibilities as an additional factor in explaining our conviction that we possess free will: "There are also the unfulfilled but possible futures to which we still like to cling in phantasy, all the strivings of the ego which adverse external circumstances have crushed, and all our suppressed acts of volition which nourish in us the illusion of Free Will" (p. 236).

Freudian Theory and Free Will

Although Freud appealed to unconscious motivation as part of his support for psychic determinism, he did not rest his conclusion about free will on any particular psychological theory. His argument is just the traditional one of the "Hard Determinist." He assumes, based partly on what he takes to be his own findings, that all actions and mental events are caused. Although he refers to this position as "determinism," it is sometimes called "macro-determinism" in that it says nothing about quantum events; consequently, it is not refuted by the finding that

there are uncaused events at the quantum level. The next step is to say that freedom of the will (and free choice and free action) is incompatible with determinism. Freud then draws the logical conclusion: There is no free will.

Because Freud does not rest his conclusion on any part of psychoanalytic theory, the falsification of that theory (excluding his thesis of psychical determinism) would not undermine his rejection of free will. Conversely, empirical support for psychoanalytic theory would not strengthen his argument, except for possibly solidifying his assumption that all human action and mental events are caused. The lesson is that psychoanalytic theory, either Freud's or one of the later versions, is not particularly relevant to the metaphysical question of whether free will exists. What matters in the debate about free will is whether human actions and mental events are always *caused* at all—not whether the causes are repressed wishes—and whether their being caused rules out free will.

Psychoanalytic theory, however, is relevant to a related issue: To what extent are we free, if we are free at all? Assume the thesis of "Compatibilism," which Freud himself rejected: that free choice and determinism can co-exist. Most compatibilists have held that although not all types of causes take away our freedom, some have that effect. For example, if behaviorists were right, and what we think, and feel, and want, and judge, made no difference to what we do, if all actions were automatic and mechanical responses to environmental events, then there would be no free choice (at least, it appears that way). It could be likewise argued that if Freudian theory is correct, then many seemingly free choices are not free because they result from motives to which we have no conscious access. Suppose, for example, that a woman has a series of bad love affairs and each time she begins a fresh affair, she believes that she gets involved for a different reason. One man is charming; another is extremely intelligent and handsome; a third is kind and loving; and so on. Unknown to her, however, none of her conscious reasons makes any difference to what she does. The real cause of her behavior is that she unconsciously views her lovers as incarnations of her father, whom she loves but also seeks to punish. Given the unconscious nature of the forces that drive her, she is not "a master of her own fate" and consequently, or so it could be argued, is not choosing freely when she chooses a lover (see Hospers, 1950).

If Freud's theory of repression is roughly right, and if our choices are unfree when they are determined by unconscious motives, then in many cases where we seem to make decisions based on rational reasons, we are, unknown to us, not making free choices. However, even if Freud's repression theory is combined with other reasonable assumptions, the combination will not support his radical conclusion that there is no free will at all. Furthermore, if psychoanalytic therapy can free a patient from the tyranny of unconscious motivation, then it is an important tool for enhancing the capacity for free choice.

So, if Freud is right both about Determinism and Incompatibilism, then psychoanalytic theory is not directly relevant to debates about free will; but if he is wrong about either—most obviously if he is wrong about Incompatibilism—then his repression theory, if correct, is relevant in deciding *when* we are free, and psychoanalytic therapy, if it is effective in making the unconscious conscious, provides, so to speak, a "remedy for unfreedom."

Freud's Incompatibilism

Freud's argument for incompatibilism rests partly on the widely held thesis that acting of our own free will equates with, or at least presupposes, the capacity to act otherwise than how we in fact act: ". . . we [i.e., those who believe in free will] would like to claim that we could have acted otherwise: that we have acted of our free—and unmotivated—will" (Freud, 1901: 254). Freud does need another assumption, one he does not spell out. He needs to assume not merely that our motives (or, in some cases, other factors) make a difference to what we do, but also that these causes, at least when combined with other factors and initial conditions, provide causally *sufficient conditions for acting*. Without the assumption of causal sufficiency, it is not clear why we would lack the capacity to act otherwise whenever we are caused to act by factors that create a propensity without necessitating our acting.

The thesis of universal causal sufficiency has been questioned by many scholars, and defended by others, but in the recent philosophic literature, it is Freud's initial assumption that has been most discussed. Compatibilists have tried to demonstrate, typically by use of either of two arguments, that there is no necessary connection between deciding or acting freely and having the capacity to do otherwise. The issue here concerns the logical implications of asserting that someone has acted or chosen freely. Freud did not, after all, appeal to empirical findings that there is a perfect correlation between acting freely and having the ability to do otherwise. Rather,

he assumed, as do most incompatibilists, that acting freely and having the power to do otherwise are one and the same thing, or at least, that a logical implication of saying that someone acted freely is that he or she could have done otherwise.

One caveat, however, is needed. It is assumed in contemporary philosophic discussions of free choice that what is being discussed is the sort of freedom required for moral responsibility.

Some compatibilists, then, argue that having the power to do otherwise and determinism are compatible; it is just that acting freely does not require that the agent have the power to do otherwise *even if everything in the universe had been exactly the same*. Rather, a hypothetical condition is all that need be met; if the universe had been different in some crucial causal respect, say, if the agent had wanted to act differently, then he or she could have done so. The attractiveness of this sort of defense of compatibilism, however, has been begun to fade because of the difficulty of specifying in any convincing way the respects in which the universe might have been different while the agent is free (see Erwin, 1997: 4–5; van Inwagen, 1983).

Consequently, some compatibilists (especially Frankfurt, 1969) rely on a second strategy; they try to show that there is there *no* necessary connection between choosing or acting freely and being able to do otherwise—at least, if we are talking about the sort of freedom required for moral responsibility.

Suppose that someone learning to drive goes through a red light deliberately and causes an accident. Assume that the driving instructor, possessing dual controls and herself being rather irresponsible, would have made the car continue its forward motion even if the client had braked, but that the client is unaware of this fact. What the driving instructor would have done, but in fact did not do, does not prevent the actual driver from freely choosing to go through the red light, nor does it absolve of her responsibility for what she did (see Fischer and Ravizza, 1998: 32). An incompatibilist can reply that the driver did have the capacity to step on the brakes, even if that act would have been ineffectual; otherwise, she is not responsible. So, she freely drove through the red light, but she also had the power to do something different. However, add another ingredient to the scenario. Suppose that the driving instructor's backup device is not a set of dual controls, but a machine hooked to the driver's brain. If the driver had, contrary to fact, decided to hit the brakes, the instructor would have pressed a button causing the driver to do exactly what she did do. The learner, therefore, could not have acted differently. She could not, let us stipulate, even have formed the intention to step on the brakes. Yet, given that the instructor never hit the button, the driver freely and deliberately chose to run the red light. If that is true, then contrary to what Freud and most incompatibilists assume, to choose freely does not logically require the freedom to do otherwise.

Both arguments for compatibilism are controversial, but even if (at least) one is rationally convincing, there is a further issue raised by some incompatibilists, although not by Freud. Even if freedom does not require the capacity to do otherwise, there is still a grave difficulty with the idea that freedom and determinism can co-exist. If Freud is right, then the events that largely determined what kind of person I have become occurred during my infancy, especially during the Oedipal period. If Object Relations theory is correct, they occurred even earlier. But I had little or no control over these events from my early life that led inevitably to my becoming neurotic or in acting in certain sorts of ways. It might be objected that even in Freud's theory, these childhood events, although they made an important difference, did not make my later actions inevitable. The childhood events talked about by Freud are causally relevant but they are not sufficient for determining what I have become. However, if determinism extends to all human behavior and our mental life, then some set of events occurring in my infancy—and in fact earlier—were causally sufficient for other events, which caused other events, which eventually and inevitably caused whatever I do today. How, then, can I ever be morally responsible if all of my actions are the inevitable result of events over which I had no control?

This last issue may be the most important in the free will debate. Some incompatibilists rest their case on what may be termed the "inevitability principle": If someone's act is the inevitable outcome of events over which the agent had no control, then the agent did not act freely and is not morally responsible for what was done (see Hospers, 1950 p. 710). Some compatibilists, however, argue that the principle is wrong. What matters to the possibility of freedom are the *kind* of causal factors that lead to the inevitable result. A severe brain injury in childhood may result in conditions that rob the adult of the capacity for free choice, but if early childhood con-

ditions (over which the child had no control) lead inevitably to the development of cognitive skills which facilitate free choice, such as the ability to process information and make reasoned judgments, then the inevitability of the act that results from the exercise of these skills does not nullify the freedom to choose (Erwin, 1997: 6–13; for an opposing view, see Inwagen, 1983; Klein, 1990).

REFERENCES

Erwin, E. (1997). *Philosophy and Psychotherapy.* London: Sage.
Fischer, J. M., and Ravissa, M. (1998). *Responsibility and Control.* Cambridge, U.K.: Cambridge University Press.
Frankfurt, H. (1969). The principle of alternate possibilities. *Journal of Philosophy,* 66: 829–839.
Freud, S. (1901). The Psychopathology of Everyday Life. S.E. 6: 1–279.
———. (1916–1917). *Introductory Lectures on Psychoanalysis.* S.E. 15–16: 9–496.
———. (1919). The 'uncanny'. S.E. 17: 219–256.
Hospers, J. (1950). Meaning and free will. *Philosophy and Phenomenological Research,* 10: 307–327.
Klein, M. (1990). *Determinism, Blameworthiness, and Deprivation.* New York: Oxford University Press.
Van Inwagen, P. (1983). *An Essay on Free Will.* New York: Oxford University Press.

EDWARD ERWIN

Freud, Anna (1895–1982)

Anna Freud, the youngest of Sigmund and Martha Freud's six children, was born in Vienna on December 3, 1895. As the youngest child, she struggled to make a place for herself in a busy household overseen by women—Martha Freud, her sister Minna, various nannies—and organized around school months in Vienna and vacation months in the Austrian countryside. Her father, who kept his consulting room in his Vienna apartment at Bergasse 19, worked long hours and was preoccupied with the development of psychoanalysis and the activities of its slowly growing band of adherents and visitors. In her own later memories, Anna Freud's childhood was dominated by her desire for her father's attention and her wish to be part of his world. As a young girl, she sat on the library steps during the Wednesday evening meeting of the Vienna Psychoanalytical Society.

Anna Freud's high school education prepared her to be a school teacher, and she took up this work just as the First World War gripped Central Europe. Following the example of other teachers who had begun to use Freud's ideas in early childhood education, such as Hermine Hug-Hellmuth, Anna decided to train as a psychoanalyst. She was analyzed by her father in the war years, and she helped found a section of the Vienna Psychoanalytical Society for child and adolescent work as the war ended. Her first publication, "Beating Fantasies and Daydreams," reports her own case in disguise.

During the 1920s, Anna Freud became involved in every facet of the growing psychoanalytic movement—building a training program, publishing journals, translating, coordinating work in Vienna, Budapest, Berlin, London—while she acted as her father's helpmate during his cancer surgeries and recuperations. She established friendships and alliances with the analysts of her father's original cohort. She also had a relationship of confidence with Lou Andreas-Salomé, and worked with all the second-generation trainees who would, eventually, carry on the psychoanalytic movement in every part of the world.

Unlike her brothers and sisters, Anna Freud continued to live at home; but she also formed a familylike relationship with an American divorcée, Dorothy Burlingham, and the four Burlingham children. The two women bought summer houses together and befriended other psychoanalyst couples: Marianne and Ernst Kris, Grete and Edward Bibring, Jenny and Robert Waelder, Annie and Maurits Katan, and Richard and Editha Sterba. During the school year, Dorothy Burlingham ran a school for her children and others along progressive, psychoanalytic lines. Erik Erikson and Peter Blos were associates in this project.

In the 1920s and 1930s, child analysis as a subspecialty of psychoanalysis became more and more important, as Freud had predicted in his 1925 preface to August Aichhorn's *Wayward Youth*, a pioneer work on juvenile delinquents: "children have become the main subject of psychoanalytic research and have thus replaced in importance the neurotics on whom its studies began" (1925, p. 273). Freud himself had proposed the idea that there are typical "lines of development" in childhood, but it was left to Anna Freud's generation to elaborate these lines on the basis of analytic work with children, not just from reconstructions of adult analyses. Differences of view arose, chiefly between Anna Freud's group and that around Melanie Klein, first in Berlin then in London after Klein's emigration there.

From the Kleinian point of view, various challenges to the convictions shared in Anna Freud's circle emerged: are adult and child analysis as different as Anna Freud thinks? can play be considered as equivalent to free asso-

ciation? is it necessary to do defense analysis as a first stage in child analysis—or can the analyst go right away for content, for active anxiety? does psychic structuration take place much earlier than Anna Freud thought? are primitive object relations also much earlier? do the instinctual drives (and with special force, the death instinct) manifest themselves in all children followed by a depressive position? is a conflict between life and death instincts, reflected in unconscious fantasy, the ultimate source of all pathology? Late in the 1920s, the groups in Vienna and London discussed these topics in exchanges of visits and papers and at international meetings. During World War II, a formal series of meetings, later called the Controversial Discussions (finally published in 1991), was organized in London.

In the late 1930s, Anna Freud and Dorothy Burlingham established the Jackson Nursery in Vienna and began to add child observation to the established research methods that had led to Anna Freud's classic *The Ego and the Mechanisms of Defense* (1936). During the war, after the Freuds and Burlinghams emigrated to England and Sigmund Freud died, Anna Freud used what she had learned in the Vienna nursery to organize care for British and emigrant children whose parents were involved in war work. From the wartime nurseries, her next organization, the Hampstead Clinic, emerged with units for therapeutic work, observation, pediatrics, and analytic training. Until her death in 1982, Anna Freud directed the Hampstead Clinic and organized there the most famous psychoanalytic center in the world, a mecca for child analysts and a meeting place for all analysts who wished to visit Freud's last home and renew themselves at Anna Freud's living legacy.

In the mid-1960s, collections of Anna Freud's books and papers began to appear from International Universities Press in New York. So it is in the eight volumes of *The Writings of Anna Freud* that her contributions, and the institutions and organizations in which they originated, can be tracked. There are two summary volumes, *The Ego and the Mechanisms of Defense* (1936) and *Normality and Pathology in Childhood* (1965), which present her two most fundamental frameworks—the first a catalog of defenses and the second a catalog of developmental lines.

Anna Freud always stressed in her work the complexity or layeredness in people's defenses. There are defenses against the id or instincts, against the superego, and against threats from the outside world; more generally, there are defenses against affects. Some defenses are typical of early childhood, some of the Oedipal period, others (which Anna Freud was the first to emphasize) of adolescence. In addition to the specific defenses Freud had considered, Anna Freud analyzed "identification with the aggressor" (turning onto others aggression experienced oneself) and "altruistic surrender" (turning over to others sexual desires or aggressive impulses felt to be unacceptable in oneself).

Anna Freud was not able to track a line of development specifically for defenses, but she did set out such lines in detail for the libido, for object relations, for ego growth, for narcissism, and for superego maturation. Looking to physical development and its mental and emotional correlates, she tracked a line of development for body control and management for play and work, for movement from passivity to activity and athleticism. These lines were then explored in their relations to cognitive development, speech development, intellectual specialization, and so forth—the domains particularly studied by Piaget.

One of the reasons for articulating so thoroughly the developmental lines was to enable analysts to be more complex in making diagnoses, or, more generally, in distinguishing pathology from normality. A diagnosis, in Anna Freud's view, should take into account a child's or adult's course along all the developmental lines, not just along one. When such a procedure—for which she wrote various guides, or diagnostic profiles—is followed, a kind of problem that is distinct from both neurosis and psychosis can show up. A "developmental disturbance" is an imbalance on the lines: normality in some areas and pathology in others; precocity in some areas and not in others; lags followed by catch-ups in some areas but not others; and so on. A developmental disturbance or a developmental disorder calls for analytic techniques different from those for neuroses or psychoses, and much of Anna Freud's attention in her last two decades went into research on alternative techniques.

In addition to the work she did with her clinic associates on defenses, on developmental lines, on diagnosis, and on techniques for developmental disorders, Anna Freud wrote many papers about psychoanalytic training and institutions (from nursery schools through psychoanalytic societies), several classic overviews of whole areas ("Notes on Aggression," 1949; "On Adolescence," 1958; "Obsessional Neurosis," 1965), a number of studies of her father's work ("A Study Guide to

Freud's Writing," 1978). In her later life, she became very interested in applying psychoanalytic insights to pediatrics, including care of children in hospitals, and to legal matters. With colleagues at the Yale Child Study Center, she coauthored three important volumes designed to show how psychoanalysis could inform legal decisions "in the best interests of the child."

REFERENCES

WRITINGS OF ANNA FREUD
Freud, A. (1925). Preface to Aichhorn's *Wayward Youth*. S.E. 19: 273–278.
———. (1928). *Introduction to the Technique of Child Analysis*. New York: Ayer Company Publishers.
———. (1935). *Psychoanalysis for Teachers and Parents*. New York: Norton.
———. (1966–1980). *The Writings of Anna Freud*. 8 vols. New York: International Universities Press.
   Vol. 1: *Introduction to Psychoanalysis: Lectures for Child Analysis and Teachers*. New York: International Universities Press (originally published 1922–1935).
   Vol. 2: *Ego and The Mechanisms of Defense*. New York: International Universities Press (originally published 1936).
   Vol. 3 *Infants Without Families: Reports on the Hampstead Nurseries* (originally published 1937–1944).
   Vol. 4: *Indications for Child Analysis and Other Papers* (originally published 1945–1956).
   Vol. 5: *Research at the Hampstead Child-Therapy Clinic and Other Papers* (originally published 1956–1965).
   Vol. 6: *Normality and Pathology in Childhood: Assessments of Development* (originally published 1965).
   Vol. 7: *Problems of Psychoanalytic Training, Diagnosis, and the Technique of Therapy* (1966–1969).
   Vol. 8: *Psychoanalytic Psychology of Normal Development* (1970–1980).
Freud, A., and Burlingham, D. T. (1944). *Infants Without Families: The Case Against Residential Nurseries*. New York: International Universities Press.

BOOKS ABOUT ANNA FREUD
Salber, W. (1986). *Anna Freud*. New York: Rowolt.
Peters, U. (1992). *Anna Freud: A Life Dedicated to Children*. New York: Schocken.
Sayers, J. (1993). *Mothers of Psychoanalysis*. New York: Norton.
Young-Bruehl, E. (1994). *Anna Freud: A Biography*. New York: Norton.

ELISABETH YOUNG-BRUEHL

Freud, Sigmund (1856–1939)

The creator of psychoanalysis and one of the most important figures in twentieth-century thought, Freud was born in Freiberg, Moravia (present-day Czech Republic), on May 6, 1856, the eldest child of Jacob and Amalie (née Nathanson) Freud. Jacob who was forty at the time of his marriage in 1855 to the nineteen-year-old Amalie, had two sons, Emanuel (b. 1832) and Philipp (b. 1836), from a first marriage to Sally Kanner. Between Sally and Amalie, Jacob was apparently also married in 1852 to a woman named Rebecca, whose existence was uncovered through archival research in the 1960s.

Early Years

Jacob Freud, an impecunious merchant, lived with his family in a single rented room. His son Sigmund, whose name at birth was Sigismund Schlomo, was followed by Julius (b. 1857) and Anna (b. 1858). Julius died at the age of eight months, but though Freud confided to his colleague Wilhelm Fliess that Julius's death left the "germ of reproaches" (Masson, 1985: 268) in him, Julius is nowhere mentioned in Freud's writings for publication. A crucial figure in Freud's household was a Catholic Czech nanny, originally thought to have been Monika Zajíc but actually probably named Resi Wittek, who took the young boy with her to church. When Freud was two and a half, the nanny was arrested for petty theft and sent to prison at his half-brother Philipp's instigation. The disappearance of his nanny coincided with Amalie's confinement at the birth of Anna. Freud's anxiety at being separated from his two mothers was conflated in a memory in which Philipp joked to him that his nanny had been "boxed up" (eingekastelt).

Implicit in Freud's memory was the fantasy that Philipp was the father of his sibling rival. The generational confusions in Freud's family were compounded by Emanuel's children John and Pauline, who lived nearby. Although they were his half-nephew and half-niece, John was a year older than Freud, and Pauline was the same age as he, just as his half-brothers were his mother's contemporaries and his father was John and Pauline's grandfather. A memory of playing in a meadow with John and Pauline, in which the two boys snatched away Pauline's flowers, surfaces in "Screen Memories" (1899) and the "non vixit" dream of The Interpretation of Dreams. In the latter, Freud refers to the fusion of "an intimate friend and a hated enemy" as "the ideal situation of childhood" and states that "all my friends have in a certain sense been reincarnations" (1900, p. 483) of John.

Because of financial pressures, Jacob Freud left Freiberg with his family in 1859, spending a year in Leipzig before settling in 1860 in Vienna, the city in which Freud would reside until 1938. While on the train journey from Leipzig to Vienna, Freud perhaps saw his mother naked, a reconstruction reported to Fliess in October 1897 using the Latin phrase matrem nudam. Four sisters and a brother were born between 1860 and 1866. In 1866, Jacob's brother Josef was imprisoned for trading in counterfeit money, a scheme in which Jacob's older sons, who had emigrated to Manchester, were allegedly involved.

The gradual abatement of legal discrimination against Jews in the Habsburg monarchy and the election in 1867 of a liberal faction in Vienna inaugurated an era in which even a Jewish boy could hope to grow up to be a cabinet minister. This ambition, which prompted Freud to contemplate a career in law, was spurred by a prediction of an itinerant poet; this echoed a peasant woman's prophecy to Freud's mother at his birth that she had brought a great man into the world. To show how much life had improved for Jews, Freud's father told him a story about an anti-Semite who had once knocked off his cap and ordered him to get off the pavement. Jacob Freud's passivity in the face of this indignity led Freud to identify with Hannibal, whose father had made him swear "to take vengeance on the Romans" (1900, p. 197). This identification is enacted in Freud's inhibition about entering Rome, which lasted until 1901.

From the ages of nine to seventeen Freud attended the local Sperlgymnasium, where he received the standard classical education and was consistently first in his class. In addition to Latin and Greek, Freud learned French and English and taught himself Spanish and Italian. His closest friends were Eduard Silberstein, a Romanian classmate, and the somewhat older Heinrich Braun, later a prominent figure in the Social Democratic Party. With Silberstein, Freud formed the Academia Espanola, a secret society modeled on Cervantes's Colloquy of the Dogs, and corresponded in Spanish and German. In 1872, Freud returned to Freiberg. Staying with the prosperous Fluss family, Freud developed a passion not only for the daughter Gisela but also her mother. He befriended Gisela's brother Emil, with whom he likewise corresponded. In 1875, Freud visited his half-brothers in Manchester, where he reencountered his childhood playmates John and Pauline. That Freud harbored fantasies of marriage with Gisela Fluss, while his father and Emanuel had concocted a plan for him to settle down with Pauline, is suggested by "Screen Memories," where Gisela's age is reported to have been fifteen though she was in actuality only eleven at the time (Breger, 2000: 36).

The Young Physician

Freud matriculated in the medical department of the University of Vienna in 1873. He later ascribed his decision to go to medical school to hearing a lecture "On Nature," a rhapsodic tract attributed to Goethe and regarded as a manifesto of the biological sciences. In addition to courses required of medical students, Freud attended five courses in philosophy taught by the theistic empiricist Franz Brentano. His avid reading of literature and philosophy included Ludwig Feuerbach's *The Essence of Christianity* (1841), which attacked religion as a pernicious illusion. With Josef Paneth, also Brentano's student, he belonged to the nationalist Reading Group of German Students. As a student in Carl Claus's Institute of Comparative Anatomy, Freud in 1876 journeyed to Trieste, where he undertook his first research project, an attempt to confirm through microscopic examination the presence of testes in male eels.

From 1876 to 1882, Freud worked in Ernst Brücke's Institute of Physiology. With Hermann Helmholtz and Emil Du Bois-Reymond, Brücke had founded the Berlin school of medical positivism, which attacked vitalism by seeking to explain organic phenomena solely in terms of physical and chemical forces. Freud's research included an investigation of the nerve cells of the lamprey prompted by Darwin's theory of evolution. In 1879–1880, Freud completed a year of compulsory military service during which he translated four essays by John Stuart Mill, whose belief in the equality of women he derided. At Brücke's laboratory, Freud met Ernst von Fleischl-Marxow, Brücke's assistant, and Josef Breuer, one of Vienna's most eminent physicians, from whom in 1882 he first heard about the case of Anna O. (Anna O. was the pseudonym used for Bertha Pappenheim, the first patient treated with a new form of psychotherapy.)

Belatedly obtaining his medical degree in 1881, which had been delayed by his scientific pursuits, Freud heeded Brücke's advice by leaving his laboratory and taking a junior position at the Vienna General Hospital in the summer of 1882. The need to provide for his future stemmed from his meeting that spring with Martha Bernays, to whom he became engaged after two months, although the marriage would not take place for more than four years. Five years younger than Freud and raised in

an Orthodox Jewish family—her paternal grandfather had been chief rabbi of Hamburg—Martha moved back with her mother from Vienna to Wandsbek, outside Hamburg, in 1883. In the same year, her brother Eli married Freud's sister Anna. Freud's incessant letters to Martha during their betrothal show him to have been jealous and insecure as a lover. After their marriage, he forbade Martha to light the Sabbath candles.

At the Vienna General Hospital Freud worked briefly on the surgery wards, then moved to the Department of Internal Medicine as assistant to Hermann Nothnagel. In 1883, he rotated to the Department of Psychiatry, headed by the brain anatomist Theodor Meynert. After further stints in the Department of Dermatology and the Department of Nervous Diseases, Freud left the hospital in the summer of 1885, having completed a dissertation on the medulla oblongata (hindbrain, excluding the cerebellum) and risen to the rank of privatdozent.

In 1884, Freud became interested in cocaine, then a little-known drug. Burdened by a growing debt to Breuer and loans from other colleagues, he saw the alkaloid as an avenue to fame and fortune. In his essay "On Coca" (1884), he hailed its wide-ranging medicinal effects. Before leaving to visit Martha in Wandsbek in September, Freud mentioned the anesthetizing properties of the drug to Leopold Königstein, an ophthamologist. Upon his return, he found that another colleague, Carl Koller, had already won acclaim for demonstrating that cocaine could indeed be utilized as a local anesthetic in eye operations. Although Koller acknowledged Freud's contribution, Freud resented Martha for having caused him to miss the success that he thought should have been his. In April 1885, Königstein operated on Freud's father for glaucoma, using as an anesthetic cocaine administered by Koller with Freud's assistance.

As the dangers of cocaine addiction became recognized, Freud fell under attack. Although in "On the General Effect of Cocaine" (1885) Freud had urged administering cocaine by subcutaneous injection to cure morphine addiction, in the 1895 "Irma dream" in *The Interpretation of Dreams*, he denied ever having done this and omitted this paper from the list of publications submitted with his application for the title of professor in 1897. In the Irma dream he likewise inaccurately asserted that his advocacy of cocaine had begun in 1885, not 1884. In the 1885 paper, Freud misrepresented the case of his admired friend from Brücke's laboratory, von

F

Fleischl-Marxow, a morphine addict who also became addicted to cocaine after injecting it at Freud's instigation (Thornton, 1984: 26). After an agonizing ordeal, von Fleischl-Marxow died in 1891.

Unease over his advocacy of cocaine may have spurred Freud's decision, imparted in April 1885 to Martha Bernays, to destroy his records of the past fourteen years. This letter, with its avowal of the desire to confound future biographers, each of whom would be left to formulate his own "Conception of the Development of the Hero," is quoted by Ernest Jones in the preface to his biography of Freud. Regret over his infatuation with Gisela Fluss had probably led to an analogous 1877 proposal to Silberstein of an "auto-da-fé" of the archives of "Academia Espanola." He undertook a third such immolation of his papers in 1907. Freud's use of cocaine extended from 1884 to at least 1896. Reporting his father's death to Fliess in 1896, Freud vowed that "the cocaine brush has been completely put aside" (Masson, 1985: 201). His addiction to cigars, begun at twenty-four, like his passion for collecting antiquities, remained lifelong.

In June 1885, Freud was awarded a travel grant to study with Charcot at the Salpêtrière hospital in Paris, where he arrived in October. Although his neurological interests would eventuate in *On Aphasia* (1891), an important monograph in which he proposed a functional explanation of speech disorders and adumbrated the psychoanalytic theory of regression, as well as in a definitive study of infantile cerebral paralysis contributed to Nothnagel's handbook in 1897, Freud's stay in Paris occasioned a decisive reorientation in his focus from physiological to psychological problems. Smitten by Charcot's influence, he won the great man's favor by offering to translate his lectures from French into German. From Charcot's theatrical demonstrations, Freud took away two key ideas: (1) hysterical symptoms such as paralysis (which could afflict men as well as women) were not due simply to organic causes but were delimited by common concepts of the body; and (2) its symptoms could be mimicked in nonhysterical patients through hypnosis. Although Charcot's postulation of hysteria as a real disease entity has been indicted as "one of the most significant misunderstandings in the entire history of medicine" (Webster, 1995: 72), it left Freud with the conviction that mental causes could have physical effects.

Freud left Paris in February 1886, returning to Vienna by way of Berlin, where he spent a month at Adolf Baginsky's pediatric clinic. Opening a private practice in neuropathology in 1886, Freud continued to work without remuneration for the next ten years at Max Kassowitz's Institute for Children's Diseases. After completing his remaining military service in August 1886, Freud married Martha in September in Wandsbek. In Vienna, the couple settled into an apartment in a building known as the House of Atonement. Their first child, Mathilde, was born the following year. Five others followed in rapid succession: Martin (b. 1889), Oliver (b. 1891), Ernst (b. 1892), Sophie (b. 1893), and Anna (b. 1895). The family moved in 1891 to larger quarters in Berggasse 19. Freud insisted on leasing the apartment over his wife's protests because, as a university student, he had been to the building with Heinrich Braun to visit Braun's brother-in-law Victor Adler, who likewise became a Social Democratic leader and with whom Freud had clashed at the Reading Group of German Students. Also in 1891, for his thirty-fifth birthday, Freud's father gave him, rebound in leather and with an elaborate Hebrew inscription he had composed, the bilingual (Hebrew and German) illustrated Philippsohn Bible that Freud had read in his youth.

Casting himself as the Viennese apostle of Charcot's views on hypnosis and hysteria, Freud soon became caught up in conflicts with Meynert, as he did also with the French neurologist Pierre Janet, whose interests overlapped his own. In November 1887, Freud met Wilhelm Fliess, a general practitioner from Berlin who attended his lectures. This friendship, the most important in Freud's life, lasted until 1901. In an unpleasant aftermath, Fliess in 1904 accused Freud of having divulged his ideas on bisexuality to a patient, Hermann Swoboda, who passed them on to Otto Weininger. Although Freud at first denied the charge, he was forced to concede its truth. In this imbroglio, Freud turned for support to Karl Kraus, editor of *Die Fackel (The Torch)*; but in 1908 Kraus would become a critic of psychoanalysis.

Freud's letters to Fliess, sold by Fliess's younger son in 1936 to Marie Bonaparte, who refused to heed Freud's pleas that they be destroyed, were published in censored form in 1950 but not until 1985 in their entirety. Fliess's numerological determinism, stemming from his belief that human life is governed by male and female periods of twenty-three and twenty-eight days, respectively, as well as his allegation of a connection between the nose and the female genital organs, seems today to have little or no scientific merit. This has led psychoanalytic commentators to regard Freud's extravagant admiration of Fliess as evidence of a transferential relationship. In a revisionist study, Frank Sulloway (1979) has contended that Freud was drawn to Fliess because of their shared allegiance to the intellectual traditions of nineteenth-century biology. Sulloway, however, conflates Darwinism proper with the theories of Lamarck (inheritance of acquired characteristics) and Haeckel (ontogeny recapitulates phylogeny), and thus perhaps minimizes the irrational tendencies of both thinkers.

The 1890s: The Evolution of Psychoanalysis

In 1889, Freud traveled to Nancy to study the hypnotic methods of Ambroise Liébeault and Hippolyte Bernheim, whose *On Suggestion* he had translated the previous year. He was accompanied by Anna von Lieben ("Frau Cäcilie M"), who, with Fanny Moser ("Emmy von N."), was one of his principal early patients. During the 1890s, Freud gradually abandoned hypnotic suggestion, including the symptom-specific cathartic method employed by Breuer with Anna O., replacing it first by the "pressure technique," in which he placed his hand on patients' foreheads and urged them to report the thought or image that came to mind in response to a question, then by the wholly nondirective technique of free association.

Breuer and Freud's "Preliminary Communication," which declared that "hysterics suffer mainly from reminiscences," was published in 1893 and reprinted two years later in *Studies on Hysteria*. Despite their collaboration, Freud chafed at Breuer's cautious temperament and his preference for a theory that explained hysteria as a result of somatic hypnoid states over his own emphasis on conversion as a defense against unacceptable ideas. Their rupture became final by 1896, as Freud turned with ever-increasing intensity to Fliess for emotional support.

In 1895, Freud sent Fliess the draft of the *Project for a Scientific Psychology*, a comprehensive metapsychology attempt to establish psychology on a neurological foundation. On July 23–24 of the same year, he dreamed the dream of Irma's injection, which became the "specimen dream" of *The Interpretation of Dreams*. The figure of Irma is a composite of Anna Lichtheim, the young widowed daughter of his erstwhile teacher of religion Samuel Hammerschlag, and Emma Eckstein, another of his patients. Earlier that year, Freud had invited Fliess to perform an operation on Eckstein's nose in the mis-

guided belief that this would alleviate her abdominal pains. Fliess had botched the operation, however, leaving a half-meter strip of gauze in Eckstein's nose that had to be removed by Ignaz Rosanes, a former school friend of Freud's. Despite this evidence of Fliess's negligence, Freud clung to his idealized image of the latter, going so far as to impute Emma's postoperative hemorrhages to "hysterical longing" (Masson, 1985: 183).

The late 1890s were the most turbulent years in Freud's life. His growing preoccupation with sexuality, and particularly his conviction that pathological states could be traced to deferred effects of childhood sexual abuse, was expressed in a series of papers culminating in "The Etiology of Hysteria" (1896). Although Freud proclaimed that he had discovered the "*caput Nili*" of pathological states, Krafft-Ebing dismissed Freud's paper as a "scientific fairy tale" (Masson, 1985: 184). The term "psychoanalysis" makes its debut in "Heredity and the Etiology of the Neuroses" (1896). In this paper, Freud distinguished between *actual neuroses*, which he attributed to unsatisfactory sexual practices that did not require psychological elucidation, and *psychoneuroses*, such as hysteria and obsessional neurosis. Hysteria was deemed to be the consequence of premature sexual arousal that had been suffered passively, while obsessional neurosis resulted if the child went on to assume a more active and pleasurable role.

Although the inception of Freud's self-analysis cannot be dated precisely, it coincides roughly with his father's death in October 1896. Freud began systematically to recover childhood memories and to interpret his dreams in letters to Fliess. His most important patient, apart from himself, was Oscar Fellner ("Herr E."). The process reached its culmination in September-October 1897, when Freud divulged his abandonment of the seduction theory and thereafter invoked *Oedipus Rex* and *Hamlet* to support the idea that the son's love of the mother and jealousy of the father comprise "a universal event in early childhood" (Masson, 1985: 272).

Freud's repudiation of his seduction theory and concomitant emphasis on the importance of fantasy constitutes a turning point in his thought. As he wrote to Fliess, "there are no indications of reality in the unconscious, so that one cannot distinguish between truth and fiction that has been cathected with affect" (Masson, 1985: 264). To his defenders, this insight into the role of unconscious fantasies beginning in early childhood is a momentous breakthrough, while to his critics it merely substituted one wrong but empirically testable theory for another wrong but unverifiable one, the data for both being contaminated by suggestion. Freud did not publicly retract his 1896 theory until *Three Essays on the Theory of Sexuality* (1905), and then only obliquely. The inconsistencies in his various accounts, especially as to whether the perpetrator of seduction could be anyone or had to be specifically the father, have been cited by Freud's detractors as evidence of his bad faith. Viewed more charitably, they reflect the natural evolution of his thought and an attempt to preserve a dialectical balance between the contributions of the internal and external worlds.

Freud's masterwork, *The Interpretation of Dreams*, appeared in November 1899 but was dated 1900. At once scientific treatise and autobiography, the book sold only 351 copies during the first six years but was widely reviewed. The second edition appeared in 1909, and six more by 1930. Freud continually revised the work, giving it the quality of a palimpsest. It argues that dreams constitute wish fulfillments and describes condensation and displacement as the principal mechanisms of the dream work. The seventh chapter reformulates the metapsychology of the *Project* while introducing the topographical division of the mind into conscious, preconscious, and unconscious strata.

Freud began to attract adherents, including Wilhelm Stekel and Alfred Adler, who collectively experienced his book as a revelation. This led in October 1902 to the formation of the Psychological Wednesday Society, which met in his apartment. In 1905 Otto Rank joined the circle, which became known in 1908 as the Vienna Psychoanalytic Society. Other Viennese recruits included Hanns Sachs and Paul Federn. Freud's routine featured weekly games of tarock in a café, excursions with his children to the woods, and biweekly attendance at meetings of the B'nai B'rith. A series of major works followed: *The Psychopathology of Everyday Life* (published as two extended essays in 1901 and as a book in 1904), the case history of Dora (completed in 1901 but not published until 1905), *Jokes and Their Relation to the Unconscious* (1905), and the *Three Essays*. In *Psychopathology* and *Jokes*, Freud extended his model of dreams and neurotic symptoms as compromise formations to ordinary social phenomena. These works also continue Freud's self-analysis, since in the former he explained several errors in *The Interpretation of Dreams* and Fliess had criticized his dreams for sounding too much like jokes. Together with *The Interpretation of Dreams*, the *Three Essays* is

Freud's most seminal work, undergoing extensive revisions in six editions over the next twenty years. It accentuates infantile sexuality and links its pregenital components to adult perversions.

Internationalization of Psychoanalysis

His long-deferred visit to Rome, the first of seven in his life, occurred in September 1901, accompanied by his brother Alexander. Another elusive goal was achieved in 1902 when Freud received an appointment as professor extraordinarius—a prestigious title that did not give him the rights of an ordinary professor—for which he had first been nominated by Nothnagel and Krafft-Ebing in 1897. Freud blamed the delay on anti-Semitism, though it may have had as much to do with his emphasis on sexuality or simply bureaucratic inertia. His success came about when he enlisted the aid of a wealthy patient, Marie Ferstel, who is said to have donated a painting to a newly opened gallery controlled by the minister of education.

The greatest enigma in Freud's life concerns his relationship to his sister-in-law Minna Bernays. She joined the Freud household in 1896, ten years after the death of her fiancé, Ignaz Schönberg. Freud and Minna traveled together in 1900 to Italy, as well as on other occasions. Linking interlocking pieces of evidence—that the *"aliquis"* parapraxis in the *Psychopathology* (which concerns the fear of having impregnated a woman) is in all probability Freud's own; Freud's avowal of a desire to enjoy a love that was "free of cost" in the "table d'hôte" dream in *On Dreams* (1901, p. 656); documentation that after their trip Minna went to a spa in Merano, where she may have undergone an abortion; and an independent report that she spoke of the matter to Jung in 1907—Peter Swales (1982) has argued that she and Freud had an affair. To many, this thesis has seemed inconceivable because it contradicts the received image of Freud's character as one of sterling probity and chastity. In recent revisionist scholarship, however, both Freud's personal and his intellectual reputation have been seriously challenged, which helps to make the thought that he thus transgressed conventional morality appear more plausible than it once did.

By 1905, the fundamental elements of the Freudian system were in place. The years 1905–1910 saw the emergence of the international recognition of psychoanalysis. In 1906 Freud received his first letter from Jung, Eugen Bleuler's assistant at the Burhölzli hospital in Zurich. In 1907, Max Eitingon, also at the Burghölzli, became the first emissary to Freud. He was soon followed by Jung, accompanied by his wife and Ludwig Binswanger, and then Karl Abraham. Sándor Ferenczi came from Budapest in 1908. The first International Psychoanalytic Congress took place in Salzburg in October 1908, with forty-two registrants. There Freud met Ernest Jones from Britain and A. A. Brill from New York. The Swiss pastor Oskar Pfister visited Vienna in 1909. The same year, Freud traveled to the United States to lecture at Clark University in Worcester, Massachusetts, where he received an honorary degree. Jung was also invited, and Freud brought along Ferenczi. Freud stayed with Clark's president, G. Stanley Hall, and James Jackson Putnam, met William James, saw Niagara Falls, and visited New York City. On their way home, Freud and Ferenczi stopped in Berlin to consult a medium, a manifestation of the latter's lifelong susceptibility to the occult. Notwithstanding his triumph, Freud returned to Vienna with an abiding antipathy to the United States.

In Salzburg Freud lectured extemporaneously for three hours on the case of the Rat Man. This case, like that of Little Hans—the first child analysis, conducted under Freud's guidance by the boy's father, the musicologist Max Graf—is integral to the unfolding of the concept of the Oedipus complex, a term first used by Freud in 1910. The fundamentals of a psychoanalytic approach to art were delineated in *Creative Writers and Day-Dreaming* (1907), *Delusions and Dreams in Jensen's "Gradiva"* (1907), and *Leonardo da Vinci and a Memory of His Childhood* (1910). By his fusion of science and humanism, Leonardo, like Goethe, became an object of identification for Freud. His fourth major case history, based on the memoirs of the paranoid jurist Daniel Paul Schreber, was begun on a trip to Sicily with Ferenczi in 1910 and published the following year. In "Formulation on the Two Principles of Mental Functioning" (1911), Freud introduced the distinction between the pleasure and reality principles. His papers on psychoanalytic technique, centering on the transference, appeared between 1911 and 1915.

Emergence of Conflict

With the expansion of psychoanalysis as practice and theory came bitter conflicts. Freud's desire to anoint Jung as his successor, in part driven by anxiety about the Jewish character of the psychoanalytic movement, aroused the enmity of his Viennese followers. At the Nuremberg Congress in 1910, the International Psycho-Analytical Association was founded, with Jung as president. Jung

retained control of the *Jahrbuch für psychoanalytische und psychopathologische Forschungen*, hatched in Salzburg. To recompense the Viennese, a new journal was started, the *Zentralblatt für Psychoanalyse*, overseen jointly by Freud, Adler, and Stekel. Adler's advocacy of the concepts of an aggressive drive and organ inferiority ran afoul of Freud's insistence on the primacy of libido, and after the 1911 Weimar Congress, Adler was forced to resign from the Vienna Psychoanalytic Society and from the editorship of the *Zentralblatt*. Stekel left the society in November 1912, but since he refused to relinquish the *Zentralblatt*, Freud, Rank, and Jones launched the *Internationale Zeitschrift für Psychoanalyse*. When Adler set up the Society for Free Psychoanalytic Research, Freud issued an edict that no one could attend meetings of both Adler's group and his own. He made an exception only for Lou Andreas-Salomé, who arrived in Vienna in October 1912.

Premonitions of the schism with Jung can be seen as early as 1909, when Freud fainted for the first time in his presence in Bremen prior to the trip to America and when, while on board the *George Washington*, he refused to allow Jung to interpret one of his dreams. Tensions mounted in 1912, following Jung's second visit to the United States, where he held forth on his revisions of Freud's sexual conception of the libido and the Oedipus complex. Matters were smoothed over until a November meeting in Munich, when Freud again fainted, this time in a hotel room where he had previously encountered Fliess. In December, Jung became enraged when Freud interpreted a slip in one of his letters. Despite the breakdown of personal relations, Jung was reelected president of the IPA at the Munich Congress in September 1913. But he presently resigned his editorship of the *Jahrbuch*, and in April 1914 also from his post. The entire Zurich group then voted to withdraw from the International Association, leaving Freud and his allies politically victorious.

Concern over the rift with Jung led, in 1912, to the formation of a secret committee of Freud's closest followers to safeguard the future of the psychoanalytic movement. Its original members were Jones, Ferenczi, Rank, Sachs, and Abraham, to each of whom Freud gave a ring. Eitingon joined the circle in 1919, and others—including Andreas-Salomé and Anna Freud—also received rings. Freud settled his scores with the defectors in the polemical *On the History of the Psycho-Analytic Movement* (1914). *The Moses of Michelangelo* (1914), published anonymously in *Imago*—a journal founded by Rank and Sachs in 1912 specializing in the cultural applications of psychoanalysis—reflected Freud's identification with the leader forced to restrain his anger against deserters. *Totem and Taboo* (1913), also published in *Imago*, challenged Jung on his own ground of mythology by speculating that an actual killing of a father by his sons in a primal horde lay at the origin of human history. This apotheosis of the Oedipus complex can be interpreted as a symbolic murder of Jung as well as a fantasy in which Freud, as the primal father of psychoanalysis, is murdered by his sons. His last and most famous major case history, that of the Wolf Man, not published until 1918, concerns an analysis conducted from 1910 to 1914. It seeks clinically to refute Adler and Jung by tracing the patient's neurosis to an infantile primal scene. Freud's vacillation as to its ontological status—whether it was a real event or only a fantasy—parallels that concerning the primal patricide in *Totem and Taboo*.

Freud spent World War I (1914–1918) almost entirely in Vienna, confident as late as September 1916 of a victory by the Central Powers. His sons Martin and Ernst served in the army, while living conditions at home became increasingly onerous. Before the outbreak of the war, Freud completed *On Narcissism: An Introduction* (1914), in which he set forth the concept of the ego ideal, later to become the superego. This paper, which continues the controversies with Adler and Jung by proposing narcissism as an alternative to both masculine protest and nonsexual libido, marks the beginning of the second major period in the development of Freudian theory. In 1915, resuming his quest for a comprehensive theoretical framework in the *Project* and Chapter 7 of *The Interpretation of Dreams*, Freud appears to have completed a series of twelve metapsychological essays, five of which were published, including *Instincts and Their Vicissitudes* (1915), *The Unconscious* (1915), and *Mourning and Melancholia* (1917). In *The Unconscious*, Freud stipulated that a complete account of a psychical process entailed description of its *dynamic, topographical,* and *economic* aspects. The other seven papers were probably destroyed, though one on the transference neuroses—a pseudoscientific amalgam of Lamarck and Haeckel that prefigures Ferenczi's *Thalassa* (1924)—was found among Ferenczi's papers and published in 1985. At the University of Vienna, Freud delivered what became the *Introductory Lectures on Psycho-Analysis* (1916–17), one of the most accessible and perennially popular of his works.

When in September 1918 forty-two psychoanalysts convened in Budapest for the first postwar congress—the dissolution of the Austro-Hungarian Empire would be sealed in November—the use of psychoanalysis in the treatment of the battle trauma of shell shock had done much to blunt the resistance of its opponents. Anton von Freund, a wealthy Budapest brewer, endowed a publishing house. Despite these favorable developments, the war left its imprint in the deepening pessimism of Freud's thought. In this trend, larger social forces were reinforced by personal tragedies. Although not experienced as a loss by Freud, Victor Tausk's violent suicide in July 1919 was a blow to the Vienna Society. Before the year's end, von Freund died of cancer. Still worse, Freud's daughter Sophie, married to the photographer Max Halberstadt, died of influenza in January 1920.

The notion of the repetition compulsion, integral to Freud's literary essay *The Uncanny* (1919), received its most systematic exposition in *Beyond the Pleasure Principle* (1920), in which he postulated a death instinct. Although Freud had begun to write the book before Sophie's death and insisted that this event had no bearing on his formulation, the term made its first appearance in a portion of the manuscript composed subsequently. Freud's theory, in which both sexuality and self-preservation are subsumed under the life instinct, now defined in opposition to a biological drive to return to an inorganic state, is a dazzling feat of philosophical speculation; but even most analysts would concede that the phenomena for which it purports to account can be better explained in less far-fetched ways. In *Group Psychology and the Analysis of the Ego* (1921), Freud treated social psychology as individual psychology writ large, attributing the deterioration in standards in group behavior to a reversion to the primal horde of *Totem and Taboo*. The leader—and again it is difficult not to think of the psychoanalytic movement as well as Freud's chosen examples of the church and the army—is ultimately the primal father, who governs the group as the ego ideal does the ego.

Final Years

The year 1923 inaugurates the final phase of Freud's life and thought. In *The Ego and the Id* (1923), he replaced the earlier topographical model with the structural division of the mind into id, ego, and superego. This schema became the cornerstone of the tradition of ego psychology. Freud took the concept of the id from Georg Groddeck, who at the 1920 congress in The Hague defiantly proclaimed himself a "wild analyst" and whose *Book of the It* also appeared in 1923; but Freud, unlike Groddeck, sought to subordinate the id to the civilizing powers of the ego. In April 1923 came the initial operation on Freud's cancer of the jaw, though his doctor, Felix Deutsch, dissembled the seriousness of his condition. Two months later, Freud suffered his most grievous personal blow when Heinz, the younger child of his deceased daughter Sophie, died of tuberculosis at the age of four. Finally informed of his cancer, Freud was operated on in October for seven hours by the surgeon Hans Pichler, who removed his upper jaw and palate on the right side, inserting a removable metal prosthesis in its place. No recurrence of cancer was found for thirteen years, though Freud underwent more than thirty operations and constant experimentation to improve his prosthesis during that time.

Freud's illness exacerbated already existing strains in the committee, whose members had been apprised of Freud's condition even before Freud himself at an August meeting in San Cristoforo. Rank quarreled with Jones and later also with Abraham. Rank and Ferenczi's joint work, *The Development of Psychoanalysis* (1923), had been written without the knowledge of other members of the committee; and Rank's *Trauma of Birth* (1924), although ostensibly an extension of Freud's thought, offended the conservatives by its challenge to the primacy of the Oedipus complex. The committee as originally constituted was dissolved by the April 1924 Congress in Salzburg, not attended by Freud. Freud was initially receptive to Rank's innovation, but his view hardened, influenced by reports from Brill of the effects of Rank's visit that summer to the United States. After protracted displays of ambivalence, Rank broke irrevocably from Freud in 1926 and moved to Paris.

Rank's defection was the most painful of Freud's career. His departure and Freud's need for care in his illness caused Freud to turn increasingly for support to his daughter Anna, who emerged after his death as the successor he had sought in vain among his male disciples. From 1918 to 1921, and again in 1924, Freud took her into analysis, an irregular proceeding even by the standards of the time. The unswervingly loyal Abraham died in December 1925, not yet fifty years of age. Freud proffered his criticisms of Rank's ideas first in *The Dissolution of the Oedipus Complex* (1924) and then again in *Inhibitions, Symptoms, and Anxiety* (1926), his last major work of theory, in which he revised his earlier conception of

anxiety as repressed libido in favor of one of anxiety as a danger signal that activates defenses. Despite his afflictions, Freud remained extraordinarily prolific. *An Autobiographical Study* appeared in 1925. The following year, he intervened on behalf of Theodor Reik, a psychologist who had been charged by Viennese authorities with treating a patient without a medical degree, and published *The Question of Lay Analysis*. The issue of lay analysis continued to polarize the psychoanalytic movement, especially in the United States, long after Freud's death.

In a 1935 postscript to *An Autobiographical Study*, Freud described himself as having made a "lifelong *détour* through the natural sciences" before returning to the "cultural problems" that had fascinated him in his youth (1925, p. 72). This cast of mind is displayed in *The Future of an Illusion* (1927), an unmasking of religion as a hollow comfort derived from childhood wishes for protection from helplessness and dependence. Freud's definitive work of political philosophy is *Civilization and Its Discontents* (1930), in which he fused his structural model of the mind with the theory of the death instinct to argue that there is an irremediable antagonism between instinctual demands and the restrictions of civilization. In 1930, while in Berlin for work on his prosthesis, Freud met William C. Bullitt, an American diplomat, and offered to collaborate with him on a biography of Woodrow Wilson, whom he blamed for Austria's plight after World War I. Not published until 1967, *Thomas Woodrow Wilson: A Psychological Study* treats Wilson's career as permutations of his conflicts with his father and younger brother and has been widely judged to be unsatisfactory. Attracting greater notice but now also generally lamented are Freud's forays into the psychology of women, from 1925 through 1933, in which he persisted in viewing gender differences through the monocular lens of penis envy.

Repeatedly disappointed in his hopes for the Nobel prize, Freud in 1930 was awarded the Goethe prize; Anna journeyed to Frankfurt to deliver his acceptance speech. His mother died the same year after reaching her ninety-fifth birthday. Ferenczi, with whom relations had grown strained, died in 1933. At their final meeting in 1932, Freud urged him not to deliver his paper "Confusion of Tongues between Adults and the Child" at the Wiesbaden Congress. Now regarded as a classic, Ferenczi's attempt to rethink the effects of childhood sexual trauma was dismissed by Freud as a regression to the seduction theory he had abandoned in 1897.

F

By 1933 the political situation in Europe had grown precarious for Jews. Hitler came to power in Germany in January, and in May Freud's books were among those burned by the Nazis in Berlin. An exchange of letters with Einstein, in which Freud countered Einstein's hope that nations would yield a measure of sovereignty to an international tribunal by asserting the impossibility of suppressing human aggressiveness, was published under the title *Why War?* (1933). Freud brought his exposition of psychoanalysis up to date by adding seven lectures to the twenty-eight he had delivered during World War I, though the *New Introductory Lectures* (1933) reached their audience only through the medium of print. Despite Freud's pessimism evinced with respect to the therapeutic aims of psychoanalysis in *Analysis Terminable and Interminable* (1937)—a paper antithetical to his belief in the possibility of permanently removing symptoms in *Studies on Hysteria* and other early works—he held out as long as possible against those who urged him to emigrate from Austria. His eightieth birthday, in 1936, was feted both in Vienna and internationally. The German writer Thomas Mann read his paper "Freud and the Future" to Freud at his home; but though the minister of education extended formal congratulations, Austrian newspapers were prohibited from reporting the event.

Hitler's triumphant entry into Austria and announcement of its incorporation into the Reich in March 1938 was commemorated in the diary Freud kept for the last decade of his life with the laconic words *"Finis Austriae."* Bullitt, now U.S. ambassador to France, drew the attention of President Roosevelt to the danger faced by Freud and his family, while Jones mobilized his highly placed friends in England. Freud finally yielded to necessity and sought permission to emigrate. Anna was interrogated by the Gestapo for a day before being released. After complying with the extortionate demands of the regime, the Freud family was granted its exit papers. A portion of Freud's library—some eight hundred items—was handed over for sale to a Viennese bookseller. These books found their way to the New York State Psychiatric Institute. The remainder, along with Freud's vast collection of antiquities, were safely transported to London.

The exodus occurred in June. After spending a day with Marie Bonaparte in Paris, Freud and his entourage arrived in England. He lived in a rented home before moving in September to 20 Maresfield Gardens, which remained the home of Anna Freud until her death in 1982. He was greeted with acclaim by high and low.

When Freud was unable to travel to the headquarters of the Royal Society to sign its Charter Book—placing his name, as he told Arnold Zweig, in the company of Newton and Darwin—its secretaries brought it to him, an honor previously reserved for the king. He summoned the strength to undertake a last new project, *An Outline of Psycho-Analysis* (1940), in which he restated the tenets of his science in apodictic fashion. He likewise brought to completion *Moses and Monotheism* (1939), a series of three essays begun in 1934. At once a reprise of his meditations on Moses and an application to religion of his thesis of a primal patricide in *Totem and Taboo*, the work aroused controversy by its contention that Moses was not Jewish but an Egyptian, and only the deferred effects of his murder—an inherited memory trace—elevated his people to monotheism. Freud's eccentric attitude to Moses is paralleled by that to Shakespeare, who, he came by 1928 to believe, was really the earl of Oxford.

In January 1939, an ominous swelling appeared at the back of Freud's mouth, and by March it was deemed inoperable. Freud refused drugs to alleviate his pain and continued to treat patients until August 1, when he closed his practice. He remained worried about his four sisters, between the ages of seventy-five and eighty, still living in Austria. All were later killed in concentration camps. On September 21, he reminded Max Schur, his physician since 1928, of a promise he had made to help him end it all when the time came. Schur administered a dose of morphine, and repeated it after twelve hours. Freud lapsed into a coma and died on September 23, 1939.

Assessments of Freud

There is probably more known—and to be known—about Freud than any other human being who has ever lived. The twenty-four volumes of the English-language *Standard Edition* will be at least doubled by the steadily increasing number of reliable scholarly editions of his correspondence. Among the still defective or unpublished sets of letters are those with Rank, Eitingon, Brill, and Martha and Minna Bernays. The countless reports of people who knew Freud personally must also be classified as primary sources. Despite a gradual policy of liberalization by the Sigmund Freud Archives, a vast repository of material remains inaccessible in the Library of Congress.

The landmarks of Freud biography include the three volumes of Ernest Jones (1953–1957), which, augmented by the moving narrative by Max Schur (1972), set forth

F

the authorized version of the story; Ronald Clark's (1980) evenhanded rendition for the general reader; Peter Gay's (1988) refurbishing of the orthodox perspective; and Louis Breger's (2000) sterner reckoning from the standpoint of contemporary relational theory. Although Jones's portrait has been accused of idealization, he took for granted that Freud's life, no less than anyone else's, could be interpreted along psychoanalytic lines. He thus inadvertently widened the door to revisionist criticism that Siegfried Bernfeld had opened when he identified Freud as the patient of "Screen Memories" and branded Freud's efforts at self-concealment as an "outright lie" (1946, p. 27). Even the abridged 1950 edition of the Fliess letters took Freud's readers behind the scenes in an unprecedented way, and though the operation on Emma Eckstein was kept under wraps, it was brought to light in a 1966 paper by Schur.

The spectrum of scholarly opinion on Freud is to some extent a matter of inevitably partial gropings of the elephant that need not be incompatible. There is Gay's secular positivist, Sulloway's biologist, William McGrath's (1985) disillusioned Habsburger, Peter Rudnytsky's (1987) heir of romantic literature and philosophy, and Sander Gilman's (1993) anxious Jewish male. But the partisans also divide into warring camps. If few would care any longer to defend Kurt Eissler's (1971) fantasy of a man of unblemished perfection, the list is considerably longer of those who have echoed Frederick Crews (1986, p.25) in quoting P. B. Medawar's denunciation of Freud as the perpetrator of "the most stupendous intellectual confidence trick of the twentieth century." Much of what Freud thought to be true has now been shown to be wrong by the advances of knowledge. His metapsychology, his account of female sexuality, to say nothing of his Lamarckism—all are, by common consent, discredited. The question is, what remains?

In psychoanalysis, as in no other discipline, the subjective and the objective realms are inextricably fused. Thus, debates over the merits of psychoanalytic theory can never be entirely separated from the ongoing reappraisals of Freud the man. What seems beyond dispute is not only Freud's brilliance as a writer but also his inexhaustible fascination. As Stephen Dedalus observes of Shakespeare in *Ulysses*, "His errors are volitional and the portals of discovery" (Joyce 1922: 190). Paradoxically, the very aspects of Freud's personality that now strike us as tragic—his anger, his quarrels, his inability to ask for forgiveness—can themselves be explained as the unconscious residues of his experiences in childhood. Thus, to see Freud in the round is also to grasp what is enduringly valuable in the new science he created.

REFERENCES

Bernfeld, S. (1946). An unknown autobiographical fragment by Freud. *American Imago*, 4: 3–19.

Breger, L. (2000). *Freud: Darkness in the Midst of Vision.* New York: Wiley.

Clark, R. (1980). *Freud: The Man and the Cause.* New York: Random House.

Crews, F. (1986). *Skeptical Engagements.* New York: Oxford University Press.

Eissler, K. (1971). *Talent and Genius: The Fictitious Case of Tausk Contra Freud.* New York: Quadrangle Books.

Freud, S. (1900). *The Interpretation of Dreams.* S.E. 4 and 5: 1–621.

——. (1901). *On Dreams.* S.E. 5: 633–686.

——. (1925). *An Autobiographical Study.* S.E. 20: 7–74.

Gay, P. (1988). *Freud: A Life for Our Time.* New York: Norton.

Gilman, S. L. (1993). *The Case of Sigmund Freud: Medicine and Identity at the Fin de Siècle.* Baltimore: Johns Hopkins University Press.

Jones, E. (1953–1957). *The Life and Work of Sigmund Freud.* 3 vols. New York: Basic Books.

Joyce, J. (1922). *Ulysses.* New York: Vintage Books, 1961.

Masson, J. M. (ed., trans.). (1985). *The Complete Letters of Sigmund Freud to Wilhelm Fliess 1887–1904.* Cambridge, Mass.: Harvard University Press.

McGrath, W. J. (1985). *Freud's Discovery of Psychoanalysis: The Politics of Hysteria.* Ithaca, N.Y.: Cornell University Press.

Rudnytsky, P. L. (1987). *Freud and Oedipus.* New York: Columbia University Press.

Schur, M. (1966). Some additional "day residues" of "the specimen dream of psychoanalysis." In R. M. Lowenstein et al. (eds.) *Psychoanalysis: A General Psychology.* New York: International Universities Press, pp. 45–85.

——. (1972). *Freud: Living and Dying.* New York: International Universities Press.

Sulloway, F. J. (1979). *Freud, Biologist of the Mind: Beyond the Psychoanalytic Legend.* New York: Basic Books.

Swales, P. J. (1982). Freud, Minna Bernays, and the conquest of Rome. *New American Review* (Spring-Summer): 1–23.

Thornton, E. M. (1984). *The Freudian Fallacy: An Alternative View of Freudian Theory.* New York: Dial Press.

Webster, R. (1995). *Why Freud Was Wrong: Sin, Science, and Psychoanalysis.* New York: Basic Books.

PETER L. RUDNYTSKY

Freud's Family

The bulk of Freud's theorizing turned out to be a challenge to traditional family life, but it requires a considerable amount of imaginative reconstruction to understand Freud's life in the context of his own times, without imposing on his experiences the hindsight that comes from all the changes that have taken place since he was born in 1856. I do not believe that our own practices and beliefs are necessarily superior to those of the past, and therefore I think we can presume that old-fashioned family life had unique strengths of its own. It is important to avoid anachronisms, and the moralizing that goes with the mistaken idea that we are somehow inherently superior to those who went before us. For example, we should not expect Freud to have behaved toward his children as one would expect a good parent to do nowadays, and the time he spent with his wife must also be understood with an anthropological-like tolerance for what would have been customary in his day.

We still do not know how Freud's own father, Jacob Freud, supported his family in Vienna. They had moved there when Sigmund was a boy of four, after his father had been financially ruined as a businessman in Moravia—later a part of Czechoslovakia. It is likely that various relatives on both sides of the family helped out; at one point Freud's parents took in a lodger.

A niece reported that as an old man Jacob spent a considerable amount of time studying the Talmud, and a literature has grown up over how much Freud knew about Jewish customs and Hebrew in particular. Freud wrote much less about his mother, Amalia, than his father, and he told us relatively little about either of his parents. His special reticence about his mother may have been in keeping with what was culturally acceptable in the society in which Freud was reared. Although Freud's father died in 1896, and Freud related his creation of psychoanalysis to Jacob's passing away, his mother lived until 1930, when she finally died at the age of ninety-five.

Most analysts have followed Freud's example by concentrating on his relation to his father and ignoring Freud's mother. But if there is one lesson that psychoanalysis should have taught us, it is that everyone necessarily suffers from self-deception. Therefore Freud's own account of his life ought in principle to be only a surface treatment, one that should be subjected to close scrutiny. Freud's autobiographical disclosures have too often been largely accepted at face value, as if they were concrete, verified facts.

We do know that Freud's mother was only nineteen when she married Freud's father, who was a mature man

of forty. Jacob's first wife, whom he had married when he was seventeen years old, died three years earlier; he briefly had a second wife. When he married Amalia, they were still living in Moravia. Jacob had two grown sons by his first wife. Freud's older half-brothers had invested in South African ostrich feathers, and when the market for them collapsed with a change in women's fashions, Jacob wrecked himself bailing them out.

For the whole of Freud's life he was enmeshed in a large family constellation. He appears to have had little difficulty in standing out amid all his family members. He was his parents' first child, and they went on to have five daughters and then another son. In championing psychoanalysis, Freud was also creating another extended family, that fostered new allegiances and responsibilities that, in the end, created most of the famous controversies now connected with his name.

After Freud married in 1886, he fathered six children within eight years. The psychoanalytic movement was like a large family, and all Freud's children's names were selected by him to commemorate people who had mattered to him. The whole household revolved around Freud's work, and he was a man with predictable rituals. Although in his youth he evidently was different, in his old age anything unexpected or out of the ordinary was apt to rouse anxiety and discomfort. This need for control extended from the most insignificant detail—the use of a particular coffee cup, for example—to the most important part of his life, his starting to write again. Each activity, which cup he favored or his having embarked on composing a book or an article, would be avidly reported within the family. His constant sending of letters, although from posterity's point of view a highly significant part of his writing, was not viewed as such within the family but simply taken for granted as a given.

Within his family circle, Freud behaved differently than one might expect of the founder of psychoanalysis. With any great figure in intellectual history one wants to be able to move from the work to the life, and then back again. So it is essential to remember that his world of old Vienna is long gone. To try to comprehend Freud without considering how radically things have changed since then—partly owing to his influence—would be historical fantasy. Freud, to the extent to which we can begin to understand him in the context of a vanished world so different from our own, becomes both more important and useful in emancipating us from preconceived notions of how life might possibly be experienced.

Freud was inevitably a man of his era; he had pulled himself up by his own bootstraps, but they were the bootstraps of someone born in 1856. He was so different from the rest of the family that his background has to be astonishing; he alone had so penetrating a mind and such unique curiosity. In a purely intellectual sense, both his parents, as well as his sisters, could be considered simpleminded. Once we see Freud in the context of his family life, we can begin to understand the human and social premises under which he worked. And we can gain some perspective on how he came to exert such an influence on his followers, who in turn were to have such an impact on twentieth-century thought.

PAUL ROAZEN

Fromm, Erich (1900–1980)

Erich Pinchas Fromm, born in Frankfurt on March 23, 1900, was descended from illustrious rabbinic families. In 1920, he helped found the *Freies Judisches Rehrhaus*, directed by Martin Buber and Franz Rosenzweig, in Frankfurt, and in 1922, he completed a doctorate in sociology on Jewish law under Alfred Weber in Heidelberg. In 1924, Fromm abandoned his rabbinic vocation to become a psychoanalyst, studying one year with Wilhelm Witenberg in Munich, another with Karl Landauer in Frankfurt, and finishing with two more under Hanns Sachs and Theodor Reik in Berlin. In 1927, Fromm, Landauer, Georg Groddeck, Heinrich Meng, and Ernest Schneider founded the Frankfurt Psychoanalytic Institute, and at Max Horkheimer's invitation, Fromm joined the Frankfurt Institute for Social Research, becoming its director for social psychology (Funk, 1982).

Fromm's first papers on psychoanalysis and society sought to effect a theoretical synthesis of Marx, Freud, and Weber, and appeared in the *Zeitschrift für Sozialforschung*, the Frankfurt School's house organ, circa 1930 to 1937 (Jay, 1973; Burston, 1991). In 1933, after a yearlong bout of tuberculosis, Fromm fled the Nazis. In 1935, now in the United States, he began publishing papers that were critical of Freud. In 1938 Fromm left the Frankfurt School, which had relocated to Columbia University, because Horkheimer refused to publish Fromm's 1929 study of pro-fascist sympathies among German workers. Published posthumously, it is the historic forerunner of Theodor Adorno's *The Authoritarian Character* (Fromm, 1984; Burston, 1991).

In 1941, Fromm published *Escape From Freedom*, his first best-seller. But his evolving critique of Freud alienated the analytic establishment. The New York Psychoanalytic Institute suspended him from supervising students in 1944, and in 1945, he was formally suspended from the the American Psychoanalytic Association (APA). Undeterred, Fromm joined Clara Thompson, Harry Stack Sullivan, and ex-wife Frieda Fromm Reichman (among others) to found the William Alanson White Institute, where he was clinical director from 1946 to 1950, when his second wife's illness prompted a move to Mexico. Shortly after her untimely death, the Mexican government invited Fromm to found the Mexican Institute of Psychoanalysis, where, in addition to the customary clinical course work and supervision, candidates study analytic social psychology, Marxist humanism, existential-phenomenology, and Zen Buddhism.

Fromm soon remarried and lived and worked in Mexico until 1976, when he retired to Locarno, Switerzerland, where he died on March 19, 1980. Prior to 1976, however, Fromm taught and had speaking engagements three months a year in the United States, and was actively involved in the civil rights movement, the nuclear disarmament movement, the anti–Vietnam War movement, and the ecology movement. During the 1950s and 1960s, Fromm was arguably the most popular and prolific analytic author in the world. However, his broad extramural appeal did not translate into influence inside analytic circles. In fact, he was dropped from the membership of the International Psychoanalytic Association in 1951.

In retrospect, his strange combination of worldly success and disdain or disinterest from his peers probably hinged on the same characteristic attitudes and ideas. Despite respect for Freud's courage and insight, Fromm was mindful of his limitations and sharply critical of ideologically rooted distortions in mainstream psychoanalytic historiography, beginning with Jones's biography of Freud (Roazen, 1990; 2000). He also transposed Freud's concept of the unconscious into a philosophical framework termed "existential humanism," though the clinical implications of this epistemic shift where not elucidated in print, an omission only partially rectified by more recent publications (Fromm, 1994; Cortina and Maccoby, 1996). Finally, his conciliatory attitude to certain religious ideas was anathema to orthodox Freudians and seemed incongruous with his radical politics to many on the left (e.g., Marcuse).

Fromm was often classed as a neo-Freudian, though he himself disliked that label. Generally speaking,

Freud's studies on "the pathology of civilized communities" focused on how civilization fosters neurotic conflicts, and yet creates social bonds by sublimating surplus libido and channeling our latent envy and aggression against out-groups. Freud said that the conflicts between Eros and aggression, society and the individual, and so on, are intractable, and he explained religion, morality, and cultural evolution as the result of the progressive elaboration, and differentiation of a single, nuclear conflict relating to the incest taboo: an Oedipal monism that was vigorously disputed by Adler, Jung, Rank, and others (Burston, 1991).

By contrast, Fromm's social psychology focused on statistically normal character traits that enhance, not hinder, the individual's adaptation to society, which diminish, not aggravate, inner conflict but which also diminish our capacity to think critically, to experience and express solidarity with out-group members, and to develop and maintain loving, intimate relationships with others. He called these "socially patterned defects." Statistical normality or cultural congruence minimize inner and interpersonal conflict but are often inimical to full human development, whose goals are articulated in the great spiritual and philosophical traditions of the East and West. Though Fromm asserted the priority of pre-Oedipal over Oedipal issues, he held that there is no single, nuclear conflict underpinning the great diversity of cultures and faiths, although economic structure and prevailing modes of authority may constrain us in our attempts to meet our material needs in ways that are dramatically at variance with our *existential* needs. This socially patterned discrepancy results in the gradual atrophy of "humanistic conscience," which in turn fosters apathy, greed, and violence. Accordingly, analysis should never treat normalization per se as a goal of treatment (Burston and Olfman, 1996).

Despite recent shifts toward a more "ecumenical" attitude in the analytic mainstream and the fact that many of Fromm's criticisms of Freud are almost commonplace by now, his writings on character and culture are still generally neglected by those who ponder the relationship between the individual and the social (or political, cultural) unconscious (Roazen, 1990; Roazen, 2000).

REFERENCES

Burston, D. (1991). *The Legacy of Erich Fromm.* Cambridge, Mass.: Harvard University Press.

Burston, D., and Olfman, S. (1996). Freud, Fromm and the pathology of normalcy. In M. Cortina and M. Maccoby (eds.). *A Prophetic Analyst.* Northvale, N.J.: Jason Aronson.

Cortina, M., and Maccoby, M. (eds.) (1996). *A Prophetic Analyst.* Northvale, N.J.: Jason Aronson.

Fromm, E. (1941). *Escape From Freedom.* Reprint, New York: Avon Books, 1965.

———. (1984). *The Working Class in Weimar Germany: A Psychological And Sociological Study.* Cambridge, Mass.: Harvard University Press.

———. (1994). *The Art of Listening.* New York: Continuum Books.

Funk, R. (1982). *Erich Fromm.* Hamburg: Rowohlt Taschenbuch Verlag.

Jay, M. (1973). *The Dialectical Imagination.* Boston: Beacon Books.

Roazen, P. (1990). *Encountering Freud: The Politics and Histories of Psychoanalysis.* New Brunswick, N.J.: Transaction Publishers.

———. (2000). *Political Theory and the Psychology of the Unconscious.* London: Open Gate Press.

DANIEL BURSTON

G

Genetics, and Psychoanalysis

Genetics has played a role in psychoanalytic thought from its earliest days. Though Freud's biological views had Lamarckian overtones—postulating the heredity of acquired characteristics—he always stressed the importance of innate factors operating together with experience. Ernest Jones (1951a), who had a special interest in genetics, wrote: "Ever since Mendel's work it has been evident that in estimating the relation of heredity to environment in respect to any character, we first have to ascertain the component units in that character; in other words what constitutes an individual gene," and (1951b) "By means of psychoanalysis one is enabled to dissect and isolate mental processes to an extent not previously possible, and this must evidently bring us nearer to the primary elements, to the mental genes in terms of which genetic investigations can alone be carried out."

The modern science of genetics spells out genes in chemical sequences that code for the building blocks of life processes. In the process of evolution, genes were selected for survival that afforded the optimal adaptation to the physical and social environments of the species. Any fears that the modern science of genetics, if viewed mechanistically, might make obsolete the developmental theories of psychoanalysis, the sense of personal self, and freedom of the will are obviated by the knowledge that gene action is regulated by environmental needs at all levels. In the living organism, genes are activated or not by a feedback mechanism responsive to the organism's needs; the expression of genes in the nervous system is modified by experience and learning (Kandel and Hawkins, 1992); in short there is continuous interaction with the outside, while even disease genes vary in degree of expression due to non-genetic influences.

Genetics today can therefore provide a framework of broad possibilities in which psychoanalysts may think about themselves and their patients. An evolutionary, genetic approach focused on survival value can offer salient clues to the development and variability of behavior. For instance, since humans require nurture from others during infancy, affect development occurs in the context of the history of interactive relations with other persons ("objects") who have provided for or thwarted such needs. Emotions such as fear, rage, depression, satisfaction, pleasure, and confidence can thus be seen as adaptive or maladaptive by-products of such personal history.

Another example relates to dream theory. Winson (1984) proposed an evolutionary role of REM sleep and dreaming as an off-line brain processing of daily experience and labeled this process the "Freudian unconscious." In this conception, dreams are seen not only as a phylogenetic mechanism for the protection of sleep but also as nonverbal, visual, metaphorical thought that sums up and reviews early experiences, using common language and images to integrate recent experience and solve current problems and conflicts in the service of adaptive functioning.

Other areas for further study are variations in drive strength and defense mechanisms, affect and pleasure potential, anxiety proneness (including separation anxiety), and capacities for identification and for gratification postponement. In such vein, scientific psychoanalysis may indeed advance Freud's legacy by furthering Ernest Jones's program—to isolate "mental genes" and study them by genetic investigation.

This broad overview, moreover, allows psychoanalysts to remain among the guardians of human freedom, dignity, and individuality. Certainly there have been instances of nefarious exploitation of pseudoeugenics, and some may still believe that genetics teaches that genes are destiny, that it aims to create and then clone the perfect human and to dictate a mechanistically based set of moral imperatives. However, a deeper understanding of the dynamic structure of modern genetics can dispel such notions and unite psychoanalysts and other biologists in a common humanistic endeavor.

REFERENCES

Jones, E. (1951a). "Mental heredity." In E. Jones, *Essays in Applied Psychoanalysis*. London: Hogarth Press.

———. (1951b). Psychoanalysis and biology. In E. Jones, *Essays in Applied Psychoanalysis*. London: Hogarth Press.

Kandel, E., and Hawkins, R. D. (1992). The biological basis of learning and individuality. *Scientific American*, 26: 78–86.

Winson, J. (1984). *Brain and Psyche: The Biology of the Unconscious*. Garden City, N.Y.: Anchor Press/Doubleday.

JOHN D. RAINER

Genital Stage See DEVELOPMENTAL THEORY.

Genitality, Theories of

Genitality is the psychoanalytic term for theories describing the nature and function of mature forms of sexuality.

Freud first wrote about genitality in *Three Essays on the Theory of Sexuality* (1905), holding that human sexual development was divided into two stages: infantile sexuality and mature, postpubertal sexuality. He initially described infantile sexuality as predominantly autoerotic and mainly concerned with the pregenital zones (mouth and anus). Freud referred to the stage of mature sexuality as the "genital phase" and the stage of "genital primacy." During the genital phase, the genitals become the leading erotogenic zone, to which the pregenital zones become subordinated. In contrast to the autoerotic character of infancy, genital sexuality seeks an object. Finally, the sexual drives are "subordinated to the reproductive function" (p. 207). This is accomplished with the help of "extremely energetic repressions" that "have been effected under the influence of education, and mental forces such as shame, disgust and morality." (1910, p. 45).

Both psychoneuroses and perversions are failures to achieve full genital primacy. Perversion is a failure to subordinate infantile sexuality: "An instinct which remains in this way independent leads to what we describe as a *perversion*, and may substitute its own sexual aim for the normal one" (Freud, 1910: 45). Freud further notes:

> We actually describe a sexual activity as perverse if it has given up the aim of reproduction and pursues the attainment of pleasure as an aim independent of it. So, as you will see, the breach and turning-point in the development of sexual life lies in its becoming subordinate to the purposes of reproduction (Freud, 1916: 316).

In the psychoneuroses, unintegrated strands of pregenital, infantile sexuality are repressed and find disguised expression in the form of symptoms (Freud, 1910). In a 1916 paper, Freud held that psychoneuroses develop when, after puberty, the preconscious system rejects unconscious genital primacy, although three years later he asserted that the Oedipus complex is unconsciously *revived* at puberty and that this causes the genital organization to regress to earlier organizations (Freud, 1919).

The concept of an *infantile* genital organization of the libido was first suggested in *A Child Is Being Beaten* (1919). In the 1915 edition of *Three Essays on the Theory of Sexuality* (Freud, 1905), when Freud introduced the idea of the convergence of the sexual drives on a single object during infancy, he included the disclaimer that "their subordination under the primacy of the genitals have been effected only very incompletely or not at all" (p. 199). In *The Infantile Genital Organization* (1923a), Freud claimed that during the period when infantile sexuality is at its height, "interest in the genitals and in their activity acquires a dominating significance which falls little short of that reached in maturity" (p. 142). Freud calls this period the "phallic phase" because "for both sexes, only one genital, namely, the male one, comes into account" (p. 142). The female genitals are as yet "undiscovered" (1924, p. 174). It is only during the genital organization at puberty that the female genitals acquire value. Central Freudian developmental concepts such as the Oedipus complex, castration anxiety, penis envy, and superego formation were reinterpreted in the context of the phallic stage (Freud, 1924). Freud's first comprehensive account of the characteristic of the girl's phallic phase was presented in *Some*

Psychical Consequences of the Anatomical Distinction between the Sexes (1925).

Freud reserved the term "phallic phase" for the infantile genital organization so as to distinguish it from the mature genital organization (1933). The process of the repression has a special connection with the genital organization. During earlier developmental phases the infant must resort to other types of defensive maneuver to keep instinctual drives at bay (Freud, 1926).

The puzzling early efflorescence of genital sexuality may be an evolutionary relic, on the assumption that our early hominid ancestors reached sexual maturity by the age of five (Freud, 1939), an hypothesis that was later independently offered by the anthropologist Margaret Mead (1963).

Several other psychoanalysts made contributions to the theory of genitality during Freud's lifetime. Among these were Wilhelm Reich (1897–1957), who wrote on the function of the orgasm; Karl Abraham (1877–1925), who formulated the concept of the genital character-structure; and Sándor Ferenczi (1873–1933), who speculated on the phylogenetic origins of genitality.

REFERENCES

Freud, S. (1905). *Three Essays on the Theory of Sexuality.* S.E. 7: 130–243.
———. (1910). Five lectures on psycho-analysis. S.E. 11: 9–55.
———. (1919). A child is being beaten. S.E. 17: 179–204.
———. (1923a). The infantile genital organization: An interpolation into the theory of sexuality. S.E. 19: 141–145.
———. (1923b). Two encyclopaedia articles. S.E. 18: 235–259.
———. (1924). The dissolution of the Oedipus complex. S.E. 19: 173–179.
———. (1925). Some psychical consequences of the anatomical distinction between the sexes. S.E. 19: 248–258.
———. (1926). *Inhibitions, Symptoms and Anxiety.* S.E. 20: 87–172.
———. (1933). *New Introductory Lectures on Psycho-analysis.* S.E. 22: 5–185.
———. (1939). *Moses and Monotheism: Three Essays.* S.E. 23: 7–137.
Mead, M. (1963). *Totem and Taboo* reconsidered with respect. *Bulletin of the Menninger Clinic,* 27: 185–199.

DAVID LIVINGSTONE SMITH

Germany, and Psychoanalysis

Vienna was the cradle of psychoanalysis, but Germany was the site of many of its most important early developments. Certain German philosophers, especially Schopen-

hauer and Nietzsche, anticipated some of the key ideas of Freud, although the degree to which they actually influenced him is still being debated. Freud was also influenced by, and often quoted, German classical writers, such as Goethe and Schiller. Other ties to Germany include the following: his wife Martha came from Hamburg to Vienna, he was married in Wandsbek, and his friend and confidante Wilhelm Fliess lived in Berlin.

As early as 1900, the senior consultants of several sanatoriums for patients with mental conditions had started to show interest in the psychoanalytic techniques of Freud, e.g., a Dr. Stegmann from Dresden, a Dr. Juliusburger from Berlin-Steglitz, W. Strohmayer and Prof. O. Binswanger from Jena, W. Warda from Blankenburg in Thuringia, as well as L. Roemheld from the sanatorium at Schloss Hornegg in Württemberg, not to mention Ernst Simmel from the sanatorium in Berlin-Tegel.

The real beginning of German psychoanalysis, however, can be traced to Karl Abraham's move from Zürich to Berlin in 1908. This move marked the beginning of the first phase of development. Three other phases can be distinguished: the Nazi period (1933–1945), the immediate post–World War II period, and the period in which Germany was divided into East and West.

The Rise of Psychoanalysis up to 1933

Before his move to Berlin in 1908, Abraham had already worked there for three years as a physician at a psychiatric clinic. Concerning the early reception of psychoanalysis in Germany, Freud wrote on October 8, 1907 in a letter to Abraham: "If my reputation in Germany increases, it will certainly be useful to you, and if I may refer to you as my pupil and follower, . . . I shall be able to back you vigorously. On the other hand, you know yourself of the hostility I still have to contend with in Germany. I hope you will not even attempt to gain the favor of your new colleagues, . . . but rather turn directly to the public."

Other important developments during this period include the holding of early psychoanalytical congresses in Germany, namely in 1910 in Nuremberg, where the International Psychoanalytic Society was founded; in 1911 in Weimar; in 1913 in Munich, where the Psychoanalytical Committee came into being; in 1922 in Berlin; in 1925 in Bad Homburg; and in 1932 in Wiesbaden.

The Berlin Psychoanalytical Training Institute began training future psychoanalysts in 1920. Abraham, Ferenczi,

Jones, Rank, and Sachs were members. According to a letter from Abraham to Freud dated November 4, 1913, of the eighteen members of the International Psychoanalytic Association, there were nine in Berlin alone. On February 16, 1920, the Berlin Psychoanalytical Association opened a polyclinic for the psychoanalytical treatment of nervous diseases under the direction of Abraham, Eitingon, and Simmel. The Teaching Committee was headed jointly by Eitingon and Müller-Braunschweig.

During the "roaring" 1920s the Berlin Psychoanalytical Institute must have been a great center of attraction both in Germany and abroad, for more and more people interested in psychoanalysis came to Berlin, among them Franz Alexander, Therese Benedek, Siegfried Bernfeld, Berta and Steff Bornstein, Otto Fenichel, Robert Fliess, Erich Fromm, Frieda Fromm-Reichmann, Angel Garma, Georg Groddeck, Alfred Gross, Karin Horney, Edith Jacobson, Werner Kemper, Hans Lampl and Jane Lampl-de Groot, Karl Landauer, Heinrich Meng, Ada and Carl Müller-Braunschweig, Sándor Rado, Anni and Wilhelm Reich, Theodor Reik, Hanns Sachs, Melitta Schmideberg, Ernst Simmel, René Spitz, and others.

Psychoanalysis in Germany was then at its peak: The Psychoanalytical Polyclinic of the Berlin Institute was working with great success. The first systematic training guidelines were laid down. Up to 1928, sixty-six analysts had been trained in Berlin, and there were also thirty-four candidates. By 1930, ninety-four analysts had carried out 604 psychoanalytical treatments. Training was already organized with the training analysis as an essential part of it. Experienced analysts supervised or controlled the psychoanalytical treatments carried out by candidates during training. Practical analytical activities were accompanied by effective public relations work. The public was very interested in the new discoveries. Psychoanalysis and German culture seemed to be starting to integrate.

In 1929, a second Psychoanalytical Institute was founded in Frankfurt, at which Karl Landauer, Erich Fromm, Frieda Fromm-Reichmann, and Heinrich Meng taught, with a department in Heidelberg.

Several analysts were politically active. Ernst Simmel attended the Conference of Social Democratic Physicians, while Wilhelm Reich, Otto Fenichel, Siegfried Bernfeld, Edith Jacobson, and Johannes Rittmeister thought and acted politically, their convictions ranging from social democratic to communist. The Frankfurt Psychoanalytical Institute collaborated intensively with the Institute of Social Research. Herbert Marcuse, Adorno, and Horkheimer even integrated psychoanalysis into what became known as critical theory. It experienced later an overwhelming revival as the Frankfurt School of philosophy during the so-called Student Movement starting in 1968.

Psychoanalysis under the Pressure of the Nazi Dictatorship

From 1930 to 1933, the two German institutes in Berlin and in Frankfurt came increasingly in the line of fire of the Nazi regime. As early as 1932, the Therapeuticum, which had been founded shortly before in 1930, headed by S. H. Fuchs (later called Foulkes, founder of the London Group Analytic Society), was closed. In 1933, the Institute of Social Research was closed, too. In Berlin, evidently under pressure from the Nazis, Felix Boehm and Carl Müller-Braunschweig were determined to expel the Jewish members from the association. According to statements made by Jane Lampl-de Groot, however, they did not receive Freud's agreement on this (Kurzweil, 1989: 47).

During Hitler's regime, attempts to discredit psychoanalysis increased, and its many Jewish practitioners were persecuted, as were other Jews, and forced to emigrate. Germany lost not only many of its most outstanding psychoanalysts but also many eminent intellectuals in other fields. That some of them perished in concentration camps during the Holocaust is the darkest chapter of German history.

The rest of the German psychoanalytic group broke away from the International Psychoanalytic Association and formed the so-called Reichsinstitut, under the chairmanship of M. H. Göring, a cousin of Reichsmarschall Hermann Göring, supported by C. G. Jung from Zürich. The majority of the members of the institute seemed obviously in agreement with the Nazi ideology and collaborated with Nazi institutions, including the army. Only a smaller "Group A" seemed to remain loyal to Freud's ideas.

Under mounting pressure from the Nazis, the German Psychoanalytical Society was forced to leave the International Psychoanalytic Association in 1936. Finally, in 1938, the German Psychoanalytical Association was struck off the list of the International Psychoanalytic Association. It is striking that in the ensuing period the term "psychoanalysis" no longer appears anywhere in

G

German publications and that, at most, psychotherapy and depth psychology are mentioned. This clearly documents the exigencies of adjustment to the prevailing political circumstances. According to Käthe Dräger, no more than 5 percent of the psychoanalysts who stayed behind in Nazi Germany were members of the Nazi Party, though Cocks (1985, p. 48) assumes a higher percentage (Kurzweil, 1989: 235).

Complicated New Beginning after World War II

After the war, Felix Boehm, Carl Müller-Braunschweig, and Harald Schultz-Hencke were still working in Berlin. These three seemed to have thought of themselves as custodians of psychoanalysis during the Nazi dictatorship. They considered themselves to be the legitimate trustees of the German Psychoanalytical Society and believed they had saved psychoanalysis all through the most terrible period of German history.

Soon after the war Schultz-Hencke and Kemper founded the Central Institute for Psychic Illnesses, with remarkable political support from the new government. They managed to receive even more remarkable financial support from the powerful Insurance Institute of Berlin. This cooperation even led to neurosis being recognized as an "illness" and psychoanalytical psychotherapy as an acknowledged method of medical treatment.

In 1947, the Institute for Psychotherapy was founded. It continued the structure of the Reichsinstitut of the Nazi period and propagated a "synopsis" between Freud's psychoanalysis, C. G. Jung's analytical psychology, and the Neo-Analysis that in the meantime had begun to crystallize around Schultz-Hencke. Its advocates came close to so-called revisionists such as Erich Fromm, Karin Horney, and others.

In 1949, the German Society for Psychoanalysis and Depth Psychology was founded as an umbrella organization of all those interested in psychotherapy. But the golden age of psychoanalysis had been replaced by a psychotherapeutic culture. The importance of the libido theory, of sexuality and aggressiveness, as well as of transference and countertransference gave way to a theory of "Antriebe" (drives) and their inhibitions. Other schools, such as those of Alfred Adler and C. G. Jung, competed with Freudian psychoanalysis.

At the Zürich Congress in 1949, members of the so-called Group A, who were convinced that they had saved Freud's psychoanalysis, applied for membership in the International Psychoanalytic Association. The hitherto latent debate between Freudian psychoanalysis, personified by Carl Müller-Braunschweig, and Neo-Analysis, personified by Schultz-Hencke, became public. In 1950, a new German Psychoanalytical Society was founded, and in 1951 it was admitted to the IPA.

Alongside the minority of the newly founded German Psychoanalytical Association, which favored Freudian psychoanalysis, the majority of the members trained at the Reichsinstitut preferred nonpsychoanalytic psychotherapy to psychoanalysis. Thus the infrastructures of the "defeated Nazi system" (Kurzweil, 1989: 295) survived for a long time.

Two Separate Developments in West and East Germany from 1950 to 1990

In West Germany, the members of the newly founded German Psychoanalytical Association created a refreshingly clear psychoanalytical atmosphere, supported by prominent psychoanalysts from abroad such as Michael Balint, Willi Hoffer, Piet Kuiper, Jane Lampl-de Groot, and René Spitz. One new institute after another was founded.

In 1956, the hundredth anniversary of Freud's birthday was celebrated in Frankfurt and Heidelberg. Psychoanalysis was no longer seen as merely a method of therapy in Germany, but rather as a cultural theory and form of social criticism, with Alexander and Margarete Mitscherlich, Horst-Eberhard Richter, and Johannes Cremerius as its outstanding figures. In 1962, an international symposium on the psychological and social preconditions of the age took place. In 1963, Alexander Mitscherlich published his ideas on social psychology in his book *Society without the Father: A Contribution to Social Psychology*. In 1967, there followed *The Inability to Mourn* with Margarete Mitscherlich-Nielsen as coauthor, which was to become the conscience of the nation (Kurzweil, 1989: 232). The majority of psychoanalysts, however, were clinically oriented. After the publication of Annemarie Dührssen's (1962) paper on the results of 1,004 psychoanalytic psychotherapies that had been empirically compared with a group of nontreated patients, the so-called psychotherapy guidelines and agreements came into being between representatives of psychotherapeutic societies on the one side and health insurance companies on the other. The result was that not psychoanalysis proper but its applications, namely, "psychoanalytical psychotherapy" and "psychotherapy based on depth psychology," could be financed by health insurance. Thus many more patients than before could be treated in a psychoanalytically oriented way. Beyond this success, however, it was often overlooked that these agreements gave the medical authorities some influence over the psychoanalytical process; for example, on its frequency and duration. This specifically West German development of psychoanalysis came in for criticism from various quarters, for example, from Edith Kurzweil (1989, p. 215). Charges were raised that psychoanalysis had "sold out" in favor of psychotherapy (Kurzweil, 1989: 215) and that the independence of its practitioners had been sacrificed for the sake of influence and power—a charge that cannot be easily denied in view of the rapid increase in membership in psychotherapeutic societies in West Germany.

In addition to the great influence of the Berlin Psychoanalytical Institute, the Sigmund Freud Institute in Frankfurt, founded in 1960, became a stronghold of psychoanalysis in West Germany. Theoretical orientation was provided by the classical Standards of Freudian Psychoanalysis. However, further international developments in theory and practice were imported from abroad, e.g., ego psychology and the separation individuation theory of Margaret Mahler. Self-psychology, developed by Heinz Kohut, also unleashed a fierce debate on the theory of narcissism. Since 1980, preoccupation with Kohut's positions has been replaced by a renaissance of Melanie Klein's and Wilfred Bion's ideas and by appreciation for Otto F. Kernberg's object relations theory. All these developments in West Germany, however, took place in close association with eminent guests from abroad, for example, at the Sigmund Freud lectures at the University of Frankfurt, as well as during the annual conferences of the association.

In East Germany, in contrast, psychoanalysis was openly suppressed by the communist authorities for forty years, in favor of Pavlovian psychology, Marxist theory, and communist practice. Only one specific method of psychoanalytically oriented group therapy could be practiced in the House of Health in East Berlin, although there was considerable research on psychotherapy using psychological instruments such as questionnaires.

Despite the attempts to suppress Freud's ideas, in the last decades of the twentieth century, a sort of "re-institutionalization of psychoanalytical therapy" took place (Geyer, 1992: 143); most psychotherapists in East Germany "kept a critical distance from the power apparatus" (p. 145), and there was a growing interest in Freud's original works.

Since the reunification of Germany in 1990, the psychotherapists of the East, through additional training, adapted to Western standards of psychoanalysis with new institutes being developed in Halle, Leipzig, Rostock, and Jena.

At present, the second-largest psychoanalytic association after the German Psychoanalytical Association—the German Psychoanalytical Society—may become another branch of the IPA. Both are subsumed in the German Society for Psychoanalysis, Psychotherapy, Psychosomatics and Depth Psychology.

The German Psychoanalytical Association has more than two hundred full members and some six hundred associate members, running thirteen institutes, while the psychotherapeutic umbrella organization including all psychotherapeutic institutions has more than two thousand members.

There are now several psychoanalytic journals such as *Psyche, Forum, Jahrbuch*, and *Zeitschrift*. Not many German contributions to psychoanalysis have been translated into English. Exceptions include Thomä and Kächele's (1987, reprinted 1994), *Psychoanalytic Practice* and Thure von Uexküll's (1997) famous textbook, *Psychosomatic Medicine*.

In conclusion, German psychoanalysts, deeply affected by the Holocaust, are fully aware of the dangers of nationalism; they see themselves as Europeans, organized in the European Psychoanalytical Federation and as a part of Psychoanalysis International (Kutter, 1992, 1995).

REFERENCES

Abraham, H. C., and Freud, E. L. (eds.). (1965). *Sigmund Freud/Karl Abraham: Briefe 1907–1926*. Frankfurt: S. Fischer, 2d ed., 1981.

Cocks, G. (1985). *Psychotherapy in the Third Reich. The Göring Institute*. New York: Oxford University Press.

Dührssen, A. (1962). Katamnestische Ergebnisse bei 1004 Patienten nach analytischer Psychotherapie. *Zeitschrift für Psychosomatische Medizin und Psychoanalyse*, 2: 94–113.

Etchegoyen, R. H. (1992). Preface. In P. Kutter (ed.). *Psychoanalysis International*, vol. 1. Hillsdale, N.J.: The Analytic Press, pp. vii–viii.

Geyer, M. (1992). East Germany. In P. Kutter (ed.). *Psychoanalysis International*, vol. 1. Hillsdale, N.J.: Analytic Press. pp. 137–149.

Kurzweil, E. (1989). *The Freudians. A Comparative Perspective*. New Haven: Yale University Press.

Kutter, P. (ed.) (1992). *Psychoanalysis International: A Guide to Psychoanalysis throughout the World*, vol. 1. Hillsdale, N.J.: Analytic Press.

———. (1995). *Psychoanalysis International. A Guide to Psychoanalysis throughout the World*, vol. 2. Hillsdale, N.J.: Analytic Press.

Mitscherlich, A. (1969). *Society without the Father. A Contribution to Social Psychology*. London: Tavistock.

Mitscherlich, A., and Mitscherlich-Nielsen, M. (1975). *The Inability to Mourn*. New York: Grove Press.

Thomä, H., and Kächele, H. (1987). *Psychoanalytical Practice*, vol. 1. New York: Springer, 2d ed., 1994.

Uexküll, T. V. (ed.) (1997). *Psychosomatic Medicine*. Munich: Urban and Schwarzenberg.

PETER KUTTER

Glover, Edward (1888–1972)

Edward Glover was born in Lesmahagow, part of the rural county of Lanarkshire, twenty-five miles from Glasgow, Scotland. His father was a schoolmaster who knew among other subjects Greek, Latin, Hebrew, and French, and taught Edward a good deal about writing English. His mother was the daughter of an old farming family and the adopted niece of a Scottish Calvinist parson; she had three sons, Edward being the last. Edward's oldest brother James preceded him as a psychoanalyst.

At the age of sixteen Glover started medical school at the University of Glasgow, as ancient a center of learning as Oxford or Cambridge. He graduated "with distinction" in 1909 when he was twenty-one. By 1915 he was licensed to practice medicine. His psychoanalytic training took place at the Berlin Psychoanalytical Training Institute during 1921; his decision to become an analyst was preceded by his first wife's death in childbirth. Glover had had to wait a year to get Karl Abraham as his analyst. Glover had heard from his brother James that Freud's list of patients was already full, and Abraham was considered by James Glover as the next best. Edward Glover was then a pacifist and in Berlin attached himself as a physician to the English Quaker Relief Commission.

On Edward's return to Britain he became a member of the British Psycho-Analytical Society. Following James Glover's death in 1926, Edward became in effect Ernest Jones's second-in-command. Glover was to serve for many years as scientific secretary of the British Psycho-Analytical Society, director of its clinic, director of research, chairman of the Training Committee, as well as

honorary secretary of the *Bulletin of the International Psychoanalytic Association*.

Today Glover is best known as the author of, among many other writings, a famous text on psychoanalytic technique (Glover, 1955), as well as of a popular book *Freud or Jung?* (Glover, 1956a). Other books by Glover include his *War, Sadism, and Pacifism* (1933), *Psychoanalysis* (1949), *On the Early Development of the Mind* (1956b), *The Roots of Crime* (1960), and *The Psychology of Fear and Courage* (1940).

While Glover's standing in the United States has always remained secure, and he was on the editorial boards of the *Psychoanalytic Quarterly* and the *Psychoanalytic Study of the Child*, in England he became demonized after having resigned from the British Society in 1944 after a frustrating public struggle with Melanie Klein and her supporters. The first biography of Klein (Grosskurth, 1986) is unremittingly hostile and unfair to Glover. And the publication of the proceedings of the *Freud-Klein Controversies 1941–45* (King and Steiner, 1991) accentuated the degree of Glover's historical isolation; he is characterized there as having been "fanatical" (p. 914), and his forecasts for the British Society supposedly "apocalyptic and ferociously one-sided" (p. 680). These charges and related issues are discussed in Roazen (1992, 2000). Glover's own indictment of Klein is contained in his 1945a and 1945b.

While the papers presented on behalf of Klein got reprinted in a book, Glover's own critiques of Kleinianism, published separately, do not even get cited in the bibliography to the *Freud-Klein Controversies*.

A central point that has so far escaped the literature is that Glover was an exceptionally kindly spirit. One obituary accurately described him as "a warm-hearted, courteous man of natural elegance and generosity." Another characterized him as an "essentially gentle and sympathetic personality." The death notices in the *Times* were almost insultingly brief. So an unusually amiable man is in danger of going down in the history books as only a partisan and dogmatist.

In reality it makes as much sense to see Glover as a historical victim of what happened. Initially attracted by Klein's originality, Glover later felt that Klein's work betrayed Freud's own conceptions; Freud himself took a similar viewpoint, although he did not want to make a fuss like that associated with the earlier so-called renegades Alfred Adler and Carl G. Jung. Once Freud came to England, having fled from Vienna in 1938 because of

Nazism, Glover's situation seemed to improve. Freud personally confirmed to Glover how intensely distasteful the founder of psychoanalysis deemed Klein's approach.

In the end, the legacy of Klein, who died in 1960, succeeded so well in enlivening and enriching psychoanalysis that few contemporary analysts in Britain are likely to want to acknowledge just how much Freud distanced himself from her ideas. Klein had rejected Freud's own view of the centrality of the Oedipus complex. It was hardly a secret, when Freud immigrated with his family, including his child analyst daughter Anna, along with other Viennese disciples, how his ardently devoted pupils felt about Kleinianism. In the 1930s, there had been formal exchanges of lecturers between the Vienna and British Societies, as the rival points of view were presented.

After Freud's death in 1939, World War II for a time took precedence over psychoanalytic politics. Jones remained president until 1944, and had tried to be protective of Klein at the same time that he sought to maintain good relations with Anna Freud. Although Anna, as did her father, felt welcome in the British Society, she had been at odds with Klein (whose specialty was also child analysis) since the mid-1920s. Freud thought that Klein's battle with Anna was a disguised displacement from real differences with himself.

Glover, having served loyally as his brother's lieutenant then Jones's, took up Freud's banner with the support of others, notably Klein's analyst daughter, Melitta Schmideberg, whom he had analyzed. But in the end it was Glover who was squeezed out. After resigning from the British Society, Glover succeeded—over Jones's objections as president of the IPA—in becoming a full member of the Swiss Psychoanalytic Society and therefore entitled to participate in IPA meetings. Glover continued to practice as an analyst in London, and Anna Freud (who succeeded Glover as IPA secretary) created her own training program within the British Society.

While both Klein and Anna Freud had their respective adherents, Glover was left historically to twist in the wind. He finally chose not to found a new group of his own. As Glover's most distinguished student, the American psychiatrist Lawrence S. Kubie, wrote (1969, p. 528): "it never tempted Glover, as so many others, to launch his own messianic school." Throughout the history of psychoanalysis, it has been those embattled enough to have had partisan followers who have been the best remembered, while the least sectarian and organizationally tenacious have tended to fall by the wayside.

So Glover, after having participated in probably the single most important defining moment in British psychoanalysis, is in danger of becoming one of the lost sheep in the story of the development of Freud's school. In addition to his extensive specialized bibliography of books, articles, and reviews, he once prolifically wrote for the *Listener, Lancet, Horizon, Spectator*, London *Times, New York Times*, and in other publications.

He was one of the great publicists for psychoanalysis in the English language and spoke on radio programs, while his books were translated into French, German, Italian, Spanish, and Chinese. In fact, an interesting history of British psychoanalysis could be written on the basis of a list of those who left or were driven out of the British Society.

The circumstances of Glover's private life also contrived to obliterate his memory. His second wife, an invalid for many years, predeceased him; and their one child was "backward." So at Glover's death in 1972, there was no one to secure his papers. Despite all the years that Glover had practiced and helped promote psychoanalysis, no effort was made to preserve his extensive literary remains.

Glover had played a central part in founding the Institute for the Study and Treatment of Delinquency (ISTD) and its clinical affiliate, the Portman Clinic, since the 1930s. The idea behind the institute was that there had to be a better way of dealing with criminals than incarcerating them. The ISTD had both humanitarian and research and scientific aims. Crime and delinquency were to be the central objects of the organization's investigative and clinical work. In 1950, the *British Journal of Delinquency* (later renamed *British Journal of Criminology*) began publication; its founding editors were Glover, Emmanuel Miller, and Hermann Mannheim. These three came from different backgrounds, were quite different from one another, yet somehow managed to function together. Glover was the Freudian, and he sometimes seemed narrowly intolerant of dissent, but he also made valuable contributions to empirical criminology.

Unlike what had happened among the analysts, Glover managed to cooperate with his colleagues at the ISTD and the Portman Clinic. He was the capable administrator, chairing meetings, organizing funds, writing introductions for annual reports, and overseeing the programs of conferences. This he accomplished in a multidisciplinary context, bringing psychiatry into contact with sociology and expanding the ISTD sphere of interest. The ISTD was "very much a place of applied psychodynamic ideas, including the practice of group therapy, with many other intellectual standpoints and disciplines playing their part. In view of Glover's ruthless orthodoxy at other times this liberality of outlook is impressive" (Cordess, 1992: 519). Glover was not only an important and successful clinician but also a pioneer in the field of forensic psychiatry, being part of a movement to bring more humanity into criminal law. The ISTD has now become the Centre for Crime and Justice Studies at King's College in London.

Glover continued to arouse the resentments of those he left behind at the British Society. Yet for other creative analysts he was a model of independence and integrity. The lessons from studying the history of psychoanalysis may lead one to question all zealotry in the humanistic sciences.

History is too often written from the perspective of the victor. Kubie (1973, p. 93) credited Glover with being an advocate of "vigorous heterodoxy," and such informed dissent added a special dimension to the history of psychoanalytic ideas. Those whom Glover wounded intellectually—Jungians as well as Kleinians—still smart from what he did. But these systems, if they deserve to survive, should be able to withstand the most rigorous scrutiny.

REFERENCES

Cordess, C. (1992). Pioneers in forensic psychiatry. Edward Glover (1888–1972): Psychoanalysis and crime—A fragile legacy. *Journal of Forensic Psychiatry*, vol. 3, no. 3: 509–530.

Glover, E. (1933). *War, Sadism, and Pacifism*. London: George Allen and Unwin.

———. (1940). *The Psychology of Fear and Courage*. London: Allen Lane.

———. (1945a). An examination of the Klein system of child psychology. London: Southern Post.

———. (1945b). An examination of the Klein system of child psychology. *Psychoanalytic Study of the Child*, vol. 1. New York: International Universities Press.

———. (1949). *Psychoanalysis*. London: Staples Press.

———. (1955). *The Technique of Psychoanalysis*. New York: International Universities Press.

———. (1956a). *Freud or Jung?* New York: Meridian Books; reprinted, with Foreword by James William Anderson. Evanston, Ill.: Northwestern University Press, 1991.

———. (1956b). *On the Early Development of the Mind*. New York: International Universities Press.

———. (1960). *The Roots of Crime*. New York: International Universities Press.

———. (1968). *The Birth of the Ego*. New York: International Universities Press.

Grosskurth, P. (1986). *Melanie Klein: Her World and Her Work*. New York: Knopf.

King, P., and Steiner, R. (eds.) (1991). *The Freud-Klein Controversies 1941–1945*. London: Tavistock Routledge, pp. 914, 680.

Kubie, L. (1969). Edward Glover. *Psychoanalytic Quarterly*, 38: 521–531.

———. (1973). Edward Glover: A biographical sketch. *International Journal of Psychoanalysis*, 54: 85–94.

Roazen, P. (1992). Book review of *The Freud-Klein Controversies* that appeared in *Psychoanalytic Books*, pp. 391–398.

———. (2000). *Oedipus in Britain: Edward Glover and The Struggle Over Klein*. New York: Other Press.

PAUL ROAZEN

Goethe Prize

The award accorded to Freud in 1930 is noteworthy for two reasons: first, its nature and the correspondence to which it gave rise; second, Freud's commemorative essay on the occasion that describes his "inner relations as a man and a scientist to Goethe." Founded in 1927 by Frankfurt, Goethe's native city, the annual prize in his honor was given to one whose creative work would be "worthy of an honor dedicated to Goethe's memory." The successive line of recipients consisted of the poet Stefan George; the musician, theologian, and medical missionary Albert Schweitzer; the philosopher Leopold Ziegler; and then Freud himself. Thus the prize, pace Schur (1972, p. 372), was given for more than merely literary achievement. After Freud, awardees included the physicist Max Plank and the sociologist Raymond Aron. Many of the trustees of the prize, however, objected to giving the honor to Freud, but they finally yielded to the combative intercession of their official secretary, the creative writer Alfons Paquet (Jones, 1957: 151). Too frail to attend the ceremonies in Frankfurt, Freud was represented by his daughter Anna, who delivered his acceptance address.

In his epistolary announcement of the prize to Freud, Paquet called attention to Freud's work in terms of its incalculable contributions to both the scientific and cultural domains. Addressing himself to other comments in Paquet's letter, Freud responded: "I have never before found the secret, personal intentions behind it [my work] recognized with such clarity as by you" (Freud, 1930b: 207). Given Freud's exceptional appraisal, Paquet's astute reflection deserves to be quoted in full: "a somewhat Mephistophelean trait favored by your investigative method in its pitiless tearing away of *all* veils is the inseparable companion of Faustian insatiability and awe before the creative powers of images that slumber in the unconscious" (G.W. 14: 546 fn., author's translation and emphasis).

Freud's address is intrinsically significant for the professional identity or persona that he assigns himself, i.e., a scientist who founded a "mental science" that explores the construction and functioning of the psyche. But never once in his essay does Freud underscore his own powers of writing qua writing; to have done so would have disrupted his strategy of self-definition. He does not compete with Goethe as a writer, but he does show that psychoanalysis can demonstrate what Goethe poetically intuited. Hence, while explicitly calling psychoanalysis a science and implicitly giving himself the restrictive title of scientist, Freud calls attention to Goethe as both scientist and artist. By integrating both roles, Goethe is held superior to Leonardo, whose scientific and artistic identities were in conflict.

Freud's commemorative address remarkably combines two different kinds of rhetoric, the eulogistic and the judicial; that is to say, Freud fuses his eulogy of Goethe with a general apologia—moved to "justify" himself before Goethe, he discusses how the German colossus would have reacted positively to psychoanalytic tenets. In fact, Goethe already places as a psychoanalytic forerunner through his insights into our first affective ties, dream dynamics, the efficacy of giving psychological assistance, and the essential unity of Eros, ranging from its primitive to its sublimated expression.

Freud also engages in a more specific apologia; fending off the reproach that analysts have been overly critical and insulting in their biographies of Goethe, Freud replies that such accounts do not "intend or signify a degradation" of their subject (G.W. 14: 549; cf. Freud, 1930: 211). Indirectly disagreeing with Paquet's tribute that he can tear away "*all* veils," Freud states that psychoanalytic biographers (including himself) are unable to explain an artist's creative gift or the aesthetic value and effect of his or her works. Positively, though, biographers fulfill our desire to get nearer to great creators whose personalities we expect to be equal to their achievements. Then in a gesture of self-contradiction, Freud adds that a biographer's making us feel closer does bring about a degradation of the great that ties in with our ambivalence toward our fathers and teachers in the past.

In the subtle ending of his essay, Freud admits his limited or veiled success in understanding Goethe, a great self-revealer as well as careful concealer. To the latter effect, he quotes the words of Mephistopheles: "The best of what you know may not, after all, be told to the boys." We know from other texts how Freud also was expert in self-revelation and concealment. And we know that Freud frequently used Mephistopheles's contemptuous words to express his own thought. Despite Freud's revolutionary contribution to human communication, he was also contemptuous of his audience, including analysts.

REFERENCES

Freud, S. (1930a). *Address Delivered in the Goethe House at Frankfurt.* S.E. 21: 208–212.

———. (1930b). *Letter to Dr. Alfons Paquet.* S.E. 21: 207.

Jones, E. (1957). *The Life and Work of Sigmund Freud*, vol. 3. New York: Basic Books.

Paquet, A. (1930). *Letter to S. Freud.* G.W. 14: 545–546 fn.

Schur, M. (1972). *Freud Living and Dying.* New York: International Universities Press.

PATRICK MAHONY

Great Britain, and Psychoanalysis

The British Psycho-Analytical Society was founded by Ernest Jones in 1919. Jones had met Freud in 1908 and was immensely interested in Freud's ideas. Trained first as a neurologist, Jones had spent some time working as a psychiatrist in Toronto. While there he had fostered the spread of psychoanalytic interests in Canada and the United States, where he helped to found the American Psychoanalytic Society (King and Steiner, 1991, p.10).

As a staunch supporter, friend, translator, biographer, and correspondent of Freud, Jones played a major part in the development of psychoanalysis in England. Under the direction of Freud, he founded the *International Journal of Psycho-Analysis* in 1920 and was its first editor. He rescued Freud, his family, and many colleagues from the Nazis and brought them to London from Vienna in 1938.

Even before that date psychoanalysts from continental Europe had found a home in England. One was Melanie Klein, well known for her work on the nature of psychic conflict, anxiety, and guilt. With considerable clinical detail derived from her psychoanalysis of children, she elaborated on the mechanisms of defense discovered by Freud, such as projection, identification, and splitting. Theories related to "introjection," a term first used by Ferenczi, was also important in her work (Klein, 1932).

Many analysts in the British Psycho-Analytical Society were analyzing children before Klein arrived in London in 1926 at the invitation of Jones. Klein had started psychoanalyzing children in Budapest, where she was in analysis with Sándor Ferenczi. She continued her work in Berlin, where Karl Abraham was a major influence. His most original contributions lay in exploring pregenital phases of development.

There was considerable contact between London and European analysts in the 1920s. Many had their training analyses on the continent: John Rickman, Joan Riviere, and James and Alix Strachey went to Vienna for analysis with Freud, while others went to Berlin to Abraham and Sachs, or to Budapest for analysis with Ferenczi, as did Jones.

Jones's theoretical interests were similar in many ways to those of Klein. He was sympathetic to her theories concerning the psychoanalysis of children and female sexuality. However, Freud's daughter Anna strongly disagreed with Klein's ideas about early development (A. Freud, 1948). These included theories concerning the origin, composition, and function of the superego, the timing of the development of the Oedipus complex, and the part played by the transference in child analysis. The variations in their approaches led to heated discussions.

Although many of the London psychoanalysts were sympathetic to Klein's ideas, some did not agree with all of them. After she published her seminal "A Contribution to the Psychogenesis of Manic-depressive States" (Klein, 1935), in which she outlined the part played by destructiveness in depression and the importance of guilt, remorse, and reparation in both normal and pathological development, some of the British analysts felt she had gone too far. Her ideas concerning the role of early sadism resulted in fierce disagreement, particularly after Freud and his colleagues arrived in London.

Debates, known as The Controversial Discussions, were held in 1943 and 1944 to attempt to resolve the disagreements in theory and practice, and in the teaching of psychoanalysis. Susan Isaacs' paper on phantasy (1952) is a clear explanation of the role of unconscious phantasy (spelled with "ph" to indicate an unconscious process and to distinguish it from conscious fantasy) in early mental life. Paula Heimann (1952) outlined the processes of introjection and projection, seen by Klein

as taking place at a much earlier age than was usually considered possible. Klein was quite convinced of the existence of the death instinct and of the part played by destructiveness in psychopathology. Some of the Viennese analysts thought her work deviated from Freud's, but she saw it as based on Freud's classical theory and technique.

These theoretical differences were not resolved but accepted and have enriched the clinical and scientific life of the British Psycho-Analytical Society. After The Controversial Discussions, a new training structure was developed to find a compromise between the interests of Klein and Anna Freud as well as of those British members not aligned on either side. A tripartite arrangement was made whereby students selected one of two main streams. One stream was for students with British or Kleinian training analysts; the other was for Anna Freud's and her colleagues' students. Over time those British analysts who agreed with Klein and/or Anna Freud on some points but not all came to be called "independents."

It is on these principles that selection, training, and supervision of candidates of the British Society exists to this day. Analysts of all three groups have made major contributions to psychoanalytic ideas and theories. The works of the Hoffers, the Sandlers, and Ilse Hellman are representative of the Contemporary Freudians, as the group who worked with Anna Freud are now called; while Donald W. Winnicott, Michael Balint, and William Gillespie were among many who showed what an independent mind can accomplish within psychoanalysis (Rayner, 1990). Of the Kleinians, Hanna Segal, Wilfred R. Bion, and Herbert Rosenfeld were among the first to treat psychotic patients in a purely psychoanalytic manner, and all have worked to define the nature of symbolic function and communication in psychosis. The theory that individuals are object seeking from birth contributes to the importance attached to the transference in Kleinian clinical practice (Spillius, E. Bott 1988a, 1988b). Betty Joseph's writings on transference and countertransference have helped this understanding.

Present-day psychoanalysis in Britain is concerned with developing and refining theory and clinical technique in the treatment of adults, adolescents, and children. The training of psychoanalysts has been extended beyond London, with candidates in the north of England, in Scotland, and in Ireland.

REFERENCES

Freud. A. (1948). *Four Lectures on Child Analysis*. London: Hogarth. Reprinted in *The Writings of Anna Freud. vol. 1*. New York: International Universities Press, 1974, pp. 3–69.

Heimann, P. (1952). Certain functions of introjection and projection in early infancy. In J. Riviere (ed.). *Developments in Psycho-Analysis*, London: Hogarth Press and Institute of Psycho-Analysis, pp. 122–168.

Isaacs, S. (1952). On the nature and function of phantasy. In J. Riviere (ed.). *Developments in Psycho-Analysis*, London: Hogarth Press and Institute of Psycho-Analysis, pp. 67–121.

King, P., and Steiner, R. (eds.) (1991). *The Freud-Klein Controversies: 1941–1945*. London: Routledge.

Klein, M. (1932). *The Psycho-Analysis of Children*. London: Hogarth. Reprinted in *The Writings of Melanie Klein, vol. 2*. London: Hogarth Press and the Institute of Psycho-Analysis, 1975.

———. (1935). A contribution to the genesis of manic-depressive states. *International Journal of Psychoanalysis*, 16: 145–174. *The Writings of Melanie Klein, vol. 1: Love, Guilt and Reparation*. London: Hogarth Press, 1975, pp. 262–289.

Rayner, E. (1990). *The Independent Mind in British Psychoanalysis*. London: Free Association Books.

Spillius, E. Bott (ed.) (1988a). *Melanie Klein Today, vol. 1: Mainly Theory*. London: Routledge.

———. (1988b). *Melanie Klein Today, vol. 2: Mainly Practice*. London: Routledge.

ATHOL HUGHES

Greece, and Psychoanalysis

The theory of psychoanalysis was first presented in Greece by the eminent linguist Manolis Triandafyllidis in 1915 to a society of scholars and writers dedicated to the advancement of progressive education, the Ekpaedefticos Omilos, with a lecture entitled "The Origins of Language and Freudian Psychology." In 1927, after a series of articles on the subject by other scholars and educators, Demetrios Kouretas, a psychiatrist, introduced Freud's theory to the country's medical profession, with a lecture entitled "Psychoanalysis, Psychology of the Unconscious." In the 1930s, along with educator Demetrios Moraitis, he practiced Adlerian psychoanalysis in Athens.

The first attempt to organize psychoanalytic training in Greece occurred shortly after the end of World War II. Kouretas, along with a child psychiatrist, George Zavitzianos, and a surrealist poet, Andreas Embirikos, all of whom had had some personal analysis in France, were recognized as a study group of the International Psychoanalytic Association (IPA) under the sponsorship of the French Psychoanalytic Association. The group had also been guided by Princess Marie Bonaparte, a member of the Greek royal family. (Celia Bertin's *Marie Bonaparte, A Life* makes only cursory mention of the princess's considerable psychoanalytic activities in Greece and her extensive correspondence with Kouretas.) The official recognition of the study group was marked by Anna Freud's visit to Greece, with a lecture at the University of Athens, in January 1949. Lectures followed by other prominent analysts from abroad, including Margaret Mahler, René Spietz, and Jean Lacan. But medical opposition to the fact that a lay analyst, Embirikos, was doing psychotherapy led to the early dissolution of the group. Embirikos left for France and abandoned psychoanalysis. Zavitzianos moved to North America, where he did considerable psychoanalytic work, becoming known for his writings on the perversions. Kouretas, the only one to remain and continue doing psychoanalysis in Greece, eventually became professor of psychiatry at the University of Athens.

A second attempt to organize psychoanalytic training in Greece was made in the early 1970s. A Committee for the Promotion of Psychoanalysis in Greece and Yugoslavia, appointed by IPA President Serge Lebovici, tried to work out an agreement with two Greek analysts, Paris-trained Panayotis Sakellaropoulos and Canadian-trained Athina Alexandris, to form a new study group, but the negotiations led nowhere. Finally, in 1981, Lebovici, who had personal knowledge of the situation in Greece, approached Peter Hartocollis, a Topeka training analyst and newly appointed professor and chairman of the Psychiatry Department of Patras Medical School, suggesting that he and Stavroula Beratis, a New York–trained analyst, recently appointed to the faculty of Patras University, along with three local analysts—Alexandris, Sakellaropoulos, and Paris training analyst Anna Potamianou—apply to the IPA to form a study group. The president of the IPA, Adam Limentani, asked Joseph Sandler to investigate conditions in Greece, and on October 11, 1982, the Hellenic Study Group received formal approval. Guided by a sponsoring committee of the IPA composed of Joseph Sandler of Israel and London, Janice de Saussure of Geneva, and Stavros Mentzos of Frankfurt, the new group began accepting candidates for psychoanalytic training.

Subsequently, two of the founders of the study group, Alexandris and Sakellaropoulos, disagreeing with the evaluation procedure of training analysts, withdrew from the group's activities. In the process, the composition of the IPA's sponsoring committee changed, Sandler being replaced by Janine Chasseguet-Smirgel of Paris; she herself was replaced later by Anne-Marie Sandler of London. De Saussure was replaced by Dinora Pines of London, with Mentzos assuming the chairmanship.

In July 1997, the Hellenic Study Group was recognized by the IPA as a provisional society, and in July 2001, as a component psychoanalytic society. By that time, the group numbered six training and supervising analysts (Stavroula Beratis, Peter Hartocollis, Nikos Kouretas, Anna Potamianou, Nikos Tzavaras, and Thalia Vergopoulo); twenty full and associate members; fourteen corresponding members (IPA analysts of Greek origin practicing abroad); one honorary member (Harold Blum); and thirty-five candidates.

REFERENCES

Bertin, C. (1982). *Marie Bonaparte, A Life*. New Haven, Conn.: Yale University Press.

Hartocollis, P. (1983). Psychoanalysis abroad: A report from Greece. *Psychoanalytical Quarterly*, 11: 250–253.

Kontos, J., Manolopoulos, S., and Kouretas, N. (1995). Greece. In Kutter, P. (ed.). *Psychoanalysis International. A Guide to Psychoanalysis Throughout the World*, vol. 2. Frankfurt: Frommann-Holzboog, pp. 288–305.

Tzavaras, T. (ed.) (1984). *Psychoanalysis and Greece*. Athens: Eteria Spoudon Neoellinica Politismou and Genikis Paedias (in Greek).

PETER HARTOCOLLIS

Groddeck, Georg (1866–1934)

A German poet, philosopher, and physician, Groddeck discovered the importance of transference and resistance independently of Freud. Groddeck was unique among the early contributors to psychoanalysis in that he maintained both an independent philosophy of treatment (*das Es*, the It) and a cordial relationship with Freud (Schacht, 1977: 6; Durrell, 1948: 390). Groddeck is credited as being the originator of both psychosomatics and countertransference, in their modern definitions (Searles, p. 446). In addition, symbolization, an enduring subject of Groddeck's interest and writing, has been proposed as a unifying theory for psychoanalysis (Aragno, 1997). Groddeck was born in Bad Kösen, Germany, into a household steeped in medicine and literature. His father, Karl, was a physician who had had an influence on Nietzsche. His maternal grandfather, August Kober-

stein, was a leader of the German literary society named for the poet, Walther van der Vogelweide (1170–1229). During Groddeck's youth, this society, the "Vogelweide," met weekly in the Groddeck home.

Upon graduating from medical school in Berlin in 1889, Groddeck became an associate of Ernst Schweninger in Baden Baden. Schweninger, who had an authoritarian manner, utilized an holistic approach in his treatment. Among his patients was Otto von Bismarck, the "Iron Chancellor," who had founded the modern German state in 1870. By 1900, Groddeck opened a sanitarium in Baden Baden, where he gave regular lectures and published his own house journal, *Die Arche*.

Starting from 1909, Groddeck developed a philosophy of treatment based on the view that it was impossible to separate the individual from his surrounding universe. Rather than referring to the illusory separate individual, or "I," Groddeck thought it was more useful to conceptualize being "lived by" an unknowable force. He struggled with what to call this secret force. Initially, he borrowed a term from Goethe: *Gottnatur* (Godnature). He even thought of using the mathematical expression X. Ultimately, he gave it the most indefinite and flexible name possible—*das Es*, the It.

The It was a theory of nonattachment that embraced a romantic naturalism common at the time. It provided a theoretical framework for Groddeck to treat physical illness in what he recognized as a unity with psychological processes. Thus, Groddeck became less interested in diagnosing disease and more interested in listening to the patient. Groddeck wrote, "Every physician needs two things: watchfulness and patience. . . . Put off action as long as you can, and watch for signs of the patient's It. Sooner or later, it will probably whisper to you advice you can pass on to the patient."

Groddeck discovered transference and resistance and understood them as unconscious expressions of the It: "The It transfers feelings both of friendship and of enmity on to the doctor, and thereby helps or obstructs his efforts. Since life is made up, more or less, of these transferences the doctor must select certain of them, if he is not to be overwhelmed by the flood of phenomena, and use them in dealing with the resistance. . . . Three-fourths of our success, if not more, rests upon the accident which gave us some sort of resemblance to the parents of our patients."

As Groddeck lectured about his discoveries, the name "Freud" was often brought to his attention.

Initially, Groddeck avoided reading Freud's work in much the same way that Freud admitted he avoided reading Nietzsche. However, on May 27, 1917, he wrote to Freud describing his concept of *das Es* and its use in his clinical work. He asked Freud whether his work was consistent with Freud's psychoanalysis. At that time, Freud was preoccupied with guarding his creation of psychoanalysis. Freud had already endured the defections of Stekel, Adler, and Jung from *die Sache* (the cause), and a secret committee had been formed to protect the future development of psychoanalysis.

Freud recognized immediately Groddeck's creativity and welcomed him enthusiastically: "I have not had a letter for a long time which so pleased, interested, and stimulated me. . . . I have to claim you, I have to assert that you are a splendid analyst who has understood forever the essential aspects of the matter. The discovery that transference and resistance are the most important aspects of treatment turns a person irretrievably into a member of the wild army. . . . I would like to hold out both my hands to receive you as a colleague" (Groddeck, 1977: 36–37). Freud wrote to Oskar Pfister, "I am not usually so taken in by anybody" (Freud, 1963: 82).

Freud identified Groddeck's work as being "very close in its ideas" to those of Ferenczi (Groddeck, 1977: 37). Freud then forwarded Groddeck's first letter to Ferenczi and instructed him, "It is in our personal interest to involve him in the circle of our collaborators. . . . It is certainly a must to meet with this man" (Dupont, 1992, p. 52). Freud and Ferenczi began writing to each other about "Groddeckian" psychosomatic symptoms. Groddeck used the early years of his correspondence with Freud as a passionate vehicle for self analysis as Freud had done with Fliess at exactly the same age of forty-two (Grossman, 1965: 202). Freud reciprocated with warmth and interest, signing his letters *herzlichst* (from the heart).

Ferenczi was initially skeptical about Groddeck's claims of treating physical illness through psychological methods. However, in 1921, Ferenczi visited Groddeck in Baden Baden on referral from Felix Deutsch for treatment of nephrosclerosis. Ferenczi was cured of this physical ailment and was greatly impressed with Groddeck. They formed a strong and lasting relationship. After this first visit, Ferenczi wrote in the guest book at the Sanitarium Groddeck, "I came to teach him but I was taught; I left enthusiastic and half-converted." In like manner, Groddeck wrote to Freud, "Ferenczi has been here . . . we profited a lot from each other."

Afterward, Ferenczi wrote Groddeck a long and intimate letter expressing "everything he was never able to tell Freud, who was a crushing paternal figure" (Dupont, 1992: 54). In addition, Ferenczi wrote to Freud that he was doing "auto-analysis in the presence and with the assistance of Groddeck" who proceeds "warily and prudently and remains loyal to the psychoanalysis for everything that is essential" (Dupont, 1992: 55). Groddeck, in turn, wrote to Freud that he had been analyzed during these visits by Ferenczi (Groddeck, 1977: 82). Ferenczi returned to Sanitarium Groddeck regularly for "therapeutic holidays" and referred his family and friends. He would also often bring his own patients with him. From 1921–1932, Ferenczi spent a total of eight months of such "therapeutic holidays" at Sanitarium Groddeck (Will, 1987).

While Groddeck maintained a correspondence with Freud for seventeen years, he became closer personally to Ferenczi. Indeed, Erich Fromm stated in 1935 that the development of Ferenczi can be understood only in the light of Groddeck's influence (Will, 1987). Groddeck provided support for Ferenczi to pursue his work on activity, relaxation, mutual analysis, countertransference, and maternal transference, despite harsh criticism from Freud and others. Groddeck became the mentor and friend that Ferenczi had wished Freud would be. Groddeck is the progenitor (in a line that extends through Ferenczi and Balint, Horney, Fromm-Reichmann, Rank, Ernst Simmel, and others) of an emphasis on the maternal and the relational in contrast and counterbalance to Freud's emphasis on the paternal and the interpretable.

In 1923, Groddeck published his humorous yet scientific classic, *The Book of the It*. Freud wrote in response, "Groddeck in vain protests he has nothing to do with pure science" (Freud, 1923: 23). In *The Book of the It*, Groddeck described what Searles later credited as the first description of countertransference in the contemporary sense: "The first writing . . . which at all explicitly describes the patient's functioning as a therapist to the doctor. . . . Even this courageously pioneering statement portrays . . . therapy *for the patient*, exclusively, in the long run" (Searles, 1979: 446).

The statement to which Searles refers reads as follows:

Certain slumbering mother-virtues were awakened in me by the patient, and these directed my procedure. . . . And now I was confronted by the strange fact that I was not treating the patient, but that the patient was treating me; or to translate it into my own language, the *It* of this fellow-being tried so to transform my *It*, did in fact so transform it, that it came to be useful for its purpose. . . . Even to get this amount of insight was difficult, for you will understand that it absolutely reversed my position in regard to a patient. It was no longer important to give him instructions, to prescribe for him what I considered right, but to change in such a way that he could use me" (Groddeck, 1923: 262–263).

Shortly after the publication of Groddeck's *The Book of the It*, Freud published *The Ego and the Id*. In it, Freud appropriated Groddeck's concept of *das Es* and radically altered it to become the id in his own structural model. Freud, most probably, adapted *das Es* to Heinroth's tripartite model (Poster, 1997: 279–280). In so doing, Groddeck considered that Freud had removed "the constructive aspect" from *das Es*, reducing it to an agency of wild forces only.

After Freud's redefinition of *das Es*, Groddeck began to refer to the unconscious as part of the psyche, and the psyche as part of the *It*. To Freud, his id was part of the unconscious, and the unconscious part of the soul of man. To Groddeck, the *It* was "all there is; whatever else there seems to be (the ego, for one thing) is only a mask, an appearance of the *It*." Yet he recommended psychoanalysis as "the best . . . closest approach to the target" of the *It* (Groddeck, 1977: 16). Indeed, Groddeck wrote that psychoanalysis was "often the only means by which to stir the man's *It* in its deepest depths into healing activity" (Groddeck, 1950b: 222).

In the *Ego and the Id*, Freud stated that Groddeck had derived *das Es* from Nietzsche. Recent scholarship (Bos, 1992: 439) has concluded that there is no evidence for this, but that Freud succeeded in placing Groddeck in a double-bind. Groddeck could neither claim originality over Freud and risk their friendship, nor deny having been generally influenced by Nietzsche who was one of the *Hausgötter* (household gods) of a whole German generation.

Freud's actions with regard to *das Es* were fueled by what Levinson has termed a "fundamental conflict" between a wish to be a scientist and a wish to build a worldwide psychoanalytic organization (Levinson, 1990: 1–2). This is where the temptation to modify Groddeck's

das Es into a concrete, named agency as part of a rational model of the mind was irresistible for Freud. However, Freud's theoretical and technical writings have been shown to have been at variance with his own clinical practice (Lynn and Vaillant, 1998: 169). Here may lie a clue to Freud's apparent fascination with Groddeck.

Grotjahn speculated that "perhaps Freud recognized in Groddeck his own inner demon, his own unconscious" (Grotjahn, 1966: 310). Both men loved literature and were steeped in Western positivist medicine from which they bravely departed to create theory and treat patients. Freud became increasingly preoccupied with his legacy, the survival of *die Sache*. Groddeck, on the other hand, explicitly discouraged such activity on his behalf: "Disciples want their master to stay put, whereas I should think anyone a fool who wanted me to say the same thing tomorrow as I said yesterday. If you really want to be my follower, look at life for yourself and tell the world honestly what you see." Similarly, Groddeck warned, "It is only he who keeps always in mind the insufficiency of his knowledge who is truly a man of science" (Groddeck, 1951: 24). As Durrell put it, "Groddeck was as different from Freud as Lao Tzu was from Confucius" (Durrell, 1948: 385).

Although Freud's id gained usage in popular culture, Grinstein's Index of Psychoanalytic Writings showed only 31 entries for "id" from 1956 to 1969 and less thereafter (Bos, 1992: 441). Freud himself, in *Analysis Terminable and Interminable*, did not conceal that his original reason for separating a realistic structure from *das Es* had turned out to be less justified than he had thought (Friedman, 1992: 20). More recently, Brenner (1994; 1998) has proposed that the structural model be relinquished. He also concluded that psychoanalysts no longer use the concepts of id, ego, or superego in their clinical work or writing (Brenner, 1998: 178).

Following a prolonged theoretical detour through Freud's structural model, a consensus has been building around the need for a new unified psychoanalytic theory of the mind. One such proposal, symbolization (Aragno, 1997), harks directly back to Groddeck's earliest and most enduring interest—the use of symbols as a key to unconscious processes. Groddeck considered the compulsion to symbolize to be a manifestation of the It: "Until the end of our lives our understanding is tied to the symbol. No matter how rational we are we cannot help it: a window will remain an eye, a cave a mother, a pole a father" (Groddeck, 1977: 18).

G

Hoffer has described the "polarities" exemplified by Ferenczi and Freud: "heart and mind, passion and reason, indulgence and frustration, mother and father, and, finally, female and male" (Hoffer, 1991: 469). The "female" side of these same polarities extends from Ferenczi back to Groddeck. Indeed, the split causing the polarities described by Hoffer can be dated from the appropriation in 1923 by Freud of Groddeck's mystical *It* and its transformation into part of his own rational model, creating what Friedman humorously called "an id with eyeballs" (Friedman, 1992: 20). Heinz Hartmann and other ego psychologists further extended this rational model. In reaction, many theories have arisen to fill the experiential, or two-person, void, e.g., object relations, self psychology, and relational and interpersonal theories.

The polarities that Hoffer described continue in psychoanalysis as expressed in different schools, lately lumped under the terms "subjectivists" and "objectivists." Interestingly, the new unified theory of psychoanalysis, symbolization, has been promoted, in part, to "put to rest schismatic arguments between hermeneuticists and hard scientists" (Aragno, 1997).

Groddeck died of a heart attack while lecturing in Switzerland. At the time, he was in danger of being arrested in Germany for openly criticizing the Hitler regime. He was mourned as "the greatest magician among the psychoanalysts and, without doubt, the most important human personality of them all" (Keyserling, in Schacht, 1977: 21). A fitting epitaph for Groddeck would be an excerpt from a statement at his Sanitarium: "The only achievement I can claim for myself, with some justification, is the introduction of a knowledge of the unconscious into the treatment of all patients."

Three years after Groddeck's death and one year before his own, Freud's *Analysis Terminable and Interminable* was published. Its pessimism about prior assertions of definitive cure through psychoanalysis may be understood as a reconsideration by Freud of some of the moderating views of Ferenczi and Groddeck. Indeed, Freud cited Ferenczi when he added "the individuality of the analyst" as a variable factor contributing to the analytic outcome (1937, p. 247). In addition, Groddeck had warned, in his sometimes provocative style, "If anybody says a patient must be analyzed 'to the end' I think he does not know what he is talking about; in fact he is talking nonsense. No analysis can be carried to the end" (Groddeck 1951a: 26–27).

Despite Groddeck's earlier objection, the Georg Groddeck Gesellschaft was founded in 1986 in Frankfurt, Germany. A fifteen-volume edition of Groddeck's works will be published by The Stroemfeld/Roter Stern Verlag. In addition to his wide-ranging clinical and theoretical contributions, these include: a "psychoanalytic novel," *Der Seelensucher* (The Seeker of Souls), named by Rank and published, with Freud's assistance, by the International Psychoanalytic Verlag; plus other poems, novels, and essays on literature, art, philosophy, and religion.

REFERENCES

Aragno, A. (1997). *Symbolization*. Madison, Conn.: International Universities Press.

Bos, J. (1992). On the origin of the Id (*Das Es*). *International Review of Psychoanalysis*, 19: 433–443.

Brenner, C. (1994). The mind as conflict and compromise formation. *Journal of Clinical Psychoanalysis*, 3: 473–488.

———. (1998). Beyond the Ego and the Id revisited. *Journal of Clinical Psychoanalysis*, 7: 165–180.

Dupont, J. (1992). Georg Groddeck entre Freud et Ferenczi. *Le Coq Heron*, 123: 51–55.

Durrell, L. (1948). Studies in genius: VI, Groddeck. *Horizon*, June: 384–403.

Freud, S. (1923). *The Ego and the Id*. S.E. 19: 12–59.

———. (1937). *Analysis Terminable and Interminable*. S.E. 23: 216–253.

———. (1963). *Psychoanalysis and Faith*. H. Meng and E. Freud (eds.) New York: Basic Books.

Friedman, L. (1992). What is the analysand supposed to be realistic about? Presentation to Psychoanalytic Society of New England, East. Cambridge: October 24, 1992: 1–25.

Groddeck, G. (1950a). *The Book of the It*. Trans. by V. Collins. London: Vision.

———. (1950b). *Exploring the Unconscious*. Trans. by V. Collins. London: Vision.

———. (1951a). *The Unknown Self*. Trans. by V. Collins. New York: Funk and Wagnalls.

———. (1951b). *The World of Man*. Trans. by V. Collins. New York: Funk and Wagnalls.

———. (1977). *The Meaning of Illness, Selected Psychoanalytic Writings of Georg Groddeck*. Trans. by G. Mander. New York: International Universities Press.

Grossman, C. and S. Grossman (1965). *The Wild Analyst*. New York: Braziller.

Grotjahn, M. (1966). Georg Groddeck. In F. Alexander (ed.) *Psychoanalytic Pioneers*. New York: Basic Books, pp. 308–320.

Hoffer, A. (1991). The Freud-Ferenczi controversy—A living legacy. *International Review of Psychoanalysis*, 18: 465–472.

Levinson, H. (1990). Freud as an entrepreneur: Implications for contemporary psychoanalytic institutes. Presentation to International Society for the Psychoanalytic Study of Organizations. Montreal: May 24: 1–51.

Lynn, D. and G. Vaillant. (1998). Anonymity, neutrality, and confidentiality in the actual methods of Sigmund Freud: A Review of 43 Cases, 1907–1939. *American Journal of Psychiatry*, 155: 163–171.

Poster, M. (1997). An hypothesis: The historical derivation of Freud's structural model of the mind. *Journal of Clinical Psychoanalysis*, 6: 279–283.

Schacht, L. (1977). Introduction. In *The Meaning of Illness, Selected Psychoanalytic Writings of Georg Groddeck*. Trans. by F. Mander, New York: International Universities Press, pp. 130.

Searles, H. (1979). The patient as therapist to his analyst. In *Countertransference and Related Subjects*. Madison, Conn.: International Universities Press, pp. 380–459.

Will, H. (1987). *Georg Groddeck. Die Geburt der Psychosomatik*. Munchen: Deutscher Taschenbuch Verlag.

MARK F. POSTER

Guilt

Freud (1914; 1923; 1924) discusses guilt feelings under very different perspectives in connection, for example, with their role in the regulation of mental processes and behavior, the formation of neurotic symptoms, and the development of the superego. To classify these rather heterogeneous formulations, in the following we rely on a more general model of the development, phenomenology, and function of emotions (Bänninger-Huber and Widmer, 1996). This model is less abstract than Freud's theory and is more easily related to observable phenomena (Bänninger-Huber and Widmer, 1996).

We start from the conceptualization widely accepted in emotion psychology: that emotions, including feelings of guilt, may be characterized as complexes consisting of several components (e.g., Scherer, 1984), including the specific situation that elicits a certain emotion, the phenomenological aspects of an emotion, and the specific intrapsychic, interactive, or behavioral processes motivated by an emotion. Emotions, in this model, are viewed as consequences of *cognitive evaluations* of specific *emotion-eliciting situations*. These cognitively evaluated situational constellations may be *intrapsychic* or part of *external reality*.

Freud conceptualized guilt feelings as manifestations of an intrapsychic conflict between impulses of the id and internalized norms of the superego. According to emotion psychology, in contrast, guilt feelings arise in connection with a comparison of one's own wishes, actions, fantasies, and the like, with the repertoire of one's own norms, values, and rules.

Guilt feelings are so-called structural emotions, i.e., emotions primarily understood as elements of intrapsychic regulatory processes. Feelings of self-esteem, narcissistic gratification, and envy are other examples of structural emotions. Use of the term "structural emotion" stresses the psychoanalytic view that the possession of certain intrapsychic structures, e.g., the superego, are a prerequisite for the occurrence of a specific emotion. Hence, structural emotions are more "complex" than so-called basic emotions as anger, fear, or sadness; they also occur only in later ontogenetic stages.

Freud describes the development of the superego structure as a consequence of the internalization of parental norms and the gradual independence of moral imperatives from the original authority figures. During this development, the infantile fear of punishment and fear of loss of love is replaced by guilt feelings. Further, Freud assumes an individual's ability of self-observation, i.e., the ability to compare one's impulses and wishes with one's internalized norms. According to emotion psychologists, self-evaluative emotions such as guilt feelings also require the development of a self-concept and the ability to compare oneself with internal social norms (Lewis, 1992).

Since the superego is formed in the context of the Oedipal conflict, its main topics are, first of all, the incest taboo and the prohibition of patricide and matricide or, more generally, the libidinous and aggressive impulses and corresponding behaviors toward others. More recent psychoanalytic authors (Sandler, 1960; Weiss, 1986) describe other guilt feeling eliciting topics, e.g., enjoyment, success, and the separation from relevant others. An empirical investigation of psychoanalytic case reports (Lüthy and Widmer, 1992) has shown that not only a misdeed but also an omission, for example, the omission of help or support, can be followed by guilt feelings. Such feelings are elicited by real actions as well as by fantasies, thoughts, or other affects. What all of these have in common is the individual's feeling responsible whether or not the feeling has any basis in external reality. In other words, guilt feelings may occur even when a person is not "objectively" guilty. On the other hand, an individual who really is guilty of having committed a crime might not experience any guilt feelings.

According to psychoanalysis and emotion psychology, the cognitive evaluation of a given situation may vary depending on an individual's *actual emotional state* and his or her *individual biography*. This variation in how

G

individuals cognitively evaluate certain situations accounts for psychoanalysts' relatively small interest in identifying universal guilt-eliciting conflicts or topics. In contrast, the understanding and resolution of *individual* neurotic guilt reactions based on the background of a patient's biography are a main focus of psychoanalytic treatment. However, recent discussions on the influence of gender on the superego and on moral values have again raised this question of universal determinants of guilt (Alpert, 1996).

The experience of guilt feelings as reported by his patients were one clue that allowed Freud to analyze their superego conflicts. He assumed that unconscious guilt feelings can influence a person's behavior without the emotion being consciously experienced and can lead to self-restrictive or compulsive behavior, or to a negative therapeutic reaction. In agreement with Freudian theory, emotion psychologists hold that consciously experienced as well as unconscious emotions can serve a *motivational function*: they can elicit specific processes that balance out perturbations in the individual's cognitive-affective regulation, as, e.g., the incompatibility of a wish with an internalized norm. With respect to the motivational aspects of an emotion, we differentiate among *intrapsychic, interactive*, and *behavioral consequences*. A guilt-ridden individual may suppress a wish, apologize, or undertake acts of restitution. Defense mechanisms such as repression, denial, or reaction formation, as conceptualized by Freud, can be understood as intrapsychic processes elicited by guilt feelings. Furthermore, Freud described a variety of behaviors, for example, acts of self-punishment or reparation, that ward off occurring guilt feelings. These observable behaviors could not be explained without the concept of unconscious guilt feelings. One of Freud's merits is his having worked out the importance of emotions for intrapsychic functioning and the regulation of relationships.

REFERENCES

Alpert, J. (1996). *Psychoanalysis and Woman: Contemporary Reappraisals.* Hillsdale, N.J.: Analytic Press.

Bänninger-Huber, E., and Widmer, C. (1996). A new model of the elicitation, phenomenology and function of emotions in psychotherapy. In N. H. Frijda (ed.). *Proceedings of the Ninth Conference of the International Society for Research on Emotions.* Toronto, pp. 251–255.

Freud, S. (1914). On narcissism: An introduction. S.E. 14: 67–104.

———. (1923). *The Ego and the Id.* S.E. 19: 1–66.

———. (1924). The dissolution of the Oedipus complex. S.E. 19: 171–179.

Lewis, M. (1992). *Shame. The Exposed Self.* New York: Free Press.

Lüthy, A. M., and Widmer, C. (1992). A model-oriented representation of superego rules. In M. Leuzinger-Bohleber, H. Schneider, and R. Pfeifer (eds.). *"Two Butterflies on my Head . . ."—Psychoanalysis in the Interdisciplinary Scientific Dialogue.* Heidelberg: Springer, pp. 197–214.

Sandler, J. (1960). On the concept of super-ego. *Psychoanalytic Study of the Child*, 15: 128–162.

Scherer, K. R. (1984). On the nature and function of emotion: A component process approach. In K. R. Scherer and P. Ekman (eds.). *Approaches to Emotion.* Hillsdale, N.J.: Lawrence Erlbaum, pp. 293–317.

Weiss, J. (1986). Unconscious guilt. In J. Weiss and H. Sampson (eds.). *The Psychoanalytic Process.* New York: Guilford Press, pp. 43–76.

EVA BÄNNINGER-HUBER
CHRISTINE WIDMER

H

Hallucinations

Freud defined "hallucination" as an experienced sensation without the concurrent presence of the stimulus. Visual and auditory hallucinations are the most common, but hallucinations can occur in all sense modalities. For example, Freud's patient, Miss Lucy R., hallucinated the smell of burnt pudding, which Freud presumed derived from a real experience in the past that had been repressed. There can also be hallucinations of bodily feeling, such as hallucinations of pain. Dora told Freud that she could still feel the pressure of Herr K.'s embrace on the upper part of her body.

Hallucinations can be positive or negative. In positive hallucinations, something is perceived that is not in the environment. In negative hallucinations, something that is in the environment is not perceived. Breuer's patient, Anna O., did not see a doctor standing right in front of her. Negative hallucinations may occur in the psychopathology of everyday life, such as in misreadings.

Freud also discussed other forms of hallucination, including zoöpsia, the hallucinations of animals. When Emmy von N. picked up a ball of wool, it appeared to become a mouse and ran away. Changes in the size of objects may also be hallucinated.

The fundamental question of how we know whether our perceptions are real or not occupied Freud throughout his career. The equation "perception = reality (external world)" does not hold for humans, since stimulation of perceptual mechanisms can occur from both internal and external events. Internal processes of the ego may acquire the quality of consciousness. Therefore, humans have had to develop a process known as *reality testing* to distinguish between the two kinds of experiences. Errors in reality testing can result in waking hallucination.

In Freud's model of the development of reality testing, there is, at first, no distinction for the infant between internally and externally caused sensations. Only when the infant learns that certain sense impressions are subject to change through motor action, and others are not, are these differentiated, respectively, into external and internal sensations.

Freud identifies a "normal" operation of the psychic system in which information flows from the perceptual system to the memory system to the motoric system. In sleep, the flow of information is shifted and partially reversed. The perceptual system's sensory input from the external world is inhibited, which allows images from the memory system to be fed back into the perceptual system. This process of reversal is called *regression*. It accounts for the hallucinations of dreaming. In regressive psychopathological states, such regression can occur during waking; the resultant vivid percepts, which originate in the memory system, are waking hallucinations.

Usually in waking hallucinations, the hallucinated image does not fill the entire sensory field but rather is superimposed on it. A man sitting in his living room may hallucinate his dead father sitting in his favorite chair. The image of the father is hallucinated, but it is inserted into the image of the rest of the living room, which is perceived normally. This is an important difference between psychopathological hallucinations and dreams, in which the entire sensory field is hallucinated.

While Freud recognized that organic syndromes can lead to hallucinations, his primary discoveries concerned the psychological determinants of hallucinations and their contents. The contents of hallucinations may derive from actual perceptions in early experience, especially traumatic ones, that have undergone repression. The emergence of these traumatic percepts is fraught with anxiety, which leads most hallucinations to be distressing and full of painful affects. A hallucination can also reflect a feared trauma. Thus, one of Freud's patients, at age five, under the influence of strong castration anxiety, hallucinated that he had cut off his little finger so that it was hanging on only by its skin.

The mechanism of hallucination may vary, depending on the type of psychopathology. Freud argued that in hysteria, hallucinations are images repeated undistorted from the repressed past. In paranoia and obsessional neurosis, an analogous modern image takes the place of the repressed one. In schizophrenia, hallucinations result from a narcissistic withdrawal, with the hallucinations representing an attempt at restitution, to restore libidinal cathexis to the world of objects.

Freud believed it was important to distinguish hallucinations caused psychodynamically from those caused by physiological disturbances, although the two factors can operate together. For example, Emmy von N. saw small animals suddenly grow enormous, which Freud first connected with her traumatic memory of a giant lizard appearing in a theatrical production. However, because of her extreme nearsightedness and astigmatism, her hallucinations may have been provoked by the unclarity of her visual perceptions.

Hallucinations, even psychopathological ones, may reflect insight into the workings of the mind. In later editions of *The Interpretation of Dreams*, Freud developed the notion of "endopsychic perception." This was his term for the potential of hallucinatory states to symbolize or represent cognitive processes that are usually unconscious. Thus a man who hallucinates someone watching over him all the time may be representing the superego in this image. Schreber's "rays of God" were, similarly, a concrete representation of libidinal cathexes. Freud believed that such psychotic experiences may visually represent the construction of the normal mind. He also believed that certain practices of mystics may lead to hallucinatory images that similarly portray mental structures.

Clinical work with hallucinations takes many forms. For Anna O., verbal expression of her hallucinations calmed her. In the hope of decreasing her hallucinations, Freud told Emmy von N. that hallucinations were had only by drunkards (knowing that she disliked drunkards

intensely). Later, Freud recognized that with hallucinations, as with delusions, it was important to identify the "kernel of truth" in the experience, and that by tracing the roots of the hallucination to a memory or trauma, the need to hallucinate could be reduced or eliminated.

Hallucinations may occur in some everyday life situations where they are not necessarily troubling. On falling asleep, we often have hypnagogic hallucinations, wherein our ideas are transformed into visual images. Hallucinations, both positive and negative, can also be invoked by posthypnotic suggestion. This fact suggested to Freud the extraordinary power of the mind over the body.

REFERENCE

Draenos, S. (1982). *Freud's Odyssey: Psychoanalysis and the End of Metaphysics.* New Haven, Conn.: Yale University Press.

MARK J. BLECHNER

Hartmann, Heinz (1894–1970)

Although certainly well within the orthodox tradition, Heinz Hartmann made contributions to psychoanalysis, metapsychology, and ego psychology that extended the Freudian views in each of these spheres; in some cases, the extension went so far that Freud himself might have cast a dubious eye on several of the developments.

One important belief of Hartmann was that object constancy begins much earlier than traditional psychoanalysts recognized. In the traditional view, the understanding that objects continue to exist even when not perceived occurs some time after a child is two years old. Clearly, this is wrong; had the earliest psychoanalysts (pre-1920) been more interested in empirical confirmation, this hypothesis would have been discarded very early on.

In contradiction to the early view, Hartmann argued that early maturation depends on the idea that the mother and other key figures in the child's life are real and that appropriate behavior on the child's part can usher them quickly into his or her presence. Oddly, however, Hartmann thought that the child must confront both the good and the bad sides of the primary caregiver and reconcile these to achieve object constancy. On the face of it, there would seem to be no connection between a need to see one's mother as neither perfect nor evil and the ability to realize she exists.

Hartmann was interested in extending psycho-analysis's concern with psychopathologies to a general theory of normal development. For him, the term "ego psychology" is precisely the development of psycho-analysis into a general psychology, but not in the sense of Gordon Allport and other pioneering psychologists who eschewed reference to "ego" and other psychoana-lytic concepts. Hartmann's work is never far from the theorizing common to Freud, but he emphasizes "sur-face" issues as well as the "depth" issues associated with instinctual drives and the unconscious mind. He insisted that the growth of the ego is not principally the outcome of conflicts with drive activity—a radical departure from tradition. He wrote of a "conflict-free sphere" in which the ego simply and naturally matures quietly outside the realm of conflict. It was precisely this concern with the surface, observable phenomena that made Hartmann so open to confirmation of psychoanalytic hypotheses via the usual channels of scientific validation.

According to Hartmann, infantile neuroses are not neuroses at all in the classical sense, i.e., stemming from the unresolved Oedipus complex and the failure to progress through the usual oral, anal, and phallic stages. Still, while Hartmann denied that childhood neuroses usually culminate in adult neuroses, he accepted the con-ventional view that adult neuroses originate in childhood neuroses.

Hartmann overlooked a deep conceptual problem. Most children, even those with infantile neuroses, do not undergo psychoanalysis; since their problems are "sur-face" ones, what else can spontaneous remission of their problems be but a "cure"? Most psychoanalysts, includ-ing Hartmann, do not admit that the elimination of symptoms constitutes a cure, but what is the alternative in cases where symptoms do not point to a "deeper" problem?

Influenced by the growth of general, normal psy-chology, Hartmann eventually defined "mental health" as learning to deal with frustrations and anxiety-producing events. In short, mental health is not leading a dysfunc-tional existence. In this view, psychoanalytic treatment may be valuable, but it does not fulfill the role of "ther-apy" in cases where the patient is merely troubled in vague ways or bothered by remote events in the past that do not keep him or her from performing social roles.

Under the influence of general, normal psychology, by the 1950s, Hartmann had not much to say about adult dreams. He has regarded them all as symbolic and as having the usual sexual interpretations. While he may have continued to analyze dreams in his clinical practice, talk of dreams contributed nothing to his construction of a theory of ego psychology.

Throughout his career, Hartmann remained mired in the conventional notions of ego, id, and superego as quasi-physical entities, as when he ponders whether some experience originated in the id or the ego. He accepted completely the ideas of his training analyst—Sigmund Freud—concerning topographic, economic, dynamic, and structural models of the mind. Hartmann never entertained the idea that the terms "ego," "id," and "superego" may be only labels for different mental func-tions, and he engaged frequently in the sort of discourse that tempts outsiders to think of the ego, id, and super-ego as little homunculi engaged in incessant warfare somewhere in the body, probably in the head.

Freud himself never used the Latin word "ego" until James Strachey introduced it in his introduction to the *Standard Edition* in 1919 as a translation for "*Das Ich*," which perhaps awkwardly is rendered more literally as "The I" or "The Me." Some writers believe that for Freud, "ego," "self," and "person" were interchange-able, and that it was not until Hartmann's work that these terms became differentiated (Van Spruiell, 1981).

Perhaps Hartmann's least "professional" book is his most interesting. *Psychoanalysis and Moral Values* (1960) provides an extraordinary survey of individual and social ethics, and it maintains that the author is merely elabo-rating and defending the views of Freud. Although brief, the book is far-ranging. Hartmann, following Freud, holds that psychoanalysis never imposes its own values on patients. He also holds that psychoanalytic therapy is only a technology for making people well; yet at the time of writing, homosexuality was universally condemned by psychoanalysts, as were a variety of other lifestyles, some of which can be maintained without loss of one's ability to function and live happily. While it was acceptable for Freud to maintain that mental health does not equate with happiness and functionality, that view was problematic for Hartmann once he became an exponent of the idea that mental health is simply learning to deal with frustra-tions and anxiety-producing events. Given his definition of "mental health," it appears that the categorizing of homosexuality as an illness was based not on an empiri-cal claim that homosexuals are incapable of dealing with frustrations and anxiety-producing events but on the sort of value judgment that Hartmann claimed to eschew.

H

Finally, a word about Heinz Hartmann, the person. One would have to look far in any field to find an individual whose ancestry and environment better prepared him or her for distinction than Hartmann's. Tracing his family roots on his father's side at least as far back as Adolf Gans, an astronomer who was friends with Tycho Brahe and Kepler, Hartmann inherited the broad interests of all the distinguished members of his family. His father and his father's father were prominent historians and academicians; his father was also the Austrian ambassador to Germany immediately after World War I. His mother's family history also was long and distinguished in the sciences and arts. Persons like Brahms were guests in the home for afternoons of music making and stimulating talk. Unsurprisingly, then, Hartmann showed great talent when he was young at a variety of musical instruments. Although he did graduate from medical school at the University of Vienna in 1920 at the age of twenty-four, he pursued several careers before settling down to psychoanalysis. He was his father's personal secretary during the period of ambassadorship, which lasted until 1924. He circulated comfortably in the cultural and diplomatic world before settling down to the serious business of undergoing his first training analysis under Sandor Rado, all the while producing his first important papers. In 1933, he collaborated with Rado in the editorship of the *Internationale Zeitschrift für Psychanalyse*, and around this time was invited by Freud himself to continue his training analysis under him. Josef Breuer, too, took a brief turn as his training analyst. It is doubtful that any other person could claim to have three training analysts of such prominence.

Hartmann married a pediatrician who became an analyst and, like so many others, fled Nazi Germany and finally settled in the United States. He served as president of the International Psychoanalytic Association before dying in 1970.

REFERENCE

Spruiell, V. (1981). The self and the ego. *Psychoanalytic Quarterly*, 50: 319–344.

SIDNEY GENDIN

Herbart, Johann Friedrich (1776–1841)

The ghost of the philosopher Johann Friedrich Herbart hovers over all of Freud's works, an inescapable albeit unacknowledged presence. Herbart, the successor to Kant at Königsberg, arguably exercised a more profound, more pervasive influence on Freud than either Schopenhauer or Nietzsche, whom many scholars regard as sources for some of his major concepts. From Herbart, Freud derived such ideas as that mental activity can be conscious, preconscious, or unconscious, that unconscious mental activity is a continuous determinant of conscious activity, and that the present is unceasingly shaped by the past, whether remembered or forgotten. From Herbart, he also borrowed some essentials of his model, the idea of conflicting conscious and unconscious psychic forces, the censorship-exercising ego, the threshold of consciousness, "resistance," "repression," and much else.

Because some of these concepts are essentially those that Freud used to bring about what has been called a "Copernican" revolution in psychology and because he mentioned no sources when he introduced them, it was suggested in the 1930s that he had slighted an important predecessor. A German scholar, comparing in detail Freud's theory with Herbart's, pointed out that only the existence of a direct influence could account for the close resemblance between them, although no such influence could be traced at the time (Dorer, 1932: 69–106). By the 1950s, when Freud's biographer Ernest Jones took up the charge that Freud had denied credit to his forerunners, the link between Herbart and Freud had been established. Jones acknowledged that Freud had studied psychology when attending gymnasium, that he had used a Herbartian textbook, and that "the main ideas in question had been familiar to Freud since his boyhood" (Jones, 1953: 377).

Among the ideas in question was the fundamental assumption that an unconscious dimension of the mind had to be postulated if conscious mental events were to be explained. Freud asserted: "the data of consciousness have a very large number of gaps in them." They remain "disconnected and unintelligible" unless unconscious links between them are inferred (Freud, 1915: 166–167). This inference, however, which Freud described as an hypothesis of psychoanalysis, "enabled psychology to take its place as a natural science like any other" (Freud, 1940 [1938]: 158).

But the hypothesis had already been affirmed by Herbart, who, in turn, had inherited it from earlier thinkers. It was Herbart's ambition to contribute to the establishment of "a research of the mind which will be the equal of natural science, insofar as this science everywhere presupposes the absolutely regular connection between appearances" (Herbart, 1850: 198). In order to do this, he had to account for the seeming "gaps" in the data of consciousness; he had to suggest how "absolutely regular" connections might exist between the apparently capricious windings and turnings of the conscious mind. He suggested that the apparent caprices vanished if it was assumed that the bulk of human thought took place outside of consciousness. He compared the situation in psychology with that of astronomy: in the pre-Copernican era, the motions of the planets had seemed irrational; every so often these heavenly bodies inexplicably seemed to reverse their courses; for this reason, they were known as the "wanderers." These peculiar paths, however, were recognized as entirely lawful as soon as the heliocentric theory was introduced. The hypothesis of unconscious thought performed the same service for the mind, Herbart maintained: "although the course of our thoughts so often seems to proceed by fits and starts and appears to be altogether irregular, this appearance deceives, like the apparent wandering of the planets." If events outside of consciousness are taken into account, then it becomes clear that "the lawfulness in the human mind is altogether equal to that of the starry skies" (Herbart, 1850: 20).

Also essentially Herbartian were the concepts that mental activity took the form of an interplay of competing forces and that these forces were of different magnitudes, or strengths. Psychoanalysts knew these concepts as the "dynamic" and the "economic" points of view. According to Herbart, every "representation," or "idea" (Vorstellung), naturally entered consciousness unless others prevented it. Because the capacity of consciousness was limited, a competition between representations ensued. Representations had "qualities," that is, they were about something and those that were alike in some way "attracted" each other and cooperated in the struggle for consciousness. Those that were incompatible "repelled" or offered "resistance" to each other and were rivals in the struggle. Representations also had "quantities" of strength; a stronger representation could prevent a weaker from entering consciousness or could "repress" it out of consciousness. Every thought therefore entered consciousness only as the end product of a preceding unconscious conflict between supporting and inhibiting forces. Herbart's hypothesis, which was very elaborate, was derived from physical science. Mathematically treating representations as quantities possess-

ing both magnitude and direction, he conceptualized opposition between them as a conflict between vector forces. Essentially the same conception served as the basis for Freudian "psychodynamics."

The model in which Herbart housed these forces, his "psychic mechanism," was clearly related to Freud's "psychic apparatus." Representations existed in three states: a few were conscious at a given moment; others were outside of consciousness but accessible to it (Freud's "preconscious"). Others were inaccessible (Freud's "unconscious"). Both Herbart and Freud compared consciousness to a sense organ, or an eye, that could perceive only a few things at a time but could rove freely over the realm of accessible mental contents. The model was pictured as a subdivided space: the "threshold of consciousness" separated the representations available to consciousness from those that were not. Because representations were forces, they were ceaselessly rising or sinking in the mind, striving to rise above the threshold or being pushed beneath it by rivals.

Consciousness, however, was more than merely an "eye," according to Herbart. It was also the ego (das Ich), which began to develop early in childhood. As the infantile ego grew and assimilated representations, an organization was formed that then determined further intake. The mass of previously integrated representations refused to accommodate new ones incompatible with those of which it was composed. It judged and then welcomed or banned new arrivals, forcing the unacceptable below the threshold. It could also alter representations, accepting them only after they were suitably changed. This function was personified by Freud as "the censor."

Both consciousness and the unconscious consisted of degrees; a representation could therefore be more or less conscious, more or less unconscious. A deeply buried representation had relatively little effect upon the conscious mind. The troublesome unconscious representations were those that were incompletely repressed. Although kept below the threshold, they were insufficiently immobilized and so produced inexplicable leaps and turns in consciousness as well as the mysterious "objectless feelings of anxiety" that sometimes troubled the mind (Herbart, 1850: 19). Yet even the deeply buried, apparently inactive representations retained their strength and continued to strive to achieve consciousness. They exercised a continuous upward pressure, and only a continuous counterpressure could keep them down. In this condition, they were indestructible, forever retaining their power, always ready to return.

Freud's acceptance of this particular Herbartian postulate had far-reaching consequences for both his theory and his therapy. On this basis, he assumed that repressed wishes were practically immortal and impervious to influence. They could be affected only to the extent that they could be raised above the threshold of consciousness. Consequently, the main aim of psychoanalytic treatment had to be the furnishing of *insight*, the bringing of what was unconscious into consciousness.

When Freud borrowed Herbart's model, he kept the framework but radically replaced the contents. Herbart's model was focused on cognition; thoughts of all kinds competed with one another for the attention of consciousness. Repression could be momentary and conflict was unavoidable. The continuous confrontation, opposition, and negotiation that took place between ideas constituted normal mental functioning. Freud adapted the model to account for the war between derivatives of the primitive instincts and the demands of civilization. The repressing force became a prudential and moral one; the repressed turned into the amoral, the libidinal and destructive urges inhibited by no considerations for reality. In Herbart's model, the mind's energies rose within the mind itself. Freud gave the mechanism a power source outside of the mind; energy flowed into it from the primordial instincts anchored in the body, and this was sexual and aggressive in nature. Thereby, a discharge problem was created; the mechanism constantly had to rid itself of this incoming energy. Since direct riddance was proscribed by society, conflict became pathogenic. Thus dramatically modified, Herbart's psychic mechanism served as underpinning for Freud's theory of neurosis.

REFERENCES

Dorer, M. (1932). *Historische Grundlagen der Psychoanalyse.* Leipzig: Verlag von Felix Meiner.

Freud, S. (1915). *The Unconscious.* S.E. 14: 161–204.

———. (1940) [1938]. *An Outline of Psycho-Analysis.* S.E. 23: 141–207.

Herbart, J. F. (1850). *Schriften der Psychologie.* Leipzig: Leopold Voss.

Jones, E. (1953). *The Life and Work of Sigmund Freud,* vol. 1. New York: Basic Books.

Lindner, G. A. (1872). *Lehrbuch der empirischen Psychologie als inductiver Wissenschaft.* Vienna: Druck und Verlag van Carl Gerold's Sohn.

Sand, R. (1988). Early nineteenth century anticipation of freudian theory. *International Revue of Psycho-Analysis,* 15: 465–479.

ROSEMARIE SAND

Heredity of Psychopathological Conditions See GENETICS AND PSYCHOANALYSIS.

Hermeneutics, and Psychoanalysis

In the 1970s, the metatheoretical interpretation of psychoanalysis as a hermeneutic discipline began to attract growing interest. G.S. Klein (1976), Donald Spence (1981), and Roy Schafer (1983) formulated systematic presentations of psychoanalytic theory and practice from the hermeneutic point of view. In Europe, such attempts had been made before by the philosophers Paul Ricoeur (1965) and Jürgen Habermas (1968). The hermeneuticist conception of psychoanalysis has been accepted by the mainstream of psychoanalysis in the last decade.

History of Hermeneutics

The *fin de siècle* witnessed a major debate in German philosophy concerning the methodological status of the *Geisteswissenschaften* (Human Sciences). It was claimed that their epistemological structure was essentially different from those of the natural sciences. The humanities created knowledge through *Einfühlung* (empathy) into unique historical phenomena (individuals, historical periods, etc.). They did not apply general causal laws in the manner of the natural sciences. Wilhelm Dilthey created the most systematic presentation of this position, which gave the humanities an independent methodology.

Heidegger (1927) created the conceptual framework needed for a sophisticated understanding of hermeneutics. *Verstehen* (understanding) is one of the most basic characterizations of human existence. Human life is always embedded in contexts of general meaning structures. Meaning is a precondition of thought rather than its result. The world of meanings is never an individual creation. Rather, the individual is born into historically determined contexts of meaning that shape every thought, every encounter with persons and objects. H.G. Gadamer's *Truth and Method* (1960) used Heidegger's philosophy to formulate what may be considered the magnum opus of hermeneutic philosophy.

The act of understanding in the humanities and social sciences cannot be formalized. It is an extension of the prereflective understanding constitutive of human existence. By interpreting a text, historical phenomenon, or individual human being, the interpreter integrates the object of study into his or her context of meaning. Interpretation is therefore essentially historical. Gadamer sees interpretation as dialogue rather than objectification—this idea is crucial to the hermeneuticist interpretation of psychoanalysis.

Psychoanalysis and Hermeneutics

One of the major motivations for reconceptualizing psychoanalysis as a hermeneutic discipline was the need for a defense of psychoanalysis against growing methodological criticism. Philosophers of science and academic psychologists attacked psychoanalysis as unscientific, either because it was considered unfalsifiable, as Popper claimed, or lacking evidence for its main theses, as Grünbaum argued.

Hermeneuticism defended psychoanalysis by arguing that clinical work does not consist in causal explanation but in ascription of meaning. Therefore the demands of scientific hypothesis testing do not apply to psychoanalysis. This position has been radicalized in Schafer's (1983) thesis that psychoanalytic interpretation is essentially a re-narration. In this view, the question of historical truth is replaced by the criterion of narrative coherence (Spence, 1981).

Strenger (1991) has argued that this criterion is problematic, because it does not differentiate between acceptable and unacceptable narratives, e.g., in the case of demonic possession. Hermeneuticism must be augmented by a criterion of external coherence, which requires that legitimate interpretations be consistent with currently accepted scientific theories. An additional consequence of the hermeneuticist view is that untested psychoanalytic theories cannot be taken for granted in clinical interpretation. Instead, psychoanalytic understanding must be construed as an extension of common-sense psychology. This derivation of psychoanalytic interpretation from culturally entrenched modes of understanding is consistent with Gadamer's conceptualization of the hermeneutic field.

Hermeneutics and Constructivism

Current psychoanalytic metatheory radicalizes hermeneuticism by becoming increasingly constructivist. Intersubjectivism (Stolorow, Brandchaft and Attwood, 1987) and the relational perspective (Aron, 1996) emphasize the ineradicability of the analyst's subjectivity. Psychoanalytic interpretation is not the formulation of preexisting psychic reality, on this view, but rather is the creation of new meaning in the patient-analyst encounter.

Dialogue, as opposed to objective inquiry, becomes the favored metaphor for psychoanalytic clinical work.

Constructivist hermeneuticism tries to come to terms with the historical phenomenon of a growing proliferation of psychoanalytic approaches. The plurality of styles and schools seems to be here to stay, and should be seen as a virtue rather than a weakness (Strenger, 1998, 2000). Psychoanalytic interpretation is a perspectival elucidation of experience (Stolorow, Brandchaft, and Attwood, 1987). Psychoanalytic theories guiding clinical work are narratives of how human beings can achieve cultural ideals of developed individuality. Different schools are guided by different ideals, e.g., stoic autonomy (Freud), spontaneity (Winnicott), or de-centeredness (Lacan). By arguing for the legitimacy of a variety of ideals, radical constructivism becomes a methodological and ethical position designed to safeguard the patient's autonomy.

REFERENCES

Aron, L. (1996). *A Meeting of Minds. Mutuality in Psychoanalysis.* New York: Analytic Press.

Gadamer, H. (1960). *Truth and Method.* Tübingen: Niemeyer. Engl. Tr. New York: Seabury Press, 1975.

Habermas, J. (1968). *Knowledge and Human Interest.* Frankfurt: Suhrkamp. Engl. Tr. Boston: Beacon Press, 1971.

Heidegger, M. (1927). *Being and Time.* Tübingen: Niemeyer. Engl. Tr. New York: Harper & Row, 1962.

Klein, G. S. (1976). *Psychoanalytic Theory.* New York: International Universities Press.

Ricoeur, P. (1970). *Freud and Philosophy.* Paris: Presses Unversitaires Françaises. Engl. Tr. New Haven: Yale University Press.

Schafer, R. (1983). *The Analytic Attitude.* New York: Basic Books.

Spence, D. (1981). *Narrative Truth and Historical Truth.* New York: Norton.

Stolorow, R. D., Brandchaft, B., and Atwood, G. E. (1987). *Psychoanalytic Treatment, An Intersubjective Approach.* New York: Analytic Press.

Strenger, C. (1991). *Between Hermeneutics and Science. An Essay on the Epistemology of Psychoanalysis.* Madison, Conn.: International Universities Press.

———. (1998). *Individuality, the Impossible Project: Psychoanalysis and Self Creation.* Madison, Conn.: International Universities Press.

———. (2000). *The Quest for Voice in Contemporary Psychoanalysis.* Madison, Conn.: International Universities Press.

CARLO STRENGER

History, and Psychoanalysis

See BIOGRAPHY, AND PSYCHOANALYSIS; PSYCHOHISTORY.

H

History of Psychoanalysis

See PSYCHOANALYSIS, ORIGIN AND HISTORY OF; PSYCHOANALYTIC MOVEMENT.

Homosexuality, Psychoanalytic Theory of

All theoretical and clinical research into the elucidation of the etiology, meaning, content, and therapy of homosexuality began with Sigmund Freud's monumental work: *Three Essays on the Theory of Sexuality* (1905). It was in Part 1, "The Sexual Aberrations," that Freud first coined the term "invert" and designated the practice of homosexuality as "inversion." He wrote that homosexuals are considerable in number but there are many obstacles in establishing the number precisely. Many homosexuals find homosexuality to be "natural" to them, while others rebel against it and consider it pathological. Homosexuality may persist throughout life, go into temporary remission (be covert or overt), or be a detour in the path of normal development. It may appear late in life after a long period of apparently heterosexual activity, and there may be oscillations between its overtness or covertness.

Freud also mentioned that a distressing or traumatic experience may lead one (especially women) into homosexual activity. He noted that many homosexuals assert they could never remember any attachment to the opposite sex from their earliest years, but he mentioned that perhaps these individuals had only repressed their positive heterosexual feelings. He remarked that many homosexuals feel both homosexual and heterosexual arousal, and only at puberty may a frail heterosexual adjustment be overrun by homosexual attachments.

Freud reviewed two conceptions that surrounded homosexuality for centuries—that it was innate or that it was a form of degeneracy—and believed both of them were untrue, for many homosexuals show a high degree of intellectual and cultural development and may distinguish themselves in life, whatever their sexual behavior. Freud asserted that homosexuality is an acquired character of the sexual instinct, and he tested this hypothesis by removing inversion by hypnotic suggestion—an event that he felt would be "astonishing" if homosexuality were truly innate or hereditary. Freud's hypothesis was that some early experience of childhood had a determining effect on the direction taken by the homosexual's libido, e.g., castration anxiety.

Addressing the question as to whether homosexuality was the expression of a "psychical hermaphroditism," he commented that all that would be required to settle the question was that homosexuality be readily accompanied by mental and somatic signs of a duality of sexes. This expectation was not realized, and he concluded that it was impossible to demonstrate a connection between hypothetical psychical hermaphroditism and the established anatomical one. He concluded that homosexuality and somatic hermaphroditism were on the whole independent of each other. The idea would have gained substance, in his opinion, if the inversion of the sexual object were at least accompanied by a parallel change of the subject's other mental qualities, instincts, and character traits into those characterizing the opposite sex. Freud commented that it was only in homosexual women that character inversion of this kind can be found with any regularity. Furthermore, in a 1915 note to the *Three Essays*, he stated that psychoanalytic research decidedly opposes any attempt at segregating homosexuals from the rest of humankind as a group with a special character. All human beings are capable of making a homosexual object choice and many have in fact made one in the unconscious. He concluded that object choice, independent of sex—freedom to range equally among male and female objects (as is found in childhood and in primitive societies in the early phases of history)—is the basis for subsequent restriction in one direction or the other in which heterosexual and homosexual types develop.

With remarkable clinical acuity, Freud offered a classification based on conscious and unconscious motivation. One: *absolute inverts*, whose sexual objects are exclusively of their own sex and who are incapable of carrying out the sexual act with a person of the opposite sex or of deriving any enjoyment from it. Two: *amphigenic inverts*, whose sexual objects may be of their own sex or of the opposite sex because this type of inversion lacks exclusiveness. Three: *contingent inverts*, whose circumstances preclude accessibility to partners of the opposite sex and who may take as their sexual object those of their own sex only to leave this object choice when the opposite sex becomes available.

In the 1910 edition of *Three Essays*, Freud stated his belief that the issue of homosexuality is a highly complex one, emphasizing a fact of sweeping importance, long ignored by many investigators of sexual behavior both then and in the present, namely, that "the connection between the sexual instinct and the sexual object" is not as intimate as one would surmise. Both are merely *soldered* together. He warned that we must loosen the bonds that exist between instinct and object, for "[i]t seems probable that the sexual instinct is in the first instance independent of its object nor is its origin likely to be due to the object's attraction" (Freud, 1905). Freud's observation as regards the independence between the sexual instinct and the sexual object further clarifies the nature of not only homosexuality but also other sexual deviations. In underscoring the interconnections among infantile sexuality, perversions, and neurosis, Freud arrived at the conclusion that the neurosis represents the negative of a perversion.

In the next five years, Freud along with Sadger and Ferenczi developed a formulation of the central developmental factors of homosexuality and several other perversions long before the advent of ego psychology. For example, he observed that the ego function of identification and repression plays an important part in homosexuality (1905), and in homosexuality, one finds a "predominance of archaic and primitive psychical mechanisms" (1905).

Foremost in Freud's discoveries in the *Three Essays* was the conclusion that in the earliest phases of childhood, future (male) inverts passed through a stage of very intense but short-lived fixation on a woman, usually their mother, and, later, continued to identify themselves with a woman and took themselves as a sexual object. They proceeded from a "narcissistic object choice" (1905, p. 146) and looked for men resembling themselves whom they might love as their mothers loved them. Freud (1905) understood that the problem of inversion indeed was a more highly complex one in men compared with women, for in women the case is "less ambiguous" (p. 146), for active female inverts exhibit masculine characteristics both physical and mental, with peculiar frequency, and look for femininity in their sexual object, although closer observation might reveal a greater variety in the female homosexual.

In the last section of the *Three Essays*, "Transformations of Puberty," Freud noted: "Where inversion is not regarded as a crime, it will be found that it answers fully to the sexual inclinations of no small number of people." He offered the following suggestions and comments as regards both sexual object choice and the possible prevention of homosexuality.

1. Where there is a lack of "an authoritative prohibition by society," the number of homosexual individuals may increase in a particular age or culture.
2. "One of the tasks implicit in object-choice is that it should find its way to the opposite sex. This, as we know, is not accomplished without a certain amount of fumbling. Often enough the first impulses after puberty go astray, though without any permanent harm resulting."
3. "No doubt the strongest force working against a permanent inversion of the sexual object is the attraction which the opposing sexual characters exercise upon one another. . . . This factor is not, in itself, however, sufficient to exclude inversion; there are no doubt a variety of other contributing factors."
4. "It may be presumed . . . that in the case of men, a childhood recollection of the affection shown them by their mother and others of the female sex who looked after them when they were children contributes powerfully to directing their choice towards women; on the other hand, their early experience of being deterred by their father from sexual activity and their competitive relation with him deflect them from their own sex. Both of these two factors apply equally to girls, whose sexual activity is particularly subject to the watchful guardianship of their mother. Thus they acquire a hostile relation to their own sex, which influences their object choice decisively in what is regarded as the normal direction."
5. "It is found that the early loss of one of their parents, whether by death, divorce or separation, with the result that the remaining parent absorbs the whole of the child's love, determined the sex of the person who is later to be chosen as a sexual object, and may thus open the way to permanent inversion" (Freud, 1905: 229–230).

In 1910, Freud explored the defensive functions of homosexuality. In his masterful study of Leonardo da Vinci, he writes of male homosexuality as due to repression of attachment to the mother colored by identification with her and the choice of an object on a narcissistic basis. He further notes that some homosexuals are fleeing women so that they are not unfaithful to their mothers. He further points out that the absence of a father and growing up in a feminine environment, or the presence of a weak father who is dominated by the mother, furthers feminine identification and homosexuality. Similarly, of course, the presence of a cruel father may lead to a disturbance in male identification.

In 1911, Freud turned his attention to the relationship between paranoia and homosexuality in *Psychoanalytic Notes on an Autobiographical Account of a Case of Paranoia (Dementia Paranoides)*.

The relationship among jealousy, paranoia, and homosexuality is further explored in 1922 in his paper *Some Neurotic Mechanisms in Jealousy, Paranoia and Homosexuality*, where Freud states: "Recognition of the organic factor in homosexuality does not relieve us of the obligation of studying the psychic processes connected with its origin." In this 1922 paper, Freud gives an account of the typical processes found in innumerable cases of homosexuality, but he concludes: "We have, however, never regarded this analysis of the origin of homosexuality as complete. I can now point to a new mechanism leading to homosexual object-choice, although I cannot say how large a part it plays in the formation of the extreme, manifest and exclusive type of homosexuality."

The observation that homosexuality is a complex psychic formation like other sexual deviations was again pointed out by Freud in *A Child Is Being Beaten* (1919). It is both a defense and an id impulse, and is related to the Oedipus complex, castration anxiety, and other perversions. Homosexual behavior and actions are, therefore, not simple expressions of a pregenital component instinct but are derived from the polymorphous perverse impulses of early childhood, and may be compared to a light ray passing through a lens and being subjected to considerable distortion and refraction. The conscious homosexual act, therefore, is only a small part of a larger system, much of which is unconscious. Significantly, homosexual acts may be classified as *ego syntonic* and pleasurable, while neurotic symptoms are *ego dystonic* and painful. An explanation of the differences and ego syntonic and ego dystonic was provided by Freud in *Two Encyclopedia Articles* (1923).

It is important to comment on the early concept of "bisexuality," which has been erroneously interpreted as designating a genetic (inborn) characteristic of attraction to persons of either sex—a constitutional neural-hormonal mechanism that dictates object choice. This was not Freud's view. He did not believe that any spe-

cific genetic (chromosomal) factor was capable of directing the sexual drive into overt homosexuality. He always believed that a number of factors determined sexual object choice, and of these the psychodynamic ones were the most important. The constitutional factors determine only the strength of the drive.

Debate continues about whether certain sexual activities, including homosexual acts, can be considered "deviant" in anything more than a statistical sense, and whether or not such acts are invariably signs of an underlying pathology. Freud's views on these matters can be found partly in his *General Introductory Lectures*, where he states: "Let us once more reach an agreement upon what is to be understood by the 'sense' of a psychical process. We mean nothing other by it than the intention it serves in a psychical continuity" (1920b, p. 40). On this view, whether or not sexual acts can be termed deviant or perverse *cannot* be ascertained by empirical findings of what is statistically normal, nor by examining merely the acts themselves. Rather, what must be studied is the conscious or unconscious motivation from which the acts issue. In his earlier *Three Essays* (1905, p. 161), Freud provides a criterion for determining when a sexual act is a symptom of pathology: "When a perversion has the characteristic of exclusiveness and fixation, then we shall be justified in regarding it as a pathological symptom."

As regards therapy, Freud wrote in 1905 that the only possibility of helping homosexual patients was by commanding a suppression of their symptoms through hypnotic suggestion, but this method led to failure. By 1910, however, he believed that psychoanalysis itself was applicable to homosexuality and other perversions (Freud, 1910), but later expressed some caution about the possibility of a complete cure (Freud, 1920b). His criterion of cure was not only a detachment of the cathexis from the homosexual object but the ability to cathect the opposite sex with love (*Psychogenesis of a Case of Homosexuality in a Woman*, 1920a). Freud further recognized that it was especially difficult to analyze an individual at "peace" with his perversion. A combination of neurotic symptoms and perversion presented a more hopeful therapeutic possibility.

In summary, Freud believed that homosexuality is caused by early accidental fixating experiences, including seductions, followed by a traumatic Oedipal period (castration anxiety). What is clear according to Freud is that homosexuality is not simply a breakthrough of id impulses unopposed by the ego or the superego, for the instinctual drives and the defenses against them as well are unconscious. And what appeared to be gratification of perverse instinctual drives actually constituted an end product of a defensive compromise (already predicted by Freud in *A Child Is Being Beaten*, 1919) in which the elements of inhibition as well as gratification were present, and the component instinct had undergone extensive transformation and disguise to be gratified in the homosexual act. This masking was conditioned by the defense of the homosexual ego, which resisted gratification of the component instinct as energetically as does the ego in the neurotic. Thus, it became readily apparent that the perverted action like the neurotic symptom resulted from conflicts between the ego and the id and represented a compromise formation that at the same time was acceptable to the demands of the superego. In homosexuality as in neurotic symptoms, the instinctual gratification takes place in a disguised form while its real content remains unconscious. The perverted action differs from the neurotic symptom in the form of gratification of the impulse: orgasm.

It is beyond the scope of this article to describe later psychoanalytic developments in the understanding of the origin of homosexuality. Foremost among these theories are those based on Gillespie's concept of Oedipal origin, Greenacre's and Socarides's clinical concepts of pre-Oedipal origin, the object relations theories of Otto Kernberg, and the application of theoretical contributions of Margaret Mahler and her associates.

REFERENCES

Freud, S. (1905). *Three Essays on the Theory of Sexuality*. S.E. 7: 125–244.

———. (1910). Leonardo da Vinci and a memory of his childhood. S.E. 11: 59–137.

———. (1911). Psycho-analytic notes on an autobiographical account of a case of paranoia (dementia paranoides). S.E. 12: 3–82.

———. (1919). A child is being beaten. S.E. 17: 175–205.

———. (1920a). Psychogenesis of a case of homosexuality in a woman. S.E. 18: 145–175.

———. (1920b). *General Introductory Lectures*. New York: Garden City Publishing, 1943.

———. (1922). Some neurotic mechanisms in jealousy, paranoia and homosexuality. S.E. 18: 221–235.

———. (1923). Two encyclopedia articles. S.E. 18: 255–263.

———. (1925). Negation. S.E. 19: 235–43.

———. (1930). Splitting of the ego in the process of defense. S.E. 23: 271–279.

CHARLES W. SOCARIDES

Horney, Karen (1885–1952)

German American psychoanalyst. Born Karen Danielsen in a suburb of Hamburg, Horney decided that she wanted to be a physician when she was thirteen and was one of the first women in Germany to be admitted to medical school. She received her medical education at the universities of Freiburg, Göttingen, and Berlin. In 1909, she married Oskar Horney, a social scientist she had met while they were both students at Freiburg. In 1910, she entered analysis with Karl Abraham, a member of Freud's inner circle and the first psychoanalyst to practice in Germany. She decided to become an analyst herself and in 1920 was one of the six founding members of the Berlin Psychoanalytical Institute. She had a second analysis with Hanns Sachs in the early 1920s. Having separated from her husband in 1926, she emigrated to the United States in 1932, when Franz Alexander invited her to become associate director of the newly formed Chicago Psychoanalytic Institute. She moved to New York in 1934 and became a member of the New York Psychoanalytic Institute. In 1941, she became founding editor of the *American Journal of Psychoanalysis* and organized the American Institute for Psychoanalysis and served as dean until her death in 1952.

Horney's thought went through three phases: in the 1920s and early 1930s, she wrote a series of essays in which she tried to modify Freud's ideas about feminine psychology while staying within the framework of classical theory. In *The Neurotic Personality of Our Time* (1937) and *New Ways in Psychoanalysis* (1939), she tried to redefine psychoanalysis by replacing Freud's biological orientation with an emphasis on culture and interpersonal relationships. In *Our Inner Conflicts* (1945) and *Neurosis and Human Growth* (1950), she developed her mature theory in which individuals cope with the anxiety produced by feeling unsafe, unloved, and unvalued by disowning their spontaneous feelings and developing elaborate strategies of defense.

During her lifetime, Horney and her work were well known, but after her death her influence gradually declined. A revival of interest began with the publication of *Feminine Psychology* (1967), a collection of her essays from the 1920s and 1930s, many of which were originally written in German. Disagreeing with Freud about penis envy, female masochism, and feminine development, these essays were controversial when they first appeared but then were largely ignored until they were republished in 1967. They have been widely read since, and there has been a growing recognition that Horney was the first great psychoanalytic feminist.

In her essays on feminine psychology, Horney strove to show that females have intrinsic biological constitutions and patterns of development that are to be understood in their own terms and not just as products of their difference from males. She argued that psychoanalysis regards women as defective men because it is the product of a male genius (Freud) and a male-dominated culture. The male view of the female has been incorporated into psychoanalysis as a scientific picture of woman's essential nature. Horney developed the concept of "womb-envy," contending that male envy of pregnancy, childbirth, and motherhood, and of the breasts and suckling, gives rise to an unconscious tendency to devalue women. She argued that men's impulse toward creative work is an overcompensation for their small role in procreation.

Horney traced the male dread of woman to the boy's fear that his genital is inadequate in relation to the mother. The threat of woman is not castration but humiliation; it is to his masculine self-regard. As he grows up, the male continues to have a deeply hidden anxiety about the size of his penis or his potency, an anxiety that has no counterpart for the female. He deals with his anxiety by erecting an ideal of efficiency, by seeking sexual conquests, and by debasing the love object.

In the second phase of Horney's thought, she maintained that culture and disturbed human relationships are the most important causes of neurotic development. As the author of *The Neurotic Personality of Our Time* and *New Ways in Psychoanalysis*, Horney is often thought of as a neo-Freudian member of "the cultural school," a group that also included Erich Fromm, Harry Stack Sullivan, Clara Thompson, and Abraham Kardiner. The critique of Freud in *New Ways in Psychoanalysis* aroused so much resentment at the New York Psychoanalytic Institute that Horney was forced to resign.

Although Horney objected to Freud's emphasis on biology and infantile origins, she always paid tribute to what she regarded as his enduring contributions. These included the doctrines that psychic processes are strictly determined and that we may be motivated by unconscious forces. She valued Freud's accounts of repression, reaction formation, projection, displacement, rationalization, and dreams; and she felt that Freud had provided indispensable tools for therapy in the concepts of transference, resistance, and free association.

Horney's first two books proposed a model for the structure of neurosis in which adverse conditions in the environment as a whole, and especially in the family, create a "basic anxiety" against which the child defends itself by developing strategies of defense that are self-alienating, self-defeating, and in conflict with each other. In a striking departure from Freud, Horney advocated starting with the current constellation of defenses and inner conflicts rather than with early experience. Our problems are the result of past experiences, to be sure, but these produce a character structure with an inner logic of its own that can be understood without reference to infantile origins. Horney's focus on the present rather than the past has led some analysts to complain that her explanations lack depth, while others feel that it is the source of her originality and power.

In her next book, *Self-Analysis* (1942), Horney presented her fullest account of how the psychoanalytic process works in terms of her structural paradigm. The object of therapy for Horney is to help people relinquish their defenses—which alienate them from their true likes and dislikes, hopes, fears, and desires—so that they can get in touch with what she called the "real self." *Self-Analysis* contains Horney's only extended case history, that of a patient named Clare, which is highly autobiographical (see Paris, 1994). The account of Clare's problems with Peter, her lover, reflects the breakdown of Horney's relationship with Erich Fromm.

In her mature theory, developed in her last two books, Horney retained the emphasis on the present and the basic conception of the structure of neurosis developed in her earlier works, but she described the defenses and the relationships between them much more systematically. According to Horney, people defend themselves against feeling unsafe, unloved, and unvalued by developing both interpersonal and intrapsychic strategies of defense. The interpersonal strategies involve moving toward, against, or away from other people and adopting a self-effacing, expansive, or resigned solution. Each of these solutions entails a constellation of personality traits, behaviors, and beliefs, and a bargain with fate in which obedience to the dictates of that solution is supposed to be rewarded. Since people tend to employ more than one of these strategies, they are beset by inner conflicts. To avoid being torn apart or paralyzed, they make that strategy predominant that most accords with their culture, temperament, and circumstances; but the repressed tendencies persist, generating inconsistencies and rising to the surface if the predominant solution fails.

In the self-effacing solution, individuals try to gain safety, love, and esteem through dependency, humility, and self-sacrificing "goodness." Their bargain is that if they are helpful, submissive people who do not seek their own gain or glory, they will be well treated by fate and other people. There are three expansive solutions: the narcissistic, the perfectionistic, and the arrogant-vindictive. Narcissists are full of self-admiration, have an unquestioned belief in their own greatness, and often display unusual charm and buoyancy. Their magic bargain is that if they hold onto their exaggerated claims for themselves, life is bound to give them what they want. Perfectionists take great pride in their rectitude and strive for excellence in every detail. They have a legalistic bargain in which correctness of conduct ensures fair treatment by fate and other people. Arrogant-vindictive people have a need to retaliate for injuries received in childhood and to achieve mastery by manipulating others. They do not count on life to give them anything but are convinced that they can reach their ambitious goals if they remain true to their vision of the world as a jungle and do not allow themselves to be influenced by their softer feelings or the traditional morality. Resigned people worship freedom, peace, and self-sufficiency. Their bargain is that if they ask nothing of others, they will not be bothered; that if they try for nothing, they will not fail; and that if they expect little of life, they will not be disappointed.

The intrapsychic strategies of defense are linked to the interpersonal. To compensate for feelings of weakness, inadequacy, and low self-esteem, people develop an idealized image of themselves that they seek to actualize by embarking on a search for glory. The idealized image generates a pride system, which consists of neurotic pride, neurotic claims, and what Horney calls tyrannical shoulds. People take pride in the imaginary attributes of their idealized selves, they demand that the world treat them in accordance with their grandiose conception of themselves, and they drive themselves to live up to the dictates of their solution. The pride system tends to intensify the self-hate against which it is supposed to be a defense, since any failure to live up to one's shoulds or of the world to honor one's claims leads to feelings of worthlessness. The content of the idealized image is most strongly determined by the predominant interpersonal strategy, but since the subordinate strategies are also at work, the idealized image is full of contradictions. As a result, people are often caught in what Horney calls a cross fire of conflicting shoulds. Since obeying the dictates of one solution means violating those of another, they are bound to hate themselves whatever they do.

Although Horney provides an analytic approach that can be found nowhere else, she deals with many of the same issues as other post-Freudians. Her "basic anxiety" is similar to Erik Erikson's "basic mistrust," and her theory illuminates many of the stages of development Erikson describes. The search for identity often involves the formation of an idealized image, and there is a crisis later in life when people realize that they cannot actualize their idealized image.

Like Heinz Kohut and his fellows, Horney is interested in problems of the self; and like Harry Guntrip, W. R. D. Fairbairn, D. W. Winnicott, John Bowlby, and other members of the British Independent School, she sees neurosis as a product of disturbed object relations, especially in childhood. She differs from self-psychologists in seeing narcissism as reactive rather than primary and from object relations theorists in her focus on present structure rather than infantile origins. Horney's "real self" bears some resemblance to Kohut's "nuclear self" and even more to Winnicott's "true self." Alice Miller's discussion of the loss of and search for the true self in childhood often sounds like Karen Horney, as does R. D. Laing's account of ontological insecurity (which is comparable to basic anxiety) and the development of a false-self system in response to it.

Horney's mature theory has helped to inspire the interpersonal school of psychoanalysis; it has provided a model for therapies that focus on the current situation, and it has influenced some of the descriptions of personality disorders in the *DSM-IV*, Axis 2. It has made an important contribution to the study of literature, biography, gender, and culture. Because of her emphasis on self-realization as the goal of life and the source of healthy values, Horney was recognized by Abraham Maslow as one of the founders of humanistic psychology. Her theory has most in common, perhaps, with the work of Erich Fromm, Ernest Schachtel, Carl Rogers, and Maslow. Many of Horney's ideas have made their way, often unacknowledged, into the array of concepts and techniques currently employed in clinical practice.

REFERENCES

Horney, K. (1937). *The Neurotic Personality of Our Time.* New York: Norton.

———. (1939). *New Ways in Psychoanalysis.* New York: Norton.

———. (1942). *Self-Analysis.* New York: Norton.

———. (1945). *Our Inner Conflicts: A Constructive Theory of Neurosis.* New York: Norton.

———. (1950). *Neurosis and Human Growth: The Struggle Toward Self-realization.* New York: Norton.

———. (1967). *Feminine Psychology.* Ed. H. Kelman. New York: Norton.

Paris, B. (1994). *Karen Horney: A Psychoanalyst's Search for Self-understanding.* New Haven, Conn.: Yale University Press.

———. (ed.) (1999). *The Therapeutic Process: Essays and Lectures.* New Haven, Conn.: Yale University Press.

———. (ed.) (2000). *The Unknown Karen Horney: Essays on Gender, Culture, and Psychoanalysis.* New Haven, Conn.: Yale University Press.

BERNARD PARIS

Humanities, and Psychoanalysis

An ideal "college of psychoanalysis," Freud believed, would offer courses in biology, sexuality, and the symptomatology of psychiatry, but also in "the history of civilization, mythology, the psychology of religion and the science of literature" (1926, p. 20). The dream of such an institution remains unrealized, except in the sense that humanities departments in universities throughout the world have in the aggregate provided a vast workshop to test, develop, and clarify psychoanalytic thought. Almost all the humanistic disciplines have fostered more or less energetic traditions of psychoanalytic work. Some few have almost died out, as in sociology and academic psychology, but most continue on despite well-publicized attacks on Freud's supposed blunders in matters of fact and scientific procedure.

Anthropology and Cultural Studies

Karl Kroeber's 1920 review of *Totem and Taboo* set the terms for how anthropologists in decades to come would regard psychoanalysis. Freud had relied too heavily on Frazer, Spencer, Crawley, Tylor, and Westermarck, the so-called armchair anthropologists of the nineteenth century, and allowed his speculations to range beyond the check of reliable ethnography. Anthropology in the twentieth century, suspicious of individualism, is almost always committed to the social construction of reality and to its familiar corollary, cultural relativism. By these standards, the earlier theorists were, like Freud, too eager to apply Western models of explanation to tribal cultures, and by defining "magic," for example, as an illusory precursor to science appealing to "primitives,"

children, and psychotics, lumbered their thinking with the prejudices of European rationality. In his influential *Sex and Repression in Savage Society* (1927), Bronislaw Malinowski maintained that the Oedipus complex may figure in the "patriarchal" families of the West but did not appear in the matrilineal cultures of the Trobriand Islanders, where the Western authoritarian father is split into the mother's brother, the main adviser in the upbringing of her children, and the comparatively insignificant biological father. Far from being universal, the Oedipus complex was the epiphenomenon of a certain set of cultural arrangements in the history of Europe.

Psychoanalysis was often discussed in attempts to decode the symbolism of tribal life, but the anthropologist most devoted to Freud, Géza Róheim, was not taken very seriously by his peers, in part because his writing was both loosely organized and dogmatic in manner. Thinkers such as Ruth Benedict and Abram Kardiner, in developing an interdisciplinary approach to culture, were more successful in integrating psychoanalysis with the Durkheimian presuppositions of anthropology. Contemporary figures like Robert Paul, Alan Dundes, and Jerome Neu, all of them working unapologetically within a Freudian framework, have demonstrated the suppleness of classical Freudian models of explanation. Melford Spiro, in his important *Oedipus in the Trobriands* (1982), brilliantly reopened the all-but-settled question of Malinowski's data on matrilineal psychology, arguing that Trobriand boys do if anything undergo a more intense Oedipus complex than in Western societies. The authors of *Oedipus Ubiquitous* (1996), Allen Johnson and Douglass Price-Williams, having collected tales from many of the world's folklores, conclude somewhat to their surprise that "there is indeed 'something there' in Freud's assertion of the universality of the Oedipus complex" (p. 7). A detailed overview of psychoanalysis in this discipline may be found in Edwin Wallace's *Freud and Anthropology: A History and Reappraisal* (1983).

History and Biography

One might be inclined to think that Freud's influence on historians has been far less decisive than that of Marx. But many are the imaginative offspring of such works as *Leonardo da Vinci and a Memory of His Childhood* (1910) and Freud and William Bullitt's *Thomas Woodrow Wilson* (1967, though Freud's contribution, fed by his anger over Versailles, was of course much earlier): psychoanalysis has become part of the prevailing intellectual climate in discussing the behavior of historical figures, indeed of the genre of biography itself in its late-twentieth-century form. The vogue for "psycho-history" initiated by Erikson's studies of Luther and Ghandi is, from this perspective, but a small academic episode in a far larger process of assimilation. Peter Gay's four-volume study of *The Bourgeois Experience: Victoria to Freud* is probably the most respected work of psychoanalytic historiography, and his *Freud for Historians* (1985) is the best single book to consult on the techniques of psychohistory and the controversies they have inspired.

Literary Criticism

Literary scholars also write biographies, and untold numbers of them contain more or less formal psychoanalytic interpretations. Until the advent of "theory" in the late 1960s, psychoanalysis in literary criticism was considered to be one of an array of "approaches" to literature. A psychoanalytic critic, it was assumed, would produce a certain sort of reading incompatible with those generated by other approaches. But the better psychoanalytic critics, even when largely concerned with the id and the unconscious, tried to integrate their interpretations with formal, generic, and historical concerns. There was also the influential example of Kenneth Burke, whose work mingles psychoanalysis and Marxism with close rhetorical analysis. In the deliberately interdisciplinary atmosphere of the "theory" decades, psychoanalysis, usually in the manner of Lacan, has merged somewhat indiscriminately with linguistic, historical, philosophical, and sociopolitical modes of analysis, to the point where Freud is just a compartment in the professional tool kit of the contemporary literary intellectual. Most of these proliferating schools of interpretation assume that literature must look to other disciplines for clarification. One of the few recent theories to assume that literature, as the height of human wisdom, can supply its own best explanation is Harold Bloom's account of influence, which reconceives the ancient topic of literary *imitatio* in the light of Freud's Oedipal fantasies and Anna Freud's mechanisms of defense.

At the level of particular authors and works, the bulk and variety of psychoanalytic literary studies cannot but impress. Although there were random suggestions here and there in the critical literature, the subject of Milton and psychoanalysis had scarcely been broached when William Kerrigan's *The Sacred Complex: On the Psychogenesis of Paradise Lost* was published in 1983.

Today's Miltonist confronts a burgeoning tradition of psychoanalytic commentary. About every poem, every novel, every story on which there is critical work at all, there is now likely to be psychoanalytic work. Distinguished recent books include James W. Earl's *Thinking about 'Beowulf'* (1994), which brings psychoanalysis to bear on heroic literature, fatedness, and the development of civilization; G. W. Pigman's *Grief and English Renaissance Elegy* (1985), which combines a groundbreaking exactitude about the shifting conventions of the elegy in the sixteenth and seventeenth centuries with a rich psychoanalytic understanding of those conventions; and Marcia Ian's *Remembering the Phallic Mother* (1993), which in the course of a wide-ranging discussion of modernism develops a fascinating view of fetishism. Work of this kind should not be thought of as "applied psychoanalysis," inasmuch as the phrase implies a fixed psychoanalysis being brought to bear on the open questions of another field. For in the best psychoanalytic literary studies the current of illumination runs in both directions.

The oldest and most coherent psychoanalytic tradition in literary criticism is devoted appropriately enough to the elucidation of Shakespeare. Inspired by Freud's observations on *Hamlet, Macbeth, Richard III, The Merchant of Venice*, and *King Lear*, as supplemented by Ernest Jones's *Hamlet and Oedipus* (1949), the tradition remains vigorous and in recent years has produced at least two indisputably major works, C. L. Barber and Richard Wheeler's *The Whole Journey: Shakespeare's Power of Development* (1986) and Janet Adelman's *Suffocating Mothers: Fantasies of Maternal Origin in Shakespeare's Plays* (1992), which is perhaps more than can be said of rival schools of Shakespeare interpretation. The early phase of this tradition, much of it written by psychoanalysts, has been usefully discussed in Norman Holland's *Psychoanalysis and Shakespeare* (1966), and may be sampled in M. D. Faber's anthology *The Design Within: Psychoanalytic Approaches to Shakespeare* (1970). Two subsequent anthologies, *Representing Shakespeare: New Psychoanalytic Essays* (1980) and *Shakespeare's Personality* (1989), reveal the eclecticism characteristic of modern literary theory. All the main movements in post-Freudian psychoanalysis—the reparation psychology of Klein; the adaptational ego psychology of Waelder, Hartmann, and Kris; the life cycle of Erikson; the individuation psychology of Mahler and Chodorov; the structuralism of

H

Lacan; the self-psychology of Winnicott and Kohut; the narrativity of Schafer and Spence—have left a mark on literary studies in general and Shakespeare studies in particular.

Film Studies

A word may be in order here on the increasing preeminence of psychoanalysis in film studies. Until recently, those in search of psychoanalytic film criticism had to make do with the incoherent ramblings of a Parker Tyler or the genre studies of Stanley Cavell, a far more impressive critic in whose work Freud is, however, as a rule presupposed rather than overtly discussed. But today this discipline, owing in part to the impact of Christian Metz's *The Imaginary Signifier* (English trans. 1982), is deeply in the grip of Lacan. While distinguished film criticism of a conventionally Freudian stamp continues to be written, as in Harvey Greenberg's *Movies on Your Mind* (1975) and *Screen Memories* (1993), Lacan's notions of "the imaginary" and "the gaze" have proven widely attractive, perhaps in part because they seem a ready-made fit with the ontology of the cinematic experience. One suspects that psychoanalysis in some form will continue to play a central role in film studies, if only because movies, for over half their history, were overtly influenced by psychoanalytic ideas, which allows film critics largely to ignore the difficult problems of method and tact, much debated among literary scholars, in applying Freud to pre-Freudian art.

Philosophy

Despite Freud's distaste for metaphysics, psychoanalysts have been from the beginning open to philosophical ideas, especially the varieties of existentialism: Binswanger, Boss, and Laing, to mention only a few. While his borrowings from Saussure have been much noted, Lacan took at least as much from Heidegger and the phenomenologists (Kerrigan, 1989). The historical process detailed in Henri Ellenberger's *The Discovery of the Unconscious* (1970), which relates Freud to the philosophers and philosophical psychologists of the nineteenth century, could certainly be continued into twentieth-century thought. It may be a cultural affinity that makes Nietzsche or Heidegger seem to spill naturally over to Freud. Lacan, exploiting this affinity, was able to adapt Hegel's master/slave dialectic—the key passage in all philosophy for Marx—to the genesis of the ego. Truth aside, the result has a pleasing coherence, as

if not just Freud but all of European thought had collectively had an idea.

Freudians have tended to ignore the British tradition of analytic philosophy, though there are signs of change in this regard. As is clear from posthumously published courses and notebooks, Wittgenstein was in fact much preoccupied with Freud, especially with how the postulate of an unconscious stood in relation to ordinary-language descriptions of action. Someone interested in how these lines of inquiry might have played out, had they ever been put into systematic form, might consult a book by one of Wittgenstein's pupils who went on to a career in psychiatry, M. O'C. Drury's delightfully sharp *The Danger of Words* (1973). Psychoanalytic theorists such as Loewald and Schafer have turned to the linguistic tradition for help in replacing the energic language of Freud's metapsychology. Interestingly, one of the main threads in Paul Ricoeur's *Freud and Philosophy: An Essay on Interpretation* (1970) is a defense of that vocabulary for manifesting "the pressure of desire." In subsequent essays, however, Ricoeur anticipated Schafer and Spence by arguing that psychoanalysis is essentially a narrative and historical discipline.

A rare example of Freud being welcomed into American philosophy occurs in Richard Rorty's *Contingency, Irony, and Solidarity* (1989). Working from distinctions found in Donald Davidson, Rorty makes a place for psychoanalysis in his broad vision of Deweyean pragmatism by proposing that Freud's is a "contingent" selfhood free from the moral universalism of Kant: when asked why one approves of certain actions and deplores others, a Freudian self will reply, not by reference to principles, but through a necessarily idiosyncratic narrative about his childhood. The idea that Freud's truth is finally a narrative one sorts well with the tendency in modern philosophy to think of morality in terms of stories and to supplant traditional "philosophical problems" with historical accounts of how such and such an issue came to seem inherently problematic. Freud becomes, for philosophers like Rorty, the originator of some truly superb stories—stories able to liberate us from the arid rigidities of traditional metaphysics.

REFERENCES

Adelman, J. (1992). *Suffocating Mothers: Fantasies of Maternal Origin in Shakespeare's Plays. Hamlet to The Tempest.* New York: Routledge.

Barber, C. L., and Wheeler, R. P. (1986). *The Whole Journey: Shakespeare's Power of Development.* Berkeley: University of California Press.

Bloom, H. (1973). *The Anxiety of Influence: A Theory of Poetry.* New York: Oxford University Press.

Bullitt, W., and Freud, S. (1967). *Thomas Woodrow Wilson: A Psychological Study.* Boston: Houghton Mifflin.

Cavell, S. (1981). *Pursuits of Happiness: The Hollywood Comedy of Remarriage.* Cambridge, Mass.: Harvard University Press.

Drury, M. O'C. (1973). *The Danger of Words.* New York: Humanities Press.

Earl, J. W. (1994). *Thinking about 'Beowulf.'* Stanford, Calif.: Stanford University Press.

Ellenberger, H. (1970). *The Discovery of the Unconscious: The History and Evolution of Dynamic Psychiatry.* New York: Basic Books.

Erikson, E. H. (1958). *Young Man Luther: A Study in Psychoanalysis and History.* New York: Norton, 1958.

———. (1969). *Gandhi's Truth.* New York: Norton.

Faber, M. D. (ed.) (1970). *The Design Within: Psychoanalytic Approaches to Shakespeare.* New York: Science House.

Freud, S. (1926). *The Question of Lay Analysis: Conversations With an Impartial Person.* S.E. 20: 183–258.

Gay, P. (1985). *Freud for Historians.* New York: Oxford University Press.

Greenberg, H. R. (1975). *Movies on Your Mind.* New York: Dutton.

———. (1993). *Screen Memories: Hollywood Cinema on the Psychoanalytic Couch.* New York: Columbia University Press.

Holland, N. (1966). *Psychoanalysis and Shakespeare.* New York: McGraw-Hill.

Homan, S., and Paris, B. J. (1989). *Shakespeare's Personality.* Berkeley: University of California Press.

Ian, M. (1993). *Remembering the Phallic Mother: Psychoanalysis, Modernism, and the Fetish.* Ithaca, N.Y.: Cornell University Press.

Kerrigan, W. (1983). *The Sacred Complex: On the Psychogenesis of Paradise Lost.* Cambridge, Mass.: Harvard University Press.

———. (1989). Terminating Lacan. *South Atlantic Quarterly,* 88: 993–1008.

Kroeber, K. (1920). Totem and taboo: An ethnologic psychoanalysis. *American Anthropologist,* 22: 48–55.

Johnson, A., and Price-Williams, D. (1996). *Oedipus Ubiquitous: The Family Complex in World Folk Literature.* Stanford, Calif.: Stanford University Press.

Jones, E. (1949). *Hamlet and Oedipus.* New York: Norton.

Loewald, H. (1980). *Papers on Psychoanalysis.* New Haven, Conn.: Yale University Press.

Malinowski, B. (1927). *Sex and Repression in Savage Society.* London: Routledge.

Metz, C. (1982). *The Imaginary Signifier: Psychoanalysis and Cinema.* Trans. Celia Britton, Annwyl Williams, Ben Brewster, and Alfred Guzzetti. Bloomington: Indiana University Press.

Pigman, G. W. III (1985). *Grief and English Renaissance Elegy.* Cambridge: Cambridge University Press.

Ricoeur, P. (1970). *Freud and Philosophy: An Essay on Interpretation.* Trans. Denis Savage. New Haven, Conn.: Yale University Press.

———. (1971). The model of the text: Meaningful action considered as a text. *Social Research,* 38: 529–562.

———. (1977). The question of proof in psychoanalysis. *Journal of the American Psychoanalytic Association,* 25: 835–872.

Rorty, R. (1989). *Contingency, Irony, and Solidarity.* Cambridge: Cambridge University Press.

Schafer, R. (1976). *A New Language for Psychoanalysis.* New Haven, Conn.: Yale University Press.

———. (1978). *Language and Insight.* New Haven, Conn.: Yale University Press.

———. (1983). *The Analytic Attitude.* New York: Basic Books.

Schwartz, M., and Kahn, C. (1980). *Representing Shakespeare: New Psychoanalytic Essays.* Baltimore: Johns Hopkins University Press.

Spence, D. (1982). *Narrative Truth and Historical Truth: Meaning and Interpretation in Psychoanalysis.* New York: Norton.

Spiro, M. E. (1982). *Oedipus in the Trobriands.* Chicago: University of Chicago Press.

Wallace, E. R. (1983). *Freud and Anthropology: A History and Reappraisal.* New York: International Universities Press.

Young-Bruehl, E. (1990). *Freud on Women: A Reader.* New York: Norton.

WILLIAM KERRIGAN

Hypercathexis See CATHEXIS.

Hysteria

The term "hysteria" has been used since ancient times. For example, Galen of Pergamon noted in the second century A.D. that the manifestations of hysteria "took varied and innumerable forms." Since the late nineteenth century, the concept of hysteria has been used to designate a psychoneurosis characterized by a variety of mental and somatic symptoms, typically emerging during adolescence or early adulthood and occurring more commonly in women than in men. The phenomena of dissociation and repression, whereby memories, ideas, feelings, and perceptions are lost to conscious awareness and become unavailable for voluntary recall, are central to an understanding of the genesis of hysterical symptoms as Janet (1907) and Freud (1905) discovered. These symptoms cluster in syndromes that consist of some dissociative psychic reactions and/or a selection of painful or otherwise altered sensations and motor disorders, the so-called conversion symptoms. A wide variety of somatic (perceptual and motor) and psychic disturbances may appear in the absence of any known organic pathology, or may accompany organic illness and grossly exaggerate its effects (Abse, 1987).

In modern usage, the term "hysterical" refers to certain character types, such as a histrionic personality, possessed by those vulnerable to, or afflicted with, hysteria. "Mass hysteria" describes forms of group excitement involving regressive phenomena such as convulsions, pareses, sensory disturbances, and alterations of consciousness that appear among participants in frenetic religious, political, or erotic aggregations.

Suggestibility factors can affect the development of hysteria, thus causing a considerable variation of symptoms. Moreover, there are variations from one subculture to another, as can be seen within the United States. LaBarre's (1962) description of the snake-handling cults of Appalachia is one among innumerable examples that show that hysterical behavior is extensively and intensively shaped by the local culture. Like Proteus, the Old Man of the Sea, hysteria has the ability to change shape, often within the life cycle of one individual. Although the term "hysteria" usually designates a type of psychoneurosis, many persons who exhibit hysterical symptoms either in a sustained and solitary fashion or more transiently within a group may also show evidence of psychotic disorder, including delusions of persecution and grandeur.

The word "hysteria" is derived from the Greek *hystera* (uterus), reflecting the ancient Greek notion of a wandering of this organ creating psychic and bodily disturbance, occurring more frequently in women, and connoting the sexual nature of the disorder. Related terms are "hysteriform" and "hysteroid," used often in an attempt at greater precision, the former to designate conditions that in some respects suggest the hysterical type of psychoneurosis but in others suggest psychotic disorder (Abse, 1966; 1987), the latter to emphasize the painful masochistic elements in the fantasies of those basically more pregenitally oriented and fixated (Easser and Lesser, 1965). Alan Krohn (1978) contends that the terms "hysteria" and "hysterical personality" should be reserved "for relatively mild or moderate forms of neurotic and/or character disturbance, characterized by a relatively intact ego, mild to moderate incapacity to handle life responsibilities, and phallic-Oedipal (as opposed to pregenital) levels of fixation."

Galen had insisted in *De locis affectis* that sexual abstinence or lack of sexual gratification frequently gave rise to hysterical troubles in women and analogous disorders in men, thus recognizing a syndrome resembling hysteria in males. Hysterical symptoms, though more commonly seen in women in peacetime, are more frequently seen in men under wartime conditions. During World War II, Emmanuel Miller (1940) noted that the problems presented by functional diseases in men stood out in bold relief from other medical conditions. Similarly, Arthur Hurst (1940) asserted that his experience in World War I provided ample opportunity to study the varying manifestations of hysteria in traumatized soldiers. Abse (1966; 1987) pointed out that in war neurosis, current conflicts play the key etiological role, whereas in peacetime, the crucial causal factor is the traumatic power of unsettled childhood experience, though one sort of factor is always related symbolically to the other. At a regrettably high cost, modern warfare, including warfare in Korea, Vietnam, and the Middle East, has facilitated the study of hysteria in both men and women, as will be evident from reviews of war neuroses, including delayed post-traumatic stress disorder (Schwartz, 1984).

Soon after returning from studies in Paris with Jean-Martin Charcot, Freud (1886) read a paper entitled "Über männliche Hysterie" (On Male Hysteria), which provoked resentment and dispute in the all-male Vienna Society of Medicine. Later in the same year, 1886, Freud published his observations of a severe case of hemi-anesthesia in a male patient. In his wide-ranging prepsychoanalytic essay "Hysteria" of 1888, he mentioned hysterical conditions in men brought about by severe bodily trauma such as those that follow railway and other vehicular accidents, as previously had been noted by Charcot (1873). Freud noted the lively opposition by German neuropsychiatrists to Charcot's inclusion of such cases in the category of hysteria, a disease confined by them to women. In more recent years, feminists have objected to the very word "hysteric," and there have been allegations of male chauvinism in propagating a pejorative label. In response to these charges, Phillip R. Slavney (1990) aptly notes: "It is not enough to extrapolate from feminist theory or even from the study of hypothetical cases, for such exercises will not provide the empirical evidence needed to establish the claim. Of course this assumes that the matter in question is whether psychiatrists can accurately assess the personalities of female patients. If the diagnostic category *itself* is thought to embody a sexist mentality, considerations other than empirical ones may be more decisive, as happened with the change from 'hysterical' in *DSM-II* to 'histrionic' in *DSM-III* [p. 155]" (pp. 119–120).

According to Anthony (1982), neurotic disorders observed in the adult, including hysteria, not only have their antecedents in childhood, but later psychoneuroses represent a more complete, more coherent, and more consolidated version of earlier, more rudimentary manifestations of disturbance. As Krohn (1978) has schematized, the development of Freud's ideas from the time of his essay on the etiology of hysteria (1896) involves a five-part process:

1. A passive sexual seduction in childhood of which a memory trace is laid down.
2. With the onset of sexual urges at puberty, the early memory is not only reactivated but now constitutes a trauma.
3. The memory has not only become extremely frightening but also unacceptable to consciousness and is thereupon repressed, thus creating a predisposition to later hysterical symptoms.
4. An adult event triggers the painful idea, bringing into association the original unconscious memory of the sexual situation, the sexual feeling that had become attached to it at puberty, and the sexual event in adult life, threatening to awaken unacceptable sexual memory and feeling.
5. Compromise occurs with symptom formation between the memory and its association with feelings and the resistances put up against it.

J. M. Masson (1984) outlines the views held by leading French authorities in Paris regarding rape and other violent acts against children when Freud studied at the Salpêtrière Hospital in 1885 as a pupil of Charcot and when he attended the demonstrations and addresses given by Professor Paul Brouardel, who had conducted forensic examinations of child rape victims. One tradition, sponsored notably by Ambroise Tardieu (1878), considered that sexual assaults on children were frequent and that children seldom imagined them. Another, developed by Brouardel, took the view that actual rape was rare but children often imagined it. In his book *Les attentats aux moeurs*, Brouardel (1909) recounted that of a hundred complaints of sexual abuse of children, sixty to eighty were unfounded (p. 52). These contending views paid no regard to the delayed effects of childhood sexual trauma in the causation of adult hysteria as Freud later discovered. However, these views must have influenced Freud's preoccupation with the seduction hypoth-

esis and his later hesitant decision that such actual seduction was certainly not an invariant in the etiology of hysteria. In this connection Ernest Jones (1954) commenting on a letter to Wilhelm Fliess of September 21, 1897, wrote: "Up to the spring of 1897 Freud still held firmly to his conviction of the reality of childhood traumas, so strong was Charcot's teaching on traumatic experiences and so surely did the analysis of the patient's associations reproduce them. At that time doubts began to creep in although he made no mention of them in the records of his progress that he was regularly sending to his friend Fliess. Then quite suddenly, he decided to confide to him 'the great secret of something that in the past few months has gradually dawned on me.' It was the awful truth that most—not all—of the seductions that his patients had revealed, and about which he had built his whole theory of hysteria, had never occurred. The letter of September 21, 1897, in which he made this announcement to Fliess, is perhaps the most valuable of that valuable series that was so fortunately preserved" (p. 265).

The case history Freud sent Fliess in a letter dated December 22, 1897, ended with his suggestion of a new motto for psychoanalysis: "What has been done to you, you poor child?" As reported by Masson (1984), it indicates clearly enough that Freud felt he had gone too far in the previous letter noted above, and that he recognized that actual traumatic seductive and sadistic events in childhood perpetrated by parents, siblings, or others were sometimes heavily involved in the etiology of adult hysteria. It is indeed remarkable that Anna Freud (1965), with her balanced view of the interplay of the inner and outer worlds of the child and the role of external stress in developmental psychopathology, should have consented to the omission of this case history from the published letters.

Whatever the shock many experience in confronting the findings of psychoanalysis, there is much less emphasis today on repressed perverse sexuality than on the elucidation of unconscious fantasy in the defense-struggle involved in adult neurosis. It was in the process of deepening understanding of hysteria and of dreams that Freud engendered the basic concepts of psychoanalysis.

REFERENCES

Abse, D. W. (1966). *Hysteria and Related Mental Disorders*, 1st ed. Bristol, England: Wright.

———. (1987). *Hysteria and Related Mental Disorders*, 2d ed. Bristol, England: Wright.

Anthony, E. J. (1982). Hysteria in childhood. In Alec Roy (ed.) *Hysteria*. New York: Wiley, pp. 145–163.

Brouardel, P. (1909). *Les Attentats aux Moeurs*. Paris: Préf. de Thoinot.

Charcot, J. (1873). *Leçons sur les Maladies du Système Nerveux Faites à la Salpêtrière*. Paris: Delahaye.

Easser, B. R., and Lesser, S. R. (1965). Hysterical personality: A reevaluation. *Psychoanalytic Quarterly*, 34: 390–405.

Freud, A. (1965). *Normality and Pathology in Childhood: Assessments of Development*. New York: International Universities Press.

Freud, S. (1886). Observation of a severe case of hemianaesthesia in a hysterical male. S.E. 1: 25–31.

———. (1888). Hysteria. S.E. 1: 41–57.

———. (1896). The aetiology of hysteria. S.E. 3: 191–221.

———. (1905). *Fragment of an Analysis of a Case of Hysteria*. S.E. 7: 7–122.

Galen. (1541). *De locis affectis*. Liber VI. Venice: Apud Junta.

Hurst, A. (1940). *Medical Diseases of War*. London: Arnold.

Janet, P. (1907). *The Major Symptoms of Hysteria: Fifteen Lectures Given in the Medical School of Harvard University*, 2d ed. New York: Macmillan, 1920.

Jones, E. (1954–1957). *Sigmund Freud, Life and Work*, 3 vols. New York: Basic Books.

Krohn, A. (1978). *Hysteria: The Elusive Neurosis*. New York: International Universities Press.

LaBarre, W. (1962). *They Shall Take Up Serpents*. Minneapolis: Minnesota University Press.

Masson, J. M. (1984). *The Assault on Truth*. New York: Farrar, Straus and Giroux.

Miller, E. (1940). *The Neuroses in War*. London: Macmillan.

Schwartz, H. J. (1984). *Psychotherapy of the Combat Veteran*. New York: Spectrum.

Slavney, P. R. (1990). *Perspectives on "Hysteria"*. Baltimore: Johns Hopkins University Press.

Tardieu, A. (1878). *Etude Médico-légale sur les Attentats aux Moeurs*. Paris.

D. WILFRED ABSE

I

Id

One of three agencies of the mind (the others being the ego and superego), the id, according to Freud, is entirely unconscious, seeks only satisfaction of instinctual needs, and is the source of much psychic conflict.

Prior to 1920, Freud distinguished three systems of the mind: the conscious, the preconscious, and the unconscious. The conscious system was said to contain what we are immediately aware of; the preconscious, all that is "latent," i.e. all that is outside of consciousness but capable of becoming conscious at any time; and the unconscious, all that is mental but incapable, at least in the absence of psychoanalytic treatment, of becoming conscious. The reason that ideas in the unconscious cannot enter consciousness is that a certain force opposes them, namely repression. What is repressed is unconscious and what is unconscious, according to Freud's view of the dynamic unconscious, is repressed. The theory, then, of the dynamic unconscious is closely linked in Freud's early writings to his theory of repression: "Thus we obtain our concept of the unconscious from the theory of repression. The repressed is the prototype of the unconscious for us" (Freud, 1923: 15).

However, on September 26, 1922, Freud read a short paper at the Seventh International Psycho-Analytical Congress, "Some Remarks on the Unconscious," in which he indicated dissatisfaction with his earlier theory. In an abstract of the paper, which may have been written by Freud himself, it is noted that the speaker, i.e. Freud, repeated the history of the development of the concept "unconscious" in psychoanalysis. The dynamic view of the process of repression, the abstract points out, made it necessary to give the unconscious a systematic

sense, so that the unconscious had to be equated with the repressed. "It has turned out, however,"—the abstract continues—"that it is not practicable to regard the repressed as coinciding with the unconscious and the ego with the preconscious and conscious. The speaker discussed the two facts which show that in the ego too there is an unconscious, which behaves dynamically like the repressed unconscious . . ." (Strachey, 1923). The two facts are: resistance proceeding from the ego during analysis and an unconscious sense of guilt.

Freud's short paper and its abstract anticipated the publication of *The Ego and the Id* (1923) in which he makes an important modification of his earlier views. Here he introduces the expression "das Es" ("the It"), which he explicitly borrows from Georg Groddeck, and is translated by Freud's English translators as "the Id." In his new theory, the structural theory, the unconscious is not equated with the repressed. All that is repressed is unconscious, but some of what is unconscious is not repressed. Some of what is in the id is repressed, but some of it is not. In addition, Freud now holds that part of the ego too is unconscious.

Freud sometimes writes as if the id were virtually unknowable, even if we know that it is unconscious; in this one respect of unknowability, it is reminiscent of Kant's noumenal self. In his *New Introductory Lectures on Psycho-Analysis* (1933), Freud (p. 73) describes the id as "the dark inaccessible part of our personality." In *An Outline of Psychoanalysis* (1940), he notes that the "sole prevailing quality" in the id is that of being unconscious (p. 163), but then asks what is the true nature of the state which is revealed in the id by the quality of being unconscious? He answers: "But of that we know nothing" (p. 163). He also refers to the id as "the obscure id" and the "core of our being" (p.197).

Despite the obscurity of the concept, however, Freud clearly attributes to the id various features that distinguish it from the ego and superego. The id is present at birth; the ego and superego develop only later: "To the oldest of these psychical provinces or agencies we give the name of *id*. It contains everything that is inherited, that is present at birth, that is laid down in the constitution—above all, therefore, the instincts, which originate from the somatic organization and which find a first psychical expression (in the id) in forms unknown to us" (p. 145).

The power of the id, furthermore, expresses the true purpose of the individual organism's life: the satisfaction of its needs. "No such purpose as that of keeping itself alive or of protecting itself from dangers by means of anxiety can be attributed to the id. That is the task of the ego . . ." (p. 198). The superego may also may make demands upon the ego, as does the id, but its main function remains the *limitation* of satisfactions.

The id is cut off from the external world, yet it is capable of a kind of inner perception: "It detects with extraordinary acuteness certain changes in its interior, especially oscillations in the tensions of its instinctual needs, and these changes become conscious as feelings in the pleasure-unpleasure series" (p. 198). Freud admits that it is hard to say by what means the id perceives—after all, it has no sense organs of its own—but he concludes that it is an established fact that self-perceptions govern the passage of events in the id.

In recent psychoanalytic writings, perhaps because Freud's structural theory is thought to be more speculative than many of his other theories or perhaps because of the obscurity of the concept of the id, there tend to be relatively few references to the id. However, the concept of the id figures prominently in Freud's theory of conflict; unless that very central theory is to be abandoned, it would appear that the idea of the id is still important for understanding Freudian theory, unless something functionally similar is found to take on its role.

REFERENCES
Freud, S. (1923). *The Ego and the Id*. S.E. 19: 12–63.
———. (1933). *New Introductory Lectures on Psycho-Analysis*. S.E. 22: 5–182.
———. (1940). *An Outline of Psycho-Analysis*. S.E. 23: 144–207.
Moore, B., and Fine, B. (eds.) (1990). *Psychoanalytic Terms and Concepts*. New Haven: American Psychoanalytic Association and Yale University Press.
Strachey, J. (1961). Editor's introduction. S.E. 19. 3–11.
                                    EDWARD ERWIN

Identification

Though Freud began to write about identification in his epochal dream book of 1900, the far-reaching conceptualization of identification as a transformative and structuralizing process began with his investigation of the role of narcissism in melancholia.

In *Mourning and Melancholia* (1917 [1915]) Freud considers identification from three perspectives: (1) as a defense (against narcissistic injury); (2) as a developmental process (the way the ego grows); and (3) as a type of regression (from object love to secondary narcissism).

Freud viewed melancholia as a response to the loss of an ambivalently loved object. Such losses occur not only because of death, but because of all sorts of interactions that result in narcissistic injury—e.g., feeling slighted, neglected, or disappointed by the love object. These are common ways in which ambivalence is reinforced or inflamed.

In *Mourning and Melancholia* Freud describes how the melancholic's self-reproaches properly belong to the lost object but have been shifted onto the sufferer's ego. When an object tie is ruptured because of hurt, disappointment, or actual loss, the libido that had been invested in the lost object is withdrawn into the ego rather than simply being displaced onto a new object. This establishes an identification of the ego with the abandoned object. "Thus the shadow of the object fell upon the ego," and the ego is now critically judged as if it were the forsaken object (Freud, 1917: 249). In this manner, the object is given up but the conflictual object relation is maintained internally through narcissistic identification This allows sadism and hatred for the lost object to be turned round upon the self, hence the melancholic's lowered self-regard and feelings of worthlessness. In Freud's view, the dramatic and often exasperating self-vilification of the melancholic reflects unconscious sadistic pleasure. The conflict between the ego and its loved and hated lost object has now become a "cleavage" between the superego (as Freud would soon come to call the ego's "critical agency") and "the ego as altered by identification" 1917, p. 249).

This dark metaphor of the shadow of the lost object falling upon the ego is deservedly famous among Freudian dicta. It has the haunting baleful sound of an elegy. Growth proceeds by loss, Freud is saying. It is among his most evocative and profound insights and marks the early intersection of ego psychology and object relations theory. The ego is built of accumulated identifications with abandoned and lost objects.

Freud extends this idea in *The Ego and the Id*, where he broadens his notion of the process of ego development to encompass character formation, stating that "the character of the ego is a precipitate of abandoned object cathexes" and that the ego "contains the history of those object-choices" (1923, p. 29). In this respect, the ego can be viewed as a palimpsest, or an embodiment of personal history.

Identification with the same-sex parent initially allows the Oedipal child to relinquish one set of erotic ties in favor of another. As the Oedipus complex unfolds, however these early identifications turn hostile and are complemented by loving and rivalrous cathexes of the opposite-sex parent as well. Identifying and dis-identifying with the parents and other important objects is a lifelong developmental task that shapes and modifies intrapsychic structures.

In *Group Psychology and the Analysis of the Ego* (1921), Freud considers identification from the point of view of group dynamics. A mere decade before the rise of the National Socialist (Nazi) Party in Germany, Freud examines the potential for dramatic alterations in super-ego functioning arising from mutual identifications between group members. Group ties are forged by a collective wish to be led and a shared predilection for exalting the group leader, who becomes the figure onto whom the group members project their ego ideals. Freud shows how group cohesion relies upon this shared craving for authority and omnipotence, and comes at the expense of mature, independent superego functioning.

Freud maintained that identification is developmentally prior to object love. Along the lines sketched by Karl Abraham before him and Melanie Klein after him, Freud saw the early ego as cannibalistic. Its first objects are incorporated, "devoured in" primal operations of attachment and appropriation that aim to move aspects of the external object across the self/not-self/ membrane. Early identifications, therefore, have the distinctive coloring of oral sadism. (Later, Fairbairn [1952] used the primary identification to denote the early ego's devouring—or, as Winnicott [1958] put it, "ruthless"— style of attachment before self and object are clearly and securely differentiated.) It is only later, once some ego growth has occurred, that it becomes possible for objects to be loved in a way that recognizes their separateness.

In Freud's view the psychopathology of melancholia involves a regression from object love to narcissistic identification. The lost, ambivalently cathected object and the ego have become one; in the language of libido theory, object libido has been transformed into narcissistic libido. This represents the reverse of what he sees as the normal developmental progression from primal identification to object love. By contrast, in hysterical identification, the object tie is maintained but in a partial and displaced version. For example, a little girl may develop her mother's cough. This could reflect a prototypical Oedipal identification signifying her wish to take the place of her mother with her father (Freud, 1921: 106).

Freud did not clearly distinguish among identification, introjection, and internalization. Subsequent theorists such as Sandler and Rosenblatt (1962), Schafer (1968), and Loewald (1973) have clarified these interrelated terms. These authors have amplified Freud's notion of identification as a basic internalizing process leading to ego change and growth.

REFERENCES

Fairbairn, W. R. D. (1952). *Psychoanalytic Studies of the Personality*. London: Tavistock/Routledge.

Freud, S. (1917 [1915]). *Mourning and Melancholia*. S.E. 14: 242–260.

———. (1921). *Group Psychology and the Analysis of the Ego*. S.E. 18: 69–143.

———. (1923). *The Ego and the Id*. S.E. 19: 12–59.

Loewald, H. (1973). On internalization. In H. Loewald (author). *Papers on Psychoanalysis*. New Haven, Conn.: Yale University Press, 1980.

Sandler, J., and Rosenblatt, B. (1962). The concept of the representational world. *Psychoanalytic Study of the Child*, 17: 128–145.

Schafer, R. (1968). *Aspects of Internalization*. Madison, Conn.: International Universities Press.

Winnicott, D. W. (1958). *Collected Papers: Through Paediatrics to Psycho-Analysis*. New York: Basic Books.

NATHAN KRAVIS

Incest

Issues about incest are important in relation to Freud's work for three principal reasons. First, Freud's own views on the subject have been extensively misunderstood and misrepresented, both by outsiders and by those within the psychoanalytic movement. Second, the apparently incestuous characteristics of much infantile sexuality raise serious difficulties. Finally, recent genetic insights into incest suggest that Freud's original findings, if properly interpreted, may be much less in conflict with biology than even he believed.

"Incest" might be defined as sexual relations between partners more closely related than first cousins. A more general term, applicable to any sexually reproducing organism, would be "inbreeding." What is and what is not regarded as incestuous varies surprisingly in human societies. For example, first-cousin marriage is criminal incest in several states of the United States but is not a crime in others. In many Third World countries, first-cousin marriage is not only very common but often regarded as the norm. Brother-sister incest is occasionally found in royal families and elsewhere.

Freud himself is often believed to have thought that the incestuous feelings of the Oedipus complex were repressed by parental or social pressure, and that the incest taboo was a cultural creation, socialized into children as a bulwark against infantile incest. It is also widely assumed that he believed that the taboo on incest created ambivalence about it; in other words, people were innately incestuous but deterred only by an imposed, cultural prohibition.

In *Totem and Taboo* (1913), Freud went out of his way to insist quite the contrary. His use of the examples of taboos relating to rulers, the dead, and enemies leaves no doubt that his finding was that taboos were created as defenses against preexisting ambivalence, not that ambivalence was created by taboos. Indeed, in the closing pages of *Totem and Taboo*, he controversially claimed that guilt about incest was an inherited trait, laid down by crucial events early in human history and now fixed in human nature, irrespective of culture.

In his paper *The Dissolution of the Oedipus Complex* (1924), Freud expressed continuing doubt about what exactly terminated the Oedipal stage. Having mentioned the possibility that "the Oedipus complex would go to its destruction from its lack of success, from the effects of its internal impossibility," he immediately adds a further consideration: "Another view is that that Oedipus complex must collapse because the time has come for its disintegration, just as the milk-teeth fall out when the permanent ones begin to grow. Although the majority of human beings go through the Oedipus complex as an individual experience, it is nevertheless a phenomenon which is determined and laid down by heredity and which is bound to pass away according to program when the next preordained phase of development sets in. This

being so, it is of no great importance what the occasions are which allow this to happen, or, indeed, whether any such occasions can be said to happen, or, indeed, whether any such occasions can be discovered at all."

If we add the point that Freud makes a few pages later, that the dissolution of the Oedipus complex also constitutes the basis of the "prohibition against incest," we can see clearly that the preceding quotation refutes those who have interpreted Freud as a believer in a purely environmental, acquired mechanism of incest avoidance. On the contrary, Freud remarks: "There is room for the ontogenetic view"—that is, personal experience—"side by side with the more far-reaching phylogenetic one," and refers to the whole process as an "innate program."

Freud concludes: "But this does not dispose of the problem; there is room for a theoretical speculation which may upset the results we have come to or put them in a new light." Although Freud himself took the matter no further, today our understanding of the biology of incest may provide a theoretical speculation that would indeed put his results in a new light.

A major shortcoming of twentieth-century views of incest was that they stressed only the genetic costs of inbreeding. These are certainly real but not always as great as they have been portrayed. For example, studies of first-cousin marriage in the Third World show that although inbreeding may impose some genetic cost in terms of death and abnormality, it is more than offset by the greater fertility of these marriages (Bittles et al., 1991).

Inbreeding confers social benefits to the extent that genes sacrifice for one another. An individual who loses his life saving three siblings sacrifices 100 percent of his genes for such altruism but saves 150 percent because each sibling would normally share half the altruist's genes. However, if altruist and siblings were related by more than 50 percent of their genes thanks to inbreeding by their parents, only two would have to be saved. This is the case in termites and the one mammal to have a social insect-style society—the naked mole rat—and results from incestuous matings between parents, offspring, and siblings. In human societies, the social benefits of inbreeding are chiefly seen in royalty, where access to wealth, power, and privilege is often restricted by intermarriage within the royal family.

Freud's fundamental discovery, set out in *Totem and Taboo*, was that human beings are ambivalent about incest and that taboos are defenses against this innate ambivalence. If, following Freud's lead, we were prepared to attribute ambivalence about incest to our evolutionary past, we might today be able to explain it somewhat better than he could. All we would have to propose is that inbreeding has both genetic costs and social benefits. Given that these costs and benefits will vary widely from individual to individual, time to time, and place to place, no single optimal solution is applicable to all societies and all persons. The consequence is likely to be chronic ambivalence about the whole issue, and this, essentially, was Freud's finding (Badcock, 1994).

REFERENCES

Badcock, C. (1994). *PsychoDarwinism: The New Synthesis of Darwin and Freud.* London: HarperCollins.

Bittles, A., Mason, W., Greene, J., and Rao, N. (1991). Reproductive behavior and health in consanguineous marriages. *Science,* 252: 789–794.

Freud, S. (1913). *Totem and Taboo.* S.E. 13: 1–161.

———. (1924). The dissolution of the Oedipus complex. S.E. 19: 173–179.

CHRISTOPHER BADCOCK

Incorporation See IDENTIFICATION.

India, and Psychoanalysis

After a dramatic and promising start in 1920, psychoanalysis in India suffered through a period of relative intellectual stagnation. There has been a recent resurgence of interest, however, and many prominent Indians, living both in India and abroad, are making significant contributions to the field.

The beginnings of psychoanalysis in India can be traced as far back as 1920. In December of that year, a thirty-three-year-old Calcutta psychiatrist named Girindrasekhar Bose began a correspondence with Freud. Bose sent Freud his recently published monograph, *Concept of Repression,* adding that he had been a "warm admirer" of Freud's theories. The subsequent Freud-Bose correspondence extended, albeit haltingly, over the next seventeen years.

Their dialogue, involving both organizational and theoretical matters, reveals that the Indian Psychoanalytic Society was founded, with the assistance of Ernest Jones, in 1922. Formal analytic training began to be offered in 1930 under the auspices of the Indian Psychoanalytic Institute, organized with the guidance of Max

Eitingon of the International Training Commission. A psychoanalytic journal in english, *Samiksa,* began publication in 1947 and has appeared regularly since then. The Freud-Bose correspondence also gives an endearing account of the remittance by the Indian Psychoanalytic Society of an ivory statuette to Freud on his seventy-fifth birthday and the latter's giving it "the place of honor on [his] desk" (Freud-Bose correspondence; Freud's letter of December 13, 1931, quoted in Ramana, 1964).

Among the theoretical matters brought up by Bose were his theory of opposite wishes, which stipulated that a trauma inherently gratifies passive wishes and leads to an "identification with the offending agent" and an active wish for mastery; this explains the coexistence of a series of passive and active wishes in the human mind. Bose also suggested that the castration threat owes its efficacy to a deeper, preexistent, and warded-off wish in the male to be a female. Freud's response to both these ideas was lukewarm, assigning the former idea to formal differences of theorizing and the latter to the realm of cross-cultural variations. (The contemporary psychoanalytic hypotheses of "primary femininity" and the boy's need to step away from mother to consolidate his masculinity might actually support Bose's second notion.)

It is ironic that such a propitious start did not lead psychoanalysis in India to grow by leaps and bounds. The small cadre of European analysts who had been practicing (or attempting to practice) psychoanalysis in India gradually left the country after its independence from England in 1947. The Indian Psychoanalytic Society, though founded by both psychologists and physicians, never gained a significant foothold within academic medicine. Mainstream Indian psychiatry, under the aegis of the Indian Psychiatric Society, did not develop any ties with the Indian Psychoanalytic Society, which remained limited to a relatively unknown and marginalized group of psychologists in Calcutta. The reasons for such lack of acceptance of psychoanalysis in India remain unclear. The medical orientation of Indian psychiatry, the pervasiveness of religious thought in the culture at large, the widespread poverty leading to a preoccupation with external realities, and the enmeshed nature of the individual Indian's psychological self might all have played a role in creating this state of affairs.

In contrast to the relative intellectual stagnation that occurred within the country, a few Indians living abroad who chose psychoanalysis as their vocation made outstanding contributions to the field. Prominent among this group were Prakash Bhandari, Narain Jetmalani, Masud Khan, and Hawrant Singh Gill in England and C. V. Ramana in the United States.

Recently, however, a new spark of interest in psychoanalysis has developed even within India. Sudhir Kakar, a European-trained psychoanalyst practicing in New Delhi, has made many significant contributions to the psychoanalytic understanding of the Indian psyche. Ashis Nandy, one of India's leading intellectuals, has also relied considerably on psychoanalytic thought in his essays on Indian society and culture. The orientation of these two influential individuals and a handful of their followers is largely Eriksonian. In contrast, the small group of psychoanalytically inclined clinicians that has emerged in Bombay is influenced more by the writings of the British psychoanalysts Melanie Klein and Wilfred Bion. Preceding both these developments somewhat was the creation of the B.M. Institute of Mental Health at Ahmadabad, which, under the directorship of B. K. Ramanujam, has made considerable contributions to psychoanalytic psychotherapy with individuals, families, and children. This has been funded by the Sarabhai family and has been overseen by the institute's current director, the psychoanalyst Kamalini Sarabhai.

The overseas scene also appears promising. There are a few practicing psychoanalysts of Indian origin in England including Baljeet Mehra and Kamal Mehra, and at least one, Tapasi Gupta, in Germany. In the United States, there are seven such psychoanalysts: Salman Akhtar, Saida Koitta, Purnima Mehta, Dwarkanath Rao, Satish Reddy, Bhaskar Sripada, and Dushyant Trivedi. In Canada, there are three such psychoanalysts: Jaswant Guzder, Madhu Rao, and Dushyant Yagnik. Many others of Indian origin are pursuing psychoanalytic training both in England and in the United States. Together with those already practicing psychoanalysis, these young men and women are keeping alive the tradition set in motion in 1920 by Bose.

REFERENCES

Akhtar, S. (1997). Book review of *All the Mothers Are One: Hindu India and the Cultural Reshaping of Psychoanalysis* by Stanley N. Kurtz. *Journal of the American Psychoanalytic Association*, 45, no. 2: 1014–1019.

Kakar, S. (1981). *The Inner World: A Psychoanalytic Study of Childhood and Society in India.* New York: Oxford University Press.

Nandy, A. (1995). *The Save Freud and Other Essays on Possible and Retrievable Selves.* Princeton, N.J.: Princeton University Press.

Ramana, C. V. (1964). On the early history and development of psychoanalysis in India. *Journal of the American Psychoanalytic Association*, 12: 110–134.

Roland, Alan (1988). *In Search of Self in India and Japan: Toward a Cross-Cultural Psychology.* Princeton, N.J.: Princeton University Press.

SALMAN AKHTAR

Infantile Neurosis See CHILDHOOD NEUROSIS.

Infantile Sexuality

Freud's first interest in sexuality goes back to his idea that what he called "actual neuroses" are the result of sexual frustration. When, still early in his career, references to sex made their appearance in his patients' associations as these led back to their past life, he became convinced that they were remembering experiences in which they had been a witness and, in some cases, victim of the sexuality of other people, notably that of their parents. When later he was persuaded that these associations were mostly false memories, he concluded that they were fantasies—not present fantasies projected into the past, but past fantasies that had come to be repressed and so continued to be active in the feelings of his patients without being recognized by them "in their unconscious mind." Freud hoped that their recollection would clear the air for them, mentally speaking, enable them to dispense with their defenses, and so come to terms with these experiences from the past, alive in their present life.

Freud thus concluded that his patients had been sexually active in their imagination, wishful thinking, or fantasy in their early childhood. In other words, as young children they were capable of sexual thoughts and found pleasure in these thoughts. This meant that the idea that human sexuality begins at adolescence with puberty was false and a prejudice. Freud attributed it to the same resistance his patients showed in analysis to recognizing their own sexual fantasies rooted in their childhood. He argued, in his *Three Essays on the Theory of Sexuality*, that sexual activity and pleasure in human beings, however much physical, cannot be separated from affective fantasy, which is the life of the imagination. The very significance of what a person engages in in his or her sexual activities is to be found in his or her fantasies.

Freud then reflected on the ways in which sex enters into "sexual aberrations"—inversions and perversions, sadism and masochism. These, he argued, can be seen to be phenomena of sex in their relation to what is to be found in "normal" adult sexuality. In perversions, we have sexuality deviated from its normal aim, namely, copulation; and in inversions, we have sexuality directed to an object other than an adult person of the opposite gender. In other respects, they resemble the phenomena of adult sexuality and they lead to orgasm. Furthermore, they are clearly regarded as phenomena of sex by those who engage in these "aberrant" activities.

Freud next focused on the resemblance between these activities and fantasies clearly found in childhood so as to establish the sexual character of the latter. He argued that in the "aberrant" sexual activities a person continues to indulge in sexual activities from early childhood and relives their fantasies. As Freud puts it in his *Introductory Lectures on Psycho-Analysis*: "Perverted sexuality is nothing else but infantile sexuality, magnified and separated into its component parts" (Twentieth Lecture).

Early infantile sexuality, Freud argued, is "auto-erotic" and "pleasure-seeking," that is, here the child seeks pleasure in the erotogenic zones of his or her own body. These are the same bodily zones the stimulation of which forms a part of the activity leading to adult sexual intercourse. But in this phase of sexual development, the child's sexual activity is not directed to a person. When, fairly soon, it is so directed, it takes the form of love and as such the mother or a surrogate becomes its object—that is, after a short narcissistic phase.

Freud thus argues that the boy's love for his mother is sexual in character. This is the "Oedipus phase," which brings him into conflict with his father—at least in his imagination. The sexual character of the young boy's love for his mother can be seen, Freud argues, in the way it duplicates itself in his sexual loves during and after adolescence. As he puts it, the characteristics of his early love are "transferred" into his later sexual loves. The French novelist Marcel Proust has given us imaginative examples of such "transference" in his novel *A la Recherche du Temps Perdu (Remembrance of Things Past)*. There he brings out how much the desire to possess the beloved, the tendency to be jealous of her intimacy with others, and the anguish that the possibility of losing her arouses, all characteristics of sexual love, come from the lover's early relationship with his mother. In Marcel's feelings, Albertine, the beloved, is, as Proust puts it, "at once a mistress, a sister, a daughter, and a mother too, of whose regular goodnight kiss I [Marcel,

the narrator] was beginning once more to feel a child-like need."

But is the fact that sexual love reduplicates the young child's love for his mother, the fact that much that is found in it has "migrated" there from the lover's childhood love for his mother, sufficient to establish that his early love for his mother was a form of sexual love? Surely *more* is needed to establish this claim of Freud. This is not to say that Freud has not successfully argued for the existence of a form of sexuality in childhood. He has. His claim is that infantile sexuality is transformed after puberty and goes on changing character in the course of the individual's affective development. It does so hand-in-glove with the change in character of one's capacity for love and of the ability to give of oneself to others in the love of which one becomes capable. But these changes may come to a standstill; one's sexuality and capacity for love may not change completely. The early forms of that sexuality may in part survive unchanged and, in certain circumstances, they may surface to reappear in the adult person's fantasies, responses, and behavior.

In what sense, then, is the young boy's love for his mother meant to be sexual? Not in the sense that he, the young child, wants to have sexual intercourse with her, but in the sense that he wants to be kissed and fondled by her, to kiss and fondle her, and to keep her all to himself. His love, that is, is meant to be sexual in character in that it craves for physical intimacy with his mother of an exclusive kind. Freud's claim is that the pleasure the young boy finds in his intimacy and the thoughts surrounding it give it an aspect reminiscent of the sexual love we find in older people. In Freud's terminology, "the sensual current" of the child's sexuality is active in his love for his mother. But, to repeat, the sexuality that belongs to such love is not adult sexuality—even though it is to be found in adult sexuality and in the adult's sexual love. It may, however, in some cases, combine with what belongs to adult life and genital sexuality to make it possible for the thought of incest to cross the adult man's mind. As Jocasta, Oedipus's mother and wife, puts it in Sophocles' play *King Oedipus*: "Nor need this mother-marrying frighten you; Many a man has dreamt as much."

In short, then, Freud's claim is that sex, as most of us in fact understand it, is not confined to sexual intercourse between adults of opposite genders. It is wider than that. In this wider everyday conception, what belongs to sex is to be found in the child's life, thoughts, and wishes. The transition from the kind of sexual activity and fantasies to be found in the young child, through puberty, to adult sexuality is part of a person's affective development as an individual. But there are psychological obstacles to such a development and most people overcome them only in some degree. Hence, with most people, their childhood sexuality does to some extent remain unchanged. Some of it survives to color their adult sexuality and loves. Infantile sexuality is thus to be seen not only in the young child but also in the adult.

REFERENCE

Freud, S. (1916–1917). *Introductory Lectures on Psycho-Analysis*, S.E. 15, 16.

                                        ILHAM DILMAN

Insight, Role of in Therapy

Insight has long been considered to be a central, if not the most important or even exclusive, change process in clinical psychoanalysis. The term refers to the activity wherein the patient becomes aware of the meaning and purpose of his or her unconscious psychological activity. This learning is of a specific sort: the patient becomes aware of some wish, emotion, motive, fantasy, or memory that has been influencing his or her mental life in covert, powerful ways. Complete insight also contains the entrance into awareness of the ways in which the patient kept himself or herself unknowing (resistances, defense mechanisms, inhibitions, and character traits). The final component of insight involves learning about the anxieties, painful affects, and anticipated interpersonal consequences that led to the warding off of the particular issue.

Insight sometimes occurs spontaneously as the patient associates freely in the presence of the therapist. Most often, insight follows some interpretation offered by the psychoanalyst, in which the patient is told about the contents of the unconscious conflict, its historical roots, and present-day manifestations. An accurate interpretation leads to the recovery of memories, to affective arousal, and to awareness of hidden feelings, desires, and perceptions of self and others. There follows a decrease in the consequent anxiety, guilt, shame, or other correlates of those inner states. As insight occurs with regularity during therapy, the patient is freed of the burdensome task of limiting his or her intrapsychic life through defenses, symptoms, and distortions of behavior.

During Freud's career, insight was assumed to be the admission to consciousness of the remnants of child-

hood sexual urges; today, psychoanalysis has expanded its understanding of unconscious mental life to include such phenomena as representations of the self and of others, and of internalized relationships with significant persons from the past. These psychic contents become accessible to awareness through psychoanalytic treatment as well.

Freud's view on the role of insight in psychoanalytic treatment changed as his clinical technique matured and as the theoretical foundations of psychoanalysis changed. Freud (1906, p. 159) first suggested that any repressed wish, memory, or motive could be the source of neurosis, and that the task of treatment was the abreaction (release) of the affect that accompanied the unconscious cognitive contents. Insight, or conscious acknowledgment of those contents, was the necessary precursor to this experience.

Freud (1905, p. 130) later placed exclusive emphasis upon the patient's awareness of repressed childhood sexual wishes and the associated anxieties that were the results of these wishes. Freud wrote as if insight and recollection were equivalent, often referring to the task of psychoanalysis as filling in the gaps in the patient's memory. What was to be remembered was not that which had occurred but, rather, those sexual pleasures that had been wished for, feared, and repudiated in the earliest stages of life (Freud, 1914: 147). The therapeutic benefit of becoming conscious of these wishes was the chance to discharge some small amount of the sexual energy that had been kept in stasis through repression, and the detachment (decathexis) on the part of the person from the wish. As insights accrued and wishes were recovered, integrated, and renounced, the person might abandon childhood erotic desires and move toward mature sexuality.

Freud's conceptualization of the therapeutic role of insight changed as his theory was expanded to include a focus on character, resistance, and transference. Freud moved to a view of insight that is strikingly prescient of the writings of contemporary psychoanalysts with regard to the centrality of the transference to the analyst, and in his discussion of resistance to the uncovering of unconscious material.

Freud (1914, p. 147) identified the central clinical task of psychoanalysis as the recovery in memory of those repressed childhood desires that the patient was unknowingly repeating in a variety of symbolic ways. Only by first identifying the sources of resistance to conscious recollection of wishes could the patient move from repression, through intellectual acceptance, to the fully lived, affectively charged experience of the memory that was necessary for its integration. Freud (1914, p. 147) indicated that insight was possible only in the context of this erotically colored recollection. Insight thus was equated with overcoming and modifying the resistances against complete recollection of one's childhood erotic desires.

Freud's concern with the need to bring resistance into awareness as a precursor to the awareness of unconscious wishes was a central theme through his writings. He cautioned that intellectual understanding of the unconscious life of the analysand would not lead to change, for resistances against the acceptance of repressed material are not influenced by the naming of what is repressed (Freud, 1915: 159).

Freud (1910, p. 221) warned against the dangers of "wild" analysis in which the patient was quickly informed about the contents of the unconscious, noting that this did not lead to useful insight. He advanced the notion that the patient must attain awareness of the resistances to the acceptance of unconscious material before being able to assimilate awareness of repressed memories: "The pathological factor is not his ignorance in itself, but the root of this ignorance in his inner resistances; it was they that first called this ignorance into being, and they still maintain it now" (Freud, 1910: 225).

Freud also repeatedly stressed his finding that mutative insights occurred within the context of the transference to the analyst. The transference was portrayed as the analysand's primary way of resisting the recall of childhood sexual fantasy, as forbidden wishes and the resistances against these wishes are unconsciously brought forward into the relationship with the analyst. Only by separating past from present, and by recalling what was repressed, can change occur. Freud described the process by noting: "The patient cannot remember the whole of what is repressed in him, and what he cannot remember may precisely be the essential part of it. . . . He is obliged to repeat the repressed materials as a contemporary experience" (Freud, 1920: 18).

In response to this repetition, the analyst must seek to keep this transference neurosis within the narrowest limits: to force as much as possible into the channel of memory and to allow as little as possible to emerge as repetition (Freud, 1920: 19). Freud described the analyst's task as follows: "He must get him to re-experience

some portion of his forgotten life, but must see to it, on the other hand, that the patient retains some degree of aloofness, which will enable him, in spite of everything, to recognize that what appears to be reality is in fact only a reflection of a forgotten past" (Freud, 1920: 18–19).

The analysand's newly acquired capacity to know that which was previously repressed allows the past and its desires and fears gradually to be left behind.

REFERENCES
Freud, S. (1896). Further remarks on the neuropsychoses of defense. S.E. 3: 15–185.
———. (1905). *Three Essays on the Theory of Sexuality.* S.E. 7: 130–243.
———. (1910). "Wild" psychoanalysis. S.E. 11: 221–227.
———. (1914). Remembering, repeating, and working through. S.E. 12: 147–156.
———. (1915). Observations on transference-love. S.E. 12: 159–171.
———. (1920). *Beyond the Pleasure Principle.* S.E. 18: 7–64.
                                    JEROLD R. GOLD

Instincts, Theory of See DRIVE THEORY.

Intellectualization

Freud did not use the term "intellectualization" in any of his writings, but his awareness that the intellectual functions may be used for the purpose of defense shows in many places. In *Negation* (1925, p. 320 ff.), Freud wrote of the uses of the function of judgment as the intellectual substitute of repression, and references to this idea appear as early as 1905 (Freud, 1905).

Anna Freud (1946, p. 172 ff.) included intellectualization among the recognized mechanisms of defense, but she used the term primarily for the way adolescents, faced with the resurgence of instinct, deal with their unruly affects by using their intellectual powers of abstraction. Their intellectualization differs from ordinary intellectual activity by being motivated not to accomplish realistic planning but for defensive purposes. It stands for the adolescent's efforts to master the instincts by means of thought, "by connecting them to ideas which can be dealt with in consciousness" (p. 178).

Most authorities would regard intellectualization as a secondary defense, one that makes use, for instance, of isolation, negation, and denial in addition to exploiting the powers of the intellect. In this sense, intellectualization also describes a mode of resistance commonly seen during psychoanalytic treatment. By generalizing rather than speaking of direct experience, or by burying the emotional meaning of experiences by belaboring pointless detail, or by speaking abstractly rather than concretely, the patient attempts to keep the analyst from disturbing the status quo and also reduces the threat of instinctual pressure.

REFERENCES

Freud, A. (1946). *The Ego and the Mechanisms of Defense.* New York: International Universities Press.

Freud, S. (1905). *Jokes and Their Relation to the Unconscious.* S.E. 8: 3–237.

———. Negation. S.E. 19: 235–239.

HERBERT J. SCHLESINGER

Interpretation

Interpretation 1

Interpretation is an attempt by the analyst to find a (usually implicit) meaning in the patient's associations and, where possible, link it to current themes in the treatment. Sharpe (1937, p. 23) describes a patient who dreamed: "I take a piece of silk from a cupboard and destroy it." To an Englishman, the phrase "take silk" means "to be called to the bar," and Sharpe, with this phrase in mind, managed to uncover hostile feelings toward the patient's father (a lawyer). A patient of Viderman's (1979, p. 265) reported the following dream: "My father and I are in a garden. I pick some flowers and offer him a bouquet of six roses." Viderman, knowing that the father had died of alcoholism, made the following interpretation: "Six roses ou cirrhose?" He took advantage of the homophone to bring together the positive connotations of the gift (six roses) with the negative feelings the patient may have had about his father's illness and death (i.e., cirrhosis of the liver).

In both examples, the interpretation functions as a kind of rhetorical device, similar to simile or metaphor, which is intended to produce a certain response in the listener. At its best, it alerts the patient to a fresh range of associations that may produce a new understanding of the dream or piece of behavior being analyzed and a new awareness of linkages to other themes in the treatment. A good interpretation, in common with arresting metaphors and similes, brings together separate ideas and opens up new possibilities for inspection. Whether it is a true reading of the material (i.e., a reconstruction) or a plausible reading (construction) seems to matter less than the permission it grants the patient to bring disparate associations to mind and in this and other ways enrich the patient's contents of consciousness.

While the traditional interpretation was aimed at unearthing unconscious ideation, current practice seems to focus more on the surface of the ego in an "attempt to read the text as written by the patient" (Busch, 1997: 410). It has been argued that interpretations that stay close to the surface of the patient's awareness are more easily tolerated and more likely to engage the patient in an ongoing dialogue. To work in a more investigative (and often arbitrary) manner, possibly suggesting linkages that appeal primarily to the analyst, runs the risk of reducing the patient to a passive observer, increasing unnecessarily the authoritarian presence of the analyst and significantly raising the chance of major errors because the patient's context of consciousness is largely ignored. To work in a more collaborative fashion leaves room for negotiations along the way as both parties work together to further refine the emerging interpretation and its conceptual surround; in the long run, the final product is more apt to describe the underlying phenomena (and in some cases prevent its future occurrence; whether an interpretation is successful because it tallies with the repressed conflict is still a matter of debate).

This more egalitarian way of thinking about interpretations is a plausible, even persuasive argument that is steadily gaining popularity but it remains, at bottom, little more than a hypothesis because we are still missing the necessary evidence that would rule in its favor. Supporting anecdotes that favor surface over depth continue to multiply, but we are still waiting for a systematic research program to settle the issue. We are still looking for the kind of detailed, context-specific evidence that we are beginning to provide to patients and that can be separated into ostensive and conjectual levels of argument (see Ahumada, 1997, for definition of these terms). It can be seen that the logic of interpretation in a clinical session can also apply to larger questions of metapsychology.

A similar ambiguity surrounds the question of impact. A close reading of the literature on interpretation reveals relatively few useful clinical specimens and even fewer examples of persuasive outcomes. Scarcity of data has not lessened the popularity of interpretation as one of the analyst's more important tools, but it leaves open the possibility that a good interpretation may function largely as a piece of constructive analysis—an attempt to formulate a cluster of ideas that help to advance the analytic process. In the most skillful hands, an interpretation is often hedged about with such provisos as "Had you considered that . . ." or "One way of looking at this . . ."; these disclaimers are intended to engage the patient's curiosity and increase her readiness to accept new formulations.

Good interpretations seem most enabling when they bring together productive clusters of associations readily available to the introspecting patient. In common with good metaphors, they help us link ideas that are usually kept separate and, in the process, open the door to new ways of seeing the world. But just as overused metaphors quickly become dead and useless, having lost forever their power to startle and surprise, so overused interpretations can easily lose their therapeutic power. While it is sometimes true that mislaying your car keys was caused by not wanting to pick up your mother-in-law at the station, the routine use of this interpretation (forgetting = repressed wish) quickly dulls its edge. The best interpretations, like the best metaphors, are invented on the spot and probably have a fairly short half-life.

Interpretation 2

Interpretation also refers to a construing of the mind, defined by psychoanalytic theory, that mediates (largely unwittingly) between observation and understanding of any particular clinical happening. Hesitations in the associative process, for example, are traditionally recognized as pointing to a resistance; specific reactions toward the analyst are traditionally construed as manifestations of transference. Knowledge of the theory and experience in its application lead to the automatic translation of certain kinds of clinical data into their recognized latent meanings. Interpretation in this second sense is constantly at work in the consulting room, even when the analyst is only listening silently. We know very little about the overall influence of this belief system on our understanding of clinical material because the majority of case studies are rendered in a standard, interpretative language and not in the raw data of the patient's original utterances.

For holders of this belief system, the practice of psychoanalysis with its emphasis on free association, interpretation (as in no. 1 above), and the traditional use of the couch follows directly from Freud's theory and is no longer in need of investigation. Psychoanalytic theory, by this view, is no longer one hypothesis among many but an accepted (and largely proven) account of human behavior and its remediation. It is assumed that the history of psychoanalysis has supplied us with more than ample documentation of the basic aspects of this world view; as a result, no general research program is under way to systematically accumulate confirming and disconfirming data. Interpretation based on standard theory is automatic and almost never open to question; research in general is seen as a minor and largely optional activity. As a result, the rationale for the Basic Rule of free association is more problematic than assured, nor is there good evidence that by following the Basic Rule we can uncover the essential features of the patient's contents of consciousness.

Belief in a psychoanalytic world view is shared by most practicing psychoanalysts and provides the underpinning for intelligible discussions of theory, clinical evidence, and the like. But the uniformity of these beliefs tends to be exaggerated, and increasing evidence suggests that there are real differences in how graduates of different training programs come to understand particular pieces of clinical material (see Hamilton, 1996). The variability of these grounding belief systems has never been systematically studied.

In its reliance on an unproven belief system, psychoanalysis may be closer to religion than to science, and the key role played by our interpretative apparatus in making sense of our clinical observations is only gradually being recognized. Conspicuously missing is a clear understanding of the personal variable that the gifted clinician brings to his or her practice and that enables him or her to apply standard theory and achieve impressive results. This mysterious addition is not documented in any standard account of the theory and is not explicitly described in any case presentation, yet all practicing clinicians are aware of its importance and of how it spells the difference between treatment success and failure. When this personal variable is present, an interpretative view shaped by standard theory seems to give a wholly adequate account of the workings of the mind and its repair; when this variable is absent (or only partially present), the theory seems a poor guide to practice. Standard theory thus provides a necessary but not sufficient interpretation of mind and behavior, and we need to know more about the boundary conditions that make the theory true and worthy of respect.

I

REFERENCES

Ahumada, J. L. (1997). Toward an epistemology of clinical psychoanalysis. *Journal of the American Psychoanalytic Association*, 45: 507–530.

Busch, F. (1997). The patient's use of free association. *Journal of the American Psychoanalytic Association*, 45: 407–423.

Hamilton, V. (1996). *The Analyst's Preconscious*. Hillsdale, N.J.: Analytic Press.

Sharpe, E. F. (1937). *Dream Analysis*. London: Hogarth Press.

Viderman, S. (1979). The analytic space: Meaning and problems. *Psychoanalytic Quarterly*, 48: 257–291.

DONALD P. SPENCE

Introjection See IDENTIFICATION.

Involutional Depression See DEPRESSION.

Irrationality

Any account of irrationality assumes and implies a conception of rationality. Philosophical tradition typically understands it in something like this way: the capacity to recognize and to draw the relevant consequences of one's beliefs, to reconsider those that conflict with other things one holds true, and, in the practical sphere, to arrive at and act on an all-things-considered judgment about what to do in a given circumstance. This conception of rationality underlies Freud's two different models for explaining irrationality. One also finds in his works, however, a certain ideal of *thinking* against which both irrationality and rationality look rather different. This ideal is briefly discussed at the end.

The first of Freud's explanatory models is a modified version of our familiar "folk-psychology" according to which we understand actions—things done intentionally—in terms of the agent's reasons. In this version, irrationality is within the domain of the rational; irrational processes depend on rational processes, which have somehow been subverted. The second model, deriving from Freud's drive theory, invokes processes that are intrinsically irrational, or prerational. (Freud defines "*Instinkt*" or "*Trieb*"—drive—as "a concept . . . lying on the frontier between the mental and the physical" [1905, p. 168].) On this second model, "unconscious" does not merely describe some mental states or processes that could under some circumstances also be conscious; instead, a hypostatized Unconscious (Freud refers to it as "the system *Ucs.*") names a particular psychical system, governed by its own peculiar laws (1915, p. 187).

We will call the first model the reasons-explanation model and the second, the drive-theory model.

On the reasons-explanation model, we understand an action in terms of beliefs and desires that have meshed to form an intention: Odysseus wanted to listen to the Sirens yet not be seduced by them; he believed Circe when she told him he might satisfy both desires by having his sailors lash him to the mast; so he acted on the tactic she had suggested. The sense of Odysseus's orders to his sailors is apparent in the beliefs and desires that motivated him. In this way, Freud's interpretive strategy in the case histories is to find the motivating beliefs and desires of which the agent him- or herself is unconscious and which supply the missing sense in his or her behavior.

For example, Freud's patient, "the Rat Man," plays out a ritual in which he works late at night, gets up and opens the front door at midnight, returns and masturbates in front of the mirror—a ritual that to the patient himself seems senseless (1909, p. 10). Freud interprets the act against the background of the man's conscious fantasy that his dead father is still alive, together with the man's unconscious wishes simultaneously to please the father—by working late—and to defy him. In the context of certain of the patient's childhood conflicts, the act makes sense; its irrationality is a function of the perseverance of these conflicts, despite their inappropriateness to his adult life, and of the way in which the conflict is (unconsciously) handled: instead of genuinely resolving it, or moving past it, or even accepting it as irresolvable, the man acts out both the conflicting desires.

In another case, five-year-old Hans is so fearful of horses, though he has never been harmed by one, that he refuses to leave his house (1909). Freud understands the child's fear as a displacement onto horses of his fear of castration at the hands of his father, a fear that has been repressed. In a late work (1926 [1925]), Freud returns to this case, asking: Just what is the symptom? or in other words, What is it in the child's thinking that is irrational? Freud answers: not the fear of castration itself, which is appropriate to beliefs and desires that a child of Hans's age would normally have; nor the child's wish not to want to be aware of the true object of his fear, his father. The irrationality lies rather in the way in which repression of the fear displaces it onto horses.

In light of Freud's use of the reasons-explanation model, it might seem that he regards repression as an intentional act: not wanting to know what one wants or fears, one represses the knowledge. This would be a misreading of Freud; for though he relies on the reasons-explanation model, he also substantially modifies it (Hopkins, 1982; Wollheim, 1984; Cavell, 1993), as his concept "mechanisms" of defense suggests. Repression, along with more specific defense mechanisms like displacement, consists of purposive, quasi-automatic, nonintentional mental acts. One of the functions of the drive-theory model is to give a fuller picture of the arational drives in which reason, on Freud's view, is embedded.

How, for example, can something like displacement happen? As early as the *Project* (1950 [1887–1902]), Freud distinguished between a primary and a secondary psychical process. Tolerant of delayed gratification, secondary process is oriented to reality and recognizes such principles of logic as the law of noncontradiction. Neither is true of primary process, which completes in the shortest way the circuit from need, or wish, to fulfillment. This primary process "thinking" is imagistic rather than conceptual and propositional, and it is characterized by what Freud calls condensation—the fusing of a number of disparate meanings onto a single object or idea—and displacement, in which the significance belonging to one idea is given to another. (For a discussion of Freud's views about "the system *Ucs.*" and primary process, see Cavell, 1993: 161–191). In Freud's view, primary process "thinking" comes developmentally first; it surfaces throughout life in dreams (1900, ch. 7) and in the creative process; and it is also summoned into play by repression, creating symptoms like Hans's phobia. In *Inhibitions, Symptoms and Anxiety* (1926 [1925]), Freud fundamentally revises his earlier accounts of both anxiety and repression, without considering the implications of these revisions for his earlier views about primary process.

The distinction that Freud so insistently draws between conscious and unconscious mental processes has obscured an equally important contrast that cuts across it, a contrast implicit throughout his case histories and in such theoretical works as *Mourning and Melancholia* (1917 [1915]) and *Remembering, Repeating and Working-Through* (1914). The contrast is between knowing and acknowledging, "knowing in one's head" or in one part of one's mind, and knowing with the appropriate feelings; between seeing that something is the case, and fully accepting that it is. In exploring this contrast, one would need to call on many of the ideas that Freud uses to describe irrationality, for example, the "splitting of the ego" (1940 [1938]). One can assent in all sincerity to a proposition, yet hold on to many beliefs and other attitudes that it calls into question. Mourning is the long, painful process it is because the mourner is continually confronted with new, affective implications of facts that in an obvious sense he or she already knows.

On Freud's view, many thinking processes that may pass as "rational" in daily life, and even in traditional philosophy, are misuses of the thinking process, or cases in which it has been unable to come into full play. Knowing in the absence of acknowledgment, and also an intolerance of ambiguity, are such cases. Free association is both a technique for developing the capacity for thinking and, understood correctly, one of the criteria for its presence, since thinking requires the ability to make various kinds of connections among one's own experiences, connections that are not only of an inductive or a deductive nature. Inimical to thinking, at its best, is the need to exert control over what one finds or sees. In this sense, thinking requires an openness to reality.

REFERENCES

Cavell, M. (1993). *The Psychoanalytic Mind: From Freud to Philosophy*. Cambridge, Mass.: Harvard University Press.

Freud, S. (1900). *The Interpretation of Dreams*. S.E. 4 and 5.

———. (1905). *Three Essays on the Theory of Sexuality*. S.E. 7.

———. (1909). Notes upon a case of obsessional neurosis. S.E. 10: 155–318.

———. (1914). Remembering, repeating and working through. S.E. 12: 147–156.

———. (1915). The unconscious. S.E. 14: 166–215.

———. (1917) [1915]. Mourning and melancholia. S.E. 14: 243–260.

———. (1926) [1925]. *Inhibitions, Symptoms and Anxiety*. S.E. 20: 87–172.

———. (1940) [1938]. *The Splitting of the Ego in the Process of Defence*. S.E. 23: 23–273.

———. (1950) [1887–1902]. *Project for a Scientific Psychology*. S.E. 1.

Hopkins, J. (1982). *Introduction to Philosophical Essays on Freud*. R. Wollheim and J. Hopkins (eds.). New York: Cambridge University Press.

Wollheim, R. (1984). *The Thread of Life*. Cambridge, Mass.: Harvard University Press.

MARCIA CAVELL

Isolation

Freud used the term "isolation" in his earliest writings to describe clinical and social phenomena (e.g., Freud, 1894; 1900). He first used the term to refer to a defense mechanism in 1926 (Freud, 1926). In the post-Freud literature, one finds "isolation" used as often in its everyday, descriptive and allusive senses as in the more restricted, technical sense of a mechanism of defense.

Freud linked isolation as a defensive operation to the other newly named defense mechanism, "undoing," as a "motor technique of defense" (1926, p. 120). He proposed that when an unpleasantness has occurred or some act of significance to the neurosis has been performed, the person "interpolates an interval during which nothing further must happen—during which he must perceive nothing and do nothing" (ibid.). Unlike repression, isolation accomplishes defense without amnesia; "the experience is not forgotten, but instead is deprived of its affect, and its associative connections are suppressed or interrupted so that it remains as though isolated and is not reproduced in the ordinary processes of thought" (ibid.). It is a less expensive way of defending than repression.

Freud proposed that isolating is involved in the normal exercise of concentration, the faculty that permits one to keep at bay what is irrelevant or unimportant to one's central concern. It is especially useful to keep elements apart that once belonged together but that became separated in the course of psychosexual development. In preventing thoughts from connecting, Freud suggested that "the ego is obeying the taboo on touching," one of the oldest and most fundamental commands of obsessional neurosis, "because touching and physical contact are the immediate aim of the aggressive as well as the loving object-cathexes" (ibid., 121–122). By interpolating an interval between the expression of thoughts that for neurotic reasons must be kept apart, they effectively become isolated.

Anna Freud (1946, pp. 36–37, 46 ff.) noted that severing of links between associations also isolates ideas from affects. This technique of defense, characteristically used in the obsessional neuroses, gives rise to the affective blanching of much of experience and the inordinate emphasis on behavior that has magical significance in severe cases. Eissler (1959, p. 43) proposed that isolation has two forms, one in which both of the separated ideas remain in consciousness, the other in which an idea can remain in consciousness only as long as its affective charge is not. He also described several ways in which a motor act effectively can bring about isolation of ideas. Later authors, when using the term to describe a mode of defense, have tended to imply isolation of the affect from the idea to which it belongs rather than to refer to the defensive separation of ideas.

Fenichel (1945) cited instances of usage of "isolation" to refer to the separation of the sensual and tender components of sexuality and to the splitting of good and bad selves and good and bad objects.

REFERENCES

Eissler, K. (1959). On isolation. *Psychoanalytic Study of Children*, 14: 29–59.

Fenichel, O. (1945). *The Psychoanalytic Theory of Neurosis*. New York: Norton.

Freud, A. (1946). *The Ego and the Mechanisms of Defense*. New York: International Universities Press.

Freud, S. (1894). *The Neuro-Psychoses of Defense*. S.E. 3: 45–61.

———. (1900). *The Interpretation of Dreams*. S.E. 4 and 5.

———. (1926). *Inhibitions, Symptoms and Anxiety*. S.E. 20: 87–172.

HERBERT J. SCHLESINGER

Italy, and Psychoanalysis

Psychoanalysis came to Italy with the writings of Freud and through the personal relationship between Freud and two Italian psychiatrists. One was Edoardo Weiss in Triest. Weiss had direct contact with Freud's circle in Vienna and had been analyzed by Paul Federn. The other, working in the central Italian city of Teramo, was Marco Levi Bianchini.

In 1925, in Teramo, Levi Bianchini founded the Italian Psychoanalytical Society. The society was to be a scientific and cultural association. It did not require all its members to be psychoanalysts, nor was it concerned with the training of new analysts. Freud was informed of the initiative and approved of it, although the project was incomplete and, in Weiss's view, premature.

In 1932, the Italian Psychoanalytical Society was transferred to Rome and reorganized as a formal institutional group of psychoanalysts with its own training institute. The society counted among its members the first Italian psychoanalysts, who had undergone training with Weiss. This group of "pioneers" included Cesare Musatti, Nicola Perrotti, and Emilio Servadio. In 1943, they were joined by Allessandra Tomasi, from the Institute of Psychoanalysis in Berlin, who came to Italy after marrying the nobleman and writer Tomasi di Lampedusa, author of *The Leopard*. The following year the Italian Psychoanalytical Society was admitted to the International Psychoanalytical Association.

The pioneers of Italian psychoanalysis were few but active. In 1932, they founded the *Rivista di Psicoanalisi*. Emilio Servadio, a man of considerable learning, was one of the few Italians to publish in the journal *Imago*. He was a member of the editorial board of the prestigious *Enciclopedia Italiana Treccani* and author of the entry "Psychoanalysis." The intellectual climate of the country, however, was not favorable. The prevailing orientation in philosophy—and consequently in psychological, literary, and cultural circles—was idealist and thus opposed the central tenet of psychoanalysis: the existence of the unconscious. Psychoanalysis also encountered resistance from the organicist views of doctors and psychiatrists, and from the Roman Catholic Church as well. The early psychoanalysts engaged in lively debates with prominent exponents of the dominant culture. Ultimately, however, it was the political situation that was decisive. The Fascist government opposed movements with an international character and prohibited the publication the *Rivista di Psicoanalisi*. When the anti-Semitic racial laws were passed, a group of psychoanalysts, including Weiss and Servadio, were compelled to leave the country, while those who remained during the years immediately preceding the outbreak of World War II were unable to continue their work.

Once the war was over in 1945 and civil liberties were reinstated, psychoanalysts resumed their activity, growing considerably both in number and in national distribution during the 1950s and 1960s. The *Rivista di Psicoanalisi* began publishing again, thanks to the efforts of Cesari Musatti, and a second journal appeared in 1948, *Psiche*, founded by Perrotti. The Italian Psychoanalytical Society began to lead a normal, active life, organizing conferences and national congresses. Many fundamental books of psychoanalysis were translated, among them, most notably, the complete works of Sigmund Freud, edited by Musatti at the head of a team of accomplished translators, and published by Boringhieri in Turin from 1967 to 1980.

The second generation of psychoanalysts was a time marked by a ferment of initiatives and aspirations. In the 1960s, the most important authors of the British School were translated and studied. Among them, the work of W. Bion aroused considerable interest, especially his innovative approach to the psychoanalytic experience of small groups. Italian psychoanalysis laid particular emphasis on institutional situations. Not surprisingly, another author to attract considerable attention in Italy was D. W. Winnicott.

By the 1970s, psychoanalysis as a doctrine and as an instrument had achieved respectable status on the Italian cultural scene. Many analysts now teach at universities; others direct psychiatric wards in hospitals. There are numerous publications and psychoanalysis and series devoted to the field. Two congresses of the International Psychoanalytic Association were held in Rome in 1969 and 1989. Moreover, books by Italian psychoanalysts have begun to appear in translation.

The development and history of psychoanalysis in Italy has been the subject of numerous volumes. The most noteworthy of these are by David (1966), Vegetti Finzi (1982), Novelletto (1989), and Di Chiara and Pirillo (1997). Also of interest are the entries on the most important Italian psychoanalysts written by Anna Maria Accerboni for the *Dictionnaire de la Psychanalyse*, edited by de Mijolla (2001).

The psychoanalytic movement in Italy has had beneficial effects on other fields thanks to the works of psychoanalysts themselves and to the efforts of all those who have worked with them. Today, there are many groups of psychoanalytical psychotherapists, both group and individual, who have profited from the contribution of institutional psychoanalysis.

The distinguishing concerns of Italian psychoanalysis include a keen interest in narratology, hermeneutics, and epistemology. The psychoanalytic treatment of so-called serious disorders is also emphasized, as is the constant monitoring of psychiatric teams through the psychoanalytic experience of the small group in mental health clinics. Finally, psychoanalysis is widely employed and psychoanalysts are directly involved in interdisciplinary debates concerning the other sciences and the arts.

There are about 600 Freudian psychoanalysts in Italy today, gathered in two societies—the older Italian Psychoanalytical Society and the more recently formed Italian Association of Psychoanalysis. Many of these practitioners are also active in the numerous associations and schools that base their work on psychoanalysis (individual and group, child and adolescent psychotherapists).

REFERENCES

David, M. (1966). *La Psicoanalisi nella Cultura italiana*. Turin: Boringhieri.

De Mijolla, A. (2001). *Dictionnaire de la Psychanalyze*. Paris: Calman-Levy.

Di Chiara, G., and Pirillo, N. (1997). *Conversazione sulla Psicoanalisi*. Naples: Liguori.

Freud, S. (1967–1980). *Opere di Sigmund Freud*. Edizione Italiana Completa, diretta da Cesare L. Musatti. Turin: Boringhieri.

I

Novelletto, A. (ed.) (1989). *L'Italia nella Psicoanalisi (Italy in Psychoanalysis)*. Italian-English ed. Rome: Instituto della Enciclopedia Italiana.

Vegetti Finzi, S. (1982). *Storia della Psicoanalisi*. Milan: Mondadori.

GIUSEPPE DI CHIARA

J

Janet, Pierre (1859–1947)

Pierre Janet claimed that he became interested in psychology at an early age and that he tried to resolve the conflict between his interests in the natural sciences, particularly botany, and his religious sentiments, by becoming a philosopher. On enrollment at university his uncle, the philosopher Paul Janet, encouraged him to combine his philosophical studies with the study of medicine. This was at a time when psychology was escaping from philosophy, and the appeal to Janet's dual interests transformed him into a psychologist. Janet was graduated from the École Normale Supérieure in April 1881 and was placed second in the *Agrégation de Philosophie* later that year. After a short appointment in Berry, he took the chair of philosophy at the Lycée at Le Havre 1883 where he remained for more than six years until defending his doctorate in 1889.

On arrival at Le Havre, Janet decided to work on perception in relation to hallucinations for his doctorate, and asked a local physician, Dr. Joseph Gibert, for suitable subjects. Gibert offered him, instead, in their original mesmeric form, the remarkable phenomena of hypnosis, including hypnotic somnambulism with clairvoyance and hypnotism from a distance, together with Léonie, an equally remarkable magnetic subject. Janet's experiments with Léonie seemed to confirm that hypnosis could be induced from a distance, a result that was communicated by his philosopher-uncle to the Paris *Société de psychologie physiologique* in November 1885. The *société* had been founded by Jean-Martin Charcot and Charles Richet, whom Janet then met. In 1885, he conducted more such experiments under the scrutiny of the Society for Psychical Research (London). While still at Le Havre, Janet had access to hysterical patients in the local hospital, and his experiments on them and Léonie formed the major part of his doctoral dissertation, which he completed December, 1888, and defended in June, 1889, just before its simultaneous publication as *L'Automatisme psychologique*.

Janet then moved to Paris where, while teaching philosophy at Lycée Louis-le-Grand, he undertook the medical studies that he completed in July, 1893. After he had been graduated in medicine, Charcot placed the Psychological Laboratory at Salpêtrière under his supervision. By that time, his work at Le Havre led to the discovery of the role of psychological trauma in producing hysterical symptoms and the usefulness of a novel variation of hypnotic therapy to remove them. This work led to his giving a paper at Salpêtrière on March 11, 1892, devoted to the nature of hysterical anaesthesia. In it he advanced the entirely original thesis that the details of hysterical symptoms were determined by the popular idea of the organ or function affected. The anaesthesias were only the first of an interrelated series of clinical presentations covering practically the whole range of hysterical phenomena, and published later that year as *L'etat mental des hystériques*.

In 1896 or 1897 Janet gave a series of lectures on clinical psychology to colleagues and students at Salpêtrière which formed the basis for an annual series at the College de France, where he was appointed in 1902 after substituting there over some years for Théodule Ribot, the father of French psychology. These lectures were later the basis for a monumental two-volume survey of practically all forms of psychological therapy, *Medications Psychologiques*, published in 1919. Between these two publications, Janet extended his interest from hysteria to other neuroses, summarizing his theses in *Les Névroses et les idées fixes* (1898), *Les Obsessions et la psychasthénie* (1903), and *Les Névroses* (1909). In the 1920s more of his work began to reflect his interest in normal psychology, especially the psychology of religion, personality, and conduct. His later works include *De l'Angoissel à l'extase* (1926), *La Pensée intriure et ses troubles* (1927), *L'Evolution de la mémoire et la notion du temps* (1928), *L'Evolution psychologique de l'personalité* (1929), *Les Débuts de l'intelligence* (1935), and *L'Amour et la haine* (1937).

Throughout his life, Janet remained very active in clinical psychology by visiting clinics regularly, by lecturing on clinical topics, and by participating with "passionate interest" in discussion at the lectures of others.

Janet and Depth Psychology

Toward the end of the nineteenth century a new kind of psychology called "depth psychology" came into being. It is now almost forgotten that Pierre Janet's contributions to the new discipline were once regarded as being of at least the same importance as Sigmund Freud's.

Depth psychology was not a monolithic psychology, but rather a loose movement grouped around the central proposition that aspects of mental life relevant to understanding unusual mental states, including the psychopathological, were set apart from normal consciousness. The various depth psychologies were different in three fundamental ways. First, they conceptualized nonconscious mentation very differently. For some, these nonconscious mental processes were like their conscious counterparts, or even superior to them, but for others they were inferior. Second, and related to the first difference, there was profound disagreement over what was hidden in the depths. Was it another kind of self, an essentially normal but subconscious personality, or was it material disavowed by normal consciousness organized according to principles very different from those of waking life? Lastly, what caused the mentation to be lost to consciousness? Had the normal ego been unable to prevent an almost passive fragmentation of itself because of some weakness or did the loss from consciousness result from an active process the ego had initiated?

Whereas the arguments among most of those who contributed to the debate never amounted to much more than polite expressions of disagreement, the public disputation between Janet and Freud, more correctly between Janet and Freud's followers, had the characteristics of a war. Janet was eventually defeated so profoundly that even as late as a few years ago it proved impossible to find a publisher anywhere, including France, for a volume of essays marking the one-hundredth anniversary of the appearance of his seminal *L'Automatisme psychologique*.

Hysterical Symptoms from Memories

Prior to the work of Janet and Freud, little attention seems to have been paid to the possibility that hysterical symptoms might be caused by unconscious memories of traumatic events. Although the notion of unconscious mentation was well known, and it was widely believed that hysterical symptoms could be caused by the patient deliberately withholding knowledge from others, especially guilty knowledge, there does not seem to be a literature of any size relating those two notions to one another or to psychopathology.

The first case of hysteria that Janet attributed to a traumatic event is that of Lucie, reported in three papers between 1886 and 1888. Lucie's hallucinatory terrors were traced to a sudden fright she had had at the age of nine years. At that time a second personality (Adrienne) began to form and Lucie's symptoms appeared each time Adrienne "emerged."

Marie, a second case of Janet's, suffered from recurrent hysterical crises with deliria, hallucinations, and violent bodily contortions beginning two days after the onset of each of her menstrual periods. Concurrently with the attack, menstruation was suppressed. Janet hypnotized her and found her first menstruation to have been an entirely unexpected event to which she reacted with shame. She made an attempt to stop the menstrual flow by immersing herself in cold water. Menstruation ceased, but she then had a severe attack of shivering followed by several days of delirium. Menstruation did not recur until five years later and, when it did, the symptoms came with it. Marie also had minor hallucinatory attacks of terror, which were repetitions of feelings she had experienced after seeing an old woman fall down a flight of stairs and die, as well as a left-sided facial anaesthesia and left-eye blindness, which had appeared after she had been forced to sleep with a child who had impetigo on the left side of her face.

Janet treated Lucie by giving Adrienne, the secondary personality, the direct suggestion under hypnosis not to have hallucinatory attacks, whereupon Lucie, the primary personality, was freed of the symptom. Marie's treatment was slightly different. Janet decided to modify the memory of the immersion by age-regressing her to thirteen and convincing her that her period had lasted three days and been normal. He similarly "returned" her to the time of the old woman's death and changed the memory from one of her being killed to one of her merely stumbling. Likewise he regressed her to the time when she had had to share her bed with the child with impetigo and made her believe the child was nice and without impetigo. All the symptoms disappeared after Janet had so effaced or removed the memories from the somnambulistic consciousness.

Janet and the Restriction of Consciousness

In 1886, in separate papers, both Alfred Binet and Pierre Janet described how a secondary consciousness formed. Experiences occurring in a somnambulistic state formed a focus to which later experiences occurring in the same state became connected. The term Binet and Janet used for the totality of the memories occurring in this other state was "condition seconde." Its fully developed form was a dual consciousness, or double conscience, and it had been a secondary consciousness of that type which had been the repository of Lucie's and Marie's memories. Whenever the secondary consciousness returned completely, it necessarily carried the ideas appropriate to it. If the secondary state manifested itself less than fully, its ideas might simply appear to intrude into the primary consciousness. Where the memories were of events that had caused symptoms, the symptoms would also return.

Charcot's experiments producing symptoms under hypnosis were at one with this explanation. Direct verbal suggestion generated symptoms having the same characteristics as the hysterical. Charcot attributed the similarity to the peculiar consequence of hypnosis that a suggested idea or a coherent group of associated ideas could lodge in the mind "like a parasite" out of the control of the collection of ideas constituting the ego. He had also sometimes caused paralyses by unexpectedly hitting his hypnotized subjects on the arm or leg. Charcot thought the slight traumatism produced a sense of numbness and a slight indication of paralysis. As a consequence of these sensations, the idea of paralysis arose and the rudimentary paralysis then became real through autosuggestion. Charcot's chain of reasoning required there be a similarity between the hypnotic and real traumatic states. He argued that emotion, nervous shock, or "intense cerebral commotion" experienced at the moment of a real trauma annihilated the ego in the same way as in hypnosis.

But what of those many hysterical symptoms which did not arise from trauma? To explain them Janet proposed that a restriction of consciousness had produced a defect in what he called "personal perception." According to Janet, elementary sensations produced by stimulation of the sense organs were subconscious, isolated, and lacked integration with the idea of personality. These elementary phenomena had to be synthesized into perceptions and then assimilated into the personality before one could truly say "I feel." Janet proposed the term "personal perception" for this type of perception and claimed it led to a more complete consciousness than did the isolated elementary sensations. Hysterical symptoms formed when what Janet called "the extent of the field of consciousness" was not wide enough to allow all the sensations to be assimilated in the act of personal perception. Patients who did not attend to their sensations in one or other modality would not be able to recall them as part of their personal perceptions and would become anaesthetic if, for example, sensations of touch were not attended to.

Janet accounted for the sudden development of symptoms as well as the development of symptoms other than anaesthesia in the same way. He proposed that traumatic situations produced a similar restriction of the field of consciousness. Ideas occurring in it were cut off from the dominant consciousness and formed a second consciousness that intruded its contents into the primary consciousness as symptoms.

Janet and Freud

There were marked similarities in the contributions that Janet and Freud made to the central ideas of depth psychology, but Janet should be given much more credit for them:

1. Both Janet (and Delboeuf) reported on their pioneering use of hypnotic suggestion to modify or remove pathogenic memories in early 1889, before Freud incorporated it into his version of "Breuer's method."
2. Janet was responsible for the thesis that ideas determined the details of hysterical symptoms. Until Janet formulated it, Freud had been able to characterize hysterical symptoms only negatively;

after it he adopted Janet's positive characterization as part of his own etiological framework. He later denied Janet any credit for the notion.

3. Janet was one of those who helped formulate dissociation theory and one of the first to use it to explain the formation of hysterical symptoms. Freud's (and Breuer's) early explanations also drew on the central concepts of dissociation theory, as did Freud's early formulation of repression in hysteria. For him the splitting of consciousness in the form of double conscience was always present and was he said, explicitly concurring with Binet and Janet, "the basic phenomenon" of this neurosis.

4. Although Breuer had noted the role of traumatic memories as causes of hysteria some five years before Janet, he was unable to explain their mode of action. It seems unlikely that he tried to do so until well after concluding his therapeutic work with Anna O. and after Janet and Delboeuf had implicated memories in the pathogenesis of hysteria in 1886, possibly after Freud returned from Paris in that year.

Freud's early theory and practice thus owes a greater debt to Janet than is usually acknowledged. Eventually the theoretical and practical differences between Janet and Freud became very marked. In two of the three differences considered here, Janet was clearly correct. The other, the apparent advantage of repression over personal perception, is not well founded.

Janet and Freud both commenced with the belief that psychological phenomena of the kinds emerging in hypnotic experiments were not affected by those expectations of the investigator that the subject had discerned, and were determined solely by processes internal to the subject. In Janet's view the processes were psychological, in Freud's they were physiological. Janet eventually realized his error and came to the conclusion that external determinants like expectations were at least as powerful as internal. Freud not only never altered his position, but went on to base his methods of gathering data in the therapeutic situation on it.

Emotion and abreaction in the formation and removal of symptoms was important only to Freud. In the very situations where Janet (and Delboeuf) might have been expected to confirm them, they failed even to observe the effect of abreaction. It is also worth remembering that the affective interpretations of Breuer's case of Anna O. and of Freud's early cases are actually reinterpretations. Emotion is not among the necessary and sufficient conditions for either symptom formation or symptom removal.

Freud's mechanism of repression is not very different logically from Janet's mechanism of personal perception. One is uncharacterized and the other rests on uncharacterized theoretical terms. There is therefore little basis for choosing between them.

REFERENCES

Ellenberger, H. (1970). *The Discovery of the Unconscious: The History and Evolution of Dynamic Psychiatry.* New York: Basic Books (especially Chapter 6).

Janet, P. (1930). Psychological autobiography. In C. Murchison (ed.). *A History of Psychology in Autobiography*, vol. 1: 123–133. Worcester, Mass.: Clark University Press.

Jones, E. (1953). *The Life and Work of Sigmund Freud*, vol. 1. New York: Basic Books.

Macmillan, M. B. (1997). *Freud Evaluated: The Completed Arc.* Cambridge, Mass.: MIT Press (especially Chapters 1–4 and 6).

MALCOLM MACMILLAN

Japan, and Psychoanalysis

Unlike other Asian countries, Japan offered a firm footing to Freud's ideas. A small group of Japanese analysts can boast of a psychoanalytic association for training and teaching, some acceptance of Freudian psychology in medical schools and other university departments, and some historical links to Freud himself.

As with China, papers on psychoanalysis began appearing in Japan in the second decade of the twentieth century, ahead of any translation of Freud's works. Marui Kiyoyasu, who had studied under Adolph Meyer at Johns Hopkins University in Baltimore in 1918, offered the first formal instruction in psychoanalysis at Tohoku University. He met some resistance from the medical establishment, which held the orthodox view, inherited from Germany, that mental dysfunction was an "illness" for which physical forms of treatment were appropriate. He himself did not feel qualified to teach therapy and confined himself to theory. His student Kosawa Heisaku, frustrated by this, visited Vienna in 1932 to seek training from Freud himself. Freud took him under his wing, but Heisaku was eventually trained by Richard Sterba and supervised by Ernst Federn. He left Vienna the following year to return to Japan to open a clinic in Tokyo. Ironically, in that same year, his teacher, Marui Kiyoyasu, visited Vienna, was granted an interview with Freud, and was also supervised by Federn. Marui asked Freud for permission to set up the first Japanese branch of the International Psychoanalytic Association, only to be told that Freud had already granted the honor to another—Yabe Yaekichi—a psychologist who had visited Vienna in 1930. Yabe, in conjunction with a literary scholar, Ohtsuki Kenji, established the Tokyo Institute of Psychoanalysis, which comprised literary scholars and interested lay people. Marui founded the Sendai branch of the International Psychoanalytic Association, and its members were all medical practitioners.

From their inception until the early fifties, the two groups were essentially rivals—a situation that Freud inadvertently initiated by allowing Yabe's group to proceed even after Marui had made an early overture in the late 1920s (Blowers and Yang, 1997). Each group published a journal and both groups set about translating all of Freud's works and bringing out at almost the same time through different publishing houses two rival sets of translations. Marui's medical group translated primarily from German, Ohtsuki's literary circle from English. As with the translation of Freud's works into Chinese, there were no standard terms, and a certain free rein in the use of symbols matched to either the meaning or the sound of the foreign term prevailed. In Japanese, the sound/meaning distinction has been achieved through the development of *kana*, or writing systems that express the sounds of words, and *kanji*, or characters that originated in Chinese that express the meaning of terms. While these systems can be used separately, they are often used in combination, and have been for Freud's translations. In spite of some differences in the relative use of kana over kanji among various translators, on the whole the rival translations of Freud's works bore a good deal of similarity in their attempts to transcribe the meanings of psychoanalytic terms. Some differences were inevitable, given that some translations were taken from English versions while others came directly from German.

By the early fifties, Marui's group effectively amalgamated with a study group, begun in the post–World War II period by Kosawa, to form the Japanese Psychoanalytic Society for medically qualified and practicing analysts, and the Psychoanalytic Association for lay analysts and other interested parties (Blowers and Yang, in press). For a number of years following Kosawa's death in 1969, training analyses were not conducted in Japan, which

may account for the small number of analysts. In 1996, there were eighteen active members and thirteen associate members (Fisher, 1996). Other reasons for the small number of analysts point to a clash of Eastern and Western fundamental understandings of the individual. It has been argued that because of the rigidly hierarchical nature of Japanese society with its stress on the need for individuals to live harmoniously with others rather than develop individual freedom and independence, a therapy stressing autonomy becomes unviable. This has echoes in Buddhist philosophy, which has influenced many systems of thought in Japan, and, notably, the work of Ohtsuki and Kosawa. The latter developed his own cultural variant on the Oedipus theme—the Ajase complex (Okonogi, 1995)—much to the indifference of Freud, to whom he first presented this idea.

The counter to this view is that analysis in Japan *is* possible, although the terms of the analytic relationship are different from those in the West. The less clearly defined ego boundaries between analysts and their clients (a "we" rather than an "I" and "you") and a mutual sensitivity to the value of the demands and requirements of the other makes communication possible and allows for the expression of conflict and the possibility of change (Roland, 1988). However, the prevailing stigma attached to the reporting of mental illness in Japan makes it difficult, if not impossible, to discuss it with candor. This presents an obstacle not only to psychoanalysis in particular, but to the open discussion of mental disorders and their treatment in general.

Although Kosawa continued to teach and train analysts with his own blend of psychoanalysis and Buddhism, one of his students, Doi Takeo, trained at the Menninger Clinic, was to make the major impact on the general field of Japanese psychotherapy with his work on *amae*, the Japanese cultural concept of dependence, and lead it away from psychoanalytic orthodoxy, although that is still practiced today by a small, dedicated group led by Okonogi Keigo (Doi, 1973).

REFERENCES

Blowers, G. H., and Yang, S. H. C. (1997). Freud's *Deshi*: The coming of psychoanalysis to Japan. *Journal of the History of the Behavioural Sciences*, 33: 115–126.

———. (In press). Ohtsuki Kenji and the beginnings of lay analysis in Japan. *International Journal of Psychoanalysis*.

Doi, T. (1973). *The Anatomy of Dependence*. Tokyo: Kodansha International.

Fisher, C. P. (1996). Panel report: Psychoanalysis in the Pacific Rim. *International Journal of Psychoanalysis*, 77: 373–377.

Okonogi, K. "The Ajase Complex." Paper read at the 39th International Psychoanalytic Conference, San Francisco. August 1995.

Roland, A. (1988). *In Search of Self in India and Japan: Towards a Cross-cultural Psychology.* Princeton: Princeton University Press.

                                                GEOFFREY H. BLOWERS

Jewishness, Freud's See JUDAISM, AND FREUD.

Jokes and Humor

Freud was always interested in Jewish humor and started assembling his own collection of Jewish jokes before the end of the nineteenth century. An important influence in his life at that time was Theodor Lipps, a Munich professor of philosophy. Freud heard Lipps present a paper on the unconscious at a psychology congress in 1897. A later reading of Lipps's 1898 work, "Komik und Humor," encouraged Freud to think about the possibility of producing his own study in this area (1905, p. 9 footnote).

In 1905, Freud published two major works, *Three Essays on the Theory of Sexuality* and *Jokes and Their Relation to the Unconscious.* The two works were evidently written simultaneously. According to Ernest Jones, Freud kept the manuscripts on adjoining tables, writing now in one, now in the other, as the mood took him. "It was the only occasion I know of when Freud combined the writing of two essays so close together, and it shows how nearly related the two themes were in his mind" (Jones, 1964: 315).

The immediate source of inspiration leading Freud to commence a book on jokes was Wilhelm Fliess. Reading proofs for *The Interpretation of Dreams* (1900), Fliess remarked that Freud's dream analyses were surprisingly full of jokes. Freud looked into this, began to investigate jokes, and found that their essence lay in the inner processes involved. He wrote: "these were the same as the means used in the 'dream-work'—that is to say condensation, displacement, the representation of a thing by its opposite or by something very small, and so on" (1925, pp. 65–66).

Freud was intrigued by the resemblance between "dream-work" and "jokework," although he went on to draw distinctions between them as well. A dream is more disguised and tends to take over a passive ego. A joke can also come from nowhere, like a dream, but the ego is more in charge of the situation and quickly regains access to secondary process thinking. "Dreams," Freud wrote, "serve predominantly for the avoidance of unpleasure, jokes for the attainment of pleasure; but all our mental activities converge in these two aims" (1905, p. 180).

Freud recognized that good humor produces a few moments of highly valued pleasure, a brief triumph of the psyche over the forces of repression or the pain of reality. He separated out "innocent" jokes, puns, and jests from what he called "tendentious" jokes, implying in the latter the presence of an obscene or hostile purpose.

A joke arises involuntarily; we do not know beforehand what joke we are going to make. A train of thought is dropped and enters the preconscious. There it is given over momentarily to unconscious revision, and the joke then emerges spontaneously. After the train of thought is dropped, an "indefinable feeling" is experienced, which Freud compared to an "absence." There is a sudden release of intellectual tension, and all at once the joke is there, "ready-clothed in words." The whole sequence enables a partial, transient, and involuntary release of some impulse or feeling ordinarily, or currently, repressed.

Freud concluded that with innocent jokes, puns, and jests, the humorous pleasure connects with the reduction in psychical expenditure that results from a temporary lessening in the need for repression. An example (1905, p. 16): A poet introduces a character who tells of how he sat beside Baron Rothschild, "and he treated me quite as his equal—quite famillionairely."

Freud shows how this joke conveys, in an amusing way, something not quite pleasant evoked by a rich man's condescension.

Whereas such an "innocent" joke raises no more than a smile, an effective "tendentious" joke usually produces laughter. In Freud's view, the slight pleasure deriving from the verbal technique of a joke is a form of fore-pleasure. Acting as an incentive bonus, it can relax the hearer and thereby prepare that person to experience some deeper sexual or aggressive prompting ordinarily kept hidden. In this way, it facilitates new pleasure by momentarily lifting suppressions and repressions, enabling a more orgasmic release of affect in the form of laughter. An example (1905, p. 74): Two somewhat unscrupulous businessmen have amassed a large fortune and are trying to invade high society. They have their portraits painted by a celebrated artist, arrange a large evening party, and lead the most influential connoisseur and art critic up to where the two portraits are hanging side by side, in order to extract his admiring judgment. He studies the portraits for a long time, and then shaking his head, points to the gap between the pictures and quietly asks, "But where's the Savior?"

Freud returned to the subject of humor in his 1927 paper (1927, pp. 162–163). Here he points out that we already know the superego as a severe master, but in humor we find something very different—a superego comforting an intimidated ego by repudiating reality and serving up an illusion. He adds that if the superego tries in this way to console the ego and protect it from suffering, this does not contradict its origin in the parental agency.

In the paper, Freud also states that humor is not resigned but rebellious. He sees humor as a triumph of narcissism, "a victorious assertion of the ego's invulnerability," a triumphant reassertion of one's narcissism via an adaptive regression. Freud was clearly influenced here by his interest in the history of Jewish humor and its gradual evolution as an adaptation to centuries of persecution. Reik (1962) and Meghnagi (1991), among others, have developed further this theme of Jewish humor as a creative form of pseudomasochistic self-assertion.

REFERENCES

Christie, G. (1994). Some psychoanalytic aspects of humour. *International Journal of Psychoanalysis*, 75: 479–489.

Freud, S. (1905). *Jokes and their Relation to the Unconscious.* S.E. 8: 3–237.

———. (1925) *An Autobiographical Study.* S.E. 20: 7–74.

———. (1927). *Humour.* S.E. 21: 161–163.

Jones, E. (1953). *Sigmund Freud. Life and Work*, vol. 3. London: Penguin Books, 1964

Meghnagi, D. (1991). Jewish Humour on Psychoanalysis. *International Review of Psychoanalysis*, 18: 223–228.

Reik, T. (1962). *Jewish Wit.* New York: Gamut Press.

GEORGE L. CHRISTIE

Jones, Ernest (1879–1958)

Jones was born in Gowerton Galles, Wales. Upon finishing his studies at the University of Cardiff, he became interested in medical studies, went to London, and became a pupil of J. Hughlings Jackson. Together with his friend W.B. Louis Trotter, he became interested in Freud in 1906 and started studying German to read Freud's work, particularly *The Interpretation of Dreams*. For various reasons, he emigrated to Canada. He met

Freud at the Salzburg Congress in 1906, where he gave his first, and perhaps his most famous, paper, "On Rationalization in Everyday Life." Immediately after the meeting in Salzburg, Jones met Freud in Vienna together with Brill. It was during these meetings that Jones and Brill discussed with Freud the problems related to the English translation of Freud's works.

After spending five years in Toronto, Jones returned to London and started practicing psychoanalysis in 1912, after founding the American Psychoanalytic Association and contributing to the diffusion of Freud's work in America. In 1913, at Freud's suggestion, Jones had a brief personal analysis with Sándor Ferenczi in Budapest that lasted two months but had deep personal repercussions in Jones, who being already a difficult character, although an extremely gifted organizer and skillful politician, remained ambivalent toward Ferenczi for the rest of his life. In 1919, Jones founded the British Psychoanalytic Society, and in 1920 he became president of the International Psychoanalytic Association (IPA). He remained in the latter office during two crucial periods of the history of psychoanalysis: from 1920 until 1924 and from 1934 until 1949.

In 1920, Jones founded the *International Journal of Psychoanalysis*, which, after the World War II, became the official organ of the IPA. It was in the 1920s that Jones, together with J. Riviere, A. and J. Strachey, J. Rickman, and others, started the project of creating a systematic, standard translation of Freud's work into English. Jones was the chairman of the famous Glossary Committee, which established the rules of Freud's translation; he published the first English glossary of Freud's work in 1924.

Through all his activities, Jones wanted to become the most prestigious and scientific representative of psychoanalysis in the English-speaking countries, trying to counteract the translations of Freud done in America, particularly those by A. Brill. In spite of Freud's original perplexities toward him, Jones gradually managed to persuade Freud of his capacities and to obtain the exclusive rights to translate Freud's works into English.

The publication of the five volumes of Freud's collected works by the Hogarth Press in London during the 1920s and 1930s was carefully controlled by Jones, who also partially translated them. Jones has to be considered the most responsible for the "scientificization" and "medicalization" of Freud's language as translated into English. These five volumes were the starting point for the standard edition of Freud's work, mainly translated and edited by J. Strachey and his collaborators after World War II. However, the original idea for the standard edition came from Jones, who incidentally went on discussing with J. Strachey the various problems of translating Freud's language into English until the end of his life.

It was also during the early 1920s that Jones created the International Psychoanalytic Library, always in collaboration with the Hogarth Press, founded by Leonard and Virginia Woolf. Jones was also instrumental in helping Melanie Klein settle in London in 1926. Jones aided her in developing her ideas about child development. He also had in mind a cultural hegemonic project: that of creating a British school of psychoanalysis based on the discoveries coming from child analysis as theorized and practiced by Klein, with its own theoretical and clinical identity *vis-à-vis* Vienna, Budapest, Berlin, and the United States. Of course, he had to face the criticisms of Freud, who supported his daughter Anna against Klein.

During the 1920s and 1930s, Jones published several clinical, theoretical papers on psychoanalysis. And he was instrumental in showing the usefulness in applying psychoanalysis to literature, the social sciences, and politics. Of fundamental importance was his essay on Hamlet, the final version of which was published in 1951 but the origins of which date to the beginnings of Jones's career as a psychoanalyst. Extremely important, besides his paper on the theory of symbolism (1916), were his papers on aggression (although he never accepted Freud's ideas on the death instinct) and his papers on female sexuality (1927, 1935), written more and more under the influence of Klein. All his papers were collected in several editions, including his "Papers on Psychoanalysis," originally published in 1912.

Jones played a fundamental role as president of the IPA, particularly in the discussions of lay analysis in the late 1920s. He supported lay analysis but with enormous caution, owing partly to the pressures of the British medical and scientific establishment during this period. Nevertheless, from the beginning of the British Society of Psychoanalysis, Jones accepted several nonmedically trained analysts, including women, besides supporting Melanie Klein and Anna Freud.

In spite of his authoritarian manner, his manipulative way of handling institutional matters, and his competitiveness with Freud's other pupils, in particular Sándor Ferenczi and Otto Rank, Jones's golden years as

president of the IPA were during the 1930s and 1940s, starting when Hitler came to power in Germany and the German Jewish psychoanalysts emigrated to escape Nazi persecution. Jones tried to help all these refugees; yet some of his political compromises with those non-Jewish psychoanalysts who supported the Nazis regime in Berlin and other cities in order to go on teaching and practicing psychoanalysis are rather questionable. It was nevertheless because of Jones that Freud and his family managed to be persuaded to emigrate to England in 1938, when they had to leave Vienna owing to the *Anschluss* between Austria and Germany. Jones was also of enormous help to many other Viennese and Hungarian analysts who had to leave their countries.

After World War II, having played a pivotal role during the famous Anna Freud–Melanie Klein Controversial Discussions, which lasted in London from 1941 to 1945, Jones tried to mediate between A. Freud's followers and Klein's. Jones gradually retired from the institutional life of the British Psychoanalytic Society and of the IPA. Yet besides supporting the publication of James Strachey's standard edition of Freud's work into English, Jones started what probably can be considered his magnum opus, his major contribution to psychoanalysis as a clinical, theoretical, and cultural discipline—the biography of Sigmund Freud. This work, written and published between 1953 and 1957, became a cornerstone in biographical studies even outside of psychoanalysis. Owing partly to the enormous control exercised over him by Anna Freud, Jones's *Sigmund Freud: Life and Work* in three volumes is inevitably a partisan biography at times. Yet because of his prodigious capacity for work and his total dedication to his task, Jones created one of the most important and even moving intellectual monuments to the work and life of Freud, by one of the most important representatives of the first generation of Freud's pupils and followers. Jones's ashes are interred at the crematorium of Golders Green not far from those of Sigmund Freud.

RICARDO STEINER

Judaism, and Freud

Freud was quite ambivalent about his Judaism. He was intensely proud of his Jewish ethnicity, but when it came to religion, he exercised the obverse side of his identity with utter rebelliousness and antipathy. What may have started with hostility to the religion of his ancestors spread to all religions. Most of his intellectual and emotional life was devoted to separating the "religious" from "religion," making the former the foundation stone of humans' relationship to one another. The pursuit and translation into action of ethical values totally severed from their anchor in formal, institutional religion became the goal toward which all therapeutic activity should strive.

Sigmund Freud (1856–1939) was born into what now appears to have been an Orthodox Jewish family (Rice, 1990, 1994; Yerushalmi, 1991). His parents had originally come from Galicia, a part of the Austrian Empire that was perceived by the intelligentsia as being primitive, unlettered, impoverished, and uncultured. They emigrated westward to the city of Freiberg in what is now the Czech Republic. This move was in large measure due to financial considerations as well as to the dramatic political changes that resulted from the Emancipation Act of 1848. Much of what was strictly prohibited was now permitted. Among other onerous restrictions in place until 1848, Jews were not allowed to dwell permanently in cities, attend public schools, have professions, or hire non-Jewish servants. Jews were also subject to a special tax solely for reasons of their religious and ethnic identity. Emancipation was further elaborated upon when the liberals assumed political power to the point where the civil rights granted were almost equal to those of the non-Jew. The Austro-Hungarian Empire, formed in 1868, would nevertheless still not permit any Jew, for example, to be appointed to a full-time, paying position in any government institution, be it in the university, diplomatic area, judiciary, or any other civil service entity without conversion to Christianity. Thus, it turned out that more than one-half of the medical faculty were Jewish but they all had to have converted to Christianity before being appointed. The same percentage pertained to the judiciary (Beller, 1989). Physicians with scientific achievement, like Freud, could be appointed to the ultimate honorary rank of professor extraordinarius, but no Jew could ever attain the rank of professor ordinarius, a full-time, salaried position with teaching responsibilities. If one may be permitted a pun, for a nonconverted Jew in Austria to be extraordinary was easy but to be ordinary was impossible.

The near-total emancipation of 1868 had little effect upon the prevailing anti-Semitism. However, Jews were now able to enjoy a degree of comfort and prosperity hitherto unknown to them. Freud's parents moved to Vienna in 1860 and their son, Sigmund, soon realized that he was up against a glass ceiling of religious bigotry. Austria-Hungary was officially a Roman Catholic empire and the Catholic hierarchy held a tight grip on all aspects of everyday life. It is not difficult to imagine the resentment that Freud, confronted by a religious authoritarianism that restricted his upward mobility, must have accumulated since childhood. Jewish students at the university suffered the indignity of verbal and physical abuse by their anti-Semitic classmates. Their shouts of "*Juden heraus*" (Jews, get out) remained loud and clear until the outbreak of World War II. Freud was also witness to the vicious scapegoating of Viennese Jews by the gentile community. The stock market crash of 1873, for example, was blamed on Jewish bankers. Jews were perceived as perverse, disease-ridden, and malformed human creatures whose males even menstruated. Whatever feelings of inferiority and underlying perversity that the prejudiced Austrian may have had was projected onto the demonized Jew. This defense mechanism allowed the persecutor to get rid of those very same qualities, wishes, impulses, and fantasies that he unconsciously felt to be residing within himself.

This prejudice permeated the thinking and behavior of many non-Jewish intellectuals as well. As noted, with political emancipation came a massive influx of eastern European Jews into Vienna and subsequently a huge increase in the student population at the university. Jewish medical students, however, were not yet home free. For example, the famous surgeon Theodor Billroth was commissioned to do a study of medical education at the university and subsequently issued a report that further inflamed the passions of the anti-Semites (Klein, 1985; Rice, 1990). His romantic perception of the German character led to the conclusion that people such as the Jews could not be sensitive to the influence of the medieval romanticism upon which German sensibilities were based and that they could not possibly share in the beauty of the German Middle Ages.

The overwhelming presence of such a political and intellectual climate had its effect on the ambitious, upwardly mobile Freud. It led to an aversion toward religion that was to remain with him for the rest of his life. Pride in his Jewish ethnicity did lead to his active participation in the secular brotherhood of the B'nai Brith, a fraternal organization of like-minded Jews. However, he remained distinctly aloof from any religious affiliation or activity.

Like most second-generation progeny, Freud resented nearly everything associated with his father. Those whose origins lay in eastern Europe, like his parents, were, as noted, considered primitive and uncultured by the established middle class. The elder Freud's poverty and lack of formal secular education and cultural acclimation certainly did not augment his son's self-esteem. Judaism, for Sigmund Freud, became the obstacle to full acceptance by the non-Jewish community. For most of his life Freud did not desist from being critical of religion. Though his feelings about Catholicism may have motivated much of his criticism of religion, his father's version of Judaism was not spared.

From a psychoanalytic perspective, whenever a personal, aggressive rebellion occurs, be it on a religious or a social level, an essential ingredient of such aggression is the underlying ambivalent emotional conflicts felt toward one's parents or their surrogates. In the sphere of religion, Freud's aversive confrontation with the body of its theological beliefs and ritual practices had much to do with his feelings toward the Judaism of his own father. Such an idiosyncratic approach obviously does not necessarily negate the validity of the arguments set forth in the actual criticisms of religion.

Freud's rebellious journey began, as it frequently does, in adolescence. At about the age of twelve, he remembered, with a seeming intense vividness, his father telling him that when he was a young man taking a Sabbath stroll, a gentile man came over, cursed him, and knocked his hat off his head. The elder Freud thought it the better part of wisdom not to confront his attacker and submitted to his humiliation. In a letter Freud wrote to his friend in his adolescence, he was highly critical of an Orthodox Jewish family that he encountered on the train back from his visit with him in Freiburg. The descriptive abuse of this family that Freud verbalized in this letter would have made an anti-Semite proud. Just prior to his marriage, he mentioned to his friend and mentor, Josef Breuer, that he would have preferred to convert to Christianity rather than go through with a religious wedding ceremony. Breuer very quickly and easily dissuaded him from such a rebellious course of action.

A brief glance at Freud's experiences with Judaism reveals a familiarity with religion that would give some meaningful content to his aversiveness. It was a requirement in the Austro-Hungarian school system that instruction in their own religion be given to all students from ages six through eighteen. The curriculum for this program has been found, and if Freud was the best student in his class, which he was, he must have imbibed a good dose of knowledge pertaining to the subject (Rice, 1990). His father, Jacob, was a student of the Talmud, and Freud himself owned complete sets of the twenty-one volumes of the Vilna edition of the Talmud in both the original Aramaic and German translation, though it is most unlikely that he ever studied the Aramaic version. He remained close to his teacher of religion, Samuel Hammerschlag, and his scientific mentor and initial collaborator, Josef Breuer, one of the most prominent physicians in Vienna and a man most active in the Jewish community. Freud's wife, Martha, was the granddaughter of the chief rabbi (Orthodox) of Hamburg, and she herself was strictly Orthodox in belief and ritual practice until her marriage to Freud. Upon the occasion of Freud's thirty-fifth birthday his father wrote a most loving poem, in Hebrew, for the occasion (Rice, 1990). Much of the content of this poem was taken from various parts of the Bible and Talmud.

In 1907, Freud published his first essay on religion, *Obsessive Actions and Religious Practices*, in which he provided a striking similarity between religious ritual observance and the compulsive, ritualistic behavior of the obsessive-compulsive neurotic. In *Totem and Taboo* (1912), he utilized the findings of both psychoanalysis and current anthropology to trace the origins of religion and morality back to its earliest roots, where rebellious sons slew the tyrannical father so that they could have access, hitherto forbidden, to the women of the primal horde. This slaying and subsequent cannibalization was a primal crime that was to be repeated in different guises and disguises down through the millennia. The totem animal, which subsequently took the place of the primal father, was destined for the same fate: it, too, was slain and eaten during an annual religious festival. This trend eventually culminated in the crucifixion of Jesus. The plot line remained the same but the scenery and cast of characters underwent constant alteration. This reenactment is seen clearly in the ritual of Holy Communion in which the body and blood of Christ are symbolically swallowed. Freud's most extensive criticism of religion was expressed in *The Future of an Illusion* (1927) and, to a lesser extent, in *Civilization and Its Discontents* (1930). During the last decade of his life, he journeyed back to his own religious roots in *Moses and Monotheism* (1939), in which he elaborated upon what he believed to be the origin of Judaism.

J

Moses and Monotheism is, at its core, an autobiographical love story between father and son but dressed in aggressive garb. According to Freud, Judaism had its origins in the monotheism of the iconoclastic Egyptian pharaoh, Akhenaton. Freud dethroned the biblical Moses from the position of Judaism's most favored native son and made him a non-Jewish Egyptian who was a prominent member of its aristocracy. This Moses took it upon himself to take charge of the unlettered, enslaved, and primitive Hebrews and founded a new religion based on a belief in an invisible and intangible monotheistic godhead. The centrality of this theological revolution was the promulgation of ethical values and an enhancement of intellectuality and spirituality. This primal prophet, Moses, was subsequently slain and probably cannibalized by the rebellious, idol-worshipping Hebrews during their sojourn in the desert. This was the ultimate price that Moses paid for his unrelenting efforts to turn the Hebrews away from their idol-worshipping behavior and all that it entailed. He was replaced by another Moses, this time a Hebrew, who stressed ritual worship rather than ethics. This endured for almost a half millennium until the arrival of the Hebrew prophets whose endeavor was to return the Jews to the religion of the first Moses.

The subtext of *Moses and Monotheism*, in the light of psychoanalytic knowledge, reveals an identity by Freud with Moses and, at times, between his own father and Moses. There is also an identity between the perceived primitiveness of the Galician Jews, of which Freud's parents were representative, and the horde of Egyptian Hebrews.

"But it is not easy to guess what could induce an aristocratic Egyptian [Moses]—a prince, perhaps, or a priest or high official—to put himself at the head of a crowd of immigrant foreigners at a backward level of civilization and to leave his country with them. The well-known contempt felt by the Egyptians for foreign nationals makes such a proceeding particularly unlikely" (Freud, 1939: 18).

Freud's father died in 1896 but, as with all of us, his incorporated image endured within Freud's mind for a lifetime. One need not wonder how the elder Freud would have reacted to his son's conception of the origins of his religion.

In *Moses and Monotheism*, Freud tried to discover some of the roots of anti-Semitism in Christianity itself. The unconscious origins of this unyielding prejudice were felt to revolve around the castration complex, a conflict that inheres in all of us. However, it was the idiosyncratic translation into conscious fantasy and reality of this universal conflict that particularized its unique expression, in all its perversity, in a "religious" framework. That framework was, down through the centuries, fleshed out by Christian theology and by cultural and political influences. Freud felt that it would not have been difficult to bring together a group of people, i.e., potential converts to Christianity, by the early Christian fathers so long as there remained another group of people, in this instance the Jews, who can then become the object of their hatred or aggressiveness. Saint Paul preached universal love, but for those not part of the Christian community there was only extreme intolerance. The Jew became a personification of the Devil and thus was facilitated the discharge of the believer's malevolence. As Freud noted, this technique served a most significant role in their psychic economy, thus giving this hatred its enduring quality.

The Catholic Church in Austria represented to Freud the insuperable obstacle to complete Jewish integration. The church had imposed a glass ceiling beyond which high-achieving Jews like Freud could not penetrate. This religious hatred toward the Jews stemmed from several sources. One was the theological origins of Christianity and the other was the psychodynamic constellation of the Christian believer. The former is made obvious by blaming the Jews for the crucifixion of their Savior. The latter has been expressed in projected form in that all the bigot's warded-off unconscious fantasies and desires are attributed to the Jews, e.g., effeminacy, perversity, murder, deceitfulness, and all the traits that constitute the satanic aspects of the human species.

One can justifiably conclude that Freud was indeed, to use Gay's apt phrase, a pugilistic atheist (1987). His hostility to organized religion, including his own, knew no bounds. Yet, if one takes a penetrating look through this barrage of anger, then quite a different picture emerges. Freud opposed any return to paganism and the focus upon ritualistic worship and obedience to a visible Son and imagined Father deities, given Freud's experiences with the fruits of such endeavors. He felt that Christianity was a return to premonotheistic pagan days, identical to the idol worship that predominated in Egypt prior to Akhenaton. It was prophetic religion that Freud pursued, and that was a worship based on the importance of individual responsibility and social justice. A theocentric conception of the universe would only interfere with its achievement. Blinded by his hostility, Freud could not allow himself to get a good look at the social benefits of organized religion. In his old age he returned to Judaism, but it was certainly not the Judaism of his father. It can thus be said that the first and last chapters of Freud's life were, in essence, Jewish.

REFERENCES

Beller, S. (1989). *Vienna and the Jews, 1867–1938: A Cultural History*. Cambridge: Cambridge University Press.

Freud, S. (1907). *Obsessive Actions and Religious Practices*. S.E. 9: 117–127.

———. (1912–13). *Totem and Taboo*. S.E. 13: 1–161.

———. (1927). *The Future of an Illusion*. S.E. 21: 5–56.

———. (1930). *Civilization and Its Discontents*. S.E. 21: 64–145.

———. (1939). *Moses and Monotheism*. S.E. 23:7–137.

Gay, P. (1987). *A Godless Jew—Freud, Atheism and the Making of Psychoanalysis*. New Haven, Conn.: Yale University Press.

Klein, D. (1985). *Jewish Origins of the Psychoanalytic Movement*. Chicago: University of Chicago Press.

Rice, E. (1990). *Freud and Moses—The Long Journey Home*. Albany: State University of New York Press.

———. (1994). The Jewish heritage of Sigmund Freud. *Psychoanalytic Review*, 81: 237–258.

Yerushalmi, Y. H. (1991). *Freud's Moses—Judaism Terminable and Interminable*. New Haven, Conn.: Yale University Press.

EMANUEL RICE

Jung, Carl Gustav (1875-1961)

Swiss psychiatrist, psychologist, mythologist, and founder of analytical psychology, Jung was born in Kesswil, the older of two children, son of Paul Achilles Jung, a minister who also tended to asylum inmates, and Emilie Preiswerk. Jung was prone to visionary experiences at an early age. At the same time, he was raised in a liberal religious household that fostered the intellectual cultivation of the mind, which included a knowledge of Eastern religions and an appreciation of psychic phenomena. He received his early education in Basle and resolved after the untimely death of his father in 1896 to enter the profession of psychiatry in 1898. He received a medical degree from the University of Zurich, submitting a dissertation on the psychology and pathology of so-called occult phenomena. Mirroring other single case studies of the era—Flournoy's Helene Smith, James's

Leonora Piper, and F. W. H. Myers's Stainton Moses—Jung's dissertation was an in-depth study of mediumistic phenomena, which he meant to be a further contribution to the development of a cross-cultural psychology of subconscious states just then emerging but, unknown to Jung at the time, was soon to be stifled by the rise of psychoanalysis.

In 1900, Jung was appointed assistant staff physician at the Bürgholzli Mental Clinic under Eugen Bleuler, where he worked with psychotic patients, investigated the word association test and the psychogalvanic reflex, and was first introduced to the ideas of psychoanalysis. In scope and content, however, Jung derived his dynamic conceptions of consciousness from the late-nineteenth-century psychologies of transcendence, remaining attracted to the ideas on subliminal consciousness, dissociation, and multiple personality put forward by Myers, Flournoy, and James. Because these other figures were already passing from the international scene, during the winter of 1902–1903 Jung studied with the only major figure left in their orbit, dissociation theorist Pierre Janet, a professor at the Collège de France in Paris. That same year, he also married Emma Rauschenbach (1882–1955), with whom he eventually had five children. He then went in search of contemporary colleagues of similar persuasion.

During this same period, as a student of Bleuler in the tradition of Kraepelinian psychiatry, Jung himself rose to international attention with his studies in word association—an experimental method that he applied in a psychotherapeutic setting to reveal unconscious complexes. By 1905, he had become senior staff physician at the Bürgholzli and lecturer in psychiatry at the University of Zurich. Also about this time, interested in the method of symbolism as well, he opened a correspondence with Freud, sending a copy of his newest book, *Diagnostic Association Studies*. In 1907, he published *The Psychology of Dementia Praecox*. Contrary to later interpreters, this work relied on French and Swiss psychology to reformulate a central category of Kraepelinian nosology and was not primarily a Freudian text, although it did make use of Freud's theory of symbolism in hysterics. Nevertheless, Jung offered it as a further contribution to Freud's theories. Freud and Jung met for the first time in 1907 and thereafter began a mutually dependent relationship, full of complicated projections, that lasted until 1914. During that time, Jung introduced Freud to the concept of the training analysis; he encouraged Freud to extend the interpretation of the psyche to primitive cultures; and from Zurich, Jung became the gatekeeper to Freud in Vienna and a prime mover in the internationalization of psychoanalysis. For his part, despite a close circle of disciples already ensconced in Vienna and elsewhere, Freud saw Jung as heir apparent to the psychoanalytic movement.

With Freud and Sándor Ferenczi, Jung attended the twentieth anniversary of Clark University in the United States in September 1909, where he first met William James and received an honorary doctorate. He also began an extended analysis with Medill McCormick, a member of the well-known McCormick reaper family. He later began an analysis of Harold McCormick, and his wife, Edith Rockefeller, which eventually led to extensive Rockefeller support of Jung's psychological activities, among them funds to found the Psychological Club in Zurich in 1916.

In the period immediately after the Clark conference, Jung was named permanent president of the International Congress of Psychoanalysis, his private practice continued to flourish, and, reflecting his international reputation, he was recalled to the United States in March 1910 to continue his analysis with members of the McCormick and Rockefeller families. However, after another trip to the United States in 1912 to deliver his Fordham University lectures, which were eventually published as *Transformation and Symbols of the Libido*, Jung broke with Freud over a variety issues, not the least of which was their differences in the interpretation of psychic energy. For Freud, the libidinal, erotic influences held sway, defining personality through the sublimation of the sexual instincts; for Jung, the growth and transformation of the individual's total life experience defined the core of psychic life. For Jung, psychic energy was not exclusively sexual.

After his break with Freud, Jung cut all ties to the university and entered a period of deep inward contemplation, during which he underwent a profound self-analysis, from which the basic themes of his subsequent system emerged. The Psychological Club was also inaugurated in Zurich during this period and *Transformations and Symbols of the Libido* was reissued in an English-language translation by Beatrice Hinkle under the title *The Psychology of the Unconscious* (1916), to widespread popular acclaim. With the exception of collected papers he published on analytical psychology, Jung's major work of this period appeared in 1921, *Psychological Types*, in which he first formally outlined his

growth-oriented psychology of individuation. During the 1920s, he traveled back to the United States to visit the Pueblo Indians, and also embarked upon a safari to Africa and a visit to Egypt.

Expanding his ideas about the collective unconscious from these experiences, Jung began intensive study of his examination of Chinese alchemical texts through his friend the sinologist Richard Wilhelm. The 1930s represented another major turning point in Jung's career, as his work began in earnest on the European alchemical tradition and its relation to archetypal symbolism. Jung commenced delivery of a series of papers to the now famous Eranos Conferences in Switzerland. He lectured at the Institute of Medical Psychology in London and journeyed to India at the invitation of the British government to celebrate the twenty-fifth anniversary of the University of Calcutta, after receiving an honorary doctorate from Oxford University and being elected to the Royal Society of Medicine. In addition, his Tavistock lectures in 1935, published as *Analytical Psychology: Theory and Practice*, had a major impact on the further evolution of psychoanalysis in Britain, particularly among the followers of Melanie Klein. He returned to the United States on two occasions, once to receive an honorary LLD from Harvard University in 1936 and again in 1938 to deliver the Terry Lectures on Psychology and Religion at Yale University.

This was also the period of Jung's controversial relationship to the International Society for Medical Psychotherapy, an organization controlled by the German psychotherapists. For this and other minor events, he was branded a Nazi sympathizer, and rumors spread through Europe and the United States falsely elaborating and enlarging this notion. While later admitting he had made some mistakes in his early assessments of the situation in Germany, Jung saw his reputation in the West suffer, and because of continued opposition by niche groups, has remained deeply distorted in some circles to this day. A recent example vilifying Jung based on invented scholarship is Richard Noll's *Aryan Christ: The Secret Life of Carl Jung*.

During World War II, Jung retreated to his books, his psychotherapeutic practice, and his tower on Lake Zurich at Bollingen, where he continued to write on spiritual themes, Eastern and Western religions, and the evolution of the psyche. A special chair was created for him in medical psychology at the University of Basle in 1944, but illness forced him to resign after only one year. He retired in 1947 and continued work on such subjects as synchronicity, alchemy, the *I Ching*, and the mystical union of opposites, and to articulate his conception of a cross-cultural phenomenological psychology of individuation. His wife died in 1955.

In 1958, with the assistance of Aniela Jaffe, Jung began work on a project half autobiographical and half biographical, which was later published as *Memories, Dreams, and Reflections*, an influential spiritual statement written partly by Jung and partly by Jaffe. Sections of the final version linking Jung to James, Flournoy, and others were excised by the editors and the publishers, however, so the two prevailing influences on Jung's thinking that were left appeared to be only Freud and God. More recently, building on the work of Henri Ellenberger and the so-called New Jung Scholarship, Sonu Shamdasani of the University of London has documented these and other omissions.

Other works of the later period for which Jung has become known include *Flying Saucers: A Modern Myth, The Undiscovered Self,* and *Man and his Symbols.* Jung died after a brief illness at his home in Kusnacht, Zurich, on June 6, 1961.

While historians of the twentieth century continue to remember Jung as merely an acolyte of Freud, believing Jung's was only a deviant theory of psychoanalysis, a new generation of scholars delving into the history of depth psychology have more correctly placed Jung as a twentieth-century exponent of the symbolic hypothesis, thereby acknowledging Jung's debt to Freud, while Jung's actual intellectual lineage remains the late-nineteenth-century psychologies of transcendence. To these earlier roots, we may attribute rising interest in Jungian ideas within the psychotherapeutic counterculture in Western countries. Meanwhile, credentialed Jungian analysts continue to identify their lineage as a variant of Freud and to seek legitimacy within the wider mainstream culture of psychology and psychiatry by their increased efforts to colonize the field of psychoanalysis, when they actually have an as yet unclaimed lineage of their own.

EUGENE TAYLOR

accepted views of the medical establishment and laid the essential patterns of the emerging discipline. In a series of recent studies by Bonomi (including 1998a, 1998b), it has been argued that, starting with his 1896 training with Adolf Baginsky, Freud's involvement in the question of the cause and cure of nervous diseases in children played an important role in the foundation of psychoanalysis. Traces of this interest are spread throughout Freud's writings, starting from the very symbol of the origins of psychoanalysis, the Irma dream (Bonomi, 1994).

REFERENCES

Bonomi, C. (1994). Why have we ignored Freud the paediatrician? The relevance of Freud's paediatric training for the origins of psychoanalysis. In A. Haynal and E. Falzeder (eds.) *100 Years of Psychoanalysis: Contributions to the History of Psychoanalysis*. Special Issue of *Cahiers Psychiatriques Genevois*. London: H. Karnac (Books), pp. 55–99.

———. (1998a). Sigmund Freud: Un neurologo tra sapere psichiatrico e sapere pediatrico del 19 secolo. *Psicoterapia e Scienze Umane*, 32, no. 1: 51–91.

———. (1998b). Freud and castration: A new look into the origins of psychoanalysis. *Journal of the American Academy of Psychoanalysis*, 26, no. 1: 29–49.

Jones, E. (1953). *The Life and Work of Sigmund Freud*, vol. 1. London: Hogarth Press.

CARLO BONOMI

Klein, Melanie (1882-1960)

Melanie Klein (née Reizes) has been the foremost influence on British psychoanalysis since Freud. She is responsible for many technical and theoretical achievements that have been accepted in varying degrees over the years. More recently there has been an increasing international interest in her ideas.

It is clear that she was not just an outstanding clinical observer and rigorous thinker, but she was also a profoundly impressive personality. Virginia Woolf wrote in her diary: "a woman of character and force and some submerged—how shall I say—not craft, but subtlety: something working underground. A pull, a twist, like an undertow: menacing. A bluff grey-haired lady, with large bright imaginative eyes" (Woolf, 1984: 209). And the obituary in *The Times* of London (September 23, 1960): "The power and acuity of her intellect had strength and integrity, her originality and creativeness left one in no doubt that one was in touch with an outstanding personality."

Melanie Klein was born on March 30, 1882, in Vienna, the youngest of four children. She idolized an older sis-

ter who died when Melanie was only four and a half; then a brother died when she was twenty. Her father was a doctor who practiced mostly as a dentist but was also a Jewish scholar. Her mother was the granddaughter of a rabbi. Klein's family background was clearly one of rigorous thinkers. Originally she wanted to train as a doctor herself, and entered schooling at the gymnasium to that end. However, her father died when she was eighteen and left the family with few resources. Rather than pursue a professional career, she married at the age of twenty-three. Arthur Klein, a man she tried to love, was an engineer whose work took them both, and eventually their family, to various parts of central Europe for two decades. This unsettled life took its toll on Melanie's health as she gave birth to her three children—in 1904, 1907, and 1914. On several occasions, she suffered quite severe depressions during which her mother intervened to look after the family and sent her away (Grosskurth, 1986). Despite the dominant and seemingly intrusive quality of her mother's personality, Melanie idealized her—so much so that when her mother died only months after the birth of her third child, she began to look for help for her own psychological states.

By then the family was living in Budapest, a major center for psychoanalysis. There she discovered Freud's writings. Moreover, her husband was working in the same office as the brother of Sándor Ferenczi, one of Freud's oldest colleagues, with whom Klein then had several periods of analysis during the years of World War I. Ferenczi was a strikingly gifted psychoanalytic clinician and was at that time collaborating with Freud on psychoanalytic research into child development. Ferenczi encouraged Klein to join in this research project, and she made psychoanalytic observations of her own children, leading to a paper (published 1921) that gained her acceptance as a member of the Hungarian Psychoanalytical Association.

From this moment, Klein had a passionate ambition to contribute to the fledgling psychoanalytic movement. No doubt this ambition formed a substitute for her abandoned hope of becoming a doctor, and psychoanalysis was at that time a profession more open than most to women. In 1919, however, the family left Hungary because of political turmoil, and her husband accepted a job in Sweden. By this time, Klein's interest was to pursue her career, and she left a difficult marriage, settling instead in Berlin with her children. She chose Berlin since after World War I the psychoanalytical society accepted views of the medical establishment and laid the essential patterns of the emerging discipline. In a series of recent studies by Bonomi (including 1998a, 1998b), it has been argued that, starting with his 1896 training with Adolf Baginsky, Freud's involvement in the question of the cause and cure of nervous diseases in children played an important role in the foundation of psychoanalysis. Traces of this interest are spread throughout Freud's writings, starting from the very symbol of the origins of psychoanalysis, the Irma dream (Bonomi, 1994).

REFERENCES

Bonomi, C. (1994). Why have we ignored Freud the paediatrician? The relevance of Freud's paediatric training for the origins of psychoanalysis. In A. Haynal and E. Falzeder (eds.) *100 Years of Psychoanalysis: Contributions to the History of Psychoanalysis*. Special Issue of *Cahiers Psychiatriques Genevois*. London: H. Karnac (Books), pp. 55–99.

———. (1998a). Sigmund Freud: Un neurologo tra sapere psichiatrico e sapere pediatrico del 19 secolo. *Psicoterapia e Scienze Umane*, 32, no. 1: 51–91.

———. (1998b). Freud and castration: A new look into the origins of psychoanalysis. *Journal of the American Academy of Psychoanalysis*, 26, no. 1: 29–49.

Jones, E. (1953). *The Life and Work of Sigmund Freud*, vol. 1. London: Hogarth Press.

CARLO BONOMI

Klein, Melanie (1882–1960)

Melanie Klein (née Reizes) has been the foremost influence on British psychoanalysis since Freud. She is responsible for many technical and theoretical achievements that have been accepted in varying degrees over the years. More recently there has been an increasing international interest in her ideas.

It is clear that she was not just an outstanding clinical observer and rigorous thinker, but she was also a profoundly impressive personality. Virginia Woolf wrote in her diary: "a woman of character and force and some submerged—how shall I say—not craft, but subtlety: something working underground. A pull, a twist, like an undertow: menacing. A bluff grey-haired lady, with large bright imaginative eyes" (Woolf, 1984: 209). And the obituary in *The Times* of London (September 23, 1960): "The power and acuity of her intellect had strength and integrity, her originality and creativeness left one in no doubt that one was in touch with an outstanding personality."

Melanie Klein was born on March 30, 1882, in Vienna, the youngest of four children. She idolized an older sister who died when Melanie was only four and a half; then a brother died when she was twenty. Her father was a doctor who practiced mostly as a dentist but was also a Jewish scholar. Her mother was the granddaughter of a rabbi. Klein's family background was clearly one of rigorous thinkers. Originally she wanted to train as a doctor herself, and entered schooling at the gymnasium to that end. However, her father died when she was eighteen and left the family with few resources. Rather than pursue a professional career, she married at the age of twenty-three. Arthur Klein, a man she tried to love, was an engineer whose work took them both, and eventually their family, to various parts of central Europe for two decades. This unsettled life took its toll on Melanie's health as she gave birth to her three children—in 1904, 1907, and 1914. On several occasions, she suffered quite severe depressions during which her mother intervened to look after the family and sent her away (Grosskurth, 1986). Despite the dominant and seemingly intrusive quality of her mother's personality, Melanie idealized her—so much so that when her mother died only months after the birth of her third child, she began to look for help for her own psychological states.

By then the family was living in Budapest, a major center for psychoanalysis. There she discovered Freud's writings. Moreover, her husband was working in the same office as the brother of Sándor Ferenczi, one of Freud's oldest colleagues, with whom Klein then had several periods of analysis during the years of World War I. Ferenczi was a strikingly gifted psychoanalytic clinician and was at that time collaborating with Freud on psychoanalytic research into child development. Ferenczi encouraged Klein to join in this research project, and she made psychoanalytic observations of her own children, leading to a paper (published 1921) that gained her acceptance as a member of the Hungarian Psychoanalytical Association.

From this moment, Klein had a passionate ambition to contribute to the fledgling psychoanalytic movement. No doubt this ambition formed a substitute for her abandoned hope of becoming a doctor, and psychoanalysis was at that time a profession more open than most to women. In 1919, however, the family left Hungary because of political turmoil, and her husband accepted a job in Sweden. By this time, Klein's interest was to pursue her career, and she left a difficult marriage, settling instead in Berlin with her children. She chose Berlin since after World War I the psychoanalytical society there began attracting many talented people to train as analysts and instituted the first formal requirements for training. The eminent founder of the Berlin Psychoanalytical Society, Karl Abraham, was also an outstanding clinician, and Klein went to him for a further personal psychoanalysis in 1924 at the age of forty-one. At this time many people from all over Europe went to Berlin for this training. One of these was Alix Strachey, a young woman recently married to James Strachey and therefore closely linked to the Bloomsbury group in London. She was also in Berlin because she too suffered considerably from depression. Klein and Strachey befriended each other. Klein's uncompromising clinical rigor, as well as her striking personality, appealed to the iconoclastic Bloomsbury spirit. In correspondence with her husband (in London), Alix Strachey wrote of an evening out together: "She was frightfully excited and determined to have a thousand adventures, and soon infected me with some of her spirits. . . . she's really a very good sort and makes no secret of her hopes, fears and pleasures, which are of the simplest sort. Only she's got a damned sharp eye for neurotics" (Strachey and Strachey, 1986: 193).

Klein had by then evolved her "play technique," as she called it, for the analysis of children. Unlike other pioneers of child analysis, Klein was uncompromising about giving young children straightforward interpretations of their unconscious fears and fantasies. Others were more circumspect about what they said to children. For instance, Alix Strachey commends Klein as "really the only person who's ever regularly analyzed children (Hug-Hell only fiddled about with 'Erziehungs-analyse' and never unearthed the Oedipus complex)" (Strachey and Strachey, 1986: 180).

"Hug-Hell" was Hermine Hug-Hellmuth, an aristocratic Austrian spinster who had adopted her sister's illegitimate son and brought him up according to psychoanalytic ideas. In the autumn of 1924, he had murdered Hug-Hellmuth in a quarrel over money. It was in this extraordinary context that, in December 1924, Klein was invited to give a lecture to the Viennese Psychoanalytical Society on her own method of child analysis. Her lecture may not have been received with much enthusiasm, though Klein put a good face on it.

When Klein's friend Alix Strachey suggested a lecture course might be arranged in London, Klein was undaunted and jumped at the chance. This was arranged by Strachey through her husband and Ernest Jones, the leading figure in British psychoanalysis. They had had a long interest in working with children, and there were many women analysts in London. Klein gave six lectures in July 1925 that aroused great interest—so much so that Jones invited her to return to London for a year to analyze his own children. She moved to London in 1926 and added Jones's wife to her practice as well.

The quality of her observations and her convincing manner of presentation were rewarded by a rapid assent to a leading position as psychoanalytic researcher. Analysts in London appeared to be proud of the talent in their midst, and when very shortly the Viennese Psycho-Analytical Society stood behind Anna Freud's disagreement with Klein over the practice of child analysis, London solidly supported Klein. Klein took the view that her ideas may be new but that she was merely adding to Freud's classic discoveries from the vantage point of analyzing young children. Her augmented London lectures were published as a book in 1932 and were greatly acclaimed in London, including a laudatory review by Edward Glover, then the scientific secretary of the British Psycho-Analytical Society. The book was a summation to date of her clinical applications to childhood and the theoretical developments she could make about child development from analyzing young children.

However, that preeminence she achieved so swiftly in London did not last. First, there was a small dissension led, sadly, by Klein's daughter Melitta Schmideberg. Klein had not only made her early observations on her daughter but planned a career for Melitta in her own mold. Melitta went to medical school in Berlin, where she also had a psychoanalysis first with Max Eitington and later with Karen Horney. Subsequently, she became a psychoanalyst in London. Klein herself had an extraordinary relationship with her own mother, who, with good intentions had pushed Klein aside during her depressions to take over the children. So Klein became an equally domineering force as a mother, steering Melitta into being a professional shadow.

In 1934, Melitta, then thirty years of age, embarked on a further personal analysis, this time with Edward Glover. It was then, perhaps as a bid for independence, that she began to enter into debates in the British Psycho-Analytical Society with antagonistic, even vituperative comments about her mother. In addition, Glover, her analyst, joined her in the disagreements and seemed to support her vindictiveness. (In the past Glover himself had had to emerge from being in the shadow of a brilliant older brother.)

Melitta's bid for independence coincided (and may even have been triggered by) the death of her brother Hans, Klein's second child, in a climbing accident in the same year, 1934. Klein's own reaction to her son's death was different. It provoked a very strong reaction to yet another family death, but characteristically it brought together many of her scientific ideas; these were about bereavement and depression. A little later that year, she gave her first paper on the depressive position (published 1935) to the International Psycho-Analytic Congress, in Lucerne. This made the Viennese even more uneasy about Klein. She had broken out of the confines of psychoanalysis of children to recast psychoanalytic theory in general. In this, she had abandoned her previous strategy of trying to be more Freudian than Freud. In any case, many British analysts were keen to see London move ahead of Vienna as a leading center of psychoanalysis.

But worse than her daughter's defection, in 1938 the Freud family escaped to London after Nazi Germany's *Anschluss* with Austria. Klein's disagreements with the first family of psychoanalysis, which had persisted for more than a decade, now arrived on her doorstep in London. At this point Klein's legendary determination no longer benefited her. She believed she must fight politically in the society for the survival of her ideas. This defensiveness led to many clashes and cost her many supporters. Eventually, the British Psycho-Analytical Society had to hold a wide-ranging debate of her ideas, in which Klein and her colleagues (Joan Riviere, Susan Isaacs, and Paula Heimann) were asked to defend their novel psychoanalytic developments. These Controversial Discussions occurred over eighteen months during 1943–1944; Klein was sixty when these began. By the time they had finished, the two camps—the Viennese and the Kleinians—seemed to have entrenched themselves further in their own positions. A large proportion of the society preferred to remain uncommitted. At this time, Klein was left with barely more than her three supporters and a handful of students.

Klein's determination never faltered despite this relative defeat. She set out to preserve her methods and ideas with her small group and build up their numbers. In 1946 she added the concept of the paranoid-schizoid position to the depressive position. Until her death in 1960, she reiterated over and over again in her papers the basic tenets of her ideas, evolving the notion of primary envy in 1957. That last innovation was in response to, and to combat, Winnicott's notion of primary omnipotence. Winni-

cott had been a pediatrician, attracted to Klein in the 1930s by her work with children. He had published a contrary notion, the transitional object, in 1951, which Klein believed seriously ignored the very early aggression in children and infants. Like many in the British society, Winnicott was provoked to elaborate other versions of the object relations theories that Klein had begun.

Klein's belief in research encouraged many of her students in the 1940s, 1950s, and 1960s to analyze schizophrenic patients. This gave rise to a period of unprecedented creativity in the British Psycho-Analytical Society—among the Klein group but also from outside and in reaction to it. Fundamental work on psychosis, symbol formation, borderline personality disorder, and latterly autism has left an undying mark on psychoanalysis and psychiatry around the world.

Klein never retired and was giving lectures and working on her papers until shortly before her death at age seventy-eight. However, she did seem to achieve an increasing pleasure in her family, not least her grandchildren. She was taken ill on holiday in the summer of 1960 and, after a successful operation, succumbed to postoperative complications. It is said that one of her last concerns was a crying child along the corridor from the hospital room in which she died.

REFERENCES
Grosskurth, P. (1986). *Melanie Klein.* London: Hodder and Stoughton.
Klein, M. (1921). Eine Kinderentwicklung. *Imago*: 251–309.
———. (1923). The development of a child. *International Journal of Psychoanalysis*, 4: 419–474.
———. (1932). *The Psycho-Analysis of Children.* London: Hogarth Press.
———. (1935). A contribution to the psychogenesis of manic-depressive illness. *International Journal of Psycho-Analysis*, 16: 145–174.
———. (1946). Notes on some schizoid mechanisms. *International Journal of Psycho-Analysis*, 27: 99–110.
———. (1957). *Envy and Gratitude.* London: Hogarth Press.
Strachey, J., and Strachey, A. (1986). *Bloomsbury/Freud.* London: Weidenfeld and Nicolson.
Woolf, V. (1984). *The Diary of Virginia Woolf,* vol. 5. London: Chatto & Windus.

ROBERT HINSHELWOOD

Kleinian Theory

Melanie Klein became a member of the Budapest Psychoanalytical Society in 1919. These were exciting times for the development of psychoanalysis. In 1920, Freud introduced the concept of the life and death instincts, revised his ideas about anxiety and guilt, and formulated his structural theory of the mind. This opened new vistas to psychoanalytical theory and practice.

Klein started her work with children in Budapest, in the way common at that time, by analyzing her own child. She also tried analyzing children in their own homes and with their own toys. But very soon she started developing an innovative technique that was at variance with the work of the other pioneers in the field, like Hermine Hug-Hellmuth and Anna Freud. She realized that in order to be analyzed, children must be provided with a setting similar to that obtaining in adult analysis. She saw the children regularly, in an appropriately furnished consulting room, five times a week for fifty-minute sessions. She developed a play technique, recognizing that the children's play symbolically represented their conflicts and phantasies and could be interpreted in a way not dissimilar to interpreting dreams and verbal communications. She provided each child with a box of small toys and play material most suitable for the child to express him- or herself. Unlike the others, who considered that children under seven were not analyzable, Klein found that with her technique she could analyze very small children, her youngest being between two and three years old. While the other analysts in the field used educational methods, Klein early came to the conclusion that an analytical attitude has to be maintained, that "a true analytic situation can be brought about only by analytical means"; and in such a situation, again contrary to the commonly held belief at the time, children develop a strong transference relationship. This approach led her to the discovery that children, of whatever age, have a complex internal world of fantasy that often dominates their lives. The rich clinical material that she obtained confirmed in large measure Freud's reconstruction of childhood development, particularly in relation to sexual and aggressive fantasies; but Klein mapped it out in great detail in actual child material. This work, however, also led to a certain shift of perspective, which also led to a departure from some of Freud's ideas.

For instance, she observed that children develop an Oedipal conflict much earlier than posited by Freud. Her youngest patient, Rita, under age three, manifested strong Oedipal phantasies, with associated fears of having her genitals attacked in retaliation.

Melanie Klein observed that as part and parcel of these early Oedipal phantasies, the children had a powerful sadistic superego far earlier than described by Freud, who saw the superego as a late outcome and precipitate of the Oedipus complex. According to her, the internal world was inhabited by highly idealized figures and by terrifying and monstrous figures that could be traced to a projection of the child's own Oedipal sadistic phantasies. But not only Oedipal. Klein had discovered terrifying persecuting figures that could be related to the child's earliest relation to the breast. Six-year-old Erna, who had a very long-standing obsessional neurosis, had not only sadistic Oedipal phantasies but also much earlier cannibalistic ones. This was one of the controversial points in the debate with Anna Freud. While Anna Freud at that time thought the psychoanalyst had to help build the child's superego, Klein soon came to the conclusion that, much as in the analysis of adults, the aim of the analysis was rather to diminish the severity of the superego. Klein also related the monstrous aspects of the superego less to the external parents than to the projection of the child's inner sadism. Interestingly, the only positive reference Freud made to Melanie Klein was in a footnote to *Civilization and Its Discontents* (1930), where he discusses the problem of the severity of the superego as depending on inner sources. He says: "as has rightly been emphasized by Melanie Klein and by other English writers."

From the beginning of her work, Klein concentrated on the child's anxieties and defenses. Among those, projection and introjection seemed to be particularly powerful. These were the most primitive mechanisms, preceding repression. And it is the projection and subsequent reintrojection that accounted for the child's inner world peopled by ideal and persecutory figures.

From very early on, Klein also paid a great deal of attention to the child's curiosity about the parents, the content of the maternal body, and the sexual relation between the parents. This she considered so important that she called it the epistemophilic instinct, an instinctual impulse as powerful as those of love and hatred. She discovered that children in their phantasies wanted to penetrate and to explore the maternal body and functions, and that this exploration was filled with anxieties because it was so ambivalent. It was linked with desire, greedy possessiveness, hostile impulses, and projections. And she attributed the inhibition of curiosity less to external prohibition and more to inner experience of

K

anxiety and guilt. This anxiety led the child to displace the original curiosity from the mother's body and parental relationships to the external world, thus imbuing the world with symbolic meaning. She considered the anxiety, if not excessive, to be a spur to mental development; but that excessive anxiety leads to the inhibition of interest in the external world and a failure of symbolic formation. She wrote a number of papers discussing the roots of the children's intellectual inhibitions.

These discoveries led to some differences from Freud's views of the development of infantile sexuality. It also led to a certain shift of emphasis. Klein considered unconscious fantasy as a much more fundamental part of the child's mind than did Freud. Freud considered phantasizing sets in which the reality principle has been established. In Klein's view, phantasy exists from the beginning of life, and from the beginning is attached to objects. Susan Isaacs, in "The Nature and Function of Phantasy" (1952), formulated explicitly what was implicit in Klein's view of phantasy. She considered phantasy as what Freud called "the mental correlate of instincts." In the omnipotent mind of the infant, the impulse includes the phantasy of its fulfillment; but since the impact of reality cannot be avoided, there is from the beginning a constant interplay between phantasy and reality perception, which molds the infant's and child's view of itself and the world. Fantasy is also a defense that, according to Klein and Isaacs, underlies what we see as "mechanisms"; there are detailed phantasies of splitting, taking in, expelling, and the like, that are experienced concretely and bodily. Phantasy is a way of organizing all the object relationships and the self, and it is a meeting ground of instincts, object relations, and defenses.

Since phantasy is expressed symbolically (as Klein found in children's play), this extension of the concept of fantasy is inextricably linked with an extension of the concept of symbolism. Freud discovered symbolism first in hysterical symptoms; Ernest Jones considered it specifically as a pathological phenomenon, stating that symbolism arises when sublimation is blocked. Klein, on the contrary, considered symbolism to be at the root of sublimation and a fundamental part of the development of the ego. In her paper "The Importance of Symbol-Formation for the Development of the Ego" (1930), an account of the first analysis of an autistic child, Klein demonstrates how his excessive anxiety about his phantasies in relation to his mother's body led to the complete inhibition in his relation to the external world, which he could not endow with meaning. She became increasingly convinced of the importance of the child's dependence on its primary object, the breast. She found that at the most primitive level children have complex phantasies of other part objects, such as the penis. It could be said that Freud discovered the child in the adult and Klein the infant in the child and the adult. This was a very controversial point. It has been argued that Klein attributes too many complications to the infant's immature mind. And yet, it is in those very first years, well before the full-blown genital Oedipus complex, that certain fundamental processes are developed—like the capacity for reality testing, symbolization, speech, and rationality.

Klein also paid more attention to the infantile aggressive impulses. While in her early work she tried to see the child's difficulties in terms of repression of the libido, she very soon noticed that it is aggression linked with libidinal impulses that is the source of both anxiety and guilt.

Although the concept of the death instinct had been available since 1920, Klein does not refer much to the death instinct in her early papers but speaks loosely of the infant's destructive impulses. Only in the second part of "The Psycho-Analysis of Children" (1932) does she speak of the conflict between the life and death instincts; but in the papers she wrote at the same time, she frequently refers to it, in particular in "Criminal Tendencies in Normal Children" (1927). The primitive nature of these fantasies and anxieties, the intensity of the anxiety, and the monstrous or excessively idealized figures that inhibited the child's internal world led her to revise Freud's view of childhood neurosis. She saw childhood neurosis not as originating in later Oedipal conflicts but as a defensive structure against more primitive infantile anxieties of a psychotic nature. In 1935 and 1940, Klein wrote the first papers ("A Contribution to the Psychogenesis of Manic-Depressive States" and "Mourning and Its Relation to Manic-Depressive States") in which she tries to give a more comprehensive conceptual framework for her discoveries by bringing forward her concept of the depressive position. One could look at her work until then as the first phase. In 1946, in her paper "Notes on Some Schizoid Mechanisms," Klein introduced the concept of the paranoid-schizoid position. This could be seen as the beginning of the third phase of her work, following which she gave a comprehensive theory of mental functioning. Here I present her theory in its final form, rather than pursuing further the historical development of her ideas.

The Paranoid-Schizoid Position

Klein believed that from birth the infant has a rudimentary ego. This was a conviction arising not only out of her clinical work and observation of infants, but also, in a way not usually recognized, consistent with Freud's views about the fate of the life and death instinct. Freud assumed that the "organism" deflects the death instinct outward. It is the ego that, according to Freud, is the seat of anxiety. According to Klein, from birth there is an ego capable of perception, including perception of anxiety, and of employing defenses against it. It is the ego that perceives anxiety and "deflects" the death instinct. This ego forms object relationships from the start since instinct has not only a source but also objects. The infant at birth is exposed to a welter of perceptions from external stimuli and from internal needs, like hunger and impulses and fears—and the rudimentary ego is not capable of distinguishing between the two. It operates in a primitive way, which Freud described as "THIS I SHALL TAKE IN; THAT I SHALL SPIT OUT." Gradually, the infant emerges from the state of chaos through splitting, projection, and idealization. Under the impact of anxieties, the libidinal ego aims to project outside everything that is bad and to take inside itself everything that is good. Its aim is to hold and keep inside and idealize a fantasied all-giving breast, and to project outside everything that is bad, including its own impulses, and this creates a fantasied bad breast. Hence the term "paranoid-schizoid" that Klein used for describing this phase of development: "schizoid" for splitting and "paranoid" because of the nature of the anxiety. The primordial anxiety in this situation is the fear of disintegration and annihilation; and the primary defenses create a schizo-paranoid world. But this in turn exposes the infant to paranoid anxieties: the loss of the ideal state and object through being invaded and possibly annihilated by persecutors.

In her 1946 paper, Klein devotes only a few lines to the concept that acquired an increasing importance in her later work, and that is the concept of projective identification. In Freud's view, projection comes into operation as a mechanism of defense fairly late, and he described it as only a projection of impulses or certain characteristics. Melanie Klein's concept of projective identification is more extensive than that. In projective identification, the infant not only projects impulses or characteristics, but has a phantasy of actually getting rid of parts of the ego, particularly those parts that experience anxiety, and locating them in the objects. Arising in the paranoid-schizoid position, projective identification operates throughout life but takes different forms at different stages of development, and it fulfills a double objective: that of getting rid of unwanted parts of the self and affecting and controlling the object; also, by being located in an object, it may achieve such aims as taking possession of, controlling, distorting, and attacking the object. It is the basis of hallucinations and delusions. It is a concept that has the clearest demonstration in Klein's view that the phantasy is a concept linking impulses and defenses. Projective identification is a mechanism of defense against anxiety, while at the same time being a wish-fulfilling phantasy. In the paranoid-schizoid position, there is no concept of ambivalence or frustration. Frustration is experienced as a persecution. There is no frustration but a bad internal breast. Good experiences are attached to the ideal breast, with which the infant also identifies, leading to states that used to be seen as primary narcissism. Bad experiences confirm the infant's view of the bad breast, while good experiences reinforce the infant's confidence, both in the object and in its own loving impulses. The situation of a split between the two is often confused by the operation of envy, which Klein saw as one of the manifestations of the death instinct, and which attacks the object of admiration and desire. When envy operates strongly, it is difficult for the infant to maintain an ideal object, because the good experience itself is attacked, which leads to a confusional state in which the good and the bad cannot be distinguished. In a good situation, when the confidence in a good object and the infant's own capacity to love are felt to be stronger than the bad, the frantic need to push the bad out—in order to retain the good—diminishes, and with it the bad breast becomes less terrifying. In such a situation the need to split, project, and idealize the good experience diminishes and, together with the infant's growing capacity for perceiving time, absence, and the reality of the object, slow steps toward integration take place, which eventually lead to a shift to what Klein called the "depressive position."

The Depressive Position

Klein defined the depressive position as that point of development at which the infant perceives his or her

K

mother as a whole object. By a whole object, Klein means many interconnected things. A whole object is not split into an ideal and a persecutory one. It is the same breast and the same arms, the same eyes that both gratify and can inflict pain. The different functions are those of the same person. With this is conjoined the awareness of separateness. The real mother can be seen as sometimes good, sometimes bad, present or absent; a process of reality testing sets in that leads to a differentiation between the phantasy world that is the infant's inner reality and his or her perception of outer reality. This awareness of the mother as a whole object is part and parcel of a process in which the infant recognizes him- or herself as one person, not an ideal infant, in love with, and sometimes confused with, an ideal breast; or a bad infant, hating a bad breast; but the same infant, loving and hating the same mother. Ambivalence becomes the great issue. The infant hates his loved mother and destroys her in his phantasy. This fills him with an experience of terrible loss and guilt. The fear of loss and guilt gradually replaces the dread of being persecuted by a bad object or objects.

Klein saw the roots of the persecutory superego in the paranoid-schizoid position, and those of a depressive superego giving rise to a feeling of guilt in the depressive position. This situation of extreme despair at having lost a good object, at once loved and hated, gives rise to a powerful set of defenses that she called "manic defenses." The interplay between these two, according to her, are the roots of manic-depressive illness. Since the depressive pain includes the importance of a loved and needed object not controlled by the self, and the experience of guilt about phantasies of destroying it, manic defenses are directed against dependence and guilt by an increase of omnipotence, denial of need and dependence, and hatred and contempt for the needed object, this leading to a vicious circle, since in mania the object is destroyed again, and therefore increases or brings back the depression. There is always some regression to the paranoid-schizoid defenses, a tendency to split again, to project and to idealize.

But another new mechanism mobilized by the depressive position is that of reparation. When the infant recognizes that her hatred has destroyed the loved and needed object, there is a wish to repair and regain it. It is not strictly speaking a mechanism of defense, since the defense protects one from recognizing one's anxiety and guilt, while in reparation there is a sense of inner

reality that is not denied but in need of being restored. In a good situation, the return of an absent mother, or her absent goodness, counteracts the infant's belief in his or her destructive powers and increases his or her belief in the capacity to restore and regain the situations of goodness. Klein saw reparation as a fundamental part of development, the basis of the capacity to tolerate ambivalence without hopelessness, confidence in one's own capacities, and a basis for symbolization and sublimation.

Klein connected the depressive position with the beginnings of the Oedipus complex. The infant's perception of the mother as a whole person implies a person with a life of her own and relationships of her own. She is no more an object viewed narcissistically—almost as a function of the infant—but a person with a complete life of her own and primarily a life with the father. Where, in the paranoid-schizoid position, envy plays a prominent role, since it attacks the sources of goodness, in the depressive position, Oedipal jealousy and jealousy of a fantasied and real new baby becomes an increasingly important factor. And as the father is also lovable, the ambivalence toward both parents comes to the fore, and the reparative impulse comes into play; parental intercourse is restored as an object of love and admiration, and the existence of the sexual creative act and the potential for babies is acknowledged. This gives rise to the conflict between love and admiration and the jealousy, envy, and hostile impulses it also arouses. This has to be worked through. The working through of the depressive position includes the working through of the Oedipus complex.

The Concept of Positions

The concept of the paranoid-schizoid and the depressive positions became the fulcrum of the Kleinian work. It is partly a developmental concept in that the paranoid-schizoid position begins in what Abraham called the first oral stage; and the change to the depressive position begins somewhere around the age of three to four months (Abraham's second oral stage). But it does not dominate psychic life until much later. The fundamental change gradually occurs in the state of the ego, the object relationships, the leading anxieties and defenses, and in reality testing. In the paranoid-schizoid position, the object is predominantly a part-object; in the depressive position, the ego is integrated and ambivalent, and the object is whole. In the paranoid-schizoid position, the leading anxiety is of disintegration and persecution; in the depres-

K

sive position, it is the fear of loss, and guilt. In the paranoid-schizoid position, projective identification dominates distorting perception; in the depressive position, projective identifications are gradually withdrawn, and with that a differentiation between external and internal is established. A reality testing of omnipotent fantasy against reality perception is gradually established. But the full transition between the paranoid-schizoid and the depressive position is in fact never achieved. Under stresses, regression occurs to the paranoid-schizoid level; and therefore Klein views the two positions not only as stages of development but as two modes of functioning, two ways of structuring the experience of oneself and the world in a fluctuating way. These transitions between the two states of mind are worked through throughout life. And they are the transitions that are also constantly worked through in the analytical process.

Klein's work was very influential in the development of modern psychoanalysis in a number of different ways. Her discoveries in relation to early psychotic anxieties gave a stimulus to the analysis of psychotics, particularly among her analysands, such as Hanna Segal, Herbert Rosenfeld, and, later, Wilfred Bion. They pioneered the technique for analyzing psychotics. Many others based their work on Klein's teaching, and they came to be known as "Kleinians." They developed her work with children and adults, including psychotic and borderline patients hitherto considered unanalyzable. At present, the younger generations of Kleinians have made significant contributions to the understanding of the earliest phases of the Oedipus complex, and its effect on forming the mental apparatus, and the development of thought. But Klein's influence went beyond the Kleinians; sometimes explicitly and sometimes implicitly, it can be detected in many non-Kleinian analysts. There is general agreement now about the importance of the first two years of life; and with it came an acknowledgment of the importance of an inner world of fantasy objects, including part-objects. The concepts of the depressive position and of projective identification are known and often used throughout the psychoanalytic world. Klein's play technique is the basis of much psychotherapeutic work with children. Outside analysis, it has influenced philosophers and writers on art, as well as group work, and has applications to the sociopolitical scene.

REFERENCES

Freud, S. (1930). *Civilization and Its Discontents*. S.E. 21: 64–145.

Isaacs, S. (1952). The nature and function of phantasy. In M. Klein et al. (eds.). *Developments in Psychoanalysis*. London: Hogarth Press.

Klein, M. (1927). Criminal tendencies in normal children. *The Writings of Melanie Klein*, vol. 1. London: Hogarth Press.

———. (1930). The Importance of symbol-formation for the development of the Ego. In M. Klein (author). *The Writings of Melanie Klein*, vol. 1. London: Hogarth Press.

———. (1932). The psycho-analysis of children. In M. Klein (author). *The Writings of Melanie Klein*, vol. 2. London: Hogarth Press.

———. (1935). A contribution to the psychogenesis of manic-depressive states. In M. Klein (author). *The Writings of Melanie Klein*, vol. 1. London: Hogarth Press.

———. (1940). Mourning and its relation to manic-depressive states. In M. Klein (author). *The Writings of Melanie Klein*, vol. 1. London: Hogarth Press.

———. (1946). Notes on some schizoid mechanisms. In M. Klein (author). *The Writings of Melanie Klein*, vol. 3. London: Hogarth Press.

RECOMMENDED FURTHER READINGS

Klein, M. (1975). *The Writings of Melanie Klein*, 4 vols. London: Hogarth Press.

Segal, H. (1964). *Introduction to the Work of Melanie Klein*. London: Heinemann.

———. (1979) *Klein*. London: Harvester, Fontana.

HANNA SEGAL

Kohut's Psychology of Narcissism

See NARCISSISM.

Korea, and Psychoanalysis

Colonized by Japan in the period 1910 to 1945, Korea adopted modern psychiatric thought that stemmed from the descriptive-organic models prevalent in Japan at that time. Some Korean doctors were trained in Japan, but it would appear that only one, Sung Hee Kim, trained as an analyst in the years 1940–1945 under Kosawa Heisaku (see *Japan, and Psychoanalysis*). He returned to Korea to become professor of psychiatry at Chonnam University Medical School. However, the formation of study circles and training programs was left to others. It was the outbreak of the Korean War in 1950, whose aftermath brought American psychiatrists to Korea and the teaching of depth psychology, and the return to Korea of a few of the many who had gone to the United States for further training after World War II, that led to the introduction of psychoanalysis into Korea as a formal system of thought.

The new thinking had to contend with a "repertoire of built-in socio-cultural mechanisms that had a preventative or even curative effect on man's psychological distress" (Chang and Kim, 1973). These included shamanism and the belief that human misfortune results from an improper relation to the spirit world. A qualified mediator, or *mutang*, performs the ritual of the *goot*, through which relations are harmonized. Those who have suffered psychological distress become qualified as shamans through their close rapport with spirits, and their children are said to inherit these abilities. There is also a long tradition of folk medicine, consisting of herbal remedies, acupuncture and *moxa*, introduced from China and still prevalent today.

As with other Asian cultures, the systems of thought that inform these practices profoundly affect the way members of the population typically seek help for, and report on, a variety of illnesses. These include a belief in multiple treatments for the same complaint and a tendency to somatize psychological problems. Thus in attempting to develop a culturally relevant approach to psychotherapy, the pioneering analysts devoted a good portion of their time to studying traditional cultural practices (including religions, myths, folk dramas, and literature) from the viewpoint of orthodox Freudian theory.

As with psychoanalysis in Japan, there have been attempts at formulating a revised view of the Oedipus complex, the resolution of which involves sublimation of incestuous wishes to *hyoa*, the Korean term for "filial piety." This is based upon a reciprocity between generations such that an understanding and responsibility of the parents balance respect accorded by the children (Kim, 1978). In another sphere, the prevalence of Taoist beliefs about illness being due to an excess of exertion in thought or action has led in some neo-Freudian quarters to "Taoistic psychotherapy," which emphasizes acceptance rather than struggling against one's inner conflicts, and transcending them by training the mind toward a more positive outlook.

Not until the 1970s did Korean clinicians seek formal ties with the International Psychoanalytic Association. Cho Doo-Young, trained at Cornell University in New York, organized the Korean Psychoanalytic Study Group. Orthodox Freudian in orientation, it has about fifty members. Two other organizations, the Korean Academy of Psychotherapy (neo-Freudian and Taoistic, with about eighty members) and the Korean Association of Jungian Psychology (with thirty members), are actively pursuing a culturally relevant psychoanalytic practice.

Since the 1980s, psychoanalytic interest in Korea, in line with other parts of the world, has diminished in the wake of a rising interest in biologically based explanations of psychological disturbance. Coupled with the lack of Korean training analysts, this has meant that training has continued in a foreign context where the differences in language and cultural understanding have traditionally (in the West) been viewed as resistance but that might become the wellspring for future developments in cultural psychoanalytic theory (Fisher, 1996).

REFERENCES

Chang, S. C., and Kim, K. I. (1973). Psychiatry in South Korea. *American Journal of Psychiatry*, 130, no. 6: 667–669.

Fisher, C. P. (1996). Panel report: Psychoanalysis in the Pacific Rim. *International Journal of Psychoanalysis*, 77: 373–377.

Kim, K. I. (1978). The Oedipus complex in our changing society; with special reference to Korea. *Neuropsychiatry* (Seoul), 17: 97–103.

———. (1996). Traditional therapeutic issues in psychiatric practice in Korea. Paper read in a Transcultural Psychiatry symposium of the 10th World Congress of Psychiatry, August 23–28.

GEOFFREY H. BLOWERS

Krafft-Ebing, Richard (1840–1902)

Richard Krafft-Ebing, perhaps the most prominent psychiatrist of the nineteenth century, published *Psychopathia Sexualis* in 1886, and this work went through twelve editions by the time its author died. It would not be unfair to call Krafft-Ebing the father of the study of modern sexual pathology. It is to him we owe the terms "paranoia," "sadism," "masochism," and "hermaphrodite," as well as an assortment of others. Today the book interests people mainly for its titillating, vivid accounts of two hundred case studies of what Krafft-Ebing regarded as the darkest perversions.

Because Krafft-Ebing was too much a moralizer and, when not that, primarily engaged in description and classification, it is unsurprising that Freud rapidly surpassed him in importance as well as in popular fame. Krafft-Ebing's work, like that of Havelock Ellis, was almost entirely devoid of explanatory hypotheses for the extraordinary phenomena he categorized, and, like the Englishman but unlike Freud, Krafft-Ebing had no flair for the subtle, even if speculative, structures of the human mind that Freud was to produce over the next fifty years. After attending one of Freud's earliest public lectures, Krafft-

Ebing declared: "It sounds like a scientific fairy tale." Nevertheless, relations between the two men were cordial and respectful. In a letter to Freud written in 1904, Wilhelm Fliess asked for references on bisexuality because he felt he was "not very well read in the literature," and in his reply Freud told Fliess he could certainly learn a great deal by reading *Psychopathia Sexualis*. Moreover, on a personal level, Freud liked Krafft-Ebing and was certainly indebted professionally to the older man (his senior by sixteen years), who supported Freud for at least six years in the latter's efforts to get promoted from a mere lowly paid privatdocent at the University of Vienna to associate professor. Only in 1902, the year in which Krafft-Ebing died, did Freud succeed to that rank.

Let us now take a closer look at some specifics of Krafft-Ebing's writings about sexuality. To the modern ear much of it will seem at best quaint, but Freud's own work is in part a reaction to it, and traces of it linger on in popular notions concerning perversions.

Whereas Havelock Ellis explored the sexual life of normal persons, Krafft-Ebing was almost morbidly fascinated with the sexual aberrations of criminals and the insane and had nothing to say about the development of the normal personality. Perhaps he was inspired by Goethe's observation that "nature reveals herself best in her abnormalities." It is to Krafft-Ebing (as well as to William Acton) that we owe the once popular idea that excessive masturbation leads to insanity, and it seems that many of the strange persons Krafft-Ebing studied were guilty of that "sin." He held, too, that foreplay in sex was a form of perversion, and he was particularly repulsed by cunnilingus, which he dubbed a masochistic perversion. It is not clear whether he referred to the receiver or the active participant in this way, although he generally thought that sadism was a male trait and masochism a female one. So-called fetishisms were regarded as extensions of normal sex by Ellis, but Krafft-Ebing held they were abnormal, and it seems that in this regard he had Freud on his side. Homosexuality was a type of depravity, typical of women when they reversed their common masochistic tendency into the sadistic, and typical of men when they reversed their sadistic impulses into the masochistic. Krafft-Ebing's tales of sadists are hardly common garden variety but consist of accounts of murderous degenerates. Havelock Ellis seemed to think that sadism was a form of sex play and that we could not recognize sadists in their everyday life, but Krafft-Ebing regarded them as pitiful neurotics who were obviously such.

The roots of sexual disorder run deep for the older psychiatrist, deeper than they did for Freud. For Freud, while biological factors had their role, sexual development is primarily to be traced through the events of early childhood. For Krafft-Ebing, neurosis is mainly a hereditary problem. "Degenerates" were destined to be the prostitutes they were to become, to practice the fetishisms they did, to engage in compulsive masturbation, and to commit the violence of dementia. Naturally, Freud rejected all of this and, according to him, in his "Contribution One" (of *Three Contributions to the Theory of Sex*), Krafft-Ebing also held the untenable view that a bisexual disposition supplies an individual with male and female brain centers. Freud rightly dismissed this idea on the simple grounds that we do not know that there are such things, much less what "supplies" them.

Krafft-Ebing's views are not systematically developed. They are usually side comments on the cases that fill his book. Consider just two such cases, neither of which is more remarkable than any of the others.

Case 17. "A four year old girl was missing from her parents' home on April 15, 1880. [One of the occupants] of the house was arrested. The forearm of the child was found in his pocket, and the head and entrails . . . were taken from the stove. . . . The genitals could not be found. M., when asked about their whereabouts, became embarrassed. . . . [An] obscene poem found on his person left no doubt that he had violated the child and then murdered her. His intelligence is limited. He presents no anatomical signs of degeneration. . . . [He] suffered convulsions at the age of nine months. . . . From the time of puberty he was irritable, showed evil inclinations; was lazy . . . and in all trades proved to be of no use. [After a term in the house of corrections and being made a marine] he returned home. He did not run after women but gave himself up passionately to masturbation and occasionally indulged in sodomy with bitches. His mother suffered with mania menstrualis periodica. An uncle was insane, and another an inebriate. M.'s brain showed morbid changes of the frontal lobes of the first and second temporal convolutions, and of a part of the occipital convolutions."

Case 18. "Alton, a clerk in England, goes out of town for a walk. He lures a child into a thicket, and returns after a time to his office where he makes this entry into his notebook: 'Killed today a young girl; it was fine and hot.' The child . . . was found cut into pieces. Many parts, and among them the genitals, could not be found. A. did not show the slightest trace of emotion,

K

and gave no explanation of the motive or circumstances of his horrible deed. He was a psychopathic individual, and occasionally subject to states of depression with taedium vitae. His father had one attack of acute mania. A near relative suffered from mania with homicidal impulses."

In all of Krafft-Ebing's case studies, lust is accompanied by the most bizarre degrees of cruelty, and not much more needed to be said than to give a family history as evidence of the inevitability of it all.

REFERENCE

Krafft-Ebing, R. (1886). *Psychopathia Sexualis: With Especial Reference to Contrary Sexual Instinct: A Clinical Forensic Study.* Burbank, Calif.: Bloat (1999).

                                                            SIDNEY GENDIN

Kris, Ernst (1900–1957)

Ernst Kris was born in Vienna on April 26, 1900. Intellectually curious and precocious, he attended seminars on the history of art at the Vienna University when he was only fourteen years old. At the age of twenty-two, he obtained a Ph.D. in the history of art and was appointed curator at the Kunsthistorishe Museum in Vienna, where he specialized in cameos. While thus employed, he published the "Art of Cameo Engraving during the Renaissance." In 1940, he coauthored *Caricature* with the noted historian C. H. Grombich. Another book, *The Legend of the Artist*, was published together with O. Kurz. The ideas expressed in this book were later reworked into chapter two of Kris's book *Psychoanalytic Explorations in Art* (1952).

Kris became a member of the Vienna Psychoanalytic Association in 1928 and was appointed by Freud, together with another "lay analyst," Robert Waelder, as an editor of *Imago*, a journal dedicated to the application of psychoanalysis to the humanities. On November 10, 1927, he married Dr. Marianne Rie, the daughter of Oscar Rie, Freud's pediatrician and tarok partner. Marianne Kris became a leading psychoanalyst in her own right. Ernst Kris was analyzed by Anna Freud and at the 14th Psychoanalytic Congress in Marienbad, Czechoslovakia, in 1936, he read a paper entitled "Remarks on Laughter," a contribution to the psychology of mime. A short paper entitled "Ego Development and the Comic" appeared in the *International Journal of Psychoanalysis* in 1938. In the same year, he reviewed Anna Freud's book, *The Ego and Mechanisms of Defense*. When Hitler entered Vienna, the Krises joined Freud's family in England, arriving there in April 1938.

In Great Britain, Kris worked for the British government, researching German war propaganda. His efforts culminated in a book published with H. Speier entitled *The German Radio Propaganda* (1944). The Krises arrived in New York in 1940. Kris became managing editor of the *Psychoanalytic Study of the Child*, the psychoanalytic journal that served as the mouthpiece for the Hartmann group. Kris died on February 27, 1957, of a coronary thrombosis at the age of fifty-six.

Kris's contributions to psychoanalysis fall conveniently into five groups of papers. The first combines Kris's background as an art historian with his understanding of psychoanalysis. These were gathered into a book entitled *Psychoanalytic Explorations of Art* (1952). Some of these works are technical and appeal only to specialists, but others, such as "On Inspiration" and "The Preconscious Mental Processes," are of psychoanalytic interest.

A second group of papers written during World War II is almost forgotten today but is of interest to anyone who wishes to follow the fate of Freud's ideas about *Group Psychology and the Ego* (1921). Some of these articles were reprinted as part four of Kris's selected papers published posthumously in 1975.

The year 1950 was particularly productive in Kris's life. In that year, a censored version of the Freud-Fleiss letters rescued by Marie Bonaparte appeared. Kris wrote an introduction to this correspondence that still serves as a valuable document in the history of psychoanalysis.

A third group of papers was jointly written by Hartmann, Kris, and Loewenstein. These papers inaugurated a new chapter in the history of psychoanalysis that Hale (1995) called the "era of American ego psychology." In a monograph on the same period I called it the "Hartmann era" (Bergmann, 1993). The main ideas of this group can be summarized as follows:

1. The truly great discoveries of psychoanalysis, such as the Oedipus complex, transference, and free association, are behind us, but like a conqueror who rushes forward leaving unexplored territory behind him, Freud did not stop to systematize his findings. Trained clarifiers are needed to coordinate various propositions. Psychoanalysis is in dire need of systematization. As Kris put it in 1947: "Sooner or later the ever more precise empirical test becomes an essential element in the development of any system of scientific proposi-

tions. In the development of psychoanalysis this moment seems to have arrived" (p. 14).

2. Cherished beliefs of Freud that no longer meet the test of science have to be weeded out. The two prime examples were Freud's acceptance of the Lamarckian view that acquired characteristics are inherited, and Freud's belief in the death instinct. In their paper entitled "Notes on the Theory of Aggression" (1946), Hartmann, Kris, and Loewenstein bypassed Freud's death instinct theory, maintaining that this hypothesis cannot now, or in the foreseeable future, be checked against empirical evidence. Freud thought that aggression can be mitigated by fusion with the libido. Hartmann, Kris, and Loewenstein thought that it could be accomplished through "deaggressivization," a term they coined as parallel to desexualization. The term "neutralization" was applied to both drives.

3. The area of promise for new psychoanalytic ideas will come primarily from infant and child observations, and secondarily from data obtained from child analysis.

In keeping with this program, the fourth group of papers comprises Kris's contributions to child psychology. In his "Notes on the Development of Some Current Problems in Child Psychology," Kris (1950a) introduced into psychoanalysis the systematic and longitudinal direct observation of children in order to observe how they develop, and how they solve or fail to solve phase-specific problems. Kris hoped that these direct observations would complement and supplement data observed in the "psychoanalytic interview" of adults associating to their childhood. These studies were conducted at the Yale University Child Study Center, where Kris was a clinical professor. Kris attempted to test psychoanalysis not only as a postdictive discipline but also as a predictor of future developments. Some predictions were made even before the infant was born, following interviews with the pregnant mother regarding her attitude toward her future child and by learning about her character structure.

Kris's interest in art and his commitment to ego psychology came together when he coined the term "regression under the control of the ego." Unlike the mentally ill, the regression of the artist remains under the control of the ego, and therefore can be utilized in his or her creative work. The same twofold interest is also discernible

behind Kris's 1955 paper, "Neutralization and Sublimation: Observations on Young Children." Freud spoke of sublimation consisting of the fusion of libidinal and aggressive wishes. The Hartmann school of psychoanalytic ego psychology introduced the term "neutralization" and differentiated it from sublimation. Kris attempted to create an experimental situation in which this process could be observed. He noted how preschool children approach the empty space on the easel. These children have only recently emerged from the anal phase. Kris observed how they struggled against and won victory over it in the creative process.

The fifth group of papers comprises Kris's writings on psychoanalytic technique. He observed that the function of remembering itself can become hypercathected, in which case a rich past is preferred to the drab present. Some patients have a tendency to treat their memories as treasured possessions, which they present to the analyst as a myth of their autobiography. Unless the therapist is alerted to it, such a personal myth is often strong enough to survive psychoanalysis intact (Kris, 1956a).

Kris succeeded in dethroning the central position of memories. Stress trauma, covering many years, usually appeared in memory as a single event. Conversely, traumatic events like seduction at an early age did not appear in sharp outline.

Freud had differentiated between screen memories and genuine memories. Kris coined the term "stress trauma" to explain many interactions between the child and his or her caretaker that affect adversely the child's development. Kris's approach to remembering had an effect on psychoanalytic technique. Instead of focusing on a single, often hypothetical traumatic event and reconstructing it, he directed attempts toward capturing the affective atmosphere of a whole period in the life of the child. Experiences, Kris believed, are stored as patterns, and it is with such patterns that the analyst should work.

In one case, Kris cited a three-year-old girl (1956b, p. 325). Her younger brother had been born when she was two. The relationship between her parents had been and continued to be stormy; a beloved dog had chewed the tail of her cat; a few months later this dog had been run over. Her grandfather had died. Kris questioned the probability that future analysts would be able to recover these events that in reality were discretely separated from one another. The synthetic functions of the ego will operate to amalgamate these memories in a way that is not predictable.

K

In the paper, "On Some Vicissitudes of Insight in the Course of Psychoanalysis" (1956c), Kris applied to the analytic hour an idea that he had first developed in 1935 in his studies on art. He differentiated between two types of regression. In the first, the ego is overwhelmed by regression, and the result is pathology. In the second, regression remains under the control of the ego. Artists in particular were thought to be capable of such creative regression. In this paper, Kris applied this concept to the analytic hour itself. It is related to the two previous papers by demonstrating optimal conditions under which childhood memories or fantasies emerge. In the "good hour," the analysand is not straining to find new memories; they appear unbidden. In the "good hour," memories appear in context, symbolizing significant events or changes related to the relative strength of ego, id, and superego. The capacity to uncover new memories coincides with the capacity to grasp the significance of what had been uncovered.

While psychoanalysts had known for a long time that certain analytic hours were regarded by both patient and analyst as particularly productive, no one had thought of submitting such "good hours" to scrutiny.

Kris differentiated the "good hour" from the "deceptively good hour." In the latter, the patient wishes to obtain the analyst's love and produces associations the analyst would appreciate. The "deceptively good hour" takes place when the transference is fueled by either wishes for merger with the analyst or by competitive wishes. The analysand makes his or her own competitive interpretations. Libidinal and aggressive wishes burden the process of free association, which cannot evolve autonomously. By contrast, Kris stressed that neutralization will favor the process of genuine free association and will result in the genuinely good hour.

Probably because of Kris's early death, the full implications of this paper remain unrecognized. However, he left a description of what he called the "morphology" of the "good hour." Typically, such hours do not start propitiously. Free associations are disjointed, recent experiences are recounted, and the transference manifestations are negative. However, because the analysand is free to express his or her negative feelings, a marked change occurs midway through such hours. Everything seems to fall into place. A dream is told with no resistance and is associated to. New memories become available. Often all that the analyst need to do

is ask one or two questions and the analysand sums up the work alone. In 1993, I pointed out that while neither analyst nor analysand can will the good hour, analysts by pursuing their own interests and not giving their analysands the necessary space for exploration can derail the formation of many good hours.

Few psychoanalysts cast so wide a net as did Ernst Kris. Rarer still was his gift for applying what he learned in one field to the other fields of his growing interests.

REFERENCES

Bergmann, M. S. (1993). Reality and psychic reality in Ernst Kris's last papers: An attempt to update his findings. *Psychoanaytic Inquiry*, 13: 372–383.

Hale, N. (1995). *Rise and Crisis of Psychoanalysis in the United States: Freud and the Americas, 1917–1985.* New York: Oxford University Press.

Hartmann, H. (1949). Notes on the theory of aggression. *Psychological Issues*, (1964), 4, no. 2: 56–85.

Hartmann, H., and Kris, E. (1945). The genetic approach to psychoanalysis. In *Psychoanalysis, The Psychoanalytic Study of the Child.* New York: International Universities Press, 1: 11–30. Also in *Psychological Issues* (1964), 4, no. 2: 7–26.

Hartmann, H., Kris, E., and Loewenstein, R. (1946). Comments on the formation of the psychic structure. *Psychological Issues* (1964), 4, no. 2: 27–55.

Kris, E. (1947). The nature of psychoanalytic propositions and their validations. *Selected Papers of Ernst Kris.* New Haven, Conn.: Yale University Press (1975), pp. 3–23.

———. (1950a). Notes on the development and on some current problems of psychoanalytic child psychology. *Selected Papers of Ernst Kris.* New Haven, Conn.: Yale University Press (1975), pp. 54–79.

———. (1950b). *Introduction to Sigmund Freud: The Origins of Psychoanalysis, Letters to Wilhelm Fliess, 1887–1902.* New York: Basic Books.

———. (1951). Ego psychology and interpretation in psychoanalytic therapy. *Psychoanalytic Quarterly*, 20: 15–30.

———. (1952). *Psychoanalytic Explorations in Art.* New York: International Universities Press.

———. (1955). Neutralization and sublimation: Observations on young children. *Selected Papers of Ernst Kris.* New Haven, Conn.: Yale University Press (1975), pp. 151–171.

———. (1956a). The personal myth: A problem in psychoanalytic technique. *Selected Papers of Ernst Kris.* New Haven, Conn.: Yale University Press (1975), pp. 271–300.

———. (1956b). The recovery of childhood memories in psychoanalysis. *Selected Papers of Ernst Kris.* New Haven, Conn.: Yale University Press (1975), pp. 301–342.

———. (1956c). On some vicissitudes of insight in the course of psychoanalysis. *Selected Papers of Ernst Kris.* New Haven, Conn.: Yale University Press (1975), pp. 252–271.

MARTIN S. BERGMANN

L

Lacan, Jacques (1901–1981)

Jacques Lacan is, arguably, the most important psychoanalytic theorist since Sigmund Freud himself. Lacan is best known for initiating what could be described as a "linguistic turn" in relation to Freudian metapsychology. The statement most often associated with Lacan—in the same way that the thought of Descartes is inextricably linked to the phrase "*Cogito, ergo sum*"—is "the unconscious is structured like a language" (*l'inconscient est structuré comme un langage*). However, his sizable oeuvre, spanning the years 1932 to 1980, cannot be adequately encapsulated by this single claim extracted from a particular period of his teaching. Rather than being a homogeneous set of dogmatic assertions, Lacan's work represents an ongoing, evolving interrogation of what it means to be a subject in light of the discovery of the unconscious.

Lacan's first major text to appear was his 1932 doctoral thesis in psychiatry: *De la psychose paranoïaque dans ses rapports avec la personnalité (Of Paranoid Psychosis in Its Relations with the Personality)*. In his thesis, the young Lacan (who, at this early stage in his career, was just beginning to grapple with Freud from within the context of French medical psychiatry) advanced the viewpoint that various mental pathologies are not reducible to an explanation/diagnosis based on organic criteria alone; that is to say, for certain mental illnesses, the underlying causal mechanisms are not brain lesions or any sort of physical defect. Instead, he proposed that specific pathological states are the result of certain (dys)functions in the structure of the "personality," and he proceeded to redefine the very concept of personality in conjunction with this proposal. Foreshadowing much of his later work (but couched within a prestructuralist and non-Freudian parlance), Lacan spoke of the subject's personality as a dense, multilayered apparatus constructed out of a diverse group of linguistic, imagistic, and sociocultural elements.

In 1936, one of the most famous Lacanian concepts was unveiled: the mirror stage. At the fourteenth international congress of the International Psychoanalytic Association held at Marienbad, Czechoslovakia, Lacan delivered a paper whose title, as recorded in the minutes of the congress meetings, was "The Looking Glass Phase." Evidently, as accounts have it, Lacan, ten minutes into his presentation, was interrupted by Ernest Jones (then the presiding president of the IPA). No written record remains of the 1936 version of the paper (only the 1949 version of the mirror stage essay is available, this being the one published in the 1966 *Écrits*). In the published version, drawing upon various influences (such as Freud, Henri Wallon, and Alexandre Kojève), Lacan presented a detailed account of the origins and essence of the psychoanalytically conceived ego. Supplementing Freud's own analyses of this psychical agency (most notably, as presented in such texts as *On Narcissism: An Introduction* [1914], *Mourning and Melancholia* [1917], *Group Psychology and the Analysis of the Ego* [1921], *The Ego and the Id* [1923], and *The Splitting of the Ego in the Process of Defense* [1938]), Lacan argued that the nucleus of the ego consists in the "Imaginary *imago*," namely, in the reflected images that the individual comes to identify as a "self" (i.e., the gestalt-like *moi*). This visual kernel of ego identity is subsequently taken up and codified by language; the Imaginary *moi* is transformed into the symbolic *je*. Lacan treats the ego as a "false self," as a symptomatic function of the subject's "misrecognition" (*méconnaissance*) of his or her subjectivity; this subjectivity is "mislaid," alienated in the mediating matrices of imaginary and symbolic alterity. Already in the 1930s, Lacan laid the foundations for his systematic and methodical assault on ego psychology as developed in his mature works of the 1950s through the late 1970s. In 1938, at the invitation of Wallon, Lacan contributed a piece to the *Encyclopédie Française* entitled "Les complexes familiaux dans la formation de l'individu" (The Family Complexes in the Formation of the Individual). This text, prior to (but prescient of) the later structuralist turn to Saussure inspired by the anthropological theory of Claude Lévi-Strauss, focused on the "complex," a notion defined as a constellation of sociosymbolic relations shaping the very identity and constitution of the psychical subject. It was also during this period that Lacan audited Kojève's seminars on Hegel's *Phenomenology of Spirit*. Lacan adopted many of the ideas and terms employed by Kojève, and they appear in various modified guises throughout both his writings and his seminars.

Because of the disruption of the World War II, Lacan published little in the 1940s. But, a few notable pieces were produced during that time: "Logical Time and the Assertion of Anticipated Certainty: A New Sophism," a 1945 essay using a variation on a sort of prisoners' dilemma to examine the formalizable features of imaginary and symbolic intersubjective relations in the shaping of individual identity; "Propos sur la causalité psychique" (Remarks on Psychic Causality), a 1946 piece in which Lacan displayed his growing tendency to mobilize philosophical figures and theories in his approach to the psychoanalytic domain; "La psychiatrie anglaise et la guerre" (English Psychiatry and the War), another 1946 essay, produced as a result of Lacan's brief stay as a medical observer in England; "Aggressivity in Psychoanalysis," a 1948 text in which Lacan further developed the consequences of his notion of the mirror stage as the foundation of ego-level identity, arguing in particular that the arousal of aggression is intimately linked to the individual encountering her or his "semblance" or "double," that hatred is triggered by the necessary, intrinsic subjugation of the ego to a set of ego versus alter ego rivalries whose description echoes Hegel's "master and slave" dialectic from the *Phenomenology of Spirit*; and as mentioned above, the extant version of the mirror stage essay itself (given in 1949 at the sixteenth IPA congress in Zurich). Although a few other essays were produced during this period, the ones listed above are the most important in light of later developments in Lacan's thinking.

The Lacan who is the most familiar to the reading public, especially in the English-speaking world, emerged in the early 1950s. In 1953, Lacan, along with several others, broke away from the psychoanalytic training institution to which he had previously been attached (Société Psychanalytique de Paris) owing to serious disagreements over the organization of the institution and its criteria for selecting analytic training candidates. This split was the beginning of Lacan's subsequent struggles with the institutional dimension of psychoanalytic practice in which he found himself entangled until his death. Those who left the SPP formed a new group, the Société Française de Psychanalyse (Lacan would remain with the SFP until late 1963, when a second crisis forced him to leave that training institution too). In September 1953, at a conference in Rome, Lacan delivered a lengthy talk entitled "Function and Field of Speech and Language in Psychoanalysis" (or, as it has come to be known, the "Rome Discourse"). This piece can be considered as a kind of manifesto heralding the arrival of a distinctive theoretical approach to the Freudian field now referred to as Lacanianism. Lacan introduced a range of topics associated with his thought: the primacy of languagelike functions in the structuring of the unconscious, the nature of the symbolic order, the recentering of the psychoanalytic clinic on the speech (*parole*) of the analysand, and the critique of any form of therapeutic intervention oriented around the strengthening of the patient's ego.

These same themes reverberate throughout the other writings produced during this crucial phase in the development of Lacan's own emerging brand of psychoanalytic theory: "Some Reflections on the Ego" (1951), "The Freudian Thing, or the Meaning of the Return to Freud in Psychoanalysis" (1955), "The Seminar on 'The Purloined Letter'" (1956), "On a Question Preliminary to Any Possible Treatment of Psychosis" (1957), and "The Direction of the Treatment and the Principles of Its Power" (1958). In all these texts, the central point that Lacan sought to emphasize was that the ego, rather than being a self-determining agent capable of taming and subduing the unconscious, *is* the deluded, overdetermined dupe behind whose back transpires the autonomous, playful machinations of the signifier. Borrowing from Saussure (and inspired by the then-novel structuralist approach to the human sciences), Lacan treated Freud's concept of *Vorstellung* (i.e., "presentation," as in the mnemonic, ideational materials constituting the "content" of the psyche) in terms of a revised theory of the signifier: the unconscious is portrayed as the network of shifting relations existing between a series of differentially defined operational elements. As the Lacan of the 1970s emphasized about this earlier set of structuralist assertions first laid out in the 1950s, no claim is made here that the unconscious literally is nothing more than the materials of spoken languages such as French, English, German, and so on (this being a common misreading of Lacan). Lacan's point was, instead, that the relations at work between the ideational representations of the unconscious—these representations are not simply impressions of linguistic units but include all the sensory features of mnemonic traces—can be best conceptualized through recourse to the theoretical tools initially fashioned within the discipline of structuralist linguistics. However, this is not tantamount to claiming that the unconscious is therefore reducible to the status of being a mere residue of *une langue* (a "tongue"—Lacan speaks of the unconscious as resembling *un langage*, not *une langue*).

It was also in 1953 that Lacan's annual seminar began. In its early years, the seminar was primarily attended by a group of practicing analysts, many of whom were already mature thinkers in their own right (such as Jean Laplanche, Serge Leclaire, Octave and Maud Mannoni, J. B. Pontalis, Moustafa Safouan, and others). However, over the period of its twenty-seven year existence, Lacan's seminar was transformed from a forum for practicing psychoanalysts into the centerpiece of Parisian intellectual life during the 1960s and 1970s. Some of the most prestigious names in France's recent philosophical history attended Lacan's seminar at one point or another: Lévi-Strauss, Hyppolite, Ricoeur, Foucault, Deleuze, and Kristeva, to name a few.

The first ten years of the seminar (1953–1963) were conducted under the banner of a "return to Freud." With a strong emphasis on Freud's early writings (*The Interpretation of Dreams* [1900], *The Psychopathology of Everyday Life* [1901], and *Jokes and Their Relation to the Unconscious* [1905]), Lacan sought to recover a genuine conception of the Freudian unconscious that, unlike so many post-Freudian exegetical bastardizations, was careful not to conflate the unconscious with the id (in other words, not to treat the unconscious as a hidden reservoir of libidinal energies impinging upon the conscious

mind). For Lacan, the Freudian unconscious is, rather than an obscure bundle of quasi-instinctual forces, an intricate tissue of interconnected representations (i.e., signifiers qua *Vorstellungen*) structuring all facets of subjectivity, a "symbolic order" shaping the speaking, cognizing subject. The first ten years of Lacan's seminar covered a wide range of topics central to psychoanalytic theory and practice: "Freud's Papers on Technique" (*Seminar I*, 1953–1954), "The Ego in Freud's Theory and in the Technique of Psychoanalysis" (*Seminar II*, 1954–1955), "The Psychoses" (*Seminar III*, 1955–1956), "The Object Relation" (*Seminar IV*, 1956–1957), "Formations of the Unconscious" (*Seminar V*, 1957–1958), "Desire and Its Interpretation" (*Seminar VI*, 1958–1959), "The Ethics of Psychoanalysis" (*Seminar VII*, 1959–1960), "Transference" (*Seminar VIII*, 1960–1961), "Identification" (*Seminar IX*, 1961–1962), and "Anxiety" (*Seminar X*, 1962–1963). During this incredibly productive period, a wide range of distinctly Lacanian concepts were forged: "the three registers" (the Real, the Symbolic, and the Imaginary); "foreclosure" (Lacan's account of the genesis of the psychoses); "the need-demand-desire triad" (Lacan's own dissection of the libidinal economy according to his tripartite register theory), *jouissance* (the literal but inadequate English translation of this term being "enjoyment"—*jouissance* was first developed by Lacan as a means of designating that aspect of the Freudian *Trieb* [drive] operating "beyond the pleasure principle"), and object *a* (although influenced by the notion of "partial object" as present in the work of Karl Abraham and Melanie Klein as well as the "transitional object" of D. W. Winnicott, this Lacanian concept is equally indebted to the philosophical theories of "objectivity" as found in the writings of Kant, Hegel, Heidegger, and Merleau-Ponty).

The eleventh seminar was originally supposed to be on "The Names of the Father." Only one session of this seminar was given, however, during which Lacan announced that he would no longer be teaching at Sainte-Anne hospital (where the first ten years of the seminar had been held). The reason for this seminar's termination was that the Société Française de Psychanalyse (SFP), under pressure from the International Psychoanalytic Association, voted to remove Lacan from their list of approved training analysts. For ten years, the SFP, having broken with the Société Psychanalytique de Paris (which was itself an IPA-approved training institution), lobbied the IPA for admittance. In November 1963, the

IPA, following recommendations presented by a special investigating team that had spent years scrutinizing the activities of the SFP, presented the SFP with an ultimatum of sorts outlining the conditions for it being granted membership in the international organization. The key requirement was that it remove Lacan from the list of approved training analysts. The main reason for this requirement was Lacan's practice of the "variable length session," sometimes called the "short session," although this obscures the fact that Lacan would either shorten or lengthen the time of analytic sessions depending on the specific analysand and his or her particular symptoms. The IPA refused to acknowledge the legitimacy of this technical innovation on Lacan's part, despite the persuasive justification that, by modifying the time of the sessions instead of rigidly adhering to the standard fifty-minute format of psychoanalytic sessions, the analyst would be able to thwart the frequent tactic of neurotics to "kill the hour" by filling it with trivial verbal material and thereby avoid the labor of free association so crucial to the analytic cure. As part of its banishment of Lacan, the IPA also refused to recognize his trainees as certified practicing analysts.

In 1964, Lacan was offered a refuge for his seminar at the École Normale Supérieure (ENS). He resumed his eleventh seminar under the new title "The Four Fundamental Concepts of Psycho-Analysis" (deservedly, this has become, apart perhaps from the Écrits, the best-known Lacanian text). He opened that year's seminar with a discussion of his "excommunication" from both the SFP and the IPA. He compared himself to Spinoza and accused those he had worked alongside and trained at the SFP of selling him out in a shameful bargain with the IPA for hollow institutional recognition. His teaching situation was quite different at the ENS: instead of speaking to a group of practicing analysts, Lacan found himself addressing a large, diverse audience consisting of people from various backgrounds (not only psychoanalysts but philosophers, literary theorists, historians, linguists, and other academics). With this change of audience, Lacan took the opportunity to step back from his previous detailed examinations of specific topics in the Freudian field—each year of the first ten years of the seminar tended to be devoted to a specified set of concepts in Freud's work—and to perform a sweeping reassessment of the foundations of the psychoanalytic metapsychological edifice. Focusing on each of the four "fundamental concepts" (drive, repetition, transference,

unconscious), Lacan inquired into the relation of psychoanalysis to science and sought to delineate precisely the axiomatic concepts making possible the analytic investigation into the structure of subjectivity and the unconscious.

It was also during this time that Lacan founded his own psychoanalytic school: the École Freudienne de Paris. This school would remain in existence, despite its internal antagonisms and various controversies (most notably, over the procedure of "the pass," a mechanism forged by Lacan as the means by which the École Freudienne would ascertain whether or not an analytic trainee should be promoted to the status of recognized practicing analyst, and the handling of the organization of the Department of Psychoanalysis at the University of Paris VIII at Vincennes), until just before Lacan's death, when he dissolved it and handed over authority of his "Freudian cause" to his son-in-law, Jacques-Alain Miller (Lacan met Miller in 1964 at the ENS, where Miller was, at the time, a student of the Marxist philosopher Louis Althusser; Miller became the general editor of Lacan's seminars and the head of the École de la Cause Freudienne). Lacan's annual seminar continued on through the 1960s: "Crucial Problems for Psychoanalysis" (*Seminar XII*, 1964–1965), "The Object of Psychoanalysis" (*Seminar XIII*, 1965–1966), "The Logic of Fantasy" (*Seminar XIV*, 1966–1967), "The Psychoanalytic Act" (*Seminar XV*, 1967–1968), "From an Other to the Other" (*Seminar XVI*, 1968–1969), and "The Reverse of Psychoanalysis" (*Seminar XVII*, 1969–1970—this seminar was conducted in an auditorium at the law school of the Panthéon, to which Lacan's seminar was moved from the ENS in 1969). These years saw the emergence of further distinctive Lacanian concepts: the split subject (\$), the formula of fantasy (\$ ♦ a—the relationship between the split subject and *objet petit a*), the act-action distinction, and the four discourses (the discourses of the master, the hysteric, the university, and the analyst).

In 1966, the second major published book by Lacan appeared: *Écrits*. Although Lacan published his medical thesis in 1932, he refrained from writing any other books until 1966. Following in the style of Kojève, Lacanianism was transmitted primarily through the spoken word, namely, through the lectures of Lacan's seminar. The rest was disseminated via articles published in various journals. After much coaxing by François Wahl, an editor at Éditions du Seuil, Lacan agreed to assemble a collection of his writings for publication (Lacan referred to publication as "*poubellication*," a French play on words that translates, approximately, into "trash-canning" as a homonym of "publishing"). The volume, produced after an arduous assembly and editing process, was over nine hundred pages long. Despite being stylistically difficult and conceptually complex, *Écrits* became a best-seller in France. This single book firmly established Lacan, in the eyes of the French public, as "the French Freud," the undisputed master of psychoanalysis in France.

Without doubt, the most controversial period of Lacan's teaching remains his work from the 1970s. Throughout his intellectual career, Lacan exhibited a strong interest in mathematics and formal logic (this is explicitly evident as early as the 1945 essay on "logical time," and can be seen in Lacan's recourse to complex graphs in the 1950s, as well as his invocation of topological models starting in the ninth seminar of 1961–1962). However, in the 1970s (beginning with the meditations on the "Borromean knot" inaugurated in the nineteenth seminar), the motif of the "matheme" (i.e., a formalized unit representing, in condensed form, an analytic concept) came to dominate Lacan's concerns. Fearing that his own thought might be subjected to the same sorts of distortions and misunderstandings under which he saw Freud's work suffer, Lacan believed that the means of preserving and transmitting his body of theory lay in distilling his ideas into a kind of formal language for psychoanalysis. The irony is that, instead of definitively fixing and stabilizing the meaning of his concepts, these mathemes have become, so to speak, Rorschach ink blots onto which interpreters project whatever preconceptions they already have about Lacan's work based on his other writings. Nonetheless, despite the problems and controversies generated by this last period, Lacan continued to elucidate and refine his theory of the three registers. During this time, he also engaged in the important task of reconsidering the nature of the psychoanalytic cure in light of his revised understanding of the essential features of the symptom. And he reexamined the status of sexual difference and the significance of gender, famously proposing, in the twentieth seminar: "*Il n'y a pas de rapport sexuel*" (There is no sexual relationship); owing to the centrality of *objet petit a* in the life of the drives, coupled with the mediating role of unconscious fantasies in sexual relations, Lacan concluded that individuals do not so much "relate" to each other as to the idiosyncrasies of their own libidinal economies. He conducted his annual sem-

inar up until mid-1980, when his deteriorating health finally prevented him from continuing. The seminars included "Of a Discourse That Would Not Be a Semblance" (Seminar XVIII, 1970-1971); ". . . Or Worse" (*Seminar XIX*, 1971–1972—during the same year, Lacan returned to Sainte-Anne hospital to give a seminar entitled "The Knowledge of the Psychoanalyst"); "Encore" (*Seminar XX*, 1972–1973); "The Non-Dupes Err" (*Seminar XXI*, 1973–1974); "R.S.I." (*Seminar XXII*, 1974–1975); "*Le sinthome*" (*Seminar XXIII*, 1975–1976); "*L'insu que sait de l'une-bévue s'aile à mourre*" (*Seminar XXIV*, 1976–1977); "Time to Conclude" (*Seminar XXV*, 1977–1978); "Topology and Time" (*Seminar XXVI*, 1978-1979); and "Dissolution" (*Seminar XXVII*, 1979–1980). Lacan died on September 9, 1981.

Exhaustively cataloguing Lacan's contributions to psychoanalysis would be a mammoth task. Lacan's extensive oeuvre contains a myriad number of crucial reconceptualizations of the Freudian legacy in terms of theory as well as therapy. Furthermore, Lacan's influence now extends well beyond the confines of psychoanalysis. Because of his active engagement with numerous disciplines—in his lifelong commitment to an unrelenting investigation into all the various facets and features of the unconscious, Lacan actively examined not only the texts of Freud but the history of philosophy, linguistics, mathematics, literature, and other fields—Lacan created a distinctive theoretical approach enabling those who employ it to make headway in addressing various questions at the heart of the human sciences today. Lacan has not only become a central figure in the ongoing development of psychoanalytic thought but is clearly a thinker whom no one interested in the history of ideas in the twentieth century can avoid.

ADRIAN JOHNSTON

Lanzer, Ernst See RAT MAN.

Latent Content See DREAMS, THEORY OF.

Lay Analysis

In Austria in Freud's day, to treat patients without having earned a medical degree constituted quackery and warranted punishment by law. Theodor Reik, a lawyer by training, had studied with Freud and was a practicing member of the Vienna Psycho-Analytical Society in

1926 when, at the instigation of a former analysand, he was prosecuted under this charge. Reik was exonerated eventually, but not until a number of expert witnesses had testified on his behalf, and Freud himself, having discussed the case with a high official, "had, at his request, written a confidential opinion on the subject."

Later that year, in *The Question of Lay Analysis*, Freud made public this opinion in the rhetorical form of "Conversations within an Impartial Person." There he summarized the prevailing argument against lay analysis as follows: "Neurotics are patients, laymen are non-doctors, psychoanalysis is a procedure for curing or improving nervous disorders, and all such treatments are reserved to doctors. It follows that laymen are not allowed to practice analysis on neurotics and are punishable if they nevertheless do so." Freud did not oppose this reasoning but disagreed with its major premises, arguing "that in this instance the patients are not like other patients, that the laymen are not really laymen, and that . . . doctors have not exactly the qualities which one has a right to expect of doctors and on which their claims should be based."

Freud began his discussion by noting that neurotic patients present medical-like complaints for which medical doctors can find no organic cause. He reviewed for his "Impartial Person" the psychoanalytic model of the mind and the psychodynamic theory of neurosis, concluding that neurotics are not like other patients because they suffer disturbances, not in the medical province of the body but in the separate and sovereign domain of the psyche. They differ, too, he said, because they act as if driven by a (most un-patient-like) desire to remain ill.

Freud went on to show that, for these patients, the lay analyst is not really a layperson because analytic training, by way of didactics, personal analysis, and clinical supervision, brings the analyst to proficiency in this form of therapy. Medical training, by contrast, not only omits such instruction but entirely overlooks "the mental side of vital phenomena." Worst of all, said Freud, orthodox medicine with its one-sided emphasis on objective science inculcates "a false and detrimental attitude" toward neurotic patients: the notion that, because their suffering is merely psychic, for medical purposes it is not real. He continues: "Only psychiatry is supposed to deal with the disturbances of mental functions; but we know in what manner and with what aims it does so. It looks for the somatic determinants of mental disorders and treats them like other causes of illness."

Thus without addressing it directly, Freud pointed to the split in our thinking about ourselves that divides the mind from the body and seems to necessitate separate approaches to the sufferings of the body and of the soul. While human suffering in fact defies this split, human attitudes reify it again and again. Psychoanalysis, which arose in part as an effort to redress the problems of this dualism, itself often divides along mind/body lines. Thus the field finds itself perennially plagued by controversies over the primacy of either the subjective or the objective domain of clinical theory and procedure— for example, whether it is "fantasy" or "what really happened" that ultimately explains the genesis of psychological symptoms, or whether "transference" or "the real relationship" offers the more solid foundation for therapeutic change.

Acknowledging the limits of the medical science of his day, Freud ended his essay on an optimistic note. Someday, he wrote, "the paths of knowledge and, let us hope, of influence will be opened up leading from organic biology and chemistry to the field of neurotic phenomena. That day still seems a distant one, and for the present these illnesses are inaccessible to us from the direction of medicine." Until that time, he argued, the diagnosis and treatment of neurotic suffering would remain a province far enough removed from mainstream medicine to call for its own specialized and nonmedical treatment profession. Toward that end, he proposed that neurotic patients should be screened by physicians for recognizable signs of organic illness, then referred for treatment in the hands of "secular pastoral workers" trained in psychoanalysis. "A new kind of Salvation Army!" his Impartial Person quipped. "Why not?" was Freud's reply.

The question of lay practice divides psychoanalysis to this day. The arguments for and against it remain essentially unchanged. Despite Freud's optimism, it seems, psychoanalysis has become no more scientific, nor science more psychoanalytic, through the passage of these seventy and more years.

REFERENCES

Eissler, K. R. (1965). *Medical Orthodoxy and the Future of Psychoanalysis*. New York: International Universities Press.

Freud, S. (1926). *The Question of Lay Analysis*. S.E. 20: 179–258.

Mann, D. W. (1988). The question of medical psychotherapy. *American Journal of Psychotherapy*, 43: 405–413.

[Various Authors]. (1927). *International Journal of Psychoanalysis* 8, part 2: 174–283.

DAVID W. MANN

Libidinal Stage See DEVELOPMENTAL THEORY.

Libido Theory

The libido theory occupied a central place in Freud's thinking. Indeed, in conversations with the author, Anna Freud described it as "the heart and lungs of psychoanalysis." But from the beginning, Freud's concept of the libido and his theories about it aroused considerable controversy, and continue to do so today. This article briefly reviews the history and rationale of the libido theory, its present standing, and its relation to recent developments in biological, genetic, and evolutionary thinking about sex and the issues that surround it.

To begin with, Freud used the term "libido" much as it might have been used by anyone: to denote sexual desire. Nevertheless, even here he qualified it with the adjective "psychical," and went on immediately to discuss the possibility of its transformation into anxiety (1950, p. 192). Although Freud was later to abandon the view that libido could be directly transformed into anxiety for the much more reasonable one that anxiety was a response to libidinal frustration, his first view of the matter reveals what is perhaps most fundamental and most original about the Freudian concept of libido. This is that libido is not limited to the purely reproductively, anatomically, or physically sexual, but extends the concept in three different dimensions.

First, Freud expanded the concept in the spatial and anatomical dimension by his concept of *erotogenic zones*. These were parts of the body that were not necessarily directly connected with sex and reproduction but from which pleasurable libidinal sensations could nevertheless spontaneously arise. Prime examples include the mouth, anus, and other orifices, but in principal more or less any part of the body can become an erotogenic zone in the right circumstances. To explain how regions remote from the genitals might become implicated in sexuality, Freud had to stretch the concept of the libido to include them and made subjective feelings of physical pleasure, rather than biological function, the chief criterion.

Erotogenic zones were of great importance as the physical focuses of *perversions*: a technical term in psychoanalysis (not a value judgment) denoting an organization of the libido in which something other than the genital of the opposite sex had become the prime object of satisfaction. Although anything—even an inanimate object in the case of fetishism—could qualify here, erotogenic zones typically tend to become centers of perverse satisfaction thanks to their intrinsic libidinal associations.

The second dimension in which Freud extended the concept of sexuality with the libido theory was time. Until Freud, it was universally agreed that sexual life began at puberty, but Freud's researches led him to the belief that libido was present from birth and that it went through a complex series of transformations before reaching its ostensible goal: genital sexuality. For example, Freud described the first stage of libidinal development as the *oral phase*. Freud felt justified in calling this a stage of libidinal development for three main reasons. First, common observation confirms that babies typically suck merely for the sake of sucking, independently of hunger. The fact that the reward of sucking is not food, but something intrinsic, was one of the reasons why Freud regarded the mouth as an erotogenic zone and sucking in early childhood a libidinal satisfaction. The second reason was that oral stimulation plays an important part in adult sexual life in the form of kissing, sucking, and licking. Finally, the existence of oral sexual perversions, in which the mouth alone is the focus of satisfaction and may even occasion orgasm, was conclusive proof that, in adulthood at least, the mouth could take on a sexual significance. Furthermore, there was an obvious biological rationale for the oral stage. Even though the mouth might seem remote from the purposes of adult reproduction, it was the critical organ for the survival of the newborn, thanks to its role in nutrition, and so there was a good reason why the libido should at first be focused there.

Following the oral stage, Freud distinguished an anal one, in which intrinsic libidinal pleasure was derived from excretion, and which he could justify for much the same reasons that he did the oral one. Finally in childhood came the phallic stage, in which the libido began to become focused on the genital, but only on the male one, signaling the beginning of a split in the development of the sexes. This phase coincided with the Oedipus complex, which Freud at first thought was perfectly symmetrical with regard to the sexes. But later he amended his view to accept that in the beginning the Oedipus complex of both boys and girls is much the same and focused on the mother (1931, p. 225).

One of the strangest claims of the libido theory was that in the unconscious the sexes are not represented as

L

male and female, but as male and not-male. Furthermore, Freud found that it was the possession of a penis that denoted maleness and its absence, not-maleness. This lay at the root of the differing developments of the sexes from the phallic period onward. Aware that she lacked a penis and so was not male, a little girl experienced penis envy, withdrew her libido from the mother she implicitly blamed for her lack of the penis, and instead took her father as the focus of her Oedipus complex. The little boy, untroubled by these complications, persisted with an Oedipus complex focused on his mother (1931, p. 223).

However, the libido theory, like much of Freud's thinking, was never complete and to the end contained some serious gaps. Although the facts convinced Freud that the Oedipus complex eventually was dissolved and followed by a latency period in which the libido lay dormant and attenuated until puberty, he remained unsure to the end of his life what brought this dissolution about, and speculated that innate factors might turn out to be decisive. However, he was sure that castration anxiety provided the dynamic motivation for the repression of infantile sexuality normally seen in the latency period, albeit different in the way it affected each sex (1924, p. 173).

Finally, puberty marked the second and decisive efflorescence of libido that ideally ushered in the genital phase of adult, reproductive sexuality. Nevertheless, fluctuations and changes in the libido were a normal part of life, and setbacks at certain stages could cause regressions to earlier ones. Here the pattern of infantile development was often found to be critical because a developmental arrest or peculiarity at one stage could lead to partial or complete fixation of the libido on its derivatives in adulthood. The result was that libido evolved in a complex fashion over the entirety of a person's life and was not simply confined to the period of reproductive fertility, or unilinear in its development. On the contrary, libido flowed backward and forward in time, with periods of growth, withdrawal, and resurgence sometimes occurring simultaneously in respect of different objects.

The third and last dimension in which Freud extended sexuality with the concept of the libido was in relation to its objects. In the narrow, reproductive view, sexuality has only one object, which is an appropriate member of the opposite sex. Freud's exploration of the human psyche revealed that the libido could have practically any object, including most crucially of all, the self.

This introduced the concept of *narcissism* understood as a product of *ego libido*, that is, libido invested in the individual's own body and mind (1914, p. 69). According to the libido theory, such primary narcissism gradually converts to object libido in the course of the development, with the breast and then the body and person of the mother being its original object (1940, p. 150). Because ego and *object libido* are fundamentally the same but differ only in regard to their object, Freud could explain so-called *secondary narcissism*, that is, the tendency for libido withdrawn from an object to return to the ego from whence it originally came, for example, in mourning (1917a, p. 239).

Contrary to common misunderstandings, narcissism as portrayed by the libido theory is not another term for simple selfishness or self-absorption. One of the triumphs of the libido theory was to provide an explanation of social cohesion and altruism in terms of narcissism. Freud explained group psychology by showing how members invested their individual ego libido in common ego identifications, typically with leaders or leading principles that formed the focus for group identity. Thanks to the mechanisms of identification and projection on the part of the individual members' egos, part of their ego libido could be made available to the wider group, or to other individuals with whom the subject identified (1921, p. 67).

If the libido could adopt the self as an object, it could certainly adopt others that resembled it, for example, members of the same sex. In this way the concept of ego libido in particular and narcissism in general opened up an entirely new perspective on homosexuality (1917b, p. 426). Another early insight of Freud's that became a fundamental component of the libido theory was the fact of *bisexuality*—the simultaneous presence of male and female components of the libido in the same individual (1905, pp. 141–148).

From the beginning, the libido theory appeared to make little sense in terms of the wider biological understanding of sex, as Freud himself ruefully admitted in successive prefaces to the *Three Essays on the Theory of Sexuality* (1905, pp. 130–134). In particular, bisexuality was singled out as a biological absurdity at the time Freud first put it forward. Today, however, the situation could not be more different, and even Freud's most bitter critics accept bisexuality as a biological finding of very wide relevance throughout nature (Daly and Wilson, 1983). In the human case, the fact that X chromosome genes spend two-thirds of their time in female, rather than male, bodies probably explains much about bisexuality in both sexes, irrespective of whether there is or is not a gene for male homosexuality on the X (Hamer et al., 1993).

The libido theory was a key part of Freud's wider instinct theory, which constantly evolved over his lifetime, reaching a final embodiment in his belief in universal life and death instincts (1920). Here libido was the energy available to the life instinct, Eros (a countervailing one available to the death instinct was never given a name by Freud [1940, p. 150]). This in turn raises the question of the current standing of the libido theory, given that today no credible biological basis for contradictory life and death instincts exists or is ever likely to.

In post-Freudian psychoanalysis, the libido theory has either been rejected entirely or greatly watered-down, and in general Freud is widely regarded as having exaggerated the importance of sex. However, some vindication of his belief in the primacy of the libido can be found in modern evolutionary thinking, at least as far as it applies to the reproductive function. Writing in 1914, Freud remarked:

> The individual himself regards sexuality as one of his own ends; whereas from another point of view he is an appendage to his germ-plasm, at whose disposal he puts his energies in return for a bonus of pleasure. He is the mortal vehicle of a (possibly) immortal substance—like the inheritor of an entailed property, who is only the temporary holder of an estate that survives him. (1914, p. 78).

It is notable that the translators of *The Standard Edition* use the very term "vehicle" in this context that Richard Dawkins, author of *The Selfish Gene*, was to adopt sixty-odd years later to describe the modern, Darwinian view of the organism as little more than the temporary repository of its DNA. Clearly, the prominence given to the libido in Freud's thinking is wholly compatible with this view.

Even ego libido can be accommodated here, because reproductive success—the only currency accepted by natural selection—can occur only after sexual maturity. This means that until then, survival should be the pre-eminent goal of the organism. As Freud himself pointed out, narcissism would be "the libidinal complement to

the egoism of the instinct of self-preservation" (1914, S.E. 14: 74). Again, because a woman's physical condition is much more critical to her reproductive success than is that of a man (who only has to achieve insemination, whereas she has to successfully endure a pregnancy), women should be more narcissistic on the whole than men. Interestingly, this is exactly what Freud reported (1914, pp. 88–90). Again, his finding that ego libido gradually converts into object libido, particularly after puberty, is exactly what we would predict if ego libido represented the value of the individual to the reproductive success of its genes (Badcock, 1994).

But however that may be, the greatest difficulty with the libido theory for people today is what it always has been: infantile sexuality. In many ways, this was Freud's most extraordinary and original finding, and it is still highly controversial. Nevertheless, arguments along the lines of those above suggest that, like libido in general and ego libido in particular, infantile sexuality may turn out to have an unexpected evolutionary and genetic foundation.

For example, positive emotional responses to the mother such as smiling in infancy may have been subject to arms race evolutionary escalation when they succeeded in securing preferential parental investment for the infants in question. The result would be a phase of intense emotional commitment to the mother at a time when she is the chief provider of parental investment but when the natural four-year spacing of births reported in primal populations meant that an existing child could no longer exploit oral behavior to postpone the birth of rivals, thanks to the contraceptive effect of breast feeding. If so, this would certainly explain the finding that children of both sexes have an Oedipus complex centered on the mother in the earlier part of the phallic period (Badcock, 1994).

As far as male and female Oedipus complexes later in the phallic period are concerned, the sex of a child can be critical for the level of parental investment that it receives. Given their greater variance of reproductive success (thanks to the fact that the only limit on a male's reproductive success is the number of females he can fertilize), parents whose offspring face good reproductive prospects ought to invest preferentially in males, but in females in the converse circumstances (Trivers and Willard, 1973). Preferential parental investment by mothers in "sexy sons" who showed evidence of their future reproductive potential through Oedipal behavior in childhood could pay a mother in terms of numbers of grandchildren. Given that natural selection would select the genes only of sons who succeeded in this way, sexy-son behavior could provide an evolutionary rationale for the male Oedipus complex.

Surprisingly enough, it could also do so for the female equivalent. This is because, if preferential parental investment is directed by parents to such sexy sons, daughters discriminated against on the basis of their sex should be selected, first to diagnose their own and siblings's sex reliably, and second to be motivated to compete for resources that brothers may be receiving by virtue of being male. Such might be the evolutionary basis of *penis envy*, particularly in view of Freud's report that women often link complaints about the lack of a penis with a further, surprising one "that her mother did not give her enough milk, did not suckle her long enough" (1931, p. 234).

At the very least, these suggestions are enough to show that it would be premature to write off infantile sexuality as wholly without biological justification, however strange it may seem to the minds of adults (Badcock, 1994). Certainly, it was Freud's view that "all our provisional ideas in psychology will presumably some day be based on an organic substructure" (1914, p. 78). Whether this will be so in the case of the libido theory remains to be seen, but current developments suggest that major surprises may yet be in store and that Freud's thinking on this central issue will continue to receive attention for a considerable time to come.

REFERENCES

Badcock, C. (1994). *PsychoDarwinism: The New Synthesis of Darwin and Freud*. London: HarperCollins.

Daly, M., and Wilson, M. (1983). *Sex, Evolution and Behavior*, 2d ed., Boston: Prindle, Weber and Schmidt

Freud, S. (1905). *Three Essays on the Theory of Sexuality*. S.E. 7: 130–242.

———. (1914). On narcissism: An introduction. S.E. 14: 69–102.

———. (1917a). Mourning and melancholia. S.E. 14: 237–258.

———. (1917b). *Introductory Lectures on Psychoanalysis*. S.E. 15–16: 9–496.

———. (1920). *Beyond the Pleasure Principle*. S.E. 18: 1–64.

———. (1921). *Group Psychology and the Analysis of the Ego*. S.E. 18: 1–143.

———. (1924). The dissolution of the Oedipus complex. S.E. 19: 173–179.

———. (1931). Female sexuality. S.E. 21: 223–243.

———. (1940). *An Outline of Psychoanalysis*. S.E. 23: 139–207.

———. (1950). Extracts from the Fliess papers. S.E. 1: 281–387.

Hamer, D., Hu, S., Magnuson, V. L., Hu, N., and Pattutucci, A. M. (1993). A linkage between DNA markers on the X chromosome and male sexual orientation. *Science*, 261: 321–326.

Trivers, R., and Willard, D. (1973). Natural selection of parental ability to vary the sex ratio of offspring. *Science*, 179: 90–92.

CHRISTOPHER BADCOCK

Literature, and Psychoanalysis

Whatever may be the fate of psychoanalysis as a psychological theory, literary historians of the future will surely regard its influence as one of the signatures of twentieth-century writing. Almost from the beginning of the century, the literary world greeted Freud as the bringer of revolutionary insights into the working of the mind. The enthusiasm with which Freud was received betrays the profound affinity between his point of view and the reigning assumptions of modern artistic culture; Freud did not so much change the course of literary production as crystallize and deepen its central tendencies. To illustrate the character of Freud's influence, it will suffice to examine three prominent motifs: the unconscious, the Oedipus complex, and repression.

The Unconscious

The term "unconscious," signifying a hidden order of mind, enjoyed currency more than a hundred years before the beginning of psychoanalysis. It was closely related to the romantic notion of genius—a capacity for artistic practice that, while purposeful and orderly, can give no account of itself nor be reduced to rules or intellectual principles. Post-romantic culture invested great significance in spontaneous imagination, in the mysteries of fantasy and dream. Idealist philosophers from Schelling onward glimpsed "unconscious" structures of order, or the "ruse of reason," as Hegel put it, behind the surface of appearances. The tendency to discover hidden orders took on an aggressive cast with the "unmasking critiques" of Marx, Nietzsche, and, finally, Freud, all of whom sought to show the importance of what was concealed beneath the polite surface of social existence.

For the twentieth century, Freud's conception of the unconscious provided writers with a powerful validation for the promptings of intuition, the sense of inner significance and complexity, as well as the deceptiveness of appearances. They frequently saw themselves as following Freud in a difficult, even heroic process of self-discovery and self-revelation. Getting in touch with the unconscious became a formula for literary power, and many solicited the "dark gods" D. H. Lawrence thought to dwell beneath the surface of the conscious mind. Some writers and artists, under the banner of "surrealism," attempted not only to make contact with the unconscious but to give themselves over to its logic; their method was to censor all conscious inhibitions and accustomed associations to produce an impression of liberating shock and disorientation. Thanks to their efforts, the imitation of dream logic, the disjointed logic of the unconscious, has become a common element of literary and artistic rhetoric. Since the 1960s, it has been visible through the whole range of culture, from television commercials to the "magic realism" of Latin American fiction. Twentieth-century writers could not have striven more singlemindedly to make the unconscious mind a conscious reality.

Oedipus Complex

It was by no means discouraging to the literary imagination to be told by an eminent scientist that the foundation of unconscious thought could be glimpsed in a figure out of myth—the figure of Oedipus. Eighteenth- and nineteenth-century writers of fiction had largely attempted to renounce mythology in favor of an empirical version of "realism," but Freud helped provide a basis upon which myth could be reclaimed as part of a realistic psychology. After Freud, writers of fiction could more readily gain access to mythological materials by sounding the depths of the unconscious, there to excavate the lingering effects of the Oedipal drama and the "family romance." The depiction of psychology through mythological fantasy and delusion was a technique at least as old as Cervantes—one of Freud's favorite authors—but in the hands of novelists like James Joyce and Thomas Mann it became a hallmark of modernism, the defining artistic movement of the first half of the twentieth century. Modernist writers shared with Freud the assertion of startling originality and daring, a militant emphasis on the centrality of the body to human existence, as well as the sense of having gotten down to the bottom of human nature by recovering access to its most primitive mythological and psychological strata.

Repression

It will be necessary here to distinguish between Freud's understanding of repression and the spirit in which the concept has been employed by others. Freud shared

and fostered the sense, prevalent in Western culture since Rousseau, that society and social life exact great costs from human nature. He believed that each individual, in the process of maturing, must either repress the natural force of instinct or direct it, by "sublimation," into socially approved activities. This process inevitably causes regrettable complications—a preference for public delusions like religion and metaphysics, or, where these have been discredited, a vulnerability to neurosis, paranoia, and other forms of mental illness. In spite of such complications, however, Freud does not see an alternative to repression; it is simply necessary for civilized life.

The Victorian rehabilitation of the subject of sex was already in vogue at the turn of the century when Freud was writing his early psychological studies, but he integrated it with science more persuasively than any other and gave it respectability beyond the ambit of the cultural avant-garde. For many artists and other devotees of Freud, their awareness of the concept of repression fueled the Rousseauian resentment against culture and gave rise to an ideology of sexual liberation. This ideology is a relentless element in twentieth-century literature; Lawrence, Henry Miller, Anaïs Nin, and Erica Jong are just a few of many examples. As a result, the eroticism and bodily exhibitionism of post-Freudian writing have a relentlessly moralizing, even utopian character. Up through the 1960s, its vocabulary of repression and liberation made psychoanalysis attractive to writers on the left and even to feminists, who have generally found a good deal to criticize in Freud's view of women.

Literary Criticism

Finally, Freud's way of thinking has had no less of an impact upon academic literary criticism than upon literary practice. Freud showed critics the way in a number of famous essays on artistic psychology and in ambitious attempts to bring psychoanalytic insight to bear on the works of major artists such as Leonardo, Shakespeare, and Dostoyevsky. In fact, psychoanalysis as a technique for interpreting unconscious motives largely came into being in an act of literary criticism when, in *The Interpretation of Dreams*, Freud attempted to explain the expressive power of *Oedipus the King* as emanating from an incestuous and parricidal wish that all of us share with Sophocles' hero.

Just as the psychoanalytic interpreter of dreams seeks the latent significance behind the manifest content of the dream, so psychoanalytic criticism aims to discover the latent psychological meaning beneath the surface of a literary work. As with dreams in Freud's theory, literary works reveal the fulfillment of a wish and the complications that arise from the struggle to express that wish in the face of censorship. Literature is an affair of pleasure and guilt, revelation and disguise. The psychoanalytic critic can analyze its dynamics in one of two directions. The first is to imitate Freud's analysis of *Oedipus the King* by interrogating the work itself to discover the sources of its appeal for its audience. What is involved is primarily an application of psychoanalytic theory, though some literary critics have attempted to develop their own theories of literary response based upon interpretations of Freud. The second application of psychoanalysis to literature is to use the work as a source of insight into the author's peculiar psychological complexes and neuroses, as Freud did in his studies of Dostoyevsky and Leonardo. With this type of treatment, the work becomes a repository of motifs from early childhood, and particularly a source for investigating the writer's way of coming to terms with the frustration of his or her early incestuous wishes. Often in these narratives literary achievement comes to be seen as a form of compensation for other, more basic emotional satisfactions denied early in life; the ideology of sexual liberation also plays a prominent role. It was partly because of psychoanalysis that literary biography has became such an important cultural institution in the twentieth century and that it acquired its peculiar character. It is no longer the admiring record of the genius's triumph over adversity—the narrative that gratified the sensibility of the nineteenth century—but rather the biographer's attempt to confront the public persona of the artist with the hidden motives of private life, to search behind the apparent strength, generosity, and power of the genius to discover the common psychological needs that foster the creative process.

REFERENCES

Bergler, E. (1992). *The Writer and Psychoanalysis,* 2d ed. New York: International Universities Press.

Brooks, P. (1994). *Psychoanalysis and Storytelling.* London: Blackwell.

Crews, F. (1989). *The Sins of the Fathers: Hawthorne's Psychological Themes.* Berkeley: University of California Press.

Ellmann, M. (1983). *Psychoanalytic Literary Criticism.* New York: Longman.

Farrell, J. (1996). *Freud's Paranoid Quest: Psychoanalysis and Modern Suspicion.* New York: New York University Press.

Kiell, N. (1990). *Psychoanalysis, Psychology, and Literature, a Bibliography.* Supplement to the 2d ed. Metuchen, N.J.: Scarecrow Press.

Kurzweil, E., and Phillips, W. (1983). *Literature and Psychoanalysis.* New York: Columbia University Press.

Simon, B. (1993). *Tragic Drama and the Family: Psychoanalytic Studies from Aeschylus to Beckett.* New Haven, Conn.: Yale University Press.

Wilson, E. (1947). *The Wound and the Bow: Seven Studies in Literature.* Oxford: Oxford University Press.

JOHN FARRELL

Little Hans

Little Hans, also referred to by Freud (1907) as "little Herbert," was the subject of Freud's first published case of a child psychoanalysis, *Analysis of a Phobia in a Five-Year Old Boy* (1909).

Little Hans's father wrote to Freud in 1908 that his son, then 5, had developed a "nervous disorder." The boy was afraid to go out into the street and feared that a horse would bite him. His father theorized that "this fear seems somehow to his being frightened by a large penis" (p. 22). Freud responded by laying down the general lines of the appropriate treatment, which was then carried out not by Freud but by the boy's father. Freud saw the boy but once; his analysis of the disorder is based on his interpretation of notes sent to him by the father.

The father's first reports concerning Hans date from when he was not quite three years old. Hans showed, Freud says, a lively interest in his penis, which he called his "widdler." He also asked his mother if she too had a widdler. When Hans was three and a half, his mother found him with his hand on his penis and told him "If you do that, I shall send for Dr. A to cut off your widdler. And then what'll you widdle with?" (Freud, 1909: 7–8). This was the occasion, Freud reports, when Hans acquired the castration complex (see "Castration Complex," this volume).

Approximately two years later, on January 7, 1908, Little Hans went out with his nursemaid, but began to cry and asked to be taken home to "coax" (i.e., cuddle) with his mummy. His mother took him out the next day, but he became frightened and began to cry, saying that he was afraid that a horse would bite him; after returning home, he expressed fear that the horse would come into his room.

After receiving the notes from Han's father, Freud arranged with him that he should tell the boy that "all this business about horses was a piece of nonsense and nothing more" (p. 28). Freud adds: "The truth was, his father was to say, that he was very fond of his mother and wanted to be taken into her bed. The reason he was afraid of horses now was that he had taken so much interest in their widdlers" (p. 28).

After the child was informed of this diagnosis and was enlightened about sexual matters, the father reported that he initially improved. Later, however, after spending two weeks in bed as a result of contracting influenza, his phobia worsened.

In late March, the father brought his son to visit Freud for a brief consultation. He opened the discussion by telling Freud that, despite all the enlightenment given to Hans, the child's fear of horses had not diminished. Freud responded by connecting the boy's fear of horses to fear of his father; he told the boy that he (Hans) thought his father was angry with him because he was so fond of his mother, and that, in fact, his father was not angry with him. Shortly after that consultation, in early April, the father noticed the first real improvement in his son's condition. Eventually, the boy recovered, and when Freud met him years later, in the spring of 1922, the young man was perfectly well.

In his discussion of the case, Freud concludes that Hans really was a little Oedipus who wanted his father out of the way so that he might be alone with and sleep with his beautiful mother. At first, Hans's wish was merely that his father would go away, but at a later stage, his fear of being bitten by a white horse attached itself on this form of the wish, owing to a chance impression (p. 111).

Some critics of Freud's interpretation (e.g., Eysenck, 1985, p. 111) argue that rather than castration anxiety and Oedipal dynamics being responsible for Hans's phobia, the more likely cause, and not merely the precipitating cause, was his witnessing an accident involving a horse falling down. The child himself believed that his problem started with the witnessing of the accident. His father suggested to him that his "nonsense"—which Freud and the father called Hans's fear of horses—preceded the accident, but Hans responded: "No. I only got it then [at the time of the accident]. When the horse in the bus fell down, it gave me such a fright, really! That was when I got the nonsense" (Freud, 1909: 50).

Freud anticipated, and tried to answer, this objection. First, he points out that chronological considerations make it impossible to attach any great importance to the actual precipitating cause of Hans's illness; for he

had shown apprehensiveness about horses long before he saw the bus-horse fall down (p. 136). However, as Eysenck points out, Hans had two other unpleasant experiences with horses prior to the accident that could account for that apprehensiveness. Furthermore, although witnessing the accident does not explain the child's earlier apprehensiveness, it might still have been the cause of the onset of the phobia. To this point, Freud has a second reply: "In itself the impression of the accident which he [Hans] happened to witness carried no 'traumatic force'; it acquired its great effectiveness only from the fact that horses had formerly been of importance to him as objects of his predilection and interest. . . ." What is the empirical basis for Freud's assumption that witnessing the accident, which the child described as giving him "such a fright," lacked traumatic force— which is just another way of saying that it could not have caused the phobia? He does not say.

In the "Discussion" section of his paper, Freud considers some issues of general interest about the evidential value of the Little Hans case and its capacity to contribute to our understanding of phobias or the mental life of children. One question he does not raise is this: How much evidence for general psychoanalytic propositions can be provided from a single case? Putting this issue aside, there is also the question of suggestion. As Freud puts the objection, ". . . an analysis of a child conducted by his father, who went to work instilled with *my* theoretical views and infected with *my* prejudice, must be entirely devoid of any objective worth" (Freud's italics, p. 102). At one point, Freud concedes that the fact that Hans's father had to tell him things he could not say himself detracts from the evidential value of the case, but, he notes, a psychoanalysis is not scientific investigation but a therapeutic measure (p. 104). Taken by itself, this suggests that Freud believed that the case had little or no evidential value. However, that apparently was not his view. He points out elsewhere (p. 102), ironically, that it ". . . has been discovered how great an economy of thought can be effected by the use of the catchword 'suggestion.' . . . everything awkward in the region of psychology can be labeled 'suggestion'" (p. 102). This is an important point given the history of appealing to suggestibility hypotheses, sometimes wantonly. However, in the Little Hans case, there are more concrete things that can be said then merely "suggestion was at work." A key problem is the material that Freud was forced to work with. Except for his brief single interview with Hans, he had to rely entirely for his data on the observations of the boy's father. How could Freud know what salient observations were omitted by the father from his reports because he failed to notice or because he thought them clinically irrelevant? How could he determine to what extent the boy's responses were shaped by what his father told him and how his father responded to the phobia? (For a critique of Freud's analysis, see Wolpe and Rachman, 1960; for a reply to their paper and a defense of Freud's account, see Neu, 1977: 124–135.)

REFERENCES

Eysenck, H. J. (1985). *Decline and Fall of the Freudian Empire.* New York: Viking Penguin.

Freud, S. (1907). The sexual enlightenment of children. S.E. 9: 129–140.

———. (1909). Analysis of a phobia in a five-year-old boy. S.E. 10: 5–149.

Neu, J. (1977). *Emotion, Thought, and Therapy.* Berkeley: University of California Press.

Wolpe, J., and Rachman, S. (1960). *Journal of Mental and Nervous Diseases,* 131: 135–145.

EDWARD ERWIN

M

Manic-Depressive Syndrome

See DEPRESSION.

Manifest Content See DREAMS, THEORY OF.

Marxism, and Freudianism

The convergence of Marxism and psychoanalysis in the Central and Eastern European and in North and South American centers of the psychoanalytic movement has alternately enjoyed a happy intermingling and suffered from controversy and conflict. The dialogue included psychoanalysts concerned with Marxism and the social sciences, as well as social scientists, Marxist philosophers, and cultural theorists interested in psychoanalysis. These groups were trying to illuminate various possible connections and interactions between the individual and society from the historico-materialistic and dialectical standpoint and the theories and techniques of psychoanalysis. Uncovering hidden conformities to the laws and structures of society, and researching the unconscious psychic mechanisms of the individual, were at the center of their attention, as was the rejection of any position deemed to be "dogmatic."

Especially during periods of upheaval (for example, in Central Europe after World War I until the beginnings of fascism and Stalinism, in Latin America before the establishment of dictatorships after World War II, and during the North American and European student movements of the 1960s), conflicts between the individual and society were much discussed, and possible changes in the individual were questioned.

The first "official" discussion of Marxism within the psychoanalytic movement was held at the Vienna Psy-choanalytic Society on March 10, 1909, when Alfred Adler gave a lecture entitled "On the Psychology of Marxism" (Nunberg and Federn, 1962–1975). In Vienna, Social Democrats and the political left were essential for the early psychoanalytic movement, and the psychoanalytic spirit was taken in by the Austrian Social Democratic Party. Until the end of World War I (1918), primarily among families and friends, and among professional acquaintances, a great deal of mutual understanding and trust was reached among psychoanalysts, Social Democrats, and "Austromarxists." Freud's signature on behalf of Red Vienna, which was printed in the *Arbeiter-Zeitung* (Worker's Journal) in 1927, exemplifies this mutual understanding. The pioneers of the psychoanalytic movement were liberals, mainly Jewish doctors and intellectuals, sympathetic to or members of the Austrian Social Democratic Party. After the fall of the Habsburg monarchy at the end of the war, the relationship between psychoanalysis and social democracy was widened on both an institutional and a social level. Psychoanalysts profited from the new spirit, the political and cultural milieu of social democratic Vienna, which showed its effects in several scientific developments. Apart from psychoanalysts who were Social Democrats before World War I (such as Paul Federn, Karl Josef Friedjung, Alfred Adler, Margarethe Hilferding, among others), representatives of a younger generation joined the Vienna Psychoanalytic Society. They had come of age as a part of the Vienna Youth Movement and were politically and socially sensitized during wartime. Siegfried Bernfeld, Helene Deutsch, Otto Fenichel, Anna Freud, Willi Hoffer, Annie and Wilhelm Reich, and others followed the socialist goals in building a new society and educating a "New Human Being." They tried to combine the insights of psychoanalysis and Marxism and reached out to the fields of social and welfare work and school and education, although psychoanalysts in general were pessimistic about the education of the human being, as psychoanalytic theory and practice were fundamentally opposed to directly influencing an individual. Nevertheless, a pedagogically oriented psychoanalysis was established in Vienna.

Similar developments can be observed in Budapest during a short period of the Hungarian Soviet Republic in 1919, and in Prague after 1933, where some of the Marxist psychoanalysts tried to combine psychoanalysis with the social sciences. Also, the anarchistic-utopian ideas of Otto Gross should be mentioned at this point.

Berlin was the center of the psychoanalytic movement during the Weimar Republic. The "classic" question at the time, whether or not Freud's and Marx's works could be combined, was debated by leftist Freudians, on the one side, and Soviet dogmatic party members, on the other. Wilhelm Reich, Otto Fenichel, Siegfried Bernfeld, Erich Fromm, Edith Jacobson, and others were the main protagonists in these discussions, which were aborted with Hitler's rise to power after 1933 and the exodus of Jewish psychoanalysts and political Freudians from Germany and Austria. A few analysts continued their debate in exile, and their interest in the development of critical and socially oriented psychoanalysis from 1934 until 1945 was documented in secret circular letters edited and distributed by Fenichel (Fenichel, 1998).

During the early 1920s, the relationship of Soviet psychoanalysts with the Soviet political and cultural ruling class was a singular phenomenon in the history of the psychoanalytic movement. The board of the Russian Psychoanalytic Society consisted of prominent Bolsheviks, and the society received support and protection from high functionaries, including Leon Trotsky, Adolf Joffe, Viktor Kopp, and Otto Schmidt. In Moscow, a State Psychoanalytic Institute and a psychoanalytic Child Guidance Clinic (especially for children of party functionaries) were founded. After Trotsky was removed from power in 1927, the Bolsheviks fundamentally changed their views on psychoanalysis (Etkind, 1997). In response to these developments, Freud's attitude toward Marxism and socialism remained ambivalent. His cultural theory and critique prove his socially and politically oriented way of thinking. But he rejected Bolshevism categorically; psychoanalysis was supposed

to be an apolitical science, and psychoanalytic organizations should, Freud believed, remain independent of political fights if psychoanalysis were to survive, even under fascist regimes.

Freud's political views and anxieties were influential not only for the Vienna Psychoanalytic Society but also for the International Psychoanalytic Association. His attitude determined the degree of adaptation and concessions made to politically reactionary forces, as well as the distance from leftist psychoanalysts. In the United States, the integration of psychoanalysis into medical and psychiatric professions led to theoretical superficiality concerning the connection between psychoanalysis and society. The basis of Freudian analysis, drive theory, was abandoned by many for more sociological theories (for example, the approaches of Karen Horney, Erich Fromm, and Abram Kardiner). Only a few psychoanalysts, especially the social philosophers of critical theory (Max Horkheimer, Theodor Adorno, and Herbert Marcuse), held on to the foundations of the early debate. They were also fundamentally responsible for reanimating the discussions in Central Europe after World War II. During the student movement of the 1960s, the debates found renewed vigor, as well as a different sociopolitical and ideological context.

Within the psychoanalytic movement, there have been several attempts to expand the international organizations of left-wing psychoanalysts. One, although failing in its original plan, was Fenichel's idea to create a "Marxist opposition" within the international psychoanalytic movement in the mid-1930s. The opposition's main purpose was to protect psychoanalysis as an independent science that was being threatened by fascism, both organizationally and theoretically. Another attempt was the formation in 1969 of the "Plataforma," comprising mainly Latin American and European leftist analysts. The group adopted as one goal the democratization of psychoanalytic training; its members also attacked the International Psychoanalytic Association for its perceived conformity with repressive political systems. The persecution of Argentinean psychoanalysts during the military regime in the 1970s, and the silence of the International Psychoanalytic Association, led to a spectacular resignation from the association of some prominent analysts associated with Marie Langer in 1971.

The observation and registration of the connections between psychic and social processes also has an established tradition within psychoanalysis on a theoretical level. Sigmund Freud explored this in his "Group Psychology and the Analysis of the Ego," published in 1921, which stimulated a psychoanalytically oriented social psychology. In his structural model (id, ego, superego) of 1923, the superego conveys the prohibitions and repressions originating in social reality. Some of the Communist and Socialist psychoanalysts used this model to pursue a politically motivated interest designed to better conceptualize the relationship between the individual and society. Siegfried Bernfeld published his "Sisyphus or the Boundaries of Education" in 1925, and Wilhelm Reich, "The Mass Psychology of Fascism" in 1933, two studies directly based on Freud's findings.

A related occurrence is the development of ethnopsychoanalysis, which addresses the relationship of psychoanalysis and Marxism, and the interaction between the individual and society. The observation and analysis of people from foreign cultures stimulated the study of the effects of social forces in the individual. These experiences were then incorporated into the psychoanalytic work within a culture, helping to clarify complex social processes. The ethnopsychoanalytic approach and the expansion of psychoanalytic theory gave researchers a broader psychoanalytic palette with which to examine individuals in their native culture. This attempt differed from others in its employment of psychoanalysis, the method and theory of which maintain a model of drive and conflict. Psychoanalytic psychology of the ego was developed to study the effects of social processes exactly where they reveal themselves: in the psychic life of the individual.

REFERENCES

Dahmer, H. (1982). *Libido und Gesellschaft. Studies über Freud und die Freudsche Linke.* Frankfurt am Main: Suhrkamp Verlag.

Etkind, A. (1997). *Eros of the Impossible. The History of Psychoanalysis in Russia.* Boulder, Colo.: Westview Press.

Fenichel, O. (1998). 119 Rundbriefe (1934–1945). vol. 1, *Europa* (1934–1938). J. Reichmayr and E. Mühlleitner (eds.). vol. 2, *Amerika* (1938–1945). E. Mühlleitner and J. Reichmayr (eds.). Frankfurt am Main: Stroemfeld Verlag.

Freud, S. (1921). *Group Psychology and the Analysis of the Ego.* S.E. 18: 69–143.

———. (1923). *The Ego and the Id.* S.E. 19: 12–59.

Nunberg, H., and Federn, E. (eds). (1962–1975). *The Minutes of the Vienna Psychoanalytic Society.* New York: International Universities Press.

Reichmayr, J. (1994). *Spurensuche in der Geschichte der Psychoanalyse.* Frankfurt am Main: Fischer Taschenbuch Verlag.

ELKE MÜHLLEITNER
JOHANNES REICHMAYR

Masochism and Sadism

M

"Sadism" and "masochism" are usually defined in psychoanalytic glossaries as, respectively, propensities either to inflict or to seek physical or mental suffering in order to achieve sexual arousal and gratification. However, as terms of analytic discourse their meanings are problematic. They are used in both narrow and broad senses. "Masochism," in its narrow sense, refers to sexual perversions or fantasies in which, for varying dynamic reasons, pain, suffering, or humiliation serve as conditions for the attainment of sexual pleasure. Because sexual masochism requires a real or imagined partner to play the sadistic role, and because participants may identify to some degree, consciously or unconsciously, with both the active and the passive roles, the perversion is often called "sadomasochism".

When the term "masochism" is used in its broad sense, there is much less consistency or consensus as to its meaning. It may label a wide diversity of manifestly nonsexual phenomena with little in common aside from some prominent element of suffering, self-destructiveness, or renunciation. Complicating matters further, "masochism" in both senses, narrow and broad, has been associated with a wide and often incompatible range of theoretical explanatory concepts deriving from different eras in psychoanalytic thought and from multiple levels of abstraction. Similar descriptive and explanatory variability can be found in discussions of sadism as well, although comparatively little has been written about this topic in the analytic literature, and it will not be focused upon here.

The confusion of meaning can be understood only in historical context (Maleson, 1984). Freud (1905) originally spoke of masochism in the narrow sense, that is, as a type of perverse sexuality. From the typically paired or complementary dominant and submissive forms of the perversion, he went on to hypothesize the existence of underlying, paired opposite "component sexual instincts" of sadism and masochism (1905, 1915), which he then thought of as driving the manifest perverse behavior. This theoretical notion influenced later analysts to speak of all masochism, perverse or otherwise, as universally paired with sadism—a somewhat axiomatic assumption that was not always supportable clinically.

In *A Child Is Being Beaten*, Freud (1919) had begun to speak of masochism in the broader way. He speculated that for some young women, paternal punishments stemming from provocative, "special irritability" toward father figures might represent disguised realizations of unconscious, erotic, Oedipally engendered beating fantasies. However, he conceded that he was unable to demonstrate any consistent *clinical* relationship between manifestly nonsexual masochism and underlying erotic excitement—a unifying link that clearly had theoretical appeal to him. In *The Economic Problem of Masochism* (1924), his last major work on the subject, he finally established a conceptual unity between the perverse and characterologic (i.e., manifestly nonsexual) forms of masochism, but only on a highly abstract level, and only by means of sweeping, and often strained, theoretical revisions that now placed masochism rather than sadism as the "primary" instinctual force. To summarize: Freud now thought that *all* masochism—"moral" (characterological) and perverse—was based on a primary erotogenic masochism (a supposed, biologically based, relatively direct capacity for deriving sexual pleasure from pain, which, from the theoretical standpoint, represented a fusion of the death instinct and libido). In the theory of moral masochism in particular, the superego was "resexualized"; an unconscious sense of guilt found clinical expression as an unconscious, sexualized wish to be beaten by the father. This wish to be beaten—essentially identical to the wish he thought was symbolically enacted in overt masochistic sexual perversions—was now central to Freud's understanding of masochistic character traits. The perverse and moral forms were parts of an erotically driven continuum.

These unifying formulations promoted and reinforced the idea of a driving erotic motivation whenever behavior is labeled "masochistic," regardless of whether the original supporting theory is embraced or ignored—as it often is. However, current clinical observation casts doubt on the existence of such a unity. For example, the concept of masochism as universally paired with sadism far better fits the manifest sexual perversions than it does the many nonsexual forms of either masochism or sadism. Moreover, consistent with Freud's own observation, characterological masochists do not necessarily or even routinely harbor masochistic sexual fantasies or preferences, conscious or unconscious. Conversely, those with masochistic sexual proclivities often achieve considerable real-world success, i.e., they may be far from masochistic in other realms.

As psychoanalysis moved beyond its early instinctual, sexual orientation, the literature burgeoned with descriptions of masochistic character in which nonsexual motivations clearly played the central role, further undermining any unified theory of masochism. An enormous diversity of phenomena, deemed masochistic, now came to be explored in terms of ego and superego analysis and the vicissitudes of aggression, narcissism, and early object relationships. The large number of dynamic formulations made from these vantage points vary in emphasis and often overlap. Masochism was variably seen to represent simultaneous defense against and expression of aggression (e.g., revenge through martyrdom); self-punishments for various forbidden wishes; projection of aggression, oral needs, and superego demands (manifested as habitual slavishness); an attempt to actively master passively feared dangers; the exercise of infantile, omnipotent control of others through the provoking of punishment; a means of clinging to a needed but indifferent or hurtful parental figure; an attachment to pain as a representation of such an object relationship; a means of fulfilling passive strivings; a means of repairing narcissistic mortifications or deficits. To this incomplete and daunting list one might add contributions underscoring cultural influences (for example, traditional subjugations of women that may influence the development of so-called feminine masochism), as well as descriptions of early antecedents, sometimes called "protomasochism."

Some general trends can be seen in these wide-ranging contributions. While the notion of hidden masochistic sexual excitement as the primary driving force in all characterological masochism has not been abandoned—indeed, as a seeming nod to tradition it is sometimes mentioned as a key motivational factor despite the absence of supporting clinical material—most modern scholars tend to deemphasize its role. By contrast, there has been much greater attention to underlying conflicts and compromise involving aggression in the genesis of masochistic phenomena. Adaptive, defensive, interpersonal, and narcissistic functions of masochism also have been stressed, as have its pre-Oedipal determinants. While points of emphasis vary, characterologic masochism must be understood as highly overdetermined, variable from case to case, and not reducible to any single motivational force or process. The same can be said of overt sadomasochistic sexual perversions. While their analysis typically reveals them as dramatizations of conflicts over such polarities as masculinity and femininity, castration and intactness, control and trust, these phenomena too are quite variable and overdetermined.

In view of all the blurring and dilution of meaning of the term, various scholars have pressed for a return to a narrower, more focused, and historically grounded sexual definition, in which masochism refers only to conditions derivative of some underlying erotic driving force, conscious or unconscious. However, the idea of masochism in other motivational contexts has become deeply entrenched in analytic discourse. Moreover, because underlying masochistic fantasies or erotization of pain as shapers of character may take years to be uncovered, or perhaps merely reconstructed in analysis, the term would have no immediate nosological usefulness. Thus, masochism is inevitably a nonspecific concept, loosely and simply denoting manifest phenomena in which pain and suffering, submission and defeat are especially prominent or tenacious, and seemingly driven or self-induced in the judgment of the analyst, based on his or her notions of behavioral and affective norms. Its range extends from relatively normal to clearly pathological phenomena, with variable dynamic underpinnings and gratifications. The label may tell us relatively little, but as knowledge of a patient unfolds during treatment, genetic, dynamic, and adaptive determinants as well as specific guiding fantasies—perverse or otherwise—may spell out what the manifest masochism actually means.

This broader approach lends itself to nosologic refinements from which more meaningful inferences might be drawn with respect to degree of pathology, therapy, and prognosis. For example, both Kernberg (1988) and Simons (1987) have delineated two major subgroups of characterological masochism. To review and elaborate on their contributions, depressive-masochistic character may be thought of as neurotic, or higher-level, masochism, primarily but not exclusively centered on Oedipal conflict. (Variations have been described many times under the rubric of moral masochism.) The chief issues are guilt, unconscious self-punishment, and inhibited aggression (a hallmark). Clinically such people are mildly depressed, relatively pleasureless, low in self-esteem, self-blaming, self-denigrating, self-punishing. They may be submissive or nonassertive in the face of legitimate grievances, sometimes evoking countertransference impulses to coach or rescue, as well as anger at those who are seen as exploiting the patient's masochism. Transferentially, the analyst is typically perceived as a strong superego figure; interpretations may primarily be experienced as criticisms or affirmations, and associations may reflect compliance as much as interpretive accuracy. Some may be especially cooperative or "well behaved" patients (Stein, 1981) whose very accommodation to the more demanding and painful aspects of analysis—a seemingly excellent therapeutic alliance—may conceal a masochistic transference and buried transference aggression. When aggression is finally mobilized, the analyst and others in the patient's life may experience a sense of shock or betrayal; such reactions may contribute to resistance to change. The category may include "those wrecked by success," negative therapeutic reactions, those who idealize unhappiness, and "fate neurosis" (Deutsch, 1932).

A second major subgroup, sadomasochistic character, includes those who alternate between sadistic and masochistic postures toward the same person. Such people typically feel victimized by deeply needed but disappointing figures. This perception, which may have origins in actual early trauma or deprivation, is used by a corruptible superego to justify a variety of aggressive, controlling, and provocative acts, typically designated as "sadistic" by those who experience their impact (regardless of the subjective state of the aggressor, again demonstrating the relative nature of these terms). In contrast with depressive masochistic characters, such people exhibit much less conflict over direct expressions of aggression. They tend to collect injustices and to coerce others by means of martyrdom, emotional blackmail, and accusation. They are sometimes "help-rejecting complainers." They are more likely than depressive-masochistic characters to provoke sadistic, punishing, rejecting responses in others, therapists included, thus perpetuating the cycle. (The depressive-masochistic character is more likely to serve as his or her *own* punisher, through *self*-reproach, *self*-depreciation.) The underlying dynamics vary from case to case, but in general the pathology originates earlier and is more severe; some, but not all, may have borderline personality organization. They are generally more difficult to treat than the first group, as they are prone to self-destructive acting out and are likely to perceive their sadism as emanating from outside themselves—factors militating against analytic treatment.

There is of course a continuum between these typical constellations and room for the delineation of other subtypes as well. Viewing masochistic character pathology in this way should prove useful in giving the term more meaning—there is no single "masochism"—and will help disentangle us from the legacy of the complicated evolution of the concept in psychoanalysis.

M

REFERENCES

Deutsch, H. (1932). Hysterical fate neurosis. In *Psychoanalysis of the Neuroses.* London: Hogarth, pp. 29–49.

Freud, S. (1905). *Three Essays on the Theory of Sexuality.* S.E. 7: 130–243.

———. (1915). Instincts and their vicissitudes. S.E. 14.

———. (1916). Some character types met with in psychoanalysis. S.E. 14: 117–140.

———. (1919). A child is being beaten. S.E. 17: 179–204.

———. (1924). The economic problem of masochism. S.E. 19: 19–172.

Kernberg, O. F. (1988). Clinical dimensions of masochism. In R. A. Glick and P. I. Meyers (eds.). *Masochism: Current Psychoanalytic Perspectives.* Hillsdale, N.J.: Analytic Press, pp. 61–79.

Maleson, F. G. (1984). The multiple meanings of masochism in psychoanalytic discourse. *Journal of the American Psychoanalytic Association,* 32: 325–356.

Simons, R. C. (1987). Psychoanalytic contributions to psychiatric nosology: forms of masochistic behavior. *Journal of the American Psychoanalytic Association,* 35: 583–608.

Stein, M. H. (1981). The unobjectionable part of the transference. *Journal of the American Psychoanalytic Association,* 29: 869–892.

FRANKLIN G. MALESON

Masturbation See NEURASTHENIA.

Materialism See BEHAVIORISM; MIND AND BODY.

Meaning, and Psychoanalysis

Disagreements about causal and hermeneutical interpretations of Freudian theory began early in the twentieth century and were closely connected to the question of whether psychoanalysis should be judged by the evidential standards of natural science.

Wilhelm Reich, who was a confidant of Freud and a member of the International Psychoanalytic Association until he was expelled in 1934, reports that leading psychopathologists—he mentions Karl Jaspers in particular—contended that psychological interpretations of meaning, and thus, psychoanalysis, were not within the realm of natural science. Reich writes (p. 244): "It was plainly a matter of the question whether or not psychoanalysis and its method belonged to natural science. In other words: *Is a scientific psychology in the strict sense of the word at all possible?* Can psychoanalysis claim to be such a psychology?" (Emphasis in the original). He notes that Freud avoided such methodological issues,

but that he (Reich) continued to oppose Jasper's view: "But we knew that—for the first time in the history of psychology—we were engaging in *natural science*" (Reich, p. 244, emphasis in the original).

Whatever Freud's views were of these methodological disputes, he himself made numerous causal claims in his writings (for example, in his discussion of whether Little Hans's witnessing a horse fall down was anything more than a precipitating cause of his phobia; see "Little Hans," this volume). Besides *using* causal concepts in his theorizing, he also gave sophisticated analyses of different types of causation.

One of the earliest challenges to his etiological views concerned his theory of anxiety neurosis. Ludwig Löwenfeld tried to demonstrate that Freud's theory could not account for a number of known facts about this sort of neurosis. In his (1895) reply, Freud tries to correct some of Löwenfeld's misinterpretations of the theory, but the bulk of his rejoinder employs a set of distinctions between different types of causes: (1) Predisposing causal factors; (2) Specific causes, (3) Contributory causes, and (4) Exciting or Releasing causes.

Freud downgrades the explanatory significance of (3) and (4), and argues that the more important explanatory notions are the concepts of (1) the predisposing cause and (2) the specific cause. In cases of anxiety neuroses, he argues, a hereditary disposition is the most important causal determinant, but it is not indispensable; it is missing in certain border-line cases. What is never missing when the effect occurs is the specific cause, which also suffices in the required quantity or intensity to bring about the effect when the predisposition is also present. The specific cause of anxiety neuroses is a sexual factor. Freud employs these causal distinctions to show that his theory is not required to explain some of the facts adduced by Löwenfeld and that other facts, contrary to what Löwenfeld claims, can be explained by the theory. It is striking, in view of recent attempts to give an acausal reading of Freudian theory, that at least in this early paper Freud makes no attempt to disown what clearly are causal hypotheses about the development of anxiety neuroses. Instead, he uses causal distinctions to disarm his critic.

The fact that Freud used causal notions in his theorizing, however, does not settle the issues raised by hermeneutical theorists. Some argue that in speaking of causation rather than meaning, he made a serious error; others argue that Freudian theory is really about meanings rather than causes, despite Freud's occasional use of causal notions.

Karl Jaspers takes the first position in his 1922 *General Psychopathology*; he holds that Freudian theory does make causal claims, but that this is precisely its fundamental error: "The falseness of the Freudian claim lies in the mistaking of meaningful connections for causal connections" (Jaspers, 1963 [1922]: 539). Jaspers, however, does not present any evidence that Freudian theory, when interpreted causally, is wrong, nor does he attempt to spell out an alternative theory that would explain in terms of meaning connections the phenomena of interest to Freud. Instead, he is content to give examples of what he means by "meaning connections." His main example (p. 303) is the connection Nietzsche drew between awareness of one's combined weakness and wretchedness and the development of a certain type of morality. Such a connection, Jaspers holds (p. 303), is self-evident. However, this is not a good example. Nietzsche was making a causal claim: namely, that a Judaeo-Christian morality developed *because* of a perceived weakness and wretchedness. It is also clearly false that this claim is self-evident; to support it, Nietzsche would have needed empirical evidence.

Jaspers's other two examples are: Attacked people become angry and spring to the defense; and cheated people grow suspicious. These examples are no better than his first. Neither claim is self-evident; and neither is generally true. When attacked people do become angry and when cheated people grow suspicious, this is generally no coincidence; they generally become angry *because* they have been attacked, and grow suspicious *because* they have been cheated. These latter claims are, of course, causal claims, supported by evidence from common experience.

Although Jaspers's examples do not help his case for replacing Freudian theory with one that talks of meaning connections, they do unwittingly illustrate something else: a serious problem for hermeneutical proposals, including his own. Suppose that Nietzsche were wrong and there really were no causal connection between people perceiving themselves to be wretched and weak, and their developing a Judaeo-Christian morality. In that case, he could not explain the origin of such a morality by postulating perceived wretchedness and weakness. Or, suppose that being attacked never made any difference to whether people get angry; if that were true we could not explain their anger in terms of

their being attacked. For Freud to have abandoned all of his causal claims—about dreams, neuroses, parapraxes, and sexual development—in favor of a theory talking only about meaning connections would have doomed his theory at the outset to explanatory sterility.

Jaspers's problem arises equally for contemporary Freudian hermeneuticians who, unlike Jaspers, do not want to reject Freudian theory but to protect it against critics who charge that there is a lack of supporting empirical evidence (see "Hermeneutics, and Psychoanalysis," this volume).

At first glance, there seems to be some substance to the hermeneutical reading of Freud; certain Freudian hypotheses do appear to be about the meaning of such items as neurotic symptoms, dreams, and slips of the tongue and pen. However, these hypotheses often also presuppose causal hypotheses either for their truth or their proof. If we reinterpret Freudian theory so that all of the implicit and explicit causal hypotheses vanish, then what is left, even if true, cannot explain the phenomena that Freud was trying to explain. For example, in analyzing his Irma dream, Freud notes that in the dream, Irma's problems are attributed to an injection given by Otto, who probably used an unclean syringe. He comments: "It occurred to me, in fact, that I was actually *wishing* that there had been a wrong diagnosis; for if so, the blame for my lack of success [in treating Irma] would have been got rid of (Freud's italics; 1900: 109). Freud is trying to explain here the manifest content of his dream, the part about Otto and the syringe, in terms of the causal connection between his wish and the formation of the dream content. Eliminate the causal hypothesis and you eliminate Freud's proposed explanation. Freud's general theory of dreams, moreover, although it talks about manifest and latent content, involves a central causal hypothesis: that repressed infantile wishes are the instigators of dreams. The very same point can be made about neurotic symptoms and slips of the tongue; if Freudian theory is reinterpreted so that it does not say that repression makes a causal difference to their occurrence, then the theory does not even attempt to explain the phenomena.

Some contemporary analysts in the hermeneutic tradition want to substitute references to the patient's "narrative" for causal talk, but what do these narratives typically consist of? They are stories about what certain events in a patient's life mean to the patient; but, then, in speaking of narratives, the analyst is not getting rid of causal commitments. Does the patient's attaching a certain meaning to these life events make any difference to the maintenance of the clinical problem or its treatment? To say that it does is to put forward a causal hypothesis; to refuse to say that it does is to abandon the attempt to explain the origin or maintenance of the problem or the effects of the treatment in terms of the patient's narrative. We can treat the patient's narrative as simply a story having no clinical significance, judging it merely by aesthetic criteria (see "Interpretation," this volume), but if we leave the matter there and make no attempt to determine the effects of the patient's interpretation of his or her life events, then we are not reinterpreting Freudian theory; we are merely abandoning the attempt to use Freud's theory to explain clinical phenomena.

In general, if what events mean to a patient make no difference to her behavior or to the contents of her mind, then how she interprets them does not explain anything important about her; if the interpreting does make a difference, then it is a cause. Speaking of what things mean to a patient may disguise the reliance on causal hypotheses—but it does not eliminate it.

Some philosophers and psychologists try to take a middle of the road position. They agree that Freudian theory talks about causal connections, but they claim that meaning connections (or, "thematic affinities") are a reliable sign of such connections. An example sometimes given is the "overlap in content" between one of Anna O.'s symptoms and an earlier experience. The symptom was her aversion to drinking water; the early experience, revealed under hypnosis, was Anna's watching a dog drink water from a glass, an event that apparently disgusted her. To say that there is an overlap in meaning here (a thematic affinity) is to say that the propositions describing both the symptom and experience have somewhat the same content. One proposition says that Anna O. found it disgusting to watch the dog drink water from the glass; the other says that she now finds it disgusting to drink a glass of water. Both propositions talk about disgust and drinking water. Some writers take this overlap in themes as evidence of a causal connection between Anna's experience of watching the dog and her later aversion to drinking water. The first caused the second. What, however, is the basis for this inference?

One option is to say that meaning connections *in and of themselves* are evidence of a causal connection; so, no empirical evidence is needed to show that if Anna O.'s

experience and symptom have similar meanings—or more precisely the propositions describing them do—then there is a likely causal connection between the two. But what is the basis for this claim? One could equally well assert that if there is a correlation between two types of events, say taking vitamin E and a reduction of heart disease, then that is evidence *in and of itself* of a causal connection. In both cases, the appeal to meaning connections and to correlations, it is hardly self-evident that meeting the condition is by itself grounds for support of a causal connection. It is reasonable to ask, then, what the argument is for the claim about meaning connections.

One writer claims that the finding of sense or meaning and the establishing of causal order are "one and the same" (Hopkins, 1991: 95). However, they are not one and the same. We find that there is an overlap in meaning between Anna O.'s watching the dog and then developing her symptom, but we can still go on to ask a further question: What caused the appearance of the symptom? Perhaps her experience with the dog was the cause, but then again any number of events, including physiological ones, might have been the cause. The attempts to demonstrate a priori that meaning connections are generally evidence of causal connections are reviewed in Erwin, 1996: 26–40; the conclusion is that they all fail (see as well, Grünbaum, 1993: 129–134).

Instead of relying on a priori arguments, one could appeal to empirical ones. For example, one might try to find statistical evidence that where there is a certain kind of overlap in meaning between two events (or the propositions describing them), then there is also a causal connection. One might search for evidence that it was no accident that Anna O.'s experience with the dog and her aversion to drinking water had similar content, that generally when events of this kind have similar meaning, they are also causally connected. On this empirical position, however, the concept of meaning-similarity loses its special epistemological significance. The situation is very much like the appeal to simplicity. It is very difficult to show that the mere fact that one theory is simpler than its main rival is reason to believe that the first is true. Because of that difficulty, some resort to an empirical argument: in certain domains, there is empirical evidence that a theory that postulates a single cause of a certain range of phenomena is more likely to be true than one postulating multiple causes. This sort of empirical argument, however, eliminates the alleged role of simplicity as a "tie-breaker" when two competing theories have equal empirical support. Moreover, when the empirical evidence goes the other way, when it makes it likely that the single-cause theory is wrong, then simplicity counts *against* a theory (Erwin, 1996: 54–60; Sober, 1990).

Those who have appealed to meaning connections as a reliable indicator of causal connections clearly did intend the appeal to have a special epistemic significance. The idea was that one could show that Freud's etiological hypotheses about dreaming, neuroses, and so forth could be established without obtaining experimental evidence. On the empirical view, however, appeal to meaning connections cannot play that epistemic role. It is true, quite trivially so, that if we find empirical evidence that where X is present there is a causal connection, then the finding of X warrants the inference that there is a causal connection. The "X" in this equation can denote many things: perceived self-evidence (of the sort Jaspers discussed); the finding of a statistical correlation; the fact that our causal theory would if true explain the known data and our inability to think of any other theory; or an overlap in meaning. For any of these items, the hypothetical claim that *if* we had the required empirical evidence that where X is present, one of Freud's causal hypotheses would be warranted is without interest. What needs to be shown is that in fact we actually have such evidence.

REFERENCES

Erwin, E. (1996). *A Final Accounting: Philosophical and Empirical Issues in Freudian Psychology*. New York: Cambridge University Press.

Freud, S. (1895) A reply to criticisms of my paper on anxiety neurosis. S.E. 3: 25–39.

———. (1900). *The Interpretation of Dreams*. S.E. 4–5: 1–621.

Grünbaum, A. (1993). *Validation in the Clinical Theory of Psychoanalysis*. Madison, Conn.: International Universities Press.

Hopkins, J. (1988). Epistemology and depth psychology. Critical notes on *The Foundations of Psychoanalysis*. In P. Clark and C. Wright (eds.). *Mind, Psychoanalysis and Science*. New York: Basil Blackwell.

———. (1991). The interpretation of dreams. In J. Neu (ed.). *The Cambridge Companion to Freud*. New York: Cambridge University Press.

Jaspers, K. (1963 [1922]). *General Psychopathology*. Chicago: University of Chicago Press.

Reich, W. (1967) *Reich Speaks of Freud*. New York: Farrar, Straus and Giroux.

Ricoeur, P. (1970). *Freud and Philosophy*. New Haven: Yale University Press.

———. (1981). *Hermeneutics and the Human Sciences*. J. B. Thompson (trans.). New York: Cambridge University Press.

Sober, E. (1990). Let's razor Ockham's razor. *Philosophy*, 27: 73–93.

EDWARD ERWIN

M

Melancholia See DEPRESSION; IDENTIFICATION; SUICIDE.

Memory See REPRESSION.

Mental Apparatus See EGO; ID; METAPSYCHOLOGY; SUPEREGO.

Mental Energy See CATHEXIS; BINDING.

Metapsychology

A term of an obscure past, uncertain meaning, and problematic future. Freud referred to it with a variety of metaphors—"my ideal and woebegone child" (1985 [1887–1904], p. 216), "the Witch," "the consummation of psycho-analytic research"—spoke of it as if it were the highest reach of his theoretical work, and then neglected to mention it for most of the subsequent quarter century of his life. Many psychoanalysts have viewed it with a mixture of intimidation, confusion, and boredom, generally neglecting to think much about it. Others took it up with enthusiasm and rode off on it in a variety of directions, with few followers. Perhaps its greatest champion in the era since Freud's death was David Rapaport (1911–1960), but he died before achieving his ambition to clarify, extend, and systematize it while making it scientifically respectable. His former colleagues and students, along with many others both within and outside of psychoanalysis, have subjected it to withering scrutiny, either abandoning it as useless or actively attempting to scotch or replace it.

Definition

Freud's first recorded use of the word "metapsychology" is in a letter to Fliess (of February 13, 1896), and he used it a total of eight times in that correspondence, in a number of somewhat different ways. Sometimes he identified it with psychology, sometimes contrasted the two terms; he treated it as a virtual synonym for biology and in the next breath spoke of it as his "psychology that leads behind consciousness" (1898, p. 274). The context of that and several other usages makes it clear that he had in mind his use in psychological (or psychopathological) theorizing of the evolutionary biology of Lamarck and Haeckel, and the physicalistic physiology of his teachers and research supervisors in medical school. He found these notions of the inheritance of acquired characteristics and recapitulationism more agreeable and useful than Darwin's ideas, and continued to lean on them all his scientific life. His borrowings of the then modish concepts of force and energy from the "biophysics movement" (sometimes misleadingly referred to as the School of Helmholtz; Cranefield, 1966) came to dominate most of his writings on metapsychology, however. A couple of other passages in the letters to Fliess tell us that his term connoted philosophy to Freud, also, probably because in metapsychology he came as close as he ever did to building a comprehensive, deductive system.

His first published usage of the word was in a throwaway line where he suggested that psychoanalysis might "transform metaphysics into metapsychology" without making it very plain what he meant. Then after fourteen years, the war's interruption of his practice gave Freud time to undertake an ambitious task: writing a dozen papers to make up a book, "Preliminaries to a Metapsychology."

The intention of the series is to clarify and carry deeper the theoretical assumptions on which a psychoanalytic system could be founded. The second of those he actually published contained the following sentence, which has become the received (approximation of a) definition: "I propose that when we have succeeded in describing a psychical process in its dynamic, topographical and economic aspects, we should speak of it as a metapsychological presentation" (1915, p. 181).

Dynamic, economic, and topographical *points of view* (another phrase from the just-quoted paper) are not completely self-explanatory terms, and they have been somewhat differently explicated by psychoanalytic writers. The prevailing interpretation, however, is that expounded by Rapaport, especially in one of his last papers (Rapaport and Gill, 1959): The dynamic point of view comprises conceptualizing motivational phenomena by the use of *psychic forces*. The economic point of view entails attempts to explain by quantitative variations in amounts of *psychic energies*. The topographic point of view means locating processes in the *structural elements* of the topographic model of Systems Cs., Pcs., and Ucs. In the last-mentioned paper, Rapaport and Gill argued for renaming the last "the structural point of view," replacing the outmoded topographic model by

the structural model of ego, superego, and id; there is a good textual basis for it in Freud's late remark equating metapsychology with "reference to the dynamic relations between the agencies of the mental apparatus which has been recognized . . . by us."

Rapaport and Gill also urged the inclusion of two more points of view, the genetic and the adaptive. Only a minority of analysts have followed their urging.

Several questions remain unanswered. What are the boundaries of metapsychology? Does it deal only with assumptions, or is it actually synonymous with psychoanalytic theory, or is there another possibility? How is it related to clinical work? How may metapsychological concepts be measured or at least roughly assessed? What was the subsequent history of metapsychological analysis in Freud's work after 1915?

History

To address the last question first, after publishing the five papers he called "metapsychological," Freud referred to the other seven in a letter to Abraham as "wartime atrocities. . . . Several, including that on consciousness, still require thorough revision" (Freud and Abraham, 1965: 228). A decade later, in his autobiography, he said that the published metapsychological papers "remained no more than a torso. . . . I broke off, wisely perhaps, since the time for theoretical predications of this kind had not yet come." Only one of the missing papers has been found since Freud's death, on "Transference Neuroses in General"; the others were to have dealt with Consciousness, Anxiety, Conversion Hysteria, Obsessional Neurosis, and perhaps Projection (or Paranoia) and Sublimation.

Freud made no mention of metapsychology as such in any of his major books, and in fact the word appears in only nine of his publications. When he did use it, several times he declared that, no matter how speculative it might get, it always had clinical foundations. He contrasted it with "mere description," emphasizing that he considered it an *explanatory* theory. Moreover, he did make constant use of psychic forces, energies, and the "agencies" of the structural (ego-id) model in most of his works. It is fair to say, therefore, that though Freud wrote nothing devoted primarily to this kind of theorizing after the metapsychological papers of 1915 (except, perhaps, *Beyond the Pleasure Principle*, 1920) and employed the term quite sparingly, metapsychological concepts and ways of thinking dominated his theorizing during most of his career.

Delimitation

Rapaport, a great advocate of metapsychology and believer that it had been too much neglected by psychoanalysts, devoted a number of years to its study, attempting to systematize it (Rapaport, 1959), and at his premature death had begun a program of empirical research based on it. He made the sharpest distinction between the clinical theory and metapsychology: "Books on psychoanalysis usually deal with its clinical theory. . . . There exists, however, a fragmentary—yet consistent—general theory of psychoanalysis, which comprises the premises of the special (clinical) theory, the concepts built on it, and the generalizations derived from it . . . named *metapsychology*" (p. 670).

Rapaport also claimed that "in relation to the clinical one it (i.e. the metapsychology) is a metatheory." I do not believe that any of Freud's metapsychological propositions can be shown to be statements about the clinical theory. Unfortunately, however, this obiter dictum has influenced and confused the discussion of metapsychology by a number of analysts.

In the view of Rapaport and his followers, Freud's metapsychology aimed to be a general, abstract theory of the psychological functioning of the human organism. This ambitious and incomplete undertaking was intended to be an *explanatory* conceptualization of the conscious and unconscious mental life (thinking, emotions, dreams, fantasies, etc.) and behavior of people, whether normal or abnormal and without regard to gender, ethnicity, culture, or historical era. It would specify *presuppositions* as well as theoretical propositions, and would provide a basic context and undergirding for the clinical theory. Rapaport and Gill (1959), also point out that Freud never actually attempted to state the *presuppositions* underlying psychoanalytic theory. Their own attempt to do so has not had many rivals, nor am I aware of any extended critical examination of the list of twenty they tentatively set forth. For another thoughtful attempt to extract the theory's presuppositions, see Rubinstein (1997).

The set of theoretical propositions consists of theories about the origin and structure of the various forms of psychopathology and of their therapy—a theory of normal development and pathogenesis; of neurosis, psychosis, and character disorder; and of psychoanalytic treatment. (Psychoanalytic developmental psychology is included here because it is so clinical in its focus, even though much of it does not deal with pathology. By the same token, psychoanalytic characterology may also be included in the clinical theory.) But even this elaboration of Rapaport's position does not contain precise enough definitions to enable us to say, for many specific parts of psychoanalytic theory, whether they are clinical or general.

Rubinstein (1997), however, does just that. Though he made the earliest and in many ways most sophisticated showings of the untenability of Freud's metapsychology, he argued convincingly that *some* metapsychology, or "extraclinical theory," as he preferred to call it, is indispensable if psychoanalysis is not to become a sterile, hermeneutic system that cannot make truth claims. See particularly his Chapter 7 for a demonstration that a scientific but strictly—i.e., purely psychological—clinical theory is impossible.

His simple and quite usable recommendation is to call "clinical" those psychoanalytic propositions that deal with persons and are couched in terms of ordinary language (plus certain more technical terms that have been absorbed into everyday speech). "Extraclinical" propositions, by contrast, are couched in an impersonal scientific language of processes, structures, and the like, mostly assumed to be intrapersonal. Evidently, much of what is treated by many authors as part of clinical theory is by this definition properly extraclinical, including the theory of instincts, the ego-superego-id model, and ego psychology. Even using Rubinstein's definitions, one finds it difficult in practice to separate the clinical theory from metapsychology. After an initial disillusionment in our own attempt to test metapsychological propositions in the work of the Research Center for Mental Health at New York University, George Klein and I hoped that the clinical theory might be purified of metapsychological intrusions and become the basis for a research program. It was then that we became aware how much of clinical writing is pervaded by metapsychological concepts and has no discernible basis in clinical observation. In it, for example, hypotheses about patients and events in their lives are often interwoven with allusions to innervations, defensive operations by the ego, cathexes, and the like.

Critique

As noted above, many psychoanalysts find metapsychology abstruse and confusing, and believe that they need not be concerned if it has problems, since they mistakenly believe that they do not use it. Likewise, a number of the psychoanalysts who have split from the

M

Freudian "mainstream" cite some of the difficulties of metapsychology—e.g., that it is too abstract, or too physicalistic—as reasons for introducing their own variant schools of psychoanalytic theory. Yet they, too, rarely abandon some of its key concepts, such as psychic energy or the ego, though they may replace these terms by others (e.g., tension, the self).

Several contemporary groups of psychoanalysts reject metapsychology for a variety of reasons, some valid but some off the mark. With the recognition that the dynamic and economic points of view originate in Freud's gymnasium and university education in the physicalistic physiology that was so much the rage in the 1870s came the realization that those doctrines are founded on the metaphysical assumptions of mechanistic materialism. Unfortunately, one of the main weaknesses of that philosophical position is its difficulty in conceptualizing and admitting to full reality the subjective world that is the main concern of psychoanalysis.

Schafer (1976, 1978) and his followers, and the numerous advocates of the hermeneutic approach to psychoanalysis, tend to reject metapsychology for committing its users to an inhumane and constricting set of philosophical foundations. They make the mistake, however, of assuming that these foundations are necessary to natural science (not just the science of the late nineteenth century), and that to escape stultification, psychoanalysis therefore must renounce Freud's ambition that his discipline should be recognized as one of the natural sciences. For several years, Schafer advocated a new language for psychoanalysis, action language, in place of not only metapsychology but much of the rest of its conceptual armamentarium. Some writers favored abandoning metapsychology and replacing it with a somewhat expanded clinical theory. Others, influenced by hermeneutic philosophers, called on their colleagues to renounce the effort to meet the criteria of science, which they rejected as inappropriate and unnecessary now that hermeneutics seemed to offer an alternative methodology.

During the last four decades of the twentieth century, a growing number of critics from within Freudian psychoanalysis as well as outside it have criticized metapsychology in ways that cannot so easily be dismissed.

1. Its philosophical foundations have been shown to include much more than mechanism, materialism, and related positions like reductionism: Freud's early religious and humanistic education left him with a rather inchoate mass of quite incompatible (animistic and contextualist) metaphysical assumptions. Thus, the philosophical underpinnings of metapsychology are inconsistent and incoherent.

2. Each of Freud's several attempts to develop a theoretical model of the human being contains internal contradictions, which have been refractory to attempts to remove them.

3. Its concepts are often reified, frequently in the form of anthropomorphism: Abstractions such as instinctual drives, for example, are treated as if they were concrete, observable entities with many of the attributes of persons, such as seeking expression and evading observation.

4. Its concepts are badly defined: Definitions are often lacking, or multiple and mutually inconsistent, or vague and metaphorical.

5. Its concepts overlap one another to varying degrees, so that there is an excessive number of redundant terms referring to more or less the same matters.

6. In developing his theoretical arguments, Freud made many logical errors and fallacies of reasoning, so that his conclusions do not follow from his ostensible assumptive and empirical starting points. For example, at critical points in a presentation where he encountered difficulties, Freud would often slip into metaphor or use other kinds of figurative language, diverting the reader from his failure to establish his point.

7. Many metapsychological propositions are translations into different terms of fallacious and/or empirically incorrect beliefs from outdated biological sciences, notably physiology and evolutionary biology.

8. Metapsychology is a closed system without links to the empirical world. Hence, its key terms cannot be measured, not even those of the economic (allegedly quantitative) point of view, and it can have no explanatory or predictive value.

Therefore, in its present form, the theory itself is not clear enough, not tightly enough organized, and too few of its concepts can be unambiguously linked to data to make it possible for anyone to undertake the task of systematically testing it, as can be done with ordinary scientific theories. Despite its prestige and familiarity, despite its appearance of being a serious intellectual achievement, Freud's metapsychology is scientifically trivial and useless. It merely supplies a jargon in which observations may be restated in impressive-sounding terms that actually add nothing to the original clinical formulations.

The Future

With the growing recognition of these deficiencies, fewer psychoanalysts attempt to defend metapsychology or to rebut the substantive critique. Most continue to use its concepts and propositions, sometimes in the mistaken belief that they can be linked to clinical observations and sometimes out of habit and for lack of anything better. There has been a growing recognition, both within psychoanalysis and outside, that the clinical theory has many of the same deficiencies as metapsychology, though it is closer to observation and contains numerous testable propositions. Promising beginnings have been made on the task of reformulating and systematizing the clinical theory (e.g., Rubinstein, 1997, chapter 6), demonstrating that with further work it can be salvaged and made both defensible and useful scientifically, while retaining its clinical utility.

There is still an important place for a new metapsychology. A much revised and improved clinical theory of psychoanalysis will need to have explicit links to the biological sciences, on the one hand, and the social sciences, on the other. Moreover, it must be grounded in a consistent world hypothesis or metaphysical system. It will need to make explicit its assumptions about the mind-body problem and the problem of free will, for example, ideally taking a position that is compatible with contemporary sciences of the organism and the human person as a social, cultural, political, spiritual being. Several authors have attempted to begin this task for our time, which Freud called "metapsychological," of clarifying "the theoretical assumptions on which a psychoanalytic" science could be built. None has fully succeeded, but there are promising beginnings.

REFERENCES
Cranefield, P. F. (1966). Freud and the "School of Helmholtz." *Gesnerus*, 23: 35–39.
Freud, S. (1887–1904). *The Complete Letters of Sigmund Freud to Wilhelm Fliess, 1887–1904*. Trans. and ed., J. M. Masson. Cambridge, Mass.: Harvard University Press, 1985.
Freud, S., and Abraham, K. (1965). *A Psycho-analytic Dialogue: The Letters of Sigmund Freud and Karl Abraham 1907–1926.*

(eds. H. C. Abraham and E. L. Freud). New York: Basic Books.
Rapaport, D. (1959). The structure of psychoanalytic theory: A systematizing attempt. In S. Koch (ed.). *Psychology: A Study of a Science. Study 1. Conceptual and Systematic. Volume 3. Formulations of the Person and the Social Context.* New York: McGraw-Hill, 1959, pp. 55–183. Also in *Psychological Issues*, 1960, 2, no. 2, Monograph no. 6.
Rapaport, D., and Gill, M. M. (1959). The points of view and assumptions of metapsychology. *International Journal of Psycho-Analysis*, 40: 153–162. Also in M. M. Gill (ed.). *The Collected Papers of David Rapaport.* New York: Basic Books, 1967, chapter 62, pp. 795–811.
Rubinstein, B. R. (1997). *Psychoanalysis and the Philosophy of Science: Collected Papers of Benjamin B. Rubinstein, M.D.* (ed. R. R. Holt). Madison, Conn.: International Universities Press.
Schafer, R. (1976). *A New Language for Psychoanalysis.* New Haven, Conn.: Yale University Press.
———. (1978). *Language and Insight.* New Haven, Conn.: Yale University Press.

ROBERT R. HOLT

M

Mexico, and Psychoanalysis

The revolutionary ideas of Sigmund Freud began to spread among neuropsychiatrists in Mexico during the early 1920s (López, 1990), thanks to teachers at the former mental sanatorium of La Castañeda and the General Hospital. The Mexican Society of Neurology and Psychiatry was founded in 1937, bringing together a group of neurologists and neuropsychiatrists that included professors and students interested in psychoanalysis (Dupont, 1991). Several of these young people would later spread the teachings of the International Psychoanalytic Association.

Beginning in 1947, some of the younger psychiatrists of that generation started traveling to the United States, France, and Argentina to complete their studies.

In 1952, these pioneers of psychoanalysis began returning to Mexico: Rafael Barajas from Paris, Ramón Parres from Columbia University in New York, and Santiago Ramírez from Buenos Aires. Two years earlier, the teachers and students remaining in Mexico had gathered around Erich Fromm to form a self-styled humanistic psychoanalytic group. This hampered the work of the pioneers who, in the winter of 1953, founded Mexico's first psychoanalytic group with the support of the international community, especially Jones, Garma, Nacht, Hartmann, Alvarez de Toledo, Karl Menninger, and

Bryce Boyer, with the participation of Ackerman, Rappaport, and Namun. The Mexican Group for Psychoanalytic Studies, sponsored by the Argentine Psychoanalytic Society, was approved at the Nineteenth International Congress of Psychoanalysis in Geneva in the summer of 1955. Its members were Rafael Barajas, José Luis González, Ramón Parres, Santiago Ramírez, and José Remus as analysts, and Fernando Césarman Carlos Corona, Luis Féder, Francisco González Pineda, and Estela Remus as candidates (Parres, 1987, 1995; Parres and Ramírez, 1966). In the following year, the Psychoanalytic Institute established its requirements and a program of study that emphasized (as it still does) the study of Sigmund Freud's complete works (Palacios, 1982). At first, the Institute accepted members of the nonmedical professions; it would later admit only psychiatrists. A new phase began in 1978, however, with the admission of psychology graduates holding a doctorate in clinical psychology; by 1984, the institute was accepting graduates in medicine, psychology, social work, nursing, and special education holding a master's degree in psychotherapy (Ayala and Perez de Pla, 1994; Ayala, 1995). The Mexican Psychoanalytic Association was approved as a constituent member of the International Psychoanalytic Association in 1957, at the Twentieth International Congress in Paris. It was joined at that time by Víctor Aiza and Avelino González.

From its inception, Mexican psychoanalysis received the benefit of many theoretical influences. From the United States it received ego psychology; from Buenos Aires, Kleinian theory as set forth by Rascovsky, Racker, Pichon-Rivière, and others; and from Paris, Freudian analysis. Of course, the teachings of Anna Freud also influenced child psychoanalysts, and Bion provided a useful model for the treatment of psychotic patients.

Thanks to that combination of theoretical approaches, the Mexican Psychoanalytic Association has, over the years, established its own guidelines for the teaching and practice of psychoanalysis. The Mexican school of psychoanalysis has developed a plural viewpoint by further incorporating the contributions of Winnicott, child-development theorists, Lacan, Kohut, Kernberg, and others.

The association suffered its worst setback in 1972 when, owing to ostensibly theoretical divergences and power struggles, a group of training analysts and candidates broke ranks, going on to found societies outside the International Psychoanalytic Association. The battle raged for several years, but it bolstered the association's cohesiveness and creativity. In addition, many Latin American analysts emigrated to Mexico during the turbulent years of military dictatorship in South America; several of them joined the Mexican Psychoanalytic Association.

Psychoanalysis gradually spread throughout Mexico. The northwestern region saw the founding, in 1977, of the Group for Psychoanalytic Studies of Monterrey, made up of Rubén Tamez, José Rubén Hinojosa, Diego Rodríguez, Eduardo Riojas, César Garza, and Ricardo Díaz Conty. The Institute of Psychoanalysis began operations in 1982 and was approved as a constituent society at the Amsterdam Congress of 1993. Its founding charter was signed by eleven training analysts and seven full members (Hinojosa, 1997).

Currently, there are approximately two hundred analysts approved by the International Psychoanalytic Association practicing in Mexico, as well as many psychoanalysts and over six hundred psychotherapists from other institutions. The country's major psychoanalytic centers are Mexico City, Monterrey, Guadalajara, Cuernavaca, Veracruz, Tuxtla Gutiérrez, León, and Querétaro.

A variety of activities, both within and outside the institution, began since the arrival of the pioneers. A Psychoanalytic Clinic, founded in June 1956, functioned for one year; reopened in 1960, it has been operating ever since. The Mexican Psychoanalytic Association has published a journal, *Cuadernos de Psicoanálisis*, continuously since 1965, with thirty-two volumes to date; it has also issued over 150 books. A training program for child psychoanalysts was launched in 1981 and has already produced five graduating classes (López, 1997). A Center for Postgraduate Studies was established in 1988 to train psychotherapists. Outreach activities have included events aimed at the general public, as well as courses in psychoanalytic psychiatry and psychoanalytic clinical psychology in hospitals and universities. Various associations and groups around the country now provide training in individual and group psychotherapy, and in psychotherapy for children, adolescents, and families.

Mexican psychoanalysts have also played a significant role on the international scene, through their activities within the International Psychoanalytic Association: Avelino González, Agustín Palacios, and Luis Féder have served as vice presidents, while Jaime Ayala and Eduardo Riojas have served in the House of Delegates. Mexicans also helped found the Psychoanalytic Confederation of Latin America and, subsequently, the Psychoanalytic Federation of Latin America, which has included Santiago Ramírez, Fernando Césarman, Víctor Aiza, and Alejandro Tamez among its presidents. In the academic field, prominent Mexican psychoanalysts teach seminars within training exchange programs and have sponsored study groups in South America, North America, and Europe. In recent years, they have participated in research projects on borderline patients, infants, and patients with psychosomatic disorders, among others (Ayala, 1995). The Mexican Association has cooperation agreements with Mexico's Council for Science and Technology, Cornell University in New York, and the Sorbonne in Paris. Three young analysts recently received the Sigmund Freud and Fepal awards granted by the Psychoanalytic Federation of Latin America.

REFERENCES

Ayala, J. (1995). Communication sent to the Societies Committee of the International Psychoanalytic Association.

Ayala, J., and Pérez de Pla, E. (1994). La selección de candidatos en la Asociación Psicoanalítica Mexicana (The selection of candidates at the Mexican Psychoanalytic Association). Paper presented at the Congress of the Psychoanalytic Federation of Latin America. Lima.

Dupont, M. A. (1991). Breve relación histórica del movimiento psicoanalítico en México (Brief historical overview of the psychoanalytic movement in Mexico). *Cuadernos de Psicoanálisis*, 24: 105–110.

Féder, L., and Dupont, M. A. (1987). Aspectos de la siembra y la cosecha psicoanalítica (Sowing and reaping in psychoanalysis). In Correio da Fepal, Federacion Psicoanalítica de América Latína, pp. 97–104.

Hinojosa, J. R. (1997). Personal communication.

López, M I. (1990). Historia del psicoanálisis en México. *Neurología-Neurocirugía-Psiquiatría*, 30: 17–20.

———. (1997). Personal communication.

Palacios, A. (1982). 25 años de la enseñanza del psicoanálisis en México (Twenty-five years of psychoanalytic training in Mexico). Paper presented at the twenty-fifth anniversary of the Mexican Psychoanalytic Association, Mexico.

Parres, R. (1987). Conferencia magistral sobre los treinta años del psicoanálisis en México (Lecture on thirty years of psychoanalysis in Mexico). *Cuadernos de Psicoanálisis*, 20: 11–20.

———. (1995). The Mexican Psychoanalytic Association. The American Psychoanalyst.

Parres, R., and Ramírez, S. (1966). Historia del movimiento psicoanalítico en México. *Cuadernos de Psicoanálisis*, 2: 11–20.

JAIME F. AYALA VILLARREAL

Mind and Body

Pinning Freud down on his view of the relation between mind and body has not been easy. Scholars have been able to find evidence from his writings to suggest a variety of theories, some dualistic and some materialistic.

Silverstein (1985) argues that Freud confronted the mind-body problem in his 1888 neurological paper "Gehirn" (*The Brain*) and adopted a dualistic position. Furthermore, Silverstein argues, Freud espoused an *interactive* view: the mind affects the brain (as well as bodily movements) and the operations of the brain affect the mind, without completely determining the latter.

Other writers agree that Freud committed to a dualistic position, at least prior to the development of psychoanalyis, but disagree with the attribution to him of an interactive position. Some (e.g., Andersson, 1962) hold that he was an epiphenomenalist. In this view, mind and brain are distinct, but mind has no causal powers at all; neurological and other physical events determine all behavior and mental events.

There is also reason to attribute to Freud the dualistic view known as "parallelism": the mental and the neurological are distinct but neither affects the other. For example, in *On Aphasia* (1891 [1953]), he writes: "The relationship between the chain of physiological events in the mental system and the mental procesess is probably not one of cause and effect. The former do not cease when the latter set in; they tend to continue, but from a certain moment, a mental phenomenon corresponds to each part of a chain, or to several parts. *The psychic is, therefore, a process parallel to the physiological, a dependent concomitant*" (Freud, 1891: 55, italics added).

Finally, a case could be made for saying that Freud held a "double-attribute" view of conscious processes: such processes have, in this view, both neurological attributes and non-reducible mental attributes that are the object of immediate awareness (see "Consciousness," this volume).

On the materialist (physicalist) side, several possibilities can be discounted. Given all that Freud argued about the existence of, and causal impact of, unconscious mental events, it is highly unlikely that he would have accepted "eliminative materialism," the idea that there are no mental states, events, or processes. Had he been aware of it, perhaps Freud would have found acceptable the contemporary view known as "functionalism"—what makes something a mental state or event is the causal role it plays in affecting behavior or other mental events—but there is no evidence that he was aware of it. The view became widely known only after 1970. If Freud did hold a physicalistic view, it most likely was the theory that

M

mind and brain are identical (or, rather, if he did not believe in an *entity* called the "mind," the theory that all mental events and processes are brain events or processes). Some writers argue that Freud, in fact, did hold the identity theory.

There are two obvious difficulties in interpreting Freud's views on the relation between mind and body: even writings from roughly the same period appear to commit him to divergent metaphysical doctrines on this issue and he may well have changed his mind as his work progressed. Perhaps, the best that can be demonstrated is that *at a particular time*, Freud's mind-body theory was such and such. Solms and Saling (1986; 1990, p. 96) review the various arguments on this topic and conclude that at least at the time that Freud wrote "Gehirn" (1888), he was a dualist of some sort, most likely a psychophysical parallelist. The above quotation from Freud's *Aphasia* clearly supports their position.

There are two additional questions that are often neglected in discussing Freud's mind-body views: one a causal question and the second a logical one.

The causal question is this: Which view of the mind-body relation influenced, or most influenced, his development of psychoanalysis? This topic is infected with all of the uncertainties of the initial one. If one cannot demonstrate that Freud held a particular view on the subject, even for a brief period, then clearly one cannot demonstrate that his holding the view influenced his development of any of his psychoanalytic theories. Even if one solves the first problem, there is still another step to be taken; to show that Freud's holding the metaphysical doctrine made a difference to his psychoanalytic theorizing.

The logical question is: Which mind-body theory (or theories) do his psychoanalytic theories either presuppose or contradict? Here something more definite can be said.

Some writers have tried to interpret Freudian theory in terms of the tenets of logical behaviorism: all sentences containing mentalistic terms are to be translated into purely behavioristic sentences. For example, if we use electric shock to train two albino rats to strike each other, and then substitute a small celluloid doll for one rat, we can translate "The rat is exhibiting Freudian *replacement*" as "The rat is striking the celluloid doll" (see Miller, 1948). Despite attempts to develop such translations (Dollard and Miller, 1950), the logical behaviorist view runs afoul of the fact that Freudian theory is a

causal theory, purporting to explain behavior, as well as dreams and other mental states. If someone is said to act in manner M because he has repressed certain motives, the statement that he has repressed these motives cannot be logically equivalent to one asserting that in that he is acting in manner M (for additional problems with logical behaviorism, see Erwin, 1978, chapter 2).

Because Freudian theory makes claims about how unconscious mental events affect dreams, slips, and neurotic behavior, there is also a problem in reconciling that part of the theory—an important part, indeed—with parallelism, epiphenomenalism, or eliminative materialism. All of these views are logically incompatible with the Freudian claim that mental events are causally efficacious. That does not mean that Freud did not accept one of these views; it does mean that there is an apparent inconsistency in combining any one of them with psychoanalytic theory.

One could try to argue that the inconsistency is only apparent. For example, an epiphenomenalist-Freudian could argue that for every unconscious mental event, there is a corresponding neurological event, and *it is* really the neurological event that instigates dreaming, determines the content of dreams, and causes behavior. We use psychoanalytic theory now, but only because we still know so little about how the brain works; psychoanalysis, Freudian or otherwise, has a useful role to play in guiding inquiry, but only until we obtain the requisite neurological information. This is a possible position, but it does not eliminate the inconsistency that arises in combining Freud theory and epiphenomenalism: It has the implication that Freudian theory, at least that part that attributes causal powers to unconscious mental events, is *false*. For in the view just described, it is just an illusion that any mental event causes anything.

Can the identity theory be squared with Freudian theory? There is an apparent problem if one assumes that the latter is interactionist; for how can mind and brain causally interact, as Freudian theory arguably requires, if they are one and the same thing? This problem is only apparent. A neurological event cannot cause itself, but it can cause other neurological events, some of which may be identical with mental events; and some mental events that are really brain events, if the identity theory is right, can cause other mental events (that are also brain events) and can affect behavior. The identity theory, then, can be rendered consistent with Freud's theory. The more popular sort of materialism, functionalism, is also consistent with his theory. However, Freud's theory does not presuppose either metaphysical theory, or indeed any other form of materialism. One could consistently combine Freudian theory with an interactive form of "property dualism," the theory that there is no substance or entity called the mind, but that there are mental states and events that are not identical with neurological states, although they may be causally dependent upon them (or, as philosophers of mind say, "supervene" on them).

In short, Freudian theory and more recent psychoanalytic theories are not entirely metaphysically neutral—they clash with mind-body theories that make the mental causally impotent—but they are compatible with certain forms of both dualism and materialism.

REFERENCES

Andersson, O. (1962). *Studies in the Prehistory of Psychoanalyis: The Etiology of Psychoneuroses and Related Themes in Sigmund Freud's Scientific Writings and Letters, 1886–1896.* Stockholm: Svenska Bokforlaget.

Dollard, J., and Miller, N. (1950). *Personality and Psychotherapy.* New York: McGraw Hill.

Erwin, E. (1978). *Behavior Therapy: Scientific, Philosophical, and Moral Foundations.* London: Cambridge University Press.

Freud, S. (1888). Gehirn. In A. Villaret (ed.). *Handwörterbuch der gesamten Meizin,* Volume 1. Stuttgart: Fernandand Enke Verlag, pp. 684–697.

———. (1891). *On Aphasia: A Critical Study.* Trans., E. Stengel, London: Imago, 1953.

Miller, N. (1948). Theory and experiment relating psychoanalytic displacement to stimulus-response generalization. *Journal of Abnormal Social Psychology,* 43: 155–173.

Silverstein, B. (1985). Freud's psychology and its organic foundation: Sexuality and mind-body interactionism. *Psychoanalytic Review,* 72: 203–228.

Solms, M., and Saling, M. (1986). On psychoanalysis and neuroscience: Freud's attitude to the localization tradition. *The International Journal of Psycho-Analysis,* 67: 397–416.

Solms, M., and Saling, M., Editors and Translators (1990). *A Moment of Transition: Two Neuroscientific Articles by Sigmund Freud.* London: H. Karnac (Books) Ltd.

EDWARD ERWIN

Modernism, Postmodernism, and Freudianism

To define the relations among modernism, postmodernism, and Freudianism is necessarily an exercise in equivocation, given certain ambiguities inherent in each of the three concepts at issue. Some decades ago, W. H. Auden described Freud as "no more a person now but a whole climate of opinion." Although this remains as true as ever, it must be added that Freud is currently being claimed as well as vilified in a bewildering variety of ways.

In contemporary psychology and philosophy, the term "modernism" usually refers to the trend of rationalistic and scientific thought that begins with Descartes, Galileo, Newton, and the seventeenth-century Enlightenment. "Postmodernism" denotes various anti-foundationalist and relativistic reactions against this trend that became prominent in the last several decades in the work of such thinkers as Thomas Kuhn, an historian of science, Richard Rorty, a neo-pragmatist philosopher, and Jacques Derrida, a post-structuralist philosopher and literary theorist.

Generally Freud's own characterizations portray psychoanalysis as an Enlightenment or modernist enterprise: a scientific attempt to discover and verify objective truths about the nature and functioning of the human psyche. In the Dora case, for example, Freud (1905, p. 59) denies that he is a "man of letters engaged upon the creation of a mental state . . . for a short story," insisting instead that he is "a medical man engaged upon its dissection." In the *New Introductory Lectures on Psychoanalysis*, Freud (1933, p. 159) writes that the "intellect and the mind are objects for scientific research in exactly the same way as any non-human things." He claims that "psychoanalysis has a special right to speak for the scientific *Weltanschauung* at this point, since it cannot be reproached with having neglected what is mental in the picture of the universe. Its contribution to science lies precisely in having extended research to the mental field." This vision of psychoanalysis as an Enlightenment enterprise has been emphasized in recent years by the philosopher Adolf Grünbaum (1984). Grünbaum, however, goes on to argue that Freud's modernist project was largely abortive, since he failed to support his psychological hypotheses with credible empirical evidence.

A rather different view of the real import of the psychoanalytic project has been adopted by various writers who focus on Freud's characterization of his prime object of study. Psychoanalysts often describe the unconscious as a nearly all-determining force—a force so elusive and mysterious that it might well seem to frustrate any attempt to pin it down or to formulate general laws of its functioning. In *The Interpretation of Dreams*, for example, Freud (1900, p. 525) speaks of the "dream's

M

navel," "the spot where it reaches down into the unknown," and where the "tangle of dream-thoughts" is so richly intertwined as to be impossible to unravel. Emphasis on the self-deluding, infinitely elusive nature of the unconscious can seem to bring the psychoanalytic conception of the psyche rather close to that of post-modernists who are inclined to deny the very possibility of true insight, objective knowledge, or verifiable truths. Freud's characterization of meandering chains of association in unconscious, primary-process thinking has, for example, been likened to Jacques Derrida's quasi-linguistic vision of the infinite deferral and elusiveness of meaning (e.g., Barratt, 1993).

For Derrida, a poststructuralist and postmodernist philosopher, the real lesson of Freud's discoveries and of his actual interpretive practices (which can be fanciful in the extreme, as both critics and admirers have noted) is rather different from the claims to scientific objectivity made by Freud and other "purveyors of truth." For Derrida (1978, p. 211; Megill, 1985: 330), Freud's interpretive method and discoveries show not merely that human beings are necessarily self-deluding, but that interpretation is something that, in some sense, might as well go on forever; that, in fact, there is no original unconscious text, such as the true and original wish underlying a dream, which is lying there waiting to be discovered. Those who take such a view have sometimes preferred to see psychoanalysis as a mythopoeic rather than a scientific system—a system that should devote itself less to the attempt to discover historical or psychological truth than to the creation of useful, inspiring, or liberating narratives.

The relationship between Freudianism, modernism, and postmodernism must also be considered in light of how the terms "modernism" and "postmodernism" have been understood in fields outside psychology and philosophy. In literary studies and in the history and criticism of art, aesthetics, and cultural sensibility, "modernism" refers not to Enlightenment rationalism and science but, rather, to the innovative, often avant-garde, and not infrequently anti-scientistic developments in art and culture in the early decades of this century—developments exemplified in the work of Joyce, Kafka, Proust, T. S. Eliot, Matisse, and Picasso. In this aesthetic and cultural context, "postmodernism" refers to more recent (post-World War II, and usually post-1960s) developments epitomized by such artists as Andy Warhol, Thomas Pynchon, and John Cage (but prefigured by Duchamp and

the Dada-ist movement). Although aesthetic modernism and postmodernism have much in common (see Sass, 1992: 28–38, 343–351), postmodernists do reject what they see as the post-romantic valorization of uniqueness, individuality, and psychological depth that was so important to such modernist writers as Virginia Woolf and Marcel Proust. The postmodernists favor more depersonalized, even mechanical conceptions that view human consciousness and expression as the product of impersonal social and linguistic factors; and they are dubious of the aspiration toward aesthetic stasis, autonomy, and self-containment that are inherent in the modernist ideal.

Perhaps the richest portrayal of a Freud who is modernist in this second sense of the term is to be found in Philip Rieff's book, *Freud: The Mind of the Moralist* (1979). Rieff portrays Freudian psychoanalysis as articulating a post-religious morality for the era of "psychological man"—an inward-focused morality that encompasses both the autonomous and expressivist ideals of modern humanism by advocating the self-actualization that comes from exploring and expressing one's unique past and individual unconscious, as well as the self-control that comes from the ability to clarify and manipulate the inner life. Readings of Freud more consistent with the vision of aesthetic postmodernism often draw on Jacques Lacan (1977). Lacan views the unconscious not as a source of all that is most passionate or personal (the aesthetic modernist, post-romantic reading), but as the locus of an impersonal, symbolic network which, as he says, "is structured like a language" (see Silverman, 1983: 149–193). Lacan also ridicules belief in the possibility of an undivided or autonomous ego. Whereas Rieff portrays a Freud who democratized the ideals of aesthetic modernism, offering authentic self-knowledge and self-control as the potential reward for those willing to take up the challenge of psychoanalysis, Lacan offers a Freud more consistent with the anti-humanist aspects of postmodernism: a Freud who teaches us to search within not to discover our uniqueness, authenticity, or self-control, but to acknowledge the profoundly determinative forces of language and the social order.

These two visions of Freud's significance can perhaps be summed up as two differing readings of the famous line from Freud's (1933, p. 80) *New Introductory Lectures:* "Wo es war, soll ich werden." In the Anglo-American world, Freud's line has generally been understood to mean that, where the id once reigned, in darkness and unreason, there the ego shall come to be, exercising rationality, insight, and self-control. But Freud's line can also be heard in ways that are more congenial to the followers of Lacan (1977: 128 and passim.) as well as Derrida, for example, as meaning: Where the "it" (das Es) was, there the ego or the "I" shall go—there to wander and there perhaps to lose its illusions of autonomy and self-control.

REFERENCES

Barratt, B. (1993). *Psychoanalysis and the Postmodern Impulse.* Baltimore, Md.: Johns Hopkins University Press.

Derrida, J. (1978). Freud and the Scene of Writing. In J. Derrida, *Writing and Difference*, A. Bass (trans.). Chicago: University of Chicago Press, pp. 196–231.

Freud, S. (1905). Fragment of an analysis of a case of hysteria. S.E. 7: 7–122.

———. (1933). *New Introductory Lectures on Psycho-analysis.* S.E. 22: 5–185.

———. (1900). *The Interpretation of Dreams.* S.E. 4–5: 1–621.

Grünbaum, A. (1984). *The Foundations of Psychoanalysis: A Philosophical Critique.* Berkeley, Calif.: University of California Press.

Lacan, J. (1977). *Ecrits.* A. Sheridan (trans.). New York: Norton.

Megill, A. (1985). *Prophets of Extremity: Nietzsche, Heidegger, Foucault, Derrida.* Berkeley, Calif.: University of California Press.

Rieff, P. (1959). *Freud: The Mind of the Moralist*, 3rd ed., 1979. Chicago: University of Chicago Press.

Sass, L. (1992). *Madness and Modernism.* New York: Basic Books. Paperback ed.: Cambridge, Mass.: Harvard University Press, 1994.

Silverman, K. (1983). *The Subject of Semiotics.* New York: Oxford University Press.

LOUIS A. SASS

Monotheism See RELIGION, AND PSYCHOANALYSIS.

Mood See AFFECT.

Morality, and Psychoanalysis

This article examines the psychoanalytic explanation of the psychological origins and functions of morality, including the ethical implications of this account for the justification of normative standards and judgments.

A key issue in the continuing debate about the psychoanalytic view of morality revolves around the definitional question: What is morality? In some places, Freud implies that morality is synonymous with the injunctions and prohibitions of the superego (1924, pp. 167–168, 170; 1930, pp. 136–137). The superego, or "conscience," is formed at the conclusion of the Oedipal crisis through "identification" with and "introjection" of the standards of parents and other authorities, alongside imagined punishments and rewards. The "ego ideal" component of the superego consists of ideals and values modeled after people the growing child would like to be like, while the second component, "conscience," representing the internalized critical voice of parental prohibition, creates the subjective experience of "thou shalt not." Failure to live up to the ego ideal engenders shame, while disobedience of a moral prohibition produces guilt. "In this way," Freud writes, the superego "proves to be . . . the source of our individual ethical sense, our morality" (1924, pp. 167–68).

If this were Freud's entire account, morality, like the superego, would be no more than a set of purely arbitrary standards, since it would rest finally on nothing more than irrational respect for whatever maxims parents and other authority figures happened to teach or to practice. The ethical relativist thesis that conflicting ethical claims are equally valid would be entailed by such an account, since there would be no basis to argue for or against differing moral standards, if all standards were equally arbitrary. Additionally, the inhibiting and punitive functions of the archaic superego would appear to make morality itself unreasonable from the standpoint of the egoistic individual seemingly implied by Freud's account of the deepest springs of human motivation in terms of instinctual drive satisfaction.

Despite widespread acceptance of this standard account of the psychoanalytic perspective on morality, a careful reading of Freud shows that the technical concept of the superego is both broader and narrower than the ordinary concept of morality, not only in everyday speech but in Freud's own usage. The superego is broader than "morality" because it includes ideals and standards that relate not to moral right and wrong but to standards of beauty, etiquette, social status, and economic success. One might feel badly about not living up to one of these nonmoral standards, but one would not be likely to feel *moral* guilt or *moral* shame. Conversely, the superego is narrower than the ordinary concept of morality insofar as morality is normally understood to encompass not only conscience but affective dispositions or virtues, like sympathy and benevolence, that develop and function somewhat independently of the injunctions and prohibitions of conscience. Freud makes it clear that authentic moral motives are not to be confused with egoistic motives for obeying the superego, such as fear of punishment or anticipation of a reward. At its foundations, genuine morality rests on the authenticity of other-regarding motives, which spring from the "heart," that is to say, from deeply grounded "affects," rather than from self-alienating commandments (see, e.g., 1915, pp. 275–300; Wallwork, 1991: 160–190).

Once morality is no longer identified with the archaic superego, the way is clear to formulate an "ego ethics" that escapes the punitive moralism of the superego with its relativistic ethical implications. Fromm (1947, 1956) and Erikson (1964) are well known for distinguishing "mature" or "healthy" ego ethics from superego moralism, but Freud was the first to formulate the distinction, without explicitly designating a name for the alternative ethic that he found compatible with psychoanalytic theory and practice. Whereas superego moralism rests on threats of punishment, that is, on guilt or shame, mature ethics for Freud as for Fromm and Erikson represent the realization of the highest potentiality of human development.

Freud's constructive moral alternative to superego moralism has not been appreciated, partly because the myth is widespread in contemporary culture that Freud was committed to a form of psychological egoism. Thus Fromm answers the question "Did Freud recognize the moral factor as a fundamental part of his model of man?" thus: "The answer to this question is in the negative. Man develops exclusively under the influence of his self interest, which demands optimal satisfaction of his libidinal impulses, always on the condition that they do not endanger his interest in self-preservation" (Fromm, 1973: 52). Similarly, Ian Gregory declares that Freud sees the human being as "wholly subject to the dictates of the pleasure principle. . . . His end is always the same, his own gratification. He is in short, wholly self-absorbed, utterly selfish, not capable of forswearing instinctual satisfaction" (Gregory, 1975: 102).

Yet, when Freud turns to the genuinely moral aspects of human nature, he makes it plain that psychoanalysis acknowledges the authenticity of nonegoistic, other-regarding motives. Surprisingly for someone for whom the dark side of human nature is so prominent, Freud asserts that most humans possess a core of genuinely other-regarding motives, grounded in Eros, that, with proper environmental nourishment, provide a basis for moral conduct independently of the superego. There is, Freud argues, an inborn, hereditary "tendency (disposition) towards the transformation of egoistic into other-regarding social instincts" (1915, p. 282). This naturally occurring transformation of the child's egoism into genuine other-regard is not be confused with externally good conduct that is a product of rewards and punishments, as meted out by the superego and external authorities. The "person who is subjected . . . [only to external rewards and punishments] will choose to behave well in the cultural sense of the phrase," Freud writes, but "no ennoblement of instinct, no transformation of egoistic into altruistic inclinations . . . [will have] taken place in him" (1915, pp. 283–284). There is a world of difference, Freud states, between the person who "acts morally" only for egoistic reasons, because "such cultural behavior is advantageous for his selfish purposes," and the person who acts morally "because his instinctual inclinations compel him to" (1915, p. 284; Wallwork, 1991: 169). The latter has undergone "the transformation of instinct" that differentiates the "truly civilized" from the "cultural hypocrites," who may act correctly but only to avoid superego condemnation or to gain some intrapsychic or interpersonal reward.

Of course, Freud is suspicious of any claim to pure altruism. The best in human nature is always intertwined with base inclinations. In Freud's own words: "It is not our intention to dispute the noble endeavors of human nature, nor have we ever done anything to detract from their value. On the contrary . . . [w]e lay a stronger emphasis on what is evil in men only because other people disavow it and thereby make the human mind, not better, but incomprehensible" (1915, pp. 146–147). Not only is there a conflict between the ego and others—that is, between egoism and altruism—there is also a conflict between the primal instincts of Eros and aggression deriving from the death instincts (1930, p. 141). The moral point Freud makes about the inevitable mixture of good and bad motives is not that we are ultimately evil or amoral, but that we are more likely to act morally if we "own" and take responsibility for our base motives than if we spend our energy erecting fruitless defenses against their recognition. As he puts it, "Obviously one must hold oneself responsible for [one's] evil impulses . . . [I]f, in defence, I say that what is unknown, unconscious and repressed in me is not my 'ego', then . . . I shall perhaps be taught better by the criticisms of my fellowmen, by the disturbances in my actions and the confusion of my feelings. I shall perhaps learn that what I am disavowing not only 'is' in me but sometimes 'acts' from out of me as well" (1923a, p. 133). It is by owning up to our base motives, Freud contends, that we gain leverage over them and are better able to guide their expression along less destructive paths. In his famous retake of Plato's equestrian metaphor for the self (1923a, p. 25; 1926, p. 95), the self-aware moral agent is like the skilled rider who is capable of guiding the powerful raw animal instincts symbolized by the horse in the direction of sublimated goals that are satisfactory to the self as a whole and to the community with which he or she is identified, that is, toward such sublimated, intrinsic goods as mutual love, creativity, freely chosen productive work, the pursuit of knowledge, and aesthetic enjoyment. (For discussion of Freud's treatment of these various intrinsic goods and their connection to "happiness" and the goals of psychoanalytic treatment, see Wallwork [1991, pp. 244–259]).

Pursuit of these intrinsic goods, which provide Freud with an implicit evaluative yardstick for evaluating less flourishing paths to happiness, is too often inhibited by culturally sanctioned repressive moralisms that suppress human vitality in the name not of the highest ethical values but irrational niggardly authority. "This [moralism] is to the advantage neither of morality nor of the person concerned," Freud (1930, p. 169) observes. It is disadvantageous to morality, because "moral masochism" actually spawns immoral behavior by flaming disavowed desires to violate moral standards in order to elicit the punishment the masochist believes irrationally she or he deserves for unknown "sinful" behavior, which may be for a mere wish. Moral maschoism is disadvantageous to the individal because the need for punishment interferes with wholehearted pursuit of vital interests or wrecks truly successful accomplishments. Even worse consequences flow from moral sadism, which commonly involves projecting onto others one's worst fears about oneself and then cruelly punishing, possibly even killing, others for what one needs to repudiate in oneself. Freud cites, in this connection, the extreme intolerance shown Jews by Christians, noting ironically that the massacres of the Jews in the Middle Ages failed to make Christians feel any more secure (1930, p. 114).

Morality need not have these deleterious consequences, however. An ethic focused on humane respect for everyone, truthfulness, and love may, in fact, contribute to the happiness, in the Aristotelian sense of the "well-being," of both the individual and the community,

as long as it is combined with a healthy suspicion directed at all sanguine illusions about our superior moral goodness and moral purity.

Psychoanalysis fosters genuine morality insofar as it frees the patient's autonomy, honesty, and capacities for respect and care for others from the debilitating constraints of intrapsychic conflict. Then, Freud writes, psychoanalytic "treatment . . . find[s] a place among the methods whose aim is to bring about the highest ethical and intellectual development of the individal" (Freud, Letter #80 in Hale, 1971: 170).

REFERENCES

Erikson, E. H. (1964). *Insight and Responsibility.* New York: Norton.

Freud, S. *Thoughts for the Times on War and Death.* 1915 S.E. 14: 275–300.

———. (1923a). *The Ego and the Id.* S.E. 19: 10–59.

———. (1923b). Some additional notes on dream-interpretation as a whole. S.E. 19: 127–138.

———. (1924). *The Economic Problem of Masochism.* S.E. 19: 159–70.

———. (1926). *Inhibitions, Symptoms and Anxiety.* S.E. 20: 77–172.

———. (1930). *Civilization and Its Discontents.* S.E. 21: 64–145.

Fromm, E. (1947). *Man for Himself.* New York: Holt, Rinehart, and Winston.

———. (1956). *The Art of Loving.* New York: Harper and Row.

———. (1973). Freud's model of man and its social determinants. In P. Roazen (ed.) (1973). *Sigmund Freud.* Englewood Cliffs, N.J.: Prentice-Hall, pp. 45–48.

Gregory, I. (1975). Psycho-analysis, human nature and human conduct. In R.S. Peters (ed.). *Nature and Conduct.* New York: St. Martins Press, pp. 99–120.

Hale, N. G., Jr. (1971). *James Jackson Putnam and Psychoanalysis.* Cambridge, Mass.: Harvard University Press, 1971.

Wallwork, E. (1991). *Psychoanalysis and Ethics.* New Haven, Conn.: Yale University Press.

ERNEST WALLWORK

Mourning See DEPRESSION; IDENTIFICATION; SUICIDE.

Multiple Personality (Dissociative Identity Disorder)

In the American Psychiatric Association's fourth edition of the *Diagnostic and Statistical Manual of Mental Disorders* (*DSM-IV*, 1994), the concept "dissociative identity disorder" (DID) replaces the concept "multiple personality disorder" (MPD) on the grounds that a person with one brain can have but one personality, though this single personality may be dissociated into more or less distinctly experienced identities. This view, however dubious, is supposed to clarify the forensic concept of dissociation and to combat the belief that different people or entities occupy one body in rotation. In this essay, the newer terminology, "dissociative identity disorder," will be used interchangeably with "multiple personality disorder."

Janet and Freud

The most important part of Pierre Janet's (1907) work in abnormal psychology was his remarkable series of studies on the dissociations of hysteria, especially those massive dissociations that become manifest as somnambulisms, fugues, and multiple personalities. In *The Ego and the Id*, Freud suggests a psychoanalytic explanation of such dissociative phenomena:

> Although it is a digression from our theme, we cannot avoid giving our attention for a moment longer to the ego's object identifications. If they obtain the upper hand and become too numerous, unduly intense, and incompatible with one another, a pathological outcome will not be far off. It may come to a disruption of the ego in consequence of the individual identifications becoming cut off from one another by resistances; perhaps the secret of the so-called multiple personality is that the various identifications seize possession of consciousness in turn (Freud, 1923: 30–31).

In this same work, Freud (1923, pp. 51–52) also points out the following:

> The hysterical type of ego defends itself from the painful perception which the criticism of its super-ego threatens to produce in it by the same means that it uses to defend itself from an unendurable object—cathexis—by an act of repression. It is the ego, therefore, that is responsible for the sense of guilt remaining unconscious. We know that as a rule the ego carries out repressions in the service and at the behest of its super-ego; but this is a case in which it has turned the same weapon against its harsh task-master.

One form of multiple and alternating personality shows just this kind of superego cleavage exemplified by the well-known literary fictional model of Robert Louis Stevenson (1886) in *The Strange Case of Dr. Jekyll and Mr. Hyde*. In this dual personality type, the ego oscillates from a position of major defense against unruly and unwelcome id impulses to a position of major defense against overly strict superego pressures. The person exhibits unique and complex behavior patterns and social relationships that contrast sharply with each other.

Dissociation and Repression

In differentiating dissociation proper, or "splitting," from the repression that Freud usually discussed, but continuing in the vein of Freud's spatial metaphor of the mental apparatus, Henry V. Dicks (1939, p. 99) notes that a whole side of someone's personality may be segregated by a more sudden and even more rigorous and effective force than repression from the main stream. We may perhaps speak, Dick notes (p. 99), of repression as a "horizontal barrier interposed between instinct impulse and its expression in egoic consciousness." Dissociation, in contrast, might then be visualized as a "vertical barrier," or perhaps cleavage, within the repressed material itself.

Multiple Personality and Child Development

Jeanne Lampl-de Groot (1981) relates multiple personality to phases of human development. Progression in the development of a child, she asserts, is not continuous but instead alternates with regressive attitudes. Some residues of each developmental phase are preserved in the psychic depths. "These remnants are," she writes, "the constituents of the multiple personality of human beings" (p. 620). A few examples of the more adaptive utilization of something like multiple personality are as follows:

1. A mother, nursing her baby, is able to revive the experiential world of her own infancy, so that her empathy is enhanced with benefit to her own well-being and for the baby's basic trust.
2. An adult playing with a toddler returns in some measure to his own state of mind as a toddler, thus being able to respect the toddler's needs for autonomy and for closeness (refueling).
3. A teacher who switches sometimes from her adult attitude to the still retained facets of her

own latency or puberty will promote her pupils' capacity for and wish to learn. Here, too, flexibility is an essential condition for optimal functioning. (Lampl-de Groot, 1981: 620)

Psychopathology

As Lampl-de Groot recognized, in its flagrant forms, multiple personality proper is the expression of severe psychopathology. These flagrant forms show a lack of flexibility in dealing with early unresolved and traumatic conflicts. Here splitting takes on a more fixed pattern, one that may prevent, at any rate temporarily and sometimes permanently, the personality's molecular disintegration (Abse, 1983). Not only does the patient lose the flexibility of switching from one facet of his or her personality to another; he or she also becomes altogether immersed in one personality when the other now confronts him or her with an unbearable strain. In multiple personality proper, the patient switches from one fixed pattern of personality, comprising a gestalt (a superego-ego pattern) in its own right, to another without later adequate progressive integration of these patterns. Moreover, the individual is lost episodically in an alternate identity in a way that crosses the border into delusions. The victim of multiple personality is periodically obliged to desert completely his or her usual identity.

But there is a condition that hovers between the complete desertion of one identity for another and one that is so common that it is apt to be taken too much for granted, namely, the gross change in personality that may occur in episodic alcoholism. In Stevenson's fictional model of alternating personality, a chemical agent periodically transforms Dr. Jekyll into Mr. Hyde. Who can doubt that this story was partly based on Stevenson's observations of alcohol abuse? The fictional model accurately portrays a kind of superego cleavage, a strict internal regulation, resulting in a commonplace respectability being replaced, following chemical ingestion, by the emergence of sadistic behavior.

Among the simplest dissociated responses are so-called absences that comprise amnesia gaps, filled often by altered states of consciousness, which interrupt the continuity of a patient's history. When these absences are lengthy, and there is a conspicuous and frightening experience of lost time, an incoherence of personality becomes a serious clinical problem, an existential disruption that Putnam (1989) rightly emphasizes.

Braun (1988) notes four interrelated processes typically involved in dissociative episodes, operating along a continuum from full waking awareness to an extreme splitting off from it. The processes include changes in behavior, affect, sensation, and knowledge. All four processes are utilized in the organization of memory; when there is a disruption, compartmentalism of memory and identity results.

Kluft (1984) in his study of thirty-three cases of multiple personality disorder (also see Kluft, 1985) showed that the encoding, storage, and retrieval of memories are state-related inasmuch as the intense emotion aroused at the time, or even toxemia, may be influential in the organization of memories for traumatic events. The emotions aroused by traumatic events are, of course, entangled in exuberant sadomasochistic fantasy as are the memories that are later recalled.

Multiple personality is the most dramatic and potentially incapacitating dissociative disorder. Its origins are embedded in physical and sexual child abuse often in the context of the family, and sometimes in that of multigenerational satanic ritual abuse (Driscol and Wright, 1991). There is burgeoning evidence linking multiple personality disorder with sexual abuse in childhood (Putnam, 1989). Van der Kolk (1988) has noted that severe dissociative disorders such as that of multiple personality are psychobiologically related to post-traumatic stress disorder that follows, sooner or later, other causes of psychic trauma. Horowitz and Solomon (1978) emphasize that the florid manifestations of stress response syndromes may not appear until after termination of environmental stress events, and sometimes only after a latency period of apparent abatement of acute symptoms of anxiety. Post-traumatic stress disorders (PTSD) may thus be more or less delayed. Whenever they arise, the symptoms fall into two categories, though some symptoms are composed of both intertwined. One category consists of intrusive ideas related to the precipitating situation, compulsive repetition of trauma-related behavior, and attacks of related stormy affects. Contrarily, there is a negative category of symptoms consisting of emotional avoidance, denial, splitting, and repression, in a massive unconscious attempt to conceal underlying conflicts and to protect against the arousal of primitive destructive impulses and terror. In discussing the "psychical mechanism of hysterical phenomena," Breuer and Freud (1893) had already pointed out these two categories of symptoms, often simultaneously present. They

M

write: "Both of these conditions, however, have in common the fact that the psychical traumas which have not been disposed of by reaction cannot be disposed of otherwise by being worked over by means of association" (p. 11), adding: "It may therefore be said that the ideas which have become pathological have persisted with such freshness and affective strength because they have been denied the normal wearing-away processes by means of abreaction and reproduction in states of uninhibited association" (p. 11).

In treating multiple personality disorder, remembering, repeating, and working through childhood traumata, including cumulative trauma (Khan, 1963), are important dimensions to consider. However, a broadening of the analytic approach, through an understanding of working with psychotic transference and resistance, becomes necessary to promote adequate integration (Hedges, 1994; also see Abse, 1982).

One of the problems involved in treating multiple personality disorders is the evocation of intense positive and negative countertransferences in the primary therapist. Where there is a team approach, as in a hospital, noxious staff countertransferences can become highly contagious. In instances of aroused hostility, sometimes exploited by a malicious alter personality, disagreements will often occur about the correct assessment of the clinical picture. Staff members may divide into two groups, one supporting and the other being antagonistic toward the patient. Confusion thus often occurs among attendants, including social workers and nurses, some of whom may indeed become victims of group hysteria.

Criminality

An angry and aggressive alter personality sometimes figures prominently in dissociative identity disorder with occasional facilitation of periodic criminality. Allison (1981) performed forensic evaluation on eight male felons, one of whom confessed to the murder of several women.

Michael J. Rostafinski (1955) studied eleven felons with dissociative identity disorder. Among these eleven inmates of the prison in Virginia where Rostafinski's observations were made, the possible existence of a causative relation between the DID and the criminal offense was not taken into account in rendering the verdict of guilty as charged, nor in setting the sentence. In another such case in another jurisdiction, the psychiatric report rendered resulted in some mitigation in sentencing and a recommendation for further treatment fol-

lowing probation from imprisonment for embezzlement. Adequate psychotherapeutic intervention is the only possible preventive measure against recidivism in such offenders. Fink (1991) has discussed the similarity of the dissociative antisocial identity of some multiples and antisocial personality disorder.

REFERENCES

Abse, D. W. (1982). Multiple personality. In A. Roy (ed.). *Hysteria* (chapter 13). New York: Wiley.

———. (1983). Multiple personality. In S. Akhtar (ed.). *New Psychiatric Syndromes: DSM III and Beyond* (chapter 14). New York: Jason Aronson.

Allison, R. B. (1981). Multiple personality and criminal behavior. *American Journal of Forensic Psychiatry*, 2: 32–38.

Braun, B. G. (1988). The BASK model of dissociation. *Dissociation*, 1: 4–23.

Breuer, J., and Freud, S. (1893). *On the Psychical Mechanism of Hysterical Phenomena: Preliminary Communication*. S.E. 2: 3–17.

Dicks, H. V. (1939). *Clinical Studies in Psychopathology*. London: Arnold.

Driscol, L. N., and Wright, C. (1991). Survivors of childhood ritual abuse: Multigenerational satanic cult involvement. *Treating Abuse Today*.

Fink, D. (1991). The comorbidity of multiple personality disorder & D.S.M. II-R Axis II Disorders. *Psychiatric Clinics North America*, 14: 547–566.

Freud, S. (1923). *The Ego and the Id*. S.E. 19: 12–59.

Hedges, L. E. (1994). *Remembering, Repeating and Working Through Childhood Trauma*. Northvale, N.J.: Jason Aronson.

Horowitz, M. J., and Solomon, G. F. (1978). Delayed stress response syndromes in Vietnam veterans. In C. R. Figley (ed.). *Stress Disorders Among Vietnam Veterans: Theory, Research and Treatment*. New York: Brunner/Mazel.

Janet, P. (1907). *The Major Symptoms of Hysteria*. New York: Macmillan.

Khan, M. M. R. (1963). The concept of cumulative trauma. *Psychoanalytic Study of the Child*, 18: 286–306.

Kluft, R. P. (1984). Treatment of multiple personality disorder: A study of 33 cases. *Psychiatric Clinics of America*, 7: 9–29.

———. (1985). *Childhood Antecedents of Multiple Personality Disorder*. American Psychiatric Press.

Lampl-de Groot, J. (1981). Notes on "Multiple Personality." *Psychoanalytic Quarterly*, 50: 620.

Putnam, F. W. (1989). *Diagnosis and Treatment of Multiple Personality Disorder*. New York: England.

Rostafinski, M. J. (1955). Dissociative identity disorder: Observations of a prison psychiatrist. (personal communication).

Stevenson, R. L. (1886). *The Strange Case of Dr. Jekyll and Mr. Hyde*. London: Longmans.

Van der Kolk, B. A. (1988). The biological response to psychic trauma. In F. M. Ochberg (ed.). *Post-traumatic Therapy and Victims of Violence*. New York: Brunner/Mazel.

D. WILFRED ABSE

Myths

Freud never composed any single substantial piece of work devoted to mythology, although he was acutely aware of such potential application of psychoanalysis. He said in *An Autobiographical Study*: "I have taken but little direct part in certain . . . applications of psychoanalysis, though they are none the less of general interest. It is only a step from the phantasies of individual neurotics to the imaginative creations of groups and peoples as we find them in myths, legends, and fairy tales" (1925, p. 69). Freud was fascinated by myths, punctuating his entire corpus with explicit and implicit references to them. One can identify three interrelated aspects of Freud's interests, some of which were more fully developed by his followers. The first relates to the definition of myth as a type of symbolic phenomenon; the second to the relationship between myth and history; and the third to the relationship between myth and psychoanalytic theory and practice.

Myths and Symbols

In his preface to the third edition of *The Interpretation of Dreams* (written in 1911), Freud stated that further expansion of the work would "have to afford closer contact with the copious material presented in imaginative writing, in myths, in linguistic usage and in folklore" (1900, p. xxvii). This shows how his early forays into the analysis of dreams had become the catalyst for expanding psychoanalysis into the broader cultural arena, with dream analysis becoming the prototype of an investigative mode capable of extension into all areas of mental life associated with the imagination. Myths, then, were to be interpreted like dreams, with the symbolisms of both emerging out of common unconscious processes. "Dream-symbolism," said Freud, "extends far beyond dreams: it is not peculiar to dreams, but exercises a similar dominating influence on representation in fairy-tales, myths and legends, in jokes and in folk lore" (1901, p. 685).

When Freud took an analytical excursion through Shakespeare, European fairy tales, and classical mythology in *The Theme of the Three Caskets* (1913, pp. 289–301), demonstrating that a set of related motifs (to do with femininity, impoverishment, and silence) had an invariant meaning (death) throughout diverse narrative modes, he assumed that the motifs were the effect of the same universal unconscious processes ("displacement, condensation and dramatization"—1901, p. 685) that were originally discovered in dream work. He did not subscribe to the view that myth and associated narrative forms (legends, fairy tales, and folklore) originated from dreams, although he clearly believed that dreams and myths were identical in their obscure relationship to repressed thoughts. "We can," he said in connection with myths and fairy tales, "only hold firmly to the suspicion that there is a specially intimate relation between true symbols and sexuality" (1916–1917, p. 166). This "intimate relation" was revealed, for example, when the symbol of Oedipus's blinding was shown to signify castration (1900, p. 398). In that sense, myths (or legends or folktales) are just one repository of "true symbols" among others: "it was only through the knowledge of infantile sexuality that it became possible to understand mythology and the world of fairy tales" (1926, p. 211).

Myths and History

Freud ascribed a more specific character to myths when he described them as conveyors of "obscure information . . . from the primeval ages of human society" (1900, p. 256). Myths, in common with other symbolic phenomena, were seen as an archaic mode of thought (1908, p. 174), but they were also seen as the "precipitate" of "the imaginative activities of primitive man" (1926, p. 212) and as "our chief witness in matters concerning primeval times" (1926, p. 214). Myths, therefore, were to be seen as a window on history, and this line of thought was most famously developed in Freud's anthropological works. In *Totem and Taboo* (1913, pp. 1–161), Freud posited the famous historical scenario of the murder of the father in the "primal horde," which he saw as being symbolized and recapitulated in the rituals and myths of contemporary "primitive" religion. Similarly, in *Moses and Monotheism* (1939, pp. 1–137), he traced links among history, Judeo-Christian traditions, and the contemporary character and fate of the Jewish people. Such relationships among myth, history, and the present were succinctly captured by Freud when he wrote that "myths . . . are distorted vestiges of the wishful phantasies of whole nations, the *secular dreams* of youthful humanity" (1908, p. 152, original emphasis). Underlying the project of psychohistory was an assumption that the development of humanity could be treated as the history of the individual writ large. For Freud, myths were collective fantasies akin to individual delusions, providing social solutions to the same problems that also caused neurotic symptoms and dreams (1913, pp. 185–186).

Myth and Freudian Theory

One matter remains unresolved in Freud's approach to myth. In the first place, Freud was drawn to mythology for inspiration in his work. Not only are his writings replete with allusions to myths, legends, and fairy tales, but certain myths clearly inform some of his key theoretical constructs, such as the Oedipus complex, narcissism, and Eros (the life instinct). The question thus arises as to the extent Freud could be said to have placed his trust in mythology as a solution to human problems. On the one hand, Freud was highly dismissive of religious thought and practice and understood psychoanalysis to be a science devoid of illusions (1927, pp. 1–56); yet he could also refer to the key section of *Totem and Taboo* as "the scientific myth of the father of the primal horde" (1921, p. 135).

This remark was more than idle usage, since Freud similarly categorized aspects of his metapsychology. "The theory of the instincts," he said, "is so to say our mythology. Instincts are mythical entities, magnificent in their indefiniteness" (1933, p. 95). Statements like these suggest that Freud was at least partially aware of the continuity of his "scientific" project with the form and function of myth, a view supported by the way in which he referred to "the psyche" as *die Seele* (the soul) in his original writing in German (Bettelheim, 1985: 70–78). While Freud may not have comfortably accepted the idea that psychoanalytic theory and practice gain their symbolic power by engaging "living myth" (Lévi-Strauss, 1972: 202), it is ironic that, in an era when his corpus is often dismissed as "myth," we find that Freud apparently retained some grudging acceptance of the legitimacy of what he called "psycho-mythology" (1913b, p. x).

REFERENCES

Bettelheim, B. (1985). *Freud and Man's Soul.* London: Fontana.

Freud, S. (1900). *The Interpretation of Dreams.* S.E. 4–5: 1–627.

———. (1901). *On Dreams.* S.E. 5: 629–686.

———. (1908). Creative writers and day-dreaming. S.E. 9: 141–153.

———. (1908). Character and anal erotism. S.E. 9: 167–175.

———. (1913). The theme of the three caskets. S.E. 12: 289–301.

———. (1913). *Totem and Taboo: Some Points of Agreement between the Mental Lives of Savages and Neurotics.* S.E. 13: 1–162.

———. (1913). The claims of psycho-analysis to scientific interest. S.E. 13: 163–190.

———. (1916–1917). *Introductory Lectures on Psycho-Analysis.* S.E. 15–16: 1–463.

———. (1921). *Group Psychology and the Analysis of the Ego.* S.E. 18: 65–143.

———. (1925). *An Autobiographical Study.* S.E. 20: 1–74.

———. (1926). *The Question of Lay Analysis.* S.E. 20: 177–258.

———. (1927). *The Future of an Illusion.* S.E. 21: 1–56.

———. (1933). *New Introductory Lectures on Psycho-Analysis.* S.E. 22: 1–182.

———. (1939). *Moses and Monotheism: Three Essays.* S.E. 23: 1–137.

Lévi-Strauss, C. (1972). The effectiveness of symbols. In *Structural Anthropology 1.* Harmondsworth: Penguin, pp. 186–205.

JOHN MORTON

N

Narcissism

The concept of narcissism is used both to describe and to explain certain human attributes and behavior. Derived from analogy to Narcissus in Greek mythology, the term still conveys the implication of self-love, but there is no general agreement among analysts about whether it refers to an individual trait, to an aggregate of traits reflecting disturbances in self-esteem and in the relations between self and object, or to the underlying cause of these traits. Freud's *On Narcissism: An Introduction* (1914) marked an important step in the subsequent development of psychoanalytic theory, and the concept he introduced in that paper has proved useful in explaining many psychopathological syndromes—neuroses, borderline conditions, psychoses, and sociopathological conditions, as well as narcissistic personality disorders.

Despite theoretical differences, there is remarkable unanimity among analysts about the clinical features regarded as narcissistic. An insufficient differentiation of the mental representations of self and objects (other persons) results in instability of self, identity, and esteem, and poor relations with objects. There is a hunger for object attention, doomed by past experience to an expectation of disappointment; a compensatory defensive delusion of self-sufficiency; and affective lability. Guilt and shame are especially frequent affects; depression and even manic denial or projection can sometimes be observed as well. Particularly in borderline conditions, there may be a painful sense of emptiness, aloneness, or isolation, at the same time that closeness may be a threat defended against by coldness and detachment. Sexual aberrations are frequent, hypochondriasis is common,

and in the borderline conditions there are occasional lapses in reality testing. The association of masochism with narcissism has been noted to be frequent, perhaps invariable. Striking, though sometimes covert, features of narcissism include a grandiosity that is compensatory for feelings of inferiority or inadequacy, and a sense of entitlement representing the wish for reparation for real or fantasied injury. Humiliation and rejection constitute the major narcissistic injuries; they often elicit rage and are manifested in the wish for revenge and the desire to undo a hurt. Despite these liabilities, most likely to be evident in intimate private and personal relationships, narcissistic individuals frequently possess considerable talent and charm and may function very well in social, business, and political settings where relationships are relatively superficial (see Akhtar, 1989).

In 1898, Havelock Ellis drew a parallel between the taking of one's own body as a sexual object and the myth of Narcissus. In the ensuing years, the term "narcissism" came to refer not only to a perversion but also to a stage of normal development, and to traits not overtly sensual that served a defensive function, such as vanity and self-admiration, and to primitive aspects of thinking and feeling, such as animism, magic, and the belief in one's own omnipotence. In his seminal 1914 paper, *On Narcissism: An Introduction*, Freud went beyond this way of thinking about narcissistic traits. He postulates an undifferentiated psychic energy that at first cathected (invested) the ego (self), a state he called "primary narcissism." Freud theorizes that some of this energy is later directed to objects (persons), but such *object libido* can be drawn back to the ego, resulting in a *secondary narcissism*, setting up an antithesis between ego libido and object libido, so that more of one means less of the other. Freud then describes two main types of choice of love objects. First, there is a *narcissistic type* of choice: a person may choose to love someone like himself, or someone he wishes to be, or someone who was once part of herself, such as a child. In fact, Freud concluded, parental love "is nothing but the parents' narcissism born again . . . transformed into object love" (Freud, 1914: 91). Second, there is an *anaclitic type* object choice, one influenced by the woman who feeds him or the man who protects him, and the succession of others who take their places. As a person matures, Freud said, he can no longer retain the narcissistic illusion of omnipotence and perfection characteristic of early childhood, and part of his narcissistic libido is redirected to an *ego ideal* that embodies the subject's cultural and ethical ideas, and is the means by which he measures his actual self.

The formation of this ego ideal provides the basis for repression of ideas inconsistent with it. Freud at this time also advanced the idea of a special agency of the psyche, later called the "superego," that watches the ego (self) and censures behavior inconsistent with the ego ideal. The ego ideal is often based on an idealized person but not in all cases; a revered leader, an idea or cause, an abstraction, or a particular aspiration may all become elements of a shared ideal, the binding force for the cohesiveness of a group. Finally, Freud postulated that self-regard (self-esteem) derives from three sources: a residue of infantile narcissism; a sense of omnipotence based on fulfillment of the ego ideal; and satisfaction of object libido.

Freud's 1914 paper was one of his major theoretical contributions and has had far-reaching influence. It was transitional in nature, with old and new conceptualizations intermingled, presaging the changes to follow. Though dissatisfied with the paper, Freud made no attempt to revise it or to integrate narcissism with some of his later concepts. Nevertheless, his introduction of the concept of narcissism contributed to his formulation of a metapsychology, led to a deeper understanding of the mechanisms of identification in relation to melancholia, pointed the way to the second dual instinct theory, and played a pivotal role in the development of the structural theory. It therefore provided the matrix for the construction of a major part of psychoanalytic theory, heuristically useful to this day.

In the light of later clinical and theoretical developments, however, a number of problems became evident. The concept of narcissism was formulated in terms of Freud's libido theory, based on a psychic energy now questioned in the light of modern neurobiology. Further, his essentially economic conception of narcissism as a libidinal investment of the ego (self) was so nonspecific that the term "narcissism" came to be applied to many different categories, including a wide variety of aspects of human behavior (biological, psychological, individual, social, normal, and pathological); pathological syndromes; and even abstractions, such as other theoretical concepts of varying significance. Its explanatory value was thereby reduced. Moreover, in applying the concept of narcissism, analysts often overlooked the aggression that appears rampant in many of the phenomena described. These phenomena, as well as the theoretical concepts previously adduced to explain them, are now considered to be extremely complex and beyond comprehension on the basis of instinctual drives alone. Even the so-called psychic structures—id, ego, ego ideal/ superego—have been shown to have developmental stages; regression in one may seriously affect others and the consequent attitude toward the self and objects, including self esteem and empathy (see Pulver, 1970).

Freud's later papers utilized his theory of narcissism to show that the ego (system) takes into itself, or "introjects," the objects presented to it that are a source of pleasure and expels what is unpleasurable (1915, p. 136), a first identificatory stage that establishes memory traces or mental representations of the object. Freud derives a second stage from his reasoning in his study of mourning (1917). He argues that the loss of a sexual object is made easier when it is installed within the ego, altering the self representation permanently so that it becomes as acceptable for loving as the object. In his definitive work on the structural theory, *The Ego and the Id* (1923), Freud concluded that object cathexis may be replaced by identification and thus can regress to narcissism, and that this transformation of object libido into narcissistic libido implies an "abandonment of sexual aims, a desexualization—a kind of sublimation" (1923, p. 30). It followed that the character of the ego could be seen to be "a precipitate of abandoned object cathexes and . . . contains the history of those object choices." Hence, in this stage of secondary narcissism, the cathexis attached to the precipitates of lost objects installed within the ego provide the ego, ego ideal, and superego with the energy for their development and functioning.

For the most part, Freud's followers have continued to adhere to his ideas about the development of the various psychic agencies. Although Freud was the first to emphasize the importance of early internal object relations in normal and pathological development, the works of Melanie Klein and Edith Jacobson have made the study of object relations a major current-day trend. Jacobson (1964) pointed out that maturation is another important factor in the development of the psychic structures and extended Freud's theory to embrace not only drives but also affects, internal objects, and their integration in the functioning of the psychic structures. Various types of narcissistic characters have been described as well as pathologic forms of self-esteem regulation (Reich, 1960).

The pathogenesis of narcissism has attracted particular attention. Loss of the object or a disturbance in the relationship in the pre-Oedipal period, especially the rapprochement phase of separation individuation, when the cathexis is primarily narcissistic, results in an identification that is ambivalent and weighted in favor of sadism. Forbidden, unconscious fantasies regarding the child are reflected in inhibitions of motherliness, projected onto the child as a devalued image of the mother, so that the child invests her libido in her self. Identification with narcissistic parents is common. When body attributes and ego functions of young children are made to serve their parents' narcissistic and partial instinctual needs, the child is robbed of her own accomplishment and regresses to narcissistic satisfactions whenever the object becomes disappointing. However, each successive libidinal stage may make its own narcissistic contribution to ego development. The genitals receive the greatest cathexis, and there is a close connection between the constancy of the self frame of reference and sexuality that simultaneously contributes to intense self-feeling and threatening oscillations.

The role of the development of the ego ideal in respect to narcissistic disorders has been found to be of major import. There is general agreement that the ego ideal is an earlier, more narcissistic structure, based at first on the earliest identifications with the mother, and that the superego is a later, more reality-syntonic one, initiated by castration fears and involving identification with the father at the time of the Oedipus complex. Both structures include identification with each parent, and the intermediary stages in development are important. Early identifications, expressed in imaginary wish fulfillments or masturbation fantasies, or as a permanent part of the personality, may undo a narcissistic hurt. The

ego ideal has magical thought among its precursors and embodies the idealization of power before that of moral behavior. The mature ego ideal tends to function antithetically to the narcissistic entitlements of the pregenital era. Failure of its proper development in severe neuroses is therefore reflected in the persistence of pregenital characteristics, especially sexual aims. These are the result of incomplete structural formation and narcissistic wounds (rejections, humiliations, etc.). Frustrations may contribute to a compensatory cathexis of precursors of the mature ego ideal (for example, images of persons representing power or pregenital sexual gratification) and lead to regressions involving pregenital sexual acting out of an exhibitionistic or sadomasochistic nature.

Chasseguet-Smirgel (1976) says that when the child gives up his narcissistic omnipotence to the object, his first ego ideal, "he senses within himself a gap which he will seek to fill throughout his life . . . [and which] cannot be closed except by returning to a fusion with the primary object [via her successors]. This hoped for fusion may be transformed into the incessant desire to enter the mother's [substitute's] body through genital coitus" (p. 348). This hypothesis provides an explanation for Fairbairn's observation that throughout life the fundamental issues for narcissistic patients are independence versus dependence, and separation versus fusion. Though there is the wish for fusion, there is the threat of maternal engulfment and a structureless state; merging precludes separation between the ego and the ego ideal, thus eliminating development and preventing differentiation of the psychic systems and the different ego functions.

When there is an affectively distressing discrepancy between the self representation and the wishful concept of the self represented in the ego ideal, there is poor self-esteem and the basis for narcissistic disorder—manifested either directly or by traits that defend against conscious awareness of the discrepancy or the affective reaction to it. Such discrepancy is probably ubiquitous, present to varying degrees in everyone, but should be considered pathological only when it seriously interferes with affective stability, reality testing, adaptation, and harmonious relations between the self and objects in particular. Hence, since the term "narcissism" connotes pathology, it is an oxymoron and confusing to regard minor deviations from arbitrary norms as "normal or healthy narcissism." Despite such deviations a person is usually regarded as "normal and healthy" who has stable

N

affects, good cognitive and self-critical functioning, satisfying object relationships, and a sense of pride in his or her accomplishments—in short, a person who has good self-esteem. This state is brought about by a harmonious integration of the functions of the psychic structures, for which both libidinal and aggressive expression must be satisfying.

Many authors have made significant contributions to the theory of narcissism and narcissistic disorders, and are cited in the references given at the end of this article. Only the work of two of the foremost recent theorists will be mentioned here.

Heinz Kohut (1966, 1971) came to regard the instinctual drives as constituents of a superordinate self and aggression as a normal assertiveness that has degenerated as a result of frustration. "Primary narcissism," he said, refers to the psychological state of the infant before differentiation from the primary object. A residue of primary narcissism remains throughout life and ultimately becomes differentiated into the "narcissistic self" (later called "grandiose self") and an "idealized parent image," the latter invested with both narcissistic and object libido.

The transformation of narcissistic libido into "idealizing libido" is a unique maturational step that differentiates it from the development of object love. If deprived of instinctual gratification, the psyche changes the object image into an introject, a structure that takes over the functions previously performed by the object. Its projected external counterpart is what Kohut calls a "selfobject." In his view, the narcissistic libido imbuing these structures has an independent line of development from object cathexis and ideally undergoes transformations throughout life that endow the individual with mature attributes such as creativity, empathy, the capacity to contemplate one's own impermanence, humor, and wisdom. Normally, both the grandiose self and the idealized object are phase-appropriate and gradually become integrated in the adult personality, but narcissistic trauma can cause both to remain unchanged. Unempathic parental care, producing injury to the child's self-esteem, is the usual cause of such interference, leading to repression of grandiose fantasies and vacillation between irrational overestimation of self and feelings of inferiority and shame. Exhibitionistic wishes are the predominant drive aspect of the grandiose self. Kohut uses the term "bipolar self" to emphasize the structure derived from two sectors of the self: a pole of goals and ambitions from which emanate basic strivings for power

and recognition, and a pole that maintains the guiding ideals and standards. An arc of tension between the two poles activates the basic talents and skills. Kohut worked primarily with narcissistic personality disorders within a psychoanalytic situation and largely ignored empirical criteria, basing his diagnosis on the nature of the spontaneously developing transference. He found the idealized parent image to be activated in an "idealizing transference," and the grandiose self in the "mirror transference." He uses the terms "guilty man" and "tragic man" to epitomize the difference between the conflict formulations of classical psychoanalysis and the defect conceptualization of his self psychology. In his view, the most positive changes in such patients occur as a result of the analyst's empathy and the patient's "transmuting internalization," a form of idealized identification with the analyst. This process is brought about by the analyst's optimal, nontraumatic frustration of the patient.

As an analyst working within hospital settings, Otto Kernberg (1975) has had the opportunity to observe, describe, and treat a wide variety of narcissistic disorders. His theory of narcissism attempts to integrate classical Freudian, Kleinian, Bionian, and object relations theories, linking drives, affects, and self and object representations into functioning units under the sway of the traditional agencies of structural theory—id, ego, ego ideal, and superego. He believes that narcissistic pathology is the result of abnormal mental structures, fixated in early childhood—a specific pathological formation rather than a type of developmental arrest. The grandiose self is formed by fusion of aspects of the real self, the idealized self, and an idealized object representation. Although he agrees with Kohut that narcissistic patients have been mistreated by their parents, Kernberg does not attribute their pathology directly to this development, but emphasizes the mistrust, hunger, rage, and guilt induced by such mistreatment and the pathognomonic condensation of Oedipal and pre-Oedipal conflicts under the overriding influence of pregenital aggression. The inflation of the grandiose self is not merely reactive; chronic envy underlies scorn for others, and devaluation, omnipotent control, and narcissistic withdrawal are defenses against such envy.

Kernberg sees the pathology of narcissistic personality disorders and borderline personality disorders as similar but of varying severity. The individual having a narcissistic personality disorder has a cohesive, even though pathological, grandiose self that hides an inner identity diffusion and aimlessness; but that disorder, as well as the borderline disorder, shows a predominance of splitting of the self and objects. Obsessional and hysterical personalities are organized around repression rather than splitting and have better organized superegos and a greater capacity for genuinely reciprocal object relations.

Regardless of the usefulness of Freud's energic concept of narcissism and the shortcomings of his paper *On Narcissism: An Introduction*, it is apparent that his 1914 paper presented a conceptual framework still useful for the understanding of a significant group of psychic disorders. Serious physical or psychic trauma, including abuse, humiliation, and even unempathic handling by the parents in the pre-Oedipal period interfere with the internalization of nurturing parental objects needed for the maturation of psychic structures able to regulate and control instincts, stabilize affects, deal with reality, and adapt to the vicissitudes of human relationships. These psychic structures may be further damaged in the Oedipal period, leading to regression to earlier stages in the development of the self and ego ideal/superego. Failure of the self to meet the standards of the ego ideal results in low self-esteem and a split in the ego whereby both derogatory and compensatory defensive ideas are simultaneously entertained, either consciously or unconsciously. Because of this double view of the self, there is extreme sensitivity to other persons and a need to project self criticisms. The objects are also split into good and bad, leading to strong attraction and yet fear of involvement, so that there may be withdrawal or intense sadomasochistic activity, contributing to poor object relations. The self-love implied in the term "narcissism" now seems to be the result of desperate attempts to cope with the consequences of the individual's damaged psychic structures.

REFERENCES

Akhtar, S. (1989). Narcissistic personality disorder. *Psychiatric Clinics of North America*, 12: 505–529.

Chasseguet-Smirgel, J. (1976). Some thoughts on the ego ideal. *Psychoanalytic Quarterly*, 45: 345–373.

Freud, S. (1914). On narcissism: an introduction. S.E. 14: 73–102.

———. (1915). Instincts and their vicissitudes. S.E. 14: 109–140.

———. (1917). Mourning and melancholia. S.E. 14: 237–260.

———. (1921). *Group Psychology and the Analysis of the Ego*. S.E. 18: 67–143.

———. (1923). *The Ego and the Id*. S.E. 19: 3–66.

Jacobson, E. (1964). *The Self and the Object World*. New York: International Universities Press.

Kernberg, O. (1975). *Borderline Conditions and Pathological Narcissism*. New York: Aronson.

Kohut, H. (1966). Forms and transformations of narcissism. *Journal of the American Psychoanalytic Association*, 14: 243–272.

———. (1971). *The Analysis of the Self: A Systematic Approach to the Psychoanalytic Treatment of Narcissistic Personality Disorders*. New York: International Universities Press.

Moore, B. E. (1995). Narcissism. In B. E. Moore and B. D. Fine (eds.). *Psychoanalysis: The Major Concepts*. New Haven, Conn.: Yale University Press, pp. 229–251.

Moore, B. E., and Fine, B. D. (1990). *Psychoanalytic Terms and Concepts*. New Haven, Conn.: American Psychoanalytic Association.

Pulver, S. E. (1970). Narcissism: The term and the concept. *Journal of the American Psychoanalytic Association*, 18: 319–341.

Reich, A. (1960). Pathologic forms of self-esteem regulation. *Psychoanalytic Study in Children*, 15: 215–337.

BURNESS E. MOORE

Netherlands, and Psychoanalysis

Psychoanalysis in Holland went through four different stages: first, laying the foundation and finding an identity, and solving ensuing problems including a splitting tendency (1917–1938); second, unification and reactions to German occupation (1938–1945); third, the Golden Age of pure psychoanalysis (1945–1980); finally, the development of psychotherapy embedded in a social health system (1977–present).

The interest in psychoanalysis in Holland developed from 1905 onward and came from three different sources. 1. Psychiatrists fascinated by Freud's papers: August Stärcke, who corresponded with Freud, and J. van Emden, who had an analysis with him, both became members of the Viennese Society in 1911. 2. Psychiatrists who went to Carl Gustav Jung in Zürich for analysis between 1911 and 1913. 3. The university: Gebrandus Jelgersma's rectorial address in 1914 at Leiden University was the first official recognition of psychoanalytic science in Europe. Thirteen representatives of these three groups founded the Dutch Society of Psychoanalysis on March 24, 1917, the seventh branch society of the International Psychoanalytic Association (IPA). The sixth IPA congress in 1920 took place in The Hague, since Dutch neutrality during World War I facilitated the reunion of analysts who had been enemies during the war.

N

After this start, there followed a period of unproductive quarreling. The main points of controversy were the question of lay analysis—until 1938 only medical doctors were admitted—and the introduction of the tripartite training system, especially the obligation of personal analysis. The opponents in the conflict were the society's president, Van Ophuijsen, in favor of lay analysis and the tripartite training model (he was treasurer and later vice president of the IPA) versus the theoretically oriented psychiatrists of the university, supported by Westerman Holstijn. These conflicts led to a split when in 1933 four Jewish analysts emigrated from Germany to Holland: Landauer, Reik, Levy-Sühl, and Watermann. The poorly trained Dutch analysts with only few patients felt threatened by the arrival of four more competent analysts. Anti-Semitism played a minor role. Van Ophuijsen, however, arranged for Landauer's participation in psychoanalytic training to improve the quality of psychoanalysis in Holland. After the resulting uproar by the Dutch Society's members, Van Ophuijsen resigned as president and member and founded, in 1933, with Van Emden, Maurits Katan, and a few others, including the German immigrants, a new society, the Society of Psychoanalysts in the Netherlands. The diplomatic analyst Westerman Holstijn put much energy into the reconciliation of the old and new societies and succeeded in 1937. However, he himself resigned out of discontent with the regulations.

In 1938, after Nazi Germany's *Anschluss* with Austria, Jeanne Lampl-de Groot, a Dutch psychiatrist who had lived since 1923 in Vienna and Berlin for analytic training and practice, and Hans Lampl came from Vienna to Amsterdam. They started to reform the Dutch training program according to Viennese standards in cooperation with two members, Rik Le Coultre and Katan. Both the tripartite training model and lay analysis were finally accepted. In May 1940, Holland was occupied by the Germans. When in November 1940 Jews had to resign as society members, as required by German law, the non-Jewish psychoanalysts resigned as well in an act of solidarity. Lampl-de Groot and Le Coultre managed to continue psychoanalytic training underground; the Jewish analysts went into hiding. In November 1945, the society was refounded.

In 1947, Holstijn and some other colleagues, who had left the society, founded the Dutch Psychoanalytical Association. Initially, the association was meant to be a forum where one could discuss psychoanalysis in a free atmosphere without the stress of training. Soon, however, a training program was organized with much less rigorous requirements than those of the society. Three successive presidents of the association—Jan Groen, Poslavsky, and Stufkens—managed to raise the quality of training gradually to the IPA level. By 1997, the association had become a provisional society within the IPA. After a period of great hostility, both societies began to cooperate in their institute and scientifically. Both the society and the association had an institute, an ambulatorium where patients were treated at low cost. As of 1995 these institutes were fused into one, the Dutch Psychoanalytical Institute (NPI), which serves all Dutch analytical candidates.

From 1945 until 1975, psychoanalysis blossomed in Holland. The number of candidates increased; there were ample patients for analysis; and there was an active scientific life. Three IPA congresses were organized in Amsterdam, in 1951, 1965, and 1993. Van der Leeuw became vice president of the IPA in 1963 and president from 1965 to 1969. Montessori was secretary from 1965 to 1969 and vice president after that until 1975. Lampl-de Groot was honorary vice president from 1963 until her death in 1987. Several Dutch held an office in the European Psychoanalytical Federation: Thiel and Dalewijk as vice president, Mekking as treasurer, Groen-Prakken as president.

In 1966, a child analytic training was organized within the society by Teuns, with great support especially from Frijling-Schreuder, who attracted teachers from the Hampstead clinic. They came to Leiden or Amsterdam for theoretical and technical seminars and supervision. Also in 1966, the government started to subsidize psychoanalytical treatment if the patient needed it. In 1980, therapies at the institutes for mental health, including the analytic institutes, became virtually free, requiring no payment. The important chairs in psychiatry, child psychiatry, and clinical psychology at the universities were mainly occupied by psychoanalysts.

During the 1980s, there was a decline in interest in psychoanalysis as in most other Western countries. In Holland, the tightening grip of the authorities on psychoanalytic practice, the near disappearance of private practice, and the replacement of psychoanalytically oriented university teachers by biologically oriented ones were important factors. At the same time, however, there is a mounting interest in the application of psychoanalysis to other fields, such as psychotherapy and art.

Symposia and lectures for a broad public are attracting many people. Several Dutch analysts are involved in teaching programs in countries situated behind the former Iron Curtain.

The frame of reference in Holland is mainly influenced by and comparable to British neo-Freudian and British independent schools (Treurniet). The influence of child analysis is considerable (Lampl-de Groot, Frijling Schreuder). Important work has been done on the sequelae of the Holocaust (Keilson, Sarphatie, and De Wind).

REFERENCES

Brinkgreve, C. (1984). *Psychoanalyse in Nederland.* Amsterdam: De Arbeiderspers.

Bulhof, I. N. (1983). *Freud en Nederland.* Baarn: Ambo.

Freud, S. (1914). *On the History of the Psychoanalytic Movement.* S.E. 14: 7–66.

Freud/Jung letters (1974). *The Correspondence between Sigmund Freud and C. G. Jung.* Ed. by W. Mc Guire. Trans. by R. Manheim and R. F. C. Hull. Princeton, N.J.: Princeton University Press.

Groen-Prakken, H. (1993). The psychoanalytical society and the analyst, with special reference to the history of the Dutch Psychoanalytical society 1917–1947. In H. Groen-Prakken and A. Ladan (eds.) *The Dutch Annual of Psychoanalysis.* Lisse: Swets and Zeitlinger, pp. 13–38.

Groen-Prakken, H., and Nobel, L. de (1992). The Netherlands. In P. Kutter (ed.). *Psychoanalysis International. A Guide to Psychoanalysis Throughout the World,* vol. 1. Stuttgart-Bad Canstatt: Frommann-Holzboog, pp. 217–242.

Spanjaard, J., and Mekking, R.U. (1975). Psychoanalyse in den Niederlanden. *Die Psychologie des 20.* Jahrhunderts. Zürich: Kindler.

HAN GROEN-PRAKKEN

Neurasthenia

The starting point of Freud's sexual theory was the discovery that repressed sexual experiences were responsible for the symptoms of many hysterical patients. However, it was rather for neurasthenic symptoms that Freud first claimed an *exclusively* sexual etiology (Sulloway, 1979: 103; Macmillan, 1991: 123). "Beard's neurasthenia" was the most important nervous disease Freud saw in the first years of his medical practice. The American nerve specialist George M. Beard (1839–1883) had defined neurasthenia as an "exhaustion" of the nerves, expressing itself in a multitude of symptoms, ranging from blushing, fatigue, insomnia, and headaches to phobias and obsessions. Beard believed that neurasthenia was an American disease, caused by the various excesses of modern life (Drinka, 1984: 192). Another American doctor, S. Weir Mitchell (1829–1914), devised the standard therapy for neurasthenics; it was given the nickname "method of Dr. Diet and Dr. Quiet" (Bromberg, 1959: 154).

Neurasthenia quickly traveled to the Old World. This new clinical entity aroused the interest of influential psychiatrists in France and in the German-speaking countries (Macmillan, 1991: 131; Shorter, 1992: 221). Beard's notion that "sexual excess" could sometimes play a role in the genesis of neurasthenia must have strongly appealed to Freud. From the so-called Fliess Papers (Draft B), we know that Freud was convinced already in the early 1890s that *all* neurasthenics were the victims of "abnormal" sexual practices, notably masturbation and coitus interruptus (1893, pp. 179–184). These sexual customs were at the basis of Freud's refinement of the broad concept of neurasthenia. According to Freud, patients practicing coitus interruptus (or who lived in abstinence) were predominantly tormented by symptoms grouped around anxiety attacks; he decided to speak in these cases of "anxiety neurosis" (1895, pp. 91, 101). Patients reaching orgasm through excessive masturbation (or suffering from frequent spontaneous nocturnal emissions) were ascribed the symptom complex of what he called "neurasthenia proper": fatigue, headaches, constipation, spinal paresthesia, and weak potency (1895, p. 90; 1896, p. 150).

Both genuine neurasthenia and anxiety neurosis were termed "actual neuroses" by Freud (1898, pp. 270, 279), because they were associated with the individual's current sex life (the German *"aktuelle"* means "present-day"). In contrast with the actual neuroses, the symptoms of the so-called psychoneuroses (hysteria, obsessions) were related to sexual experiences in the subject's past life (1898, p. 268). The actual neuroses were seen as being organically conditioned; their etiology did not involve the psychical mechanisms underlying the symptom formation of the psychoneuroses (or "neuropsychosis of defense"). In spite of this sharp distinction, Freud thought it likely that psychoneuroses may have an actual neurotic nucleus (1906, pp. 278–279; 1916–1917, p. 390).

In Freud's explanation of the symptoms of both forms of actual neurosis, the assumption that sexual energy was inadequately discharged played a major role. Applied to neurasthenia, the explanation ran as follows (see Macmillan, 1991: 190–191). Masturbation lowered the threshold for the discharge of somatic sexual excitation; repeated discharge at low levels depleted "the sexual substances," causing general weakness and the other typical symptoms of neurasthenia. Later, Freud formulated that in cases of coitus interruptus as well as in cases of masturbation, there was "an insufficient libidinal discharge" that had a poisoning effect on the organism, in other words, neurasthenia was the result of (auto-)intoxication (1905, p. 216; 1906, pp. 272, 279; 1916–1917, p. 388).

In Freud's opinion, only the symptoms of the psychoneuroses were removable by psychotherapy; the symptoms of neurasthenia (and of anxiety neurosis) were not, because they were somatically determined (1893, p. 183). Kneipp cures (natural, herbal remedies developed by a Bavarian priest named Sebastian Kneipp) and the like were dismissed because they did not take account of the fact that neurasthenics were "crippled in sexuality" (1898, pp. 274–275). Neurasthenia could only be prevented, not cured. Incipient neurasthenics had to be persuaded to adopt "normal" methods of sexual discharge. Society had to permit its adolescents to have premarital heterosexual intercourse using condoms (1898, p. 278; cf. 1893, p. 184).

Already about the time Freud first began to attract disciples, there was disagreement with the master on his views on the etiology of neurasthenia. Wilhelm Stekel (1868–1940) maintained that masturbation as such did not cause physical damage resulting in neurasthenia; if masturbation was harmful at all it was because of a psychic conflict only. Moreover, Stekel declared that all neuroses develop as the result of a conflict between a repressed urge and human conscience.

On several of their Wednesday evening gatherings (1910–1912), Freud, with his fellow members of the Vienna Psychoanalytical Society and some guests, debated the issue of masturbation. Stekel doggedly upheld his view of the unharmfulness of autoeroticism. In his evaluation of the *Onanie-Diskussion*, Freud declared that Stekel was wrong in denying the toxic effects of masturbation and, indeed, the existence of neurasthenia (1912, pp. 248–250). This unresolved controversy was one of the reasons for Stekel's departure from the society in 1912 (Groenendijk, 1997).

Freud never recanted his views about the pathogenic relationship between masturbation and neurasthenia that he had developed during the 1890s. "The observations which I made at the time still hold good," he wrote thirty years later (1926, p. 110). The majority

of his successors, however, denied a direct or simple causal link between masturbation and neurasthenia. Otto Fenichel (1897–1946), in his authoritative handbook on the neuroses, maintained that masturbation played a role in the etiology of neurasthenia only in those cases where "the satisfactory character" of this sexual practice was disturbed by feelings of guilt (Fenichel, 1946: 188; see also Jones, 1920).

The once popular concept of "neurasthenia" has become obsolete in Western psychiatric discourse; complaints formerly linked with neurasthenia are now diagnosed as depression (Wessely, 1995: 518). Today, depression and related affective disorders are conceived by biologically oriented investigators as resulting from neurohormonal disturbances. The particulars of Freud's (toxicological) explanation of neurasthenia were undoubtedly wrong (Macmillan, 1991); nevertheless, from the viewpoint of modern biological psychiatry, he was basically right in associating "neurotic" symptoms with abnormalities in the neurochemical infrastructure. Freud's views on masturbation, however, were not just wrong, they were reactionary as well, not adding to his reputation as the fearless critic of "Victorian" sexual morality (Sulloway, 1979: 185; Webster, 1995: 4).

REFERENCES

Bromberg, W. (1959). *The Mind of Man. A History of Psychotherapy and Psychoanalysis*. New York: Harper and Row.

Drinka, G. F. (1984). *The Birth of Neurosis. Myth, Malady, and the Victorians*. New York: Simon and Schuster.

Fenichel, O. (1946). *The Psychoanalytic Theory of Neurosis*. London: Routledge and Kegan Paul.

Freud, S. (1893). Letter 14. Coitus interruptus as an aetiological factor. S.E. 1: 184.

———. (1894). *Draft B*. The aetiology of the neuroses. S.E. 1: 179–184.

———. (1895). On the grounds for detaching a particular syndrome from neurasthenia under the description "anxiety neuroses." S.E. 3: 90–117.

———. (1896). Heredity and the aetiology of the neuroses. S.E. 3: 143–156.

———. (1898). Sexuality in the aetiology of the neuroses. S.E. 3: 263–285.

———. (1905). *Three Essays on the Theory of Sexuality*. S.E. 7: 7–122.

———. (1906). My views on the part played by sexuality in the aetiology of the neuroses. S.E. 7: 271–279.

———. (1912). Contributions to a discussion on masturbation. S.E. 12: 243–254.

———. (1916–1917). *Introductory Lectures on Psycho-Analysis*. S.E. 15–16: 9–496.

———. (1926). *Inhibitions, Symptoms, and Anxiety.* S.E. 20: 87–122.

Groenendijk, L. F. (1997). Masturbation and neurasthenia: Freud and Stekel in debate on the harmful effects of auto-erotism. *Journal of Psychology and Human Sexuality*, 9: 71–94.

Jones, E. (1920). *Treatment of the Neuroses. Psychotherapy from Rest Cure to Psychoanalysis.* London: Baillière, Tindall, and Cox.

Macmillan, M. (1991). *Freud Evaluated: The Completed Arc.* Amsterdam: North-Holland.

Shorter, E. (1992). *From Paralysis to Fatigue. A History of Psychosomatic Illness in the Modern Era.* New York: Free Press.

Sulloway, F. J. (1979). *Freud, Biologist of the Mind. Beyond the Psychoanalytic Legend.* New York: Basic Books.

Webster, R. (1995). *Why Freud Was Wrong. Sin, Science and Psychoanalysis.* London: HarperCollins.

Wessely, S. (1995). Neurasthenia and fatigue syndromes. In G. E. Berrios and R. Porter (eds.). *A History of Clinical Psychiatry. The Origin and History of Psychiatric Disorders.* London: Athlone, pp. 508–532.

LEENDERT F. GROENENDIJK

Neuroscience, and Psychoanalysis

See APHASIA; BRAIN SCIENCE, AND PSYCHOANALYSIS; PROJECT FOR A SCIENTIFIC PSYCHOLOGY.

Neuroses

In current psychoanalytic usage, the term "neurosis" defines an illness in which there is not an organic cause and in which the symptoms of the illness can be explained as a compromise resulting from a conflict and its displeasure brought about by a forbidden wish and the defense against that wish. Confusion about the term "neurosis" has occurred because the term has changed meaning, both within and outside of psychoanalysis, in general psychiatry. William Cullen was the first to use the term "neurosis" in his *First Lines of the Practice of Physick* in 1777. The term "neurosis" was applied to all diseases not accompanied by fever or localized pathology (Alexander and Selesnick, 1966).

Originally, Freud distinguished between actual neuroses and psychoneuroses, which he further divided into transference and narcissistic neuroses. He believed that the actual neuroses resulted from a buildup of sexual tensions—a belief he never modified in later writings. Modern analysts no longer find this theory of actual neurosis to be correct.

Freud reserved the term "narcissistic neuroses" for those patients incapable of investing libido in the ana-lyst to form a transference; an example he used was schizophrenia. The libido is directed inward, resulting in symptoms such as hypochondriasis and delusions of grandeur. Clinical evidence does not support this view. In fact, patients with schizophrenic illnesses are quite capable of forming very intense transferences to their therapists. What they lack, especially in the acute phase of the disorder, is the ability to step back and work productively with the transference because of the disorganizing effect of the illness.

In 1924, Freud continued to hold on to the term "actual neuroses" but divided the psychoneuroses into neuroses, narcissistic neuroses, and psychoses. He used narcissistic neuroses to cover manic depressive illness that conformed to the then current psychiatric nomenclature. In 1924, Freud was more concerned with the outcome of conflict and less in how libido was directed, and thus he dropped the term "transference neuroses." Modern psychoanalysis makes a distinction between symptom neuroses and character neuroses (personality disorders). This article focuses on symptom neuroses but later contrasts these with character neuroses or personality disorders.

General psychiatry has also contributed to the confusion. In the *DSM-I*, the neuroses had a similar meaning to what was understood by the term in psychoanalysis, but the *DSM-I* also gave it an additional meaning to signify degree. For example, if a patient had a few symptoms of depression, he was diagnosed as having a neurotic depressive reaction, and if he had more symptoms of depression, he was diagnosed as having a psychotic depressive reaction. In 1979, with the publication of the *DSM-III*, the term "neuroses" was dropped entirely and has not been replaced in subsequent nomenclatures. Under the *DSM-IV*, anxiety, phobic, and obsessive-compulsive neuroses are found among the anxiety disorders. Hysterical neurosis, conversion-type, and hypochondriacal neuroses are under the somatoform disorders and the hysterical neuroses; dissociative-type are under the dissociative disorders.

Nineteenth-Century Theories of Neuroses

Now let us focus more in detail on the development during Freud's time. Wilhelm Griesinger's ideas held sway during the middle and late nineteenth century. According to him (Kaplan and Sadock, 1986), mental disorders such as the neuroses are caused by the degeneration of nervous tissue, which is caused by constitutional factors. Such problems are irreversible, and there is nothing to do for patients but to diagnose and classify them. The German diagnostician Emil Kraepelin came from this school of thought. Treatments were nonspecific (rest, hydrotherapy, and good nutrition). There was no reason to talk to a patient other than to make a diagnosis, since the patient's thinking was viewed as nothing more than the rambling of a madman whose neurons were degenerating.

Griesinger influenced Theodor Meynert and Meynert taught Freud. After medical school, Freud had training in neurology and received a traveling fellowship to Jean-Martin Charcot's clinic in Paris. Charcot was the leading neurologist of his time, and in his clinic Freud witnessed something that must have been, for him, extremely remarkable. Charcot took patients with degenerative mental disorders, hypnotized them, and made the symptoms disappear. Therefore, Freud had to rethink his conception of mental illness.

Pierre Janet offered an alternative explanation. He postulated that there was a split in the mind, that certain aspects of the psyche operated unbeknown to other aspects of it. Janet believed that this property of mental functioning was constitutionally determined.

Around the same time, in Vienna, Joseph Breuer was treating neurotic patients with hypnosis. Breuer told Freud about a patient, Anna O., whom he had treated with such a method, and they began treating similar patients and writing up their cases. These cases appear in the first volume of the standard edition of Freud's work. Freud and Breuer devised a new theory of psychopathology. This is a "hydraulic" model in which the mind is conceived as if it were a pressure cooker: A person comes upon an upsetting event in her current life. She is unable to react to it emotionally, and the memory of the event (with its concomitant feelings) is split off from consciousness. The unreleased energy, unable to be expressed, is bottled up in the system and exerts itself as a physical symptom. Freud hypnotized such patients, got them to remember the traumatic event in their current life, then had them "abreact" (see the article, Abreaction) to it. The symptom would then subside. Freud found that it was not necessary to induce hypnosis because he could accomplish the same goal by having patients recline on a couch and say whatever came into their minds. So he had a traumatogenic theory for neurosis: The neurosis was a reaction to an upsetting external event. Freud

never gave up the notion of constitutional factors but considered them to be predisposing rather than precipitating. For the first time, physicians had a medical reason to listen to their patients do more than describe their symptoms.

Freud's Topographical Model

When Freud realized that actual traumatic events did not always precede the onset of neurosis, he needed to revise the hydraulic model. There is currently a misunderstanding of Freud's position on trauma. Some writers, such as Masson and Miller, accuse Freud and psychoanalysts in general of denying that real traumas are causative factors of illness. But one must remember that Freud was writing about neurosis, and now, just as then, some neurotic patients have endured trauma prior to the onset of their neurosis, but some have not. Thus, external real trauma is not a necessary condition of all neuroses.

Freud's second theory of neurosis is an intrapsychic one. Here he divides the mind into conscious, preconscious, and unconscious. The conscious part is that of which we are immediately aware; the preconscious contains those things that we are not aware of immediately, but that we can call to mind easily; and the dynamic unconscious is that part of the mind that is cut off from consciousness, but which continually presses for expression. The function that cuts off the unconscious from the system conscious-preconsciousness was called "repression." When unconscious impulses that are sexual in nature cross the repression barrier, they cause neurotic symptoms (as the conscious part of the mind tries to bind the unpleasure released by the impulses). Freud called this the "topographic" model of the mind.

Using this model, Freud faced a problem that did not make sense clinically. His patients were not always conflicted on the one hand by the unconscious wish and on the other hand by something conscious. More often both parts of the patient's conflict were unconscious. Freud then devised the structural theory of the mind described earlier, namely, the mind was divided into functions: id, ego, and superego (Sandler, Dare, and Holder, 1973).

The Structural Theory and Anxiety

Anxiety has always been the hallmark of the neuroses, and the various defense mechanisms employed to deal with anxiety give each neurosis its unique form. Anxiety is a subjective sense of apprehension with a concomitant activation of the autonomic nervous system. Some authors make a distinction between fear and anxiety. Fear, according to this view, is the affect state reserved for an anticipation of an external danger, whereas anxiety is the affect state of an internal danger. These internal dangers, which relate to the calamities of childhood, include the loss of a need-fulfilling person or object, loss of love, castration anxiety, and superego anxiety (Brenner, 1982).

Neuroses are unique to the human condition for two reasons. One is that the human has a relatively long period of dependence on parents as compared with other species. In early development, the individual must be able to master his instinctual needs in relationship to the adults who raise him. This sets up a situation in which a sense of helplessness is created when the needs come in opposition to her internal representation of the early caregivers.

Second is the human's capacity for language, meaning, and symbolism. Here the child, because of faulty cognitions and magical thinking, has the capacity to distort both drive derivatives and the mental representations that oppose the drives. The first basic anxiety of the child is the loss of the object. Around the age of one to one and a half, the baby appreciates, at some level, that she desperately needs the mothering person to relieve tension, and without this she will be overwhelmed by her own needs. Around the age of two to two and a half, a more sophisticated step is reached in which the child realizes not only that the parents' care is required, but also their love. Without that love, the child feels alone, abandoned, and unloved. The toddler must learn to relinquish that which is pleasurable to win the parent's love. Toilet training is the prototype for this conflict. Thus, the second basic anxiety is the loss of love.

Between the ages of two and a half to six, the child is preoccupied with physical injury, especially to the genitals. During this stage, the child is masturbating and fantasizing about an exclusive intimate relationship with the parent of the opposite sex and has aggressive feelings for the parent of the same sex. Because of magical thinking (the attribution of magical powers to the parents), the child believes that the parent of the same sex knows what she is thinking and will retaliate. The anxiety during the Oedipal stage is called "castration anxiety."

During the ages of five to seven, there is an internalization of the conscious with the resolution of the Oedipal stage. Now the child fears punishment from her own internalized parental images. This is called "superego anxiety."

These traumatic states have in common an overwhelming sense of helplessness. Until about seven, the child does not have sufficient ego development (an example is cognitive development) and is too dependent to consider other options.

The classic psychoanalytic view postulates that the neurotic core conflict occurs during the Oedipal period with the consolidation of the superego as an internal agency. However, the core conflict is colored by the pre-Oedipal stages; for example, individuals who have the most intense separation anxiety have the greatest amount of castration anxiety. The theory postulates that this childhood neurosis is repressed, but not without a heavy toll paid by the person because the neurotic needs and wishes continue to press for discharge. The person will tend to turn her reality into the image and likeness of her Oedipal struggles. This is what Freud called the "repetition compulsion."

The person then goes through life eventually encountering an external situation that reverberates intrapsychically with her past. When this occurs, as the old infantile wishes and the archaic prohibitions are about to come into play, the ego signals with anxiety. The ego must then satisfy the wishes of the id and the prohibitions of the superego, yet temper the anxiety. This is called a "compromise formation." Defensive or adaptive mechanisms are used to effect such compromise formations. The type of defensive mechanism employed gives the neurosis its form. Repression alone can be employed. The person still experiences anxiety but unconsciously blocks out the ideational outlet of the wish. This is called an "anxiety neurosis." Repression is viewed as the primary defense mechanism in all the neuroses, and the other defense mechanisms are so-called second-line defense mechanisms. If repression is used and symbolic displacement is added, this results in a hysterical neurosis such as conversion disorder. In other words, the person blocks out the ideational content of the wish but the wish is deflected to a body part or function. The result is a paralysis of that body part or function that may be understood also as a punishment for the wish. For example, when a person has unacceptable aggressive impulses that are only partially repressed, the mind tries to bind the anxiety by deflecting the aggressive wish onto a body part; the hand, say, may be curled into a fist. The hand is involuntarily rigid and paralyzed in that position (as a punishment for the wish).

In phobic neurosis repression is employed, but when it begins to fail, other defenses are added: externalization, displacement, or avoidance. In other words, a current situation in the patient's life stimulates unacceptable aggressive wishes. The ego tries to repress these wishes but is only partially successful. The aggressive wish is deflected outside of the individual. For example, in Freud's case of Hans (a boy with a fear of horses), the aggressive wish is externalized to Hans's father. The maneuver is unsuccessful because his father is often present, so Hans must deflect the wish from father to horses, which are less a part of Hans's immediate environment. Then Hans uses the defense of avoidance to distance himself further from horses, which now contain his original aggressive impulses (Freud, 1909).

Obsessive-compulsive neuroses are the most complex. Again, a current situation calls forth an unacceptable hostile wish. Repression is deployed, but again it is only partially successful. A host of secondary and tertiary defenses come into play; reaction formation, undoing, magical thinking, and intellectualization. For example, a harried mother's child becomes sick, which stimulates certain unconscious death wishes toward her own younger siblings. Her ego attempts, unsuccessfully, to repress the wishes, but anxiety breaks through, and she automatically employs reaction formation and becomes overly solicitous toward her ill child as a way of warding off her hostile feelings. She may, for example, be unable to sleep at night because she believes she left the gas stove on. She goes to the kitchen and turns the gas on (an expression of her hostile wish) and turns it off as a way of undoing her wish. She must do this ten times as a way of binding her anxiety. It is as if this is a magical ritual to ensure her child's safety—a derivative of omnipotent magical thinking she explains to herself (intellectualization) as behavior that demonstrates her concern for her child.

In each of these examples, aggressive wishes are used for simplicity, clarity, and consistency. Sexual wishes could have been used, and clinical experience has shown that wishes are often a mixture of aggressive and sexual impulses.

In summary, this presents the structural theory of neurosis, which postulates that the functions of the mind are the result of component forces. In neuroses, these component forces are drives, governing forces, and the adaptive forces. In the structural theory these are associated with, respectively, the id, the superego, and the ego. The interpretation that one gives to external reality can also be included as a causal factor.

Salient Characteristics of Neuroses

In classifying neuroses, a useful approach is first to differentiate the symptom neuroses from the functional psychoses and the character neuroses, or personality disorders, then differentiate the symptom neuroses from each other. To differentiate the neuroses from functional psychoses and personality disorders, one can ask about a number of aspects of each type of disorder, as noted below.

1. How do others view the patient? Vaillant once remarked that a patient with a neurosis is like someone who gets on an elevator with a pebble in her shoe—she is uncomfortable, but no one else on the elevator notices. Whereas the patient with a personality disorder is like someone who enters an elevator smoking a smelly cigar—he is content, but everyone else on the elevator is uncomfortable. In other words, the person with a neurotic illness suffers in silence for the most part, as if the disorder were well encapsulated and hidden from the world, and the person may be seen as "normal" by others. Whereas the patient with a personality disorder (or a functional psychosis) is disturbing and viewed by others as unusual.

2. How does the patient view her own symptoms? Often the neurotic patient is embarrassed by her symptoms and views them as foreign. This often results in the patient's having difficulty in volunteering information in the interview. A patient embarrassed by his phobic reaction to driving across bridges may tell the psychiatrist that he has not taken a driving vacation for years. Only later in the interview are the true symptoms revealed. The term for this attitude on the patient's part is called "ego-alien" or "ego-dystonic." In contrast, the patient with a personality disorder is unaware of his psychopathology. It is actually lived out in his relationship to others. He is blind to his disorder. It is as if the psychopathology is woven into the fabric of the personality. This attitude is called "ego systonic." We can apply this

term to patients with functional psychoses. A psychotic patient who is delusional and believes that the D.A.R. is plotting to kill her is unable to step back and view this belief as unusual. In fact, she may take measures to protect herself from the D.A.R. Thus, for a functionally psychotic patient symptoms are ego systonic.

3. How accurate is the patient's perception of reality? For patients with either a neurosis or a personality disorder, reality testing is intact. For the patient with functional psychoses, reality testing is impaired by delusions and/or hallucinations.

4. Does the patient exert appropriate control of impulses? Neurotic patients struggle with—and are conflicted over—their impulses and often appear inhibited. Impulse control may be impaired in the personality disorders for example, in borderline and antisocial personality disorders. Impulse control can be affected in the psychoses; for example, because of a delusion of persecution a psychotic patient may attack someone to protect himself.

5. Does the patient have in-depth object relations? The patient with a neurosis is involved with others, but uses his neurosis to manipulate others. For example, an agoraphobic patient might exploit her illness by insisting that her husband accompany her every place she goes. The person with a personality disorder has disturbed object relations, as if the personality disorder is acted out in her relations with others. On the other hand, the psychotic patient has withdrawn from others and will isolate himself, consumed with his delusions or hallucinations.

Depressive and anxious affect can be found in each disorder. In the neuroses, depressive and anxious affect can signal defense. Patients with a personality disorder can become depressed or anxious secondarily to how others react to or disappoint them. Patients with a psychosis are overwhelmed with anxiety or depression and attempt to bind these affects with primitive defenses.

6. What defense mechanism does the patient use? Vaillant's hierarchy of defenses is useful here. The patient with a neurosis uses the so-called neurotic defense such as repression, reaction formation, intellectualization, or undoing. In the personality disorders, the patient employs the so-called immature defenses such as acting out. The psychotic patient uses the so-called narcissistic or psychotic defenses such as denial and delusional projection (Vaillant, 1977).

Within the class of neuroses, each neurotic illness can be differentiated primarily by the cluster of defenses used. In anxiety neurosis, one sees the defense of repression that is only partially successful. For the phobic neurosis, the cluster of defenses includes externalization, displacement, and avoidance. In hysterical neuroses, dissociation type, the defenses include repression and dissociation. For hysterical neuroses, conversion type, one sees repression, somatic displacement, and identification. The obsessive-compulsive neuroses contain the largest cluster of defenses: isolation of affect, magical thinking, undoing, reaction formation, and intellectualization. The source of the anxiety or depressive affect does not differentiate the various neuroses since any one or combination of the calamities of childhood can trigger these effects, which in turn trigger the defenses.

7. How does the patient's superego function? In the neuroses, superego functions are rigid and harsh; as a consequence, neurotic patients suffer greatly. In the personality disorders, the superego functions vary from lax in the antisocial personality disorder, to harsh in the obsessive-compulsive, to self-defeating in masochistic personality disorder. In psychotic patients, superego demands are projected and can cause delusions in which the patient believes that the police are watching him.

8. Finally, can the patient develop a transference and observing ego? Patients with neuroses are capable of developing a transference in psychotherapy and are capable of developing an observing ego to explore the transference in treatment. The ability of patients with personality disorders to do so depends on the strength of their ego functions. For example, a person with a high-functioning histrionic personality disorder is able to, but a patient with a severe borderline personality disorder may quickly form a transference but initially lack the capacity to step back and examine it. Freud believed that psychotic patients were incapable of forming a transference, but clinically this has not proved to be

so. These patients can develop very intense transferences that are greatly distorted by primitive defenses, and the transference can quickly lose its "as if" quality. For example, a psychotic patient may develop a delusional transference and believe that the therapist has hypnotized her.

REFERENCES

Alexander, F. G., and Selesnick, S. T. (1966). *The History of Psychiatry*. New York: Harper and Row.

Brenner, C. (1982). *The Mind in Conflict*. New York: International Universities Press.

Freud, S. (1909). Analysis of a phobia in a five year old boy. S.E. 10: 5–149.

Kaplan, H., and Sadock, B. (1986). Historical and theoretical trends in psychiatry. In H. Kaplan and B. Sadock (authors). *Modern Synopsis of the Comprehensive Textbook of Psychiatry*, 3d ed. Baltimore: Williams and Wilkins.

Sandler, J., Dare, C., and Holder, A. (1973). The clinical situation. In J. Sandler, C. Dare, and A. Holder (authors). *The Patient and the Analyst, The Basis of the Psychoanalytic Process*. New York: International Universities Press, pp. 18–19.

Vaillant, G. (1977). *Adaptation to Life*. Boston: Little, Brown.

GERALD A. MELCHIODE

Neutrality, Therapist's

See PSYCHOANALYTIC TECHNIQUE AND PROCESS.

Nietzsche, Friedrich Wilhelm (1844–1900)

Nietzsche was educated as a classical philologist, and he created a good deal of controversy with his first book, *The Birth of Tragedy Out of the Spirit of Music* (1872). Through the 1870s, he moved more expressly into the fields of philosophy and psychology. He held the discipline of psychology in high regard and on many occasions referred to himself as a psychologist. Regarding his historical (later genealogical) inquiries into origins, he stated that such inquiries should not be separated from the natural sciences. Nietzsche was familiar with the work of a number of nineteenth-century authors, such as Schopenhauer, Herbart, Fechner, Wundt, Hartmann, Taine, Ribot, and others who made contributions to the development of a psychology of dynamic unconscious mental processes. He was also aware of mesmerism, magnetism, and somnambulism. He was familiar with the diagnosis of hysteria, and was concerned throughout his work with the ways in which the multiplicity of our psychic selves can function in healthy, creative ways rather than lead to exhaustion and breakdown.

During Freud's years at the University of Vienna in the 1870s, Nietzsche was a prominent presence for Freud's friends and acquaintances. These admired individuals, such as Viktor Adler, Heinrich Braun, Sigfried Lipiner, and Joseph Paneth, were deeply involved with Nietzsche's writings of the period, particularly *The Birth of Tragedy* and the essays later collected in the volume *Untimely Meditations* (1873–1876). By 1875, Freud was familiar with the first of the *Untimely Meditations*, "David Strauss, the Confessor and the Writer" (1873). Freud's fellow students were discussing Nietzsche, lecturing on him, and writing to him. In his writings of this period, Nietzsche wrote of the illusion-creating functions of dreams, the instinctual and revelatory substratum beneath individuated form, the importance of creatively integrating the more primitive aspects of our nature, the importance of integrating our past and making it our own as well as the importance of forgetting, the nature of the intellectual hero, idealization of a group leader, ideas approaching the concept of resistance, the importance of incest in the Oedipus myth as portrayed by Sophocles, and how even the quest for truth can be prompted by the drives. Unlike Freud, Nietzsche wrote of many drives, but he emphasized the erotic and aggressive drives, both implicated in the will to power. He wrote of aroused drives as well as inherent, internal drives that press for discharge. The concept of the sublimation of drives was a particularly important one in his psychology. Freud followed Nietzsche's use of *Triebe* (drive) and employed other significant terms used by Nietzsche.

In the 1880s, Freud's friends and acquaintances continued to read and discuss Nietzsche. Berggasse 19, Viktor Adler's Vienna residence before Freud moved in, was a place of gathering at which Nietzsche was often a topic of conversation (Venturelli, 1984). There was also a direct link between Freud and Nietzsche in the person of Joseph Paneth, who met in Nice with Nietzsche on a number of occasions from December 1883 through March 1884. Late in his life, Freud recalled that Paneth had written much to him about these meetings, and that at the time Nietzsche was a remote and noble or distinguished figure to him (E. Freud, 1970: 78). Paneth's letters to Freud have not survived, but during this period Paneth also wrote about these meetings to his future wife, Sophie Schwab. In these letters Paneth expressed

N

his high regard for Nietzsche and wrote of their discussions on philosophy and science, the work of Meynert on moods, Schopenhauer, the importance of unconscious mental processes, and much more (Godde, 1991; Hemecker, 1991; Krummel, 1988; Lehrer, 1995: 44–48).

Nietzsche's writings in the late 1870s and early 1880s include *Human, All Too Human* (vol. 1, 1878, with two subsequent works of 1879 and 1880 added as two divisions of vol. 2 in a second edition of 1886), *Daybreak* (1881), and *The Gay Science* (1882, second expanded edition 1887). These works contain many explorations on the relationship between conscious and unconscious mental functioning, the nature of instincts and drives, dynamic psychic conflict, the development of conscience, sublimation, the nature of dreams, emotional states and actions being determined by multiple motives, and much more. In pointing to our tendency to refuse to take responsibility for thoughts and wishes expressed in dreams, Nietzsche (1881, pp. 78–79) even refers to the same lines in Sophocles' *Oedipus* that Freud will later refer to in *The Interpretation of Dreams* (1900, p. 263).

There is little information available on Freud's exposure to Nietzsche from the late 1880s to mid-1890s. However, in his last productive years (before he became permanently insane in January 1889, probably owing to having contracted syphilis), Nietzsche wrote, as did Freud in the early to mid-1890s, of the problems that arise when a quantum of damned-up energy or force that demands discharge or release does not find it, that a distinction should be made between a drive seeking, so to speak, discharge or release and the particular manner in which the quantum of energy or force is discharged, that both remembering and forgetting (as inhibition or repression) are necessary for psychic functioning, and that certain kinds of psychological trauma can prevent the normal wearing away of memories. Nietzsche even suggested that psychology *as a science or discipline* has to contend with the unconscious resistance of the investigator.

In very Nietzschean style, Breuer and Freud write in the "Preliminary Communication" (1893, included as the first chapter in *Studies on Hysteria* [1895, pp. 3–17]), of the importance of "an energetic reaction to the event that provokes an affect" for the normal wearing away process of forgetting. In particular, they note "acts of revenge . . . in which affects are discharged" (1895, p. 8). They refer to the consequences of "an injury that has been repaid" in implicit contrast to one that has not been repaid (1895, p. 8). Breuer writes: "To defend oneself

against injury . . . to injure one's opponent is the adequate and preformed psychical reflex. If it has been carried out insufficiently . . . it is constantly released again by recollection, and the 'instinct of revenge' comes into being" (1895, pp. 205–206). This description has strong affinities with Nietzsche's man of *ressentiment*, and echoes passages in Nietzsche such as the following: "the ressentiment of natures that are denied the true reaction, that of deeds, and compensate themselves with an imaginary revenge . . . the submerged hatred, the vengefulness of the impotent" (1887, pp. 472–473). Freud probably heard about Nietzsche from Breuer, who read widely in philosophy, as well as from Paneth, who probably introduced Freud to Breuer.

After the late 1890s and the turn of the century, there is never much time that goes by without Nietzsche coming up in Freud's life and work in one way or another. For example, on February 1, 1900, as Freud is depressed and somewhat in crisis over what he regards as the lack of enthusiastic reception of his dream book (which shares much with Nietzsche on dreams), he writes to Fliess that he has just acquired Nietzsche, in whom he hopes to find much that remains mute in him, but that he has been too lazy to open him (Masson, 1985: 398). It is significant that Freud would turn to Nietzsche in such a way at such a time.

Many of Freud's early disciples, such as Rank, Adler, Jung, Graf, and Jones, were familiar with, and in a number of cases deeply influenced by, Nietzsche's writings. At two 1908 meetings of the Vienna Psychoanalytic Society, Nietzsche's *On the Genealogy of Morals* (1887) and *Ecce Homo* (1908 [1888]) were discussed. Paul Federn exclaimed: "Nietzsche has come so close to our views that we can ask only, 'Where has he not come close?'" Adler stated: "Nietzsche is closest to our way of thinking," and Rank (who took the minutes) suggested that Nietzsche "explored not the external world, as did other philosophers, but himself" (Nunberg and Federn, 1962: 358–359). Freud insisted, as he always would, that Nietzsche had no influence on him. In the *Genealogy*, Nietzsche wrote of the role of aggression turned inward upon the self in the development of bad conscience and the role of the latter in the development of civilization. These ideas are related to Freud's concept of the superego as well as, more generally, to his more social and anthropological works, a fact noted by many, including Jones (1957, pp. 283–284). Remarkable, particularly in light of Freud's heroic self-analysis, is Freud's statement during the discussion of *Ecce Homo* to the effect that the degree of introspection achieved by Nietzsche had never been achieved before and was unlikely to be achieved again (Nunberg and Federn, 1967: 31–32). Perhaps this is one of the reasons that led Freud to regard Nietzsche as one of a handful of truly great individuals (Jones, 1957: 415).

In 1911, Jones and Hanns Sachs visited Nietzsche's sister, Elisabeth Förster-Nietzsche, to share with her the psychoanalytic ideas that were close to the psychological explorations of her brother. In 1912, Lou Andreas-Salomé, a strong and emotionally charged link to Nietzsche, joined the psychoanalytic movement and developed a very close relationship with Freud. In the 1920s, Freud was reading Nietzsche and appears to have again been looking over the *Genealogy* (E. Freud, 1960: 350; Wittels, 1924: 62). Even in tributes to Freud on the occasion of his eightieth birthday, Arnold Zweig, Thomas Mann, and Ludwig Binswanger all paired Freud with Nietzsche (Lehrer, 1995: 222, 224; 1996: 373). Only two years earlier, Zweig had written to Freud of the Freud-Nietzsche cycle and how Freud had completed what Nietzsche set out to accomplish but could not (E. Freud, 1970: 23–24). Freud was directly and indirectly exposed to Nietzsche's ideas and frequently had his ideas and even his position in intellectual history compared to the work and figure of Nietzsche. At times, Freud was willing to concede priority to what he regarded as the remarkable intuitive anticipation of psychoanalytic ideas by such thinkers as Schopenhauer and Nietzsche, and that it was one of the achievements of the science of psychoanalysis to have independently demonstrated the validity of such remarkable intuitions. Yet he would never allow that Nietzsche had any influence on his thought or reveal what he read of Nietzsche and when he read it.

REFERENCES

Breuer, J., and Freud, S. (1895). *Studies on Hysteria.* S.E. 2: 19–305.

Freud, E. L. (ed.) (1960). *Letters of Sigmund Freud.* Trans. Tania Stern and James Stern. New York: Basic Books.

———. (1970). *The Letters of Sigmund Freud and Arnold Zweig.* Trans. Elaine Robson-Scott and William Robson-Scott. New York: New York University Press.

Freud, S. (1900). *The Interpretation of Dreams.* S.E. 4–5: 1–621.

Godde, G. (1991). Freuds philosophische Diskussionskreise in der Studentenzeit. *Jarbuch der Psychoanalyse,* 27: 73–113.

———. (1993). Wandlungen des Menschenbildes durch Nietzsche und Freud: Eine vergleichende Interpretation aus philosophiegeschichtlicher Perspektive. *Jarbuch der Psychoanalyse,* 30: 119–166.

Hemecker, W. W. (ed.) (1991). *Joseph Paneth—ein Gelehrtenleben zwischen Freud und Nietzsche. Autobiographie-Essais-Briefe.* Amsterdam: Rodopi.

———. (1991). *Vor Freud. Philosophie geschichtliche Voraussetzungen der Psychoanalyse.* Munich: Philosophia Verlag.

Jones, E. (1957). *The Life and Work of Sigmund Freud,* vol. 3. New York: Basic Books.

Kaiser-El-Safti, M. (1987). *Der Nachdenker. Die Entstehung der Metapsychologie Freuds in ihrer Abhängigkeit von Schopenhauer und Nietzsche.* Bonn: Bouvier Verlag Herbert Grundmann.

Krummel, R. F. (1988). Dokumentation: Joseph Paneth über seine Begegnung mit Nietzsche in der Zarathustra-Zeit. *Nietzsche-Studien,* 17: 478–495.

Lehrer, R. (1995). *Nietzsche's Presence in Freud's Life and Thought: On the Origins of a Psychology of Dynamic Unconscious Mental Functioning.* Albany: State University of New York Press.

———. (1996). Freud's relationship to Nietzsche: Some preliminary considerations. *Psychoanalytic Review,* 83: 363–394.

Masson, J. M. (ed.) (1985). *The Complete Letters of Sigmund Freud to Wilhelm Fliess,* 1887–1904. Trans. J. M. Masson. Cambridge, Mass.: Belknap Press of Harvard University Press.

McGrath, W. J. (1974). *Dionysian Art and Populist Politics in Austria.* New Haven, Conn.: Yale University Press.

Nietzsche, F. W. (1881). *Daybreak: Thoughts on the Prejudices of Morality.* Trans. R. J. Hollingdale. New York: Cambridge University Press, 1982.

———. (1887). *On the Genealogy of Morals.* In W. Kaufmann (trans. and ed.). *Basic Writings of Nietzsche.* New York: Random House, 1968, pp. 449–459.

Nunberg, H., and Federn, H. (eds.) (1962–1967). *Minutes of the Vienna Psychoanalytic Society,* vols. 1–2. Trans. M. Nunberg. New York: International Universities Press.

Venturelli, A. (1984). Nietzsche in der Berggasse 19. Über die erste Nietzsche-Rezeption in Wien. *Nietzsche-Studien,* 17: 448–480.

Wittels, F. (1924). *Sigmund Freud: His Personality, His Teaching and His School.* Trans. C. Paul. London: George and Urwin.

RONALD LEHRER

Nineteenth-Century Precursors of Freud

While Freud's ideas have encountered different degrees of resistance throughout the twentieth century, and are today perhaps more under attack than ever before (see "Critique of Psychoanalysis," this volume), there has always been a rather firm belief in the profound originality of Freud's theoretical edifice. For example, the headline of a recent issue of *Time Magazine* on the twenty most influential intellectual figures of the twentieth century stated that Freud, who is the very first presented, "opened a window on the unconscious" (*Time Magazine*, March 29, 1999, p. 36). This widespread evaluation is difficult to reconcile with the fact that nineteenth-century philosophers had elaborated psychological theories, which took unconscious processes explicitly into account. Although historians have occasionally pointed to these pre-Freudian theories of the unconscious (e.g., Dorer, 1932; Ellenberger, 1970; Whyte, 1960), a coherent picture of the extent of these anticipations did not emerge until recently. Thus, for many decades the general view that most of Freud's ideas regarding unconscious mental functioning represented a radical departure from earlier conceptions of the mind, prevailed. The aim of this entry is to draw attention to the multifaceted philosophical determinants of Freud's creation, by providing an integrative view of different philosophical figures and traditions taken together. In doing so, particular care shall be devoted to bridging the gap in the relevant literature between the German and English speaking communities.

We should start by pointing out that the young Freud was not only interested but also quite versed in philosophy. He had studied a textbook on Herbartian psychology in high school (see below), and at university, he not only took several courses with Franz Brentano but also planned to obtain a double Ph.D. in zoology and in philosophy. In addition, he was member of the *Leseverein der Deutschen Studenten Wiens* from 1873–1878, an intellectually active student organization in which Schopenhauer's, Nietzsche's and von Hartmann's ideas were regularly discussed (McGrath, 1967; 1986). In the 1880s Freud had accumulated sufficient competence in philosophy to consider writing a general introduction entitled a "philosophical A.B.C." (Jones, 1953: 172). In preparation for the *Interpretation of Dreams*, Freud went once again through extensive readings of the philosophical literature—now on the unconscious (Gödde, 1999). Thus, there is no reason to question the authenticity of Freud's statement to W. Fliess of April 2, 1896: "As a young man I knew no longing other than that for philosophical knowledge, and I am now about to fulfill it as I move from medicine to psychology" (Masson, 1985: 159).

After the *Interpretation of Dreams* was published, however, Freud's attitude to philosophy changed, becoming increasingly sarcastic and denigrating. For example, Freud now compared philosophical works to the constructions of the mentally ill (1919, p. 261; see also 1925, pp. 59–60; 1900, p. 490; 1933, p. 161). Apart from ridiculing philosophers because of their speculative tendencies (e.g., 1933, p. 161), he now began to claim that nineteenth-century philosophy refuted the concept of the unconscious: "The philosophers' idea of what is mental was not that of psycho-analysis. For them the world of consciousness coincides with the sphere of what is mental. . . . Or, more strictly speaking, the mind has no contents other than the phenomena of consciousness" (1925, p. 216). Hence, believing that philosophical psychologies were utterly speculative and had nothing to offer to a new psychology of the unconscious, there was apparently not much Freud could have learned or taken over from them: "Even when I moved away from observation, I have carefully avoided any contact with philosophy proper" (1925, p. 59).

This anti-philosophical image Freud carved out for himself and for posterity set the stage for a number of influential biographies refining and cultivating Freud's image as a scientist/clinician who was neither interested in nor indebted to the philosophical psychologies preceding his creation (e.g., Bernfeld, 1949; Jones, 1953). Thanks to a number of contributions that were all published in the 1990s (Gasser, 1997; Gödde, 1999; Hemecker, 1991; Lehrer, 1995; Zentner, 1995), we are finally able to document what seemed plausible for many decades: Namely that the fundamental hypotheses of psychoanalysis—usually referred to as Freud's metapsychology—are an *extension* of theorizing about the unconscious that did not start, but was taken an enormous step further during the nineteenth century, in particular by two philosophers, A. Schopenhauer (1788–1860) and J. F. Herbart (1776–1841). While Schopenhauer and his followers F. Nietzsche and E. von Hartmann focused on the *contents* of unconscious activity, in particular its affective and irrational nature, Herbart and his school were primarily concerned with the formal properties of unconscious functioning which they primarily saw as cognitive activity. Freud's metapsychology can be seen as a hybrid of both strains.

Arthur Schopenhauer (1788–1860)

The parallels between Schopenhauer and Freud have been noted frequently. Yet, it is only recently that Schopenhauer's early clinical experiences with psychiatric

N

patients have been discovered (Zentner, 1995). More-over, the true extent of Schopenhauer's contribution to Freud also came to light only gradually, following a number of publications that extensively addressed the relationship between these two authors (Gödde, 1999; McGrath, 1986; Young and Brook, 1994; Zentner, 1995). Freud left little doubt that the most important discovery he made concerned the process of repression. As he tells us, "The theory of repression is the cornerstone on which the whole structure of psycho-analysis rests. It is the most essential part of it" (1914, p. 16). Consequently, we are to regard Freud's theory of repression as his most fundamental discovery. In his *Autobiographical Study* he solemnly emphasizes its innovative character: "I named this process repression; it was a novelty, and nothing like it had ever been recognized in mental life" (1925, p. 30). What has later been specified as innovative about Freud's view of repression is not the bare existence of the psychic mechanism of repression, but its causal role as a pathogen (Grünbaum, 1984, p. 188). In fact, that we tend to avoid unpleasant thoughts is a trivial observation that was articulated already by ancient philosophers, such as Marcus Aurelius who writes: "How easy a thing it is to put away and blot out every impression that is disturbing . . . and to be at once in perfect peace" (Aurelius, 1961: 101). What stands out as innovative in Freud's view of repression is the idea that this seemingly innocent avoidance can be the starting point of a process leading to mental illness.

Between 1811–1813, the philosopher Arthur Schopenhauer observed patients in the psychiatric ward of the Berlin Charité Hospital, also called the "Melancholic Station." Schopenhauer was particularly intrigued by two patients, whose names could be identifed as Ernst Hoeffner and Traugott Schultze. Schopenhauer regularly visited, observed and tried to understand them. In return, the patients wrote poems and essays for Schopenhauer. After the fall of the Berlin wall, some of the relevant materials could be found and Schopenhauer's experiences in the Charité reconstructed (Zentner, 1995).

The central motivation for Schopenhauer's visits was a dissatisfaction with the psychiatric theorems of the time, dominated by biological determinism or moral condemnation (e.g., Dörner, 1969; Marx, 1990; 1991): "Nowhere did I find a clear and satisfactory explanation of the nature of madness. . . . Thus, I had to search for such information in the madhouses myself, and think to have found a largely satisfactory account" (V, 390. Unless

otherwise indicated, all translations are my own). In contrast to the prevalent theories of his day, Schopenhauer's empirical approach allows him to conceptualize mental illness as being the result of trauma. In particular, three hypotheses characterize Schopenhauer's theory of mental illness: First, at the core of mental illness there are gaps and interruptions in the thread of memory. Second, the difficulty of many psychologically disturbed patients in remembering important events in their lives is not due to a dysfunctional memory, but to repression of traumatic events. Third, the repressed events and the resulting gaps in the thread of recollection are replaced by innocent but false memories. The accumulation of such protective but fictitious memories progressively leads to a disturbed perception of reality resulting in psychosis. In a passage from the yet untranslated lectures of 1820, the young philosopher summarizes the insights he gained through his visits to the Melancholic Station: "The origin of madness is to be found in violent mental pain, pride that is unexpectedly hurt, intense love which is rejected, of unexpected and terrible events of all sorts. My explanation goes as follows: . . . If such a sorrow reaches the point where it becomes unbearable . . . and the individual would succumb to the pain, then life would be jeopardized: In this case the scared person seizes on madness as the last means of saving life: it shakes off the thought that undermines the life of the individual; tears it out of consciousness . . . the mind, tormented so greatly, destroys the thread of memory and the gap, which is brought about, is filled with fictions" (V, 395; see also WI, 228; WII, 457).

In addition to this key insight, at least three further distinctive aspects of Freud's theory of repression can be found in Schopenhauer's theory of mental illness: First, that the mechanisms of repression and substitution are due to a tendency to avoid the overwhelming displeasure caused by traumatic events. According to Schopenhauer, the traumatized mind "escapes from the overwhelming mental pain into madness—as one removes a burnt limb and replaces it with a wooden one" (WI, 228; see also HN, 146; WII, 458). Second, the pain leading to repression may be due to intra-psychic conflict between a real and an ideal self: "Whenever a painful memory comes to mind, *but particularly one that hurts our pride*, we try to chase it away mechanically and immediately" (V, 396; see also WII, 235, 243, 457). Third, repression is not a distinctly psychopathological phenomenon, but occurs in everyday life. Thus, mental illness lies on a continuum with normal mental functioning (see WI, 228, and Zentner, 1995 for an elaboration for these anticipations).

When Freud declared that the concept of repression constituted the basic building block of the psychoanalytic edifice, this is particularly true of the successive models of the structure and function of the psychic apparatus propounded in 1895, 1900 and 1923, and often denominated as the "metapsychology" of Freud's theoretical edifice (Laplanche and Pontalis, 1973: 250). Its perhaps most distinctive feature is a bipartite model of the psyche within which what is instinctual, blindly self-centered, immediately demanding, and largely unconscious is considered *primary* and what is rational, controlled, and adult *secondary*. Indeed, according to Freud, we would not even have developed the skills needed to engage in cognitive activities, if it had been possible to gratify our instinctual needs without reliance on these cognitive skills. A look at the following tables reveals where Freud derived this deeply irrationalist view of human nature:

These tables provide unequivocal evidence for the striking overlap in Schopenhauer's and Freud's models of the psyche. Indeed, not only the general idea that the rational, conscious part of our mind is nothing but a *derivative* of a blindly self-centered unconscious repository of instinctual urges, but also a whole array of specifications that have been listed in the tables according to different criteria (structural, dynamic, functional, qualitative, and metaphorical) are of Schopenhauerian origin (see Zentner, 1995: 78–111 for details and Schopenhauer's sources of this view).

Schopenhauer believed that his model could serve as a theoretical framework for discovering and organizing *psychological* facts about the "inner man." Indeed, conceiving the human mind as he did, Schopenhauer was prepared to detect phenomena that come close to what Freud later described as defense mechanisms or parapraxes, although he did not use these terms, of course. For example, in the following passage, Schopen-

Table 1. Schopenhauer's predicates of the Will—Freud's predicates of the Id

Predicates of Schopenhauer's Will (1844)	Predicates of Freud's Id (1923)
Structural	**Structural**
• Core, foundation, inner part of our being (*WII: 148, 224, 228, 252, 270, 336*) • Primary part of mental life *(224–)* • First part of the self to appear, present at birth *(236, 265–267)*	• Core, original, deeper part of our being *(S.E.: 20: 195; 23: 163, 197)* • Primary process *(10: 285; 23: 198)* • Oldest portion of the psychical apparatus, present at birth *(23: 145)*
Dynamic	**Dynamic**
• Untiring drive *(407, 409)*	• Filled by instincts *(20: 196, 200; 22: 73)*
Qualitative	**Qualitative**
• Unconscious *(313)* • Locus of wishes, passions and affects *(252)* • Strives for immediate gratification of drives *(237)* • Strives for complete pleasure *(656, 669)* • Its clearest expression is the sexual drive *(268, 588)* • Has laws which are fundamentally different from the laws of the intellect *(231–232, 253)* • Not subject to causality and time *(568)*	• Unconscious *(19: 23; 22: 72; 23: 163)* • Stands for untamed passions and instinctual needs *(22: 73, 76)* • Striving to bring about immediate satisfaction of instinctual needs *(20: 201; 22: 73)* • Governed by the pleasure principle *(20: 200)* • Reservoir of libido *(18: 257; 19: 46)* • Rules governing the course of mental acts are different in the ego and the id *(20: 196)* • Logical laws of thought do not apply. There is nothing in the id that corresponds to the idea of time *(22: 72–73; 23: 198)*
Metaphorical	**Metaphorical**
• Can be described only metaphorically *(370)* • Untamed horse *(238)* • Master *(243)*	• We approach the id by analogies *(22: 73)* • Horse *(19: 25; 22: 77)* • Master *(22: 77)*

Table 2. Schopenhauer's predicates of the Intellect—Freud's predicates of the Id

Predicates of Schopenhauer's Intellect	Predicates of Freud's Ego
Structural	**Structural**
• Derivative of the will *(WII: 323)* • Arising from the will *(572)* • Is subordinate to the will *(236)* • Secondary to the will *(228)*	• Portion of the id *(S.E.: 22: 76)* • Developed from id's cortical layer *(23: 129)* • Id is more extensive, imposing than Ego *(20: 195)*
Dynamic	**Dynamic**
• Stimulated by the will *(230)* • Without own sources of energy *(238)*	• Borrows its energies from the id *(22: 77)*
Functional	**Functional**
• Serves the survival *(229)* • Serves the will to communicate with the external world *(253)* • Is the department of the exterior *(272)*	• Task of self-preservation *(23: 199)* • Mediator between the id and reality *(22: 78–79)* • Relation to external world as its decisive factor *(22: 75)*
Qualitative	**Qualitative**
• Enables to reason and good sense *(229)* • Time is one of its perceptive features *(549)*	• Stands for reason and good sense *(22: 76)* • System that provides the origin of the idea of time *(22: 76)*
Metaphorical	**Metaphorical**
• Servant of the will *(233)* • Tool of the will *(253)* • Slave of the will *(238)* • Rider *(460)*	• Servant of the id *(22: 78)* • Helper of the id *(19: 56)* • Slave of the id *(19: 56)* • Rider *(22: 77)*

hauer not only illustrates the process of repression; he also astutely observes that the repression happens outside of the awareness of the person: "We often do not know what we desire or fear. For years we can have a desire without admitting it to ourselves or even letting it come to clear consciousness, because the intellect is not to know anything about it, since the good opinion we have of ourselves would inevitably suffer thereby. But if the wish is fulfilled, we get to know from our joy, not without a feeling of shame, that this is what we desired; for example, the death of a near relative whose heir we are. Sometimes we do not know what we really fear, because we lack the courage to bring it to clear consciousness. In fact, we are often entirely mistaken as to the real motive from which we do or omit to do something. . . . In individual cases this may go so far that a man does not even guess the real motive of his behavior, and in fact believes himself to be incapable of being moved by it" (WII, 235; see also WII, 224).

Given Schopenhauer's *habitual and systematic* qualification of our behaviors and beliefs as motivationally

opaque rather than transparent, Freud's verdict that "the ego is not master in its own house" can hardly be considered "Copernican" (1917, p. 143; Zentner, 1995, chapters 4–6 for Schopenhauer's influences on other parts of Freudian theory, such as sexuality, pessimism, and critique of religion).

Friedrich Nietzsche (1844–1900)

Although Schopenhauer is at the source of the modern inclination to look for meanings beneath the surface of behavior, it was his pupil Nietzsche who carried the tendency to be always on the alert for the "real" but hidden significance of our beliefs and behaviors to the extreme. Thoughts, moral beliefs and overt behaviors in general, are systematically mistrusted and are seen as the mere deceiving surface of a psyche that is dominated by an unconscious struggle between instinctual urges. This position is already fully developed and articulated by the late 1870s and early 1880s, notably in "Human, All Too Human" (1878–1880), "Daybreak" (1881) and "The Gay Science" (1882). This *Entlarvungspsychologie* (psychology of unmasking) not only appears throughout Nietzsche's works, but is quite explicitly formulated: "With regard to everything man expresses, one can ask: what is it supposed to mask? What should it deflect our attention from? Which prejudice is it supposed to elicit?" (1880–1881, § 523, p. 305). Furthermore: "I am not interested to show what effects this [ascetic] ideal has had; rather . . . what it *means*, what it leads us to suspect, what is behind it, under it, what is hidden in it, what . . . it is expressive of" (1886–1887, § 23, p. 411). This is what Nietzsche has in mind when he refers to himself as a psychologist: "That a psychologist speaks in my writings . . . is perhaps the first insight to which a good reader comes to" (1888–1889, § 55 p. 303). Many of Nietzsche's texts analyze psychological processes by which "hidden" motives are transformed into conscious beliefs, attitudes and actions that are often opposed to their motivational origins: "Good actions are sublimated evil ones" (1876–1878, § 107, p. 102). The different processes by which such transformations are brought about include what Freud in his terminology later labeled as reaction formation, displacement, rationalization and so forth. Not suprisingly, in one of the sessions of *The Vienna Psycho-Analytical Society*, A. Adler comes to the conclusion: "Nietzsche is closest to our way of thinking" (Nunberg and Federn 1962–1975, I, pp. 358–359).

Although most of Nietzsche's texts *are* examples of a "psychoanalytic" way of thinking, the *Genealogy of Morals* (1887) is perhaps the most perfect example. Nietzsche explains that aggression was primary at the beginning. Civilization was then built on the basis of conscience and morality. The latter two are conceived as resulting from aggression turned inward upon the self. Referring to the same phenomenon on the level of the individual, Nietzsche had noted already earlier that "some people have such a strong need to express their violence . . . that, because they lack more appropriate objects or because of chronic failure, they finally end up tyrannizing parts or strata of themselves." This tendency, Nietzsche explains, is attributable to a "tyrannizing demanding something" within the self (Nietzsche, 1876–1877, § 137, p. 131). These ideas about the role of aggression in the development of civilization, conscience and morality are related to Freud's concept of the superego as well as to his anthropological works, in particular *Civilization and its Discontents* (1930, p. 21). It is often overlooked that Nietzsche's insights, rather than arising from solitary moments of illumination, were increasingly embedded in extensive readings of the psychiatric research literature of his day. This is shown in Nietzsche's growing use of psychiatric jargon during the 1880s (see Lampl, 1986; 1988).

While much more could be said obviously about the relation of Nietzsche to Freud (see Gasser, 1997; Gödde, 1999; Lehrer, 1995; Venturelli, 1984), my aim here was primarily to put Nietzsche's role in perspective *vis-à-vis* the contributions of other nineteenth-century philosophers. This perspective should not overlook a number of significant differences between Nietzsche's and Freud's views. In contrast to Freud, who abandoned physiology in order to acquire a new identity as psychologist, Nietzsche moved progressively first from philology to psychology, and then from psychology to physiology. After having evoked the perspective of a new "psychophysiology" (*Physio-Psychologie*) in "Beyond Good and Evil" (1886, p. 32), his late fragments document an increasing concern with a physiologically based psychology. Another important difference concerns Nietzsche's emphasis of the power motive in contrast to both Schopenhauer and Freud who focused on the sexual motive. Again like Schopenhauer, Freud tended to be a pessimist who only half-heartedly believed in the possibility of change. Nietzsche, on the other hand, was an optimist who believed in the change of character through insight. Overall, however, the works and ideas I have traced so far substantiate Ellenberger's general conjecture that "the closest approach to psychoanalysis is to be found in the philosophers of the unconscious . . . particularly Schopenhauer and Nietzsche. For those familiar with the latter two philosophers, there cannot be the slightest doubt that Freud's thought echoed theirs" (1970, p. 542).

Eduard von Hartmann (1842-1906)

Von Hartmann is the author of the *Philosophie des Unbewussten* (1869). This work is remarkable due to the simple fact that virtually everything that had ever been written about the unconscious in the nineteenth century, including facts regarding the association of ideas, perception, affective and instinctual life, was compiled in Hartmann's opus. The enormous popularity and pervasive influence of this work during the last decades of the nineteenth century has been well described elsewhere. As a best seller, it was a subject of discussion among intellectuals and students at parties and in the cafes of Vienna during the 1870s (see Ellenberger, 1970; Hemecker, 1991).

N

In the foreword to its seventh edition (that appeared just seven years after the original publication), Hartmann conceded that the success of his book was in part due to its Schopenhauerian orientation. Moreover, it did not take commentators long to realize this. Hermann Ebbinghaus, who wrote his doctoral thesis on the "Philosophy of the Unconscious" (1873, p. 67), stated: "What is true is not new and what is new is not true: the essential can be traced back to Schopenhauer." Similarly, Nietzsche talked about the philosopher of the unconscious in relation to Schopenhauer as a mere imitator.

Several authors have hypothesized indirect and direct influences from Hartmann to Freud. According to Shakow and Rapaport (1964), for example, Freud was introduced to Hartmann's book already during adolescence, but ultimate proof is lacking (see also Dimitrov, 1971; Nitzschke, 1983; Riese, 1958). What we know for sure is that Freud cited from the *Philosophie des Unbewussten* in the original publication of the *Interpretation of Dreams* and then again in a later edition (1900, p. 134; 528n). In the footnote to the later edition, Freud acknowledges that Hartmann anticipated the notion or law of free association, even if only by stressing that Hartmann "was unaware of the scope of the law."

A closer look at Hartmann's work reveals that key technical terms of psychoanalysis were first coined or popularized by Hartmann. This is of course the case with the "unconscious," a more appropriate term for what others had called "will." However, it was also Hartmann who was the first to use the particular term *Das Es* ("the it") as an expression for the unconscious: "This 'Id' lies . . . in the unconscious" (Hartmann, 1871: 34). A few features highlight the close resemblance of Hartmann's "unconscious" and Freud's "id" (*Es*). A fabric of desires, the unconscious "never tires, but all conscious mental activity tires." Exemplary in this regard is the dream that can be characterized by an "untiring persistence of affective life." This is related to the fact that the unconscious is "timeless." The unconscious "does not need time to think . . . the thinking of the unconscious has no relation to time" and "it never doubts or hesitates." Furthermore, "the unconscious attempts to perform its acts with a minimum of effort" (see Hartmann, 1871: 375–379). Finally, the unconscious is not only "omnipresent" but also "omniscient" (p. 620).

Although most of these predicates replicate Schopenhauer's qualifications of the will (see Table 1), the last reveals the influence of C. G. Carus, Schelling and Hegel. In contrast to Schopenhauer's irrational *will*, Hartmann's unconscious is, like the unconscious of a number of romantic German philosophers, intelligent. In discussing the cognitive, intelligent aspects of the unconscious, Hartmann not only extensively wrote about the association of ideas but also attributed particular importance to the "abbreviation of the association of ideas" the result of which he called *Verdichtung* (condensation). Hartmann considered this process to be "one of the most important processes in the whole field of psychology" (Hartmann, 1890: 193). Another term introduced by Hartmann is the "preconscious" (*vorbewusst*), a term that bears more than just formal resemblance to Freud's concept of the preconscious. In fact, the preconscious is understood by Hartmann as what "lies beyond consciousness in a preconscious process of emergence," and, therefore, has to be defined in "conceptual contrast" to what is empirically given in consciousness (Hartmann, 1890: 207–208).

J. F. Herbart (1776–1841)

Among the key traditions that prepared the ground for Freud's theory, Herbart's school has so far received surpisingly little attention, especially in the United States (but see Sand, 1988; this volume, for an exception). Yet, Herbart initiated a current of psychological theorizing that was extremely influential throughout the Austro-Hungarian Empire for several decades. Between 1845–1875, it enjoyed a popularity comparable to that of behaviorism in the United States between 1925–1955. Several theorists that are recognized as Freud's forerunners were educated in Herbartian psychology. For example, in the preface to his *Elements of Psychophysics* (1860), Gustav Theodor Fechner (1801–1887) acknowledged his debt to Herbart in unequivocal terms.

In two major works, *Lehrbuch zur Psychologie* (1816) and *Psychologie als Wissenschaft* (1824), Herbart introduced three notions which are difficult to underestimate in the context of a historical analysis of Freud. First of all, he developed the notion of psychology as a quantitative science, and more importantly, the notion that such a scientific psychology could only be developed by resorting to the assumption of unconscious processes. Secondly, he propounded the conception of mental events as lying on a continuum ranging from conscious to unconscious—a conception that was intimately linked to a dynamic view of the psyche. Indeed, for Herbart, ideas and representations are quantities that have both magnitude and direction, sometimes resulting in conflict among them. Thus, a stronger representation can prevent a weaker one from accessing consciousness or can repress it altogether: "First: one of the older ideas can be completely repressed out of consciousness by a new one. . . . Thereafter, the striving of the latter can not be considered ineffective . . . it works with full strength against the ideas that lie in consciousness" (Herbart, 1816: 106–107; see also Herbart, 1824 §§ 41–73). In accordance with his conception of the mind as a balance of forces, Herbart posited a "law of conservation" according to which mental events can be transformed, but never "lost." Third, Herbart was concerned with what happened to mental events once outside of conscious awareness. This led him to an examination of the laws governing the reproduction of unconscious ideas. For example, he devoted a lengthy analysis to "spontaneously recurring representations" (*Von spontan steigenden Vorstellungen*)—ideas that were too "strong" to be successfully repressed and therefore kept reappearing in consciousness (see Herbart, 1851: 388–446).

Herbart's psychology was carried further and disseminated by his students and followers among which Gustav Adolf Lindner (1828–1887) deserves particular attention in the present context. Lindner was the author of a popular textbook of Herbartian psychology, entitled *Lehrbuch der empirischen Psychologie als inductiver Wissenschaft*, whose third edition (Lindner, 1872) was mandatory reading for Freud in his last year at the *Leopoldstädter Gymnasium* (1872–1873) (Hemecker, 1991; Jones, 1953: 377).

Following the importance Herbart attributed to the "threshold of consciousness," this concept reappears in Lindner's book. Representations can lie either above or below the threshold of consciousness, thus be conscious or unconscious. The former are referred to as "clear" the latter as "dark" representations. The process by which clear representations turn into dark ones is what Lindner calls inhibition (*Hemmung*). Alternatively, Lindner refers to same process as "repression" (§ 29, p. 67; § 36, pp. 81–82). Inhibition or repression results when a representation is opposed by another representation of equal or superior force. When discussing the properties of representations lying below the threshold of consciousness Lindner proposed a further distinction among dark or unconscious representations. Dark representations can be either simply "inhibited" (*gehemmt*), or they can be "darkened" (*verdunkelt*). In the former

case, representations are merely pushed down towards the threshold of consciousness. In the latter case, representations fall far below the threshold of consciousness (pp. 98–99). In sum, then, representations can assume three degrees of consciousness—they can be completely conscious (*klar*), somewhat unconscious (*gehemmt*) and completely unconscious (*verdunkelt*) (Lindner, 1872, § 44, pp. 98–101).

Adhering to Herbart's model, Lindner stressed that unconscious ideas retain their effectiveness and continue to exert a pervasive influence on whatever goes on above the threshold of consciousness. Even in their darkened or unconscious state, ideas continue to be "part of the potential consciousness of the mind, which comprises all ideas that once were in the mind and of which the actual consciousness . . . is only a minor fraction" (Lindner, 1872, § 44, p. 101).

The concept that unconscious ideas continue to exert their influence on the mind is intimately linked to the assumption of a law of conservation for representations: "For representations the law of constancy (*Beharrungsgesetz*) applies, according to which once they are stimulated, they will tend to persist in their action. If they are darkened by other, new representations, they will continue to exist in a bound state and can, under favorable circumstances, be reproduced. Through this permanently existing possibility of reproduction they [darkened representations] participate significantly in the vicissitudes of the mind" (Lindner, 1872, § 46, p. 103). Due to the law of conservation, one "can say of no representation that it is completely forgotten . . .; although working the representation back again to the surface is difficult, it is not impossible" (Lindner, 1872, § 36, p. 81). Reproduction of unconscious representations is possible if—be it by their own force or by means of "aids of reproduction" (*Reproduktionshilfen*)—such repressed representations acquire sufficient strength "to overcome the resistance of all the representations opposing them" (Lindner, 1872, § 44, p. 100; similarly, § 29, p. 67; § 36, p. 81).

According to Lindner there are two primary "aids of reproduction" which allow access to the unconscious part of the mind: associations and dreams. First of all, "reproduction" or the "return of darkened ideas into consciousness" (Lindner, 1872, § 29, p. 66), can be achieved by means of association. There are four laws of association, two of which follow logical, and two of which follow rather illogical paths (Lindner, 1872, § 30,

N

p. 68). The latter ones, the *Gesetz der Gleichzeitigkeit* (the law of simultaneity) and the *Gesetz der Reihenfolge* (the law of succession) are related to Freud's concepts of condensation and displacement—two mental operations that are characteristic of unconscious mental functioning, and are sometimes also referred to as primary processes. Lindner states that "this type of mechanical association of representations, which can never be found in pure form in a waking and healthy state, is most clearly expressed in the phenomena of the dream . . . and of madness" (Lindner, 1872, § 47, p. 105).

The dream is seen as the second major road to the unconscious: "During sleep, when the opposing forces of the awaken psyche are lifted, such 'forgotten representations' often reemerge with surprising clarity" (Lindner, 1872, § 36, p. 81). The final chapters in Lindner's book are devoted to mental illness, where the dream is again discussed in relation to mental illness and defined as the "model of mental illness": "It is particularly the state of sleep . . . that presents us temporarily with phenomena such as they appear in permanent manner in mental illness" (Lindner, 1872, § 101, p. 220). In addition, he also stressed the link between normal and abnormal mental life: "Mental disturbances seem to be of a miraculous and inexplicable nature only as long as they are not placed in analogy with the phenomena of normal mental life. On the basis of a more detailed examination one will be persuaded that the beginnings of mental illness can often been found in mental life that is considered normal and that the full-blown mental illnesses only show on a large scale what we can observe in ourselves and in others in daily life" (Lindner, 1872, § 101, p. 220).

Many of these ideas, which Freud studied in preparation for his high school diploma, were not specific to Lindner's textbook. Much of what Lindner had to say can also be found in other textbooks of Herbartian psychology (see for example: Moritz Wilhelm Drobisch's *Empirische Psychologie nach naturwissenschaftlicher Methode* [1842], Theodor Waitz's *Lehrbuch der Psychologie als Naturwissenschaft* [1849], Wilhelm Volkmann's *Lehre von den Elementen der Psychologie als Wissenschaft* [1850], Robert Zimmermann's *Philosophische Propädeutik* [1867] which included a section entitled *Empirische Psychologie*, and Mathias Amos Drbal's *Lehrbuch der empirischen Psychologie* [1868]). In these works one will find discussions of concepts such as the "threshold of consciousness," "clear," "dark," or

"repressed" representations, "repression," "resistance," "conflict among representations," as well as "reproduction or return of inhibited or repressed representations." Especially in his early works, Freud not only used Herbartian ideas but also terms (e.g., 1894, pp. 43–61, where he regularly used the terms of "contrasting" or "incompatible representations"—*kontrastierende, unverträgliche Vorstellungen*—which would lead to their "repression"; see also the passages about the "strength" or "intensities of representations" in the *Interpretation of Dreams*, 1900, pp. 588–621).

The presence of these connections should not prompt us to overlook significant differences. The most important difference lies in Herbartian psychologists' indifference about the qualitative aspects of psychological states, in particular motives. Although Herbartians recognized that unconscious representations influence conscious mental states in lawful ways, the question about why certain representations are weaker than others, why they are repressed, was stated in consistently quantitative, not in qualitative terms.

Franz Brentano (1838–1917)

Among the philosophers discussed in this entry, Brentano occupies a special place. For not only did Freud follow Brentano's lectures and seminars during four semesters, he also had personal contact with Brentano. In a letter to E. Silberstein from the beginning of his first university term (October 22/23, 1874) Freud described what major fields of study the various members of the Gymnasium had chosen. Despite their diverse choices and course schedules, Freud wrote that "we all meet together at Brentano's lectures. He is teaching two courses which we attend regularly: Wednesday and Saturday evenings, selected metaphysical questions, and Friday evenings a work by Mill on the utility principle" (Freud, 1989: 78). Two meetings at Brentano's house brought him directly under the spell of the latter's magnetic personality. In his letter of March 7, 1875, he characterized Brentano as a "remarkable man and in many respects ideal human being" (Freud, 1989: 109), and, by the end of the semester, he was caught up in the intellectual problems raised by the man that he considered altering the framework of his professional education. The change consisted in abandoning one of his most cherished dreams, the idea of spending a year in Berlin taking courses with Helmholtz, Du Bois-Raymond, and Virchow and instead pursue a double Ph.D. in philosophy and medicine (Freud, 1989: 109; see also McGrath, 1986: 113).

Freud's plan for a double Ph.D.—which was never realized—matched Brentano's concern with the "noteworthy trend which is now bringing philosophy and the natural sciences together" (Brentano, 1874: 16). According to Brentano "just as the natural sciences study the properties and laws of physical bodies, which are the objects of our external perception, psychology is the science which studies the properties and laws of the soul, which we infer by analogy, to exist in others" (Brentano, 1874: 8). He underlined that the "phenomena revealed by inner perception are also subject to laws. Anyone who has engaged in scientific psychological research recognizes this" (Brentano, 1874: 17). In the spring of 1875, Freud looked forward to taking further courses with Brentano, one on logic and one on psychology entitled "philosophical reading." Brentano had taught the latter course in Würzburg two years earlier (1872–1873), and the lecture notes of that course have survived. As McGrath points out, "even though the course Freud took two years later may not have been identical, it is very likely that many of the same topics were covered" (McGrath, 1986: 122). One of the most important topics of the course concerned the association of ideas, which for Brentano represented an important alternative explanation to the assumption of unconscious ideas (see Brentano, 1874: 155–160). It is interesting that Brentano, not unlike Lindner, carried his discussion of association into the area of dreams, insanity, and other bizarre mental phenomena (see McGrath, 1986: 122–124).

If we consider the important role Brentano played in Freud's life as a student, it is surprising how little the young Freud seems to have derived from Brentano's ideas. This becomes clear when we turn our attention to the fundamental differences between Brentano's and Freud's conceptions of the mind. First of all, Brentano defended a strictly rationalist, Cartesian model of the mind, in which representations are considered far more basic than instinct or affect (Brentano, 1874: 109–120; Brentano, 1889: 16–18). More important, and in even starker contrast to the philosophers discussed earlier, Brentano was very firm in denying the possibility of unconscious mental activity (Brentano, 1874: 143–194). Indeed, at the end of a thorough analysis Brentano came to the key conclusion: "The question: Is there an unconscious consciousness . . . has thus to be answered with a decisive No" (Brentano, 1874: 194).

Brentano's impact on Freud, then, was of a different, more general nature than the influence of the philosophers I traced beforehand. Clearly, he boosted Freud's emerging interest in philosophy and psychology, and impressed him with his general framework and direction of thinking about psychology. However, Brentano's rationalism and, in particular his refutation of unconscious mental activity were later opposed and even caricaturized by Freud as typical examples of the philosopher's limited view of the mind (but see Fancher, 1977 for a different opinion).

Conclusion

According to Freud's account, nineteenth-century philosophy refuted the concept of the unconscious and regarded it as absurd. Thus, when psychoanalysis introduced its concepts of unconscious functioning, according to its founder, these were "bound to seem very strange to ordinary modes of thought" and to "fundamentally contradict current views" (1940, p. 282). Although *some* philosophers, like Brentano, indeed rejected the notion of an unconscious, several others did not. In fact, when Freud received his education in high school and at university, philosophical conceptions of unconscious functioning were fairly current, and Freud was aware of at least some of them. Thus, it is not surprising to find that, from the beginning of the nineteenth century onwards, one can trace the development of a psychology of the unconscious that is *continuous* with the fundamental principles laid down in Freud's metapsychology. Although I believe that the authors covered in this entry were the most important forerunners of Freud in the nineteenth century, they were by no means the only ones. Carl Gustav Carus (1798–1869), Gustav Th. Fechner (1801–1887), Hermann von Helmholtz (1821–1894), Theodor Meynert (1833–1892), Theodor Lipps (1851–1914), Wilhelm Jerusalem (1854–1923), and Johannes Volkelt (1848–1930) all made additional contributions that can be placed on this same continuum of theorizing about the unconscious (see Ellenberger, 1970; Gödde, 1999; Zentner, 1995).

Specifically, while Freud's view of the unconscious as a repository of instinctual urges, as "hot and wet," is rooted in a Schopenhauerian conception of the mind, the formal framework for his mechanistic notion of the interplay between conscious and unconscious representations and affects was provided, or at least prepared, by Herbartian psychology. In a sense, then, while the *formal*

N

characteristics of Freud's "mental apparatus" seem to be borrowed from the Herbartian school, the specific *contents* of his metapsychology are indebted to the Schopenhauerian conceptions of the unconscious. This can be briefly exemplified with reference to the process of repression,—a process that was recognized and extensively described by both schools. Schopenhauer and Nietzsche proposed that painful memories and socially undesirable instinctual urges were most likely to be repressed, and Schopenhauer also attributed a pivotal role to this process in the etiology of mental illness. However, Schopenhauer did not scrutinize what happened to mental contents once repressed (nor did Nietzsche or Hartmann). In contrast, Herbart and his school introduced the view that repressed thoughts and affects have a life of their own. Exponents of this psychology held that what is repressed is subject to a law of conservation. Thus, it remains effective in its repressed and unconscious state and continues to influence conscious mental processes in lawful ways. A number of Freud's most fundamental hypotheses, then, may be characterized as a hybrid of both views.

Why, then, was Freud so adamant about denying the significant philosophical contributions to his creation? He certainly recognized that his theories were not direct abstractions from sensory information. In the opening page of his paper entitled "Instincts and their Vicissitudes," Freud notes that scientific theories are in general empirically underdetermined, pointing out that "even at the stage of description it is not possible to avoid applying certain ideas to the material in hand, ideas derived from somewhere or another but certainly not from the new observations alone" (1915, p. 117). Although these concepts "appear to have been derived" from the material of observation they have "in fact . . . been imposed" on it (1915, p. 117).

Very clearly, however, Freud refuted the possibility that the ideas he admittedly "imposed" on his material of observation were nineteenth-century philosophy ideas. One possibility is that Freud was unaware of the philosophical influences. This is not entirely impossible, since ideas are sometimes so well known, so "universal" in a historical period, that they become "invisible." This was true for both philosophical traditions Freud drew from. In his memoirs Wilhelm Jerusalem, a contemporary and friend of Freud, remembers of "having been raised, as it were, in the traditional Herbartian psychology. In high school and at the university I had not heard

anything else" (Jerusalem, 1925: 6). The same "invisible pervasiveness" characterized the ideas of the Schopenhauerian tradition as is well exemplified by a statement the German novelist Theodor Fontane made in a letter to friends in 1873, the same year Freud joined the *Leseverein*: "People descend into the depths of Schopenhauer, and will and representation, instinct and intellect have become part of the household vocabulary, well-known even to children" (Fontane, 1925: 312).

A second explanation for Freud's possible unawareness relies on the possibility of *cryptomnesia*, which is defined as "hidden or unconscious memory; generally used for ideas and thoughts (often apparently creative and novel) that are memories of past experiences and events that the individual does not (consciously) recall" (Penguin dictionary of psychology, 1985, p. 169). Indirectly, this is conceded by the father of psychoanalysis himself: "I can never be certain, in view of the wide extent of my reading in early years, whether what I took for a new creation might not be an effect of cryptomnesia" (1937, p. 245).

Yet, although plausible at first sight, the unawareness-hypothesis fits poorly with what Freud conceded later in his life: "The 'unconscious' had, it is true, long been under discussion among philosophers as a theoretical concept; but now for the first time, in the phenomena of hypnotism, it became something actual, tangible and subject to experiment" (1923, p. 192). This suggests that Freud was at least partly aware of philosophical anticipations of his theories. The closeness between Freud's views on the unconscious and its philosophical antecedents, however, represented a double threat: On the one hand, it was a threat to the recognition of his theory as a natural science; on the other it was a threat to its recognition as truly innovative (see also Sulloway, 1979, chap. 13). To avert this danger, Freud and his followers set out to profess what may be labeled a *methodological separatism*: Psychoanalysis was a natural science, but philosophers based their theories on speculations and intuitions. Thus, any results between the two were not really comparable, and if they were incommensurable, there was also no reason or need to acknowledge them. Indeed, while philosophy had merely "toyed" with the concept of the unconscious, psychoanalysis had "taken it seriously" (1940, p. 286).

While created by Freud, the habit of contrasting the "careful empirical observations" of psychoanalysis to the untrustworthy "speculations" or "intuitions" of its philosophical forerunners soon became standard practice in manuals, textbooks and historical accounts of psychoanalysis (see Zentner, 1995). Schopenhauer's observations of psychiatric patients, Nietzsche's extensive integration of the psychiatric research of his day as well as Herbart's goal to establish psychology as a natural science, however, shows how misleading this simplistic separatism is in truth. Indeed, in the light of the recent sobering assessments of the empirical merits of Freud's *own* theories (e.g., Grünbaum, 1984; Erwin, 1996; MacMillan, 1991; Sulloway, 1992), any distinction between Freud's views of the unconscious and their philosophical anticipations, which is drawn on purely methodological grounds, strikes us as obsolete today.

This being said, it may not be unnecessary to specify what these critical conclusions do *not* imply. First of all, it is Freud's *metapsychology* that grew out of the two strains of philosophical theorizing about the unconscious reported here. Other influential parts of his creation, such as his theories of psychosexual development as well as the entire domain of psychoanalysis as a therapeutic method fall outside the realm of the influences treated here. Secondly, the fact that a number of Freud's most fundamental views of the mind lie on a continuum with nineteenth-century philosophical conceptions of the unconscious does not mean that they are redundant with them. The exotic synthesis of Schopenhauerian and Herbartian ideas which characterizes Freud's metapsychology already proves this point, reminding us of the crucial difference between prediction and reconstruction: Now that we know exactly how Freud carried further certain concepts of nineteenth-century philosophers, we can easily trace the final product back to them. But how much more difficult would it have been to know what shape these concepts would take in Freud's mind during the 1890s? Incidentally, a brief but pregnant description of this problem has been put forward by the father of psychoanalysis himself: "So long as we trace the development backwards, the connection appears continuous, and we feel we have gained an insight which is completely satisfactory and even exhaustive. But if we proceed the reverse way, if we start from the premises . . . and try to follow these up to the final result, then we no longer get the impression of an inevitable sequence of events, which could not have been otherwise determined. We notice at once that there might be another result, and that we might have been just as well able to understand and explain the latter" (1920, p. 167). Although nobody liv-

ing in the last decade of the nineteenth century could have guessed how Freud would transform the concepts I traced in this entry, it is nevertheless important to appreciate the strong continuity between these conceptions and Freud's extensions of these ideas. For one thing, such recognition will facilitate and enrich understanding of psychoanalytic theory. Also, critiques of psychoanalytic theory remain inevitably incomplete without consideration of the philosophical foundations upon which it was built. Finally, current research on unconscious processes often takes Freud as a classical point of reference (see Kihlstrom, 1999; Westen, 1999 for recent reviews). But, with a certain distance, we are able to see that this point of reference turns out to be rather arbitrary.

REFERENCES

Aurelius, M. (1961). Communings with himself. Transl. by C. R. Haines. Cambridge, Mass.: Harvard University Press.

Bernfeld, S. (1949). Freud's scientific beginnings. *American Imago*, 6: 163–196.

Brentano, F. (1874 [1973]). *Psychologie vom Empirischen Standpunkt*. vol. 1. Hamburg: Meiner.

———. (1889 [1969]). *Vom Ursprung sittlicher Erkenntnis*. Hamburg: Meiner.

Dimitrov, Ch.T. (1969). E. von Hartmanns "Philosophie des Unbewussten" und Freuds "Tiefenpsychologie". *Zeitschrift für Psychosomatische Medizin und Psychoanalyse*, 15: 131–146.

Dorer, M. (1932). *Historische Grundlagen der Psychoanalyse*. Leipzig: Meiner.

Dörner, K. (1969). *Bürger und Irre. Zur Sozialgeschichte und Wissenschaftssoziologie der Psychiatrie*. Frankfurt: Europäische Verlagsanstalt.

Ebbinghaus, H. (1873). Über die Hartmannsche Philosophi des Unbewussten. Dissertation. Düsseldorf: Dietz.

Ellenberger, H. F. (1970). *The Discovery of the Unconscious*. New York: Basic Books.

Erwin, E. (1996). *A Final Accounting: Philosophical and Empirical Issues in Freudian Psychology*. Cambridge, Mass.: MIT Press.

Fancher, R. (1977). Brentano's psychology from an empirical standpoint and Freud's early metapsychology. *Journal of the History of the Behavioral Sciences*, 13: 202–227.

Fontane, T. (1925). *Briefe an seine Freunde*. O. Pniower and P. Schlenther (eds.), vol. 1. Berlin: Fischer.

Freud, S. (1894). The neuro-psychoses of defence. S.E. 2: 43–61.

———. (1900). *The Interpretation of Dreams*. S.E. 4–5: 1–621.

———. (1914). On the history of the psycho-analytic movement. S.E. 14: 7–66.

———. (1915). Instincts and their vicissitudes. S.E. 14: 111–140.

———. (1917). A difficulty in the path of psycho-analysis. S.E. 17: 137–144.

———. (1919). Preface to Reik's ritual: Psycho-analytic studies. S.E. 17: 259–263.

———. (1920). The psychogenesis of a case of homosexuality in a woman. S.E. 18: 147–172.

———. (1923). *The Ego and the Id*. S.E. 19: 3–66.

———. (1923). A short account of psycho-analysis. S.E. 19: 191–209.

———. (1925). The resistances to psycho-analysis. S.E. 19: 213–222.

———. (1925). An autobiographical study. S.E. 20: 7–74.

———. (1933). *New Introductory Lectures on Psycho-Analysis*. S.E. 22: 5–185.

———. (1937). Analysis terminable and interminable. S.E. 23: 209–253.

———. (1940). An outline of psycho-analysis. S.E. 23: 141–207.

———. (1940). Some elementary lessons in psycho-analysis. S.E. 23: 281–286.

———. (1989). *Jugendbriefe an Eduard Silberstein, 1871–1881*. W. Boehlich (ed.). Frankfurt: Fischer.

Gasser, R. (1997). *Nietzsche und Freud*. Berlin: De Gruyter.

Gödde, G. (1999). *Traditionslinien des Unbewussten. Schopenhauer, Nietzche, Freud*. Tübingen: Diskord.

Grünbaum, A. (1984). *The Foundations of Psychoanalysis: A Philosophical Critique*. Berkeley: University of California Press.

Hartmann, E. von (1871). *Philosophie des Unbewussten*. 3d ed. Berlin: Duncker.

———. (1890). *Philosophie des Unbewussten (Dritter Theil: Das Unbewusste und der Darwinisums)*. 10th edition. In *Ausgewählte Werke*, Bd. 9. Leipzig: Wilhelm Friedrich.

Hemecker, W. (1991). *Vor Freud. Philosophische Voraussetzungen der Psychoanalyse*. Munich: Philosophia Verlag.

Herbart, J. F. (1816). *Lehrbuch zur Psychologie*. Königsberg: Unzer.

———. (1824 [1825]). *Psychologie als Wissenschaft*. Königsberg: Unzer.

———. (1850). Schriften zur Psychologie. Erster Theil. In G. Hartenstein (ed.). *Sämtliche Werke*, Band 5. Leipzig: Voss.

———. (1851). Schriften zur Psychologie. Dritter Theil. In G. Hartenstein (ed.). *Sämtliche Werke*, Band 7. Leipzig: Voss.

Jerusalem, W. (1925). Selbstdarstellung. In W. Jerusalem, *Gedanken und Denker. Neue Folge*. Wien: Braunmüller, pp. 1–25.

Jones, E. (1953). *Sigmund Freud, Life and Work*, vol. 1. London: Hogarth Press.

Lampl, H. E. (1986). Ex oblivione: Das Féré-Palimpsest. *Nietzsche-Studien*, 15: 225–264.

———. (1988). *Flair du livre. Friedrich Nietzsche und Théodule Ribot*. Zürich: Nyffeler.

Laplanche, J., and Pontalis, J. B. (1973). *The Language of Psychoanalysis*. New York: Norton.

Lehrer, R. (1995). *Nietzsche's Presence in Freud's Life and Thought: On the Origins of a Psychology of Dynamic Unconscious Mental Functioning*. Albany: State University of New York Press.

Lindner, G. A. (1872). *Lehrbuch der empirischen Psychologie als inductiver Wissenschaft*. 3d ed. Wien: Gerolde.

Macmillan, M. (1991). *Freud Evaluated: The Completed Arc*. New York: North Holland.

Marx, O. (1990). German romantic psychiatry. Part 1. *History of Psychiatry*, 1: 351-381.

———. (1991). German romantic psychiatry. Part 2. *History of Psychiatry*, 2, 1–25.

Masson, J. M. (trans. and ed.)(1985). *The Complete Letters of Sigmund Freud to Wilhelm Fliess 1887–1904*. Cambridge, Mass.: Harvard University Press.

McGrath, W. J. (1967). Student radicalism in Vienna. *Journal of Contemporary History*, 2, 183–201.

———. (1986). *Freud's Discovery of Psychoanalysis*. Ithaca: Cornell University Press.

Nietzsche, F. (1967). *Kritische Gesamtausgabe Werke (KGW)*. G. Colli and M. Montinari (eds.). Berlin: DeGruyter.

———. (1876–1878). *Menschliches, Allzumenschliches*, vol. 1, in: KGW, 4th section, second volume, 1–375.

———. (1881). *Morgenröthe*, in: KGW, 5th section, first volume, 15–335.

———. (1882). *Die fröhliche Wissenschaft*, in: KGW, fifth section, second volume, 11–335.

———. (1884–1885). *Nachgelassene Fragmente Frühjahr 1884– Herbst 1885*, in: KGW, seventh section, fourth volume.

———. (1886–1887). *Zur Genealogie der Moral*, in KGW, sixth section, second volume, 258–430.

———. (1888–1889). *Ecce Homo*, in: KGW, sixth section, third volume, 253–372.

Nitzschke, B. (1983). Zur Herkunft des Es (I): Freud, Groddeck, Nietzsche-Schopenhauer und v. Hartmann. *Psyche*, 37, 769–804.

Nunberg, H., and Federn, E. (1962–1967). *Minutes of the Vienna Psycho-Analytical Society*. vols. 1–2. New York: International Universities Press.

Penguin Dictionary of Psychology (1985). A. S. Reber (ed.). London: Penguin Books.

Riese, W. (1958). The pre-Freudian origins of psychoanalysis. In J. H. Masserman (ed.). *Science and Psychoanalysis*, vol. 1. New York, London: Grune & Stratton, pp. 29–72.

Robinson, P. (1993). *Freud and His Critics*. Berkeley: University of California Press.

Sand, R. (1988). Early nineteenth century anticipation of Freudian theory. *International Review of Psychoanalysis*, 15: 465–479.

Schopenhauer is quoted after the following editions:

I. Historisch-kritische Ausgabe: Sämtliche Werke. Ed. A. Hübscher. 7 volumes. Mannheim: Brockhaus, 1988, using the following abbreviations: WI = *Die Welt als Wille und Vorstellung* (Vol. 1, 1819). WII = *Die Welt als Wille und Vorstellung* (Vol. 2, 1844).

II. *Vorlesungen*, part I: Theorie des gesammten Vorstellens, Denkens und Erkennens. München: Piper, 1990, using the abbreviation: V.

Shakow, D., and Rapaport, D. (1964). The influence of Freud on American psychology. *Psychol. Iss. Mon. IV*. New York: International University Press.

Sulloway, F. (1979). *Freud, Biologist of the Mind*. New York: Basic Books.

Sulloway, F. (1992). Reassessing Freud's case histories. The social construction of psychoanalysis. In: T. Gelfland and

J. Kerr (eds.). *Freud and the History of Psychoanalysis* (pp. 153–192). Hillsdale, N.J.; London: The Atlantic Press.

Venturelli, A. (1984). Nietzsche an der Berggasse 19. Ueber die erste Nietzsche-Rezeption in Wien. *Nietzsche Studien*, 13: 448–480.

Whyte, L. L. (1960). *The Unconscious Before Freud.* New York: Basic Books.

Young, C., and Brook, A. (1994). Schopenhauer and Freud. *International Journal of Psychoanalysis*, 75: 101–118.

Zentner, M. R. (1995). *Die Flucht ins Vergessen. Die Anfänge der Psychoanalyse Freuds bei Schopenhauer.* Darmstadt: Wissenschaftliche Buchgesellschaft.

MARCEL R. ZENTNER

Norway, and Psychoanalysis

Psychoanalysis, throughout its history in Norway, has had strong connections both with the psychiatric healthcare system and with academic psychiatry and psychology. It has also played a central role in cultural life, especially in the 1930s. In 1907, Ragnar Vogt, who was to become the first professor of psychiatry in Norway, discussed Freud's psychocathartic method in his psychiatric textbook, *Psykiatriens Grundtræek (An Outline of Psychoanalysis)*. Freud (1914, p. 91) mentioned this as the first textbook of psychiatry to refer to "psychoanalysis." It was not until the 1920s, however, that psychoanalysis was practiced in Norway, first and foremost under the leadership of Harald Schjelderup, from 1928 onward professor in psychology at the University of Oslo.

Schjelderup and several others went to Central Europe for training, and psychoanalysis was established as a clinical discipline in the 1930s, although there were intense debates and at times heavy opposition from the medical and clerical establishment. In the cultural field, psychoanalysis was well received and had a decisive influence on several writers. On the political scene, psychoanalysis was discussed both theoretically (e.g., the Freud-Marx debate) and on a practical-political level. An example of the latter is the contribution by analysts to the struggle for healthier attitudes toward sexuality, partly through publications in the journal *Sexual Information*, published by Karl Evang, later the surgeon general of Norway.

In 1931, a group of Scandinavian psychoanalysts gathered in Stockholm to establish a study circle of psychoanalysis with the aim of affiliation with the International Psychoanalytic Association (IPA). In 1933, a Nordic Psychoanalytic Society was formed with Alfhild Tamm

of Sweden as president and Harald Schjelderup of Norway as vice president. At the Lucerne congress in 1934, a decision was made to establish a Danish-Norwegian and a Finnish-Swedish society; this was decided after heated debate on the subject of wild analysis, caused partly by the fact that Wilhelm Reich had arrived in Oslo in 1934 at the invitation of Schjelderup. Ernest Jones, then president of the IPA, set the condition that Reich was not to become a member of the Danish-Norwegian society. This condition was not accepted at the time but, nevertheless, at a vote by the society, Reich was not accepted as a member. But he gave seminars and supervisions attended by members. The Danish-Norwegian society (soon renamed "Norwegian-Danish" because of Denmark's negligible participation) was then established with Schjelderup as president and Otto Fenichel as secretary.

Fenichel had arrived in Oslo in 1933 and stayed until 1935. The first years of organized psychoanalysis in Norway were thus marked by the influence of Fenichel and Reich, but also by the struggle between their powerful personalities. This created lots of tension in psychoanalytic circles but also led to increased creativity. The controversies around psychoanalysis, which engaged the medical establishment and the public as well, were concentrated mainly on Reich's transformation of character analysis into vegeto-therapy and his quasi-scientific "discoveries" of the energy of life.

Partly because of his wild practice, Reich's stay in Norway was terminated in 1939; he then left for the United States. His works on character analysis, however, have influenced psychoanalysis and psychiatry in Norway, especially child psychiatry through the work of Nic Wall, who later laid the foundation for a psychoanalytically based education in child psychiatry in Norway.

When German troops occupied Norway in 1940 after the start of World War II, a temporary dissolution of the psychoanalytic society was decided to avoid interference from the Nazi-imposed government, as had been the case in Germany. Most members of the society participated in the resistance movement or war activities. Schjelderup, leader of the resistance at the University of Oslo, was interned in the concentration camp of Grini in Norway, and several other analysts had to flee the country. Landmark died in war activities in northern Norway and P. Bernstein perished in a German concentration camp.

Yet the temporary dissolution of the society during wartime was treated by the IPA authorities as a permanent withdrawal, and the Norwegian society was denied status as a component society after the war. The pioneers Schjelderup, Braatøy, and Simonsen reestablished the Norwegian-Danish society in 1947 as a study group. It existed until 1953, when the Danes started their own study group. The Danish group was accepted as a component society in 1957, but it was not until 1975 that the Norwegian society received this status. The reason for its wartime exclusion has not been established, and there is no official documentation that an exclusion occurred. But it was obvious that the supposed influence of Wilhelm Reich on the society's members was a disadvantage in the eyes of the IPA. An application made at the eighteenth congress in London in 1953 was turned down on the basis that a few of the group's members did not practice psychoanalysis; this rejection obviously referred to members seen as followers of Wilhelm Reich. The Norwegian group argued that it was impossible to break from colleagues with whom one had fought during the war. There followed a long struggle for recognition with applications made at different congresses. One problem was the practice of Schjelderup after the war; he used fewer (two to three) sessions a week in training analysis with the purpose of raising the educational capacity (he also claimed to show good results).

In 1971, the Norwegian society was given status as a study group, and it finally gained status as a component society in 1975 (Alnæs, 1994).

The Norwegian Psychoanalytic Institute had been established in 1967 under the leadership of Peter Andreas Holter. The formal recognition granted by the IPA gave impetus to an expansion of its activities, with the responsibility for psychoanalytic education being at their center. In later years, the institute has taken on other activities, such as research and external teaching/lecturing.

As of May 2001, the society had 66 members and 73 candidates. There is an active child-analytic group and a group working on psychoanalytic research. The main trend in its program is a broad object relational approach with emphasis on the analysis of character, with some inspiration from ego psychology (Anthi and Varvin, 1993). The society is characterized by an open-minded attitude toward current developments in psychoanalytic theory and practice.

Important Individuals in the History of Psychoanalysis in Norway

Harald Krabbe Schjelderup (1895–1974), professor of philosophy in 1922 and professor of psychology beginning in 1928, was the main pioneer of psychoanalysis in Norway. He was responsible for numerous publications on psychoanalysis, among them: *Neurosis and the Neurotic Character* (1940) and "Lasting Effects of Psychoanalytic Treatment" (1957), the latter being a retrospective follow-up of psychoanalytic treatments.

Trygve Braatøy (1904–1953) trained in Berlin and worked at the Menninger Clinic in 1949–1951. He was clinical director at a main psychiatric hospital in Oslo and had numerous publications on psychoanalysis and literature, e.g., his *Foundation of Psychoanalytic Technique* (1954). Hjørdis Simonsen (1899–1980) also trained in Berlin; he was a training analyst and a central figure during the 1930s and after World War II. Nic Waal (1905–1960) received his training in Berlin and practiced as a child psychiatrist. Finn Hansen (1918–1996), as did the others, trained in Berlin, and worked as a training analyst. Peter Andreas Holter (1927–1998), a training analyst, was the first leader of the institute and was an honorary member.

REFERENCES

Alnæs, R. (1994). Psychoanalysis in Norway. History, training, treatment, research (in Norwegian). *Nordic Journal of Psychiatry*, 48, supl. 32.

Anthi, P. R., and Varvin, S. (1993). *Psykoanalysen i Norge.* Oslo: Universitetsforlaget.

Braatøy, T. (1954). *Fundamentals of Psychoanalytic Technique.* London: Wiley.

Freud S. (1914). On the history of the psycho-analytic movement. S.E. 14: 7–66.

Schjelderup, H. K. (1957). Lasting effects of psychoanalytic treatment. *Psychiatry*, 18: 109–133.

Vogt, R. (1907). *Psykiatriens Grundtræek.* Christiania, Norway: Steenske Forlag.

SVERRE VARVIN

O

Object

The term "object" first appears in Freud's writings in 1891, in *On Aphasia: A Critical Study*, as a component of "object representation" (*Vorstellung*). The notion applied to the cortical sensory derived associative psychic construction of the perception of a "thing" existing in reality (*Gegenstand*). At that point, Freud was concerned with understanding the process of giving psychic representation to things perceived by the senses: "In what manner is the body reproduced in the cerebral cortex" (Freud, 1891: 50). He concludes that the complex associative process leading to the formation of an object representation gives it a richness that exceeds that of its source, the "thing" itself. This object representation leaves a modification in the cortex, thus making possible its later reactivation as memory (p. 55). This first use of the term establishes a clear distinction between the thing perceived and the associatively organized psychic object representation.

Freud (1905) introduced two technical terms in *Three Essays on the Theory of Sexuality*: "Let us call the person from whom sexual attraction proceeds the *sexual object* and the act towards which the instinct tends the *sexual aim*" (pp. 135–136). He does not connect the term "object of the instinct" to the object representation notion of 1891. The context suggests that the object, as Freud is conceiving it in his 1905 paper, is the actual person, not the psychic representative of its perception.

The choice of a sexual object, Freud holds, is diphasic: "The first of these begins between the ages of two and five [Oedipal period], and is brought to a halt or to a retreat by the latency period; it is characterized by the infantile nature of the sexual aims. The second wave sets in puberty and determines the final outcome of sexual life" (Freud, 1905: 200). This second stage, puberty, is the stage of development when the "finding of an object, for which preparations have been made from earliest childhood, is completed. . . . The finding of an object is in fact a refinding of it" (p. 222).

In normal development, the pregenital "preparations" include a sequence: The first sexual object is linked to nourishment and finds its sexual object of instinctual satisfaction in the maternal breast. The erotogenic oral zone coincides with the organ that obtains the food needed for survival. The sexual satisfaction obtains from the appropriate stimulation of the erotogenic oral zone. The object as such is not differentiated: it is only that which provides oral erotic satisfying stimulation. The satisfaction becomes autoerotic: "The need for repeating the sexual satisfaction now becomes detached from the need of taking nourishment" (p. 182). Thumb sucking is the prototype of infantile sexuality characterized by attaching itself to one of the vital somatic functions; having no sexual object; being autoerotic. The developmental change of erotogenic zones moves the satisfaction to the consecutive stimulation of the oral, anal, and genital organs (p. 182). In the course of these developments, the choice of a sexual object (person) may have been established as a result of bodily ministrations that excite and satisfy the erotogenic zones: "that is to say, the whole of the sexual currents have become directed towards a single person in relation to whom they seek to achieve their aims" (p. 199), even when there is not yet a subordination to the primacy of the genitals. This subordination occurs in puberty when a true object choice is possible.

The question is, what is the drive's object in the human object? The actual person who offers satisfaction? The combination of the memories of previously satisfying objects and the present object in the "refinding of an object"? The representation of a previous object projected onto the actual object? This question has not yet been answered in psychoanalysis. Strachey, in a footnote in *Three Essays on the Theory of Sexuality*, affirmed: "in speaking of the libido concentrating on 'objects,' withdrawing from 'objects,' etc., Freud has in mind the mental representations (Vorstellungen) and not, of course, objects in the external world" (p. 217). In contrast to Strachey, Melanie Klein held that what matters is the construction of the internal object by means of projection and introjection, whereas Winnicot affirmed the importance of the real mother and the child's internalization of the maternal function mediated by his creation of a transitional object that stands for the mother. British object relation theorists generally favor the importance of the actual mother. However, whatever her importance, the child cannot relate to her without the mediation of the active construction of her psychic representation, which never fully coincides with the actual mother. The issue that still requires clarification is the connection between internal representations of objects as guidance for seeking satisfaction and the actual person (object) that seems to provide it.

REFERENCES

Freud, S. (1905). *Three Essays on the Theory of Sexuality*. S.E. 7: 120–243.

———. (1953 [1891]). *On Aphasia: A Critical Study*. Trans. E. Stengel. New York: International Universities Press.

Jacobson, E. (1964). *The Self and the Object World*. New York: International Universities Press.

Rangell, L. (1985). The object in psychoanalytic theory. *Journal of the American Psychoanalytic Association*, 33: 301–335.

Sandler, J., and Rosenblatt, B. (1962). The concept of the representational world. *Psychoanalytic Study of the Child*, 17: 128–145.

ANA-MARÍA RIZZUTO

Object Libido See DRIVE THEORY; OBJECT RELATIONS THEORY.

Object Relations Theory

Freud and Contemporary Psychoanalysis

From the classical Freudian emphasis on the instinctual basis of development, contemporary psychoanalysis diverged in various directions, including self psychology, intersubjectivity, relational psychology, and Kleinian and object relations theories. These new developments reflect the sociocultural diversity, philosophical influences, and scientific advances of the twentieth century. They derive from but also challenge the original psychoanalytic findings and theories discussed by Freud. They build upon and elaborate aspects of psychology that Freud identified but did not take further, possibly because of the inevitable constraint on the outer limits of his thinking owing largely to his gender, his ethnicity, and his historical period (J. Scharff and D. Scharff, 1992).

Freud and the Roots of Object Relations Theory

Antecedents of object relations theory can be found in Freud's work, even though object-relational views are incompatible with some central parts of his theories in that they reject the instinctual basis of development and posit the need to relate as the fundamental drive for development. I reserve the term "object relations theory," a term coined by Fairbairn, for the body of work contributed by British analysts such as Fairbairn himself, Balint, Winnicott, Guntrip, and Sutherland. More recent contributors include Bollas, Ogden, D. Scharff, and J. Scharff.

The term "object relations theory" has also been used in the United States to refer to the work of American theorists in the tradition of Jacobson, Mahler, and Kernberg, but since they accept Freud's drive/structure models rather than developing a purely object-relational model, they are not covered by the definition of object relations theory used for the purposes of this entry. Similarly, American usage of the term may at times include the theory of Melanie Klein, whose focus on internal objects as a function of unconscious fantasy illuminates and adds to the aforementioned object relations theories, most usefully in understanding aggression through projective identification. Since Kleinian theory, however, retains a primarily instinctual basis for development, it remains fundamentally distinct, and so Kleinian theory and its relation to Freud is not addressed here (see "Kleinian Theory," this volume).

Object relations theory holds that the infant is motivated by the need to relate to another person, not by the wish for instinctual gratification. This is a radical revision of Freud's theory, yet one that builds on his concepts of object, libido, narcissism, group psychology, repetition compulsion, identification, splitting of the ego, and structural conflict. From study of the therapeutic relationship rather than the analysand alone, an understanding of the here-and-now effects of the patient's personal history of dealing with the vicissitudes of infantile independence led to the formulation of the theory of object relations. According to this theory, how the infant manages the early years, helped or hindered by the mothering person, is as crucial as the resolution of the Oedipus complex in determining personality development.

Instinct Theory and the Pleasure Principle

Freudian instinct theory (Freud, 1910; 1915) holds that instincts (also referred to as "drives") are biological givens, consisting of impulses of energy that seek expression and gratification and are opposed by countervailing instinctual forces. For instance, the libidinal (sex) instinct may be opposed by the self-preservative instinct or the death instinct, so that the organism can return to the resting, nonexcited state in keeping with the principle of entropy.

When unsuitable instincts are successfully opposed, they do not invade consciousness in which rational thinking takes place. They are given acceptable expression by the pre-conscious or remain in the unconscious, a seething mass of instinctual energy where thinking is not rational but is governed by the primary process. Conceptualizing the mind in layers from surface to depth, Freud's theory at this stage has also been called the *topographic theory.*

In Freud's theory of early development, the infant is not looking for a mother, a relationship, or food. The infant is driven by the libido (the sexual instinct) to seek satisfaction through stimulation of the oral orifice that happens to occur during feeding. The mother is the *object that the drive attaches to,* but she is *not the object of attachment* for her infant. In object-relations theory, however, the infant's need to be in a relationship is primary. The infant finds security and meaning in the loving arms and eyes of the mother and other family members, and in the predictable rhythm of stimulation and rest, togetherness, and tolerable separation.

Freud's instinct theory presupposes the *pleasure principle.* The libido seeks expression by being gratified at the site of the pleasure zone that predominates at the different psychosexual stages—oral, anal, phallic, and genital. In emphasizing the source, expression, and control of the pleasure-seeking libido as it meets an envi-

ronment experienced as hostile to its aims, instinct theory minimizes individuals and their families, even though in practice Freud was well aware of the importance of family relationships, as his case histories show. Unconscious sexual and opposing aggressive instincts give rise to impulses for pleasure, survival, and destruction. These impulses are in conflict as they compete for expression along the reflex arc to consciousness and their associated affects compete for release. This conflict is experienced as anxiety, a *discharge affect.*

Freud hypothesized that this anxiety is a fear of the consequences of not being able to tame the instinct, these consequences being loss of the object, love of the object, or love of the self. Here the theory begins to require an object relational focus to explain why the instincts have to be opposed. And, indeed, as Freud developed his ideas on the Oedipus complex and explored mourning reactions to lost objects, the objects of the drives acquired an increasingly *personal* significance for personality development, but he never gave up the instinctual basis for development in favor of an object-relational motivating drive.

Freud on the Object

The Infantile Narcissistic Object. Freud introduced the term "object" to refer to the *object of the drives* that are aimed at it. In the beginning, he thought, there is no external object in the environment, human or nonhuman. The libido is directed internally and finds its primary object in itself. In Freud's words, the internal object is infused with "narcissistic libido," meaning that infants look to their own bodies for stimulation, gratification, and soothing. Freud called this the stage of *primary narcissism.*

Gradually, the libido develops *object cathexis,* that is, energy is aimed outside the self: Infants reach out when their mothers seem to promise gratification of their libidinal aims. When the mother proves disappointing, hurtful, rejecting, or traumatic in response to the baby's needs for pleasure, the baby stops looking to her for gratification. In Freud's words, the infant retreats to using the self as the primary object after the external object fails to gratify the libido. Freud called this the stage of *secondary narcissism.*

Object relations theory follows Freud in postulating withdrawn ego states but regards them as secondary phenomena, not as a retreat to an original condition. It holds that the infant is not motivated by sexual and aggressive instincts—and, therefore, it has no id—and has a pristine whole ego at birth. It further views narcissism as always secondary to frustration owing to lack of fit between the infant's constitutional ego capacities for expressing need and tolerating organismic distress and the quality of maternal response.

The Anaclitic Object. The ego may look to the external object, not just for gratification but for support, when the ego seems weak and the object is viewed as strong. Freud (1917) introduced this view in his paper "In Mourning and Melancholia" to explain the depression of bereaved adults who have relied so heavily on the presence of their loved ones that they are devastated by their departures. But dependency was a pathological condition in Freudian theory, not a natural condition for development, as it is in object-relations theory. Freud recognized the importance of the parents as objects of the drives, but he did not focus on the child's ego in relation to its objects until the Oedipal stage. Even then, when he took the family dynamics into account, he retained a drive-oriented approach. Although he said that "it is inevitable and perfectly normal that a child should take his parents as the first objects of his love," he nevertheless revealed his commitment to an instinct-based view of the object, when he continued "But his libido should not remain fixated to these first objects; later on, it should merely take them as a model" (Freud, 1910: 48).

The Lost Object. Freud studied the effect of the loss of the object on development. He saw the *lost object* as an important stimulus to thinking. In its absence, the person learns to hallucinate the missing object to secure wish fulfillment. In this way, *the person has the object*. When the person identifies with the lost object that is being hallucinated, he or she *becomes the object*, so to speak. The ego is then divided into two parts, one of which rages against the part that is identified with the lost object. In this way, *the ego is split by its relation to the lost object*.

From Objects to Identification. From studies of narcissistic, anaclitic, and lost objects, Freud developed his theory of *identification*, which he acknowledged as the original form of emotional tie to the object. He thought that identification could operate regressively—so that the object was introjected into the ego as a substitute for a libidinal object tie—or could operate to enrich the personality when the ego identifies with a person with whom it shares a quality and who is not an object of the libido. This line of thinking led to the idea

of the *splitting of the ego*, a concept that was further developed by Fairbairn, who saw splitting occurring in degrees as a response to the temporarily or chronically unresponsive external object, and by Klein, who saw it as a response to perceptions of the object colored as good or bad by projective identification under the force of the life or death instincts.

Intrapsychic versus Relational Perspectives in Freud

The State of Being in Love. Freud noted that adults in love do not see each other's characteristics objectively. Instead, they overvalue each other because each of them needs to see the other as a wonderful object in order to gratify the libido. The object (i.e., the other person) is used to aggrandize the ego instead of loving and appreciating it for its unique characteristics, its otherness. In Freud's way of putting it, the new love object is overvalued by being infused with "narcissistic libido." The new object has to be glorified so that it can serve as a successful substitute for the unattainable Oedipal object. Only if it serves this purpose can it satisfy the narcissistic aims of the libido.

When falling in love, the lover may become so preoccupied with the loved one that he or she may lose the sense of being a separate person or, by idealizing the love object, may diminish the individuality of the loved one. In either case, to use Freud's language, the loved object may consume the lover's ego, or the ego may "consume" the object, when the choice is dominated by the narcissistic aims of the libido. In contrast to Freud's view, the object-relations view of marriage uses Fairbairn's theory of the individual personality, which holds that a personality is composed of parts—of ego, object, and affect connected in internal object relationships. It is held that the internal object relationships of one spouse communicate with the other spouse's internal relationships through the Kleinian mechanism of projective identification. As a result of this reciprocal process, a joint marital personality is created. In the healthy marriage, this has a beneficial effect on each spouse's internal world, but in marriages that typically come to treatment, it cements faulty internal constellations (Dicks, 1967).

Group Psychology. In his (1921), "Group Psychology and the Analysis of the Ego," Freud again seems to be moving toward a relational approach. He notes that, "in the individual's mental life someone else is invariably involved, as a model, as an object, as a helper, as an opponent; and so from the very first individual psychology is at the same time a social psychology as well" (p. 69). He observes that human beings tend to want to live and work in groups and establish emotional ties to others in the group even if only to avoid a conflict between following the leader or acting for oneself. Freud found that the human being is a social animal. This was quite a move beyond his intensely intrapsychic, drive-motivated view of development, but, not surprisingly, Freud had to find an instinct to explain social relations. He named it *the social instinct*. But instead of giving it a solely biological basis, he looked for its origin in social terms. He said that "the social instinct may not be a primitive one and insusceptible of dissection, and that it may be possible to discover the beginnings of its development in a narrower circle, such as that of the family" (p. 70). Freud acknowledged the family as the possible source of the human tendency to want to live and work in groups.

Freud, however, abandoned his move toward an object-relational approach based on the psychology of family, social, and individual development, perhaps because he was horrified when the social instinct, augmented by the death instinct, led to group efforts at mass destruction in World War I. Drawing on his study of primary and secondary narcissism, identification in loss and mourning, and his watershed discovery of Oedipal fantasy, Freud produced the concept of parts of the ego and object in a structural relationship; by 1920, he had prepared the way for an object relations theory of the dynamic, intrapsychic relation between these parts of the self and also their continuing development in interaction with significant others throughout the life cycle. Perhaps Freud could have moved more solidly in this direction, but his concept of identification received too little attention from his colleagues and from himself. In any case, he could not pursue every theory at once, and he made his choices according to personal inclination, scientific credibility, and political implications.

Freud on Psychic Structure

In Freud's account, as the infant matures and mental functioning comes under the force of the reality principle, the instincts undergo delay, detour, binding, and neutralization of their energy. The drives that are constantly pressing for gratification can be persuaded to hold off until a later date, when their eventual satisfac-

tion can be confidently expected with greater personal pleasure. The absence of the object and the resulting delay in instinctual expression leads to a formation of mental structure that is then capable of securing further delays. Conflict is then experienced between the id, where the drives are located, and the reality-oriented ego formed from identification with the lost objects. In other words, Freud now viewed *the conflict as structural*, occurring between parts of the self. The conflict is experienced as anxiety, now in the form of *signal affect*. To account for this capacity for managing delay, Freud postulated the existence in consciousness of the ego, the conscious executive part of the mind, in which lost objects are represented and which can respond to the signal affect by alerting the mind's defenses against the threat of instinctual energy release.

Instead of giving up his topographical theory of the broadly based realms of consciousness and unconsciousness, Freud superimposed his new structural theory on his earlier one. He still held that the infant progresses along a predetermined time line, relating to its objects because they satisfy instinctual demands specific to each psychosexual stage, and experiencing them progressively through the oral, anal and phallic routes, with Oedipal-level renunciation of the object as the ultimate renunciation.

The structural theory took account of childhood misperceptions of parent figures and the role of the family as the culture carrier and shaper of human ideals and behaviors. Freud's (1905) *Three Essays on the Theory of Sexuality* and his case histories demonstrate his understanding of the infant's need for holding and handling, and as well as the older child's need for family support and validation. In his (soon to be abandoned) seduction theory, Freud's emphasis on family influence was clear when he claimed that neurosis was caused when seduction by a family member overwhelmed a young person's capacity to oppose the demands of the libido to seek such gratification (see "Seduction Theory," this volume). But in his more mature and most developed theory, Freud gave less attention to the influence of family relationships on the child's developing personality structure than to the impact of the child's inherent constitutionally and phylogenetically predetermined characteristics. Although he outlined the way in which the child selectively identifies with or creates reaction formations against the character traits of the parents in the Oedipal phase, and although he said that the ego is filled with the lost objects, Freud mainly claimed that the ego formed out of the id, the cauldron of instinctual energy.

Fairbairn followed Freud in being interested in internal conflict, but he did not agree that it occurs among the agencies of id, ego, and superego. In his theory, there is no id; the nucleus of the superego is an internalized accepted object shorn of its troublesome libidinal and antilibidinal features (it resembles Freud's ego ideal); and the central ego is subdivided into parts that relate to the accepted, libidinal, and antilibidinal objects. Conflict may be experienced between parts of the self at many points in the dynamic system of partly conscious, and—depending on the degree of the trauma and the strength of the constitution—partly repressed, and partly dissociated, ego, parts of objects, and affect.

Conclusion

To the object relations theorist looking back, Freud's structural theory seems to hold within it the potential for developing an object relations view of the mind. But his structural theory remained a biologically centered, intrapsychic, individually oriented theory of linear and deterministic type, in keeping with the scientific influences of the time. It stood in contrast with the diverging ideas and methodologies of Ferenczi (1933) that later influenced his analysands, Balint and Klein, to develop the object relations perspective that flourished later in the twentieth century (Falzeder, 1994). In addition, Freud's translator's choice of Latin terminology—"id," "ego," "superego"—had the unfortunate effect of reifying Freud's central structural concepts. Bruno Bettelheim (1982) has made the point that in the original German, Freud had used the highly personal term "I" (translated as "ego") and the impersonal "it" (translated as "id"). "Ego" seems to suggest a rather mechanistic, reflexively operant management function, as opposed to what Freud may have intended—a proactive, personal, executive structure for receiving affect signals and managing affect states, integrating experience with the objects, selecting object qualities to identify with or defend against, and, in general, dealing with internal and external reality. Perhaps Freud's concern for the person's self—as opposed to his ego structures—expressed in his German theory-building was not evident to his English-language followers, and may have contributed to delaying the emergence of an object relations perspective. For various historical, personal, and professional reasons, the radical, redefining potential of this set of Freud's ideas

remained undeveloped. This is because he continued to subscribe to his model of the mind as one that generated its own form and did so under pressure from the instincts as the driving force that governed development. It was not until new information infused the culture that disparate and overlooked elements in Freudian theory led to a radical revision according to the object relations perspective. The crucial new influences not available to push Freud in this direction were studies of attachment by Bowlby and others, group reactions of dependency, fight/flight, and pairing in response to task and leader (Bion, 1959, 1962), war neuroses resulting from unresolved infantile dependence (Fairbairn, 1943), and cybernetic systems (Bertalannfy, 1950). In the twenty-first century, the cultural effects of feminist theory, the scientific advances in chaos theory, the communication explosion, and whatever the future may bring, will move Freud's invention of psychoanalysis in yet new directions.

REFERENCES

Balint, M. (1952). *Primary Love and Psychoanalytic Technique.* London: Tavistock, 1965.

———. (1968). *The Basic Fault: Therapeutic Aspects of Regression.* London: Tavistock.

Bertalanffy, L. von. (1950). The theory of open systems in physics and biology. *Science,* 111: 23–29.

Bettleheim, B. (1982). Reflections: Freud and the soul. *The New Yorker,* March 1, pp. 59–93.

Bion, W. (1959). *Experiences in Groups.* New York: Basic Books, 1961.

———. (1962). *Learning From Experience.* New York: Basic Books.

Birtles, E. F., and Scharff, D. E. (eds.) (1994). *From Instinct to Self: Selected Papers of W. R. D. Fairbairn,* vol. 2. Northvale, N.J.: Jason Aronson.

Bollas, C. (1987). *The Shadow of the Object.* New York: Columbia University Press.

———. (1989). *Forces of Destiny: Psychoanalysis and Human Idiom.* London: Free Association Books.

———. (1992). *Being a Character: Psychoanalysis and Self Experience.* New York: Hill and Wang.

———. (1995). *Cracking Up.* New York: Hill and Wang.

Bowlby, J. (1958). The nature of the child's tie to his mother. *International Journal of Psycho-Analysis,* 39: 1–24.

———. (1969). *Attachment and Loss, Volume 1.* New York: Basic Books.

———. (1973). *Attachment and Loss, Volume 2. Separation: Anxiety and Anger.* New York: Basic Books.

———. (1980). *Attachment and Loss, Volume 3. Sadness and Depression.* New York: Basic Books.

Dicks, H. (1967). *Marital Tensions: Clinical Studies Towards a Psychoanalytic Theory of Interaction.* London: Routledge and Kegan Paul.

Fairbairn, W. R. D. (1943). The repression and return of bad objects (with special reference to the "war neuroses"). In *Psychoanalytic Studies of the Personality*. London: Routledge, pp. 58–81.

———. (1952). *Psychoanalytic Studies of the Personality*. London: Routledge.

Falzeder, E. (1994). The threads of psychoanalytic filiations or psychoanalysis taking effect. *Cahiers Psychiatriques Genevois*, Special Issue, pp. 169–194.

Ferenczi, S. (1933). Confusion of tongues between the adult and the child. In *Final Contributions to the Problems and Methods of Psychoanalysis*. London: Hogarth Press, 1955, pp. 156–167.

Freud, S. (1905). *Three Essays on Sexuality*. S.E. 7: 130–243.

———. (1910). Five lectures on psycho-analysis. S.E. 11: 9–55.

———. (1911). Two principles of mental functioning. S.E. 12: 218–226.

———. (1915). Instincts and their vicissitudes. S.E. 4: 109–140.

———. (1917). Mourning and melancholia. S.E. 14: 243–258.

———. (1920). *Beyond the Pleasure Principle*. S.E. 28: 7–64.

———. (1921). *Group Psychology and the Analysis of the Ego*. S.E. 18: 69–143.

———. (1923). The Ego and the Id. S.E. 19: 12–66.

Greenberg, J. R., and Mitchell, S. A. (1983). *Object Relations in Psychoanalytic Theory*. Cambridge, Mass.: Harvard University Press.

Guntrip, H. S. (1961). *Personality and Human Interaction*. London: Hogarth Press.

———. (1969). *Schizoid Phenomena, Object Relations and the Self*. New York: International Universities Press.

———. (1986). My experience of analysis with Fairbairn and Winnicott. In P. Buckley (ed.). *Essential Papers on Object Relations*. New York: New York University Press, pp. 447–468.

Jacobson, E. (1964). *The Self and the Object World*. New York: International Universities Press.

Jones, E. (1955a). *The Life and Work of Sigmund Freud 1856–1900. The Formative Years and the Great Discoveries*. New York: Basic Books.

———. (1955b). *The Life and Work of Sigmund Freud 1901–1919. The Years of Maturity*. New York: Basic Books.

———. (1955c). *The Life and Work of Sigmund Freud 1919–1939. The Last Phase*. New York: Basic Books.

Kernberg, O. (1976). *Object Relations Theory and Clinical Psychoanalysis*. New York: Jason Aronson.

———. (1979). An overview of Edith Jacobson's contributions. *Journal of the American Psychoanalytic Association*, 30: 793–819.

———. (1980). *Internal World and External Reality*. New York: Jason Aronson.

Klein, M. (1955). *New Directions in Psycho-Analysis*. London: Tavistock.

Mahler, M., Pine, F., and Bergman, A. (1974). *The Psychological Birth of the Human Infant*. New York: Basic Books.

Mitchell, S., and Black, M. (1995). *Freud and Beyond*. New York: Basic Books.

Ogden, T. (1982). *Projective Identification and Psychotherapeutic Technique*. New York: Jason Aronson.

———. (1986). *The Matrix of the Mind: Object Relations and the Psychoanalytic Dialogue*. Northvale, N.J.: Jason Aronson.

———. (1989). *The Primitive Edge of Experience*. Northvale, N.J.: Jason Aronson.

———. (1994). *Subjects of Analysis*. Northvale, N.J.: Jason Aronson.

Rapaport, D. (1960). The structure of psychoanalytic theory. *Psychological Issues*, 2, no. 2, Monograph 6. New York: International Universities Press.

Scharff, D. E. (1981). *The Sexual Relationship*. Northvale, N.J.: Jason Aronson, 1998.

———. (1996). *Object Relations Theory and Practice*. Northvale, N.J.: Jason Aronson.

Scharff, D. E., and Birtles, E. F. (eds.) (1994). *From Instinct to Self: Selected Papers of W. R. D. Fairbairn*, vol. 1. Northvale, N.J.: Jason Aronson.

Scharff, J. S. (1992). *Projective and Introjective Identification and the Use of the Therapist's Self*. Northvale, N.J.: Jason Aronson.

———. (1994) (ed.). *The Autonomous Self: The Work of John D. Sutherland*. Northvale, N.J.: Jason Aronson.

———. (1998). *Object Relations Individual Therapy*. Northvale, N.J.: Jason Aronson.

Scharff, J. S., and Scharff, D. (1992). *A Primer of Object Relations Therapy* (formerly Scharff Notes). Northvale, N.J.: Jason Aronson.

Shapiro, R. (1978). Ego psychology: its relations to Sullivan, Erikson and the object relations theorists. In J. Quen and E. Carlson (eds.). *American Psychoanalysis*. New York: Brunner Mazel, pp. 162–179.

Sutherland, J. D. (1980). The British object relations theorists: Balint, Winnicott, Fairbairn, Guntrip. *Journal of the American Psychoanalytic Association*, 28, no. 4: 829–860. In J. S. Scharff (ed.). *The Autonomous Self: The Work of John D. Sutherland*. Northvale, N.J.: Jason Aronson, pp. 25–44.

Winnicott, D. W. (1958). *Collected Papers: Through Pediatrics to Psycho-Analysis*. London: Tavistock. (Reprinted by Hogarth Press, 1975).

———. (1965). *The Maturational Processes and the Facilitating Environment*. London: Hogarth Press.

———. (1971). *Playing and Reality*. London: Tavistock.

Yankelovich, D., and Barrett, W. (1970). *Ego and Instinct*. New York: Random House.

JILL SAVEGE SCHARFF

Obsessional Phenomena

"Obsessional neurosis is unquestionably the most interesting and repaying subject of analytic research," or so Freud claimed in 1926. He also noted that as a problem it was not yet mastered and that the effort to penetrate more deeply into its nature required that one rely on "doubtful assumptions and unconfirmed suppositions" (1926, p. 113). This article examines how efforts since the publication of *Inhibitions, Symptoms and Anxiety* have added both to the understanding of the etiology of the obsessional neurosis per se and, more important, to the clarification of the more general problem, that is, the propensity to obsessional behavior in whatever form or context it may occur. This distinction is made repeatedly but not always adhered to, especially in the discussions of etiology. The *Glossary of Psychoanalytic Terms and Concepts* (Moore and Fine, 1967), for example, has separate entries for obsessions and the obsessive-compulsive neurosis, but it offers an etiologic hypothesis only for the latter.

The vagueness and imprecision to which Freud alluded has to do with the origins of obsessional phenomena, not with their manifestations in neurosis. That he made this distinction is clear from his characterization of Dora's mother. He wrote: "this condition, traces of which are to be found often enough in normal housewives, inevitably reminds one of forms of obsessional washing and other kinds of obsessional cleanliness. But such women . . . are entirely without insight into their illness, so that one essential characteristic of obsessional neurosis is lacking" (Freud, 1905: 20).

With regard to the etiology of the neurosis, he was quite certain. He wrote that it "originates in the same situation as hysteria, namely the necessity of fending off the libidinal demands of the Oedipus complex." With equal apparent certitude he goes on to say, "Every obsessional neurosis seems to have a substratum of hysterical symptoms that have been formed at a very early stage. But it is subsequently shaped along quite different lines owing to a *constitutional* factor. The genital organization of the libido turns out to be feeble and insufficiently resistant, so that when the ego begins its defensive efforts the first thing it succeeds in doing is to throw back the genital organization (of the phallic phase), in whole or in part, to the earlier sadistic-anal level. This fact of regression is decisive for all that follows" (1926, p. 112). With few if any modifications, this etiologic hypothesis has continued to enjoy close to universal support among analysts. Thus, in 1965, at the international congress devoted to obsessional neurosis, Anna Freud wrote that obsessional defenses occur when the ego matures more rapidly than the drive "with the result that anal-sadistic traits only come to the height of their expression after the ego

and superego are too far advanced in their development to tolerate them" (1966, p. 117). Again, Munich (1986), in discussing brief episodes of a specific form of compulsive behavior in a man with significant chronic obsessional character traits, uses essentially the same formulation— with the addendum that the exacerbation of symptoms may have been precipitated by the implied threat of separation.

Accounting for obsessiveness, outside the context of a neurosis, is not so clear-cut. In this area, confusion, doubtful assumptions, and unconfirmed suppositions appear to be rampant. It is not at all clear, for example, whether we have the same event or state in mind when we talk about obsessional thinking, obsessional character, or being obsessed with something. It is also questionable whether, when we use the adjective "obsessive" in these various contexts, we are characterizing the same "thing." As Sandler and Hazard (1960) have observed, we use the word "obsessional" alternatively as a term of opprobrium and one of approbation. Indeed, one is hard put to state in clear defining terms what that something, to which we allude as obsessional, is. Is there a common referent that includes all the already enumerated uses and also makes sense in relation to Freud's (1905) characterization of religion as a group obsessional neurosis and the obsessional neurosis as a private religion?

The very breadth of the word's use leaves open the possibility that what we refer to as "obsessional" is some generalized form of behavior or character structure, the various manifestations of which share only a final common path. Is it possible, in other words, that to characterize someone as obsessional has no more etiological significance than to say, "He has a headache"? Could it be that just as the symptom headache may derive from a multiplicity of entirely independent antecedent circumstances, so may instances of obsessiveness have in common only some behavioral manifestations that we designate "obsessional"? Although this position would not be very popular among analysts, it does have some historical as well as contemporaneous empirical support. Paul Schilder (1938) proposed to regard the dyskinesia of individuals with post-encephalitic Parkinson-like disease as obsessional. Zohar and Insel (1988) have more recently reviewed efforts to treat obsessional disorders pharmacologically. There appears to be a developing consensus that troubling symptomatology may be beneficially affected by monoamine reuptake inhibitors. According to these authors, this is most impressively the case with respect to serotonin. It would appear, however, that we are looking at a very general effect. Drugs that can alleviate as many symptoms as these synaptic reuptake blockers can hardly be assumed to be affecting specific etiologic complexes with laserlike precision. In this regard, too, a review of the anatomic organization of serotonergic neural systems (Molliver, 1987) makes it clear that they are widely distributed throughout the forebrain and the limbic cortex. In a commentary on the use of serotonin reuptake inhibitors, Pigott and Murphy have observed that effective treatment is characterized by only partial remission of symptoms. A parsimonious conclusion would be that the serotonergic system is somehow involved in the mechanism of expressing obsessional phenomena but does not help us understand why such phenomena occur.

Many years ago, Abraham (1921) pointed out that when they are euthymic, individuals who suffer from major affective disorders are characterologically obsessional. Much more recently it has been pointed out by many observers (e.g., Molliver, 1987) that pharmacologic agents and electroconvulsive therapy, which are effective in the treatment of affective disorders, also block serotonin reuptake. The belief that obsessional symptoms are associated with the propensity to experience major affective disorders has, in other words, been endorsed on both psychodynamic and neuropharmacologic grounds.

But to return to more immediate psychological problems, it is self-evident that an hypothesis that will account for obsessional neurosis cannot be sufficient to account for all obsessional phenomena as they are seen in individuals who, like Dora's mother, did not, according to Freud, suffer from a neurosis. It is also clear, from his writings about religion (Freud, 1905b) and taboo (Freud, 1913), in which he drew parallels between widespread and highly adaptive models of behavior and obsessional phenomena, that Freud recognized the importance of not confusing a clinical syndrome, in which obsessive modes of adaptation are prominent, with obsessive phenomena per se.

For the neurosis, Freud emphasized a predisposition, perhaps in his view, constitutional, that must be present. As has already been noted, the importance of the libidinal fixation, in the face of Oedipal conflict, on regression to anal phase modes of adaptation was emphasized not only by Freud but also by most early analytic writers. Some of the latter (e.g., Abraham, 1921; Landauer, 1939;

Weissman, 1956), however, also noted the importance of the compliance of the child and the imperative that he or she accommodate parental demands—the making, in Abraham's words, of a virtue out of a necessity. All also stressed that the imperative to comply with parental demands and strictures was by no means restricted to bowel function. The metaphorical quality of the phrase "anal phase" is well attested to by such alternative characterizations of the same period as Mahler's practicing subepoch of separation individuation, Erickson's autonomy vs. self-doubt, and Spitz's third organizer, "No."

Most psychoanalytic writings about obsessions unfortunately ignore the cognitive limitations of youngsters at this stage of their development. This subject was addressed by Sandler and Joffe (1965). Regrettably, little attention has been paid to it since. Children, in Piaget's terms, are "pre-operational"; they live in an egocentric, animistic, and phenomenalistic world in which their idea of causality is pretty much limited to the assumption that when something good or untoward happens, it is a consequence of their behavior. The differentiation between these alternatives is, of course, the prerogative of the parent. Children can know only *after the fact* whether their acts are blameworthy or praiseworthy. The level of the cognitive competence of youngsters of this age is indicated by such widely prevalent convictions as that a "hole is to dig," "that it gets dark at night because it is time to go to bed," and so on. In brief, toddlers live in a very different cognitive world from that of their parents. Adults are both indispensable and inscrutable. Consequently, toddlers' understanding of their communications, including both their strictures and their approbations, may have little to do with the parents' intentions. Because the youngsters are of the age to be phenomenalistic in their interpretation of events, if a particular piece of behavior seems to have a consistent relation to a particular outcome, they accept their causal connections both as self-evident and as requiring no further investigation. At least from the perspective of the observing adult, children of this age function as though they are believers in and practitioners of magic. To achieve their ends, toddlers must carry out rituals, i.e., behaviors that are required by the adult if their desires are to be requited. How or why particular behaviors are required by adults and what makes them important is beyond chilren's ability to understand. That it should bring a particular reaction, whether positive or negative, is a parental decision, a decision by the same inscrutable authority who will define, however clearly or vaguely, what is bad and indifferent as well as what is good and praiseworthy. A child's impossible task is to anticipate what the parent's definition of "good" at any given point will be. Furthermore, because this is not a sharply defined parent with whom the child has a simple "whole object" relation, the youngster is not able to anticipate such vagaries of parenting as might derive from adult concerns or changes in physiologic state that may make the loving parent of yesterday an irritable and critical parent today. How, for example, is the toddler to understand the change in behavior of a mother who is suffering from premenstrual stress disorder?

If their efforts to achieve approbation fail, toddlers try harder to do what they understand is required. Ultimately, these efforts may lead to a despairing state, a state that in its adult incarnation was epitomized by a woman who, when she failed to win my approval, would say, "I can't get it right, I can't get it right." Her conviction that I had a criterion for "right" and that once she figured it out she would be able to bask in my continuing approval was, at that time, unshakable. It is of more than passing interest that the theme of "getting it right," the axiom (or better, the pseudoaxiom) that there is a right way, a way to do things that will ensure approbation or protect against an adverse outcome, is a repeated theme in behavior we regard as obsessional. Not the least of the questions this patient presented was to explain the persistence of such an infantile, "magical" conviction, especially as she was a highly sophisticated professional person who had long since transcended the more naive use of magical connections. Her problem was certainly not unique. Circumscribed mini-obsessions are ubiquitous. They range, after all, from knocking on wood to the evocative use of prayer. The origin of such behavior in the turbulent pre-Oedipal years seems fairly straightforward. Not so clear is how to explain the persistence of adult obsessional phenomena observed in most of us.

The foregoing alluded to the numerous contexts in which the word "obsession" is used. Now let us turn to a consideration of the conceptual underpinning that makes it possible to apply this designation to so many apparently diverse phenomena. It is with this objective in mind that a consideration of the word's etymological origins is relevant. The *Unabridged Oxford English Dictionary* (1933) tells us that the word "obsess" derives from the Latin verb *"obsidare,"* and that it meant in its original usage "to sit at or opposite to, to beset or besiege," as in a military

operation; that is, it explicitly referred to an external, alien, threatening force with respect to which one might say a community was compelled to take defensive action, otherwise stated to make adaptations. With time, the obsession agent became less precisely defined as to location, and the objective of the obsession also became less narrowly defined. By the mid–sixteenth century, the very specific meaning "siege" in a military sense had been extended to include, and was ultimately replaced by, the connotations of "to haunt or to harass as by evil spirits." Pari passu, to be obsessed also came to be an experience to which an individual as well as a community could be subject. As recently as during the mid–nineteenth century, the word was still used to refer to being "beset by foreign, backstairs and domestic influences, by obsessions at home and abroad." It is only in the Supplement (vol. 3, 1982) that the word, both by definition and by illustrative example, takes on the primary connotation of a process going on within the psyche of an individual. Not surprisingly, it is also at this time that the illustrative examples come from the psychoanalytic literature. That this derivation from a word, which in its original meaning had to do with the imperative to respond to an external force, is no mere vagary of its Latin origin is indicated by the fact that the German equivalent, *"Zwang,"* has a similar derivation. The conceptual similarity of their origins to the adaptive exigencies that confront the pre-Oedipal child vis-à-vis his or her parents should be clear.

It is evident, however, that throughout its etymological history the term "to obsess" has referred to the influence of an agency to whose intentions, however inscrutable, originally a community and, later, an individual is constrained to make "appropriate" responses. Since "appropriate" in this context is knowable only after the fact and in the form of the reaction of the obsessing agency, doubt and uncertainty is inevitable as inherent properties of obsessional behavior.

REFERENCES

Abraham, K. (1921). Contributions to the theory of the anal character. In E. Jones (ed.). *Selected Papers on Psychoanalysis.* London: Hogarth Press, 1949, pp. 370–392.

Chekov. A. (1897). *Uncle Vanya.* In *Uncle Vanya and Other Plays by Anton Chekov.* Trans. Betsy Hulick. New York: Bantam Books, 1994.

Freedman, D. A. (1971). On the genesis of obsessional phenomena. *Psychoanalytic Review,* 58: 367–383.

Freud, A. (1966). Obsessional Neurosis: A summary of psychoanalytic views as presented at the Congress. *International Journal of Psychoanalysis,* 47: 116–122.

Freud, S. (1905a). Fragment of an analysis of a case of hysteria. S.E. 9: 15–122.

———. (1905b). Obsessional acts and religious practices. S.E. 9: 117–128.

———. (1913). *Totem and Taboo.* S.E. 13: 1–162.

———. (1926). *Inhibitions, Symptoms, and Anxiety.* S.E. 20: 77–178.

Ishiguro, K. (1989). *Remains of the Day.* New York: Vintage International.

Landauer, K. (1939). Some remarks on the formation of the anal-erotic character. *International Journal of Psycho-Analysis*, 20: 418–425.

Molliver, M.E. (1987). Serotonergic neuronal symptoms: What their anatomic organization tells us about function, *Journal of Clinical Psychopharmacology* (Supplement), 3S: 245.

Moore, B. E., and Fine, B. D. (1967). *Glossary of Psychoanalytic Terms and Concepts.* New York: American Psychoanalytic Association.

———. (1990). *Psychoanalytic Terms and Concepts.* New York: American Psychoanalytic Association.

Munich, R. L. (1986). Transitory symptom formation in the analysis of an obsessional character. *Psychoanalytic Study of the Child*, 4: 515–536.

Piaget, J. (1932). *The Moral Judgment of the Child.* Trans. Marjorie Gabain. London: Kegan Paul.

Sandler, J., and Hazari, A. (1960). The obsessional: On the psychological classification of obsessional character traits and symptoms. *British Journal of Medical Psychology*, 33: 113–122.

Sandler, J., and Joffe, W. G. (1965). Obsessional manifestations in children. *Psychoanalytic Study of the Child*, 20: 425–438.

Schilder, P. (1938). The organic background of obsessions and compulsions. *American Journal of Psychiatry*, 94: 1398.

The New Compact Oxford Unabridged Dictionary (1971). "Obsession." Oxford: Oxford University Press, 1933.

The New Compact Oxford Unabridged Dictionary, Supplement (1982). "Obsession," vol. 3.

Weismann, P. (1956). On pregenital compulsive phenomena and the repetition compulsion, *Journal of the American Psychoanalytic Association*, 4: 503–510.

Zohar, J., and Insel, T. R. (1988). Diagnosis and treatment of obsessive-compulsive disorder. *Psychiatric Annals*, 18: 168–171.

DAVID A. FREEDMAN

Occult, and Freud

In spite of his philosophical commitment to materialism and scientific naturalism, Freud had a long-standing interest in extrasensory perception. Although he rejected belief in disembodied spirits and clairvoyance, Freud came to believe in the reality of telepathic thought transference.

A number of Freud's distinguished contemporaries such as James, Myers, Bleuler, Charcot, Richet, Schrenck-Notzing, Bergson, Hall, Dessoir, and Flournoy were involved in the investigation of occult phenomena during the closing decades of the nineteenth and the early years of the twentieth century (Shamdasani, 1994). Freud's earliest direct exposure to the scientific study of extrasensory perception may have occurred during his stay in Paris in 1885–1886, when Paul Janet read two papers at a meeting of the Société de Psychologie Physiologique, with Charcot in the chair, reporting on his nephew Pierre's experiments using long-distance telepathic suggestion with his hysterical patient Léonie. In 1889 he mentioned Forel's discussion of telepathy in his review of the latter's *Hypnotism* (Freud, 1889).

In the 1907 edition of *The Psychopathology of Everyday Life*, Freud (1901) expressed a skeptical but open-minded attitude toward occult phenomena. On March 4, 1908, Freud presented three cases of apparent telepathy to the Vienna Psychoanalytic Society, and demonstrated that each instance could be satisfactorily explained without recourse to the idea of extrasensory perception. The subject was again discussed in 1910 (Nunberg and Federn, 1962).

In 1909, on the way back from their lectures at Clark University in the United States, Freud and Ferenczi stopped to visit a medium in Berlin (Jones, 1957). This led to a series of letters between Freud and Ferenczi concerning extrasensory perception (Brabant, Falzeder, and Giampieri-Deutsch, 1993). Freud expressed skepticism and stated that if experimentation were to establish the existence of telepathy, the phenomenon must have a materialistic explanation. Freud was finally convinced by Ferenczi's report of an experience with one of his patients that seemed to him to have "shattered the doubts about the existence of thought transference" (p. 211). Freud was concerned that Ferenczi's ideas would bring psychoanalysis into disrepute and asked him to keep them secret. On November 23, 1913, a séance was held in Freud's home with a medium, but neither Freud nor the analysts in attendance were favorably impressed. Freud and Ferenczi's shared interest in extrasensory perception eventuated in three-way telepathic experiments involving Ferenczi, Freud, and Freud's daughter Anna (Jones, 1957). Freud found these convincing but dissuaded Ferenczi from publicly reporting on them.

Freud became a member of the English Society for Psychical Research in 1911. He accepted honorary membership in the American Society for Psychical Research in 1915 and the Greek Society for Psychical Research in 1923 (Jones, 1957). In a 1935 letter to Weiss (1970), Freud referred to the "fact" of thought transference. In a 1921 letter to Hereward Carrington, Freud wrote that if he were at the beginning of his career, he might choose the investigation of "so-called occult psychic phenomena" as his field of research (E. L. Freud, 1970: 339).

Freud expressed greater conviction about telepathy privately than he did publicly. This was in large measure due to his fear that an avowed interest in occult phenomena would call psychoanalysis into disrepute and provide ammunition to its enemies.

Freud's paper on *Psycho-analysis and Telepathy* was based on a presentation that he gave to the so-called Central Executive Committee of the International Psycho-Analytic Association (consisting of Freud, Rank, Ferenczi, Jones, Abraham, Eitingon, and Sachs) at a meeting in Germany's Harz Mountains in 1921. The presentation addressed the question "If we had to accept the phenomena summarized under the term 'telepathy,' how would it influence the theory and practice of psychoanalysis?" (Grosskurth, 1991: 107). The written version of the paper (Freud, 1941) was posthumously published in 1941b. It is more cautiously worded than the original presentation (Jones, 1957). Freud is careful to stress that telepathic phenomena must be given a naturalistic explanation. He then goes on to give three putative examples of thought transference.

Freud's first *published* work devoted to telepathy was his paper on *Dreams and Telepathy* (Freud, 1922), which was written shortly after the publication of a psychoanalytic study of telepathic dreams by Wilhelm Stekel. Freud presents and analyzes two accounts of ostensibly telepathic dreams provided by correspondents, and concludes that telepathic messages, if real, do not play a role in the formation of dreams but may become incorporated into the structure of a dream in much the same way as other stimuli. Freud also asserts "the incontestable fact that sleep creates favorable conditions for telepathy" (p. 219).

In the 1924 edition of *The Psychopathology of Everyday Life* (Freud, 1901), Freud confessed that "in the last few years I have had a few remarkable experiences which might easily have been explained on the hypothesis of telepathic thought-transference" (p. 262). This is almost certainly a reference to the experiments conducted by him, his daughter Anna, and Ferenczi.

Freud used some of the material from the 1921 presentation for his discussion of "The Occult Significance of Dreams" in a paper on *Some Additional Remarks on Dream Interpretation as a Whole* (Freud, 1925). A year before, in the 1924 edition of *The Psychopathology of Everyday Life*, Freud had given his first published endorsement of telepathy. In the 1925 paper, Freud asserts that "it may well be that telepathy really exists" (p. 136). He suggests that "thought-transference . . . comes about particularly easily at the moment at which an idea emerges from the unconscious, or, in theoretical terms, as it passes over from the 'primary process' to the 'secondary process'" (p. 138). Apparently referring to the experiments with Anna and Ferenczi, Freud writes: "I have often had an impression, in the course of experiments in my private circle, that strongly emotionally colored recollections can be successfully transferred without much difficulty" (p. 138).

Freud's final published work on telepathy was the chapter on "Dreams and Occultism" in the *New Introductory Lectures on Psycho-analysis* (1933). Freud once again used material from the 1921 presentation. A new theme in this paper is the idea that telepathic communication may have been the "original, archaic method of communication between individuals" (p. 55) that has been overlaid by the more effective method of sensory communication. This in turn leads to the hypothesis that telepathy should be particularly evident in the mental life of children. Freud goes as far as to suggest that the common childhood anxiety that one's parents can read one's mind may be related to childhood telepathy.

Freud states in the 1933 work:

> The telepathic process is supposed to consist in a mental act in one person instigating the same mental act in another person. What lies between these two mental acts may easily be a physical process into which the mental one is transformed at one end and which is transformed back once more into the same mental one at the other end. The analogy with other transformations, such as occur in speaking and hearing by telephone, would then be unmistakable. (Freud, 1933: 55)

Anna Freud, wrote to Ernest Jones that "I never could see that he [Freud] himself believed in more than the possibility of two unconscious minds communicating with each other without the help of a conscious bridge" (A. Freud, cited in Gay, 1988: 445). In fact, Freud's telephone metaphor first appeared in his writings in the context of a discussion of unconscious communication. Freud wrote:

> To put it in a formula: he [the analyst] must turn his own unconscious like a receptive organ towards the transmitting unconscious of the patient. He must adjust himself to the patient as a telephone receiver is adjusted to the transmitting microphone. Just as the receiver converts back into sound waves the electric oscillations in the telephone line which were set up by sound waves, so the doctor's unconscious is able, from the derivatives of the unconscious which are transmitted to him, to reconstruct that unconscious, which has determined the patient's free-associations. (1912, pp. 115–116)

This paper was written during the height of Freud's correspondence with Ferenczi concerning telepathic events in the psychoanalytic situation. It is possible that Freud believed the derivatives of the patient's unconscious are "transmitted" *telepathically* to the unconscious of the analyst.

REFERENCES
Brabant, E., Falzeder, E., and Giampieri-Deutsch, P. (eds.) (1993). *The Correspondence of Sigmund Freud and Sándor Ferenczi.* Trans. Peter T. Hoffer. Cambridge, Mass.: Harvard University Press.
Eisenbud, J. (1953). Psychiatric contributions to psychiatry: A review. In G. Devereux (ed.). *Psychoanalysis and the Occult.* New York: Basic Books.
Freud, E. L. (1970). *Letters of Sigmund Freud: 1873–1939.* Trans. Tania Stern and James Stern. London: Hogarth Press.
Freud, S. (1889). Review of Forel's *Hypnotism.* S.E. 1: 91–102.
———. (1901). *The Psychopathology of Everyday Life.* S.E. 6: 1–279.
———. (1912). Recommendations to physicians practicing psycho-analysis. S.E. 12: 111–120.
———. (1922). Dreams and telepathy. S.E. 18: 196–221.
———. (1925). Some additional notes on dream-interpretation as a whole. S.E. 19: 125–138.
———. (1933). *New Introductory Lectures on Psycho-analysis.* S.E. 22: 5–185.
———. (1941a). A premonitory dream fulfilled. S.E. 5: 623–625.
———. (1941b). Psycho-analysis and telepathy. S.E. 18: 177–193.
Gay, P. (1988). *Freud: A Life for Our Time.* London: J. M. Dent and Sons.
Grosskurth, P. (1991). *The Secret Ring: Freud's Inner Circle and the Politics of Psychoanalysis.* Reading, Mass.: Addison-Wesley.
Jones, E. (1957). *The Life and Work of Sigmund Freud, Vol. 3.* London: The Hogarth Press.
Nunberg, H., and Federn, E. (eds.) (1962). *Minutes of the Vienna Psycho-Analytic Society, Vol. 1.* New York: International Universities Press.
Paskauskas, R. A. (ed.) (1993). *The Complete Correspondence of Sigmund Freud and Ernest Jones, 1908–1939.* Cambridge, Mass.: Harvard University Press.
Shamdasani, S. (1994). Introduction to T. Flournoy. *From India to the Planet Mars.* New Haven, Conn.: Yale University Press.
Weiss, E. (1970). *Sigmund Freud as a Consultant: Recollections of a Pioneer in Psychoanalysis.* New York: Intercontinental Medical Book Corporation.

DAVID LIVINGSTONE SMITH

Oedipal Stage See OEDIPUS COMPLEX.

Oedipus Complex

"Oedipus complex" designates a complex emotional content, rooted in parental love and hate as a child's dynamics of wishes and anxieties, that brings about in an adult's life concerns and inhibitions inaccessible to consciousness but that play an important part in determining the child's intentions, actions, and judgments.

According to Freud's theory of development, every child passes through an Oedipal phase between its third and fifth year. I shall demonstrate how Freud makes a connection with the myth of Oedipus and interprets it, and how he elucidates the Oedipal dynamics, whose primary existence he dates from the early emotional development of the child, a development that its discoverer credits with central effects on an adult's capacity for love and work.

The Murder-Incest Catastrophe

From the outset, Freud's theory refers explicitly to a famous figure of Greek mythology and ancient tragedy. The Oedipus complex, which derives its name from Greek mythology and drama, is named after King Oedipus. In his writings, Freud refers more than twenty times to the legend and to the tragedy by Sophocles; a particularly detailed discussion may be found in his *Interpretation of Dreams* (1900, pp. 261–264). Beginning with his first mention of the Greek legend in a letter to his friend Wilhelm Fliess (Freud, 1954; 1962, p. 238), dated October 10, 1897, Freud expressed particular interest in the emotional reaction of the public to Sophocles' play. Freud speaks as a reflective "recipient," i.e., he puts himself in the place of either the spectator or the reader, and argues on the basis of his emotional reaction. Boldly seizing hold of the literary pattern, he believes he can assume that the material substance of the Oedipal fate is the source of its fame, and he consequently treats the Greek prototypes in rather loose fashion. It cannot always be determined whether he is dealing with the Greek drama or merely with a traditional figure from a legend. Freud discerns in the fate of Oedipus an otherwise mute dynamics anchored in key elements of the scenario: Oedipus eliminates his own father by murdering him and takes his own mother as a wife. Oedipus is not sure that the person he marries is his mother or that the man he slays is his father. Having once been abandoned by his biological parents and raised under the royal care of others, he acts with no knowledge of his family situation.

Oedipus and the Involved Recipient

According to Freud, the fate of King Oedipus has involved the public from the very beginning, because (1) every son once wanted to remove his father and win his mother; (2) these powerful childhood wishes are obsolete and yet insuperable; (3) the powerful influence of the wishes that have become unconscious precludes the possibility of free action with informed responsibility. Freud emphasizes these aspects of the material and yet keeps returning to the example of a literary form, the tragedy of Sophocles, often without explicitly announcing or clearly demarcating it. Thus the perspective of Freud, the recipient—the reader or witness of the events—remains opaque because he does not distinguish between the traditional material and the poetic laws of the Sophoclean dramaturgy, even though he reacts to the latter very astutely and with great literary understanding.

The dramaturgy of Oedipus's lack of knowledge, the rhetorical function of which Freud does not explain, is indispensable for producing the public's positive reaction to the figure of Oedipus. This fact of nonknowledge permits us to depict this figure as a positive character. Portraying Oedipus as knowing what he was doing, for example, in slaying his father, would make the protagonist a villain. However, the dramaturgy of not knowing is merely an unspecific technique of producing sympathy (as presented by Aristotle in his *Poetics*; Fuhrmann, 1996: 39). It does not explain the special substance of tragic entanglement. According to Freud, Oedipus's fate is touching because he represents a central human concern that crystallizes within an individ-

ual's developmental history as a core conflict—a human concern that is generally subject to moral opprobrium. The point is that through his deeds the Oedipus figure obtains the right to rule as well as sexual rights that are extraordinarily attractive. In Freud's view, the reaction of shocked interest in a dramatic constellation that effectively shows Oedipus as a victor over a father who abandoned him as a helpless infant and in productive union with his mother/spouse derives from the fact that, prior to the catastrophe, the listeners are gripped by a wish fulfillment that causes them to side with Oedipus as a man who has been thrown off the victory track by preordained forces (Freud, 1900: 261ff.).

The Sophoclean Dramaturgy

Oedipus the King is constructed as an analytical drama— the play concentrates on a topical problematical situation that needs a solution. There have been relevant occurrences in prehistory, and these are represented on the stage and integrated into the action through the explicit introduction of characters as well as reports, particularly those given by messengers. The timely problematic situation that requires a solution is made clear as early as line forty-six. The plague is raging in Thebes. An aged priest, the spokesman of a group of supplicating inhabitants, begs Oedipus, the ruler, to save the city and consult the Delphic oracle for that purpose. The supplication already introduces Oedipus as a man of the highest reputation and an extraordinary bearer of hopes who is capable of interpreting a divine judgment and acting in accordance with it vigorously and responsibly. After all, he freed the city from the Sphinx solely by virtue of his intellectual superiority.

Creon, Oedipus's brother-in-law, conveys the Delphic judgment, which demands that the murderer or murderers of Laios, the former regent of Thebes, be apprehended and punished by being outlawed or killed. This is the start of the hero's well-thought-out investigation. He begins by inquiring why the bloody deed is still unsolved and learns that this has been prevented by the Sphinx's admonishment to let the matter rest. In line 262, the seer Teiresias, who has been summoned by Oedipus, announces after considerable reluctance that Oedipus is the man being sought. Oedipus at first denies the accusation and suspects that this outrageous defamation was part of an intrigue by the power-hungry Creon, who had induced Teiresias to lie in order to overthrow Oedipus. The rest of the play, which totals 1,530 lines, deals with the continued investigation by the hero. The evidence piles up in his disfavor. Gripped by an awful presentiment, Jocasta, the wife/mother, hangs herself and Oedipus blinds himself with her brooches. Creon becomes his lawful successor, and Oedipus humbly requests his protection for his two daughters, Ismena and Antigone, freedom for his sons Eteocles and Polyneices, and banishment for himself. Creon does not immediately grant this last request but wants to make his agreement dependent on the pronouncements of the oracle.

Emotion and Trembling

The principle of denied information, which is part of the dramaturgy of nonknowledge, removes the possible odor of reprehensibility from Oedipus's intentions. His enthronement and wedding took place in good faith as far as everyone was concerned. Everyone was willing to have the hero, a man unequaled in bravery, strength, and intellect, receive the deserved distinction and advancement.

The Oedipus of Sophocles' play is never suspected of having desired sexual union with his mother and of having actively pursued the elimination of his father. For that reason the public is able to feel the emotion of "*eleos*" (pity) for him and be shaken by "*phobos*" (fear) of that which befalls him (based on the sixth chapter of Aristotle's *Poetics*, cited by Steinmann, 1989: 76). Yet long before the development of the actual catastrophe, Oedipus knew himself as someone to whom the later fate of marriage and elimination was ascribed via divine prophecy. He does not regard this attribution as absurd. On the contrary, as Freud pointed out, he takes it seriously as a threatening possibility and attempts to take remedial action. He outwardly distances himself from the persons whom he regarded as his parents, but he does not try to escape physical clashes or marriage projects. In a fight with an older man, he displays no inhibition of the aggressive impulse. Nor does he recognize his mother in his (older) bride, and he is not inhibited in consummating the marriage. Thus the countermeasures taken by Oedipus are not effective.

Freud's View of Oedipus's Programmatic Unawareness

Freud sees the essence of the tragedy in the formation of an Oedipal wish scenario that conflicts with the taboo nature of this wish (Freud, 1916–1917: 331ff.). The tragedy begins with the open presentation of a masculine-Oedipal situation of wish fulfillment. Its forbidden nature determines the course of the action, and it does so without affecting the dignity of the hero or trivializing him as the victim of unfavorable accidents. This evidences, for one thing, a determination to punish himself that should not be misinterpreted as a masochistic impulse, for it is explicitly confessional in nature. Then, too, the Oedipus figure articulates itself in a central entanglement: This protagonist can be seduced by a momentary situation. Both in Sophocles' play and in the myth, he is carried away by anger. However, he may also be considered sexually seduceable, for he blinds himself with his wife's brooches, which accentuated her charms and "blinded" him. At the same time this protagonist is introduced as a man of extraordinary mental powers. By dint of his cerebral and deductive faculties, his detective work succeeds, but because of his instincts, he is partially blind about the nature of his actions.

At the same time, the Oedipus figure's plan of action is determined by partial recognition and avoidance of risks. When it becomes evident at the end of his investigative work that it has not been possible to avoid risks, Oedipus hastens not only to accept severe sanctions but to mete out punishment to himself, spurning any excuses.

Triumph of the Superior Man and Horrors of Punishment

The actions of the Sophoclean Oedipus figure may be understood as having been favored by silent accessories and fed by unstated interests of the protagonist. There are three factors:

1. Acclaim of the Thebans for the social and sexual successes of the hero.
2. Acceptance by the hero of the attribution of murder and incest.
3. Acclaim of the Thebans for the male superiority of the hero.

These three factors make a case for an identification with the hero on the basis of a specific motivation that is bound to weigh in the balance for the hero as well as the public because of its taboo nature. This taboo assumes graphic form in the general catastrophe of the plague (Freud, 1912–1913: 80) in Thebes, which the hero is politically responsible for combating.

If the fate of this tragic hero has a lasting emotional effect on the reader, this is, in Freud's view, because of the following:

1. Oedipus gets plaudits for perfectly attaining the sexual and assertive goals of a grown man.
2. The public appreciates that Oedipus gives credence to the judgment passed upon him—not only because of time-bound cultural and religious standards (which would concern only the form of the prophecy and not its specific contents), but because Oedipus considers this action possible in himself and the public shares his conviction.
3. That Oedipus slays Laios not only shows him as the man who acted but also demonstrates his superior manliness.

Wish Versus Objective Logic

In Freud's view (Freud, 1908: 146), the structure of the dramatic plot does not obey the laws of objective logic but the interest of the wish. In that sense, the recipient, who identifies with the Oedipus figure, enjoys the triumph of the superior man and at the same time experiences the terrors of the legal prohibition (Freud, 1916–1917: 331). In light of the latter, the man is to be expelled from human society, but the structure of the tragedy does not affect his attractiveness or diminish the admiration for his achievements as a ruler, husband, and father. The tragedy is able to have this effect because the core conflict, relating to the elimination of the father and the incestuous union with the mother, is so well established that all concerned evoke this ideational circle in the interplay between approach and distancing.

The Perspective of the Man and the Perspective of the Child

Why should the wish for elimination be directed precisely against the biological father and interest in a sexual conflict precisely at the biological mother? A complete analysis would take account of both the perspective of the child and that of the mature man represented in the tragedy. The perspective of the child is articulated in the fateful verdict that determines that Oedipus shall pursue the goal of murder and incest. The perspective of the mature man is articulated in the presentation of the protagonist's rationality. The reader commits himself emotionally on the basis of an attitude that, according to Freud, reflects the perspective of the child who knows what it means to desire the sexual conquest of the mother (who, to the child, is young and has certainly not aged—Freud, 1905: 178), as well as the elim-

ination of the father and exposure to the horror of a mutilating punishment.

Oedipus: The Material and the Drama

The juxtaposition of the Oedipus material and the Oedipus drama is theoretically significant. The material itself does not have either a positive or a negative resonance; only the communicative content of its dramatic adaptation invites an emotional response. If Freud attributes the enduring popularity of *Oedipus the King* to the content of the play, he is evidently guided by the idea that this subject has been prepared in the psyche of the recipient as a scenario or an "ideational complex" and, as it were, finds its counterpart in the foundation of the tragedy as freed from the scenery. In this view, the material or the "ideational complex" constitutes the causally effective core and the communicative structuring of the vehicle that is replaceable, exchangeable, and capable of being presented to the public.

The Oedipal Core

Thus the "material" must be viewed as the linguistic substitute for a psychic dynamics. From this it may be concluded that wherever thematically related configurations, "reworkings in the imagination" (Freud, 1918: 29), may be encountered in the world of individuals, psychic dynamics are kindled and the individual reacts emotionally.

With this Freud postulates a psychic core as a motivated configuration of wishes and anxieties in relation to a love-filled and hate-filled triad of parents and child. This motivated configuration is preserved in psychic latency and makes itself felt in traces or indirectly when it encounters thematically congenial configurations. Freud takes another step and speculatively identifies a phylogenetic source for the infantile Oedipal dynamics in possible real events of a prehistoric period. Thus that which now enjoys a singular right to existence in the world of wishes and anxieties (if one disregards familial murders and sex offenses) was "once reality in the primeval times of the family of man" (Freud, 1916–1917: 371; 1918: 191). In *Totem and Taboo* (1912–1913), Freud constructs a prehistoric deed of a primal horde, a collective parricide and maternal incest, as a myth of origin that, according to him, is the source of relevant primal fantasies in ontogenesis (Freud, 1918: 193).

Freud's conception opens up a prospect of comprehending central forms of human living arrangements and human productivity as motivated. Nevertheless, the question of the relationship between "material" and "form," "scenario" and "drama," psychic configuration and life scene remains unclarified.

Emotional commitment, identifying role playing, exciting, lustful, or anxiety-laden involvement with what happens on the stage materializes neither as a reaction to the mere material nor to any specific arrangement of it. Not every parricide on the stage moves the audience, not every Oedipal fate of a young man that is given literary expression prompts suicidal decisions, as a reading of *The Sorrows of Young Werther* did; not every triumphant lover of women fascinates like Don Giovanni.

In the Freudian conception, the Oedipal motivation of an individual is unconscious after the "destruction and elimination of the complex" in early childhood (Freud, 1924a: 177). Only its return—in fact, its fresh experience in the framework of an analytic treatment—gains it articulation, while a sober explanation by itself would remain wholly ineffectual. This viewpoint was current as early as 1895: "Affectless remembrance is almost always completely ineffective; the psychic process that originally ran its course must be repeated as vividly as possible" (Breuer and Freud, 1893–1895: 6).

If the analyst insists that the Oedipal situation newly experienced in analysis is only a new version of an infantile precoinage, he will have little with which to counter the reproach that what he observes is the product of his own implicit suggestions (Grünbaum, 1984: 218).

The thematic core of the Oedipus legend has no emotional resonance. Nevertheless, this psychologically interesting question remains: What motivates readers or viewers to concern themselves with *Oedipus the King*, and why do Oedipus scenarios enjoy particular prominence?

Conditions of a Primary Object Choice
In the play, Oedipus is predestined to have sexual and aggressive encounters as an adult with his parents. The reader or witness to the play, when a child, unconsciously wanted to encounter the parents in this way. This desire is explained by psychoanalytic premises:

1. The parents enjoy the (temporal and psychic) primacy of the child's attention.
2. The child has a primary developmental task of organizing and regulating its instincts.
3. The phallic stage of organization requires the choice of a partner for the satisfaction of instincts.
4. The choice is the mother figure as a familiar guarantor of solicitous and partially exciting intimacy.

5. As a result, there has to be a rebellion against the father's claim to exclusive intimacy with the mother.
6. The child fears being exposed to the sanctions of the father and the parents.

Active Establishment of the Oedipal Triad
The child enters the Oedipal conflict in the course of the development of its partial phallic impulses. There develops a dynamic configuration between the child and its sexual options, which are determined primarily by the partial phallic impulse, the mother, who is the object of choice, and the father as the privileged sexual partner of the mother. The chosen one is the mother figure as the person familiar to the child from the very beginning, the caring, nurturing, protective, calming, and stimulating companion in physical contact (Freud, 1925a: 249). The past closeness (Freud, 1905,: 223ff.) is to enter into a new phase. Its distinguishing feature is that the child, which was once the recipient of tender and sensual devotion, now becomes an active wooer. Its partial phallic impulse constitutes a physical experience that offers new chances.

Oedipal Triads
In connection with Sophocles' tragedy, Freud postulates a constellation of relationships that includes two parents and a son in a conflictual motivation situation. The son desires sexual intimacy with the mother to the exclusion of the father. He wishes to abandon the position of the child and to assume the position of the father. This constellation is regarded as the classical male positive Oedipus complex.

The classical male negative Oedipus complex involves the son's wish to produce sexual intimacy with the father to the exclusion of the mother.

The classical female positive Oedipus complex is characterized by the girl's wish to establish sexual intimacy with the father to the exclusion of the mother. However, unlike the male child, the girl desires the father in hope for compensation and hates the mother out of disappointment (Freud, 1924a: 178ff.).

Freud is skeptical about the possibility of a negative female Oedipus complex, pointing out that the daughter's motivational situation does not fit: While the little girl remains attached to her mother intensively and for a long time, in this attachment she is dependent and hopes for a better physical (phallic) equipment. According to Freud, the desire to assume the position of a privileged parent figure does not play an important part for the female child, and neither does the desire, in contrast to the male child, to impress and lure the mother with the child's own sexual potency and competence. If the founder of psychoanalysis clung to this viewpoint, however, this would lead to a demand to take back the generalization that the Oedipus complex is the kernel of the neuroses (Freud, 1931: 226). Consequently, Freud resorts to a terminological stretch, albeit a vague one, in the face of the "intensity and passionate nature" of lengthy phases of "exclusive attachment to the mother" (1931, p. 226) in which "the father is for the girl not much more than a burdensome rival" (1931, p. 248).

Oedipal Triads from a Paternal or Maternal Perspective

Freud sketches Oedipal constellations almost exclusively from the perspective of the child. However, different perspectives are possible. For example, from the father's viewpoint, the position of the child can appear as specifically privileged. The father may feel that he is barred from an exclusive mother-child communal relationship with its unmistakable pleasure premium. Or the father might devalue the status and attractiveness of his adult love partner in favor of the child as a love object—for instance, in enthusiastic affection for the figure of a little son in the role of the radiant, promising male hope that the father would have liked to play in the past. He may also sexually privilege a little daughter figure; this would have the advantage of freeing him from a confrontation with well-developed primary and secondary female sexual characteristics.

Female and Male Oedipus Complex

Freud assumes a primary parallelism in the psychic development of both genders. The forms of satisfaction of drives, the object relationships, and the conflict dynamics of the first developmental phase, which organizes itself around orality, are basically the same for both genders. Following the process of ingesting food through breast feeding or bottle feeding, both genders experience a first sexual satisfaction through sucking, with the lips as the first erogenous zone (Freud, 1905: 180).

Freud defines "sexuality" as a pleasurably stimulated corporeality that runs parallel for both genders. This means that the differentiation between organ erotism and specifically sexual hedonic gain is not possible in the earliest phase of human development and does not become differentiated until the time of physical maturity, the point at which it is possible to distinguish for the first time between the pleasure of sexual excitement and that of sexual satisfaction. In this way, Freud expands the meaning of "sexuality" and also detaches it from object relationships (Freud, 1905: 183). At first, a child's sexual object is only a sexually indeterminate aid to fulfillment of its instinctual needs, a substitute for autoerotic activity, and a mere object of frustration or gratification. In the oral phase, the goal is incorporation of this object. The second phase of the anal (and subsequent anal-sadistic) organization requires seizure and subjugation of the object. Activities of tension and relaxation, control and submission, are prominent in the child's sphere of pleasurable activity. Added to this are rubbing up against the object, a testing of its strength and stability, pleasurable resistance and pleasurable submission, the aggressive pleasure of expulsion, and the titillating perseverance of retention. Freud emphasizes that in the anal phase the first clear outlines of "masculine" and "feminine" are equated with an active and a passive attitude and that "the sexual polarity and the outside object are already demonstrable" (Freud, 1905: 199).

In the development of both genders, gratification of the instincts, the realm of object relationships, and conflict dynamics revolve around the "phallus." Objects are classified according to whether or not they have an appropriate physical attribute. Both the female and the male child believe that every fully equipped individual must possess a clearly visible, generously proportioned, erectable stimulation center at the appropriate place. If this organ of extreme pleasure is missing, the child believes that it can only have been lost or become the victim of a punishment. This assumption causes girls to react with penis envy. In a formulation consistent with this, Freud should have spoken of envy of a phallic equipment that was deemed superior. Boys, fearing the loss of their phalluses struggle with castration anxiety. The use of the word "phallus" rather than "penis" emphasizes the product of an infantile fantasy in accordance with which in the framework of the child's physical image the erogenous zone is highly appreciated without consideration of the real biological differences between the genders. Freud believes that even girls unacquainted with the sexual anatomy of a male do not escape penis envy. What he has in mind is not only the child's observation of the genital equipment of pets, but also an association of size and strength, be it male or female, with phallic size and superiority (Freud, 1923; 1924a: 178).

In the phallic phase, infantile ideas and ideal conceptions of the sexual achievements of the phallic pleasure giver play the decisive role. (Freud speaks of specific childhood sexual theories, here the theory of "phallic primacy"—1925b, p. 36). According to Freud, a serious differentiation between male and female drive destinies does not appear until the phallic phase (Freud, 1918: 155):

> The boy enters the Oedipal phase and begins the manual handling of his penis, at the same time fantasizing about some sexual application of the penis to the mother until the combination of a threat of castration and the sight of a female's lack of a penis makes him experience the greatest trauma of his life, which initiates the latency period with all its consequences. After a futile attempt to emulate the boy, the girl experiences the recognition of her lack of a penis, or, rather, the inferiority of her clitoris, with lasting consequences for her character development. As a consequence of this first disappointment in rivalry, she frequently turns away from sex life in general. (p. 155)

The phallic phase also appears as a factor in the initial integration of the earlier sexual endeavors, and with the primacy of a sex organ. However, a young person does not exhibit a marked interest in the instruments of procreation and birth until puberty. This is in keeping with a fourth phase, which now really is genital:

> Firstly, some earlier libidinal cathexes have been retained; secondly, others are integrated into the sexual function as preparatory and auxiliary acts, the gratification of which produces what is known as forepleasure; thirdly, other urges are excluded from the organization and are either completely suppressed [repressed] or are employed in the ego in another way, forming character traits or undergoing sublimation with a displacement of their aims. (p. 155)

When a young person enters the Oedipal phase, the phallic desire is directed toward a love object with whom intimacy and community are to be established. At

this point, the girl experiences the futility of her courtship of the mother. The availability of a large, demonstrable pleasure organ is the supposed guarantee of an impressive equipment, but this "pleasure machine" has an object-related purpose as well. It is to be not merely evidence of the young person's own magnificence but also a lure for the desired partner in intimacy. The good fortune of an exclusive mother-daughter relationship to the exclusion of the world of fraternal competitors and paternal rivals would constitute the quintessence of a female negative Oedipal wish fantasy. However, as stated above, it remains unclear whether Freud views the existence of a negative Oedipus complex in girls as a regular phenomenon of early childhood, or whether he believes that the girl clings to the mother in a pre-Oedipal attachment for an indeterminate period of time then leaves her in favor of the father—perforce and reproachfully, so to speak, under the influence of a phallic hurt.

This is the key to the recording of a female's fate of dependency: While for a boy the Oedipus conflict fades to a distant future through an identification with the father and the postponement of the project "Find a wife like my mother," a girl, who has been disappointed by her mother, has no choice but to foster the object relationship with her father so as not to lose him as a donor of phallic goods. Related to this is the girl's dependence on outer limitations in place of the demands of the superego. While fear of a paternal castration threat causes a boy to identify with the father's prohibitions and commands at the end of the Oedipal development, it is the girl's aim to win the father over, to preserve her relationship with him, but not to internalize a paternal law-giving function (Freud, 1925a: 255ff.). This produces an inhibition of the girl's aggressive-expansive sphere, because the latter conflicts with fundamental dependency interests. Thus the development of female identity particularly favors the formation of those capacities that regulate a fundamental object dependence (on the love partner, the child, the mother) in the interest of one's own psychic equilibrium.

Decentering of the Primary Objects

In the service of parental approbation, a child accomplishes a "decentering" in the course of its growth to adulthood (Freud, 1918: 426). This achievement prompted Freud to assume that a girl has strong psychic interests to fight it. Decentering is a withdrawal of desire from the parental partners, an avoidance of the intimacy of love and hate with them, and a transformation of the affectionate and sensual parent-child relationship into a gentle and submissive familiarity (on the part of the child) with tactile limitations. This development, which should be imagined as long-term, includes the treatment of a child's individual early history.

Shared memories give the impulses of the first year the character of expressions and actions for which the individual is not responsible. These expressions and actions are not attributed to him, nor are the child's verbalizations interpreted as ways of expressing genuine desires. Utterances of a little boy to his mother indicating that he wants to marry her later; jealous attachment to her; a tendency to show off for her and woo her; a marked preference for her company to that of the father—all these things can be observed in the daily life of a child without the assumption of an incest motive or an intention to eliminate the father, and are not the occasion for calling the child to account. The Oedipal stirrings of the child are not regarded as intended actions or plans for action, but as evidence of the play character of a child's activities and expressivity (Freud, 1908: 144).

Wishes from a Psychoanalytic Point of View

Freud includes in his Oedipal theory the concept of "hallucinatory wish fulfillment." This concept refers to a primitive psychic activity, a primary form of psychic life. It serves as a hedonic tension regulator with limited effect in a deficit situation. Its principle is the temporary epistasis of an unpleasant condition by a hedonic "key." The temporary positive change in this condition that is effected by the hedonic correction of wish fulfillment appears sometimes with a concrete prospect of real gratification but, when there is no prospect of such gratification, in compensatory form (Freud, 1900: 550ff.).

Wish fulfillment constitutes a psychic evocation of hedonic experience, in such a way that the person involved fashions and enjoys a scenario of fulfillment with the resources of the imagination. Fashioning a wish-fulfilling scenario in one's imagination signifies not only a mere activity of imagining and picturing something, but also extends to the stage-managing of what exists. This means that an actual event presents itself as a candidate for the production of a wish fulfillment, provided that at least one of those involved evaluates what exists from the perspective of his or her wish, welcomes it, and

enjoys it. In this process of enjoyable appropriation, the actual event gains the character of a game or a feast (Freud, 1924b: 207). Thus this conception of wish and wish fulfillment explains neither an intentional nor a planned action in everyday life, nor does it clarify the development and organization of life goals. On the contrary, wish and wish fulfillment have no future perspective; they are decidedly oriented toward the present and exhaust themselves in the fantasy-produced enjoyment of the moment. If a boy says, "I want to marry you some day, mommy," he does not announce an intention but rather acts in his role as a love partner in the Oedipal drama and lures the person he is facing into it. Most of the time, the parents join in the playacting for a while as they emphasize and even demonstrate the playful elements.

REFERENCES

Breuer, J., and Freud, S. (1893–1895). *Studies on Hysteria*. S.E. 2: 19–305.

Freud, S. (1900). *The Interpretation of Dreams*. S.E. 4–5: 1–621.

———. (1901). *The Psychopathology of Everyday Life*. S.E. 6: 1–279.

———. (1905). *Three Essays on the Theory of Sexuality*. S.E. 7: 130–243.

———. (1908). Creative writers and day-dreaming. S.E. 9: 141–156.

———. (1912–1913). *Totem and Taboo*. S.E. 13: 1–161.

———. (1916–1917). *Introductory Lectures on Psycho-Analysis*. S.E. 15–16: 9–496.

———. (1918). From the history of an infantile neurosis. S.E. 17: 7–123.

———. (1920). The psychogenesis of a case of homosexuality in a woman. S.E. 18: 147–172.

———. (1923). *The Ego and the Id*. S.E. 19: 12–59.

———. (1924a). The dissolution of the Oedipus complex. S.E. 19: 173–179.

———. (1924b). A short account of psycho-analysis. S.E. 19: 191–209.

———. (1925a). Some psychological consequences of the anatomical distinction between the sexes. S.E. 19: 248–258.

———. (1925b). *An Autobiographical Study*. S.E. 20: 7–74.

———. (1931). Female sexuality. S.E. 21: 225–243.

———. (1940). *An Outline of Psycho-Analysis*. S.E. 23: 144–207.

———. (1954). *The Origins of Psycho-Analysis*. New York: Basic Books.

———. (1962). *Aus den Anfängen der Psychoanalyse, 1887–1902. Briefe an Wilhelm Fliess*. Frankfurt: Fischer.

Fuhrmann, M. (ed.) (1996). *Aristoteles. Die Poetik*. Stuttgart: Reclam.

Grünbaum, A. (1984). *Foundations of Psychoanalysis: A Philosophical Critique*. Berkeley: University of California Press.

BRIGITTE BOOTHE
TRANSLATED BY HARRY ZOHN

Oral Character

All theories of personality must somehow account for developmental changes throughout the life span. Freud's training as a physician made him sensitive to bodily structure and function during the course of physical and psychological maturation. Indeed, his theories have been called theories of the body.

He named the stages of development after body parts and body functions, beginning with the two pre-genital stages, the oral and the anal, then phallic, latency, and finally genital. These stages are not distinct but over-lap and merge, behavior at any one stage reflecting the presence of all that went before it. Freud used the metaphor of an army forced to leave troops behind at each obstacle encountered as it advances from its initial starting place, birth, to old age to explain the lasting effects on adult development of the pleasures and frus-trations encountered at each of the first four stages. Fix-ation, i.e., failure to move on to the next phase, can result for either of two reasons—excessive indulgence of the needs at that stage or frustration so extensive that the needs are not met.

The oral stage begins at birth and continues for the first year and a half or so. During this time, the infant is connected to the world by its mouth, and its existence is maintained only through the intervention of others, a circumstance deeply understood by both the child and its caretakers. These two characteristics—concern with the pleasures and frustrations experienced in the mouth and dependence on the goodwill of others for survival—mark the oral character. For this reason, the oral phase of development is frequently called the "oral dependent" stage, because both the satisfactions and the demands of orality and of dependency are experienced and need to be resolved. An early distinction between oral eroticism, marked by sucking, and oral sadism, marked by biting, has not received empirical support and is no longer made. Similarly disused is the once common theoretical separation of the stage into two parts—oral optimism, said to result from indulgence of oral needs, and oral pessimism, thought to result from frustration of oral needs—again because the distinction has failed to receive consistent confirmation from the empirical literature.

A number of personality measures, both objective and projective, have been used to assess orality. The most frequently used projective tests have been Blum's Blacky Test (Blum, 1949) and Masling et al. (1967) Rorschach measure, while Fisher (1970) and Lazare et al. (1966, 1970) have developed frequently used objective meas-ures of orality. The system for scoring Rorschach responses for oral-dependent content (Masling et al., 1967), the most widely used of these tests, provides one point each for any response mentioning oral activity; any body part connected to oral activity; any food source, food provider, or food object, any passive act or passive person, nurturers, and gift givers; any negation of oral percepts (e.g., empty cupboard, thin man, woman with no breasts); and baby talk (e.g., "bunny rabbit," "teeny weeny") in the speech of the test subject.

Empirical research results are consistent with many psychoanalytic hypotheses about oral dependence. As might be expected, food and alcohol abusers as well as ulcer patients report more oral images than control sub-jects. High oral scores are also reported in those who show such dependent behaviors as yielding in a group conformity situation, being compliant and "good" sub-jects in an experiment, praising authorities for their efforts, and looking for guidance when attempting a complex task. Oral people tend to be dutiful, partici-pating in required classroom experiments early in the semester rather than waiting until later. More than those with less pressing oral needs, they tend to believe in a kind, nurturing God and in a life after death. Because they are so needy themselves, demands made on them by children for nurturance are met more often by physical abuse than is true for nonoral parents.

For the oral person, the source of all good is exter-nal. As the infant needs the mother to survive, the oral person needs harmonious relationships with others to retain a constant source of support. As empirical research has demonstrated, to maintain good relations with others, the oral person develops greater skill in read-ing interpersonal cues than is true for nonorals. Oral clients can predict the values and attitude of their ther-apists more accurately than nonoral clients. Oral people manifest less autonomic nervous system arousal in stress-ful situations when another person is present than when they are alone, in contrast to nonoral people, for whom the presence of others does not ameliorate physiological arousal.

Although a large number of investigators have attempted to discover a link between early feeding prac-tices and later personality characteristics, the results defy a simple conclusion. Some research has found links between infant care and later personality but others have not. The best that can be said is that while it is likely that such a relationship exists, the specific, consistent details have yet to be discovered.

What remnants of the oral stage can be found in adults? Dependency, helplessness in difficult situations, a desire to please others, discomfort in having to nurture others, conformity and compliance, considerable participation in such oral behaviors as eating and drinking, and careful attention to interpersonal cues.

REFERENCES

Blum, G. S. (1949). A study of the psychoanalytic theory of psychosexual development. *Genetic Psychology Monographs*, 39: 3–99.

Fisher, S. (1970). *Body Experience in Fantasy and Behavior.* New York: Appleton-Century Crofts.

Lazare, A., Klerman, G. L., and Armor, D. J. (1966). Oral, obsessive and hysterical personality patterns. *Archives of General Psychiatry*, 14: 624–630.

———. (1970). Oral, obsessive and hysterical personality patterns: Replication of factor analysis in an independent sample. *Journal of Psychiatric Research*, 7: 275–290.

Masling, J. M., Rabie, L., and Blondheim, S. H. (1967). Obesity, level of aspiration, and Rorschach and TAT measures of oral dependence. *Journal of Consulting Psychology*, 31: 233–239.

                                JOSEPH M. MASLING

Oral Stage See DEVELOPMENTAL THEORY.

Overdetermination

A distinct kind of causal process associated with the productions of the unconscious, overdetermination functions through psychical conflict and the interaction and convergence of often contradictory forces.

The process of overdetermination is a dynamic one, tied up with the act of repression and the compromise between preconscious and unconscious forces in the production of psychical phenomena. For example, a dream or a symptom, each of which is a manifestation of this process, expresses both an unconscious wish and the repression of that wish. The forces at work in producing an overdetermined instance do not stand in an additive relation; they are, rather, interactive and cooperative, as well as opposed. A single element derived from this process will hence serve or represent multiple, and often contrary, purposes and meanings. "Overdetermination" hence refers to a process of nonlinear causality where the provoking causes of psychical phenomena such as

dreams and symptoms are neither individually necessary nor sufficient. Freud claims at one point in *Totem and Taboo* that "psychical acts and structures are invariably overdetermined" (1912–1913, p. 100), maintaining that the origin of complex psychical phenomena cannot be traced to a single source. The overdetermined instance is variously referred to by Freud as a nexus or a nodal point; we say that an instance (e.g., a symptom or a dream) is overdetermined if it represents more than one cause (idea, thought, affect, or force). A nodal point thus indicates the site where numerous trains of thought converge, and in this context Freud uses the metaphor of a "weaver's masterpiece" (1900, p. 283), indicating that the various ideas are knit together or interwoven. Freud most frequently uses the word "overdetermination" to describe the distinct kind of causality at work in the formation of dreams and symptoms.

Freud's most sustained account of overdetermination is to be found in *The Interpretation of Dreams*. In dreams, "overdetermination" denotes the process by which the dream is constructed, the development from the dream thoughts to the manifest content of the dream. Freud writes that "[n]ot only are the elements of a dream determined by the dream-thoughts many times over, but the individual dream-thoughts are represented in the dream by several elements" (1900, p. 284). In referring overdetermination to a nodal point that unites and relates diverse elements, Freud allies its processes to those of condensation and displacement (the primary processes of the unconscious). "Condensation" refers to the process by which many elements are combined into one that represents (and substitutes for, or "sacrifices") the others; "displacement" refers to the process by which meaning or affect is shifted from one idea to another (or a number of others). Together condensation and displacement guarantee that there will be numerous associative connections between the different elements at work in the creation of a dream or symptom. Freud clarifies this operation by stating that we ought not to think of the dream work as though each individual thought could find its own separate and individual representation; a thought is only represented, and a dream constructed, "by the whole mass of dream-thoughts being submitted to a sort of manipulative process in which those elements which have the most numerous and strongest supports acquire the right of entry into the dream-content" (1900, p. 284). At the same time, the wishes expressed in a dream are subject to censorship, and the dream must be understood as answering or representing both demands, that of the wish and that of censorship.

Freud also makes use of the concept of overdetermination in his early writings on hysteria in *Studies on Hysteria* (Breuer and Freud, 1895) to explain the formation of hysterical symptoms, and later develops and refines this concept in his analysis of Dora. In the instance of symptoms (especially hysterical symptoms, where psychical conflict is converted into somatic expression), we can clarify the meaning of overdetermination by observing its work in the production of a compromise formation. This production is evident in the case history of Dora, where each of her symptoms is found to have more than one exciting cause. Freud understands a compromise formation to be a reconciliation between competing forces that function in the establishment of a symptom. A symptom arises through "the mutual interference between two opposing currents" and represents "not only the repressed but also the repressing force" (1916–1917, p. 301). A symptom is hence the "outcome of a conflict," a more or less stable convergence of opposing determinants, each of which is condensed and displaced, so that the symptom might represent (and to some extent, satisfy) all of them. Because "it is supported from both sides" (p. 359), the symptom is particularly resilient: compromise formations are stable in that they signify, in repressed form, the ideas and affects that would otherwise remain only in tension with one another but are hereby able to reinforce one another. (They are, however, also unstable insofar as they represent a multiplicity of determinants, none of which is openly or fully represented; since the symptom does not entirely satisfy either force independently, and requires that each renounce some of its demands, it is not a final solution.) In the production of a compromise formation, as in all its productions, overdetermination operates not only by the accumulation of causes but, more important, by their conjunction and entanglement, i.e., according to "the principle of the complication of causes" (1901, pp. 60–61), as Freud writes in *The Psychopathology of Everyday Life* (which moreover indicates that jokes and slips of the tongue are also to be understood as instances of overdetermination).

The forces at work in the production of an overdetermined instance are not only numerous but may often be contradictory as well, and yet it is precisely for this reason that they are able to sustain that instance. Dreams and symptoms are therefore a site not only of stability but also of instability, contention, and crisis; they are ambiguous, representing both conscious and unconscious determinants, and since it is likely that the conscious element will efface or conceal the unconscious one, the analytic process requires "over-interpretation." To uncover the various meanings of a dream or symptom, the analyst must keep in mind that the product of overdetermination is an ambiguity whose meanings might well be in complete contradiction. The process of condensation indicates that there will likely be multiple meanings, and that these meanings will be layered as well as possibly oppositional (i.e., some layers will be hidden or concealed). Interpretation continues, therefore, until the point at which multiple lines of association become so dense that further elaboration would provide no additional access into unconscious meaning.

REFERENCES

Breuer, J., and Freud, S. (1895). *Studies on Hysteria.* S.E. 2: 19–305.

Freud, S. (1900). *The Interpretation of Dreams.* S.E. 4–5: 1–621.

———. (1901). *The Psychopathology of Everyday Life.* S.E. 6: 1–279.

———. (1912–1913). *Totem and Taboo.* S.E. 13: 1–161.

———. (1916–1917). *Introductory Lectures on Psycho-Analysis.* S.E. 15–16: 9–496.

EMILY ZAKIN

P

Pankejeff, Sergei See WOLF MAN.

Pappenheim, Bertha See ANNA O.

Paranoia

Freud was long aware that paranoia posed difficult theoretical and clinical problems. His writings focus largely on psychotic disorders that we would now term schizophrenia and delusional disorder. On January 24, 1895, Freud wrote Wilhelm Fliess describing paranoia and suggesting a psychological explanation, although, in that same letter, he described his own use of cocaine, which offers a potential biological cause that he did not note (Masson, 1985: 106.) Freud considered that "people became paranoid over things they cannot put up with" (p. 108). In other words, paranoia was a defense against painful experiences. Describing a clinical situation, he focused on embarrassment or humiliation as a painful experience that paranoia defensively avoids. He succinctly explains this mechanism by noting that, when an internal change is perceived, a choice must be made as to whether the cause is internal or external. The paranoid person focuses on the external, "what people know about us and . . . what people have done to us" (pp.109–110). Freud emphasizes that projection is overutilized in paranoia.

Throughout this letter, Freud implies that a problem with self-esteem is an important part of paranoia. He notes that grandiosity in the paranoid is defensive (Masson, 1985: 110–111). A draft, also sent to Fliess, describes paranoia as an aberration of mortification. (p. 162). Later, he states that the primary symptom of paranoia is distrust that permits the avoidance of self-reproach (p. 167). The paranoid person maintains a chronic focus on the faults of the external world so that he or she does not have to be consciously aware of feelings of internal deficiency. This defensive focus leads to narcissism, which plays a crucial role in paranoia, as Freud emphasized in his 1911 paper on the German jurist Daniel Paul Schreber.

The paranoid's struggles with anger and aggression are frequently noted as equally important and must be addressed for a patient to progress clinically. Freud describes paranoia as one of the "psychoses of spite or contrariness" (Masson, 1985: 112). In *The Origins of Psychoanalysis*, obstinacy and defiance are noted to play important clinical roles in paranoia (Bonaparte et al., p. 115).

The Schreber case represents Freud's attempt to keep paranoia within the libido theory. Initially, in his failed seduction hypotheses, Freud had speculated that paranoia was caused by sexual abuse that occurred some time between the ages of eight and fourteen (Masson, 1985: 209). However, when he recognized that not every patient had been abused and that a person's own internal world played a crucial role in the origin of neuroses, he was left without a sexual etiology for paranoia. He believed that Judge Schreber's memoirs offered insight into paranoia originating in unconscious homosexuality. He saw Schreber's love for his psychiatrist Flechsig as reversed and then projected. "I love him" became "I hate him" and then "He hates me." While modern definitions of homosexuality may well differ from Freud's, which seems to have included stereotypic gender role behavior rather than just sexual arousal patterns, Freud certainly points to the idea of maintaining a relationship through hostile attachment. In 1915, he published on a case of a paranoid woman without apparent homosexual conflicts, which contradicted his theory. However, he believed that she had a repressed infantile homosexual attachment to her mother. He continued to point to the idea of the origin of paranoia in repressed homosexuality in a 1922 paper (Freud, 1922).

In Freud's description of the Wolf Man (1918), he focused on the association between beating fantasies and paranoia. This anticipates the connection between paranoia and sadomasochism. The paranoid patient anticipates and perceives attack when none was intended, often counterattacking in response to the falsely perceived attack. This pattern can lead to cycles of abusing others and then being attacked and of maintaining attachment through this pattern.

Freud made numerous contributions to the understanding of paranoia including his elucidation of projective mechanisms and aggressive motivations. He provides important ideas about the relevance of self-esteem regulation and sadomasochistic patterns.

REFERENCES

Bonaparte, M., Freud, A., and Kris, E. (eds.) (1954). *Origins of Psycho-analysis. Letters to Wilhelm Fliess. 1887–1902.* New York: Basic Books.

Freud, S. (1911). Psychoanalytic notes on an autobiographical account of a case of paranoia (dementia paranoides). S.E. 12: 3–82.

———. (1915). A case of paranoia running counter to the psycho-analytic theory of the disease. S.E. 14: 263–272.

———. (1918). From the history of an infantile neurosis. S.E. 17: 1–122.

———. (1922). Some neurotic symptoms in jealousy, paranoia and homosexuality. S.E. 18: 225–230.

Masson, J. (ed.) (1985). *The Complete Letters of Sigmund Freud and Wilhelm Fliess. 1887–1904.* Cambridge, Mass.: Belknap Press of Harvard University.

STANLEY BONE

Parapraxes See SLIPS, THEORY OF.

Penis Envy

Among the most controversial terms in psychoanalysis, "penis envy" refers to three related phenomena also known collectively as the female "castration complex": 1. Shocklike reactions that commonly occur in little girls between the ages of eighteen and thirty months when they discover the difference between male and female genital anatomy. These reactions, which may include sad-

ness, inhibited motility, increased inner fantasy life, diminished autoerotic activity, and verbalized wishes to be like a boy (Galenson and Roiphe, 1976), were interpreted by Freud as indicating that little girls "at once recognize [the penis] as the superior counterpart of their own small and inconspicuous organ [i.e., the clitoris]. . . . She has seen it and knows that she is without it and wants to have it" (1925, p. 252). 2. Symptoms and other psychological events (dreams, parapraxes, and character patterns) noted in some women that, upon analysis, are found (or inferred) to be derivative expressions of a repressed wish to be male, resentment of males, feelings of envy or inferiority related to gender, or defenses against these feelings and motives. Freud understood these as outcomes of the "ineradicable traces on . . . development and the formation of . . . character" (1933, p. 125) left by the traumatic infantile discovery of sexual anatomy (while recognizing that they may be codetermined by later social and developmental experiences [p. 126]). 3. A motivational factor to which Freud attributed great general importance in his conceptualization of female development. In both normal and abnormal women, "even after penis-envy has abandoned its true object, it continues to exist" (1925, p. 254). Transformed into an attraction to her father and a basis for rejecting her mother, the castration complex moves the little girl into the triangular conflicts of the Oedipal period. Next, it becomes an important source of the girl's developing wish to have a baby; and finally, it "changes into the wish for a man, and thus it [the unconscious motive] puts up with the man as an appendage to the penis" (1917, p. 129). Although Freud recognized that women have important rational interests in establishing relationships with men and in becoming mothers, he proposed that "the original wish for a penis becomes attached to [these impulses] as an unconscious libidinal reinforcement" (p. 130).

In the early works that drew attention to psychoanalysis and defined its general tenets, Freud assumed that boys and girls follow analogous psychosexual developmental paths (1905). In 1908, he stated for the first time that the female toddler considers herself no different from boys *until*, as commonly occurs, she happens to become interested in the penis of a male playmate or small relative. Observing a difference, she interprets her own organs as inferior, and feels "unfairly treated" (1908, p. 218), castrated and degraded. Her interest then "falls under the sway of envy. . . . When a girl declares that 'she would rather be a boy,' we know what deficiency her wish is intended to be put right" (ibid.). From then until the end of his life, especially in four classic papers (1917, 1925, 1931, 1933) Freud elaborated, sometimes in relatively concrete ways, his understanding of the wide-ranging significance—both pathological and adaptive—that penis envy has in women's lives. "The appeased wish for a penis is destined to be converted into a wish for a baby and for a husband, who possesses a penis. It is strange, however, how often we find that the wish for masculinity has been retained in the unconscious and, from out of its state of repression, exercises a disturbing effect. . . . At no other point in one's analytic work does one suffer more from an oppressive feeling that all one's repeated efforts have been in vain . . . than when one is trying to persuade a woman to abandon her wish for a penis. . . . It is the source of outbreaks of severe depression in her, owing to an internal conviction that . . . nothing can be done to help her. . . . We often have the impression that with the wish for a penis . . . we have penetrated through all the psychological strata and have reached bedrock, and that thus our activities are at an end" (1937, pp. 251–252).

As Freud anticipated, his "assertion that one-half of the human race is discontented with the sex assigned to it and can overcome this discontent only in favorable circumstances" (Horney, 1924: 51), has been hotly disputed as "decidedly unsatisfying, not only to feminine narcissism but also to biological science" (p. 51). Sometimes such criticisms have formed the nexus (and a significant motive) for efforts to discredit the entire psychoanalytic corpus, but many committed psychoanalysts have also found these formulations unsatisfactory on the logical and scientific grounds of explanatory adequacy and consonance with the data of observation.

While she did not dispute its existence, Horney (1924) understood penis envy largely as a reactive and defensive development in the woman's psyche, rather than a primary factor in its own right. She also drew attention to important areas of life in which boys have greater power and opportunity, and that contribute to the girl's feelings of disadvantage and inferiority. Similarly, Jones (1927, 1935) considered penis envy largely a defensive and secondary phenomenon, and disagreed with Freud's "phallocentric" views on the subject. Also contrary to Freud, he held that girls are psychologically feminine from the beginning.

Schafer (1974) has proposed that Freud's theoretical aims and value system motivated him to emphasize the castration complex in both sexes. This suited his predilection for seeking symmetrical, homologous developmental forces, and, Schafer asserts, it was also consonant with Freud's teleological concept that development is "biologically destined" (1933, p. 119) to fit children for "normal" male and female reproductive roles. However, in treating the child's reaction to the genital difference simply as a traumatic event rather than as the manifest content of a fantasy that can be further analyzed (How did this girl develop the notion that prominent genitals are superior? Why is it so important to her?), Freud was deviating from his own analytic procedure. "Freud was remarkably incurious about the background of these reactions. [He did not ask] why is the girl so extremely mortified and envious? [or wonder about the reasons for] the apparent precariousness of the girl's self-esteem in the face of the genital discovery" (Schafer, 1974: 473–475).

REFERENCES

Freud, S. (1905). *Three Essays on the Theory of Sexuality.* S.E. 7: 130–243.

———. (1908). On the sexual theories of children. S.E. 9: 207–226.

———. (1917). On transformations of instinct as exemplified in anal erotism. S.E. 17: 126–133.

———. (1925). Some psychological consequences of the anatomical distinction between the sexes. S.E. 19: 243–258.

———. (1931). Female sexuality. S.E. 21: 223–243.

———. (1933). *New Introductory Lectures on Psycho-Analysis.* Lecture 33. Femininity. S.E. 22: 112–135.

———. (1937). Analysis terminable and interminable. S.E. 23: 216–254.

Galenson, E., and Roiphe, H. (1976). Some suggested revisions concerning early female development. *Journal of the American Psychiatric Association,* 24: 29–58.

Horney, K. (1924). On the genesis of the castration complex in women. *International Journal of Psychoanalysis,* 5: 50–65.

Jones, E. (1927). The early development of female sexuality. *International Journal of Psychoanalysis,* 8: 459–472.

———. (1935). Early female sexuality. *International Journal of Psychoanalysis,* 16: 263–273.

Schafer, R. (1974). Some problems in Freud's psychology of women. *Journal of the American Psychiatric Association,* 22: 459–485.

FREDERIC J. LEVINE

Peru, and Psychoanalysis

Professor Honorio Delgado introduced psychoanalysis in Peru and Latin America, his influence lasting from

P

1915 to 1930. A psychoanalytical identity, however, cannot be attributed to the period that immediately followed because after 1930, the movement he initiated veered toward a radically opposing position. Moreover, Delgado did not leave disciples.

Carlos Alberto Seguin founded the first school of dynamic psychotherapy in the Psychiatry Service of the Hospital Obrero of Lima (1941), in which he gathered disciples including the pioneers of psychoanalysis in Peru, Drs. Peña, Crisanto, and Hernández, and the first Peruvian psychoanalysts. Seguin is undoubtedly the forerunner of the psychoanalytic movement in Peru.

Origins

As an associate member of the British Psychoanalytical Society, I qualified as a child psychoanalyst as of the 23rd of September in 1969. Because it was the moment to combine my analytical identity with my identity as a Peruvian, I returned to Peru in October 1969. It was a privilege to have initiated and taken part in the development of psychoanalysis. The legitimacy of my activities has been recognized by the national and international scientific community.

On the 8th of January, 1970, the Peruvian Psychiatric Association, presided over by Oscar Valdivia, gave me the responsibility for forming a study group for the foundation and development of the Peruvian psychoanalytical movement. During the first three years, I worked alone. With the arrival of Carlos Crisanto (1973) and Max Hernández (1974), we continued this work, maintaining a close bond during the training of psychiatrists at the Hospital Obrero, then in the independent London group. We formed the Centre for the Development of Psychoanalysis in Peru.

The most notable influences on Peruvian psychoanalysis have been those of Freud, Heimann, and Winnicott. My own analyst, Paula Heimann, was analyzed by Theodor Reik, who himself was analyzed by Freud. Reik analyzed Angel Garma, who in turn analyzed Arnaldo Rascovsky; both were pioneers of psychoanalysis in Argentina and Latin America. Thus, Peruvian psychoanalysis comes in a direct line from Sigmund Freud. My supervisors of adults were Adam Limentani and Charles Rycroft and of children Donald Winnicott, Marion Milner and Masud Khan. Peruvian psychoanalysis grows out of the psychoanalytical societies of London, Argentina, Frankfurt, and Venezuela.

Peruvian psychoanalytical thought has been, and continues to be, antidogmatic. We have always fought for

this and for its humanist essence, integrating medical and cultural psychoanalysis, extending to all of the disciplines of humankind: psychiatry, psychology, philosophy, anthropology, history, sociology, linguistics, literature, ethics, politics, and theology.

Our movement gives fundamental importance to clinical work, training, teaching, praxis, and applied psychoanalysis. Its stature was formally recognized by the Universidad Nacional Mayor de San Marcos by naming Alexander Mitscherlich as Professor Honoris Causa, because of his social investigations from a psychoanalytical perspective.

From those who initiated their therapeutic analysis and defined their vocation with us, there emerged a group who continued their work abroad before returning to Peru. We stimulated other analysts to return and to satisfy the requirements of an autonomous society with consistent bonds with the International Psychoanalytical Association (IPA).

The Centre for the Development of Psychoanalysis in Peru

The Centre was formed in 1974 constituted by Drs. Peña, Crisanto, and Hernandez, and professionals of diverse disciplines. This was made possible by the genuine interest, creative capacity, and profound motivation of those who participated.

The presence of Carlos Crisanto and Max Hernández was indispensable. They fortified and consolidated the movement because it required a determined number of members for its constitution, and we took the lead in supervision and seminars. Moreover, thanks to the quality and solid formation of the Centre, we could exchange ideas and deepen our knowledge of group work. The Centre's own personality, idiosyncrasy, and interests gave Peruvian psychoanalysis many varied tones.

Many foreign analysts graced us with their presence. We welcomed approximately one hundred psychoanalysts including Daniel Widlöcher, then secretary general of the IPA, Adam Limentani and Leo Rangell, both ex-presidents of the IPA, and John Bowlby, who was present at the foundation of the Peruvian Psychoanalytical Society. We fought for the Peruvian movement in all of the Latin American and international congresses.

The Formation of a Study Group

The IPA conferred upon us the category of Pre-Study Group in 1979 at the 31st Congress in New York. The first group of sponsors was formed by David Zimmermann, Chairman (Brazil), Carlos Plata (Colombia), and Guillermo Teruel (Venezuela). Their mission was to structure an institute on the lines of the IPA. Of eleven aspirants for admission to the group, five were initially accepted, and later two more were added. Owing to the high scientific level of the three pioneers, we were named didactic analysts.

At the 32nd Congress (Helsinki, 1981), we became a Study Group. A second Sponsors Committee was named chaired by Serge Lebovici, ex-president of the IPA; Willy Baranger, ex-president of the Psychoanalytical Federation of Latin America; Otto Kernberg, president of the IPA, and consultants Adam Limentani, Leo Rangell, honorary president of the IPA, and Inga Villarreal, then associate secretary for Latin America. During this first visit the Peruvian Institute of Psychoanalysis was constituted and the Joint Training Committee was made up of the sponsors and Drs. Peña, Hernández, and Crisanto, as members of the Local Sponsors Committee.

In 1979, Noel Altamirano and Gustavo Delgado arrived in Peru. Altmirano was trained in the Argentine Psychoanalytical Association and Delgado in the British Society (from the independent group); he was the first analyst not a psychiatrist.

The Peruvian Psychoanalytical Society

The Society was created on January 30, 1980. Its founding members were: Saúl Peña, Carlos Crisanto, Max Hernández, Noel Altamirano, and Gustavo Delgado. Its Executive Council was formed by Saúl Peña, president, Carlos Crisanto, vice-president, and Max Hernández, didactic co-ordinator.

Because of a problem at the Universidad Católica, there was a massive resignation of forty professors in March, 1982, causing conflict in the analytical society. The editorial regarding this in the magazine COPSI of the Psychological Consulting of the Universidad de San Marcos captures its transcendence and magnitude.

The first Psychoanalysis Conference dealt with basic concepts, such as cultural extension. In 1981, the Lima Association of Psychoanalytical Psychotherapy and the Peruvian Institute of Psychotherapy, Research, and Interdisciplinary Application of Psychoanalysis Sigmund Freud were formed. The second group trained a small number of psychotherapists and then discontinued its activity. The first group continues to exist, initiating various congresses and publications.

For 1983–1984, Dr. Hernández was elected as president; Peña, director of the Institute; Heresi, vice-president, Lemlij, scientific secretary, and Péndola, treasurer. At the 34th Congress (Hamburg, 1985), we were designated a Provisional Society of Psychoanalysis, this being agreed to unanimously by the Executive Council of the IPA. Drs. Gheiler, Cabrejos, Caplansky, Rey de Castro, Alayza, and Yori were the first psychoanalysts who trained and graduated in Peru.

At the 35th Congress (Montreal, 1987), we became a Component Society of the IPA, with the autonomy we were granted corresponding to seventeen years of work. At this Congress, Max Hernández was elected vice-president of the IPA.

On the 27th of May in 1987, with unanimous vote and by acclamation, I was conferred the honor of being distinguished as honorary president of the Peruvian Psychoanalytical Society. Also named as honorary members were Drs. Limentani, Rangell, Lebovici, Baranger, Kernberg, and as honorary executive secretary, Irene Auletta.

During 1987, fourteen candidates for the fourth training class were selected. In 1988, the first Peruvian Congress "Psychoanalysis and Identity" was held in Lima, and in 1989 in Cusco the "International Symposium of Universal, American, and Contemporary Myths." In 1989, the First Congress of Candidates of the Institute, "Training and Social Crisis" was organized by the third training class with the participation of the fourth.

For 1990–1991 were elected: Alberto Péndola, president; Hilke Engelbrecht, vice-president: Marcos Gheiler, scientific secretary; Matilde de Caplansky, treasurer; and Moisés Lemlij, director of the Institute. For 1992–1993 were elected: Carlos Crisanto, president; Pedro Morales, vice-president; Matilde de Caplansky, scientific secretary; Fernando Alayza, treasurer; and Hilke Engelbrecht, director of the Institute, carrying out the III Peruvian Congress, "From Hearing to Interpreting in Peru Today." In 1991, I was elected president of the Psychoanalytic Federation of Latin America.

I was eager to publish the Latin American Psychoanalysis Journal, knowing that there had been previous attempts that had failed. The first issue was published for the XX Latin American Congress of Psychoanalysis. The first two issues contained works of the pioneers, the most conspicuous psychoanalysts in Latin America at the moment of its foundation. Works of contemporary analysts were also included. Horacio Etchegoyen stated that the Incas began this dream of all of us, and that is

P

the principal reason for our success because it is designed to last.

The first Latin American Congress of Psychoanalysis of Children and Adolescents in Latin America was held in Cordoba, Argentina (1994) away from the head office of FEPAL, a landmark in the history of psychoanalysis in Latin America. The publication of these the papers of this Congress represents the first endeavor of this scope carried out by FEPAL.

In detailing the history of psychoanalysis in Peru, Gustavo Delgado deserves a special mention for editing the *Annual Book of Psychoanalysis* (five volumes) spreading in Spanish the most important works in other languages. He published the first book of clinical reflection in Peru, *Labyrinths of Madness.*

César Rodríguez directs the group Psychoanalysis and Society. Moisés Lemlij, director of the Peruvian Library of Psychoanalysis, has edited and published more than twenty volumes: *Between the Myth and History, Psychoanalysis and Its Andean Past.* "The return of the Indian burial ground" of SIDEA, an Interdisciplinary Seminar of Andean Studies, was formed by Max Hernández, Moisés Lemlij, Alberto Péndola, and by the anthropologist Luis Millones and the ethnohistorian María Rostworowski, et al. This interdisciplinary work is an attempt to comprehend the psychoanalytical side of our history, exploring the collective psyche.

The members and candidates of our institution have published approximately one hundred works. For example, Noel Altamirano wrote the book *Neruda, a Psychoanalytical Reading* and is working on another book, *Vallejo and the Poetry of the Body.* Alvaro Rey de Castro published the letters of Sigmund Freud to Honorio Delgado and the book *Freud and Honorio Delgado, Chronicle of a Breakaway.* I am preparing a book entitled *Unconscious Ideology.*

In the United States, there are four Peruvian psychoanalysts: Julio Morales Galarreta, Javier Galvez, Alberto Goldwasser, and Manuel Morales. In Madrid, another Peruvian, Patricia Grieve, trained in London; two Peruvian psychoanalysts belong to the British Society: León Kleimberg, honorary secretary, and Carlos Fishman. A Peruvian analyst, Alex Castoriano, trained and lived in Sweden, but unfortunately is now deceased. Five members of the Argentine Psychoanalytical Association are Peruvians: Pepa Reisfeld, Miguel Wagner, Charo Boza, Gilberto Valdez and Francisco de Zela. María Paz de la Puente returned to Peru after complet-

ing her training in Argentina, as did Carmen Labarthe of the British Society.

In 1987, the Association of Child Psychoanalytical Psychotherapy was formed after fifteen years of work, naming as honorary members Max Hernández, Moisés Lemlij and Saúl Peña. More than twenty years ago, the group of companion therapists was formed and continues its work today.

The main aim of training psychoanalysts in Peru has been met, integrating Peru's own medical, cultural, and individual aspects together with universal ones. This work was a twenty-nine-year long effort. We have the profound satisfaction of seeing our purpose fulfilled.

SAÚL PEÑA

Perversions

What is sex? Freud begins his *Three Essays on the Theory of Sexuality* (1905) by pointing out it is *not* what the person in the street might be inclined to answer (though perhaps using more vulgar terms), namely, heterosexual genital intercourse between adults. Even the person in the street knows better and is prepared to recognize a much wider range of activities as sexual: everything from homosexuality, to foot fetishism, to necrophilia. The interesting question is to what extent these sexual perversions are recognizably *sexual*, given their distance from the initial, unthinking definition. Once Freud offers his expanded definition of sexuality, the further question arises as to what of the sexual perversions are regarded as *perverse*. The distinction between the normal and the pathological becomes rather tenuous in light of the new understanding of the nature of sexuality.

Sex for Freud must be understood as an instinct, or set of instincts, but an instinct is not simply a biologically inherited pattern of behavior, as it might be for ethologists. While human biology is relatively uniform, human sexuality is wildly diverse. Sexual activities range as widely as the human imagination. For almost anything one can think of, there is someone who will find it sexually stimulating and desirable. For Freud, instincts, and the sexual instincts in particular, lie on the borderland between the mental and the physical. Whatever might be said of the sources of instincts, their objects and aims are thought-dependent, rather than being set by chemistry or biology.

Once one starts to classify the perversions systematically, one begins to see the need for distinctions, for example, between the object of the instinct and the activity aimed at. The existence of homosexuality (then termed "inversion") shows that "the sexual instinct and the sexual object are merely soldered together" (1905, p. 148). And variation in object is only one dimension of variation. For some of the perversions involve variation in aim as well. The voyeur desires to look, rather than have intercourse, and the hair fetishist may desire merely to touch the object of his or her fascination. And the genitals are not the only bodily center of arousal (what Freud terms the "source" of the instinct). The mouth, the anus, indeed the skin and almost any other part of the body can become an erotogenic zone. A systematic classification and understanding of the perversions requires that the sexual instinct be analyzed along underlying dimensions of source, object, and aim. Once one does that, homosexuality, for example, becomes recognizably sexual in virtue of underlying continuities of source and aim, despite variation in object.

That certain dimensions of sexuality become isolated and prominent in certain perversions enables one to see that they are present even in so-called normal sexuality, for example, in foreplay. That the mouth is an erotogenic zone is a fact familiar to all who kiss. What may be perverse about the hair fetishist is that he wants *only* to stroke his beloved's hair. So at one point Freud suggests "exclusiveness and fixation" as a general criterion for perversion. But so generalized, heterosexual genital intercourse between adults (the very paradigm of normal sexuality), if too exclusive an interest, might have to be regarded as perverse. As Freud puts it, "from the point of view of psycho-analysis the exclusive sexual interest felt by men for women is also a problem that needs elucidating and is not a self-evident fact" (1905, p. 146n).

The dimensions of sexuality that emerge in isolation in perversion are visible not only in foreplay but also in development. What obscures them there is that the infant is polymorphously perverse, taking pleasure in all parts of his or her body. But thumb sucking involves an erotogenic zone also important to adults (e.g., in kissing and in oral intercourse), and it involves sensual sucking—only the object (the thumb instead of, say, the penis or clitoris) is different. The broadening of the concept of sexuality made necessary by the understanding of "the sexual aberrations" (the title of the first of Freud's *Three Essays*) makes possible the recognition of infantile sexuality.

Freud came to see the psychosexual stages (oral, anal, phallic, genital) as biologically given. There thus emerges

a developmental standard for perversion: perversion is immature sexuality; its aims are nonreproductive. Perversion involves fixation at or regression to an earlier stage of development; it is an aspect of infantile sexuality persisting or emerging in an adult. But as a general criterion of perversion, if perversion is a term of reproach, this may confuse what is at least in part a social norm with what is biologically given. After all, if we live long enough, we eventually decay. Later does not necessarily mean better. And the stages of psychosexual development themselves have varying social significance. The biologically given aim of sexuality is, according to Freud himself, pleasure (discharge), not reproduction. Must heterosexual intercourse while using contraception be regarded as perverse? In an overpopulated world, must all sexual activity aim at reproduction? One should not confuse the ripening of an organic capacity with the valuation of one form of sexuality as its highest or only acceptable form.

In his *Three Essays on the Theory of Sexuality*, Freud brings forward several possible criteria of perversion. Each is problematic. The traditional content criterion, which would regard as perverse any interest in parts of the body other than the genitals or in activities aimed at something other than heterosexual intercourse, is called into question by the universality across individuals of such interests (as shown in foreplay and in individuals' responsiveness to external circumstances) and the diversity across cultures in attitudes toward such interests. Once one accepts Freud's view of the sexual instinct as complex or composite, as having dimensions, and as developing, it is no longer possible simply to privilege one set of variations as better than another. The mere fact of difference, variation in content, is no longer enough once one cannot say one set of variations is somehow natural and others are not. Once one sees sexuality as involving a single underlying instinct, with room for variation along several dimensions, new criteria for pathology are needed. And as we have noted, if one is seeking a scientifically objective, universal criterion, the various possibilities considered by Freud—exclusiveness and fixation, development and maturation (with reproduction as the ultimate marker)—are as problematic as content (with perhaps disgust, itself conventional, as the ultimate marker). One must conclude with Freud, "In the sphere of sexual life we are brought up against peculiar and, indeed, insoluble difficulties as soon as we try to draw a sharp line to distinguish mere variations within the range of what is physiological from pathological symptoms" (1905, pp. 160–161).

P

Neuroses, like perversions, have their root in infantile sexuality. The crucial difference is that the desires and fantasies acted on in the case of perversion are, in the case of neurosis, repressed. The neurotic's symptoms constitute (on at least one interpretation) his or her sexual activity. In Freud's formulation, "neuroses are the negative of perversions" (1905, pp. 165 and 231). But for Freud, so-called normal sexuality (as well as character) also has its roots in infantile sexuality, and "the finding of an object is in fact a refinding of it" (1905, p. 222). All of our complex and diverse sexual lives emerge out of the universal dispositions that make up the components of the sexual instinct, as we undergo organic changes and the experiences that make for development, inhibiting and dissociating from some components as others achieve dominance. The perversions are one constellation of variations among the many made possible by human thought and biology. If they are to be judged, it is by the same standards we judge all human thought and action.

REFERENCE

Freud, S. (1905). *Three Essays on the Theory of Sexuality.* S.E. 7: 130–243.

JEROME NEU

Pfister, Oskar (1873–1956)

Oskar Pfister fits none of the stereotypes associated with Freud's loyal followers. As a Swiss pastor in Zurich, he profoundly disagreed with Freud's most famous stated outlook on religion. And in response to Freud's *The Future of an Illusion*, Pfister published in 1928 a piece of comparable length: "The Illusion of a Future." Pfister also differed with Freud on art and morality, as he found inadequate Freud's approach to ethics, philosophy, as well as, implicitly, the practice of psychotherapy. Pfister's "The Illusion of a Future" appeared first in Freud's journal *Imago*; its publication was an unusual sign of Freud's willingness to tolerate disagreement within his movement.

When the pre–World War I difficulties between Carl G. Jung and Freud broke out, Pfister was exceptional as a Swiss in not resigning along with Jung. Freud must have appreciated this sign of Pfister's loyalty. Following World War I, Pfister and Emil Oberholzer started a new Swiss Society for Psychoanalysis, which was affiliated with the International Psychoanalytic Association.

After Freud published *The Question of Lay Analysis*, Oberholzer left to found an exclusively medical group; once again, Pfister stuck with Freud's side, and Oberholzer's Swiss Medical Society for Psychoanalysis did not survive World War II.

The 1963 edition of the letters between Freud and Pfister (1909–1939) has, like all such early collections of Freud's correspondences, been severely cut, and some day a new volume of the complete exchanges will be undertaken. Until then, it is necessary to be appropriately tentative about the relationship between Freud and Pfister. It will be particularly interesting to be able to read what they wrote each other about concrete clinical cases. We know, for example, that Pfister sent one American patient to Freud whom Freud diagnosed as a schizophrenic, yet Freud treated him in analysis for a number of years; that patient was also seen by some famous European psychiatrists and ended his days living in a private mental hospital outside Boston. We also know that in addition to what Pfister had to say on the subject of religion, he was prolific as a continental popularizer of psychoanalysis, specializing in the implications of Freud's work for early education.

By now, psychoanalysis has had a transformative impact on what the clergy know about human psychology, and Pfister has to be credited with having taken a leading role in legitimizing this whole area. Whatever eighteenth-century Enlightenment prejudices against priests Freud may have had, he could somehow make an exception when it came to Pfister. Pfister's critique of *Future of an Illusion* is not well enough known, even though by now many of our contemporary psychoanalytic thinkers would be inclined to take a favorable view of the innovations that Pfister was attempting to make. While Freud thought he was overturning many of the most central features of Western ethics, Pfister was trying to show how psychoanalysis could be used to breathe new life into some of the oldest values in Christian thought. Freud's willingness to maintain his tie to Pfister shows a very different side to Freud's convictions as expressed in *The Future of an Illusion*. And the debate over religion between Freud and Pfister retains its vitality today.

REFERENCE

Pfister, Oskar. (1999). *The Psychoanalytic Method.* (International Library of Psychology.) New York: Routledge.

PAUL ROAZEN

Phallic Stage See DEVELOPMENTAL THEORY.

Phantasy See FANTASY (PHANTASY).

Philippines, and Psychoanalysis

It is tempting to speculate that the origin of psycho-analysis in the Philippines dates to the time when Freud was studying under Charcot in Paris because the influential writer, doctor, and revolutionary, Jose Rizal, was also studying there, and imbibed the same Weltan-schaung that intrigued the European academicians—with its pertinent questions of modern psychopathology such as "hysterical neurosis," suggestibility, autosuggestion, and hypnotic phenomena. Rizal, in several important works of fiction, would go on to develop characters who, on a political reading, might be taken to represent elements of a repressed nation but in nonpoliticized form bore an uncanny resemblance to some of Freud's early case histories (Rizal, 1885, 1887; Santiago, 1966; Santiago and Rizal, 1997).

Nonetheless, the origins of Filipino psychoanalytic thought predate this period by some fifty years. In a literary work entitled *Florante at Laura*, the writer Francisco Balagtas (1788–1838) refers to some form of incest problem in the extended familial system not unlike that which occurs in Malaya-Indonesian societies (Sebatu, 1989). The perspicacity of Balagtas's work in antedating psychoanalytic discourse is evidenced by his references to Oedipus in this and other literary works, and has been taken by Freudian scholars as further proof of the universal validity of Freudian theory in the advancement of social organizations (Balagtas, 1849, 1856; Santiago and Rizal, 1997).

However, it is from the time of the American dominance of the university education system in the early decades of the twentieth century that several distinguished Filipino doctors studied in the United States and imbibed psychoanalytic theory from the American psychiatric tradition.

One of the first products of this generation was Virgilio Santiago, whose medical education at the Universidad de Santo Thomás (UST) was completed in 1949. This led him to a psychoanalytic training under Robert Waelder, a student of Freud's. He went on to study at the Menninger Clinic in Topeka, Kansas. This training distinguished him from those in the dominant, so-called organic school in psychiatry as represented by Gamez at UST. In the 1950s, the conservative Catholic clergy strictly forbade psycho-analysis. Santiago himself was discouraged by his colleagues from pursuing it. Nonetheless in a private practice Santiago found a clientele among the expatriate population, and a small number of Filipinos suffering from psychosis also consulted him. He later summarized his views of psychoanalysis in the Philippines by saying that the Filipino patient is generally found unsuitable for the psychoanalytic process, this commentary alluding as much to the level of health care in the country as to the applicability of Freudian theory per se (Crisanto-Estrada, 1977). According to Santiago, 98 percent of practicing psychiatrists in the Philippines adhere solely to drug therapy, and it cannot be categorically stated whether the latest diagnostic disease systems are enforced or even taught.

Two other early pioneers deserve mention. Baltazar Reyes, also a product of University of the Philippines and the Langley Porter Institute in California, still actively teaches and researches at the State University and has produced a brief history of psychiatry (Reyes, 1968). The other is Rodolfo Varias, who came from a long line of doctors and taught in the Luzon region. He was one of the first to be trained in classic psychoanalysis in New York, in the 1950s. He returned to practice and teach at the Institute of Public Hygiene (now the College of Public Health). He left in the 1970s to return to New York.

Of the contemporary health professionals, Lourdes Lapuz, a graduate of the UP-PGH and the Strong Medical Center in New York, practices and teaches at St. Luke's Medical Center, in Manila. Her groundbreaking *A Study of Psychopathology* (Lapuz, 1969) influenced a whole generation of psychiatrists, psychologists, and counselors—practitioners who recast the original psychoanalytic theory in which they had been instructed to suit the Filipino cultural mold with its more interactive role demanded of the doctor in view of the sociocultural expectations of the doctor as role model and authority figure. Her book *Children of Oedipus* (1973) directly addresses the Freudian theory. Her succeeding works on marital counseling gave way to couple and family therapy in the 1980s (Lapuz, 1979).

In every instance, then, psychoanalytic theory has been appropriated by practitioners who have adopted it to the needs of the prevailing Filipino culture. Here the modern mental health system is poorly understood, owing to the low level of medical awareness of the population and to the prevalence of alternatives to modern medicine, whether indigenous forms of herbal health or even cult healing practices. Coupled with a poor health

P

insurance system and the need for gainful employment, these factors have diminished the need for formal institutes of psychoanalysis, and explains why no training analysts are practicing at the moment in the Philippines. The impact of Freud's work has not hit hard in this predominantly Catholic culture, where even today the teaching of human sexuality, from the point of view of psychology, has not gained much ground in the academic world. Sex education remains basically a tool of population control.

REFERENCES

Balagtas, F. (1849). *Florante at Laura*. Nobelang Tagalog. Philippines. Reprint.

———. (1856). *Ibong Adarna*. Tagalog epic poem.

Crisanto-Estrada, T. (1977). Interview with Virgilio Santiago. November, Manila.

Lapuz, L. (1969). *A Study of Psychopathology*. Quezon City: New Day Publications.

———. (1973). *Children of Oedipus*. Quezon City: New Day Publications.

———. (1979). *Marriage Counselling*. Quezon City: New Day Publications.

Reyes, B. V. (1968). *History of Psychiatry*. History of the Department of Psychiatry in the University of the Philippines, *Manual of the Structural and Functional Organization of the Department of Psychiatry of UP-PGH Medical Center*.

Reyes, B. V., and Della, C. D. (1999). Treatment of mental illness in the Philippines: A historical perspective. *Philippine Journal of Psychiatry*, 23, 7–11.

Rizal, J. L. M. (1885). *La curacion de los Mechizados*. Apuntes hechos para el estudio de Medicina Filipina. Dapitan.

———. (1887). *Noli Me Tangere*. Novela Tagala.

Santiago, L. (1966). Psychopathology of Sisa. *Acta Medica Philippina*, 2, no. 3: 140–145.

Santiago, L., and Rizal, L. (1997). Philippine psychiatry. Paper read at the Freud-Rizal Conference of the R.I.O.P., De Meester, November 1997.

Sebatu, A. (1989). Malayo-Indonesian Incest Taboos. In Ma. Trinidad Crisanto (ed.). *Intramuros/Extramuros: A Collection of Psychological Essays*. Unpublished U.P. papers.

CHIQUIT CRISANTO-ESTRADA
GEOFFREY H. BLOWERS

Philosophy, and Psychoanalysis

There are three parts to the topic: the influence of philosophy on the formation of psychoanalysis, the philosophical views specific to psychoanalysis, and the influence of psychoanalysis on philosophy. This entry focuses almost exclusively on Freud's own thought.

Philosophical Sources

Freud seems to have studied some of Kant's philosophy in school. At the University of Vienna, he studied with Franz Brentano, and, probably through Brentano's influence, read John Stuart Mill. At one point in his student career, Freud planned to take a degree in philosophy, but of course he did not. As a student, Freud's intellectual path forked between Brentano and Ernst Brucke, professor of physiology. In the end, Freud chose Brucke's program of materialist physiology over Brentano's program of introspective psychology, but Brentano had a large influence, both positive and negative, which the mature Freud did not acknowledge. Freud assumed Brentano's criterion—intentionality—for an event or state or process to be mental and used that criterion as part of his argument for unconscious mental states. Brentano, who did not believe in unconscious mental states, introduced Freud to the very idea and provided a variety of arguments both for and against it. Freud later gave some of Brentano's arguments for the unconscious—arguments Brentano rejected in his *Psychology from an Empirical Standpoint*—that Brentano published and lectured about while Freud was his student.

Brentano introduced Freud to his own version of Aristotelian logic, which was presumably the source for Freud's use of the subject-predicate representation of "ideas" in the *Project for a Scientific Psychology* and elsewhere. Brentano was an enthusiast for Mill's philosophy, especially for his *Logic*, and arranged for Freud to translate some of Mill's essays on social topics for a German edition of Mill's works. A German translation of Mill's *Logic* had been available for some years, and it is virtually certain that Freud read it or at least learned its characteristic doctrines from Brentano. Mill's methods accorded nicely with the methods of cognitive neuropsychology that Freud learned from Theodor Meynert, who was professor of psychiatry in Vienna. Mill's methods were also consonant with the generally a-statistical reasoning by examples, nonexamples, and counterexamples of co-occurrence that was standard in experimental physiology at the time. The mode of argument is illustrated and advocated in Claude Bernard's *Studies in Experimental Medicine*. Freud employed a generally Millian form of argument throughout his career. Beginning with *The Interpretation of Dreams*, the examples and counterexamples Freud used in this form of argument were often produced through psychoanalytic interpretation. Freud's mature methods of argument in fact seem a synthesis of several strands: (1) psychoanalytic interpretation as a data-generating procedure; (2) Mill's methods; (3) Bernard's principles for reasoning about causes; and (4) a psychologized version of the cognitive neuropsychologists' strategy of inferring the mechanisms of normal functioning from features of abnormal functioning.

Attempts have been made to relate Freud's thought to Spinoza, Kant, Nietzsche, and other philosophers, but they rest chiefly on analogies or brief references, with little historical basis for postulating a direct influence on Freud's intellectual development.

Philosophical Opinions

Freud famously described himself as a determinist, by which he meant at least to deny traditional Christian doctrines of freedom of the will. Determinism, in his view, also had methodological implications, requiring that adequate theories not leave particular features of thought unexplained or indeterminate, a doctrine he used to good rhetorical effect in the critical parts of *The Interpretation of Dreams* and elsewhere. Freud's atheism is equally famous, and as gods went so too went doctrines of immortality and of souls.

Freud's views about the relation of the mental to the physical were complicated and in some respects obscure. Freud's properly psychoanalytic publications are not informative, but in *On Aphasia* and in the *Project for a Scientific Psychology*, mental states are identified with physical states, although the identification changes between the two works. (In the *New Introductory Lectures on Psychoanalysis*, Freud entertained extrasensory perception, but there is no indication that he thought that the capacity is extraphysical.) For that reason, Freud had no difficulty supposing that mental states have causal roles, but whether *conscious* mental states have any causal role except as effects of unconscious processes is unclear from the *Project*, since in that work the cells whose activation constitutes consciousness are said to be influenced by and correlated with the activation of cells that carry on ordinary mental processing unconsciously. It is unclear whether the theory entails that activation of cells of the former kind can influence cells of the latter kind. These distinctions do not survive in any straightforward way in the metapsychology.

If presented today, Freud's early models of mind would be recognized as explicitly connectionist computational architectures, with some novel twists. The theory of *On Aphasia*, for example, is very close both in

content and in style of argument to that advanced in a recent work in cognitive neuropsychology, Martha Farah's *Visual Agnosia*, and many aspects of the *Project* are paralleled in John Anderson's almost recent *The Architecture of Cognition*. Freud retained his computational model, with physiological and computational details suppressed, in the economic model in psychoanalysis. Freud's computational model, like much else, is interestingly original, involving what we would now describe as both digital and analog aspects. At some level, Freud thinks of mental computation as like a rebus, with calculation over roughly linguistic representations mixed with "mnemic images."

Psychoanalytic "moral psychology" is given first in the multiple agent theory of the metapsychology. Irrationality, weakness of will, loss of memory, many errors, and the like result from the struggle (or negotiation or compromise or combination of forces) of internal functional agents with conflicting goals. Each agent is rational given its goals, but the resulting compromise behavior is often irrational. It is not entirely anachronistic to think of Arrow's proof of the impossibility of rational collective choice as a formalization of Freud's substantive hypothesis. Freud's later theory of instincts, notably in *Beyond the Pleasure Principle*, uses a similar model, this time of conflicting drives, to account for a variety of normal and abnormal behaviors in children and adults.

Freud wrote little about ethics per se, but several ethical commitments of his views are quite clear. Freud's ethical theory appears to be original, although it has Darwinian inspirations and some Aristotelian themes. Its focus is not action but character; it is entirely naturalized, and might reasonably by described as antiexistentialist and anti-Kantian. Fundamental features of character are formed from the interaction of the universal structure of mind with the accidents of genetic inheritance and life history. No one creates his or her own character. There is a standard or normal development of aspects of character more fundamental than the usual virtues, including sexual identity and character of sexual desire, where the norm is determined both by actual frequency and (less clearly) by evolutionary role. Unfortunate genetics and unfortunate circumstances, especially childhood circumstances, combine to create deviations from the norm, which vary in kind and degree.

Psychoanalytic theory has no use for a deontic ethics of Kant's extreme kind, which locates moral action in moral motives or the very idea of moral law, since according to

P

psychoanalytic theory, action, even moral action, springs from the inner resolution of a clash of motives, some of which are not nice. Freudian psychoanalytic theory must reject retributive justice and any form of punishment founded on traditional conceptions of free will.

Unsurprisingly, Freud's few explicit remarks on philosophy of science—as distinct from whatever philosophy of science is implicit in his and others' psychoanalytic practice—address the underdetermination of theory by evidence, a problem that at times he felt keenly and personally. His account (for example, in *Instincts and Their Vicissitudes*) is that theoretical assumptions are used to interpret evidence and to form an expanding set of conclusions, until, and if, evidence can no longer be accommodated, in which case fundamental assumptions must be revised. That essay may be usefully compared with Quine's views on the methods and progress of science, but, so far as I know, Freud's views did not prompt Quine's.

The Influence of Psychoanalysis on Philosophy

There are many Freudian themes in twentieth-century philosophical discussion: Carnap and Quine on theory confirmation are at times quite close to Freud; discussions of mental representation, for example, in connectionist models, turn on issues Freud addressed, more or less in the terms he addressed them; the ethics of virtue has had a rebirth; there are theories of consciousness—albeit more often in psychology than in philosophy—that are quite close to Freud's; the doctrine of rationality as a realizable norm has been in philosophical decline, and unconscious mentation is largely taken for granted.

These connections notwithstanding, major philosophical work in the twentieth century has little traceable debt to psychoanalysis or to Freud. Psychoanalysis, and Freud's writing in particular, has had almost no influence on mainstream Anglo-American philosophy, no matter whether in ethics, metaphysics, epistemology, or philosophy of science. There are a few exceptions. Donald Davidson gave an account of weakness of will more or less deliberately modeled on the multiple internal agents of psychoanalytic theory. The psychoanalytic theory of dreams figured as a stalking horse in Norman Malcolm's much ridiculed behaviorist argument that there are no dreams. A few philosophers adopted psychoanalytic theory and attempted to explain philosophical activity in psychoanalytic terms. Karl Popper used psychoanalysis as his paradigm of an unfalsifiable theory, and Adolf Grünbaum has written at length

contending against Popper that psychoanalysis is falsifiable, and false. Glymour used the Rat Man case and some of Freud's remarks on psychoanalysis and the law as illustrations of a strategy of theory testing he endorsed. But with the exception of Davidson's moral psychology, all of this is marginal to mainstream philosophy in our time.

The reason is not simple neglect. Psychoanalytic theory was known to many philosophers in an informal way, and to many others more personally. The reasons have instead to do with the dominance of semiformal logic and probability theory as techniques for building philosophical theories, with the preeminent philosophical interest in the analysis of language, with, for much of the twentieth century, a verifiabilist epistemology, and with a deliberate separation of philosophical thought from all but behaviorist psychology. When cognitive psychology was reborn (it was alive and well in the late nineteenth century) in the middle of the twentieth century, Freud's early work, which had the most obvious bearing on the new way of looking at the mind, was largely unknown and remained unknown until Karl Pribram's study of the *Project* in the 1970s. No substantial part of mainstream philosophy became "naturalized"—engaged with psychological theories and results—until the 1980s, by which time there were more proximate sources for the ideas in psychoanalysis that are most relevant to the concerns of professional philosophy.

CLARK GLYMOUR

Physicalism See BEHAVIORISM; MIND AND BODY.

Piaget, Jean (1896-1980)

Jean Piaget was born in 1896 in the French-speaking Swiss city of Neuchâtel (Switzerland), and died in Geneva in 1980, where he had been professor at the university. He was best known for his work on the development of intelligence. The beginnings of his psychological career were marked by a strong interest in psychoanalysis, which, in his autobiography, he attributes in part to his mother's "instability." His first documented encounter with psychoanalysis took place in 1916 through a lecture by the Genevan professor of psychology Théodore Flournoy. A mentor of Carl Gustav Jung, and a major figure in the study of the "subliminal self," Flournoy compared the "schools" of Vienna and Zürich, and favored the latter as being more respectful of religious phenomena.

In his 1918 autobiographical novel *Recherche* (Research), Piaget used psychoanalysis, as understood by Flournoy and the Zürich "school," as a tool for self-understanding. He criticized the Freudian theory of sublimation, employed the Jungian notion of "complex," and branded his earlier mystical and metaphysical tendencies as instances of "autistic" thought. (The term had been coined by Eugen Bleuler, director of the Burghölzli clinic in Zürich, to designate one of the main features of schizophrenia.) At the end of 1918, after his studies in natural sciences, Piaget left for Zürich where (according to his autobiography), he attended lectures by Jung, Bleuler, and the psychoanalyst and Protestant pastor Oskar Pfister.

Early on during his 1919-1921 stay in Paris, Piaget gave a lecture on the "currents of pedagogical psychoanalysis," a topic which was at the time a Swiss specialty. The published version, "Psychoanalysis and its relationship with child psychology," was his first article in psychology. In it, he emphasized the significance of psychoanalysis for pedagogy and moral education. In line with the "Zürich school," however, he criticized the "excessively rigid distinction between consciousness and the unconscious," and asserted that "unconscious mechanisms" are only the "first stages of conscious activity." He also anticipated one of the main topics of his early research program, the "correlation" between "unconscious" and "mental development" (i.e., the development of intelligence). Reviewing the article, Pfister reported that Piaget "had energetically initiated himself into the theory and practice of psychoanalysis," emphasized "the value of [Piaget's] detailed personal research," and praised the "young scholar from whom the psychoanalytic movement is entitled to expect important contributions."

In 1921, Piaget joined the faculty of the Jean-Jacques Rousseau Institute of Geneva, founded in 1912 by Edouard Claparède to combine teacher training with experimental pedagogy and child development research. Claparède, Flournoy's successor, was strongly interested in psychoanalysis. He was president of the Psychoanalytic Group of Geneva, and wrote the entry "Psychoanalysis" for André Lalande's reputed *Vocabulaire technique et critique de la philosophie*. With his introduction to the first translation into French of a text by Freud (*Five Lectures on Psychoanalysis*), Claparède performed a pioneering task; and although he criticized psychoanalysts for their tendency to sectarianism and dogmatism, he valued the theory.

Various elements highlight Piaget's closeness to the psychoanalytic movement at the time. He became a member of the Swiss Society for Psychoanalysis in 1920. The first psychology congress he ever attended was the International Congress of Psychoanalysis (Berlin, 1922). As for practice, apart from the "young autistic person" he claimed to have successfully treated, he analyzed at least one student of the Rousseau Institute in 1924 as an educational experience; according to the recollection of his late sister Marthe (herself a psychoanalyst) he also tried to psychoanalyze his own mother.

The Russian psychoanalyst Sabina Spielrein was at the Rousseau Institute between 1920 and 1923. Piaget told Bringuier that his "didactic analysis" with her took place every morning "at eight o'clock for eight months"; he also said that he wanted to be analyzed "as a learning experience," and was "glad to be a guinea-pig." As he explained, the experience ended because Spielrein discovered that he was "impervious to the theory," and that she would never convince him. Piaget, however, regretted it, since he was "deeply interested" in the process, and found it "marvelous" to discover his complexes."

In the early 1920s, psychoanalysis remained for Piaget a major theoretical reference. He described childhood thought as characterized by "egocentrism," that is, by the inability to adopt someone else's point of view, and a tendency to regard all reality as resulting from one's own activity. The child's spontaneous thought was syncretic, animistic and magical; it therefore resembled "primitive" thought, and especially the "autistic" thought defined by Bleuler. For Piaget, dream, dementia and mystical imagination were "pre-logical" aspects of intelligence that manifested a loss of contact with reality, as well as a lack of conscious "direction" in the temporal and logical organization of judgment. It is gradually through contact with others and the "grasp of consciousness" (a key concept of Claparède's psychology) that childhood thought adapts itself to reality. Although Piaget's thinking at the time was closer to the psychology of his Paris teacher Pierre Janet than to Freud's, he felt that his description of child development was generally consistent with psychoanalytic theory. In *The Language and Thought of the Child* (1923), his first book on psychology, he drew the reader's attention to what he had "borrowed from psychoanalysis," which seemed to him "to throw new light on the psychology of primitive thought." Spielrein and Piaget planned to work together on a theory of symbolic thought.

P

Piaget established parallelisms between intellectual and affective development, but did not approach them in psychoanalytic fashion. By the early 1930s, he had criticized the Freudian conceptions of symbol, memory and the unconscious. Toward the end of his career, he integrated the "cognitive" and the "affective unconscious" into a structure made up of non-conscious elements, and therefore resembling a Freudian "pre-conscious" or a non-psychoanalytic "subconscious." Most of the attempts at articulating psychoanalysis and Piagetian psychology have focused on the parallelisms in the developmental sequences described by each theory.

REFERENCES

Amman-Gainotti, M., and Ducret, J. J. (1991). Jean Piaget et la psychanalyse: les étapes d'une réflexion. *Neuropsychiatrie de l'enfance*, 39: 83–90.

Gouin Decarie, T. (1962). *Intelligence and Affectivity in Early Childhood. An Experimental Study of Jean Piaget's Object Concept and Object Relations.* New York: International Universities Press, 1965 (English translation).

Greenspan, Stanley I. (1979). *Intelligence and Adaptation: An Integration of Psychoanalytic and Piagetian Developmental Psychology.* New York: International Universities Press.

Leuba J. (1934). Compte rendu, VIIIe Conférence des Psychanalystes de Langue Française, Revue française de psychanalyse, 7: 116–136.

Pfister O. (1920). J. Piaget, "La psychanalyse et la pédagogie" [review of Piaget, 1920], *Imago*, 6: 294–295.

Piaget J. (1920). La psychanalyse dans ses rapports avec la psychologie de l'enfant, *Bulletin de la Société Alfred Binet*, 20: 18–34, 41–58.

———. (1930). Autobiography. In C. Murchison, (ed.). *A History of Psychology in Autobiography.* Worcester, Mass.: Clark University Press.

———. (1933). La Psychanalyse et le développement intellectuel, *Revue française de psychanalyse*, 6: 405–408.

———. (1971). The affective unconscious and the cognitive unconscious. A. Sinclair (trans.). In B. Inhelder, and H. Chipman, (eds.) (1976). *Piaget and His School. A reader in developmental psychology.* New York: Springer.

Schmid-Kitsikis, E. (1990). *An Interpersonal Approach to Mental Functioning: Assessment and Treatment.* H. Sinclair (trans.). Basel: Karger.

Vidal, F. (1986). Piaget et la psychanalyse: premières rencontres, *Le Bloc-notes de la psychanalyse*, 6: 171–189.

———. (1994). *Piaget before Piaget.* Cambridge, Mass.: Harvard University Press.

———. (2001). Sabina Spielrein, Jean Piaget—going their own ways, *Journal of Analytic Psychology*, 46: 139–153.

Wolff, Peter H. (1960). *The developmental psychologies of Jean Piaget and psychoanalysis.* New York: International Universities Press.

FERNANDO VIDAL

Pleasure Principle

Humans are motivated to seek pleasure and to avoid pain. Freud, searching for a scientific explanation of this fundamental of human behavior, drew on the experimental psychology of Fechner. The mind, Freud proposed, contends with changing levels of biologically based drive tension, seeking discharge in action or in fantasy. The accumulation of this psychic energy is intrinsically intolerable to the psychic apparatus and is experienced as unpleasurable. This unpleasure then serves a hedonic motivation for action. Pleasurable need satisfaction, Freud hypothesized, is sought through the immediate reduction of unpleasurable drive tension. Through discharge, psychic equilibrium is restored.

With this conceptualization, Freud conflated the etiological and psychological, the quantitative and the qualitative, and the objective and the subjective, which would ultimately prove theoretically untenable. Initially focused on the problem of accumulating tension or energy, Freud spoke of the "Unpleasure Principle," then the "Pleasure/Unpleasure" principle, and, finally, the "Pleasure Principle."

Linked to the pleasure principle, the constancy principle, also derived from Fechner, proposes that the psychic apparatus seeks to maintain a constant or stable level of psychic energy or drive tension in the system, binding or discharging energy through action or psychic defense. For Freud, the mind is essentially an energy-processing structure, mediating the power of the biological drives with the external world. With development, the pleasure principle is influenced by reality; the psychic apparatus learns to perceive and adapt to reality in the service of need satisfaction and safety. Immediate drive discharge may have painful consequences and therefore must be delayed, repressed, or bounded by the mechanisms of defense.

In *Formulations on the Two Principles of Mental Functioning* (1911), Freud codified the pleasure principle and the reality principle as the two regulatory principles governing all mental activity, including the adaptive processes necessary for need satisfaction—the avoidance of pain and the maximizing of pleasure, now with regard for the adaptation to reality.

As governors of mental life, the pleasure principle and the reality principle would serve as the theoretical foundation for Freud's theory of modes of thinking, namely, primary and secondary process. Primary process, as the earliest and most primitive form of mentation, functions without regard to logic and reality. Intolerant of delay, it seeks immediate peremptory satisfaction of wishes. As the direct expression of the pleasure principle, primary process thinking remains largely unconscious throughout life, as unconscious fantasy. As a developmental acquisition, secondary process, the realistic and adaptive mode of conscious and preconscious thinking, expresses the influence of the reality principle on mentation, functioning along with and modifying the influence of the pleasure principle.

By 1920, with the publication of *Beyond the Pleasure Principle* (1920), Freud faced the theoretical challenges to the pleasure principle posed by the clinical problems of masochism, the philosophic dilemma of human aggression and destructiveness, and life's obvious pleasurable tensions. By proposing the death instinct as beyond the pleasure principle, he envisioned an innate motivation for the lowest level of psychic energy, for total elimination of drive tension, namely, psychic inertia, psychic (and biological) death. Freud borrowed the idea of the nirvana principle from Barbara Low. Human existence reflected, at the deepest core, the struggle of the life instinct, eros or libido, with the death instinct. Mental life reflected the efforts of the libido to fuse with and tame the manifestations of the death instinct in the fight for drive satisfaction and adaptation in life.

With establishment of the structural hypothesis, the pleasure principle, "that almost omnipotent institution" (Freud, 1926: 92), assists the ego as it gives a "signal of unpleasure" to oppose an instinctual process from the id. The pleasure principle guides the ego as it defends against the unpleasures from the superego and the external world.

REFERENCES

Freud, S. (1911). Formulations on the two principles of mental functioning. S.E. 12: 213–226.
———. (1920). *Beyond the Pleasure Principle.* S.E. 18: 1–64.
———. (1926). *Inhibitions, Symptoms, and Anxiety.* S.E. 20: 87–172.

ROBERT ALAN GLICK

Postmodernism See MODERNISM, POSTMODERNISM, AND FREUDIANISM.

Preconscious

In Freud's topographical theory, the preconscious is a system distinct from the unconscious system. According to traditional thinking, the preconscious is descriptively, but not dynamically, unconscious; that is, the preconscious contains knowledge and memories that, although not presently conscious, are in principle accessible to consciousness and not dynamically repressed.

Clinically, preconscious processes may be seen to represent the implicit, and conscious processes the explicit (LaPlanche and Pontalis, 1973).

Freud (1940) links the preconscious to the ego, to language, and to conscious processes (the system PCs-cs), just as he links the unconscious to the id. This may sound as if the preconscious is simply that which is momentarily not conscious, not in the forefront of the mind, but ready at any moment to become conscious. However, Freud suggests in several passages that the preconscious has psychic qualities of its own. For example, he speaks of the periphery of the ego as involved in perceptual and conscious processes, and the inside of the ego, comprising internal thought processes, as having the quality of being preconscious.

Further, psychic qualities and psychic processes are not as static as topographical theory may seem to represent. In attributing psychical qualities to conscious, preconscious, or unconscious processes, Freud states, "The division between the three classes of material which possess these qualities is neither absolute nor permanent. What is preconscious becomes conscious, as we have seen without any assistance from us; what is unconscious can, through our efforts, be made conscious" (1940, p. 160).

Freud alludes to the transformative function of the preconscious when be states: "material which is ordinarily unconscious [in the usual dynamic sense] can transform itself into preconscious material and then becomes conscious" (p. 161). And again, when referring to the ordinary course of development, he states, "certain contents of the id were transformed into the preconscious state and so taken into the ego" (p. 163). Although he fails to develop this notion further, later writers do so. Matte-Blanco (1975), in explicating the multiple organizations of psychic experience guided by principles of mathematical set theory, speaks of the bilogic of experience, wherein asymmetrical, conscious linear logic mixes with or interpenetrates symmetrical, unconscious, nonlinear logic. Here, conscious and unconscious experience exist simultaneously, and the preconscious serves a transformative function, linking symmetrical and asymmetrical modes. The distinction between what is repressed and unrepressed, what is dynamically unconscious and what is simply unconscious (or asymmetrical) by nature, is not necessarily clear. The preconscious, then, is not simply what is momentarily not conscious but readily recalled; it has linking and transformative functions.

Similarly, Civin and Lombardi (1990) develop Freud's notion of the preconscious into a bridging function linking unconscious and conscious processes. "If we reframe the system preconscious in terms of process (rather than topography, structure, or quality), then we have aligned the preconscious with twentieth century psychics, extricated it from mechanistic positivist science, and provided a rationale for the concept of bidirectional mapping. The preconscious and potential space can then be seen as serving bridging or linking functions between internal and external experience" (p. 577). Developmentally, preconscious experience may be seen as originating in a kind of Winnicottian transitional space (Winnicott, 1971) that the infant experiences with the holding functions of the mother (Deri, 1984), and out of which symbolization develops. Civin and Lombardi advocate a greater focus on the process of intermediation between internal and external experience in the psychic life of the individual. Precedent for such a focus is found in Freud's conception of the preconscious as "an essential third dimension whose function was to mediate between the conscious and the unconscious" (Civin and Lombardi, 1990: 584).

REFERENCES

Civin, M., and Lombardi, K. (1990). The preconscious and potential space. *Psychoanalytic Review*, 77 (4): 573–585.

Deri, S. (1984). *Symbolization and Creativity*. New York: International Universities Press.

Freud, S. (1923). *The Ego and the Id*. S.E. 19: 3–66.

———. (1940). *An Outline of Psychoanalysis*. S.E. 23: 141–208.

LaPlanche, J., and Pontalis, J. B. (1973). *The Language of Psychoanalysis*. New York: Norton.

Matte-Blanco, I. (1975). *The Unconscious as Infinite Sets: An Essay in Bi-logic*. London: Duckworth.

Winnicott, D. W. (1971). *Playing and Reality*. Harmondsworth, England: Penguin.

KAREN L. LOMBARDI

Pregenital Eroticism See INFANTILE SEXUALITY.

Preliminary Communication
See BREUER, JOSEF.

Pre-Oedipal State
See DEVELOPMENTAL THEORY.

Primal Fantasy See FANTASY (PHANTASY); PRIMAL SCENE.

Primal Repression See REPRESSION.

Primal Scene

The concept of the primal scene refers to the scene of sexual intercourse between adults—usually one's parents—that a child either witnesses or fantasizes about. Freud's first allusion to the primal scene concerns its pathogenic role in the formation of anxiety symptoms. In a letter he wrote to Wilhelm Fliess in 1893, he claims to have analyzed two cases of anxiety neurosis in virgins and explains their anxiety symptoms in terms of a "presentient dread of sexuality, and behind it things they had seen or heard and half-understood" (1893, p. 49). Two years later, in *Studies on Hysteria*, Freud again refers to reactions of "horror" in young (virginal) girls when faced with the world of sexuality for the first time. Initially, Freud refers to "sexual scenes" but does not specify that this "world" is related to parental coitus. In a footnote to the Katharina case, he presents the case of a girl who dates the onset of her anxiety attacks to a time when she was exposed to, and excited specifically by, parental intercourse (1895, p. 127).

Freud explains the explicit role the child's parents play in primal scene anxiety in *The Interpretation of Dreams*: "It is, I may say, a matter of daily experience that sexual intercourse between adults strikes any children who may observe it as something uncanny and that it arouses anxiety in them. I have explained this anxiety by arguing that what we are dealing with is a sexual excitation with which their understanding is unable to cope and which they also, no doubt, repudiate because their parents are involved in it, and which is therefore transformed into anxiety" (1900, p. 585).

Freud remarks that witnessing of the primal scene is not necessarily experienced as traumatic at the time of exposure; rather, later interpretation, deferred action (*nachträglich*), of such events is what results in trauma (1897, p. 244). In a letter from May 2, 1897, Freud attributes the deferred action causing primal scene trauma as the causative factor not only in anxiety neurosis but also in hysteria: "Everything goes back to the reproduction of scenes, some of which can be arrived at directly, but others always by way of phantasies set up in front of them. The phantasies are derived from things that have been heard but understood subsequently and all their material is, of course, genuine" (1897, p. 247). In this letter Freud employs the term "primal scene" for the first time. He describes how one must return, either directly or via fantasy, to the primal scenes of hysterics. Primal scenes are here defined as a combination of "things that have been experienced and things that have been heard, past events (from the history of parents and ancestors) and things that have been seen by oneself" (p. 248).

Fantasy and reality are not always clearly distinguished in Freud's mind, yet he claims the outcome of both to be equally traumatic in potential. He considers the primal scene fantasy a phylogenetic endowment; it is one of several primal fantasies (*Urphantasien*) common to neurotics and generally universal in nature (1916–917, pp. 370–371).

Although Freud never resolved the problem of whether actual exposure was necessary for primal scene trauma, he never relinquished his belief that the primal scene is inherently traumatic. He considered the primal scene to be traumatic because he believed the child was overstimulated to a point at which his or her defensive barrier is breached. Lacking the ability to cope when introduced prematurely to the world of adult sexuality, the child responds with a "surplus of sexuality." Following his original theory of anxiety, Freud claimed that the resultant undischarged libido creates anxiety that then results in symptom formation or psychic disequilibrium. Although he later changed his theory of anxiety, Freud continued to maintain this view insofar as it concerned the primal scene. Part of what is traumatic, he added in his *Three Essays*, is the child's perception of the sexual act as sadistic.

The case of the Wolf Man (1918, p. 17) is by far Freud's most extensive clinical investigation of the primal scene. He interpreted the famous dream, in which his patient saw wolves sitting immobile on a tree's branches, as a reversal for the violent movement associated with primal scene activity. Serious question has been raised regarding Freud's attempts to demonstrate that his patient's entire neurosis could be traced back to a single primal scene exposure at the age of eighteen months (Blum, 1974).

Freud extended the primal scene experience beyond the traditional notion of the excluded child when noting a patient's identification with her mother (1915), leading to recent literature on the subject that views primal scene fantasies as an important blueprint for internalized object relations involving multiple and shifting identifications with all dramatic personae (Knafo and Feiner, 1996).

REFERENCES

Blum, H. (1974). The borderline childhood of the wolf man. *Journal of the American Psychoanalytic Asssociation*, 22: 721–740.

Breuer, J., and Freud, S. (1895). *Studies on Hysteria*. S.E. 2: 19–305.

Freud, S. (1893). Letter to Fliess. S.E. 1: 49.

———. (1897). Letter to Fliess. S.E.1: 244.

———. (1900). *Interpretation of Dreams*. S.E. 4–5: 1–621.

———. (1905). *Three Essays on Sexuality*. S.E. 7: 130–243.

———. (1918). From the history of an infantile neurosis. S.E. 17: 7–123.

———. (1916–1917). *Introductory Lectures*. S.E. 15–16: 9–496.

———. (1915). A case of paranoia running counter to the psychoanalytic theory of the disease. S.E. 14: 263–272.

Knafo, D., and Feiner, K. (1996). The primal scene: Variations on a theme. *Journal of the American Psychoanalytic Association*, 44, no. 2: 549–569.

DANIELLE KNAFO

Primary Process See DREAMS, THEORY OF.

Project for a Scientific Psychology: Freud's Theory of Neuronal Excitation, Conveyance, and Discharge

In the autumn of 1895, Freud wrote what he referred to as a "Psychology for Neurologists," intended as an encompassing description of mental phenomena, a theory of the mind in its entirety. He sought to emphasize basic research and, within a month, filled two notebooks with his views totaling one hundred manuscript sheets that were subsequently mailed to his friend Wilhelm Fliess for study and critique. Freud retained a third notebook identified as the "Psychopathology of Repression," because he felt the work was problematic, and it was apparently left uncompleted. The contents of the third notebook remain unknown to date. Fortunately, the notebooks sent to Fliess survived, later to be published in 1950 in German after Freud's death, with the title "Entwurf einer Psychologie" (Sketch of a Psychology). The editor of the subsequent English translation, James Strachey, named the work "Project for a Scientific Psychology." As it is known today, the "Project" comprises three sections labeled (1) "General Scheme," (2) "Psychopathology," and (3) "An Attempt to Represent Normal Psychical Processes."

Freud explained the nervous system with his principle of neuronic inertia, stating that it is the natural tendency of all neurons to divest themselves of excitation.

P

Pain or unpleasure is related to a primary neuronic system having acquired excessive excitation, while pleasure results from discharge, the primary function of neuronic systems. Discharging excitation that impinges on the nervous system maintains psychic equilibrium for either internal or external sources. Specific pathways selected for such discharge are related to the development of the secondary function that controls the psychic attempt to flee from excessive/undischargeable stimuli. Because of endogenous needs, including hunger, respiration, and sexuality, the neuronic system must learn to tolerate a store of excitation that is undischargeable while still attempting to keep the quantity down. The neuronic system is thus regulated by the principle of constancy, where mental processes strive toward an equilibrium known as "homeostasis," maintaining as low a level of tension as possible. Secondary process involves levels of conscious awareness reflected in the construction of defenses.

Freud's "Project" presents three separate systems to account for perception, memory, and consciousness: the phi, psi, and omega systems. Each system has assigned physiological properties deriving from contact-barrier modifications leading to various functional aptitudes. The permeable phi neurons serve the function of perception. The psi neurons are also involved in perception, but their impermeability conveys a special capacity for retention and recollection. Memory is represented by differences in the facilitations (which serve the primary function) between the psi neurons. The third system of neurons, the omega neurons, are also excited in perception, giving rise to different qualities of conscious sensations. With unrelenting forces of experience linked by emotional association, chance association, and symbolization, a psyche with both primitive judgment and sophisticated reality testing evolves.

Additional subject matters in the "Project" include "Affects and Wishful States," "Introduction to the Concept of an 'Ego,'" "The Primary and Secondary Processes in Psi," "The Analysis of Dreams," "Dream Consciousness," and "The Psychopathology of Hysteria," all reflecting Freud's high aspirations in writing this document. Owing to the incompleteness of the perhaps critically binding final section on repression, controversy regarding the broad nature and implications of the "Project" has persisted. Various examiners have attempted to decipher the work as being either "psychological" or "neurological," only to conclude in many instances that the "Project" was written with an intricate dualist spirit. Beyond this, it can be maintained that Freud's "Project" advances a complex "neurophysiology" with constructs like local field potentials allowing for more reflexive and automatic behavior to occur in the psyche. Local field potentials translate as "cathexis." Additionally evident is a knowledge of propagated nerve impulses known as "action currents" translating as "currents in flow." The resistances at "contact-barriers" are synapses that connect the "specifiable materials" known as "neurons." The resistances can be worn down by use when both the pre- and postsynaptic sites are activated. Selective learning is ascribed to the restricted lowering of certain synaptic resistances by the absorption of energy, "precathexis," at the pre- as well as postsynaptic sites as a result of repeated activation. Freud provides exceptional detail: a double feedback system between basal forebrain and cortex to produce the attentional process necessary for reality testing, the memory-motive structure in the basal forebrain that underlies a wish, the equality of drive, self-help, and caretaker in the development of ego in the basal forebrain. Indeed, more closely examined, the profound significance of the "Project" rests with its place as a "Rosetta stone" that truly defines psychoanalysis as a natural science.

REFERENCES

Freud, S. *Project for a Scientific Psychology.* S.E. 1: 283–397.
Pribram, K. H. (1962). *The Neuropsychology of Sigmund Freud.* In A. J. Bachrach (ed.). *Experimental Foundations of Clinical Psychology.* New York: Basic Books, pp. 442–468.
Sulloway, F. J. (1992). *Freud, Biologist of the Mind.* Cambridge, Mass.: Harvard University Press.

KARL G. SIEG
KARL H. PRIBRAM

Projection

Projection, a moderately complex defense mechanism, involves the unacknowledged attribution of an individual's own unacceptable thoughts, feelings, wishes, or impulses onto another person. The individual then becomes aware of the existence of these thoughts or feelings but sees them as residing in someone else, and is thus protected from knowing about their personal origin.

The development of the concept of projection, however, leaves some unclarity concerning the role of awareness about the projected attribute. Originally, Sigmund Freud (1895) identified "projection" as a process in which the cause, or responsibility, for some unacceptable thought or behavior was attributed to another person: "He made me think (do) it." In this case, the individual is aware of the unacceptable thought but attributes the responsibility for that thought to someone else. Similarly, in "projective identification," individuals attribute to another person a thought or feeling that they subsequently recognize to exist in themselves, although that feeling is experienced as a reaction to the other person's (projected) feelings. Again, responsibility for the feeling has been placed on another person. Although the defense has been broadened to include *any* mental operation in which inner psychological phenomena are attributed to the external world, in its most pristine form, "projection" occurs with thoughts, feelings, and wishes not acknowledged as part of the self. (See Novick and Kelly, 1970, for a full discussion).

To use the defense of "projection," the individual must have reached a developmental level in which certain cognitive operations are possible. The individual must be able to differentiate between the inside and outside of the self; between the self and other; between acceptable and unacceptable, as determined by social mores; and between conscious and unconscious mental representations.

Research studies indicate that this defense is prominent among normal school-age children and early adolescents. It is only in adolescence that some individuals begin to understand how the defense works, at which time it loses its effectiveness. (See Cramer, 1991, for a review of these studies; also, Cramer, 1997; Smith and Daniellson, 1982).

In its most blatant form, "projection" may be seen in the phenomenon of hallucination. Reacting to an inner wish or need, the individual "sees" as existing in reality that which is wished for. This form of projection is generally associated with psychotic psychopathology, although such phenomena have been reported from people under extreme duress—for example, the thirst-quenched man hallucinating an oasis in the desert. Psychotic delusions may also be based on projection; the individual under the sway of such delusions may strike back at imagined persecutors, as in the psychopathology of paranoia.

One interesting aspect of projection is that it sometimes contains a kernel of truth. When people project their angry feelings onto another and then accuse that other person of being angry with them, there may be some truth in this accusation. It appears that the targets of projection are not random, and are sometimes chosen to match the projected feeling (S. Freud, 1922). Further, the ability to perceive one's own emotion in others—i.e., for projection—may also facilitate the capacity for empathy with others.

REFERENCES

Cramer, P. (1991). *The Development of Defense Mechanisms.* New York: Springer-Verlag.

———. (1997). Evidence for change in children's use of defense mechanisms. *Journal of Personality*, 65: 233–247.

Fenichel, O. (1945). *The Psychoanalytic Theory of Neurosis.* New York: Norton.

Freud, A. (1936). *The Ego and the Mechanisms of Defense.* New York: International Universities Press.

Freud, S. (1895). Draft H. paranoia. S.E. 1: 206–212.

———. (1922). Some neurotic mechanisms in jealousy, paranoia and homosexuality. S.E. 18: 221–232.

Novick, J., and Kelly, K. (1970). Projection and externalization. *Psychoanalytic Study of the Child*, 25: 69–95.

Smith, G. J. W., and Danielsson, A. (1982). *Anxiety and Defense Strategies in Childhood and Adolescence.* New York: International Universities Press.

Vaillant, G. E. (1992). *Ego Mechanisms of Defense: A Guide for Clinicians and Researchers.* Washington, D.C.: American Psychiatric Press.

———. (1994). Ego mechanisms of defense and personality psychopathology. *Journal of Abnormal Psychology*, 103: 44–50.

PHEBE CRAMER

Projective Techniques

Sigmund Freud first alerted our attention to the widespread human tendency to use the defense mechanism known as projection, in which individuals would both communicate and evacuate complicated and unwanted thoughts onto somebody else. Mindful of Freud's insight, the pioneering Swiss psychoanalyst Hermann Rorschach began to experiment with the use of inkblot pictures in the assessment of psychiatric patients. Rorschach discovered that if he showed a picture of an inkblot to a patient, that patient would then free-associate as to what the inkblot might resemble, and in this way Rorschach began to theorize that through the mechanism of the projection of internal thoughts onto the inkblot, one could begin to obtain a clearer picture of the content of the patient's mind. Although other workers had used the inkblot in research work prior to the 1910s and 1920s, Rorschach deserves credit as the first psychiatric worker to employ the inkblot in a more carefully researched and systematic form. His German-language book on psychodiagnostics first appeared in 1921. Since Rorschach's time, other techniques based on the mechanism of projection have developed, and collectively psychologists have come to refer to these as "projective techniques."

Without doubt, the Rorschach Inkblot Test remains the most popular form of projective test, and to this day the image of the inkblot is still used as a popular means of caricaturing psychologists in cartoons and other forms of popular culture. Rorschach himself began to experiment with literally thousands of different inkblot configurations, which he ultimately reduced to fifteen; but on the advice of his publisher, he then reduced that number even further to ten. Today, psychological testers still use the ten inkblot pictures first advocated by Hermann Rorschach. Essentially, the test consists of ten separate cards, each containing a symmetrical inkblot shape. Five cards are monochrome, and five cards contain various colors. The psychologist administering the test presents each card in sequence to a patient in a psychiatric setting or to a subject in a psychological experiment or assessment situation, then asks the person to free-associate verbally to the card. The investigator then records the subject's verbal responses and subsequently uses one of the many available scoring systems, in an effort to make sense of the patient's communications. The more psychoanalytically oriented scoring system focuses on such themes as the accuracy of the patient's perception and on the number of responses made to each card, as well as on the amount of time spent responding to each card. Although many critical, empirical psychologists have questioned both the utility and the validity of the Rorschach Inkblot Test, psychoanalytically trained psychologists continue to find the test a useful means of providing a sense of the patient's psychic structure.

Other well-known projective tests include the Thematic Apperception Test, first developed in the 1930s at Harvard University by the psychologist Henry Murray. Similar in style to the Rorschach Inkblot Test, the Thematic Apperception Test, commonly known as the "T.A.T.," involves thirty-one separate cards, thirty of which contain pictures of actual people, and one of which remains blank. In the administration of the T.A.T., the investigator asks a subject to free-associate and to construct a story involving the figure or figures in the picture; in this way, the subject projects some of his or her inner preoccupations onto the characters in the story. In addition to the Thematic Apperception Test, one might mention the Holtzman Inkblot Test, a variant of the Rorschach Inkblot Test, as well as the Children's Apperception Test, the Blacky Pictures, the House-Tree-Person Test, and the Lowenfeld Mosaic Test, among many others.

Projective tests tend to be administered mostly by clinical psychologists and educational psychologists, and such tests have always enjoyed greater popularity in the United States than in other countries. In Great Britain, for example, one would be hard-pressed to find more than a tiny handful of psychologists versed in the use of projective techniques. In recent years, as more and more psychologists have trained to become psychoanalysts and psychotherapists, the use of projective tests has begun to decline, and psychologists have become increasingly immersed in the rich work of ongoing psychotherapeutic treatment with patients. But as a rough-and-ready indicator of the patient's level of psychic functioning, many clinicians still find projective tests of value.

REFERENCES

Allison, J., Blatt, S. J., and Zimet, C. N. (1968). *The Interpretation of Psychological Tests.* New York: Harper and Row.

Kissen, M. (ed.) (1986). *Assessing Object Relations Phenomena.* Madison, Conn.: International Universities Press.

Kline, P. (1993). *The Handbook of Psychological Testing.* London: Routledge.

BRETT KAHR

Pseudoscience, and Psychoanalysis

One long standing issue about Freudian theory concerns its scientific status. Freud believed it to be part of natural science (1940, p. 282), but some critics have charged that it is pseudoscientific.

The best known of these critics, the British philosopher of science, Karl Popper, argued that any theory that is unfalsifiable in principle is pseudoscientific and that Freudian theory had this characteristic. One reason that Popper and his supporters give for thinking that Freudian theory is unfalsifiable is that it conflicts with no possible observations (Notturno and McHugh, 1986: 250).

The reply to this charge is now well known and requires little discussion. A particular part of Freud's theory may not *by itself* entail any observation statement (i.e, a potential falsifier), but that is true of most scientific hypotheses that talk about unobservable entities or phenomena. If a social learning theorist conjectures that a change in self-efficacy expectations often plays an important causal role in treating phobias, this theory by itself entails nothing about observable behavior. To clash with possible observations, it is sufficient that an hypothesis do so *when combined with auxiliary assumptions*, including a statement of initial conditions. If, however, auxiliary assumptions may be employed, then it is not obvious that *any* Freudian hypothesis lacks the capacity to clash with some possible observations. One might try to demonstrate for some particular Freudian hypothesis that there is *no* consistent set of auxiliary assumptions that can be combined with it to generate an observation statement, but Notturno and McHugh provide no such argument, nor has Popper or anyone else. (For an argument that for virtually any theory, even creationism and astrological theories, there is always some possible observation that would disconfirm it, see Erwin, 1960).

A more interesting argument about falsifiability concerns the logical structure of the theory, which appears to permit one part to protect another part from falsification: "Freud often puzzles us, not by putting forward claims without falsifiers, but by putting forward other claims as well whose natural force is to cancel the falsifiers of the more straightforward ones" (Cioffi 1985: 233).

Another way of stating Cioffi's point is this: Even if one Freudian hypothesis, when combined with auxiliary assumptions, entails an observation statement, the falsity of the latter can always be explained by one or more other Freudian hypotheses without rejecting any part of Freudian theory. This claim is not being made about all of Freudian theory, but only about some of it. Popper (1986) probably intends to illustrate the same point as Cioffi when he discusses the case of a man who throws a child into a river with the intention of drowning it. A Freudian could explain this event, Popper notes, by saying that the man suffered from repression of some component of his Oedipus complex. However, if another man—or even the same man—sacrifices his life in trying to save the child, the Freudian need not take this as counter evidence to Freudian theory; he can explain the behavior in terms of sublimation. He can, in Cioffi's terminology, "cancel" the alleged falsification.

How can a falsification be "cancelled"? If *H*, together with *A* (the conjunction of certain auxiliary assumptions) really does entail some observation statement O, and O is false, then either H or A is false. This result is a matter of logic, and cannot be "cancelled." What we

might do, however, is to undermine one or more of the auxiliary assumptions by appealing to the truth of some other Freudian hypothesis. To take Popper's example, the hypothesis that a certain man suffered from repression will, together with other assumptions, entail that he will try to drown a certain child; but if he does not do that, one of the auxiliary assumptions can be challenged by appealing to the hypothesis that he is sublimating his homicidal tendencies.

Popper's example may be unrealistic in that few Freudians would try to use their theory to predict whether or not a man will try to drown or save a child. To make such a prediction, we would need more information about the initial conditions than we would be likely to have. A more realistic case concerns an actual experiment that has been discussed by both Freudians and anti-Freudians. In 1957, Scodel tested Freud's orality hypothesis, which says that male preference for large female breasts results from earlier frustration of oral dependency. He tested the hypothesis by deriving from it and other assumptions the following prediction: Men preferring large breasted women will tend to show more oral dependency as measured by the TAT (the Thematic Apperception Test). Scodel then performed an experiment and found the opposite result. Men in the small breast preference group gave significantly more TAT dependency themes than both those in the large breast preference group and the no preference group. Scodel concluded that his results falsified a widely held Freudian hypothesis. His interpretation of the data, however, is rejected by Paul Kline, who tries to save the orality hypothesis by postulating reaction-formation in Scodel's small breast preference group. He even suggests (Kline, 1981: 123) that Scodel's results can be taken as *support* for Freud's orality hypothesis, on the grounds that only Freudian theory could have explained the experimental results.

The Scodel experiment, then, better illustrates the point made by Popper and Cioffi than does the made up case of the drowning child. Here we have a seemingly well-designed experiment with a negative outcome; yet, the Freudian can seemingly cope with the negative results by appealing to another Freudian hypothesis to "cancel" the falsification.

Because a Freudian can sometimes appeal to reaction-formation or other defense mechanisms to explain away seemingly negative results, parts of the theory *are* difficult to test. Freudian theory is not alone, however, in containing certain assumptions that can serve as a buffer against disconfirmation. For example, suppose that an operant conditioning theorist tries to explain the linguistic behavior of an individual in terms of reinforcement. If we find no current reinforcing stimulus, we need not take this as evidence against operant conditioning theory. Instead, we can appeal to an assumption about the history of the individual's reinforcement schedules and an assumption about response generalization. If a theory has such a "buffer" feature, severe practical difficulties may arise in trying to falsify the theory—especially, if we focus only on one case rather than examine a pattern of evidence. It is doubtful, however, that the protection offered is absolute, that it will prevail come what may (for a discussion of the case of operant conditioning, see Erwin, 1978, Chapter 3). To return to the Scodel experiment, we can agree that the appeal to reaction-formation, *if it occurred*, would explain Scodel's results. We still need to ask, however, if the reaction-formation explanation is more plausible, given our background evidence, than the one offered by Scodel: that a reinforcement hypothesis explains the preference for large breasts in the high dependency group. If we were concerned here with the practical possibility of disconfirmation, we might have to examine the actual background evidence for Freudian theory and learning theory to evaluate the merits of the rival hypotheses. Given, however, that we are talking only about the logical possibility of disconfirmation, we can avoid this issue. We are free to stipulate that we are discussing a possible world in which prior to the Scodel experiment, there is no firm evidence at all for Freud's orality hypothesis and that there is solid evidence that reinforcement mechanisms can explain the type of behavior that Scodel's subjects exhibited. Suppose, further, that we were to find a behavioral correlate of the unconscious anxiety associated with reaction formation. We might find, for example, that among adults who display extreme affection for the parent of the same sex, they always report having the same type of recurring, bizarre dream. The most plausible explanation of this finding might be that these people are expressing the "opposite" kind of emotion they consciously feel; unconsciously, they hate their same-sexed parent. This explanation might become more plausible if, after psychoanalytic treatment, such people tended to display hatred toward the parent when the bizarre type of dreaming ceased. Once behavioral indicators of reaction-formation were established in this way,

the continued failure to find them in a given case might be evidence of the absence of the activation of this particular defense mechanism in a particular individual. If only such individuals were studied in a Scodel-type experiment, then the appeal to reaction formation would not be a defensible explanation of the experimental results.

Given the stipulated background evidence, the reinforcement hypothesis would provide a more plausible explanation of the Scodel results than would the orality hypothesis. The results, then, would clearly favor the reinforcement hypothesis and would also provide *some* (not necessarily overwhelming) evidence against the orality hypothesis.

The Scodel experiment is only one experiment but it illustrates something important, something that runs exactly counter to the Cioffi-Popper thesis. No doubt Freudian defense mechanisms can often be invoked to explain away apparently disconfirming results, but what is doubtful is that such explanations will always be equal to or superior to their rivals no matter what empirical data are obtained. In the Scodel case, if our background evidence was as I stipulated it to be, then Kline's appeal to reaction formation would have been a demonstrable failure; his explanation would have been markedly inferior to Scodel's. In order to support their thesis, Popper and Cioffi have to do far more than merely point out that certain Freudian hypotheses can always be brought in to "cancel" apparent falsifications. They have to show that the attempted cancellations will always be successful no matter what the experimental evidence may be. They do not argue for this assumption. Consequently, their argument for untestability fails to show that even one Freudian hypothesis is untestable.

Even if the results of the Scodel experiment were clearly disconfirmatory (which I doubt), would Freudians acknowledge that fact? They might not, and this raises a further issue about testability. Although Notturno and McHugh (1986) give two reasons why a theory might be untestable, they appeal only to the second in discussing Freudian theory: the theory's proponents' refusal to acknowledge falsifications as such.

Suppose, contrary to fact, that Freud and all Freudians always refused to accept counter evidence to Freudian theory. Would this make all or part of their theory unfalsifiable? It would not. If an experimental result falsifies a Freudian hypothesis, then it does so whether or not Freudians agree to the falsification. The claim that

Scodel's results refuted Freud's orality hypothesis does not logically entail that Freudians will accept the refutation; their failure to accept the refutation is consistent with it being genuine. Of course, as with any experimental result, supporters of Freud might challenge Scodel's derivation of his conclusion or one of his auxiliary assumptions, and they might be right to do so. (His reliance on the TAT to measure oral dependency can be reasonably challenged.) But the mere non-acceptance of a falsification does nothing by itself to nullify it.

Instead of merely balking at the counter evidence, the Freudians may, as Notturno and McHugh put it (p. 250), use "evasive tactics." For example, they may change their original hypothesis. However, that move does not protect *it* (the original hypothesis) from the charge of falsification. They may also bring in "ad hoc" assumptions, i.e., assumptions brought in after the experiment has been completed, and use them to explain away the apparent disconfirmation. However, if the invocation of these assumptions is warranted, then the "disconfirmation" is illusory. On the other hand, an ad hoc assumption may fail to explain the data in a satisfactory manner; but, then, the disconfirmation stands whether or not the Freudian agrees. In neither alternative does his or her failure to accept the counter evidence, by itself, cancel the refutation.

The third argument of the Popperians, then, is no better than the first two. The fact that proponents of a theory refuse to accept what is apparently a disconfirming experimental result is normally no grounds whatsoever for believing that a disconfirmation has occurred.

Cioffi (1985) tries to challenge the distinction between falsifying a theory and its adherents refusing to acknowledge the falsification. Here is how the challenge goes: Freud's response to apparent falsifications of his libido theory, Cioffi claims, cannot be distinguished from "the theory-in-itself"; for his responses tell us what is meant by expressions like "narcissism" and how it is distinguished from "egoism."

Cioffi's challenge depends on an extremely dubious theory of meaning elucidation; without some support for this theory, the challenge fails. Suppose that a linguist hypothesizes that we are all born with unconscious knowledge of universal grammar, and a test of the hypothesis is devised. If the test is negative, but the linguist dogmatically refuses to accept the falsification, and instead engages in evasive behavior, his or her response does not change the meaning of the original hypothesis, nor does it necessarily tell us anything about what the hypothesis means.

Cioffi gives a case that he thinks obviously illustrates his theory. Suppose that two zoologists assert, let us say in the eighteenth century, that all swans are white. They then find out that black swans have been discovered in Australia, but they refuse to give up or qualify at all their original hypothesis. Cioffi suggests that we can take their response as an *elucidation* of their original hypothesis, but he gives no reason for what looks like an obviously wrong thing to say. If the zoologists said without any qualification that all swans are white, then their theory has been refuted; their dogmatic behavior does not change that fact. If they reply "Well, we never intended to be talking about *all* swans," that does not help their case; they said all swans are white, with no exceptions for Australian swans. Their subsequent dogmatic behavior does not clarify the meaning of their original hypothesis.

Cioffi does have another argument to show that Freudian theory is pseudoscientific; this last one does not depend on claims about testing the theory: "To claim that an enterprise is pseudoscientific is to claim that it involves the habitual and wilful employment of methodologically defective procedures (in a sense of wilful which encompasses refined self-deception)" (Cioffi, 1970). In speaking of "methodologically defective procedures," Cioffi is thinking of those used to prevent the discovery of disconfirming evidence. After stating his criterion, Cioffi tries to show, as he puts it, that there are a host of peculiarities of psychoanalytic theory and practice which are manifestations of the same impulse: the need to avoid refutation. Whatever the evidence for this charge, Cioffi's argument fails from the start. His criterion for identifying pseudoscience talks not about theories but about *enterprises*. Even if it were true that Freud had habitually and wilfully employed methodologically defective procedures, and this were sufficient to make his enterprise pseudoscientific, it would not follow that any of his *theories* were pseudoscientific; some of them might in fact be true and might be supported by reasonably firm empirical evidence, amassed after Freud had died. Without some explanation of how one can bridge the logical gap between saying that an enterprise is pseudoscientific and saying that the theory associated with that enterprise is pseudoscientific, Cioffi's argument fails.

In a more recent publication, Cioffi (1998) has refined his criterion of pseudoscience, but the new version is no better than the old (Erwin, 2001).

P

All of the arguments examined so far have failed to show that any part of Freudian theory is pseudoscientific. What are the prospects for some new argument of this sort being developed? They are not good. Popper and others who tried to demonstrate the pseudoscientific nature of Freud's theorizing were clearly trying to *discredit* his theories. But there is a deep problem with such attempts. What follows from saying that a theory is "pseudoscientific"? That may vary with the critic; not everyone uses this expression in the same way. In the 1960s, some who applied this concept to Freudian theory meant only that the key theoretical terms could not be operationally defined. An attempt was then made by some of Freud's supporters to provide operational definitions (usually by distorting the meaning of the concepts). Suppose that Freudian theory is "pseudoscientific" in this operational sense. Why would it matter? The theory, or important parts of it, might still be true, and we might know that because it might be supported by powerful evidence.

Suppose, however, that we build into the very idea of a pseudoscientific theory that it is untrue or unsupported by empirical evidence. If we do that, we are doing something obviously important if we demonstrate that in this sense Freudian theory is pseudoscientific. But we are now making a lack of truth or supporting evidence a necessary condition of being pseudoscientific; in that case, we cannot demonstrate that the theory is pseudo-scientific without first either refuting the theory or undermining the many empirical arguments, including those from over 1500 experimental studies, that have been amassed in its favor. However, this is exactly what was supposed to be avoided; the demonstration of pseudoscientificality was supposed to give us a short cut for discrediting Freudian theory.

The dilemma then is this: Saying that a theory is pseudoscientific either entails that it is *untrue or empirically unsupported* or it does not; if it does not, then a theory can be pseudoscientific and also be true and well supported by evidence. In this event, why would it matter that the theory is pseudoscientific? In the other alternative, we cannot demonstrate that the theory is pseudoscientific unless we also demonstrate that it is false or unsupported. But how do we do that without examining the empirical arguments pro and con? It might be thought that we can avoid such an examination by demonstrating a priori that there cannot possibly be supporting evidence; for the theory cannot possibly be falsified and so it cannot be supported either. However,

we have already seen that the attempt to show that Freudian theory is unfalsifiable in principle has failed.

Some theories, for example, astrological and certain parapsychological theories, are aptly called pseudoscientific. They are not only unsupported by any firm empirical evidence, and are probably completely wrong, but they also have the superficial trappings of scientific theories. To discredit them, however, what needs to be done is to show that there are no rational grounds for believing them, or better yet, to demonstrate their falsity. To do neither while trying to show that they are pseudoscientific is not going to result in effective criticism. It is fair to say that attempts to discredit what may in fact be pseudoscientific theories by taking a short cut—ignoring the complicated empirical arguments while trying to demonstrate pseudoscientificality—has proven to be not a viable short cut but an intellectual dead end.

REFERENCES

Cioffi, F. (1970). Freud and the idea of a pseudoscience. In R. Borger, and F. Cioffi (eds.). *Explanations in the Behavioral Sciences.* Cambridge, UK: Cambridge University Press.

———. (1985). Psychoanalysis, pseudoscience, and testability. In A. Musgrave, and G. Currie (eds.). *Karl Popper and the Human Sciences.* Boston: Martin Nijhoff.

———. (1998). *Freud and the Question of Pseudoscience.* Chicago: Open Court.

Erwin, E. (1960). The confirmation machine. *Boston Studies in the Philosophy of Science,* 8: 306–321.

———. (1978). *Behavior Therapy: Scientific, Philosophical, and Moral Foundations.* New York: Cambridge University Press.

———. (2001). *Review of Freud and the Question of Pseudoscience. Philosophy and Phenomenological Research,* LXII: 730–732.

Freud, S. (1940). Some elementary lessons in psycho-analysis. S.E. 23: 281–286.

Kline, P. (1981 [1972]). *Fact and Fantasy in Freudian Theory,* edition 2. New York: Methuen.

Notturno, M., and McHugh, P. (1986). Is Freudian psychoanalytic theory really falsifiable? *Behavioral and Brain Sciences,* 9: 254–255.

Popper, K. (1986). Predicting overt behavior versus predicting hidden states. *Behavioral and Brain Sciences,* 9: 254–255.

Scodel, A. (1957). Heterosexual somatic preference and fantasy dependence. *Journal of Consulting Psychology,* 21: 371–374.

EDWARD ERWIN

Psychiatry, and Psychoanalysis

The relationship between psychiatry and psychoanalysis varies considerably from country to country. There are

P

parts of the world where psychoanalysis does not yet have a cadre of educators and practitioners, and psychiatry has not been influenced significantly by the ideas of Freud. As a matter of fact, in some countries psychiatry is barely developed. In Western Europe and North America, however, the relationships between psychiatry and psychoanalysis have been intense and complex. During the two decades following World War II, psychiatry and psychoanalysis were closely intertwined theoretically and clinically; later in the twentieth century the relationship changed, and clearer lines of separation and differentiation emerged, especially in the United States. At the beginning of a new century, a pattern has evolved that is likely to persist. In this brief description of the interaction between psychoanalysis and psychiatry, it might be most useful to describe three stages of the relationship between the two during the latter half of the twentieth century in the United States. These models may be prototypic of future potential developments.

World War II had an enormous impact on American psychiatry; psychoanalysis became a central pillar of psychiatry after the war, as well as emerging in its own independent manner. The relationship between unconscious processes and psychological trauma was a centerpiece of wartime psychiatry. The large number of individuals rejected from military service because of mental illness also had a powerful impact on the attitudes of the general public. In the decade after the war, psychiatry crystallized its position in academic medicine, and within twenty years almost all U.S. medical schools had organized their departments of psychiatry. Psychoanalysts participated actively in this growth, and a significant number of those appointed to be departmental chairs in psychiatry had been trained as analysts. While nearly half of the psychiatric departments followed this pattern of leadership, many departments maintained an "eclectic" approach, and analysis was less dominant. Nevertheless, textbooks of psychiatry were heavily influenced by Freud's ideas, including emphasis on the power of unconscious forces, the dynamics of conflict, the hegemony of developmental sequences, and the need to conduct a psychodynamic formulation for each prospective patient. Psychiatry did not possess a viable clinical or theoretical alternative for psychodynamics; psychoanalysis became the central core of psychiatric education while also creating its own institutes to teach psychoanalytic practices and concepts. Several institutes developed within the administrative structure of medical

schools, and these models reflected close organizational and personal ties between analysts and their colleagues in psychiatry. Meetings of the American Psychiatric Association included many papers and symposia on analytic topics. Psychoanalysis affected psychiatric practice very deeply. Mental illness was defined broadly to include less severe personality disorders as well as the most disruptive psychoses.

During the 1970s, the close relationship between psychiatry and psychoanalysis began to weaken. Most significantly, the growth of neuroscience and psychopharmacology proceeded as a very important alternative model for psychiatric education and practice. Other diagnostic and therapeutic models also began to develop. Emerging economic pressures demanded rapid therapeutic results, and reimbursement for the practice of psychotherapy by psychiatrists became increasingly difficult in the late 1980s and early 1990s. Reimbursement for psychoanalytic work in general became constrained; many patients could be analyzed only if they paid their analyst out of their own private resources. Dire predictions of a "divorce" between psychoanalysis and psychiatry became more frequent. Decisions by the American Psychoanalytic Association to accept more nonmedical candidates for training were interpreted by many as the end of an era of special relationships between psychoanalysis and psychiatry.

During the late 1990s, however, the relationship between psychiatry and psychoanalysis began to stabilize. While more nonmedical analysts were being trained, the need for a close and continuing relationship between the American Psychoanalytic Association and the American Psychiatric Association became accepted by leaders in both groups. Common interests in economic and government affairs were acknowledged. While psychoanalysis faced competition for its curricular role in academic departments of psychiatry, that role once again began to be recognized as important even if not exclusive. The number of new departmental chairs who were analysts was reduced but not entirely eliminated. Analysts began to learn more about the utility of psychopharmacological treatment, and the combination of psychotherapy and medication became an area of increasing interest. The stabilization of the relationship between psychoanalysis and psychiatry evolved out of practical needs and was likely to survive for the next decade.

The current status of practical coexistence has both a scientific and an economic underpinning. It appears that cooperation will solidify, and both clinical and academic relationships will be maintained. Such cooperation will depend heavily on organizational interaction, but it will also involve awareness by many analysts of the role that psychiatric practice has on their work. Reciprocally, most psychiatrists will continue to rely on concepts and principles derived from the work of Freud.

MELVIN SABSHIN

Psychic Energy See CATHEXIS.

Psychic Phenomena See OCCULT, AND FREUD.

Psychical Determinism

Freud's stance with respect to determinism was deeply intertwined with his philosophical views on the nature of mind and science. During the period when Freud received his education and carried out his first psychological and neuroscientific research, the study of the mind was still very much under the influence of Descartes's heritage. Descartes had argued that the mind was made from an immaterial "substance" quite different from the gross material substance from which our bodies are formed. This position was *dualistic*, in that it held that mind and body were divorced from each other, and *antinaturalistic* in that it held mind to stand outside the material world. Freud seems to have at first adhered to this general doctrine but changed his philosophical views in the spring of 1895 when he began writing the *Project for a Scientific Psychology* (Freud, 1954). He moved to a materialist position, describing mental states and processes as activities of the central nervous system, and continued to espouse a materialist conception of mind until the end of his life (Smith, 1999).

Freud's belief that all mental events are lawfully caused, which he described as the doctrine of "psychical determinism," follows from his materialism and naturalism. If the mind is identical to the brain, it is clear that the mind is a part of nature that is probably subject to those causal processes and laws that govern the rest of the material universe. If events in the material universe are governed by exceptionless causal laws, it follows that mental events are similarly determined. According to this view, the material mind is just as much subject to deterministic laws as any other natural object. The doctrine of psychical determinism therefore holds that

"nothing in the mind is arbitrary or undetermined" (Freud, 1901: 242).

Freud believed that *any* scientific psychology must embrace psychical determinism. The opponent of psychical determinism "makes a breach . . . in the determinism of natural events" and "has thrown overboard the whole *Weltanschauung* of science" (Freud, 1916–1917: 28).

Even if mental events are strictly determined, this does not entail that they are predictable. Freud held that mental events, though determined, are largely unpredictable:

So long as we trace the development from its final outcome backwards, the chain of events appears continuous, and we feel we have gained an insight which is completely satisfactory or even exhaustive. But if we proceed the reverse way, if we start from the premises inferred from the analysis and try to follow these up to the final result, then we no longer get the impression of an inevitable sequence of events which could not have been otherwise determined. We notice at once that there might have been another result . . . in other words, from a knowledge of the premises we could not have foretold the nature of the result" (Freud, 1920: 167).

Freud (1920) argued that the prediction of mental events is not possible because psychoanalysis does not possess the resources to *quantify* the causal power of competing and confluent mental forces. This explanation is related to a second, more philosophically interesting explanation for mental nonpredictability implicit in Freud's work. This approach to the problem concerns the relationship between psychological and neuroscientific forms of explanation.

Given Freud's thesis of mind/brain identity, what was his view of the relationship between psychological and neurophysiological modes of explanation? He seems to have held that psychological explanation is in some ways misleading and does not provide us with a real grasp of the causal structure of a mental event. Freud was grappling with this problem as early as 1895 in the "Project," where he attempted to "represent psychical processes as quantitatively determinate states of specifiable material particles, thus making those processes perspicuous and free from contradiction" (Freud, 1954: 295). A year later, he claimed that so long as we do not have an understanding of the neurophysiological events corresponding to repression and symptom formation, we

P

must "be content with . . . remarks which are intended more or less figuratively" (Freud, 1896: 170); later he described psychoanalysis as comparable to primitive animism (1915). In fact, Freud seems to have been a philosophical *eliminativist*—one denies the existence of the mental—in that he did not believe that psychological discourse could be smoothly reduced to the language of neuroscience, and held that science should ultimately replace mentalistic talk with pure neuroscientific explanation: "The deficiencies in our description would probably vanish if we were already in a position to replace the psychological terms by physiological or chemical ones" (Freud, 1920: 60).

Why, then, did Freud continue to rely on a psychological vocabulary? Because he had no other option. There "still seems no possibility of approaching it from the direction of physical events" (Freud, 1913: 179). Freud said in 1909 that the problem of creating a neuroscience of mind "may be on the agenda a century after us" (Nunberg and Federn, 1962–1975: 280). He was forced to use a scientifically unsatisfactory psychological vocabulary to describe mental events, a constraint that defined "the very nature and limitation of our science" (Freud, 1940: 196). If only a neurophysiological description is able to provide a correct account of the causal processes within the mind, it follows that descriptions couched in the mentalistic language of psychoanalysis cannot be used to provide accurate predictions of mental events.

Freud's commitment to the doctrine of psychical determinism had important clinical ramifications. Chief among these was perhaps the creation of the method of free association, about which Freud wrote: "A strong belief in the strict determination of mental events certainly played a part in the choice of this technique as a substitute for hypnosis" (Freud, 1923: 238).

The notion of psychical determinism clearly has some bearing on the debate concerning the existence of "free will." Freud appears to have been a *compatabilist* with respect to free will and determinism, that is, he did not believe that there is a contradiction between strict psychical determinism and the existence of freedom of the will. He did not believe that psychoanalysis needs to "dispute the right to the feeling of conviction of having a free will" (Freud, 1901: 254), and even asserted that psychoanalysis strives "to give the patient's ego *freedom* to decide one way or the other (Freud, 1923: 50). For Freud, "free" actions are in fact determined. They are determined by motives of which one is conscious and with which one identified.

REFERENCES

Freud, S. (1896). Further remarks on the neuro-psychoses of defense. S.E. 3: 162–185.

———. (1901). *The Psychopathology of Everyday Life.* S.E. 6: 1–279.

———. (1913). The claims of psycho-analysis to scientific interest. S.E. 13: 165–190.

———. (1915). The unconscious. S.E. 14: 166–215.

———. (1916–1917). *Introductory Lectures on Psycho-Analysis.* S.E. 15–16: 9–496.

———. (1920). *Beyond the Pleasure Principle.* S.E. 18: 7–64.

———. (1923). Two encyclopedia articles. S.E. 18: 235–259.

———. (1923). *The Ego and the Id.* S.E. 19: 12–59.

———. (1940). *An Outline of Psycho-analysis.* S.E. 23: 144–207.

———. (1954). *The Origins of Psycho-Analysis.* New York: Basic Books.

Nunberg, H., and Federn, E. (eds.) (1962–1975). *Minutes of the Vienna Psycho-Analytic Society*, vol. 2. New York: International Universities Press.

Smith, D. L. (1992). *Freud's Philosophy of the Unconscious.* Dordrecht: Kluwer Academic Publishers.

DAVID LIVINGSTONE SMITH

Psychoanalysis, Origin and History of

"Psychoanalysis is my creation," Freud stated (1914, p. 7). But exactly what did Freud do, and how original and scientific were his procedures and conclusions?

In creating psychoanalysis, Freud developed a therapy for neurotic disorders and a theory of mental functioning; he also created and presided over an institutionalized psychoanalytic movement. With the development of his psychoanalytic movement, Freud used his great rhetorical skills to shape the story of the early development of psychoanalysis. His three accounts of the origins and development of psychoanalysis, *Five Lectures on Psycho-Analysis* (1910), the polemical *On the History of the Psycho-Analytic Movement* (1914), and *An Autobiographical Study* (1925), were crafted by Freud to create and perpetuate the image of himself as a heroic, completely original discoverer of a set of "facts" that, although validated by his clinical findings, nevertheless were received with hostile responses. Following Freud's lead, the movement he founded assumed the mission of defending and perpetuating his "discoveries" and his legend (Roazen, 1975; Grosskurth, 1991).

Several decades of independent historical research concerning the origins and development of psychoanalysis have succeeded in demonstrating how unbalanced Freud's own accounts were. A great deal of myth perpetuation also can be found in the most influential loyalist biographies of Freud—Ernest Jones's three-volume *The Life and Work of Sigmund Freud* (1953, 1955, and 1957) and Peter Gay's *Freud: A Life for Our Time* (1988). The following account of the origins and history of psychoanalysis incorporates the results of a considerable volume of revisionist Freud scholarship. The reader is invited to consult the works cited above for Freud's story in his own words and for histories from within the psychoanalytic movement.

While it is not possible to date exactly when the concepts of mental functioning that evolved into psychoanalytic theory first germinated in Freud's mind, the period from late 1885 to early 1886 was a major formative period in the birth of psychoanalysis. During this time, Freud, a twenty-nine-year-old Viennese neurologist, spent about four months in Paris studying with the renowned French neurologist J. M. Charcot. Freud observed Charcot's clinical demonstrations in which hypnotic suggestion was used to produce paralysis in patients' limbs. The paralyses caused by hypnotic suggestion were seen by Charcot as strikingly similar to some types of paralyses that occurred after railroad accidents, which, in the absence of observable neurological damage, Charcot attributed to post-traumatic psychological shock. Charcot reasoned that such post-traumatic cases of paralysis were caused by an autosuggestion, rooted in the mind during a self-induced hypnoticlike mental state, which was a reaction to fear and shock. He further argued that hysterical paralysis in general, that is, any case of paralysis not traceable to specific organic damage, must be due to an autosuggestion implanted in the patient's mind during a self-induced, hypnoid mental state, in reaction to some emotionally traumatic experience. Such autosuggestions of motor weakness remained active in a dissociated mental state as fixed ideas. These auto-suggested *ideas* of motor paralysis had the power to realize themselves objectively in the form of hysterical symptoms of paralysis.

Freud was profoundly influenced by Charcot. He returned to Vienna in 1886 convinced that, even in the absence of observable organic damage, hysterical paralyses and anaesthesias were a genuine form of disease. Moreover, the cause of hysterical symptoms lay in the psychological realm: ideas could cause physical symptoms. These ideas were not part of ordinary conscious experience.

Before studying with Charcot, Freud had learned from an older Viennese physician, Josef Breuer, about Breuer's treatment of a young woman, Bertha Pappenheim, between 1880 and 1882. Bertha presented a variety of symptoms that Breuer regarded as hysterical: for example, paralysis of the arms or legs, disturbances of sight and speech, nausea, and memory loss. Bertha evidenced a tendency, spontaneously, to enter trancelike or hypnoid mental states during which she reported stories and reveries. Breuer told Freud that allowing Bertha to vent fantasies and reveries while in a trancelike state brought some relief from symptoms he believed were hysterical in nature. After his return from Paris, Freud began to apply the concepts of the psychical mechanisms of hysterical symptom formation he had learned from Charcot to an evolving interpretation of the Bertha Pappenheim case.

In 1895, because of Freud's instigation, the volume *Studies on Hysteria*, by Breuer and Freud, was published. This volume contained a case history of Bertha Pappenheim under the pseudonym of "Anna O." The book also contained several other case histories of patients whom, by that time, Freud had treated for hysterical symptoms, as well as a Breuer chapter on theory and a Freud chapter on therapy. Although preceded by an 1893 preliminary communication concerning their views on psychical mechanisms in the causation of hysteria, the 1895 *Studies on Hysteria* may be called the seminal book of psychoanalysis.

By the time of the publication of *Studies on Hysteria*, Freud had developed a point of view that differed markedly from Charcot's approach to hysteria. Breuer, on the other hand, maintained an opinion much like that of Charcot. Breuer accepted that entrance into a hypnoid state, in reaction to emotional trauma, was the prerequisite condition for memories that were not available to ordinary consciousness to become pathogenic roots of hysterical symptoms. Freud saw no need to assume that an abnormal, hypnoid mental state was involved in creating hysterical symptoms. Rather, he saw memories becoming unconscious, and pathogenic, as a result of the patient being in conflict with the content of the memories. Such conflict arose because the memory content was incompatible with the patient's conscious view of self. The patient intentionally repressed or excluded from consciousness ideas incompatible to the ego, a psychical act of self-defense. In hysteria, psychic conflict over pathogenic memories involved defense and compromise formation. Nervous excitation associated with the repressed idea was channeled into a somatic innervation, which produced a physical symptom. This physical symptom was a compromise formation in that it now occupied the patient's consciousness, in place of the repressed idea, which it symbolically represented, in a manner not recognized by the ego—a poetic use of the body to represent, metaphorically, incompatible repressed ideas.

In spite of his disagreements with Breuer, it was to Freud's advantage to publish jointly with him. A joint publication put the younger Freud in company with a highly respected physician and scientist, increasing the likelihood that Freud's view would receive the acceptance that he desired.

Freud's belief that he was reporting significant discoveries concerning the cause and treatment of hysteria apparently helped him to feel justified in encouraging Breuer in presenting an untrue portrait of the Bertha Pappenheim (Anna O.) case—a presentation distorted to create, retrospectively, the myth that Anna O. was the primal psychoanalytic patient, the first patient to be cured of hysterical symptoms by a psychical treatment, in this case a cathartic method claimed to be invented by Breuer. Further, Breuer's discovery of a psychical mechanism and treatment, in a case of hysteria, was falsely attributed to a date before publication on the role of traumatic memories and the emotional reproduction of traumatic memories in the causation and treatment of hysteria by Charcot, Pierre Janet, and a few German neurologists. Comparisons of Breuer's notes on the Anna O. case from 1882, versus his 1895 account, reveal a retrospective reinterpretation of the case and treatment based on subsequent ideas published by Charcot and Janet (Borch-Jacobsen, 1996b; Macmillan, 1997).

Breuer and Freud claimed in 1895 that, using hypnosis, Breuer had successfully cured Anna O.'s hysterical symptoms. The cure was supposed to have been achieved by painstakingly tracing symptoms back to forgotten emotional traumas. Once unconscious traumatic memories were brought to consciousness and an emotional-cathartic, present reexperience of the trauma occurred, pathogenic memories were supposed to have been reunited with the nervous excitation that had been split off from them, thus allowing for a proper discharge of this energy. The claim for a successful cure was made in spite of the fact that Breuer and Freud knew that, after Breuer terminated his treatment of Anna O., some of her symptoms, believed to be hysterical, returned, and she had to be hospitalized at least four times over a six- to seven-year period (Hirschmüller, 1978).

As early as 1888, Freud believed that "conditions related *functionally* to sexual life play a great part in the aetiology of hysteria (as of all neuroses) and they do so on account of the high psychical significance of this function especially in the female sex" (p. 51). While Breuer saw sexuality playing no role in the Anna O. case, Breuer did grant sexuality a role in many cases of hysteria as a source of increased excitation in the nervous system. However, by 1895, with his new psychical-defense theory of hysteria, Freud added to this notion the centrality of the ideogenic role of incompatible ideas relating to sexuality, and hidden motives, in the genesis of a range of defense neuroses: hysteria, obsessional neurosis, and phobias.

In addition to neuroses that were psychogenic in origin, Freud proposed that there were two actual neuroses—neuroses of organic origin—that definitely had a sexual basis: neurasthenia (a general weakness) and anxiety neurosis (an overexcited condition). Each actual neurosis resulted from a failure to properly regulate the amount of sexual chemicals (hormones) in the bloodstream, through periodic, uninterrupted sexual intercourse. Thus, the actual neuroses originated in the current sexual life of the patient. In neurasthenia, the sexual dysfunction was masturbation, which depleted the body of substances required for adequate internal excitation of the central nervous system. On the other hand, anxiety neurosis was an autotoxic condition. It was the result of an accumulation of too much sexual substance —which overexcited the nervous system, producing anxiety. This neurosis was caused by sexual abstinence or coitus interruptus.

In sum, by 1895 Freud speculated that all neuroses might be sexual in origin. Hysteria, obsessional neurosis, and phobias were ideogenic. They were compromises employed in defending against exciting, conflictual memories of a sexual nature. The actual neuroses were the outcome of imbalances of internally produced sexual chemicals, affecting the level of excitation in the nervous system, resulting from disturbances in the patient's current sexual life.

The evolution of Freud's views on the role of sexuality in neuroses during the 1890s can be observed in his many letters to a Berlin physician, Wilhelm Fliess (Masson, 1985). Fliess encouraged and contributed his own ideas to Freud's speculations concerning a sexual, organic substrate for neuroses. Both Freud and Fliess drew on the 1884 work of George Miller Beard, *Sexual Neuras-*

P

thenia, which proposed that one of the causes of neurasthenia was an expenditure of "nerve force" caused by sexual problems (Macmillan, 1997). Sexuality became Freud's pragmatic link between mind and body.

In developing his view of the mind-body relationship, Freud had been influenced by his philosophy professor, Franz Brentano. Brentano taught that it was necessary to distinguish between psychical or mental processes, and physical-physiological processes. Mental phenomena represented a distinct phenomenal realm, subjective reality, with distinct properties not found in the physical realm. Motivational factors—subjective intentionality—were extremely important in determining the flow of thought. What was mental had to be understood in terms appropriate to the quality of subjective reality; the mental world could not be equated with, or reduced to, a physiological substrate. Brentano's influence was so strong that when Freud was still his student in 1875, Freud characterized himself as "a former swashbuckling stubborn materialist," even though he felt uncomfortable abandoning previously held faith in what was generally held to be correct, and he was trying to keep an open mind (Boehlich, 1990: 109).

In 1875, Freud already was familiar with the famous 1872 lecture by the eminent German physiologist Du Bois-Reymond, entitled "On the limits of our understanding of nature" (Boehlich, 1990: 107). Even though he rigorously defended the truth of a mechanistic account of the world, Du Bois-Reymond argued that there were certain limits beyond which scientific understanding could not go. Faced with the questions how are nerve processes related to conscious experience and what is the relationship between nerve processes and the qualities to which they give rise, Du Bois-Reymond would have to say, "*ignorabimus*," we will not be able to know. We will ignore it. Mindful of Du Bois-Reymond's warning that there might be limits to human cognition, Freud adopted and maintained a skepticism toward any premature uniting of the mental and the physical into a materialistic monism. He was fond of quoting the poet Heine's derisive comment on the philosopher who clings to the illusion of being able to present a coherent picture of the universe without any gaps: "With his nightcaps and the tatters of his dressing-gown, he patches up the gaps in the structure of the universe" (Freud, 1933: 160–161).

From the time that Freud wrote his 1891 neurological monograph, *On Aphasia*, it is clear that he also had been influenced by the British neurologist John Hughlings Jackson. Hughlings Jackson had insisted that it was a pragmatic, methodological necessity for neurologists to treat the mental and the physical as distinctly different phenomena. They were knowable by different methods, and they required distinct, separate mentalistic and physicalistic modes of description and explanation. Hughlings Jackson believed that neurologists had to turn to psychology to understand the rules, or organizing principles, of the ideational and linguistic accompaniments of complex nervous activities. Hughlings Jackson proposed an evolutionary, hierarchical model of the nervous system, and of mental functioning, with lower-level mental functioning dominated by a prelinguistic mode of cognition, which followed rules of association different from those found in higher-level, linguistically organized mental processes. In addition, Hughlings Jackson pictured the nervous system as functioning to dispose of excessive quantities of energy (excitation). Freud incorporated Hughlings Jackson's ideas in his evolving conceptions of the dynamics of neuroses and in his evolving topographical theory of mental functioning, which he first published in *The Interpretation of Dreams* (1900), discussed below.

Freud saw sexuality as a pragmatic link between the subjectively knowable mental world and the empirically knowable physical world. He saw apparent correlations between sexuality in the mental realm—sexual thoughts and intentions—and sexuality in the physical realm—changes in physiology and internal excitation of the nervous system. Basing his reasoning upon such considerations, Freud adopted a methodological-dualist-interactionist position on the mind-body relationship: the mental world had to be observed through inner perception and described in motivational-intentional language, while the physical world was observed empirically and described in terms from physics and chemistry. Nevertheless, he believed that the mental and the physical interacted, in that ideas could produce effects in the body, while changes in physiology could affect motivation and thought.

Even though the mechanism(s) that governed mind-body interaction remained unknown to Freud, he avoided a reductionistic position. He created a theory of mind that incorporated two fundamentally different classes of phenomena: the mental and the physical. Freud not only asserted that ideas possessed causal efficacy, but it was unconscious ideas, following their own associational rules not discoverable by simple introspection, that most powerfully affected bodily functions (although Freud regarded the puzzling leap from the mental to the physical as inexplicable). In addition, conscious mental functioning was determined by unconscious mental processes. These unconscious mental processes were intentional, but their motivational impetus originated within the body. In neuroses, the underlying organic factor was to be found in the motivational excitation resulting from sexual physiology (Silverstein, 1985). These lines of thinking were the precursors of Freud's topographical theory of mental functioning and his motivational theory of instinctual drives, discussed below.

Freud had been unhappy over Breuer's theory chapter in *Studies on Hysteria*. While he shared with Breuer an emphasis on an economics of the nerve force as a necessary part of an explanation of hysteria, Freud wanted an explanatory model that could accommodate his evolving emphases on intentions, conflicts, defense, and compromise.

In October 1895, Freud mailed two notebooks to Wilhelm Fliess that contained an elaborate account of his evolving psychology for neurologists. In these notebooks, psychical processes were represented as the buildup of quantities of energy within a number of hypothetical neuronal systems, with the intentional quality of thought represented as the discharge of quantities of energy along pathways from one structure to another (Masson, 1985). These notebooks, which Freud never published, have come to be known as *The Project for a Scientific Psychology*. After mailing the notebooks to Fliess, Freud expressed grave discontent with their contents. He also indicated that he was still working on *The Project*, but he was finding it impossible to account for the process of repression in strictly mechanical terms. Therefore, Freud abandoned the entire enterprise of representing mental processes in neurological terms. Nevertheless, dynamic, energy-force concepts employed in *The Project* can be found in Freud's subsequent models of mental functioning. Freud always depended on analogies from the physical world in his later mental models.

In his eagerness to beat Breuer at the economics of the nerve-force game, Freud seemingly ignored his own understanding that it was necessary to treat psychical processes as something distinct from neurological processes. Although his future models of mental functioning would never again be based on any specific references to a neurological substrate, Freud continued to link mental processes to an organic substrate in the form

of sexual physiology. Regarding efforts to reduce psychology to neurology, Freud told Jung that he had "absolutely forsworn the temptation to 'fill in the gaps in the universe'" (McGuire, 1974: 125).

Freud's post-project strategy of opting for a methodological-dualistic-interactionist view, with sexual processes as the indispensable organic foundation linking mind and body, was deemed scientifically acceptable in accordance with Du Bois-Reymond's 1872 pronouncement on human limits to our understanding of nature. Du Bois-Reymond had stated, "The more unconditionally the natural science researcher recognizes and accepts the limits set for him, and the more humbly he resigns himself to his ignorance, the more strongly he feels it is his right to come to his own opinion about the relationship between mind and matter, by way of his own induction, unmoved along the way by myths, dogmas and proud old philosophers" (Du Bois-Reymond, 1872: 460–461, my translation).

The development of Freud's method of psychotherapy is inextricably bound to the evolution of his psychological theories. In 1887, Freud used hypnotic suggestion as a mode of therapy. By 1889, Freud was combining hypnotic suggestion with hypnotic searching for traumatic memories (Swales, 1986; Macmillan, 1997). In 1896, Freud used the term "psychoanalysis" for the first time for the suggestive methods he was using then to trace hysterical symptoms back to their origin, combined with cathartic reliving of emotionally charged memories. By then, he believed that the origin of hysterical symptoms would always be found in some event of the patient's sexual life, appropriate for the production of a distressing emotion.

Even though by 1895 Freud had separated himself from Charcot and Breuer, he still followed their lead in searching for an actual traumatic event as the precipitating cause in hysteria. However, in 1895 Freud speculated that the traumatic event had to be sexual. Using hypnosis and suggestive, directed waking concentration, Freud guided his patients to produce memories of a sexual nature that would fit his concept of an appropriate precipitating cause.

Back in 1889, while Freud was trying to improve his skills as a hypnotist, he returned to France, but this time to Nancy, to study with H. Bernheim, an advocate for the therapeutic use of hypnosis. He insisted that hypnosis was simply suggestion and not related to any pathological mental state. Bernheim taught Freud that relaxing a patient and insisting that the patient recall some event, seemingly unavailable to consciousness, produced the desired recollection without hypnosis. When Freud had difficulty hypnotizing a patient, he insisted that his patient would recall the right memory at the moment when he laid his hand on the patient's forehead. From 1892, Freud progressively abandoned hypnosis in favor of this "pressure technique," with directed concentration in the waking state.

By 1895, Freud began to formulate what would become known as his "seduction theory." At first, he speculated that a necessary precondition for hysteria, and obsessional neurosis, must be some prepubertal sexual experience. Over a period of almost two years, Freud's speculations about what must have happened to his patients when they were children appeared to be confirmed as his patients, if often with expressions of disbelief in response to Freud's direction and "pressure," obliged Freud by telling him stories, or acquiescing to his reconstructions, that fit Freud's current version of a suspected primary cause. The blame for the prepubertal sexual abuse, which must have happened, shifted several times as Freud reformulated his etiological hypothesis. First, older children were the usual suspects; then suspicion shifted to nearby adults or parents; finally, Freud concluded that, in all cases, it was the father who "had to be accused of being perverse" (Masson, 1985: 264).

It appears that Freud's patients, if often grudgingly, may have submitted in some manner corroborating childhood sexual abuse stories that matched his current speculation concerning a necessary childhood sexual event, the memory of which could generate distressing emotions, even years after the event occurred. In 1896, Freud stated that before they came for treatment, the patients claimed to have no memories of being sexually abused in childhood: "They are indignant as a rule if we warn them that such scenes are going to emerge. Only the strongest compulsion of the treatment can induce them to embark on a reproduction of them" (p. 204). Nevertheless, by 1896, Freud believed that recovering such childhood sexual abuse memories in the context of a cathartic emotional experience was an absolute requirement to cure psychogenic-defense neuroses.

In two papers Freud sent for publication, in February 1896, he claimed to have carried out a "complete psychoanalysis" in thirteen cases of hysteria, with each case revealing early sexual traumas. In April 1896, Freud gave a lecture on his seduction theory. A written version of this lecture, *The Aetiology of Hysteria*, was mailed for publication at the end of May. In this publication, Freud put forward the thesis that, at the bottom of every case of hysteria, there were single or multiple occurrences of premature sexual experiences, dating from the earliest years. Freud (1896) now claimed that "in some eighteen cases of hysteria I have been able to discover this connection in every single symptom, and, where the circumstances allowed, to confirm it by therapeutic success" (p. 199).

Barely sixteen months after Freud's bold claims for confirmation and therapeutic success, on September 21, 1897, he wrote to Fliess: "I no longer believe in my *neurotica*," i.e., his seduction theory. Further, the first reason Freud offered for his change of mind was "The continual disappointment in my efforts to bring a single analysis to a real conclusion; . . . the absence of the complete successes on which I had counted; the possibility of explaining to myself the partial success in other ways, in the usual fashion" (Masson, 1985: 264). What is seen here is that, in private communication to Fliess, Freud indicated that he had not achieved the therapeutic success with his patients suggested in his publications of the previous year. Furthermore, Freud's understanding that he could explain his "partial successes" in "the usual fashion" suggests that he understood that his patients were responding to his suggestions, or autosuggestion, when they obliged him with stories that fit his etiological hypothesis of the moment. As Freud's critics had been charging, the childhood scenes Freud's patients had been reporting, for the most part, came from Freud; additionally, Freud's "psychoanalysis" could be seen as just a form of Bernheim's "suggestive therapeutics" (Borch-Jacobsen, 1996a).

As much as he recognized the role suggestion might have played in shaping patients' behavior toward confirming his expectations, Freud always denied that he forced seduction stories upon his patients. In his September 21, 1897, letter to Fliess, Freud conjectured: "there would remain the solution that the sexual fantasy invariably seizes upon the theme of the parents," and, "there are no indications of reality in the unconscious" (Masson, 1985: 264–265). Here is the start of a major turning point in the development of psychoanalytic theory. Freud sidestepped the dilemma of suggestion, and he protected his theories of psychic-conflict, repression, and defense neuroses by speculating that he actually had succeeded in unearthing repressed material from his patients' unconscious minds associated with early sexual trauma. However, what was repressed was childhood sexual fantasies (wishes) concerning the parents, associated with memories of overstimulating, traumatic childhood masturbation (Makari, 1998), which were experienced as reality in the unconscious, and they never overcame repression—emerging in consciousness only as derivative, defensive, compromise-formation memories of parental sexual abuse (and with later theoretical development, as disguised, fulfilled wishes, in dreams).

In the fall of 1897, Freud increasingly speculated on a point only suggested the year before: children have a sexual life before puberty, even in early childhood, which decisively influenced later sexual development. Freud's concept of childhood sexuality, which developed over the years from 1897 to 1905, derived, in part, from suggestions Freud accepted from Wilhelm Fliess, as well as from the writings of late-nineteenth-century sexologists such as Albert Moll and Havelock Ellis (Sulloway, 1979). By 1905 in Freud's hands, however, the concept of childhood sexual development would be linked to later adult characteristics in a unique, systematic fashion. By 1905, Freud no longer conceptualized childhood masturbation as traumatic and pathogenic. He reconceptualized childhood masturbation as a pregenital expression of an innate sexual drive that evolved through stages from infancy to puberty.

In 1896, Freud's father died. Freud experienced significant emotional stress in coping with his father's death, and as a result, he began to apply his evolving psychoanalytic method to himself; he started a process of self analysis. At first, he looked for evidence of childhood sexual abuse in his own case, even possibly involving his father. However, after he repudiated his theory that actual childhood sexual abuse was required in every case of hysteria, Freud examined his own childhood for evidence of repressed sexual desires that would corroborate his new hypothesis. On October 3, 1897, Freud reported to Fliess that, when he was a young boy, his "libido toward matrem" was awakened during a railway journey he took with his mother, "during which we must have spent the night together and there must have been an opportunity of seeing her *nudam*." (Masson, 1985: 268). These were not actual memories but reconstructions of what must have happened to provide data that would support Freud's new theory.

Less than two weeks later, on October 15, Freud wrote to Fleiss: "A single idea of general value dawned on me. I have found, in my own case too, [the phenom-

enon of] being in love with my mother and jealous of my father, and I now consider it a universal event in early childhood, even if not so early as in children who have been made hysterical" (Masson, 1985: 272). Now, drawing on his interpretive reconstructions of his patients', and his own, childhoods, Freud made the theoretical leap that all children experienced a sexualized love for the mother, and jealousy of the father, the precursor of what Freud, in 1910, officially named the "Oedipus complex."

Freud's putative discoveries—first, of repressed memories of childhood sexual abuse, and, second, of repressed childhood sexual wishes and fantasies—were largely based on his search for retrospective material concerning childhood that he could interpret as consistent with the hypothesis he already had in hand. In other words, Freud repeatedly found what he expected to find; his clinical data always showed him what his hypothesis predicted. While clearly, this is not an objective, scientifically valid method of clinical data collection and hypothesis testing, Freud appeared to regard his ability to find clinical data he could interpret as supporting his theories as genuine, scientific validation of them.

As Freud progressively abandoned reliance on therapeutic hypnosis, in 1892 he began to employ the method of free association in response to some patients' protestations that he should let them talk. Nevertheless, Freud still relied on the "pressure technique" and directed, waking concentration. With the collapse of his seduction theory, Freud made free association his fundamental method for gathering clinical data, since he believed that free association avoided the pitfall of the therapists's suggestions determining what the patient reported. With free association, Freud observed that patients sometimes resisted following his directive to report uncensored, whatever came to mind. He interpreted such resistance as evidence for repression, and he made analysis of such resistance a fundamental part of his (nonhypnosis-based) psychoanalytic technique.

Even after abandoning hypnotic and "pressure" techniques, Freud remained concerned with an explanation for suggestion itself; how, and why, might a patient become vulnerable to meeting demands (even if inadvertent) from a therapist? As early as 1890, Freud had speculated that a hypnotized person adopted a relationship to his or her hypnotist such as shown only by a child to a parent (Silverstein and Silverstein, 1990). Freud's adoption of the concept of childhood sexual desire for the parent enabled him to propose a new explanation for the power of suggestion (or autosuggestion) in his work with his patients. Freud (1905b) spoke of an unconscious fixation of the subject's libido to the hypnotist, as though he were the parent. In addition, Freud (1905a) used the term "transference" to refer to the inevitable arousal in the analytic patient of impulses and fantasies concerning parents that the patient directed toward the analyst, even though no hypnosis was employed. He concluded that it was necessary to resolve this "transference" in order for a patient to arrive at a sense of conviction of the correctness of the analyst's interpretations. In his *Introductory Lectures on Psycho-Analysis*, Freud (1916–1917) stated: "in our technique we have abandoned hypnosis only to rediscover suggestion in the shape of transference" (p. 446).

For Freud, "transference" referred to an actualization of unconscious wishes in a specific relationship. He believed that, in the analytic situation, the patient's childhood sexual and aggressive wishes reemerged, focused on the analyst, and they were experienced with a vivid sensation of immediacy. Not just the surfacing of previously unacknowledged childhood wishes but the acceptance and working through of such wishes, through interpretation and resolution of the transference, came to define the nature of a psychoanalytic cure.

Psychoanalytic technique came to be defined by the methods of free association, interpretations of resistance, and the establishment of a transference toward the analyst, with appropriate interpretation, working through, and resolution. The neurotic symptom had to be traced back to earliest childhood. Since Freud's evolving theories of childhood sexuality, and the Oedipus complex, attributed childhood sexual and aggressive wishes to everyone, normal development came to be seen as requiring repression and sublimation of such wishes. It was not the existence of such wishes, or repression, that now was seen as the cause of neurosis; unsuccessful repression was the cause, with neurosis breaking out when repression failed, and childhood sexual and aggressive wishes reemerged in disguised form (compromise formations) as symptoms. Traumatic memories and actual sexual abuse might play a role in some neuroses, but the primary focus in psychoanalysis became childhood wishes and fantasies, and early autoerotic activities.

With the use of free association, patients talked about their dreams. By the summer of 1895, Freud concluded that a dream was similar to a neurotic symptom: they both were compromise formations. Freud believed

that a dream was a symbolic (usually disguised) expression of fulfilled wishes. Psychoanalytic technique came to include the interpretation of dreams as "the royal road to a knowledge of the unconscious activities of the mind" (Freud, 1900: 608).

Freud had discussed the wish-fulfilling character of dreams in his unpublished *Project* of 1895. Early in 1898, Freud finished a first draft of the book, *The Interpretation of Dreams*, which would present this thesis in elaborate form. The book was completed in 1899 and published with a 1900 date of publication. Freud considered this book his greatest work. Nevertheless, Freud's claim for the complete originality of his approach to dreams is questionable. Before Freud, some of Europe's most prominent physicians anticipated him in discussing the scientific importance of dreams, and dream interpretation, for the exploration of the unconscious mind, for example, Charcot, Janet, and Krafft-Ebing (Sand, 1992).

In *The Interpretation of Dreams*, Freud presented his hierarchical, topographical model of the mind. Mental functioning was portrayed as a continuous, dynamic relationship between unconscious, preconscious, and conscious mental processes. Unconscious mental processes were based on prelinguistic, image (primary process) modes of representation. The evolutionary, higher-level, conscious-preconscious system was based on linguistically structured modes of representation (secondary process). Each level of mental functioning followed its own laws of association, as previously suggested by Hughlings Jackson. Freud portrayed consciousness as determined by unconscious mental processes, without concern for correlated neural substrates.

In his early student days, Freud had been exposed to the philosopher Herbart's topographical model of the mind, which was quite similar to the model Freud presented in *The Interpretation of Dreams* (Sand, 1988). In this book, he admitted that he followed the lead of the philosopher Theodore Lipps when Freud (1900) asserted: "the unconscious must be assumed to be the general basis of psychical life" (p. 612). Further, Freud added: "The unconscious is the true psychical reality" (p. 613). While Freud developed a systematic view of unconscious mental life linked to sexuality, he was not absolutely original in his conceptions of the unconscious. Ellenberger (1970) extensively documented the popularity of the concept of unconscious mental life in the late nineteenth century.

In *The Interpretation of Dreams*, Freud discussed the dynamic power of unconscious, childhood sexual and aggressive wishes to force their way back to consciousness. In 1905, in his *Three Essays on the Theory of Sexuality*, Freud proposed distinct pregenital stages of psychosexual development: oral, anal, phallic, and latency. During the first three stages, sexuality was expressed through particular erogenous zones, generating particular wishes for pleasure. The impact the child's pregenital experiences had on his or her evolving mental structure was seen by Freud as determining healthy or neurotic or perverse adult characteristics.

In *Three Essays on the Theory of Sexuality*, Freud also discussed the impact of anatomical distinctions on the development of boys and girls. Here, he introduced his concepts of castration complex and penis envy.

Also, in *Three Essays on the Theory of Sexuality*, Freud remained consistent in his mind-body, dualist-interactionist viewpoint when he introduced his concept of the sexual instinctual drive. Freud (1905b) explained: "By an 'instinct' is provisionally to be understood the psychical representative of an endosomatic, continuously flowing source of stimulation. . . . The concept of the instinct is thus one of those lying on the frontier between the mental and the physical. . . . The source of an instinct is a process of excitation occurring in an organ and the immediate aim of the instinct lies in the removal of this organic stimulus" (p. 168). The unconscious mind was seen as full of wishful images representing sexual, need-satisfying objects.

In 1910, Freud expanded his theory of human motivation by proposing a dualistic division of all instinctual drives into two categories: ego instincts, in the service of the preservation of the individual's life, and sexual instincts, directed toward the attainment of pleasure (and species preservation). The striving for pleasure underwent developmental transformations correlated with the development of the child's erogenous zones. Freud came to use the term "libido" to refer to the energy of the sexual instinct.

Freud bridged the gap between mind and body with his concept of instinctual drives, and he also used his dualistic drive concept to explain why, in his view, it was human nature to be in conflict with society, and, through socialization, to be in conflict with oneself. Ego instincts inevitably came into conflict with sexual instincts: the need for survival required repression of forbidden and taboo thoughts that directed us to pursue sexual pleas-

ure through the stimulation of erogenous zones. The dynamic power of unsuccessfully repressed sexual wishes was the force behind neurotic symptoms.

Freud twice revised his dualistic conception of basic human motivation. In 1914, he introduced a new division of instinctual drives: ego libido (self-love, self-preservation) versus object libido (other love, species preservation). Finally, in 1920, Freud proposed the dualism of Eros, the life instinct (including ego libido versus object libido), versus Thanatos, the death instinct (including self-directed versus other-directed aggression).

In 1915 and 1917, Freud published a series of essays on his metapsychology, his psychology of unconscious mental processes. In 1915, Freud had written a book consisting of twelve metapsychological essays, but he never published the book, choosing to publish, separately, only five of the component metapsychological essays (Silverstein, 1986). In these essays, Freud attempted to offer definitive statements on key components of his metapsychology, including instincts, repression, the unconscious, and dreams.

In 1923, Freud created his final model of the mind, the structural model. Freud supplemented his topographic model, which represented mental functioning with the spacial metaphor of levels—conscious, preconscious and unconscious—with a hypothetical set of interactive agencies: the id, the ego, and the superego. The id was the locus of wishful, image, object representations, correlated with the satisfaction of bodily needs generated by underlying biological processes. The id functioned unconsciously, following the pleasure principle—the wishful image was experienced as the real object. The ego functioned at all topographical levels. The ego utilized linguistically structured thought patterns, and it followed the reality principle. The task of the ego was to match the images (wishes) of the id with their counterparts in the real world, and to obtain satisfaction of bodily needs with minimum cost, in terms of punishment or guilt. The superego, mostly unconscious, consisted of moral dos and don'ts internalized through identification with a parent.

In 1926, Freud proposed the last major revision in his metapsychology. As we have seen, previously Freud conceptualized anxiety as resulting from undischarged sexual excitation. With his new structural model, Freud was required to make the ego the seat of anxiety. Anxiety was a warning signal of danger to the ego. The ego could experience anxiety in relation to real external

P

threat, or the possibility of the failure of repression, or the moral objections from the superego. The primary task of the ego was seen as mediating between the conflicting demands of reality, the id and the superego, while minimizing the experience of anxiety.

The ego controlled consciousness. It was unconscious ego functioning that made repression, compromise, and defense possible. The ego functioned to minimize the experience of anxiety by maximizing instinctual gratification, with the minimum cost in punishment and guilt. Neurotic symptoms were defenses against anxiety, arising from an internal conflict. Neurotic symptoms were symbolic expressions of a psychical conflict that originated in childhood: The symptoms were compromises between wish and defense.

It is now clear that many of the ideas that became the building blocks of psychoanalytic theory were part of the powerful intellectual, scientific, and medical trends of the late nineteenth century. They were not derived solely from Freud's clinical data. Freud absorbed, synthesized, and applied ideas available from a variety of sources. Nevertheless, Freud created a new explanatory system and a new method of psychotherapy. Through the volume of his publications and the rhetorical brilliance with which he gave expression to his new system and method, Freud eclipsed his sources and created his own legend.

REFERENCES

Boehlich, W. (ed.) (1990). *The Letters of Sigmund Freud and Eduard Silberstein: 1871–1881.* Cambridge, Mass.: Harvard University Press.

Borch-Jacobsen, M. (1996a). Neurotica: Freud and the seduction theory. *October,* 76 (Spring): 15–43.

———. (1996b). *Remembering Anna O.: A Century of Mystification.* New York: Routledge.

Du Bois-Reymond, E. (1872). Über die Grenzen des Naturekennens. In *Reden von Emil Du Bois-Reymond, Erster Band.* Leipzig: Verlag Von Veit and Comp., 1912, pp. 441–473.

Ellenberger, H. (1970). *The Discovery of the Unconscious: The History and Evolution of Dynamic Psychiatry.* New York: Basic Books.

Freud, S. (1888). Hysteria. S.E. 1: 39–59.

———. (1896). The aetiology of hysteria. S.E. 3: 189–221.

———. (1900). *The Interpretation of Dreams.* S.E. 4–5: 1–621.

———. (1905a). Fragment of an analysis of a case of hysteria. S.E. 7: 3–122.

———. (1905b). *Three Essays on the Theory of Sexuality.* S.E. 7: 130–243.

———. (1910). *Five Lectures on Psycho-Analysis.* S.E. 2: 9–55.

———. (1914). On the history of the psycho-analytic movement. S.E. 14: 6–66.

———. (1916–1917). *Introductory Lectures on Psycho-Analysis.* S.E. 15–16: 9–496.

———. (1925). An autobiographical study. S.E. 20: 7–74.

———. (1933). *New Introductory Lectures on Psychoanalysis.* S.E. 22: 3–182.

Grosskurth, P. (1991). *The Secret Ring: Freud's Inner Circle and the Politics of Psychoanalysis.* Reading, Mass.: Addison-Wesley.

Hirschmüller, A. (1978). *The Life and Work of Josef Breuer: Physiology and Psychoanalysis.* New York: New York University Press.

Macmillan, M. (1997). *Freud Evaluated—The Completed Arc,* rev. ed. Amsterdam: Elsevier, 1990.

Makari, G. (1998). The seductions of history: Sexual trauma in Freud's theory and historiography. *International Journal of Psychoanalysis,* 79: 857–869. Cambridge: M.I.T. Press.

Masson, J. F. (ed.) (1985). *The Complete Letters of Sigmund Freud to Wilhelm Fliess: 1887–1904.* Cambridge, Mass.: Harvard University Press.

McGuire, W. (ed.) (1974). *The Freud/Jung Letters: The Correspondence Between Sigmund Freud and C. G. Jung.* Princeton, N.J.: Princeton University Press.

Roazen, P. (1975). *Freud and His Followers.* New York: Knopf.

Sand, R. (1988). Early nineteenth century anticipation of Freudian theory. *International Review of Psychoanalysis,* 15: 465–479.

———. (1992). Pre-Freudian discovery of dream meaning: The achievements of Charcot, Janet and Krafft-Ebing. In T. Gel-Fand and J. Kerr (eds.). *Freud and the History of Psychoanalysis.* Hillsdale, N.J.: Analytic Press, pp. 215–229.

Silverstein, B. (1985). Freud's psychology and its organic foundation: Sexuality and mind-body interactionism. *Psychoanalytic Review,* 72: 203–228.

———. (1986). "Now Comes a Sad Story": Freud's lost metapsychological papers. In P. E. Stepansky (ed.). *Freud: Appraisals and Reappraisals: Contributions to Freud Studies,* vol. 1. Hillsdale, N.J.: Analytic Press, pp. 143–195.

Silverstein, S. M., and Silverstein, B. R. (1990). Freud and hypnosis: The development of an interactionist perspective. *Annual of Psychoanalysis,* 18: 175–194.

Sulloway, F. (1979). *Freud: Biologist of the Mind: Beyond the Psychoanalytic Legend.* New York: Basic Books.

Swales, P. J. (1986). Freud, his teacher and the birth of psychoanalysis. In P. E. Stepansky (ed.). *Freud: Appraisals and Reappraisals: Contributions to Freud Studies,* vol. 1. Hillsdale, N.J.: Analytic Press, pp. 3–82.

BARRY SILVERSTEIN

Psychoanalytic Movement

The term "psychoanalytic movement" refers to the development and unfolding of the psychoanalytic enterprise, in its organizational and theoretical dimensions, during

Freud's lifetime. Freud himself introduced the term in 1914 when he wrote *On the History of the Psychoanalytic Movement*, which described the growth of the enterprise from about 1895 (his early collaboration with Josef Breuer) up to that point. The intellectual and ideological capital of the movement was of course Vienna, with Budapest, Zurich, and Berlin as major satellite centers and with other Western European countries, the United States, and Canada at the periphery. South America was still psychoanalytic terra incognita. In 1925, Freud amplified and updated this history with his paper *An Autobiographical Study*, which in the view of his editor, James Strachey, is less an autobiography than "an account of [Freud's] personal share in the development of psychoanalysis" (p. 4). After Freud's death in 1939, psychoanalysis changed substantially. Its impetus *as a movement* gradually subsided as it affirmed itself worldwide and became theoretically more diversified.

Freud's (1914) essay *On the History of the Psycho-Analytic Movement* was written very soon after the defections of Alfred Adler, Wilhelm Stekel, and C.G. Jung. These occurred, in that order, between 1910 and 1913 and shook the foundations and the stability of the organization. Faced with the challenge from these competing views, Freud felt the need to give an accounting of what psychoanalysis was and stood for. He did so in his characteristically clear and theoretically cogent way, pointing out the difficulties he saw in the contributions of his erstwhile colleagues. Freud also addressed the question of how much diversity of theoretical views could be allowed while maintaining consistency with the basic tenets of psychoanalysis; he drew the line at the place to be given to the unconscious, to infantile sexuality, and to conflict and repression. Both Adler and Jung, according to Freud, had minimized the role of the unconscious and of the instinctual drives (i.e., of sex and aggression, but especially the former). Adler had given undue emphasis to the ego and to the pressure of social forces, while Jung had diminished the drives from the side of the superego, by emphasizing religious principles and ethical guidance. The problems with Stekel were less theoretical than tactical; Stekel wanted to replace psychoanalysis with his brand of brief analytic psychotherapy. Freud was at pains to spell out the divergence of these views from his own conception of psychoanalysis, which he saw as central and most valid: "I consider myself justified in maintaining that even today no one can know better than I do what psychoanalysis is" (p. 7).

Following the departure of Adler, Stekel, and Jung, Ernest Jones in London largely replaced Jung as the head of the organization. He also conceived the idea of organizing a committee of close and loyal colleagues who, like the paladins of old, formed a shield around Freud and the fledgling psychoanalytic organization and anticipated any significant theoretical or ideological controversies that might arise. In addition to Jones, the committee consisted of Hanns Sachs, Sándor Ferenczi, Karl Abraham, Otto Rank, and Max Eitingon. Each received from Freud an antique Greek intaglio that he then had made into rings, symbolic of their purpose. The committee was secret and Freud (who also received a ring) was the only one besides its members who knew of its existence. Each made a pledge that, should he at some point develop theoretical views significantly different from those of Freud and the other members of the committee, he would not declare these disagreements publicly until there had been the opportunity to discuss them thoroughly in private. The pledge, however, was not very effective in keeping the members in line. Rank, who at one time had been personally very close to Freud, eventually broke with him and left the organization. The same might well have happened with Ferenczi, had it not been for his premature death.

Jones, the prime mover in the committee, devoted himself with great energy to the myriad of organizational tasks. He developed and maintained a network of contacts among psychoanalysts in Europe, England, the United States, Canada; his initiative led to the establishment of the London (later, the British) Psychoanalytic Society, the American Psychoanalytic Association, and the American Psychopathological Association. The task of the International Psychoanalytic Association, founded in 1910, was to promote the standing of psychoanalysis, arrange biennial psychoanalytic congresses, encourage psychoanalytic presentations outside the profession, and respond to criticisms and challenges of psychoanalysis from external sources. An impressive number of psychoanalytic journals were founded to promote awareness of the clinical findings discovered by the flourishing new discipline.

In his autobiography, Jones devotes a long chapter to the psychoanalytic "movement," which he places in quotation marks. Despite his contributions on its behalf, he was not happy with some of the implications of the word "movement"; he felt that the term was more fitting to an enterprise that was ethical or religious rather than scientific. Yet, he agreed with Freud that the psychoana-

P

lytic organization was not intellectually restrictive and that a consensus about basic theoretical issues and assumptions was appropriate and consistent with the tenets of science.

Wallerstein, in his 1988 presidential address to the International Psychoanalytic Association, reviewed the development of psychoanalysis over the recent decades and in the title of his paper raised the central question—"One psychoanalysis or many?" He then gave official recognition to the changes that have taken place and emphasized how the field is now characterized by pluralism and theoretical diversity. New theoretical positions (e.g., Kleinian psychoanalysis, object relations theory, self psychology) have arisen since Freud's death, and even some of the original contributions of Adler, Jung, Ferenczi, and others gradually and unobtrusively have been reabsorbed into the psychoanalytic mainstream. The term "psychoanalytic movement" belongs to the past, when psychoanalysis spoke with one voice, Freud's, and to a time when pressures from both within and without called for a dedicated and disciplined allegiance.

REFERENCES

Ferenczi, S. (1911). On the organization of the psycho-analytic movement. S. Ferenczi (author). *Final Contributions to the Problems and Methods of Psycho-Analysis*. New York: Basic Books, 1955, pp. 299–307.

Freud, S. (1914). On the history of the psycho-analytic movement. S.E. 14: 3–86.

———. (1925). *An Autobiographical Study*. S.E. 20: 3–74.

Jones, E. (1955). *The Life and Work of Sigmund Freud*, vol. 2. New York: Basic Books.

———. (1959). *Free Associations; Memories of a Psycho-Analyst*. New York: Basic Books.

Nunberg, H., and Federn, E. (1962–1975). *Minutes of the Vienna Psychoanalytic Society*, vols. 1–4. New York: International Universities Press.

Sachs, H. (1944). *Freud. Master and Friend*. Cambridge, Mass.: Harvard University Press.

Wallerstein, R. S. (1988). One psychoanalysis or many? *International Journal of Psychoanalysis*, 69: 5–21.

Wittels, F. (1924). *Sigmund Freud. His Personality, His Teaching, and His School*. New York: Dodd, Mead.

PIETRO CASTELNUOVO-TEDESCO

Psychoanalytic Technique and Process

Introduction and History

Analytic technique begins with Breuer and Freud's terrible struggles to deal with the miseries of dysfunctional women (1893–1895). Those struggles evolved into patterns of dealing with patients and their problems. These patterns constituted a procedure or technique that yielded strange data demanding a theoretical framework to account for them. When Anna O. (Bertha Pappenheim) used the couch, her treatment with Breuer eventuated in her false pregnancy and delusion of having been impregnated by him. Freud later attributed her pseudocyesis to unrecognized sexual wishes toward the analyst. When Freud's patient Dora left her treatment, Freud attributed the premature termination to her intolerance of her erotic wishes toward him and his failure to interpret it to her in time. The most striking datum found was that when the patient lay on a couch and talked about her symptoms, sexual feelings toward the analyst could develop. It was these sexual wishes that Freud conceptualized as the transference. He noted the appearance of anxiety in his patient Dora as the sexual wishes came to awareness and patients' difficulty in talking about what was on their minds when the ideas approached the forbidden wishes too closely. Later in the history of analysis, other aspects of wishes came to be seen as engendering anxiety in patients. Aggressive wishes and such unpleasurable affects as shame and guilt were recognized as sources of neurotic misery. These data required technical changes to effect therapeutic change and to conform to ethical principles. As analytic technique changed to accommodate the data obtained in analyses, the theoretical frame has changed with it. Psychoanalysis is thus a therapeutic technique first, a method of investigation second, a body of data third, and a theory last. For this reason, theories that have technical implications spark controversy; those that allow the use of standard technique do not (Richards, A. D., 1984a). Freud's technical papers of 1904–1937 can be seen as a record of the progress he and his patients made in investigating their wishes and the associated affects and thoughts prohibiting their satisfaction.

These papers were meant as a record of progress and as a response to the difficulties encountered in analytic work. The papers are concerned less with positive injunctions than with mistakes. Removing symptoms by searching for their origins is difficult, slow, and limited to educated, nonpsychotic adults. The method in 1904 was conceived of as a way of overcoming internal resistances to awareness of forbidden wishes.

In his 1910 paper, Freud proposed a refinement in technique excluding such "wild analysis" as telling the patient directly about her wishes. Caution protects patients from too sudden awareness of the unacceptable. Treating dreams as if they were symptoms (Freud, 1912) allows deeper and sometimes less painful development of awareness. Thus listening to dreams and to patients' associations to dreams becomes part of analytic technique. Having begun analytic work with the investigation of symptoms, Freud extended it to the exploration of dreams. While symptoms were clearly the province of doctors, dream interpretation widened the range of appropriate interpreters. Dreams were normal phenomena, but with roots in the hidden part of mental functioning from which symptoms sprang. In this sense, dreams were the way into the unconscious. Freud used his interpretations of his own dreams to demonstrate what could be found through psychoanalysis and to convey the method and the data to others. At the end of *The Interpretation of Dreams* (1900), Freud used the data and the demonstration of his method of thinking about those data to construct a theory. Thus, the tripartite structure of psychoanalysis as a technique, a body of data, and a theory was established.

It became evident to Freud by 1905 that the most difficult yet imperative part of psychoanalytic technique was the analysis of the transference. Now understanding of the term "transference" was broadened to include hateful "negative" as well as affectionate "positive" transference manifestations. Transference became the battleground on which victory over neurosis could be achieved. "For when all is said and done, it is impossible to destroy anyone in absentia or in effigie." (Freud, 1912: 108). With respect to analysis of the transference, Freud admonished analysts to pay equal attention to anything the analysand says or does, avoiding note taking during the sessions or conceptualizing the case too quickly, and minimizing self-disclosure and the expression of the analyst's own wishes. Being content with the patient's own goals rather than setting standards for cure became a touchstone for analytic termination.

Freud used the clinical phenomenon of the patient insisting that he had already told the analyst something that the analyst believes to be new as a clue to the gradual process of making the unconscious conscious. He remarks that those who wish to put off beginning the treatment are unlikely ever to start it. He notes that it is not a good idea to treat one's own friends or relatives. Skepticism is seen as a better prognostic sign than uncritical belief in the analytic method. Arrangements about time and money are regularized in the beginning of the treatment. A particular hour is to be set aside for each patient, every day, six days a week. Duration of the work is left up to the patient, with the analyst advised to refuse predicting how long it may take. Fees are to be set so as to allow the analyst to live comfortably from earnings. The analyst has to be willing to talk about fees in order to demonstrate to the patient that shame is not allowed to stifle discussion. As an expansion on the idea of avoiding "wild analysis," the patient is to be understood at the beginning of the treatment, not confronted with interpretations. The interpretations made later in the treatment are to be as close as possible to what the patient is already aware of but can be useful even when they are ahead of the patient's awareness, even if they must be denied when first offered. Timing is everything. Premature interpretations cause patients to bolt treatment not only because such interpretations arouse resistance but also because patients obtain relief from them. Intellectual understanding is no longer valued because it is not therapeutically efficacious.

After replacing intellectual understanding and abreaction as goals of technique, removal of resistances became the primary aim of the psychoanalyst (Freud, 1914). Once the resistances were removed, it was the patient who would recall and articulate lost memories. Now ideas and connections, fantasies and impulses were more important to recollect than events. The analyst has to guard against the repression of these memories, since failure to recapture them leads to acting them out in current life. Once the repressed mental processes are recovered, a long period of alternately wrestling with resistances and recapturing the memories in new contexts ensues. It is this working through that Freud now considers the essence of analytic therapy. Such treatment is dangerous because it can evoke wishes and impulses in the analyst, especially the wish to love and be loved by the patient: countertransference (Freud, 1915).

By 1919, Freud advocated carrying out analytic treatment in a state of abstinence. A certain amount of educative exhortation may be needed, for example, to approach the phobic object. But the patient is not to be induced to be like the analyst in philosophy or way of life. The patient is to fulfill his or her own potential. In a not very often remembered passage, Freud describes the ideal of free analysis to be provided in clinics for the poor.

By the time of *Analysis Terminable and Interminable* (1937), Freud had come to focus on problems of how long analysis should last and on issues of what happens after analysis. Symptom removal and sufficient self-understanding for belief that the symptoms will not recur became criteria for the termination of analysis. Understanding that it was impossible for analysis to prevent new illness when new life circumstances stirred up conflicts that had never surfaced before, Freud had to conclude that complete prophylaxis cannot be achieved in any analysis. In the end, curative value was attached especially to constructions in which the analyst told the patient some piece of his or her own history that connected affects, events, object relations, and fantasies. The patient was to judge whether such a construction rang true or not. Then the analyst would evaluate the patient's response. A simple yes or no would have little evidential value. More important was the production of new material that would indirectly confirm the construction by building on it or disconfirm it by producing no noticeable change in the patient. From these beginnings, a standard technique has been built up over the years.

Beginning, Middle, and End Phases of Analysis

The Beginning Phase. How to begin an analysis is a question of interest to the novice analyst. One can be an analyst for years before facing the need to terminate an analysis. But it is sometimes only in the termination of an analysis that one learns of the impressions left on the patient in the earliest phases, and only after the completion that one understands the significance of the early interviews. A preliminary consultation or series of consultations is used to determine whether the patient wants or can tolerate the analytic process, to set the fee, to determine the hours, and to decide whether patient and analyst are suited to each other. Following Freud, Fenichel (1941) and Glover (1940) place little emphasis on attempting to get a history, seeing the analysis as the process of uncovering what will turn out to be the true history.

The beginning phase of analysis is the time from the first meeting until analyst and analysand agree to work together. History taking, setting the schedule and fee arrangements, and a variety of interactions may take place before the pair feel settled in enough to have completed the beginning phase. Often a consultation period of several sessions serves as the beginning phase, but it may take weeks or months. Sometimes a phase of psychotherapy precedes the analysis proper, and that can constitute the beginning phase.

The major controversy about the beginning phase of analysis is whether the analyst must try to establish a "therapeutic" (Zetzel, 1956) or "working" (Greenson, 1965) alliance, or should simply use listening and interpretation from the start. Some symptoms can be removed only by insight. And attaining insight is always painful, inducing self-doubt as well as temporary lowering of self-esteem as the patient recognizes that she has not known herself as well as she thought. Attaining insight requires tolerating this loss of self-esteem, thus requiring the analyst to support and bolster the patient. This kind of support is what Greenson and Zetzel believe necessary to produce the alliance that allows the patient to tolerate the pain of interpretations.

In opposition to Greenson and Zetzel, Brenner (1983) points out that such an alliance would always be understood by the analysand in terms of the same transference he or she brought to other personal relationships. In Brenner's view, the possibility of distinguishing between the alliance and the transference is obviated by the patient's perceptual distortion of what the analyst intends to convey in the relationship exactly because the patient is neurotic. Forming a therapeutic or working alliance may be seen as an attempt on the part of the analyst to counter the effect of confrontation and interpretations. Such interventions would not give the patient hope or comfort but would be aimed at depriving her of defensive distortions and misrepresentations in that world that she had constructed as comforts (Richards, A. D., 1984b). According to Buie et al. (1983), aggression is required to make interpretations because overcoming resistance in the analytic situation is aggressive. Interpretations always hurt.

Brenner (1979) contends that the concept of establishing an alliance by means of nonanalytic interventions in the first phase of treatment is not worthwhile. For Brenner, the most comforting thing the analyst can do for a patient is to make a good interpretation. Poland (1985) describes his own practice of using the consultation to demonstrate to the patient his belief that present troubles are connected to past relationships and events by asking the patient to describe himself and his history. He then decides whether he believes the patient can use the kinds of insight analysis has to offer. Once analysis is decided on as the method of treatment, he explains that it works best if the patient tries "to put into words all thoughts, feelings, body feelings, dreams, ideas, or whatever as they come up" (p. 153). Poland's contemporary view thus emphasizes Freud's original instruction on how to begin an analysis.

The Middle Phase. No criteria for when the middle phase of the analysis begins have been established, but the instruction to the patient to say everything that comes to mind is one convenient marker. After this instruction is given, anything that is said is part of the process of trying to free-associate and of the resistance to doing so. A. Kris (1982) explored the vicissitudes of the attempt to free-associate, concluding that the entire analytic process is the struggle to do that impossible task. The other possible analytic goals follow from it. Thus, insight, symptom reduction, and analysis of transference all follow when the analyst deals with the resistances that prevent the patient's associations from being truly free.

Friedman (1991) has shown that the attempt to free-associate inevitably calls up resistance, and that Freud's technical papers are a manual for dealing with this resistance. According to Friedman, the analyst is taught to seduce the patient into wishing for what the analyst will ultimately not give. The seduction animates the analytic work, and the interpretations allow self-observation on the patient's part. The fundamental rule now demands that the patient express desire without expecting it to be satisfied and the analyst courts desire without allowing it satisfaction. The patient must frustrate the very wishes the analyst elicits in order to please the analyst. Friedman regards later formulations of the splitting of the ego and theraputic alliance as evasive maneuvers meant to minimize the perception of analysis as dangerous and unfair.

Fenichel (1941) attempted to fill in the gap between the opening phase and the concluding one by talking about some typical problems in analytic technique. Like Freud, Fenichel believed that there was no way to prescribe positively what to say, what to focus on, or what to do. All that could be said is that the analyst should listen. The technique is simply to keep listening until the patient gets into trouble. Therefore, all that can be taught is troubleshooting.

But how to troubleshoot? Alternate intuition with understanding in the analyst; attend alternately to emotion and rational thought in the patient. "The subject matter, not the method of psychoanalysis, is irrational" (Fenichel, 1941: 13). Psychoanalysis allows the analysand to become increasingly tolerant of the awareness of forbidden wishes. As these wishes are better tolerated, they become less distorted. The analyst is continually making

connections: Connecting feeling with thought, past with present, the contents of the analytic hour with the events of everyday life, love with hatred, and desire with aggressive, destructive wishes.

The wish to act out rather than understand is the primary problem and disrupter of the transference. Thus the importance of not gratifying the transference wishes and maintaining the tension in the transference is balanced by the need to allow realistic gratification of the libidinal needs of the patient outside the transference. Early in the treatment, the analyst attempts to arouse the patient's curiosity about the symptom or character trait, isolating it from the experiencing ego. Then it is understood as an activity of the ego rather than as an intrusion from the outside. Motives for this activity are then elucidated. Other spheres of life in which similar traits or events are found are then connected to the event that has already been understood. Then the infantile origins of these current manifestations are made clearer. By continually going through the stages of this process, the patient gradually attains greater comfort and ease with the original wishes. The patient accepts interpretations by recognizing their connection with what he or she already knew, because of positive feelings toward the analyst for having already helped the patient and because of identification with the interpreting analyst.

The End Phase. Analysts have considered when to terminate analysis since the earliest days. Most of the early patients broke off their analyses with symptom remission, changed life circumstances, or some breach of the analytic relationship. Breuer broke off his treatment of Anna O. when the transference love eventuated in her false pregnancy and delusion of having been impregnated by him. Dora left because of her intolerance of the transference to Freud. The Rat Man had both symptom remission and military call-up to end his analysis. Freud got into trouble with the Wolf Man when he believed that the treatment had bogged down in the middle phase as the Wolf Man seemed content to go on for years without changing his life and without recovering the infantile memories believed to be necessary for his cure. Freud attempted to resolve the impasse by imposing an outside time limit, allowing a final year in which the transference was to be resolved and the infantile memories recaptured. This is somewhat analogous to the preanalytic way of thinking in which the therapist "forced" the process by hypnosis or by pressure on the forehead. Since the Wolf Man was followed for the remainder of his life,

P

analysts reclaimed the later idea that the process had to take as long as the patient took for it. In fact, Firestein (1974) found that most analytic patients in a clinic also interrupted their treatment for reasons similar to those of Freud's early patients. Issues of analytic termination are still worth study for those patients who can and do stay with it.

Fenichel took up the question of the completion of analysis in terms of the transference. He thought that the dissolution of the transference was not a special phase at the end of the treatment but was, rather, a gradual process beginning with the first transference interpretation. His view of this process was that each interpretation removed a bit of libido from the analyst and returned it to its true connection. Analysis was thus a process of continually analyzing and dissolving "libidinal" transference.

Yet negative transference had to appear and be dissolved as well. Negative transference appeared when the patient was irrationally angry at the analyst. But not all such anger was negative transference. While Fenichel was not willing to include all negative feelings toward the analyst in the category of negative transference, he accepted the grain of negative transference in any anger at the analyst. "Negative transference" was a term reserved for those situations in which the immediate interaction was such that the average or normal person would not get angry. It was only the irrational negative transference that could be analyzed. Fenichel emphasized the importance of inquiring about negative feelings when they were not directly expressed.

Analysis originally had the goal of symptom removal. When the original symptoms were gone, treatment would logically end. When the treatment extended into attempting to strengthen the patient against relapse, and the idea of working through superseded the goal of symptom removal, analysts began to question how much analysis is enough. What goals should be met? If a patient came into treatment to deal with fears of being unable to find a mate, should treatment continue until he or she got married? If the complaint was work inhibition, should treatment go on until the person established a satisfying career? Ticho (1972) pointed out that meeting such goals could make analysis truly interminable. He distinguished life goals from analytic goals. Life goals are criteria of professional and personal achievements. Analytic goals include increased self-esteem, self-acceptance, and freedom to define life goals.

When the patient was comfortable with his or her wishes and fears and was willing to explore and attempt to understand any aspect of his or her own personality, then the treatment goals had been met. If life had not yet provided opportunities to achieve the person's life goals, the analysis could not make up for that. What the patient had to do was live, not continue analysis.

In the early days of analysis, it was common practice for the analyst to decide that the patient was ready for a termination of the analysis and to announce this to the patient (Glover, 1940). Shake her hand and be done with it. The patients' negative reactions to such endings made it clear that there had to be more effort put into termination. The patient needed the opportunity to talk to the analyst about feelings engendered by the wish to terminate, by the actual plans to terminate, and by the analyst's acceptance of the inevitability of termination. When the patient seemed to be ready, the analyst would agree to the patient's request that treatment end. The patient and analyst together would agree on a termination date weeks or months ahead.

Technique now included a definite phase for termination. As the idea of a termination phase was absorbed into technique, some authors believed that the termination phase should consist of weaning the patient from dependence on the analyst, while others considered it important to continue the analytic work on the same level as it had been done during the middle phase, allowing the patient to examine his or her affects, wishes, moral prohibitions, and fears as the date for termination approached. A consensus about strategy included agreeing on the idea of termination, setting a definite date for termination, and, finally, talking about the feelings evoked by the termination process.

In an attempt to pinpoint more precisely the indications for agreeing to a termination phase, a pretermination phase has been postulated (Van Dam et al., 1975). In this phase, analytic work has reached a level at which the patient is able to understand and interpret his or her own dreams and symptoms, has a realistic view of the analyst as neither omniscient nor uncaring, and has a reasonably optimistic life plan. When the analyst believes the patient to have attained such a state, the next mention of an idea of termination by the patient should be agreed to by the analyst, and the termination phase will have begun. This pretermination phase is an attempt to push the specification of technique one step further back from the actual termination than had been done before.

It extends what Freud had likened to the closing moves of a chess game by specifying one prior move. Bond and Richards (1992) have specified one aspect of the pretermination phase by showing how it can be inferred from analysis of a patient's dreams.

Countertransference, Transference, and Interpretation

Definitions of countertransference have been controversial from the beginning of analytic thinking. When Breuer left Anna O. to take a vacation with his wife, he was clearly running away from an intolerable (to him) situation. He had understood his relationship with his patient to be a therapeutic effort; she thought of it as a love affair. What went wrong between them could be seen as due to her transference to Breuer of loving feelings originally directed at her father. In his management of the case, Breuer behaved in ways that she understood to be seductive. Was his behavior due to his having transferred onto her loving feelings originally directed toward his parent? Or was it due to his response to her feelings toward him? Analysts have argued on both sides of this issue. Self-analysis is required of the analyst to figure out which parts of her or his past and current wishes, fears, and superego prohibitions have been aroused by the patient. This work is clearly the analyst's burden, and the classical position is that it is not to be shared with the patient.

Beginning with Strachey's (1934) assertion that transference interpretations are the only mutative ones, there has been controversy about what else besides mutative transference interpretations can make a difference in analysis. Strachey himself was clear. Other kinds of interventions were necessary and proper to make the analytic work tolerable to the patient. Extra-transference interpretations, suggestion, reassurance, and abreaction are among the interventions Strachey put forth as analytic even if not mutative examples.

Gill (1982) insists on the priority of transference interpretation over all other modes of understanding patients. Introducing a twofold meaning for analysis of transference, he distinguishes between analysis of resistance to the awareness of transference and analysis of resistance to understanding the meaning of the transference. Thus, a patient who does not acknowledge that he feels sad at the thought of an impending vacation because he anticipates missing the analyst is resisting awareness of the transference. But a patient who will not

acknowledge that he is vulnerable to feeling this because he felt abandoned by his mother when she was hospitalized in his childhood is resisting the meaning of the transference, keeping out of awareness the psychic equivalence of analyst and mother.

Gill believes that resistance is always manifested in the transference. But reluctance to talk about a painful issue may reflect reluctance to recall it rather than to discuss it with the analyst (Richards, A. D., 1984b). Thus, resistance may be outside the transference but still available for analysis. For example, if the patient suddenly cannot remember her dreams when the analyst announces an impending break in the treatment, it is not necessarily a wish not to tell the analyst what she feels about the announcement, but it may be a wish to protect herself from knowing what she feels. Similarly, the patient who has a reaction to the here-and-now behavior of the analyst may be reacting for realistic rather than transferential reasons. If the analyst wishes to charge the patient for missed sessions and has not notified the patient in advance that this would be the policy of the treatment, the patient may react with anger even without a strong genetic reason for this. Or if the analyst is late, or nags about some issue, or is overly apologetic, the patient may react to these distortions realistically; the feelings he has may be more significantly related to the here and now than to transference from a there and then.

Opinions on the possibility of altering the transferential distortions vary widely. Gill (1980) believes that the analyst should encourage the transference to expand by interpreting resistances to awareness of transference. By contrast, Weinshel (1992) suggests: "In psychotherapy I would probably be tempted to interpret transferences earlier than I would in an analytic situation where it would be advantageous to let the transference deepen and 'ripen.'" Where Gill seems to be saying that the transference will grow with interpretation, Weinshel implies that interpretation will have the opposite effect. Strachey (1934) had noted this paradox and resolved it by remarking that interpretation of the transference has two phases. In the first phase, the analysand becomes aware of libidinal and/or aggressive impulses toward the analyst. In the second phase, the analysand becomes aware that these impulses derive from similar impulses toward the parents or caretakers of infancy. Strachey believes that the first-phase interpretations intensify the transference while second-phase interpretations diminish it. If Gill meant interpretations leading to awareness of feelings toward the analyst and Weinshel had the latter-phase complete interpretations in mind, Strachey's observation reconciles the two.

As we see it, even if transference analysis is the most powerful tool in psychoanalytic technique, it would be a mistake to make it the only tool, because doing so would reduce it to a boring formula, unlikely to convince the patient or serve as an impetus for psychic change. Rather, using transference together with understanding the patient's situation in life outside the analytic situation and affective life in the past is likely to provide a convincingly full picture so that the patient recognizes herself or himself in the analysis.

Transference analysis can be conceived of as the most superficial of all possible understandings of the patient's communications; it is the surface in that it is closest in space and time to the patient's perceptions. If analyzing infantile wishes and fears is working at the deepest level, analyzing the derivatives of these fears and wishes and the prohibitions against them is the middle layer. In most instances, the analysis of transference begins when the patient is still barely acquainted with the analyst. It involves the least intense relationship the patient has at the time. Often, patients find it trivial or "picky" and complain that it sounds to them as if the analyst is interested only in herself or in the patient's reactions to the analyst's every vacation, every absence, every bill paid late, or new bit of office decor. Only by making the connection between the transference situation in the office and the transference situation in the patient's current life and the early experiences can this reaction to transference be countered.

Analytic interventions may require challenging the analysand's view of what has happened, of what is felt, or of what is remembered. When the analyst hears a contradiction between what happened and what was felt, that may need to be pointed out to the analysand. Otherwise, two versions of the same story may be told at different junctures in the analysis, and the analysand may be confronted with the discrepancy between them. One kind of confrontation has been emphasized by Kernberg (1974) in his treatment of narcissistic personalities. He advocates early confrontation, even in the first session of the patient's negative transference. He points out the ways in which the patient attempts to humiliate the analyst. This is confrontation of the object relation as Kernberg sees it. It can be used in analysis, but, unlike interpretation, is equally appropriate as part of a diagnostic process or a psychotherapy.

Once it is agreed that the distinctive technique of analysis is the interpretation, the question becomes when and how to make an interpretation. Strachey (1934) asserted that the interpretation will be mutative only when the id impulse to be interpreted is active at the moment in the transference when the interpretation is given to the patient. According to Strachey, interpretations are vague and general at first, but they can be made more and more concrete and specific as the analytic work goes on and the patient recalls and recounts more of the details of early life. For example, a patient who announces that she wishes to cut back her hours after each session in which the analyst believes that they have made progress might be told that she seems to be afraid of some consequence of the last session. When this happens several times, she might be told that it seems to be a regular pattern. When she replies that the reason she wants to cut back on her sessions is that they are too early in the morning and she wants to sleep, she might be told that her pattern may have to do with fears that the analyst is invading her sleep. Eventually, such a line of interpretation might develop into an exploration of childhood wishes to have someone come to sleep in her bed. More specifically yet, a parent or sibling may have been the object of such a wish.

Glover (1931) warned that the interpretation must be exact to have analytic effect. He believed that the blatantly inexact or incorrect interpretation will have no effect, but that an almost correct one will have an antianalytic effect that is still therapeutic. Resulting in more effective repression, it would alleviate symptoms, but it would be antianalytic in that it would do so at the cost of decreasing self-awareness. While Glover seemed to be in favor of the grand, exact, and encompassing interpretation as the therapeutic instrument, Strachey preferred the idea of many tiny steps in which interpretations inched closer to the exact and comprehensive. Reik (1933) regarded the element of suddenness and surprise as essential in getting through the defenses. This position contrasts with Strachey's gradualness. For Strachey, the modifications brought about by interpretation were modifications of the superego, generally modifications in the direction of loosening its prohibitions to allow more sway to the rational.

Ego psychologists established the idea of an *order* of interpretation. Kaiser (1976), writing in the same era, believed that interpretations of resistance were the only necessary and appropriate interventions in analysis. Interpreting the defense before the id wish, the negative transference before the positive transference, and

P

surface before depth became shibboleths in ego psychology. Poland (1975) linked timing with tact. Putting off an interpretation until the patient is able to accept it, using indirection, waiting for the previous interpretation to be assimilated are all aspects of tact. He also cautioned against the pseudotact of avoiding all confrontation. This avoidance of aggression on both sides, Poland observes, leads to mutual admiration and failure to analyze.

Tact may also involve prefacing a potentially humiliating interpretation with a disclaimer. Such phrases as "I could be wrong, but here is what I think . . ." or "I may be off the mark here, but . . ." give the patient the idea that she is free to disagree. They provide a model of openness and hypothesis testing on the part of the analyst. In this way, they invite ego functions such as judgment and self-observation to be brought to bear by the analysand.

Analytic Process and Technique

What has been called the "analytic process" is the central phenomenon that provides the basis for the mode of treatment, the investigative procedure, and the body of knowledge and theory that constitute psychoanalysis. Like Winnicott's "transitional space," it is an illusion, a phenomenon within both the mind of the analyst and the mind of the analysand that links them in a common task. It is the result of intrapsychic responses to interpersonal interchanges. The actions and words of the analyst contribute to it; the initiatives and responses of the patient, both in words and in action, contribute to it. Transference wishes, fantasies, prohibitions, and fears come into play in the analytic situation, and countertransference counterparts spring to life there as well. One way of conceptualizing the analytic alliance may be this: a fit between transference and countertransference may be the beginning of the possibility of initiating the analyzing process.

A comprehensive survey of the concept of analytic process was attempted in an issue of the *Psychoanalytic Quarterly* dedicated to that topic (1990). In that journal, Arlow and Brenner (1990) assert that there is no difference between the technique and process. They see the process as the interplay between the unconscious of the analysand and the interventions of the analyst. This view is a corollary of their idea that psychoanalysis is the analysis of the dynamics of psychic conflict. To the extent that others believe that there is more to analysis than

conflict, they also see process as different from technique. Arlow and Brenner believe that pre-Oedipal, developmental, and relational theories are the basis for distinguishing psychoanalytic process from psychoanalytic technique.

In describing what the analyst brings to the analytic situation, Isakower (New York Psychoanalytic Institute, 1963) delineated a process of using the unconscious as an "analyzing instrument." He considered it to be composed of two complementary halves. One half is the speaking patient in the act of free-associating, the other half is the listening analyst in the act of imaging the patient's utterances. By imaging in this way, the analyst creates a picture of the analysand's inner world of memory and fantasy that is corrected and amplified as the partners in the enterprise communicate with each other. Salter et al. (1980) amplified this idea, suggesting that the instrument consists of similarly regressed portions of the egos of the analytic pair.

Meissner (1991) summarizes current thinking that analysis can be viewed as an interactive process in which the two participants are constantly refining their understanding of the process by generating hypotheses and producing disconfirming data, thus stimulating the formation of new and more nearly correct ones, which lead again to producing more data in the form of memories, affects, or interactions.

REFERENCES

Arlow, J. (1991a). Methodology and reconstruction. *Psychoanalytic Quarterly*, 60: 539–563.

———. (1991b). Conflict, trauma and deficit. In S. Dowling (ed.). *Conflict and Compromise Formation*. Madison, Conn.: International Universities Press.

———. (1991c). *Psychoanalysis: Clinical Theory and Practice*. Madison, Conn.: International Universities Press.

———. (1991d). Changing perspectives in psychoanalytic technique. Unpublished paper.

Arlow, J., and Brenner, C. (1990). The psychoanalytic process. *Psychoanalytic Quarterly*, 59: 678–693.

Bach, S. (1985). *Narcissistic States and the Therapeutic Process*. New York: Aronson.

Baranger, M., and Baranger, W. (1964). Insight in the analytic situation. In R. E. Litman (ed.). *Psychoanalysis in the Americas*. New York: International Universities Press.

Blanck, G., and Blanck, R. (1980). Separation-individuation. In R. Lax, S. Bach, and J. Burland (eds.). *Rapprochment*. New York: Aronson.

Blum, H. (1980). The prototype of pre-Oedipal reconstruction. In R. Lax, S. Bach, and J. Burland (eds.). *Rapprochment*. New York: Aronson.

Bond, A., Franco, D., and Richards, A. K. (1992). *Dream Portrait*. Madison, Conn.: International Universities Press.

Brenner, C. (1979). Working alliance, therapeutic alliance and transference. *Journal of the American Psychoanalytic Association*, 27: 137–153.

———. (1983). *The Mind in Conflict*. New York: International Universities Press.

Breuer, J., and Freud, S. (1893–1985). *Studies in Hysteria*. S E. 2: 19–305.

Buie, D., Meissner, W., and Rizutto, A. M. (1983). Aggression in the psychoanalytic situation. *International Review of Psychoanalysis*, 10: 159–170.

Dowling, S. (ed.) (1991). *Conflict and Compromise Formation*. Madison, Conn.: International Universities Press.

———. (1992). The impact of infant research on clinical work with children and adults. Paper presented at IPTAR, March 1992.

Etchegoyen, H. (1991). *The Fundamentals of Psychoanalytic Technique*. London: Karnac Books.

Fenichel, O. (1941). *Problems of Psychoanalytic Technique*. New York: Psychoanalytic Quarterly.

Firestein, S. (1974). Termination of the psychoanalysis of adults: Review of the literature. *Journal of the American Psychoanalytic Association*, 22: 873–894.

Freud, S. (1900). *Interpretation of Dreams*. S.E. 10: 4–5.

———. (1910). "Wild" psycho-analysis. S.E. 11: 219–227.

———. (1911). The handling of dream interpretation in psychoanalysis. S.E. 12: 89–96.

———. (1912). The dynamics of transference. S.E. 12: 97–108.

———. (1914). Remembering, repeating and working through (Further recommendations on the technique of psychoanalysis II). S.E. 12: 145–156.

———. (1915 [1914]). Observations on transference-love (Further recommendations on the technique of psycho-analysis III). S.E. 12: 157–171.

———. (1937). Analysis terminable and interminable. S.E. 23: 209–254.

Friedman, L. (1991). A reading of Freud's *Papers on Technique*. *Psychoanalytic Quarterly*, 60: 564–595.

Gill, M., (1980). The analysis of transference. *Journal of the American Psychoanalytic Association*, 27 (Supplement): 263–288.

———. (1982). *Analysis of Transference, Vol. 1: Theory and Technique*. New York: International Universities Press.

Glover, E. (1931). The effects of inexact interpretation. *Journal of Psychoanalysis*, 12: 397–411.

———. (1940). *An Investigation of the Technique of Psychoanalysis*. London: Baillie're, Tindall and Cox.

Greenson, R. (1965). The working alliance and the transference neurosis. *Psychoanalytic Quarterly*, 34: 155–181.

Jacobs, T. (1991). *The Use of the Self*. Madison, Conn.: International Universities Press.

Kernberg, O. (1974). Contrasting viewpoints regarding the nature and treatment of narcissistic personalities: A preliminary communication. *Journal of the American Psychoanalytic Association*, 22: 255–267.

Kohut, H. (1979). The two analyses of Mr. Z. *International Journal of Psychoanalysis*, 60: 3–27.

Kris, A. (1982). *Free Association: Method and Process*. New Haven, Conn.: Yale University Press.

Meissner, W. (1991). *What Is Effective in Psychoanalytic Therapy?* Northvale, N.J.: Aronson.

New York Psychoanalytic Institute. (1963). Minutes of Faculty Meeting. November 20. Unpublished.

Poland, W. (1975). Tact as a psychoanalytic function. *International Journal of Psychoanalysis*, 56: 155–162.

———. (1985). At work. In J. Reppen (ed.). *Analysts at Work: Practice, Principles and Techniques*. Hillside, N.J.: Analytic Press.

Racker, H. (1968). *Transference and Countertransference*. London: Hogarth. (Reprinted, London: Karnac Books, 1982).

Rangell, L. (1990). *The Human Core*. Madison, Conn.: International Universities Press.

Reik, T. (1933). New ways in psychoanalytic technique. *International Journal of Psychoanalysis*, 14: 321–334.

Richards, A. D. (1984a). The relationship between psychoanalytic theory and psychoanalytic technique. *Journal of the American Psychoanalytic Association*, 32: 587–602.

———. (1984b). Transference analysis: Means or end? *Psychoanalytic Quarterly*, 4: 355–366.

Schwaber, E. (1990). Interpretation and the therapeutic action of psychoanalysis. *International Journal of Psychoanalysis*, 71: 229.

Shane, M., and Shane, E. (1989). The struggle for otherhood: Implications for adult development. *Psychoanalytic Inquiry*, 9: 466–481.

Steingart, I. (1983). *Pathological Play in Borderline and Narcissistic Conditions*. New York: Spectrum.

Strachey, J. (1934). The nature of the therapeutic action of psychoanalysis. *International Journal of Psychoanalysis*, 15: 127–159.

Ticho, E. (1972). Termination of psychoanalysis: Treatment goals, life goals. *Psychoanalytic Quarterly*, 41: 315–333.

Van Dam, H., et al. (1975). On termination of child analysis. *Psychoanalytic Study of Children*, 30: 3–474.

Wallerstein, R. (1990). Psychoanalysis: The common ground. *International Journal of Psychoanalysis*, 71: 3–348.

Weinshel, E. (1992). Therapeutic technique in psychoanalysis and psychoanalytic psychotherapy. *Journal of the American Psychoanalytic Association*, 40: 327–348.

Zetzel, E. (1956). Current concepts of transference. *International Journal of Psychoanalysis*, 37: 369–376.

ARNOLD DAVID RICHARDS
ARLENE KRAMER RICHARDS

Psychoanalytically Oriented Psychotherapy

The psychoanalytically oriented psychotherapies are those talk therapies that have developed out of psychoanalysis and accept Freud's conception of the dynamic unconscious as central to an understanding of intrapsychic life and therefore to effective psychotherapeutic treatment.

Before he became the first psychoanalyst, Freud was a psychotherapist. Like generations of physicians before him, he used the authority delegated to him by patients to effect change with forms of suggestion, including direct advice and manipulation of events of the patient's life (Bibring, 1954). While this approach apparently succeeded with some hysterical patients, Freud was not satisfied with the efficacy of suggestion and hypnosis, and his continuing efforts to understand and treat formerly untreatable patients laid the foundation not only for the theory and practice of psychoanalysis, but also for the subsequent evolution of psychotherapeutic approaches based on psychoanalytic principles. Freud's primary interest was in developing and refining the technique of psychoanalysis. Nevertheless, in 1919 he stated: "It is very probable too, that the large-scale application of our therapy will compel us to alloy the pure gold of analysis freely with the copper of direct suggestion; and hypnotic influence, too, might find a place in it again, as it has in the treatment of war neuroses. But, whatever form this psychotherapy for the people may take, whatever the elements out of which it is compounded, its most effective and most important ingredients will assuredly remain those borrowed from strict and untendentious psycho-analysis" (pp. 167–168). The prescient statement indicates his recognition of the enduring value of earlier techniques, but also provided a precedent for regarding psychotherapy as a less valuable form of treatment than psychoanalysis.

Although techniques vary, all forms of psychoanalytically oriented psychotherapy take account of the existence of transference, as well as the defense mechanisms and resistance. But systematic interpretation of the transference from a position of technical neutrality is the essential feature of psychoanalysis proper and the one that most distinguishes it from other psychotherapies, even those that are psychoanalytically oriented (Gill, 1954). In contrast to psychoanalysis proper, in the psychotherapies the transference may be left alone or utilized manipulatively. When transference is interpreted in psychotherapy, it is not a systematic interpretation of a transference neurosis. Usually such transference interpretation occurs in psychotherapies in which sessions are frequent, the period of treatment is not limited, and the patient is especially psychologically minded. It is

obvious that in such cases the psychotherapy comes close to being analysis. However, the line dividing psychoanalytically oriented psychotherapy from psychoanalysis is not now as clear to all authors, even to Gill, as it was to him in 1954. For an extensive scholarly overview of the history and current state of the psychoanalytic psychotherapies, the reader is referred to Wallerstain's (1995) *The Talking Cures* (see as well the references and discussion in Seelig, 1995).

Psychoanalytic psychotherapies can be subdivided by duration, focus, and the extent to which they are exploratory (uncovering) or supportive (suppressive). Most long-term psychotherapies are open-ended and nonfocal, in contrast to short-term (time-limited) treatments, which are generally "focal," i.e., they focus on specific problems. Free association may take place in some of the open-ended uncovering therapies, but unlike in psychoanalysis, it is not encouraged. Sessions are less frequent in therapy than in analysis. Regression is discouraged.

At the beginning of a focal treatment, the therapist decides what specific issue(s) to address; the number of sessions is determined; and termination issues are present throughout the treatment. Limiting the time available is used to actively overcome resistance and push treatment forward. This is in sharp contrast to the open-ended, nondirective psychoanalytically oriented psychotherapies, whether short- or long-term, which resemble analysis proper in this respect.

Expressive psychotherapies foster the uncovering of unconscious conflicts and their exploration. Interpretation is central, as it is in analysis. Acquisition of insight and ventilation of repressed affects are encouraged. In contrast, insight is not sought in supportive psychotherapies, which aim to seal over conflict. Ventilation of conscious affects is encouraged, but no effort is made to uncover repressed affect in purely supportive treatment. The therapist doing supportive treatment aligns her- or himself strongly with the demands of reality and makes efforts to strengthen the ego and assist the patient in employing healthier mechanisms of defense. Manipulation of the patient's environment, advice giving, and various forms of suggestion to be effective.

Analysis will generally be the treatment of choice if a person's neurotic difficulties are serious and appear to be affecting most areas of life, as it is also for some borderline patients who have access to higher-level defenses. Psychoanalytically oriented psychotherapy with a com-

P

bination of expressive and supportive techniques is the appropriate treatment for most borderline patients. When a person's difficulties appear to be circumscribed, acute, or mild, analysis is generally not needed and exploratory psychotherapy is indicated. Supportive psychotherapy, often in conjunction with pharmacotherapy, is generally the treatment(s) of choice for psychotic as well as the most severe borderline individuals.

Short-term, analytically oriented psychotherapy is the treatment of choice for mildly neurotic patients with circumscribed acute problems. Frequently, such difficulties develop in response to a life crisis. Generally, short-term treatment is not suitable for chronic pervasive characterologic difficulties. If the acute problem is embedded in a seriously neurotic or borderline character, the likelihood is small that a short-term approach will be adequate, although it might be attempted initially, with the understanding that the goals must be limited and that more extensive treatment will probably be needed later on.

The goals of any psychotherapy involve decreasing neurotic suffering and improving functioning. The psychotherapeutic approach chosen will vary with the severity and nature of the psychopathology, the time and financial resources available for treatment (an increasingly significant factor in these days of managed care), and the patient's inclination, which is often influenced by resistance.

REFERENCES

Bibring, E. (1954). Psychoanalysis and the dynamic psychotherapies. *Journal of the American Psychoanalytic Association*, 2: 745–770.

Freud, S. (1919). Lines of advance in psycho-analytic therapy. S.E. 17: 159–168.

Gill, M. (1954). Psychoanalysis and exploratory psychotherapy. *Journal of the American Psychoanalytic Association*, 2: 771–797.

Seelig, B. (1995). Psychoanalytically oriented individual psychotherapy. In B. Moore and B. Fine (eds.). *Psychoanalysis: The Major Concepts.* New Haven, Conn.: Yale University Press, pp. 46–60.

Wallerstein, R. (1995). *The Talking Cures: The Psychoanalyses and the Psychotherapies.* New Haven, Conn.: Yale University Press.

BETH J. SEELIG

Psychohistory

Psychohistory is the application of psychoanalysis to the study of history. Psychohistory is an interdisciplinary, innovative approach to the study of history, and it has enriched our understanding of the past, adding a more insightful perspective on the role of the individual, the group, and society.

The traditional approach, which neglects the psyche, or the inner life of the individual, emphasizes political, military, social, and economic factors as the sources of causation. Traditional historians assess historical developments on the basis of intuition. They claim that they are objective because they base their work on verifiable documentary sources, such as government documents, memoirs, newspapers, and other such data. Psychohistorians use the same sources but look at the evidence in a more comprehensive manner illuminated by the use of psychoanalytic theory (Loewenberg, 1996: 15). The psychohistorian seeks to understand *why* something happened, not just *what* happened (Binion, 1982: 7). The psychohistorian seeks to detect the unconscious motivations of the actors of history, the individual, and the group, seeking a more textured and insightful reconstruction of individual and group historical events. The use of psychoanalytic concepts to deepen the understanding of history and society is also referred to as "applied psychoanalysis."

Sigmund Freud was the first psychohistorian. After having developed the main tenets of psychoanalytic theory, Freud turned to applying his theories and clinical experiences to historical figures, culture, and society. In numerous works, he demonstrated how psychoanalysis could be utilized as an investigative technique. As Freud recognized, psychoanalysis and the study of humankind's past have much in common. They have many parallels in that they both take a genetic approach. In 1910, he published his first biographical study, *Leonardo da Vinci and a Memory of His Childhood.* In his study of the great artist, Freud explored Leonardo's artistic creativity, his sexual inhibitions, and the role of his narcissism, and traced it to the circumstances of his childhood. Another historical figure Freud studied and admired was the biblical Moses. In *Moses and Monotheism*, published in 1939, Freud explored the role of the "Great Man" in history, the distinctive characteristics of the Jewish people, and the roots of anti-Semitism.

The cornerstone of psychoanalysis is the Oedipus complex, which Freud used to explain how civilization originated. In *Totem and Taboo*, Freud advanced the thesis that civilization started with a murder—parricide—because the sons, or the primal horde, wanted to depose the father. But the commission of such an act led to feelings of guilt on the part of the group, then to the development of conscience, and ultimately to the organization of society, which could exist only if hostility and violence were curtailed.

Also of importance to the study of psychohistory is the role of groups, which Freud pioneered in his work *Group Psychology and the Analysis of the Ego* (Freud, 1921). In this work, Freud discussed how groups achieve cohesiveness. To illustrate these concepts, Freud examined two institutions, the army and the church, depicting the nature of the relationship that binds a group and its leader. In one of his last works, *Civilization and Its Discontents*, first published in 1930, Freud finds that all societies are aware of human aggression and therefore try to curb aggressive drives. In this respect, he considers the role of nationalism in achieving this end, which is an attempt to channel destructive drives toward another group by making it a target. Freud further broke the ground for psychohistory as an interdisciplinary field of research by founding, with Hanns Sachs, the journal *Imago*. Since 1939, this journal has been published in the United States and is now known as *American Imago*. As a journal of applied pychoanalysis, *American Imago* publishes articles on culture, society, the arts, and psychohistory.

Psychohistory received a fillip in the late 1950s from two closely related occurrences. One was the presidential address by William Langer, the eminent historian and president of the American Historical Association, who spoke at the banquet of the organization's annual meeting in 1957. Langer emphatically recommended that historians avail themselves of psychoanalysis to study historical figures and group behavior. For example, he said that a fitting subject of study would be the mass hysteria exhibited by people during the period of the Black Death, in the fourteenth century. He said that at this time there was a striking collective mentality that exhibited a sense of guilt and fear of retribution. Langer's address, appropriately entitled "The Next Assignment," became a clarion call to the historical profession to deepen its understanding of the past by employing psychoanalysis. When Langer delivered this apparently radical address, observers at this meeting noted that the participating historians reacted with consternation. Nevertheless, Langer's challenging address has become celebrated and a touchstone of the field.

The other significant event was the publication of Erik H. Erikson's *Martin Luther: A Study in History and Psychoanalysis*, in 1958. Ignored at first, this psychodynamic work on Luther eventually became a best-seller, and for many years was a paradigm for psychohistorical biographies. In line with psychoanalytic theory, Erikson attempted to answer two basic questions about Luther: what his unconscious motivation was and what the reasons for his success were. Exploring his childhood conflicts, which Erikson traced to his troubled relationship with his father, and his becoming a priest, which his father opposed, Erikson found that Luther eventually repudiated the authority of the pope. Luther's success in propagating the Protestant movement made him the preeminent revolutionary of his era. Like Freud, Erikson explored the role of the great man in history. And Luther's success as a leader was realized because in working out his own problems, what Erikson calls his "identity crisis," he was also helping to resolve problems of a religious nature that people had at this time. Although the focus of Erikson's work was on Luther, he also illuminated the historical interplay between leader and led.

As psychohistory is interdisciplinary, there is the question of what is required to be a competent practitioner of this relatively novel field. Erikson came to psychohistory as a practicing psychoanalyst. Preponderantly, however, psychohistorians come from the ranks of academic historians, who in various degrees have acquired a knowledge of psychoanalysis. The extent of their expertise and training varies. Some are self-taught, others additionally undergo a personal analysis, and still others receive clinical training at a psychoanalytic institute. Even if training in an institute to become a practicing psychoanalyst is not currently the norm as an education for psychohistorians, it has become, since the 1970s, more commonly practiced and recognized as an optimum goal. Indeed, a compelling case can be made for clinical training, because it brings enhanced empathic understanding, greater self-analytical abilities, and methodological acuity.

At the present time, nearly one hundred years after the publication of Freud's momentous *The Interpretation of Dreams*, psychohistory is far less controversial than it was in the 1950s and 1960s. Psychohistory is now more accepted in academic circles, as measured by its being taught in many colleges and universities, and by the abundance of psychohistorical publications. Psychohistory has been in the vanguard of historical scholarship and has provided a more profound, insightful, and scientific method of studying historical developments (Szaluta, 1999: 227–240).

P

REFERENCES

Binion, R. (1982). *Introduction à la psychohistoire*. Paris: Presses Universitaires de France.

Erikson, E. H. (1962). *Young Man Luther: A Study in Psychoanalysis and History*. New York: Norton.

Freud, S. (1921). *Group Psychology and the Analysis of Ego*. S.E. 18.

———. (1953). *The Interpretation of Dreams*. S.E. 4–5.

———. (1910). Leonardo da Vinci and a memory of his childhood. S.E. 11: 63–137.

———. (1912–1913). *Totem and Taboo*. S.E. 13: 1–161.

———. (1930). *Civilization and Its Discontents*. S.E. 21: 64–145.

———. (1939). *Moses and Monotheism*. S.E. 23: 7–137.

Langer, W. L. (1958). The next assignment. *The American Historical Review*, 63, no. 2: 283–304.

Loewenberg, P. (1996). *Decoding the Past*. New Brunswick, N.J.: Transaction Publishers.

Szaluta, J. (1999). *Psychohistory: Theory and Practice*. New York: Peter Lang.

JACQUES SZALUTA

Psychoneuroses See ANXIETY NEUROSIS; CHILDHOOD NEUROSIS; NEUROSES; PSYCHOPATHOLOGY.

Psychopathology

"Psychopathology" refers to the study, manifestations, and classification of disturbances of behavior assumed to have significant psychological causes or precipitants. Historically, there have been two principal lines of study. The first is descriptive and sets itself to define and classify groups of psychopathological symptoms under specific names (nosology). This endeavor, generally atheoretical, seeks primarily to refine both the reliability with which a psychopathological entity (e.g., "depression") can be identified and the validity with which a specific morbid state can be denoted. This is a categorical effort whose aim is nomothetic, that is, to study behavior in order to find lawful regularities, relationships, and principles in large numbers of cases. The second line of study, driven by specific theories of etiology and pathogenesis, seeks to define and clarify the specific meanings that psychopathological symptoms and behaviors represent in a person's life. This line is clearly committed to studies of individuality, and its aim is idiographic, where the focus is on the individual and the factors that produce uniqueness in a particular person. Freud began his scientific efforts as a descriptive psychopathologist, which followed from his neuroanatomical work in Meynert's laboratory in the 1870s and 1880s, where he studied and

wrote about the commonalities and the differences between nervous pathways, such as the dorsal roots of petromyzon (a type of eel). Freud's focus changed in the first decade of the twentieth century, when he began to probe more profoundly into the individuality and uniqueness of psychological dynamics.

In the 1880s and 1890s, Freud was concerned with the description and classification of psychopathological conditions such as hysteria, obsessions, and phobias, which, in earlier times, had been labeled as "demonic possession" (Kramer and Sprenger, 1971 [1486] *The Malleus Maleficarum*) or regarded (e.g., by Charcot) as a "congenital constitutional degeneracy." Freud began his psychoanalytic efforts as a search for a rational treatment for these psychopathological conditions, each of which he presumed had a specific psychological etiology: the persistence in memory of sexual conflicts that were, however, barred from consciousness by psychological mechanisms (repression, isolation, or displacement, for example). The characteristic psychological mechanisms, not the sexual etiology, defined the differences between the conditions.

Freud's therapeutic method, however, showed itself to be less than optimal for curing many of these conditions, and his interests then shifted toward exploring the individual variation in the meanings of behaviors that were more decisively expressive of all human development and especially of character. Hence, he became concerned with individual conflict, wishes, methods of coping with conflict (ego defenses), developmental shifts in sexual and aggressive motivation of behavior, and the nature of relations with other people (including the psychoanalyst). Thus, Freud replaced his early interest in specific neurotic syndromes and the categories of psychopathological symptoms (e.g., "actual" versus "transference" neuroses) with probing explorations into the unique, personal meanings that underlie habitual and even commonplace behaviors. Papers such as *Some Character-Types Met in Psycho-analytic Work* (Freud, 1916) and psychobiographical essays such as his writings on Leonardo da Vinci and Michelangelo were more characteristic of Freud's output than writings on diagnosis and psychopathology.

This change in Freud's interest increased the isolation of psychoanalysis from descriptive psychiatry. The isolation, however, had little practical consequences on the practice of psychiatry, inasmuch as there was no scientific consensus about the efficacy of rational treatments for specific psychopathological conditions. Whatever the diagnosis, the prescriptive treatment was generally the same: psychoanalysis or a variant of it. Psychoanalysts continued to focus on individuality, such as character (how this particular person got that way and what purposes some behaviors fulfill) and the amenability of certain character types to change by psychoanalysis. General psychiatry, on the other hand, continued to focus on classification and nosology. In some instances, there was a confluence of interests, as in the issue of borderline and narcissistic personalities.

Nevertheless, Freud and other psychoanalysts attempted to describe the putative underlying and motivating conditions of several psychological disorders. These formulations appeared in the five case histories (Dora, the Rat Man, the Wolf Man, the Schreber Case, and the study of female homosexuality). The most complete attempt to produce a psychoanalytic canon of psychopathology was the work of Otto Fenichel (1945), which summarized in encyclopedic fashion all the relevant formulations on neurotic, psychotic, and character disturbances and even included some organic conditions, such as disorders of the respiratory and cardiovascular system. The essential approach was to identify the specific drive conflicts underlying each pathological condition, then to correlate for each condition the specific drive-defense conflict with particular psychosexual developmental phases. From this matrix he offered a generalized reconstruction of the circumstances that shaped neurotic fixations during childhood.

In discussing obsessions and compulsions, for example, Fenichel argued that these phenomena may be regarded as direct or indirect manifestations of urges by drives; compulsions represented urges in behavior and obsessions represented urges in thought. The illustrations, in case vignettes and patients' free associations, were the evidence for the formulations. Hypothetical dynamics such as fixation at a particular phase of psychosexual development and regression to that phase were considered to be decisive for the emergence of a psychopathological condition. This model of psychopathology directed the psychoanalyst to identify the drive elements in the symptom, the anxiety that triggered the regression to the earlier drive expression, the nature of the drive-defense compromise, and the reasons for the regression and the earlier fixation. The principal problem with these formulations was the failure to ground them in observable, if not measurable, phenomena that diagnosticians could agree were either present or absent.

Fenichel's compendium, with its attempts to fix etiological and dynamic specificity, appears to be quite different from Freud's view of psychopathology. For Freud, after the first decade of the twentieth century, the separation of the normal from the pathological became much less of a concern. Indeed, his concept of psychopathology placed neurotic disturbances on a continuum with normal character and left out of consideration the clearly categorical differences between normal and psychotic conditions. Even in his last writings on the subject, he eschewed specific etiological events and conditions, which were so much a part of Fenichel's canon, written just a few years after Freud's death. Unlike infectious diseases, Freud wrote in *An Outline of Psycho-Analysis* (1940), neurotic conditions have no specific determinants, either in the environment or within the person. He stated that these conditions easily shade into normality, and in normal conditions "there is scarcely any state . . . in which indications of neurotic traits could not be recognized." Those who receive the diagnosis of "neurotic" have the same innate dispositions and life experiences as those who are termed normal. He then asked why they suffer so much more pain, anxiety, and simple lack of pleasure. His answer was a quantitative one. "The determining cause of all the forms taken by human mental life is, indeed, to be sought in the reciprocal action between innate dispositions and accidental experiences. Now a particular instinct may be too strong or too weak innately, or a particular capacity may be stunted or insufficiently developed in life. On the other hand, external impressions and experiences may make demands of differing strength on different people; and what one person's constitution can deal with may prove an unmanageable task for another's. These quantitative differences will determine the variety of the results" (Freud, 1940: 183–184). His view of psychosis, particularly schizophrenia, however, was different, inasmuch as he believed that there were etiological, pathogenic, and pathophysiological conditions, as yet unknown but discoverable, that characterize those with schizophrenia, for example ("dementia praecox," as this condition was usually referred to in the early part of the twentieth century), and that those with this psychotic disorder were not amenable to psychoanalytic treatment.

This situation, in which categorical diagnoses were of little importance for treatment recommendations,

P

changed abruptly in the 1950s when chlorpromazine was introduced for the treatment of psychoses like schizophrenia. Pharmacologic agents such as the monoamine oxidase inhibitors and tricyclics became widely useful for the treatment of major depressions. Lithium salts were found to be uniquely beneficial for the treatment of manic psychoses. With the choice of these pharmacotherapies, diagnosis moved once again to center stage in the concerns of psychiatry. It made a difference whether a psychotic condition was thought to be schizophrenic or manic. The former would receive a phenothiazine, the latter lithium. No longer was there one treatment for all psychiatric illnesses. The reliability of diagnosis became a prominent consideration; validity could be decided by treatment response. This turn of events occurred almost simultaneously with a curious observation: there was a discrepancy between diagnostic standards in the United Kingdom and in the United States with respect to the prevalence of schizophrenia and manic depressive illness. Schizophrenia was diagnosed several times more frequently in the United States than in Britain, and the reverse was true for manic depressive illness. The awareness of this difference led to a major diagnostic collaborative study between the two countries, which revealed that different diagnostic approaches to these two illnesses were used in the two countries. The American Psychiatric Association followed with a sponsorship of a canon containing operational definitions of various diagnoses: the *Diagnostic and Statistical Manual of Mental Disorders*, third edition (*DSM-III*, now in its fourth edition). This manual was avowedly atheoretical, particularly with respect to the etiology of the psychopathological conditions, and was crafted to be clearly in the mold of the classical descriptive psychiatrist Emil Kraepelin.

Beginning in the mid-1950s, therefore, a major shift occurred in how the psychiatric profession viewed and valued the diagnosis of psychopathological conditions. With the advent of pharmacologic agents that targeted specific diseases (like schizophrenia, bipolar affective disorder, obsessive-compulsive disorder, monopolar depression, and post-traumatic stress disorder, for example), there concurrently appeared psychological treatments that were applied along with drug treatments. Some of these psychological treatments were psychoanalytically based, but most were strictly focused on the alleviation of symptoms, as in behavior modification, cognitive therapy, and interpersonal therapy. For the treatment of clearly defined disorders (the Axis I and Axis II conditions), objective criteria for improvement could now be established. Objective methods for evaluating the efficacy and safety of the pharmacologic treatments established their usefulness and limitations. The same objective evaluations were now demanded of the psychological treatments, including psychoanalysis. But objective standards cannot be reliably established for authenticating the existence of putative entities such as "regressive flight from Oedipal relationships," or "a condensation of aggressive and antiaggressive forces."

The contemporary psychoanalyst, following Freud, does not think in the categorical terms of diagnosis. Rather, psychoanalysts are interested in the uniqueness of their patients' lives, a uniqueness that denotes the meaning of particular symptoms to the patient, the special significance of events and people that give pain or pleasure, why the patient works against his or her best self-interests, and how the patient's character can aid or impede the treatment of a condition that is a diagnosable illness. At this time, the categorical approach and the individual dynamic approach appear to be complementary rather than opposed to each other.

REFERENCES

Fenichel, O. (1945). *The Psychoanalytic Theory of Neurosis.* London: Routledge and Kegan Paul.

Freud, S. (1916). Some character-types met with in psychoanalytic work. S.E. 14: 309–333.

———. (1940). *An Outline of Psycho-Analysis.* S.E. 23: 144–207.

Kramer, H., and Sprenger, J. (1971 [1486]). *The Malleus Maleficarum [The Witch Hammer].* Trans. with introductions, bibliography, and notes by Rev. M. Summers. New York: Dover. First edition (estimated date) 1486.

PHILIP S. HOLZMAN

Psychoses See PARANOIA; SCHIZOPHRENIA.

Psychosexual Development

See DEVELOPMENTAL THEORY; INFANTILE SEXUALITY; LIBIDO THEORY.

Psychotherapy

See PSYCHOANALYTIC TECHNIQUE AND PROCESS; PSYCHOANALYTICALLY ORIENTED PSYCHOTHERAPY.

R

Rank, Otto (1884–1939)

Otto Rank was the youngest member of Freud's inner circle and the most important writer on the applications of psychoanalysis to literature and myth. Born April 22, 1884, Rank, the younger of two brothers, was forced by his alcoholic father to attend a trade school. In 1905, Alfred Adler, Rank's physician, introduced him to Freud. The autodidact's manuscript, *The Artist*, impressed Freud, who supported his studies at the university in Vienna, where Rank received a doctorate in 1912 for a thesis on the Lohengrin legend.

From 1905 through 1924, Rank was one of Freud's most brilliant and loyal followers. His prolific publications during this period include *The Artist* (1907); *The Myth of the Birth of the Hero* (1909); his magnum opus, *The Incest Theme in Literature and Legend* (1912); *The Double* (1914); and *The Don Juan Legend* (1922); as well as essays on the play-within-the-play in *Hamlet*, Homer's epics, and nakedness in literature and myth. From 1906 through 1915, Rank served as secretary of the Vienna Psychoanalytic Society; the four volumes of minutes are his work. From the fourth (1914) through the seventh (1922) editions of *The Interpretation of Dreams*, Freud incorporated Rank's "Dream and Myth" as sections of Chapter 6.

In 1909, Rank, whose family name was Rosenfeld, legally adopted the non-Jewish pen name he had begun to use in 1903 and changed his religious registration to "unaffiliated." With Hanns Sachs, Rank became editor in 1912 of *Imago*, a journal of applied analysis, and published *The Significance of Psychoanalysis for the Mental Sciences* (1913). During World War I, Rank was stationed in Kraków, where he edited the newspaper of the Aus-tro-Hungarian armed forces. There, in November 1918, he married Beata ("Tola") Mincer, who later became a psychoanalyst. A daughter, Helene, was born the following year. After the war, Rank, who was never analyzed, began the clinical practice of psychoanalysis and solidified his position as Freud's lieutenant and the only member of the secret committee of his chief disciples living in Vienna. Rank formed a friendship with Sándor Ferenczi but clashed with Ernest Jones over matters of publication at a time when Austrian currency had lost its value.

Although Rank's importance to Freud is often underestimated, in a letter of August 4, 1922, Freud regrets that he had not urged Rank to study medicine, because "under those circumstances I would not now be in doubt as to whom I would leave the leading role in the psychoanalytic movement" (Taft, 1958: 77). Rank's expectation that he would be Freud's successor, coupled with the discovery of the cancer in Freud's jaw in the spring of 1923, led to a crisis following the publication of Rank's *The Trauma of Birth* (1924). Although cast as an extension of Freud's theories, Rank's emphasis on the birth trauma challenged the primacy of the Oedipus complex; and Freud's doubts about the book, as well as about the modifications of psychoanalytic technique proposed by Rank and Ferenczi in their joint work, *The Development of Psychoanalysis* (1923), grew under the pressure of the objections of Jones and Karl Abraham. When Rank failed to gain his father surrogate's unqualified approbation, the negative pole of his ambivalence manifested itself. After protracted turbulence, the breach between Freud and Rank became complete in May 1926, when Rank settled in Paris.

Rank's career after *The Trauma of Birth* can be divided into two subphases: from 1924 to 1927, in which he no longer considered himself Freud's disciple but continued to work along psychoanalytic lines; and from 1927 to 1939, in which he renounced psychoanalysis completely in favor of "will therapy." The former of these subphases, during which Rank published the first parts of *Technique of Psychoanalysis* (1926) and *Genetic Psychology* (1927)—works that remain untranslated into English—anticipates the direction of contemporary psychoanalysis (Rudnytsky, 1991). Rejecting Freud's libido theory, Rank stresses the pre-Oedipal mother-child bond and defines anxiety in terms of experiences of separation. He likewise conceives of transference in maternal terms and highlights the emotional aspects of the therapeutic relationship. Although Ferenczi has often been considered the first object relations psychoanalyst, Rank was the dominant figure in their intellectual partnership, and it is he who properly deserves this appellation.

Rank's defection from psychoanalysis dealt a grievous blow to Freud, who repeatedly criticized him in his later writings. The view of Rank as a heretic was consolidated by Jones, though his aspersion that Rank was "wrecked" by mental illness (1957, p. 77) is now discredited. On an intellectual plane, however, Rank came to espouse a quasi-religious perspective resembling that of Jung. In the books translated by Jessie Taft as *Will Therapy* and *Truth and Reality*—actually portions of *Technique of Psychoanalysis* and *Genetic Psychology* published between 1929 and 1931—Rank rejects the concept of the unconscious and the utility of understanding the present in terms of the past. A mainstay of his mature thought is the typology of artistic, average, and neurotic characters. The vicissitudes of the creative impulse and the human longing for immortality are traced in *Psychology and Soul-Belief* (1930), *Modern Education* (1932), *Art and Artist* (1932), and the posthumous *Beyond Psychology* (1941). This phase of Rank's work has found a receptive audience among social workers, gestalt therapists, and cultural critics, such as Ernest Becker in his Pulitzer Prize–winning *The Denial of Death* (1973). There are excellent biographies of Rank by Jessie Taft (1958) and E. James Lieberman (1985), and a sympathetic critical study by Esther Menaker (1982). A valuable compilation of texts mainly from Rank's 1924–1927 period has been edited by Robert Kramer (1996).

While in Paris, Rank was visited by Henry Miller after he and Anaïs Nin had read *Art and Artist*. Nin, who as an adult committed incest with her father, entered analysis with Rank in November 1933 and became his lover in May 1934, the same month that he took her husband, Hugh Guiler, into treatment. Prior to departing for the United States in October 1934, Rank offered Nin the ring he had received from Freud (Nin, 1992: 394). In America, Rank lived in New York City and taught chiefly at the Pennsylvania School of Social Work. In 1939, he planned to move to California with his new wife, Estelle Buel, an American who had been his secretary since 1932. At the age of fifty-five, some five weeks after Freud's death, Rank died in New York on October 31, 1939, from an antibacterial drug administered for an infection following the removal of a kidney stone.

REFERENCES

Jones, E. (1957). *The Life and Work of Sigmund Freud*, vol. 3. New York: Basic Books.

Kramer, R. (1996). *A Psychology of Difference: The American Lectures of Otto Rank*. Princeton, N.J.: Princeton University Press.

Lieberman, E. J. (1985). *Acts of Will: The Life and Work of Otto Rank*. New York: Free Press.

Menaker, E. (1982). *Otto Rank: A Rediscovered Legacy*. New York: Columbia University Press.

Nin, A. (1992). *Incest: From "A Journal of Love." The Unexpurgated Diary of Anaïs Nin. 1932–1934*. New York: Harcourt Brace.

Rudnytsky, P. L. (1991). *The Psychoanalytic Vocation: Rank, Winnicott, and the Legacy of Freud*. New Haven, Conn.: Yale University Press.

Taft, J. (1958). *Otto Rank: A Biographical Study*. New York: Julian Press.

PETER L. RUDNYTSKY

Rapaport, D. See EGO PSYCHOLOGY.

Rat Man

The third of Freud's major case histories. Before publishing it, Freud had already published his first major case about hysteria, the Dora case (Freud, 1905a), and his second, about phobias, the Little Hans case (1909a). In the case of the Rat Man, Freud returned to a subject that had interested him more than a decade before: obsessional neurosis. At that time, Freud had dealt with obsessional neurosis in three papers (1894; 1895; and 1896) and returned to it one more time (1907) before this case. In his discussion of the Rat Man (1909b), Freud indicated that he hoped to make disconnected statements about the *genesis and finer psychological mechanisms of obsessional processes* and to develop his first observations on the subject, which were initially published in 1896. Such an update was necessary because these first observations were written while he still believed in the seduction theory. After changing his mind about the seduction theory, he shifted his thinking toward the pivotal role of the unconscious (1900) and instincts (1905b).

As with most of Freud's major case histories, the identity of the Rat Man is known. He was Ernst Lanzer, a twenty-nine-year-old Viennese lawyer who came for treatment on October 1, 1907. His treatment lasted less than a year. A footnote added in 1923 indicates that Lanzer died during World War I. What is remarkable about this case is that it is the only one for which Freud's original records of the early part of the treatment exist. (These consisted of the daily records Freud wrote about the case.) These records made it possible for future commentators to go back to the original record to draw their own conclusions about the dynamics and the treatment method.

The case presentation alternates between clinical and theoretical material. During the first session, the patient indicated that he had suffered from obsessional neurosis since childhood, but that the intensity had increased in the past four years. His major concerns were fears that something terrible might happen to a woman whom he loved and to his father; compulsive impulses such as cutting his throat with a razor; and prohibitions, sometimes in connection with unimportant things. After a few associations, Freud soon discovered that the patient was under the domination of a component sexual instinct, scopophilia; he had an intense wish to look at naked women. The fear that something dreadful would happen to beloved persons was intimately connected with this wish. Subsequently, the great obsessive fear was revealed: that rats would bore into the anus of his lady friend and his father—hence the name "Rat Man," a name that Freud used in an endearing way to refer to the patient. The bizarre nature of the fear was further illustrated when the patient revealed that his father had died nine years earlier.

The genesis of the rat obsession occurred during military maneuvers in which the Rat Man participated as an officer. He heard about the rat punishment from a cruel captain who approvingly described a Turkish torture in which a pot containing rats is turned upside down and tied onto the buttocks of the victim; eventually, the rats bore their way into the victim's anus. This same cap-

tain, of whom he had a "kind of dread" (Freud, 1909b: 166), told him that a "Lieutenant A" had paid for a pince-nez the Rat Man had ordered by mail from his opticians in Vienna, and that the Rat Man must pay him back. The Rat Man immediately developed both a "sanction" and a vow: the sanction was not to pay the money back, because if he did, the rat punishment would befall a woman he loved and his father; the vow was that he must pay back the 3.80 kronen to Lieutenant A. However, Lieutenant A denied that he had paid the money, indicating instead that a Lieutenant B had paid. To fulfill his vow, the Rat Man developed a complex plan: Lieutenant A would pay the 3.80 kronen to the woman working at the post office, who would then pay this sum to Lieutenant B; the Rat Man would, in turn, repay Lieutenant A. Later, the patient revealed that he had known all along that the post office woman had paid for the pince-nez to curry favor with him.

Subsequently, the Rat Man revealed extensive infantile sexual activities involving his governess and his sisters. By age six, he felt that he must prevent these sexual activities or his father would die. Freud concluded that although age six was not the beginning of the Rat Man's illness, by then he had developed a complete obsessional neurosis.

During the Rat Man's treatment, Freud was very active and educational. He realized that there were no rational explanations for the Rat Man's fears. Instead, Freud tried to decipher the unconscious meanings of these fears. He told the patient about the archaeological metaphor of the unconscious, that the material in the unconscious is preserved and is destroyed only when it becomes conscious. Freud pointed to old figurines in his office and explained that objects in Pompeii had been preserved by being buried; now that they had been uncovered, they were being destroyed. Freud concluded that love and hate, particularly for the father, had coexisted in the Rat Man since his childhood. The repressed and disavowed sadism reflected his interest in and horror of cruelty. The cruel captain's story about the rat punishment stimulated the Rat Man's ambivalence about this father, who was the prohibitor of sexual pleasure and had to be gotten rid of. However, he also loved his father. This was his dilemma of ambivalence. This tormenting ambivalence characterized his relationship with his love objects, particularly his woman friend and his father. Moreover, these two objects were inversely coupled: the more he loved one, the more he hated the other.

The Rat Man also identified with his father. Freud found that the Rat Man used rats as symbols for many things: gambling, penises, children, his mother, and money. Of significance was the image of his father as a gambling rat who once got into gambling debts in his youth during military maneuvers. The father could not pay back his debt because he could not find his benefactor. Thus, the military setting of the pince-nez incident re-created in the patient's mind a sense of identification with his father: the Rat Man's attempts to pay his own debts reflected his attempts to pay his father's debt. Yet, the complications he set up that made the payment of the loan impossible also reflected his ambivalence toward his father. Once he understood and accepted the meanings of his behavior, the rat delirium disappeared.

In addition to deciphering the unconscious meanings of the Rat Man's bizarre symptoms, Freud provided a firsthand view of the technique he used at that time, which was very different from that which he espoused a few years later in his papers on technique. This technique is also different from the practice of most analysts today. Freud was very active, educational, and confrontational, but he was also warm and friendly. Much has been said about an entry in the process notes not mentioned in the case history, the entry, "He was hungry and was fed." Most remarkable was the attitude that resistance should be actively removed, not analyzed, and that transference should be used positively, not analyzed. One explanation for Freud's style could be that this was a transitional period in his thinking about technique, which was later replaced by the ideas expressed in the papers on technique. Another possible explanation is that the records accurately represent Freud's actual style (this is supported by the reports of analysands who saw him in subsequent years), implying that Freud meant his technical papers to be general guidelines, not descriptions of specific techniques.

REFERENCES

Freud, S. (1894). The neuropsychosis of defence. S.E. 3: 51–58.
———. (1895). Obsessions and phobias. S.E. 3: 74–82.
———. (1896). Further remarks on the neuropsychosis of defence, section II. S.E. 3: 168–174.
———. (1900). *The Interpretation of Dreams*. S.E. 4–5: 1–625.
———. (1905a). Fragments of an analysis of a case of hysteria. S.E. 7: 3–122.
———. (1905b). *Three Essays on the Theory of Sexuality*. S.E. 7: 125–243.
———. (1907). Obsessive actions and religious practices. S.E. 9: 115–127.
———. (1909a). Analysis of a phobia in a five-year-old boy. S.E. 10: 3–149.
———. (1909b). Notes upon a case of obsessional neurosis. S.E. 10: 153–318.

GEORGE A. AWAD

Reaction Formation

"Reaction formation" is the cathartic transformation of an impulse that causes intrapsychic conflict into an exaggerated and opposite impulse. The affect associated with the original impulse is also reversed. This catharsis allows the ego to defend against the impulse without directly experiencing the adverse consequences associated with the original impulse.

Freud first described reaction formation in his *Three Essays on the Theory of Sexuality* (1905), where he discussed the nature and characteristics of the sexual instinct (libido), deviations of the libido, and the mental forces that control sexual instincts. It is within the context of describing the mental functions that impede libidinal energy that Freud first mentioned reaction formation. He postulated that barriers restricting the flow of sexual instinct are constructed during the period of sexual latency of childhood. These barriers include disgust, feelings of shame, and the claims of aesthetic and moral ideals (morality). Freud further suggested that it is through reacting impulses (reaction formation) of sexual instincts that these barriers are built up: "on the one hand, it would seem, the sexual impulses cannot be utilized during these years of childhood, since the reproductive function has been deferred ... on the other hand, these impulses would seem in themselves to be perverse—that is, to arise from erotogenic zones and to derive their activity from instincts which, in view of the direction of the subject's development, can only arouse unpleasurable feelings. They consequently evoke opposing mental forces (reacting impulses) which, in order to suppress this unpleasure, effectively build up the mental dams that I have already mentioned—disgust, shame, and morality" (Freud, 1905).

In his *Character and Anal Erotism* (1908), Freud further elaborated his concept of reaction formation in relation to character formation. He described orderly, parsimonious, and obstinate character traits as originating in the conflicts that surround psychosexual development leading up to the latency period. He further stated that these traits develop as a result of erotic fixation. It is within the context of discussing erotic fixation that Freud discussed reaction formation. Drawing from his theory of sexuality, Freud described erotogenic zones and postulated that excitation coming from these zones is partially channeled into libidinal energy and partially deflected from sexual aims. Anal eroticism particularly leads to the development of the character traits of orderliness, parsimony, and obstinacy through the counterforces (reaction formations): "during the period of life which may be called the period of 'sexual latency' . . . reaction formations . . . are actually formed at the expense of the excitations preceding from the erotogenic zones. . . . It is therefore plausible to suppose that these character traits—traits of orderliness, parsimony, and obstinacy, which are so prominent in people who were firstly anal erotics, are to be regarded as the first and most constant result of anal eroticism" (Freud, 1908).

Thus in both *Three Essays on the Theory of Sexuality* and *Character and Anal Erotism*, reaction formation is tied to the latency period and to the redirection of sexual drives. Although it was Freud's daughter Anna who subsequently compiled a compendium of defense mechanisms and discussed their various manifestations (A. Freud, 1937), it was Freud who introduced the concepts of defense mechanisms and ontogeny of defense mechanisms. He postulated that defense mechanisms occur not only along a continuum of psychopathology, but also along a continuum of ego development. Freud fully anticipated the importance that defense mechanisms would play in our understanding of psychopathology: "further investigations may show there is an intimate connection between special forms of defense and particular illness, as, for instance, between repression and hysteria" (Freud, 1926).

REFERENCES

Freud, A. (1937). *The Ego and the Mechanisms of Defense.* London: Hogarth Press.
Freud, S. (1905). *Three Essays on the Theory of Sexuality.* S.E. 7: 130–243.
———. (1908). Character and anal erotism. S.E. 9: 169–175.
———. (1926). *Inhibitions, Symptoms, and Anxiety.* S.E. 20: 87–172.

MICHAEL WM. MACGREGOR
KARINA DAVIDSON

Reality Testing

The capacity to judge whether one's ideas conform to reality. This capacity has been variously described as the ability to distinguish ideas from perceptions, or fantasy from reality, or the capacity to determine whether a mental image or sensation arises from within oneself or from a percept in the external world. The term "reality testing" was coined by Freud (1911, p. 225), who imagined it as developing from a primitive state in which no such distinction exists. Early life experience provides occasions to differentiate between those sensations that could be obliterated by motor activity (e.g., flight) and those that could not (1915, p. 119): the former would ultimately be understood as originating in the external world and the latter in the internal world. As development proceeds, the capacity to test reality becomes a matter of the application of attention, judgment, and memory to compare ideas or images to percepts in the real world.

Reality testing plays a crucial role in pathogenesis and in treatment, in that ideas actively kept out of conscious awareness (repressed) are not subject to judgment about their accuracy, i.e., they are not tested against reality. Ideas that are repressed at a point in psychological development when the distinction between fantasy and reality, between thought and deed, is not yet well established are not available for reality testing, and so they may function as unexamined, unrealistic assumptions: thoughts, wishes, or desires related to a repressed idea may be experienced with a sense of danger or guilt as if imagining an act had the same consequences as committing the act. Coming to awareness of such chronically avoided ideas and the imagined danger associated with them, so that they may be reconsidered (tested) in light of reality, is an important component of psychoanalytic therapy.

The concept of reality testing has been used in the differentiation of psychosis from less severe pathology; for example, hallucinations were said to represent a failure of reality testing, in that an endogenous mental image was experienced as a perception of something external. In this usage, reality testing was assessed either as grossly impaired or relatively intact. This coarse distinction must be qualified when one looks more closely at mental processes. It is clear, for example, that perception is not an objective yardstick against which the reality of a thought may be judged, because perception is constantly colored by psychological need and expectations, including the unconscious fantasies about how the world operates that are part of all mental functioning (Arlow, 1969: 29–30). Furthermore, it is often the case that a person will have the capacity to test reality, i.e., to use rational judgment to assess the accuracy of certain convictions, but will refrain from doing so to avoid awareness of something upsetting. In such cases it would not be accurate to say reality testing is "impaired" so much as suspended more or less willfully (Grossman, 1996: 512).

One often refrains from testing reality in the course of daily life. The most dramatic instance of a normal neglect of reality testing is dreaming (Freud, 1917: 234), in which the unrealistic, timeless, hallucinatory mentation that underlies all thought is allowed to emerge, in large measure because the sensory input against which the dream ideas could be tested is diminished. In the waking state, one often has no cause to exercise reality testing for periods of time, and at certain times one voluntarily suspends the capacity to test reality, e.g., while daydreaming or watching a play. In the psychoanalytic situation, the analyst creates conditions that facilitate the relative suspension of reality testing by encouraging the patient to try to notice and report all thoughts and feelings, regardless of how unrealistic, i.e., to attend to mental activity before it is tested against reality. The position of the analyst out of sight limits perceptions that the patient might use to test the reality of his or her expectations of the analyst's reactions. These conditions make it easier for both parties to notice the patient's underlying fantasy life, which reality testing would otherwise help keep out of awareness.

One might object that the psychoanalytic view of reality testing presupposes a naive definition of reality as an independent, external, passively perceived landscape. We have already remarked on the inevitable coloration of perception by psychological need; from a psychoanalytic perspective, the idea of a literally accurate, value-free perception may not make sense. Many contemporary psychoanalysts are taking up the implications of a view of reality as socially constructed. But these considerations do not materially alter the clinical utility of the concept of reality testing if one takes into account that, for the nonpsychotic patient, the "reality" against which ideas are tested is the subject's own; in other words, when a patient's fantasy comes to awareness for consideration, the patient him- or herself usually judges it to be unrealistic (Grossman, 1996: 511). Of course the analyst's view of what is real comes into play as well; if patient and analyst disagree about what is real, the analyst has no special claim of authority on the subject. And if patient and analyst tacitly agree on a point of reality, that is no guarantee that a third party would share their view.

REFERENCES

Arlow, J. A. (1969). Fantasy, memory, and reality testing. *Psychoanalytic Quarterly*, 38: 28–51.

Freud, S. (1911). Formulations on the two principles of mental functioning. S.E. 12: 213–226.

———. (1915). Instincts and their vicissitudes. S.E. 14: 109–140.

———. (1917). A metapsychological supplement to the theory of dreams. S.E. 14: 217–235.

Grossman, L. (1996). "Psychic Reality" and reality testing in the analysis of perverse defences. *International Journal of Psycho-Analysis*, 77: 509–518.

                                                    LEE GROSSMAN

Reception of Freud's Ideas

Psychoanalysis came to the United States with Freud in 1909 and with the European émigrés fleeing Nazism in the 1930s and 1940s. Each time, supporters explored psychoanalysis's scientific and curative potentials while appealing, also, to a larger public. This dual reception engendered ambiguities and misunderstandings, and threatened entrenched beliefs and careers. And when expectations remained unfulfilled, disappointment ensued.

Freud's "Introductory Lectures"—which stressed the scientific exploration of the unconscious, its eventually liberating benefits for humanity, and the roles of sublimation, trauma, and catharsis—were tailor-made for his American audience. And the sensationalist coverage by the American press appealed to a broad segment of the public, which, in turn, envisioned psychoanalysis as the road to happiness. Subsequently Freud was displeased with the Americans' simplifications, while also criticizing the physicians' decision to allow access to their associations to doctors alone. He wanted them also to train lay analysts. Eventually this led to the rift between European and American Freudians, since the latter prohibited inclusion of lay analysts in the American Psychoanalytic Association (APA).

After the Austrian *Anschluss*, in 1938, European émigrés—sponsored by American Freudians over many objections by the American Medical Association—swelled the American analysts' ranks. Many worked in hospitals, where they soon demonstrated the efficacy of the "talking cure" to their colleagues. By 1942, textbooks for medical students included a section about the influence of unconscious factors on their patients' behavior. Many of these students later became psychoanalysts. And the émigrés, who were seeing patients and enlarging Freud's structural theory, became training analysts and started institutes around the country. Although disagreements about restricting the practice of psychoanalysis to physicians remained unresolved, physicians accepted Freud's lay disciples as honorary members of the APA. But Freud's death in September 1939 and the outbreak of World War II in Europe on September 1 took precedence over the business of the International Psychoanalytic Association (IPA).

By the time the IPA again met, in 1949, associations by so-called deviants had begun to form. For instance, Karen Horney, whose books had become best-sellers, started the Association for the Advancement of Psychoanalysis; Theodor Reik had begun to train psychologists; and similar efforts occurred throughout the country. Moreover, Horney's *The Neurotic Personality of Our Time* (1937) and Erich Fromm's *The Fear of Freedom* (1942) and *Man for Himself* (1947) introduced psychoanalytic concepts to a broad public—a public that did not really care about the disputes over theories and clinical methods. Though not simplistic himself, Fromm appealed to the American propensity to believe in quick fixes and to the native optimism about the malleability of human nature. Now, the links between psychological and societal phenomena also were being investigated by such social scientists as the Harvard sociologist Talcott Parsons and the political scientist Harold Lasswell—in line with Freud's postulates in *The Ego and the Id*. Literary scholars such as Lionel Trilling and art critics like E. H. Gombrich and Clement Greenberg responded to the intellectual challenges of psychoanalysis and began to introduce students in the humanities to psychoanalysis.

The émigrés' experiences—resettlement in a new country, delegitimation as psychoanalysts, functioning in a new language, and reestablishing themselves after their experiences with a virulent, racially based anti-Semitism and sudden poverty—turned the psychoanalysts into their own foremost subjects and expanded their knowhow. By 1946, Heinz Hartmann, together with Ernst Kris and Rudolph Loewenstein, summarized the many theories Freudians had derived from their research and speculations, from clinical work and cooperation with intellectuals, and from increasingly differentiated observations of infants and children. By then, they even had been invited by the U.S. government (together with some of the country's best minds) to advise on reeducating the German populace after the end of the war; to cure war neuroses; to provide a psychoanalytic portrait of Hitler;

and to assess leadership qualities among American recruits in the armed forces. The questions these projects raised would guide their research for the coming years. So when the IPA reconvened in Europe after the war, these Americans inevitably insisted on imposing their theories and clinical methods.

Success brought prestige and research moneys to the profession, and ego psychology remained the leading theory. By 1970, individuals and groups outside the APA and the IPA increasingly were chafing at the bit. Having grown in numbers and experience, they resented the privileged status enjoyed by insiders. "Defectors," such as Horney, William Silberberg, Clara Thompson, Harry Stack Sullivan, Fromm, and Reik, and their students, were doing much therapy with patients. In sum, as Philip Rieff already noted in *The Triumph of the Therapeutic* (1966), America had become the therapeutic society par excellence.

By that time, patients no longer were suffering from hysteria, or even from obsessions and phobias, but from malaise and a variety of neuroses. Thus the clinical techniques based on the structural theory were being questioned and no longer seemed to be as effective as they had been before. Soon, Heinz Kohut furthered his so-called self-psychology, and Otto Kernberg advanced Melanie Klein's object relations approach, as practiced in London. Whether or not these and other new approaches developed because of changing symptomatology alone or because classical psychoanalysis had made promises for cures it could not achieve, is a debatable issue. Certainly, changing cultural trends and contact with European and South American analysts contributed to the development of clinical theories and methods in the United States. The psychoanalysts themselves were both products and creators of their culture.

Ultimately, the reception of psychoanalysis went through many phases, in line with changes in the culture, breakthroughs in drug and behavioral therapies, and advances in psychoanalytic knowledge. Throughout all the shifts, there has been a constant tension—and much misunderstanding of the connections—between what practicing analysts do and the place accorded Freud's ideas either in the culture at large or in academia. The various aspects of psychoanalysis that are being stressed or denied keep changing, so that its first and second major receptions have been followed by smaller waves of reaction and adoption. Though what the next major wave will be remains to be seen, Freud has irrevocably altered Western tradition.

REFERENCES

Freud, S. (1910). Five lectures on psycho-analysis. S.E. 11: 1–55.

———. (1923). *The Ego and the Id.* S.E. 19: 1–66.

Fromm, E. (1942). *The Fear of Freedom.* London: Routledge and Kegan Paul.

———. (1947). *Man for Himself.* London: Routledge and Kegan Paul.

Hartmann, H., Kris E., and Loewenstein R. M. (1946). Comments on the formation of psychic structure. *Psychoanalytic Study of the Child,* 2: 11–38.

Horney, K. (1937). *The Neurotic Personality of Our Time.* New York: Norton.

———. (1939). *New Ways in Psychoanalysis.* New York: Norton.

Reiff, P. (1966). *The Triumph of the Therapeutic.* New York: Harper/Torch.

EDITH KURZWEIL

Regression

The word "regression" is defined in the following ways by the Oxford English Dictionary (1971): the act of going back; a return or withdrawal to the place of origin; a previous state or condition; back in thought from one thing to another; from an affect to a cause; relapse; reversion to a less developed form.

One implication of this definition concerns the undoing of progress, sometimes reflecting a possible deterioration. Yet there is a second possibility: the return to fundamentals and origins that might facilitate a potential reorganization leading to better integration. It seems paradoxical that we are dealing with a process often considered to be a central factor in the most serious psychopathology, and yet many acknowledge regression to be a most potent therapeutic opportunity. Do patients really show signs of such a process? Are there observations to be made in practice or in the experimental laboratory that can be related to this idea?

Freud proposed several theories of regression. His first view (1900) was that regression is related to Hughling Jackson's (1888) hierarchical-evolutionary neurological schema. Freud applied these ideas in his study *On Aphasia* (1891). He later extended his theory and introduced the concept of "temporal regression." His underlying assumptions were that there had been a gradual psychological development from simpler, primitive stages toward a more complex, organized level, and that a process of undoing these advances is embodied in regression. Freud utilizes this theory in his *The Interpretation of Dreams* (1900). The concept of reversal of genetic development became one of the cornerstones of psychoanalytic theory.

Another concept of regression also appears in *The Interpretation of Dreams*: the notion of "topographic regression." To explain the hallucinatory quality of dreams, Freud adapted the reflex-arc model. He proposed that in waking states excitation ordinarily begins as sensory stimulus, which passes from unconscious through preconscious, with the conscious thought terminating in motor action. In dreaming, the regression toward the unconscious sensory imagery accounts for the hallucinatory nature of dreams. Originally "borrowed" from biology, regression has gradually developed meaning as a defensive and adaptive mechanism (dreaming, avoiding stress) and as an element in pathogenesis (hallucinations, symbolic expressions, infantile behavior). The issues regarding therapeutic use will soon be explored.

In retrospect, Freud (1914) came to realize that during his early studies on hysteria, the backward turning in time of patients' associations was a characteristic feature of neurosis: "Psychoanalysis could explain nothing in the present without referring back to something in the past" (p. 10), and thus analytic technique that neglected regression would render scientific study of neurosis impossible. Temporal and topographic regressions gradually found their way into theory and technique in psychoanalysis. As Freud formulated newer *theoretical* constructs involving progressive developmental aspects, still other forms of "backward movement" could also be conceptualized. Consequently, as Freud's psychosexual theory evolved, instinctual or libidinal regression was postulated. Similarly, energic structural and ego regressions have been described.

Peto (1967) refers to the first relevant case in the history of psychoanalysis (Anna O.) as having shown both the dangers and the benefits of regression. Problems associated with regression led Breuer to abandon his patient. Only much later did Freud recognize the Scylla and Charybdis of "good" and "bad" regression. He sensed that the regressed form of transference could be a most potent type of resistance. And yet, he acknowledged that certain patients repeated their forgotten past in the transference, and that this material had somehow become inaccessible by any other means. This repetition was partly induced by the "new" technique of free association in the analytic situation. And so, Freud referred to regression as an ally in analytic treatment. In 1914, looking back at the earlier Dora analysis, he noted that direct attempts to resolve the pathological effects of a recent trauma had failed, and that Dora had to make "a long detour, leading back over her earliest childhood" (Freud, 1914: 10). Furthermore, he warned against the neglect of regression in analytic technique!

The tragic Freud-Ferenczi controversy that developed over sixty-five years ago concerning the use of regression in treatment shocked the psychoanalytic community (Balint, 1968; Lorand, 1965). Sándor Ferenczi (1930, 1931) had proceeded with his experiments of "active technique." At first, Freud (1919) supported this work. Ferenczi elicited the reactivation of what he considered to be vivid infantile traumas that apparently involved significant child-rearing persons: His patients craved reparation, comfort, and understanding. Ferenczi then experimented further. He wondered whether the neutrality of the analyst might not repeat the attitudes of indifferent or neglectful parents. Therefore, he explored the possibility of reducing the tensions of these longings by responding positively and called his new procedure "relaxation technique" (Ferenczi, 1932). Furthermore, the technical possibilities of countertransference interpretations and the importance of the analysts' reactions opened up a new area for consideration by Ferenczi in 1932 and was further explored in his "Clinical Diary" paper published posthumously (Dupont, 1988).

Freud, on the other hand, changed his mind about Ferenczi's research. He became distressed about the dangerous possibilities of arousing incessant cravings and frustration rather than "working them through" in accordance with the classical position (Peto, 1967). This clash between the "father" of the field and a brilliant pioneer—who died before the issues were clearly resolved—seems to have discouraged conservative analysts from further study of the potential in Ferenczi's work. An exploration of the therapeutic use of regression in analysis was suspended, especially by "classical" analysts.

Ferenczi's student Michael Balint pursued this subject in relative isolation, remaining in contact with several of Ferenczi's former patients. Balint (1968) refers to Ferenczi's eventual awareness of the hazards and failings in his research; however, there were also great theoretical benefits. By obtaining data from patients when the analyst did not maintain "classical" neutrality, evidence was elicited that illustrated the effects the classical analytic attitude can have on the particular transferences that are encouraged to develop.

Kris (1952) was one of the very few among classical analysts to formulate a new and important idea about regression, mainly during his investigations of artistic creativity. He distinguished two forms: one where the ego is overwhelmed by regression, and the other where regression is "manifested in the service of the ego." In this instance, a well-integrated individual who regresses has the capacity to regulate and utilize some of the primary processes creatively. There appears to be a relation between the two forms of regression described by Kris and the sort of regression studied by Balint. Yet there is a vital difference in their concerns, namely, Kris was interested in sublimation and artistic creativity as an intrapsychic one-person psychological act, whereas Balint refers to a therapeutic regressive process occurring in a two-person, therapeutic relationship. Furthermore, although Kris's contributions involve some concern with the therapeutic uses of regression, he was primarily interested in intrapsychic aspects and brief regressive episodes of relatively resilient personalities or creative artists.

Balint (1968) carefully studied the value and dangers of regression, conceiving of regression as benign and beneficial in treatment when the analyst provides an accepting atmosphere in which the patient feels safe enough to regress "for the sake of recognition" and understanding and shared experiencing. In contrast to this, a malignant regression occurs when the aim is libidinal gratification, which, Balint (1968) proposed, is quite similar to regression that "overwhelms the ego" (Kris, 1952).

Thus, the first task of the understanding analyst, who has determined that therapeutic regression is indicated, involves the facilitation of a trusting therapeutic partnership that encourages the dissolution of resistances to that regression. Once this is accomplished, the function of the treatment is to allow the patient to experience acceptance and recognition. In this way, the treatment provides what was unavailable during the patient's early life. Balint (1968) became the major advocate of this approach and has been joined by other contemporary analysts who have become proponents of making therapeutic use of a regressive opportunity in treatment. The focus is on the analytic atmosphere and the crucial dyads of (1) caretaker-child in early life, and (2) analyst-patient in treatment. In summary, the skillful acceptance of regression to the traumatic developmental phase where something needed for growth was missing, and then facilitating understanding and growth from that point forward, via an analytic relationship that has transitional,

R

mirroring, nonautocratic, nonintrusive, and synthetic qualities along with play and experimentation, are necessary steps in such treatment if healthy individuation is to occur (Winnicott, 1960; Mahler, 1973). The analytic use of interpretation and empathically facilitated regression-reconstruction is utilized in, one hopes, appropriate combination by effective practitioners working with the severely disturbed patient. The interpretive-neutral model alone cannot, in my opinion, operate in the treatment of severe character disorders or borderline and psychotic patients without generating overwhelming resistances. For example, a theory that focuses upon the patient's split-off rage, aggression, and hate would, perhaps inevitably, arouse tendencies of guilt, resentment, perhaps a masochistic stance or a sadistic "counterattack." This would most likely occur when such a patient is projecting unconscious rage while in a state of self-object confusion regarding the "bad." All too often *such a patient experiences the doctor's interpretation about "split-off" rage as if* the analyst were saying: "Patient, you are bad. The hate is in you, while I am knowing and good! You, patient, want to devour and kill, and then blame it on me—the good, innocent doctor." Thus we become trapped in a vicious cycle: the patient projecting hate, envy, and rage onto the patient! A less verbal, less interpretive focus at certain times might aid in resolving such stalemates. One might, for example, listen quietly when acknowledging the patient's aggression, interpreting—if this is necessary—but with an understanding emphasis. The analyst could empathize with the patient's predicament and rage relating to experiences of discomfort and despair from the past and present. In conclusion, it has been my experience that regression in treatment affords many patients a new chance to make crucial material accessible to consciousness—to the "observing self" that is developing in alliance with the analyst. As a consequence, a productive experience often ensues. Both participants cope with "the unfinished business" of fragmented precepts and primitive longings, hurt and rage, anxious confusion and early-life maladaptive coping patterns. Here is the opportunity for a more true self (Winnicott, 1969) to emerge.

REFERENCES

Balint, M. (1968). *The Basic Fault: Therapeutic Aspects of Aggression.* London: Tavistock

Ferenczi, S. (1930). The principle of relaxation and neo-catharsis. In S. Ferenczi (author). *Final Contributions.* London: Hogarth Press; New York: Basic Books, 1955.

———. (1931). Child analysis in the analysis of adults. In S. Ferenczi (author). *Final Contributions.* London: Hogarth Press; New York: Basic Books, 1955.

———. (1932). Notes and fragments. In S. Ferenczi (author). *Final Contributions.* London: Hogarth Press; New York: Basic Books, 1955.

Freud, S. (1891). *Zur Auffassung der Aphasien (On Aphasia).* Vienna. New York: International Universities Press, 1953.

———. (1900). *The Interpretation of Dreams.* S.E. 4–5: 1–621.

———. (1914). On the history of the psycho-analytic movement. S.E. 14: 7–66.

———. (1919). Lines of advance in psycho-analytic therapy. S.E. 17: 157–168.

Jackson, J. H. (1888). Remarks on the diagnosis and treatment of diseases of the brain. In *Selected Writings of John Hughlings Jackson,* vol. 2, pp. 365–392.

Kris, E. (1952). *Psychoanalytic Explorations in Art.* New York: International Universities Press.

Lorand, S. (1965). *Psychoanalytic Pioneers.* New York: Basic Books, pp. 14–35.

Mahler, M. et al. (1975). *The Psychological Birth of the Human Infant.* New York: Basic Books.

Oxford English Dictionary. (1971).

Peto, A. (1967). Differentiations and fragmentations during analysis. *Journal of the American Psychoanalytic Association,* 15: 534–550.

Winnicott, D. W. (1960). Ego distortion in terms of true and false self. In D. W. Winnicott (author). *The Maturational Process and the Facilitating Environment.* New York: International Universities Press.

———. (1969). The use of an object and relating through identification. In D. W. Winicott (author). *Playing and Reality.* New York: Basic Books, 1971, pp. 86–94.

SAUL TUTTMAN

Reich, Wilhelm (1897-1957)

Wilhelm Reich was born in Dobrzanica, Galicia (then a part of the Austro-Hungarian Empire), on March 24, 1897. He grew up on the country estate of his assimilated Jewish parents, Leon Reich and Cecilia Roniger, in Jurinetz, Bukovina. His mother committed suicide in 1909.

Reich received his elementary school education from tutors before attending the German gymnasium in Czernowitz, where he completed his studies in 1915. During World War I (1914–1918), Reich was drafted into military service. At the end of the war, he and his younger brother Robert moved to Vienna. In the spring of 1918, he began his studies at the Vienna Medical School. Reich contributed with lectures to establishing the Wiener Seminar für Sexuologie (Vienna Seminar for Sexology), initiated by Otto Fenichel in the beginning of 1919. In

October 1920, Reich—still a medical student—was accepted by the Vienna Psychoanalytic Society following his lecture on libido conflicts and phantasms in Ibsen's "Peer Gynt" ("Libidokonflikte und Wahngebilde in Ibsen's 'Peer Gynt'"). In 1922, Reich received a medical degree and, in the same year, married the medical student and later psychoanalyst Annie Pink, who had been in analysis with him prior to their engagement (they separated in 1933). In the same year, Reich became an assistant doctor at the newly founded outpatient clinic (Ambulatorium) of the Vienna Psychoanalytic Society. In 1928, he became its second director. From 1925 on, Reich was a member of the training institute of the society and from 1924 to 1930, he was head of the technical seminar. Reich also worked at the Wagner-Jauregg Psychiatric Clinic under Paul Schilder and had completed analyses with Isidor Sadger and Paul Federn.

In 1927, Reich published "Die Funktion des Orgasmus" (The Function of Orgasm). His theory of orgasm was considered to be the natural continuation of Freud's libido theory and was the foundation for all Reich's further works. In the same year, at the 10th International Congress of Psychoanalysts in Innsbruck, Reich lectured for the first time on the notion of character armor. Together with Marie Frischauf-Pappenheim, Reich founded the Socialist Society for Sexual Counselling and Sexual Research in Vienna in 1929, which experienced its most active period until Reich moved to Berlin at the end of 1930. The Viennese sexual counseling centers, mass events, and popular brochures were designed to inform the public on practical items such as contraceptives; as well, Reich spoke on the political aspects of sexual suppression. In Berlin, he founded the Deutscher Reichsverband für Proletarische Sexualpolitik (German Association for Proletarian Sexual Politics—Sexpol) and the Verlag für Sexualpolitik (Press for Sexual Politics). He became a training analyst at the Berlin Psychoanalytic Institute and a member of the German Psychoanalytic Society. In 1933, "Charakteranalyse" (Character Analysis) was to be published with the International Psychoanalytic Press (Verlag), but the book was rejected for political reasons; it was finally printed by the author himself. Reich was a member of the German Communist Party and visited the Soviet Union. With "Dialektischer Materialismus und Psychoanalyse" (Dialectic Materialism and Psychoanalysis), he tried to establish a link between Marxism and psychoanalysis. In 1933, Reich was expelled from the German Communist Party.

After Hitler came to power in 1933, Reich fled for a brief period to Vienna. He moved to Copenhagen a month later, where he continued to work as a training analyst. His visa was not renewed after six months, and he was compelled to settle, under difficult circumstances, in Malmö, Sweden. When his work permit was not renewed, he finally emigrated to Oslo, Norway.

At the 13th International Psychoanalytic Congress in Lucerne, Switzerland, Reich appeared as a guest speaker, giving his last lecture before the International Psychoanalytic Association on "Psychischer Kontakt und Vegetative Strömung; ein Beitrag zur Affektlehre und Charakteranalytischen Technik" (Psychic Contact and Vegetative Flow; A Contribution to the Theory of Affects and Character-Analytic Technique). Previously, he had been excluded from the German Psychoanalytic Society and the International Psychoanalytic Association.

In Oslo, Reich had contact with Otto Fenichel and was a member of the group that received Fenichel's circular letters (Fenichel, 1998). Theoretical and political disagreement led to a distancing from each other, and Fenichel stopped sending the newsletters to Reich in 1935. In 1936, Reich founded the Institut für Sexualökonomische Lebensforschung (Institute for Sexual Economic Life Research). Under the pen name Ernst Parell, he edited the *Journal for Psychology and Sexual Economy* and began his own biological-physiological studies on the connection between fear and sexuality.

In 1939, Reich accepted a teaching assignment at the New School for Social Research in New York City. He married Ilse Ollendorf that same year. In the United States, he worked mainly on his orgone theory, and in 1940 he constructed the first orgone-accumulator, a machine that was supposed to store vital energy then release it for therapeutic purposes. At his country home in Maine, he constructed a laboratory and an observatory, and founded a publishing company, Orgone Press. "He claimed that his discovery of biones had fundamentally advanced a theory concerning the origin of life, and that it was also related to the cancer problem. Going beyond his theory of biones, Reich claimed that he had discovered a method for gathering cosmic radiation that, with a device he used on patients, had therapeutic value. But these claims brought him into legal difficulty with the U.S. Food and Drug Administration (Briehl, 1966: 436n). In 1954, he was indicted in connection with the sale of orgone-accumulators. He pleaded not guilty but was sentenced to two years in

R

jail. Reich died in prison in Lewisburg, Pennsylvania, on November 3, 1957.

REFERENCES

Briehl, W. (1966). Wilhelm Reich 1897–1957. Character Analysis. In F. Alexander, S. Eisenstein, and M. Grotjahn (eds.). *Psychoanalytic Pioneers.* New York: Basic Books, pp. 430–438.

Fallend, K. (1988). *Wilhelm Reich in Wien. Psychoanalyse and Politik.* Vienna: Geyer.

Fenichel, O. (1998). 119 Rundbriefe (1934–1945), vol. 1, *Europa* (1934–1938). J. Reichmayr and E. Mühlleitner (eds.), vol. 2, *Amerika* (1938–1945). E. Mühlleitner and J. Reichmayr (eds.). Frankfurt am Main: Stroemfeld Verlag.

Reich, W. (1988). *Passion of Youth. An Autobiography 1897–1922.* New York: Farrar, Straus and Giroux.

———. (1994). *Beyond Psychology. Letters and Journals 1934–1939.* M. Boyd-Higgins (ed.). New York: Farrar, Straus and Giroux.

Sharaf, M. (1983). *Fury on Earth. A Biography of Wilhelm Reich.* New York: St. Martin's Press/Marek.

ELKE MÜHLLEITNER
JOHANNES REICHMAYR

Reik, Theodor (1888–1969)

Theodor Reik was a disciple of Sigmund Freud, secretary of the Vienna Psychoanalytic Society, author of more than twenty books and hundreds of papers on literature, music, religion, analytic technique, and masochism, founder of the National Psychological Association for Psychoanalysis (NPAP) in New York, and an analyst in four major cities who wrote in a confessional way about his life, loves, failures, and triumphs. He occupies a unique place in the history of psychoanalysis.

Reik was born on May 12, 1888, in Vienna, the third child of four born to the cultured, lower-middle-class Jewish family of Max and Caroline Reik. Reik's father was a low-salaried government clerk who died when Reik was eighteen. Freud became a father figure for the rest of Reik's life. He attended public schools in Vienna and entered the University of Vienna at eighteen, where he studied psychology and French and German literature. He received a Ph.D. in 1912, writing the first psychoanalytic dissertation, on Flaubert's *The Temptation of Saint Anthony.* He met Freud in 1910 and two years later became a member of the Vienna Psychoanalytic Society. From 1914 to 1915, he was in analysis with Karl Abraham in Berlin and, with the outbreak of World War I, served as an officer in the Austrian cavalry from 1915 to 1918, seeing combat in Montenegro and Italy. He was decorated for bravery.

Following the resignation of Otto Rank, Reik became the secretary of the Vienna Psychoanalytic Society. For ten years he practiced in Vienna and began to write so extensively that Freud asked him: "Why do you pee around so much? Just pee in one spot" (Natterson, 1966: 254).

Freud wrote *The Question of Lay Analysis* in defense of Reik, who was prosecuted under the quackery laws of Austria for practicing medicine. Reik moved to Berlin, where he lived and practiced from 1928 until 1934 and again became a celebrated teacher at the Berlin Psychoanalytic Institute. Fearing the rise of the Nazis, he moved to The Hague in the Netherlands, where he continued practicing and teaching. During this time, his first wife, Ella, mother of his son Arthur, died and he married Marija. There were two children born of this marriage, Theodora and Miriam. Still fearful of the Nazis, Reik moved with his family to New York, where, as a nonmedical analyst, he was denied full membership in the New York Psychoanalytic Society. Reik would not accept the position of research analyst, although he could have made a "charade" of agreement and practiced, as many did. Reik experienced financial difficulties for many periods in his life. He was treated gratis by both Karl Abraham and Freud and for a time he received financial support of two hundred German marks per month from Freud. Writing to Freud for help in 1938, Freud wrote back: "What ill wind has blown you, just you, to America? You must have known how amiably lay analysts would be received there by our colleagues for whom psychoanalysis is nothing more than one of the handmaidens of psychiatry" (Hale, 1995: 129). He persevered, however, in building a practice, and soon a group of colleagues gathered around him and, in 1948, the National Psychological Association for Psychoanalysis (NPAP) was founded.

Reik's influence on the development of nonmedical analysis in the United States is great. Not only did his many books have a profound effect on the general reading public, but his influence, through NPAP and the several institutes that split from it, suggests that Reik is the major promulgator of nonmedical analysis in the United States.

Reik's psychoanalytic studies include such writers and composers as Beer-Hofmann, Flaubert, and Schnitzler as well as Shakespeare, Goethe, and Gustav Mahler, to name a few. He had a (unique way of) communicating, and his writing and conversational style was free-associational. His autobiography is to be found in his many works. Among his better known are *Listening with the Third Ear* (1948); the monumental *Masochism in Modern Man* (1949); *Surprise and the Psychoanalyst* (1935); his recollection of Freud, *From Thirty Years with Freud* (1940); an autobiographical study, *Fragment of a Great Confession* (1949); applied psychoanalysis of the Bible in *Mystery on the Mountain* (1958); anthropology in *Ritual* (1958); sexuality in *Of Love and Lust* (1959), *Creation of Woman* (1960), and *The Psychology of Sex Relations* (1961); and music in *The Haunting Melody* (1960).

Toward the end of his life Reik, who grew a beard, resembled the older Freud and lived modestly, surrounded by photographs of Freud from childhood to old age. He died on December 31, 1969, after a long illness. According to Natterson, "In many ways, Reik is the epitome of the sensitive aesthete, the pleasure-loving, erotic, highly intellectual, secular Jewish scholar. These characteristics are to be treasured" (Natterson, 1966: 263).

REFERENCES

Hale, N. G., Jr. (1995). *The Rise and Crisis of Psychoanalysis in the United States.* New York: Oxford University Press.

Natterson, J. M. (1966). Theodor Reik: Masochism in modern man. In F. Alexander, S. Eisenstein, and M. Grotjahn (eds.). *Psychoanalytic Pioneers.* New York: Basic Books, pp. 249–264.

JOSEPH REPPEN

Religion, and Psychoanalysis

Freud made many interesting contributions to the psychoanalytic explanation of cultural phenomena, including art, literature, and religion but his account of the latter remains troublesome, not only in terms of his negative assessment of religion, but also because of questionable methodological issues raised by his agnostic convictions. However one adjudicates those complex issues—and the variants in the sixty-odd years following Freud's death have been considerable—it was an aspect of Freud's genius that, even when he miscalculated or went astray in his efforts to bring the resources of psychoanalytic method to bear on cultural phenomena, he managed to open new vistas and perspectives, and to bring new questions into focus that inevitably enriched and deepened the inquiry. This was prototypically the case in relation to religion (Meissner, 1984).

The evolution of Freud's views on religion can be cast in four stages, marked by successive pivotal works—first his *Totem and Taboo* (1912), second *The Future of an Illusion* (1927), then *Civilization and Its Discontents* (1930), and finally *Moses and Monotheism* (1939). These works reflect both progressive aspects of Freud's thinking and his tenacious clinging to core convictions regarding dynamic processes and developmental configurations, particularly those reflecting Oedipal dynamics.

Totem and Taboo (1912) arose out of the combination of Freud's extensive anthropological interests and his previously formulated idea that religious thinking and behavior were essentially related to the same mechanisms as obsessive-compulsive disorders (1907). Freud translated the behavioral analogy between obsessional rituals and religious ceremonials into an identity, focusing particularly on pangs of conscience resulting from omission of the act, the need to protect against external interruption, preoccupation with detail, and the propensity for increasing complexity and esoteric significance in such rituals. On Freud's account, religion was a thing of infantile conflict and superstition, of emotion and passivity—a view he had inherited from Schleiermacher and Feuerbach.

In attempting to explain how these primitive mechanisms came into play in the origins of religious experience, Freud relied on the analogy assumed in *Totem* between the mind of the primitive human and the obsessional. He traced the origins of totemism with its associated taboos, including the incest taboo and exogamy, to an imaginative fiction of the primal horde. The primitive tribe, according to this anthropological fantasy, was organized under dominance of the tribal leader or father figure. To escape repressive domination of the leader, particularly the repressive and controlling prohibition of sexual access to the females of the tribe, the younger males banded together to murder the leader. This parricide was the primal crime. The guilt felt because of this original misdeed led to erection of the totem animal as substitute for the primal father, worship of which brought with it prohibitions against killing or eating the totem animal and against incestuous relations with the women of the totem clan. The origins of sacramental killing and communal eating of the totem animal are derived from this source. Thus the totem phenomenon and related sexual taboos are rooted in primitive Oedipal dynamics inherent in the primal horde, based on the primitive impulse to kill the father and have sex with the mother. Veneration and fear of the totem ancestor was further displaced into elevation of the father totem into a divinity.

Freud took the next step in *The Future of an Illusion* (1927). In this work, the seeds that had been germinating in previous efforts came to full fruition. What emerged was a magisterial statement of Freud's mature thinking about religious experience—with the full force of agnostic and antireligious conviction and bias. *Future*, however, cannot be read in isolation; it should be read in conjunction with a second current of dialogue found in the correspondence between Freud and his Swiss Lutheran pastor, friend, and devoted follower of over thirty years, Oscar Pfister (Meng and Freud, 1963) and in Pfister's rejoinder published on Freud's invitation, "The Illusion of a Future" (1928). Not only did Pfister's rejoinder point in the direction of much of post-Freudian thought about religion, but it underlined the fact that Pfister was indeed the unnamed protagonist of *Future*.

The argument of *Future* did not deviate much from earlier directions. Religion was rooted in essential human weakness and dependence and in our helpless longing for the father of infantile need, displaced onto the figure of a divinity. We have learned to survive the terrors of a hostile world by a dependent and supplicating attachment to the all-powerful and protecting father-god or gods of religious belief systems. The gods held sway over the universe and its laws, but they have withdrawn to leave humans to fend for themselves in the face of forces that determine their destiny. The onus to placate the gods and find the way to salvation issued in a divinely determined morality and a set of divinely ordained commandments, to which one must submit and accommodate. Thus the helplessness and dependence of childhood, and fears of punishment and disfavor from the powerful father, are carried into adult life and displaced into the relation of the individual believer and his or her god. Even the sting of death is mitigated by promises of an afterlife and obliteration of the misery and pain of this life by the promise of blessed bliss in the next.

Freud regarded such ideas as illusions, wish fulfillments corresponding to the oldest, strongest, and most urgent of human desires and needs. Persistence of this sense of helplessness and vulnerability throughout life leads us to cling to the father in infantile terms, and to his substitute, the belief in an all-powerful, loving, and protecting father in heaven. Thus belief in the benevolent rule of divine providence protects us against the

assaults afflicting us in this world. Religion offers reassurance that to the extent that we obey the divine commandments and rely on the goodness and love of the heavenly father and his promises, we shall survive the rigors of fate and find that ultimate justice and love that escapes us in the here and now. Freud translated these needs and wishes into infantile derivatives that reflected basic wishes, but nothing more. To the extent that such wishes found no correspondence in reality, Freud tended to see them as beyond illusion, as forms of mass delusion shared by communities of believers.

Freud made it clear that if he was going to put his trust in anything, it was to be in science. He wrote: "I know how difficult it is to avoid illusions; perhaps the hopes I have confessed to are of an illusory nature, too. But I hold fast to one distinction. Apart from the fact that no penalty is imposed for not sharing them, my illusions are not, like religious ones, incapable of correction. They have not the character of a delusion. . . . If this belief is an illusion, then we are in the same position as you. But science has given us evidence by its numerous and important successes that it is no illusion" (pp. 53–54).

In Pfister's rejoinders, he stressed the distortions Freud brought to his understanding of religion, limited for the most part to one pathological variant rather than the full spectrum of religious endeavor, including thoughtful and reasoned efforts of serious theologians to explore and understand the complexities of religious experience and the dimensions of authentic belief—an endeavor that could in no way be charged with avoidance of the demands of reason and reality. Needless to say, the views of the two men regarding religion were diametrically opposed: if Freud saw it as a matter of infantile needs and weakness, Pfister saw it as the repository of the noblest striving and the highest ideals of the human condition; if Freud tried to insist on a radical differentiation between religion and psychoanalysis, Pfister saw them as mutually supportive and oriented toward similar goals and truths; if Freud's outlook was basically pessimistic and fatalistic, Pfister's was strikingly optimistic and hopeful. One can read the debate between these two protagonists as foreshadowing much of the thematic currents that continue to swirl around the discussion of the relation of psychoanalysis and religion ever since.

Not long after, Freud returned to some of the same themes in his *Civilization and Its Discontents* (1930). The motifs that had found such powerful expression in the

Future were extended to embrace the full range of human civilization and culture. Freud posed an irremediable antagonism and opposition between instinctual demands on one side and demands of civilized life on the other. Inhibition of the sexual drive was essential for adaptation of the child to society, a task largely accomplished during the latency period. But Freud was more concerned with vicissitudes of aggression and the requirements for restraint and control of its destructive dimension. Freud had only begun to recognize aggression as an independent drive in *Beyond the Pleasure Principle* (1920) rather than as a modification of libidinal (sadism) and self-preservative drives. Freud thought of aggression as derived from the death instinct and thus as inherently destructive and self-destructive. Humans seek happiness, driven by the search for pleasure and the avoidance of pain and unpleasure. The harsh necessity of life and reality does not allow us to satisfy these needs so that we are forced to find fulfillment in illusion. This theme connects with the argument of the *Future* but at the same time extends it to include other aspects of culture and social integration. The cost at all points in this effort is stifling and repression of basic human drives and needs. The prime exemplar of this process is found in religious illusions, yet these illusions do not arise from the "oceanic feeling" described by Romain Rolland (Freud, 1936) but from the feelings of infantile helplessness and dependency that lie at the core of human experience.

Freud's last major work on religion was *Moses and Monotheism* (1939). Writing at the end of his life, Freud returned once more to the themes first enunciated in *Totem and Taboo* and tried to apply them to the roots of the Judeo-Christian tradition. Freud argued that Moses was really an Egyptian prince in the court of Akhenaton—the pharaoh who came to the throne about 1375 B.C. and brought with him sweeping religious reforms, including the monotheistic worship of a single god, Aten. Moses then extended this religious vision to the Hebrews in the form of the worship of Yahweh. But, as the story goes, the Jews, unable to tolerate this spiritualized and restrictive religion, rebelled against and murdered the prophet who had tried to impose it on them. Later, in the face of a need for tribal unity and a common religion, the Jews returned to the religion of the murdered prophet and the worship of one all-powerful deity. In Freud's words, "the central fact of the development of the Jewish religion was that in the course of time the

God Yahweh lost his own characteristics and grew more and more to resemble the old god of Moses, the Aten" (p. 63).

This historical fiction was buttressed by the familiar Freudian appeal to a neurotic model. The history of childhood is marked by repression of early traumas resulting in infantile amnesia and subsequent latency that ultimately gives way to return of the repressed in fragmented and transformed expressions of sexual, aggressive, and narcissistic derivatives. These expressions carry a characteristic compulsive stamp that isolates them from the requirements of logic and reality. Freud then makes a great leap in logic to suggest that the history of the individual finds a parallel in the history of the race. Once again, the murder of the father of the primal horde sets the stage for emergence of forms of social organization and renunciation of instinctual urges. The memory of the father-prophet lives on in the totem, which is then elevated to divine status. The murder of Moses lies at the root of the worship of Yahweh and determined the further evolution of religious practice in forms of sacrifice (Bergmann, 1992) and sacramental rites of consuming the totem-god substitute, as in the Christian eucharistic liturgy.

The Freudian argument about the nature and origins of religion rests on slender reeds at best, and critics have not been slow to point out its flaws and inadequacies. Freud's effort to translate an analogy between religious ceremonial and obsessional devices into an identity takes a limited aspect of relatively pathological religious expression for the whole and thus leaves out of consideration the multiple aspects of religious belief and cult that are most meaningful to the religious mind. The analogy thus becomes reductionistic in the worst sense, and in the end contributes little to the understanding of authentic faith and religious practice. As Ricoeur (1970) pointed out, the analytic approach can only illumine that aspect of religious experience found in the "birth of idols." The analogy is not invalid, but it raises the further question whether religious thought is condemned to endless repetition of archaic patterns to the exclusion of progressive or epigenetic developments that leave open the possibility of transcending such archaisms.

The argument of *Totem* has met particularly trenchant rejection, particularly from anthropologists. Despite the efforts of some scholars to argue the contrary, there is simply little or no evidence to support Freud's postulation of the primal horde in human prehistory (Bad-

R

cock, 1980, 1983). Even so, one can argue that Freud's ingenious approach raises important questions that deserve continued exploration. Undoubtedly, unconscious dynamics and residues of infantile experience play a central role in the genesis and persistence of religious beliefs and commitments. If appeal to an archaic substratum on Freudian terms falls short, we are left with a significant problem that continues to challenge our understanding and imagination.

Similar objections have been brought against *Civilization*, since Freud's view of civilization, and especially culture, is cast in limited and negative terms that may not do justice to the rich complexity and multifaceted reality. If enculturation requires a degree of regulation and mastery of instinctual forces, there is also an important gain in the process. It is through the civilized organization of society and the development of cultural resources that human existence is illumined, ennobled, and rendered increasingly able to transcend and sublimate archaic determinants and forces, thus providing meaning and purpose to human life and experience. As Pfister (1928) argued, without art and religion, along with the many other avenues of cultural expression, human life would be bleak and unsatisfying. Culture and civilization, then, can mean much more and much different from the Freudian supposition.

By the same token, *Moses* has been much taken to task (Meissner, 1984). Our ability to read it critically has been considerably enriched by recent research (Rice, 1990; Yerushalmi, 1991). Freud's reading of the Old Testament was framed by the Hegelian views of Julius Wellhausen, whose work was to influence a generation of biblical scholars. The view of religious origins evolving through stages of development in Hegelian progression suited Freud's views well. But more recent archaeological and textual research has cast much of the Wellhausen approach into doubt. Greater attention and weight have been given to the Mesopotamian origins of Hebrew religious traditions than to Egyptian. The upshot is that the Freudian construction, including the idea that Moses was an Egyptian, is no longer tenable. Moreover, from the perspective of current psychoanalytic thinking, perhaps a major flaw of Freud's perspective is that it is trapped within a basically Oedipal frame of analytic reference, with the effect that it ignores broader and deeper strata of dynamic influence and developmental transformation, and in this sense totally ignores the influence of the mother in contributing to religious motivation as well as other more feminine determinants of religious experience.

Despite the weakness of the underpinnings of Freud's view, and its obvious connection with his own religious conflicts and agnosticism (Meissner, 1984), it would be a mistake to disregard or undervalue Freud's contribution, because it opens the way to profoundly meaningful issues that remain to be resolved and understood. The openness of the Freudian critique of religion to a deeper and more meaningful understanding of religion was captured by Ricoeur (1970):

> Psychoanalysis is necessarily iconoclastic, regardless of the faith or nonfaith of the psychoanalyst, and this "destruction" of religion can be the counterpart of a faith purified of all idolatry. Psychoanalysis as such cannot go beyond the necessity of iconoclasm. This necessity is open to a double possibility, that of faith and that of nonfaith, but the decision about these two possibilities does not rest with psychoanalysis. (p. 230)

REFERENCES

Badcock, C. R. (1980). *The Psychoanalysis of Culture.* Oxford: Blackwell.

———. (1983). *Madness and Modernity.* Oxford: Blackwell.

Bergmann, M. S. (1992). *In the Shadow of Moloch: The Sacrifice of Children and Its Impact on Western Religions.* New York: Columbia University Press.

Freud, S. (1907). Obsessive acts and religious practices. S.E. 9: 115–127.

———. (1912). *Totem and Taboo.* S.E. 13: vii–162.

———. (1920). *Beyond the Pleasure Principle.* S.E. 18: 7–66.

———. (1927). *The Future of an Illusion.* S.E. 21: 1–56.

———. (1930). *Civilization and Its Discontents.* S.E. 21: 57–145.

———. (1936). A disturbance of memory on the acropolis. S.E. 22: 237–248.

———. (1939). *Moses and Monotheism: Three Essays.* S.E. 23: 1–137.

Meissner, S. J., W. W. (1984). *Psychoanalysis and Religious Experience.* New Haven, Conn.: Yale University Press.

Meng, H., and Freud, E. L. (eds.) (1963). *Psychoanalysis and Faith: The Letters of Sigmund Freud and Oskar Pfister.* New York: Basic Books.

Pfister, O. (1928) The illusion of a future: A friendly disagreement with Prof. Sigmund Freud (with an introduction by P. Roazen). *International Journal of Psychoanalysis,* 74 (1993): 557–579.

Rice, E. (1990). *Freud and Moses: The Long Journey Home.* Albany: State University of New York Press.

Ricoeur, P. (1970). *Freud and Philosophy: An Essay on Interpretation.* New Haven, Conn.: Yale University Press.

Yerushalmi, Y. H. (1991). *Freud's Moses: Judaism Terminable and Interminable.* New Haven, Conn.: Yale University Press.

W. W. MEISSNER, S.J.

Repetition Compulsion

Neurotic suffering develops without apparent organic cause. To understand and treat it, therefore, we must search beyond the body into the broader domains of human psychic and social experience, where cause and effect find expression through unconscious and symbolic means. The covertness of its cause, however, is not what brings neurotic pain to clinical attention. Neurotics seek help because their discomfort does not cease but repeats in subjectively meaningless and vicious cycles that limit their freedom and stereotype their lives. Neurotics are not unintelligent but they fail to learn from painful experience, which they repeat as if compelled. A neurotic symptom, whether somatic, psychic, or social in its domain of expression, always appears to express a compulsion to repeat. To repeat what? In what form? And compelled by what forces? From his earliest clinical encounters to his final theoretical musings, Freud struggled with these questions but never fully answered them.

From its outward presentation as symptom, Freud traced the repetition compulsion to its vanishing point at the threshold of consciousness. Here the symptom's loss of apparent meaning marked the intervention of repression, a process to which Freud ascribed a protective function. Thus from his reflection on the clinical phenomenology of repetition, Freud's topographical theory arose, with its conscious, preconscious, and unconscious theaters of expression. So, too, came a general theory of symptom formation: instinctual drives, abrupted prior to awareness, find conscious expression in symbolic form. But the symbolic "solution" cannot resolve the actual conflict, so that it (the symptom) repeats with futile and frustrating results, in the process preventing more tangible success. The symptom, in short, is a symbol that does not satisfy, but instead inhibits the resolution of conflict between the self and its surround. To an observer, the symptom arises at the border between action and symbol, calling for help from either side, as if pleading, "How do I translate these impulses into action, or these actions into words?" Because the symbolic solution brings no fruition, the neurotic activity is repeated: A tiresome, irrational expression of covert and conflicted, emotionally laden biological drives.

What makes biological drives so problematic? They interfere with the demands of social life. Humans must simultaneously possess themselves and belong meaningfully to their world. From this line of thought, Freud developed his structural and economic theories. The demands of nature (biology) versus nurture (society) create conflict. In response, the human mind splits into the id, ego, and superego. Repetitions in clinical psychopathology as well as in everyday life result from repeated efforts to resolve such discord in ways that are not optimal. Thus from the literal to the symbolic to the underlying biological, Freud traced the "what" of repetition, but in doing so only changed his level of discourse, not yet explaining the "why" of the compulsion to repeat.

If we seek pleasure ultimately, why do people keep doing what hurts? Explaining why neurotic suffering occurs posed perhaps the most obdurate challenge of Freud's career as a theoretician. From his earliest writings to his last, he tried to find a motive for repetition in the pleasure principle, generally by reducing all habitual—but unsatisfying—action to "the one major habit, the primal addiction," namely, masturbation—the symbolic coition, that does not satisfy (Freud, 1897: 272). Yet Freud balked at the fact that repetition, on balance, compels more suffering than it dispels—it is, after all, what defines the neurotic's suffering, brings him or her into treatment, and generates the transference that resists a cure. To explain this, we must go "beyond the pleasure principle." In his essay by that name, Freud found in the repetition compulsion evidence of a second instinctual prime mover operating alongside, at times even prevailing beyond, the demands of Eros. The death instinct, Thanatos, he felt forced to conclude, also rules human destiny. Despite the apparent contradictions that this solution entails (e.g., it appears inconsistent with his masturbation theory), Freud held fast to this conclusion until the end of his writing career, even though, he confessed, "I am not convinced myself." Since Freud's time, other writers have tried to resolve its paradoxes—by positing an urge for active mastery, for example, or a drive toward self-possession, or a halting growth toward affect-competency. Regardless of theoretical perspective, the repetition compulsion remains among the most vexing problems of psychoanalysis.

REFERENCES

Freud, S. (1897). Letter 79. Masturbation, addiction and obsessional neurosis. S.E. 1: 272.

———. (1914). Remembering, repeating and working-through. S.E. 12: 147–156.

———. (1920). *Beyond the Pleasure Principle*. S.E. 18: 7–64.

———. (1926). *Inhibitions, Symptoms and Anxiety*. S.E. 20: 87–172.

———. (1928 [1927]). Dostoevsky and parricide. S.E. 21: 175–198.

———. (1937). Analysis terminable and interminable. S.E. 23: 216–253.

———. (1941. [1938]). Findings, ideas, problems. S.E. 23: 299–300.

Loewald, H. (1980). Repetition and repetition compulsion. *Papers on Psychoanalysis*. New Haven, Conn.: Yale University Press, p. 94.

Mann, D. (1994). *A Simple Theory of the Self*. New York: Norton.

Russell, P. L. (2001). Trauma, repetition and affect. Unpublished.

Szasz, T. (1968). Hysteria. *International Encyclopedia of the Social Sciences*, ed. David L. Sills. New York: Macmillan, pp. 47–52.

DAVID W. MANN

Repression

Freud's Account of Hysteria: The Emergence of Repression

"The essence of repression lies simply in turning something away, and keeping it at a distance, from the conscious" (Freud, 1915: 147). It is understandable that Freud (1914a) referred to repression as the "cornerstone" of psychoanalysis (p. 16). For it is with his introduction of the concept of repression that Freud's theorizing becomes distinctively psychoanalytic. The concept of repression constitutes a dividing line between Freud's prepsychoanalytic and psychoanalytic writing. Prior to his introduction of repression, Freud's account of hysteria was not essentially different from Janet's (1889) and other representatives of "dynamic psychiatry" (Ellenberger, 1970). Indeed, in the introduction to *Studies on Hysteria*, the editor acknowledges in a footnote Janet's priority regarding a number of concepts and formulations that Breuer and Freud employ in that work. Undoubtedly partly reflecting the influence of Breuer, terms such as "*condition seconde*," "hypnoid states," "absences," "double conscience" (dual consciousness), and "splitting of consciousness"—all of which evoke the concept of dissociation—are used to describe and account for hysterical phenomena. For example, in their *Preliminary Communications*, Breuer and Freud (1893–1895) write that:

> the longer we have been occupied with these phenomena the more we have become convinced that the splitting of consciousness which is so striking in the well-known cases under the form of "double conscience" [dual consciousness] *is present to a rudimentary degree in every hysteric and that a tendency to such a dissociation, and with it the emergence of abnormal states of consciousness (which we shall bring together under the term "hypnoid") is the basic phenomenon of this neurosis*. In these views we concur with Binet and the two Janets, though we have had no experience of the remarkable findings they have made on anesthetic patients (p. 12, emphasis in original).

At other points, too, in *Studies on Hysteria*, Breuer and Freud indicate their general agreement with Janet. For example, Breuer writes: "In one way or another there comes into existence a region of mental life . . . our knowledge of which we owe, above all, to Binet and Janet. The splitting of the mind is the consummation of hysteria" (p. 249). There is one point, however, on which Breuer and Freud disagree with Janet. Freud states that "Janet, to whom the theory of hysteria owes so very much and with whom we are in agreement in most respects, has expressed a view on this point which we are unable to accept" (p. 230). That view is Janet's claim that at the core of hysteria is a constitutional weakness. Thus, Freud argues that "it is not the case that the splitting of consciousness occurs because the patients are weak-minded; they appear to be weak-minded because their mental activity is divided and only a part of its capacities at the disposal of the conscious thought. We cannot regard mental weakness as the *typus hystericus*, as the essence of the disposition to hysteria" (p. 231). In his case study of Frau Emmy von N. Freud also registers his disagreement with Janet, noting that the patient shows no evidence of "psychical inefficiency."

Although Breuer and Freud reject Janet's idea of constitutional weakness, as we have seen, they seem to agree with him on virtually all other aspects of his account, including the appeal to dissociation as the primary mental mechanism to account for hysterical phenomena. Indeed, Anna O.'s description of her own state and Breuer and Freud's discussion of her condition suggest multiple personality more than any other diagnosis. For example, Breuer refers to Anna O.'s description of herself as "two selves, a real one and an evil one which forced her to behave badly" (p. 211). In his summation of her case, Breuer writes, "It is hard to avoid expressing the situation by saying that the patient was split into two personalities of which one was mentally normal and the other insane" (p. 45).

Despite the apparent general agreement with Janet in *Preliminary Communication*, when Freud presents his own cases in *Studies on Hysteria*, the concept of repression comes to the fore in his explanatory accounts. For example, in the case of Miss Lucy R., Freud declares, "Now I already know from the analysis of similar cases that before hysteria can be acquired for the first time one essential condition must be fulfilled: an idea must be intentionally *repressed from consciousness* and excluded from associative modification" (Breuer and Freud, 1893–1895: 116, emphasis in original). In discussing the same case, he boldly claims, "It turns out to be a *sine qua non* for the acquisition of hysteria that an incompatibility should develop between the ego and some idea presented to it" (p. 122). He goes on to describe the "advantage" of conversion symptoms as the fact that "the incompatible idea is repressed from the ego's consciousness" (p. 122). In the case of Elisabeth von R., after referring to her conflict between her guilt at leaving her sick father for an evening in order to meet a young man, and her "blissful feelings she had allowed herself to enjoy" that evening, Freud writes, "The outcome of the conflict was that the erotic idea was repressed" (p. 146).

In the theoretical section of *Studies on Hysteria* entitled "Psychotherapy of Hysteria," Freud states, "I have shown how, in the course of our therapeutic work, we have been led to the view that hysteria originates through the repression of an incompatible idea from a motive of defense" (p. 285). Although he seems to refer to all cases of hysteria in the preceding assertion, Freud comments that, "Breuer and I have repeatedly spoken of two other kinds of hysteria, for which we have introduced the terms 'hypnoid hysteria' and 'retention hysteria'" (p. 285). With regard to hypnoid hysteria, Freud notes Breuer's view that "no psychical force has . . . been required in order to keep an idea apart from the ego and no resistance need be aroused if we introduce it into the ego" (p. 285) and observes that "Anna O.'s case history in fact

shows no sign of any such resistance" (p. 286). Despite Freud's apparent acceptance of the category of hypnoid hysteria (he states that "I willingly adhere to this hypothesis on there being a hypnoid hysteria" [p. 286]), he observes that "any [case of hypnoid hysteria] that I took in hand has turned into a defense hysteria" (p. 286). He finally concludes that "I am unable to suppress a suspicion that somewhere or other the roots of hypnoid and defense hysteria come together and that the primary factor is defense" (p. 286). Freud then adds the somewhat disingenuous last sentence of the paragraph: "But I can say nothing about this" (p. 286).

As for retention hysteria, here, too, Freud writes, "I . . . suspect though once again subject to all the reserve which is proper to ignorance, that at the basis of retention hysteria, too, an element of defense is to be found which has forced the whole process in the direction of hysteria" (p. 286). His final comment on this topic is a seemingly open-minded hope "that fresh observations will soon decide whether I am running the risk of falling into one-sidedness and error in thus favoring an extension of the concept of defense to the whole of hysteria" (p. 286).

In *The Neuro-Psychoses of Defense*, Freud (1894) highlights the concept of repression and explicitly contrasts his account of at least one form of hysteria with Janet's (1889) account of hysteria. Even here, however, the divergence is only a partial one. In seeking an understanding of the general nature of hysteria, he continues to refer to the "splitting of consciousness, accompanied by the formation of separate psychical groups" (p. 46), although he argues that such splitting is not, as Janet claims, primary, but rather secondary to the existence of "hypnoid states," the latter described as the *sine qua non* of hysteria. According to the latter view, the splitting of consciousness comes about because the ideas that emerge in hypnoid states are cut off "from associative communication with the rest of the content of consciousness" (p. 46). Freud goes on to "bring forth two other extreme forms of hysteria in which it is impossible to regard the splitting of consciousness as primary in Janet's sense" (p. 46). One of these Freud calls "defense hysteria," claiming that in this form of hysteria he "was repeatedly able to show that *the splitting of consciousness is the result of an act of will on the part of the patient*" (p. 46, emphasis in original). He maintains that there is no evidence of a "hereditary trait" in these patients, thereby again rejecting Janet's attribution of some constitutional weakness to all patients suffering from hysteria. Patients suffering from defense hysteria, Freud writes, enjoyed "good health up to the moment at which an *occurrence of incompatibility took place in their ideational life*," that is, "until their ego was faced with an experience, an idea, or a feeling which aroused such a distressing affect that the subject decided to forget about it" (p. 44, emphasis in original). Here we have a description of the essence of repression: the banishment of mental contents from consciousness in order to avoid distressing affect.

At this point in his writings, Freud thinks of repression as voluntary and conscious. For example, he refers to patients' ability to recall their intention of "pushing the thing away" (p. 47). Although "pushing the thing away" succeeds in freeing the ego from a contradiction, "it has burdened itself with a mnemic symbol, 'lodged in consciousness' like a sort of parasite, either in the form of an unresolvable motor innervation or a constantly recurring hallucinatory sensation" (p. 49). The consequence is that "the memory trace of the repressed idea . . . forms the nucleus of a second psychical group" (p. 49). Freud's description of the consequences of repression, even the language he employs, is very similar to Janet's language and conception of the pathogenic effects of mental contents isolated from consciousness and the rest of the personality. Freud's reference to "a sort of parasite" is paralleled by Janet's description of "an idea excluded from personal consciousness" as "a virus, [which] develops in a corner of the personality inaccessible to the subject, works subconsciously, and brings about all disorders of hysteria" (Janet, 1889, quoted in Ellenberger, 1970: 149). Freud's reference to a "second psychical group" suggests the kind of dissociative process emphasized by Janet.

Thus, although Freud and Janet disagree regarding the means by which the isolation of a mental content from "personal consciousness" comes about, they agree regarding the pathogenic potential of such isolated mental contents. Indeed, it is accurate to say that this idea—that is, the potential pathological effects of mental contents isolated from personal consciousness—is the single most continuous idea running from prepsychoanalytic to classical psychoanalytic to contemporary psychoanalytic theorizing. With regard to more contemporary psychoanalytic theories, consider Fairbairn's (1952) formulation of the pathological influences of internalized objects and ego structures that are not assimilated by the central ego,

and Kohut's (1984) discussion of the pathological nature of archaic grandiosity that is not integrated into a mature self structure.

As to the *means* by which the isolation of a mental content occurs, for Janet it is mainly a constitutionally based "result of mental weakness" (cited in Ellenberger, 1970: 366), whereas, for Freud, once the concept of repression has been formulated, the isolation of a mental content from "the rest of the content of consciousness" is an "act of will" that is motivated by the aim of avoiding distressing affect. Furthermore, the distressing affect, which prompts the need for repression, is a function of a "psychical incompatibility" (p. 51) between the ego and the mental content that needs to be repressed. Freud then carries his discussion beyond hysteria and examines the central role of the incompatible idea in obsessional and phobic symptoms, adding that it is the patient's sexual life that is inevitably the source of incompatible ideas—although he seems to leave room for the role of other factors, such as "the common fears of mankind" (e.g., animals, thunderstorms) that are "seized upon" in phobias, and feelings of loss in "hallucinatory psychosis" (p. 59). With regard to the latter, in an early expression of the distinction between denial and repression (although Freud does not make this explicit), Freud observes that in denial the ego rejects not only the incompatible idea and its affect, but also that piece of reality to which the idea is connected. His poignant example is of a mother who, following the death of her child, rocks a piece of wood as if it is her child.

To recapitulate, one finds in *The Neuro-Psychoses of Defense* an early form of some of Freud's most important and central ideas and concepts: the rejection of Janet's emphasis on constitutional weakness; repression defined as the forgetting of incompatible ideas that is motivated by the need to avoid the distressing affect produced by the ideas; the continued active status of repressed contents (e.g., they bring about "the formation of separate psychical groups" [p. 46]); the pathogenic potential of repression (e.g., the repressed remains "lodged in consciousness" and operates "like a sort of parasite"); and, by implication, the idea of inner conflict (i.e., between the ego and an incompatible idea).

Repression and Pathology

Freud's formulations regarding the role and influence of repression have varied considerably in his writings and are not free of certain inconsistencies. The main source of inconsistency lies in the apparent contradiction between, on the one hand, the idea that repression is inherently pathogenic and, on the other hand, the idea that it is not repression itself that is pathological, but rather the return of the repressed that results from the failure of repression. Indeed, in his later work, Freud (1930) suggests that renunciation of instinct through repression or "some other means" is necessary for adaptive living in society (p. 97).

The Pathogenic Nature of Repression. The first question, then, is how and why is repression pathogenic? There are a number of interrelated reasons that Freud provides.

SPLITTING OF CONSCIOUSNESS. As we have seen in Freud's early writings, repression is viewed as pathogenic because it isolates mental contents from consciousness and leads to such consequences as the splitting of consciousness and the formation of a second psychical group. According to this formulation, the pathogenic nature of repression lies in its capacity to bring about dissociations in the personality, an idea not essentially different from Janet's formulation of the pathogenic effects of mental contents excluded from personal consciousness, or from what Fairbairn (1952) referred to as "splits in the ego." Freud (1938) referred to the splitting brought about by defense in one of his last papers, titled *Splitting of the Ego in the Process of Defense.*

PREVENTION OF DISCHARGE OF AFFECT AND EXCITATION. Another reason given in Freud's early writings for the pathogenic potential of repressive processes has to do with his assumption that every experience is accompanied by a "quota of affect" that needs to be discharged and is normally discharged through action, including speaking (Breuer and Freud, 1893–1895: 166). With certain people, and in certain circumstances, particularly when an experience is accompanied by a large amount of affect, affect does not get discharged and remains in a "strangulated" state. The reasons for the failure of discharge of the affect is that the experience took place while the person was in a hypnoid state or that the experience was "incompatible" with the person's ego.

As Strachey asks, however, in the editor's introduction to *Studies on Hysteria,* "Why should affect need to be 'discharged'? And why are the consequences of its not being discharged so formidable?" (p. 19). The answer to these questions, Strachey notes, is found in Freud's "principle of constancy," which was first stated in an 1893 lecture by Freud and more fully stated in *Beyond the Pleasure Principle* (Freud, 1920). In the former, Freud (1893) writes, "If a person experiences a psychical impression, something in his nervous system which we will for the moment call the sum of excitation is increased. Now in every individual there exists a tendency to diminish this sum of excitation once more in order to preserve his health" (p. 36). Freud continues, "If, however, there is no reaction whatsoever to a psychical trauma, the memory of it retains the affect which it originally had" (pp. 36–37). In other words, when an adequate reaction does not occur, as when the memory of the trauma is repressed, the sum of excitation fails to be diminished and will find expression in a variety of pathological ways (e.g., conversion symptoms).

Later in Freud's writings, when his drive theory has been formulated, instinctual wishes and impulses, rather than trauma, constitute the main sources of potentially excessive increases in the sum of excitation and therefore are the main threat to the integrity of the nervous system (or the mental apparatus). One can see a direct link between the early 1893 formulation of the "principle of constancy" and the later central role given to instinctual wishes and impulses. What remains unchanged is the idea that increases in the "sum of excitation"—whatever their source—and the need to reduce excitation in some fashion play a central role in the formation of neurotic symptoms. The pathogenic potential of repression lies in its prevention of an adequate discharge and reduction of the "sum of excitation."

PREVENTION OF ASSOCIATIVE RECTIFICATION. Still another reason for the pathogenic potential of repression—one that has not received adequate attention—is that it prevents mental contents from entering "the great complex of associations" (Breuer and Freud, 1893–1895: 9) and thereby being worked over and being subjected to the normal "wearing away" process (Freud, 1893: 37). Normally, when an idea does enter "the great complex of associations, it comes alongside other experiences, which may contradict it, and . . . subject [it] to rectification by other ideas" (Breuer and Freud, 1893–1895: 9). Because repression prevents this wearing away and rectification process, a repressed idea (e.g., a memory of a trauma) retains its "freshness and affective strength" (Breuer and Freud, 1893–1895: 11), with the result that "psychical traumas which have not been disposed of by reaction [Freud is referring here to an adequate reaction or abreaction] cannot be disposed of either by being worked over by means of association" (Breuer and Freud, 1893–1895: 11). Although affective abreaction

R

and the associative wearing away process are related to each other (e.g., the associative wearing away process also reduces an idea's affective strength) and have similar consequences, Freud clearly views them as somewhat separate processes and repeatedly distinguishes between them. For example, at one point he writes that "even if [a psychical trauma] has not been abreacted," there are other methods of "dealing with the situation . . . open to a normal person" (Breuer and Freud, 1893–1895: 9); the method that he identifies is the associative wearing away and rectification process.

In most accounts of early Freudian theoretical formulations, primary attention is usually paid to his concepts of "strangulated" affect and abreaction. However, as I have tried to show, Freud gives equal importance to the normal corrective and wearing away function of a mental content being associatively linked to other mental contents and becoming part of a "great complex of associations," and to the pathological consequences of the failure of an idea to come into "extensive associative connection" (Breuer and Freud, 1893–1895: 11) with other ideas—in short, to the pathological consequences of the isolation of a mental content from "personal consciousness." (Here again, we see the similarity between Freud's and Janet's formulations regarding the pathological consequences of mental contents "dissociated" from consciousness and from the ego.)

Although Freud does not make it entirely explicit, he identifies two adaptive components of the associative wearing away process. One is its capacity to reduce the affective strength of an idea, even when, or particularly when, abreaction does not occur. The other adaptive component is what one might call its cognitive *rectification* function. Freud clearly has in mind this latter function when he talks about the memory of a trauma coming "alongside other experiences, which may contradict it, and . . . subject [it] to rectification by ideas" (Breuer and Freud, 1893–1895: 9). In effect, Freud is referring to what we would normally call putting an experience or mental content into perspective. As noted, one consequence of wearing away and rectification, of putting an experience into perspective, is that it also reduces the affective intensity of the experience or memory, although in a manner and through a process that is different from a direct abreaction of affect. One might say that whereas abreaction of affect directly addresses the "quantitative" factor—that is, it reduces the "sum of excitation" of the "quota of affect" through direct expression of affect—

the wearing away and rectification process focuses on the cognitive and meaning aspects of mental contents and modifies the "affective charge" of an experience through cognitive means.

As noted, it is surprising that near exclusive attention has been given to concepts such as "strangulated" affect and abreaction and so little to the process of associative correction and wearing away in the usual histories of early psychoanalysis. Whereas the concept of abreaction was soon discarded (largely because of the failure of abreaction to bring about lasting therapeutic change), the concept of associative correction contained the seeds of, and was assimilated into, later formulations regarding the therapeutic value of insight and making the unconscious conscious and, in that sense, had a more important and lasting influence on psychoanalysis.

DIVIDING AND WEAKENING THE PERSONALITY. One consequence of the "splitting of consciousness" and "the formation of second psychical groups" is that they "weaken" the personality to the extent that they entail the presence of a set of mental contents, including aims and motives, that, at best, are irrelevant to one's central conscious aims and, at worst, are contrary to and undermine these aims. In the latter case, the personality structure is weakened by internal divisions and rifts. Surely this is the sort of thing Freud has in mind when he employs such terms as "separate psychical groups," and a "parasite" that is "lodged in consciousness" to describe mental contents, or when Janet compares "an idea excluded from personal consciousness" to a "virus . . . that brings about all disorders of hysteria" (Janet, 1889, quoted in Ellenberger, 1970: 149). As noted earlier, one finds a version of this basic idea in Fairbairn's (1952) comment that although repression of the bad object protects the individual from experiencing the original bad object situation (i.e., from experiencing the original trauma), it results in splits in the ego and the presence of an "internal saboteur" lodged in the mind that becomes part of one's personality structure. Thus, once again one sees the basic idea of an unintegrated "foreign body" weakening and undermining the personality.

It should be noted that the pathogenic potential of repression discussed here exists independently of its presumed consequence of preventing the discharge or reduction of the sum of excitation. That is, even if repression did not (presumably) interfere with the normal reduction in the sum of excitation or the "quota of affect" accompanying an experience, insofar as it entails "splits in consciousness" brought about by the isolation and sequestering of mental contents, it would neverthe-less possess pathogenic potential. (Note that Fairbairn's [1952] discussion of the pathogenic nature of "splits in the ego" is entirely devoid of reference to such matters as increases in the sum of excitation or quota of affect.)

Up to this point, the reasons for the pathogenic potential of repression have to do with the process of repression itself, or at least the consequences of repression. However, at a later point in his writings, Freud (1950) states that it is not repression itself that is pathological, but *the return of the repressed*, that is, the *failure* of repression (as well as other defenses).

Return of the Repressed

What is the reasoning behind the move from Freud's view of repression as inherently pathological to a view that it is a normal process and that it is primarily the return of the repressed that is pathological? Are there any inconsistencies or contradictions involved in this shift? There are complex issues involved in attempting to respond to these questions. One can attempt to clar-ify at least some of them. Even in Freud's early discus-sions of the consequences of repression, where it is viewed as inherently pathogenic (e.g., repressed contents remain "lodged in consciousness" and operate "like a sort of parasite"), he comments that repression itself need not be pathogenic, but is so only in those people who are predisposed to hysteria. He also suggests the adaptive function of repression by commenting that when someone "decide(s) to forget" an incompatible idea, the "distressing affect" that is aroused by the "occurrence of incompatibility" (Freud, 1894: 47) is no longer experienced.

Quite early in his writings, Freud (1892–1899) observes that it is not repression itself that is pathologi-cal, but rather *the return of the repressed* (p. 222). This idea remains essentially constant in Freud's writings and is then linked to his later theory of anxiety and his con-ceptualization of the formation of neurotic symptoms. As is well known, according to Freud neurotic symptoms are formations that represent a *compromise* between the repressed contents that threaten to reach consciousness and gain access to motility (action) and the forces of repression (as well as other defenses). As early as 1896, Freud writes that obsessional ideas and affects are "a compromise between the repressed ideas and the repress-ing ones" (p. 170). Thus, the development of neurotic symptoms bespeaks a partial failure of defense and a par-

tial and disguised return of the repressed. One can under-stand neurotic symptoms as a second line of defense inso-far as, although they entail partial gratification of the repressed wish, the repressed content remains disguised and does not appear in consciousness in undisguised form. Another way to put this is to say that when repres-sion (and other defenses) fails to prevent any trace of repressed content from emerging into consciousness, neu-rotic symptoms "guarantee" that the expression of such content will be limited (i.e., partial) as well as disguised.

One already sees the basic idea that symptoms serve defensive functions formulated in Freud's (1894) early discussion of conversion symptoms. As noted earlier, in *Studies on Hysteria*, Breuer and Freud (1893–1895) write about the "advantage" that conversion symptoms pro-vide in freeing consciousness from the incompatible idea. "The incompatible idea is rendered innocuous by its sum of excitation being transformed into something somatic" (p. 49) (i.e., a conversion symptom). Alternatively, the affect of the incompatible idea is displaced or "attaches itself to other ideas which are not in themselves incom-patible" (p. 52) and takes the form of an obsessional symptom. As can be seen, Freud is pointing here to the adaptive function of both repression and symptom for-mation. However, Freud also notes the maladaptive aspects of both repression and symptom formation. The maladaptive nature of symptoms is obvious and needs no further discussion. As for the maladaptive nature of repression, I have already noted Freud's discussion of this issue. For example, Freud observes that although repression succeeds in relieving the ego of distressing affect, the memory trace of the repressed idea "forms the nucleus of a second psychical group" (Freud, 1894: 49). At another point, in referring to the combination of repression and conversion, Freud (1894) writes that although the ego has freed itself of a contradiction, "it has burdened itself with a mnemic symbol, 'lodged in consciousness,' like a sort of parasite" (p. 49). As a final example, in the case of Lucy R. Breuer and Freud (1893–1895) write that

the incompatible idea . . . is not annihilated by a repudiation of this kind [i.e., by repression], but merely repressed into the unconscious. When this process occurs for the first time there comes into being a nucleus and center of crys-tallization for the formation of a psychical group divorced from the ego—a group around which everything which would imply an acceptance of the incompatible idea subsequently collects. The splitting of consciousness in these cases of acquired hysteria is accordingly a deliberate one (p. 123).

In his later work, where Freud (1915) discusses psychoneuroses, a similar point is made regarding the pathogenicity of repression, but this time in the context of instinct theory. He writes that the "instinctual representative develops with less interference and more profusely if it is withdrawn by repression from conscious influence. It proliferates in the dark . . . and takes on extreme forms of expression" that are alien to and terrify the individual because it gives "him the picture of extraordinary and dangerous strength of instinct. This deceptive strength of instinct is the result of an inhibited development of it in phantasy and of the damming-up consequent on frustrated satisfaction" (p. 149).

Let me return now to Freud's later idea that it is the return of the repressed that is pathological. How does one reconcile the apparent inconsistency or even contradiction between the ideas that repression is pathogenic and that repression is normal and between the ideas that repression itself is pathogenic and that it is the return of the repressed that is pathological?

The short answer to this question is that repression is both normal and pathogenic. Given the logical structure of Freudian theory, there is little doubt that repression is potentially pathogenic insofar as it is understood as increasing the sum of excitation (in both pre- and post-drive theory) and thereby carrying the risk of a traumatic "damming-up" of excitation. Freud never relinquished the constancy principle, and it is a clear implication of that principle that any factor, including repression, that interferes with the adequate discharge of excitation possesses pathogenic potential insofar as it entails the risk of producing a traumatic level of excitation. It also follows that other factors, such as an intensification of drive, that increase excitation beyond a tolerable level are also potentially pathogenic.

Repression and Repressivelike Defenses as Adaptive

If repression is both pathogenic and normal, in what way is it a normal process? As a corollary question, why and in what way is the return of the repressed a pathological phenomenon? In order to answer the first question, one

must take into account two related factors: (1) the role of social prohibitions, punishment, and threats of punishment in relation to certain wishes, thoughts, desires, and behaviors; and (2) Freud's move from his first ("toxic") to his second ("signal") theory of anxiety. The increased role of social-interpersonal factors in defense and the development of the "signal" theory of anxiety are intimately linked in the following way: Certain wishes, ideas, and actions come to be associated with anticipated "danger situations" (i.e., loss of object, loss of object's love, danger of castration, and later, superego anxiety), that is to say, they come to be associated with *anxiety*. Incipient experiences and expressions of these forbidden mental contents generate small doses of anxiety (i.e., anticipation of danger), which functions as a "signal" for the triggering of repression (and other defenses). When repression is successful, that is, when it succeeds in banishing danger-associated mental contents from conscious experience, anxiety is dampened or extinguished rather than intensified. In short, it functions as a negative feedback system, similar to a thermostat device, in which a signal triggers a mechanism that serves to dampen or "correct" the intensity of the triggering signal.

When repression fails—when the anxiety-laden mental contents are not successfully banished from consciousness—what may have originally been a small dose of signal anxiety becomes *amplified and intensified*, often to the point of a full-blown anxiety attack. In other words, we now have a positive feedback system in which the mechanism that, when it functions adequately, would dampen the triggering signal, now, by virtue of its failure intensifies the signal. Furthermore, if one keeps in mind that the anxiety, which has become intensified due to failure of repression, elicits further anticipatory anxiety, one can understand how the original failure of defense, and its consequent failure to keep the original signal anxiety in check, can lead to an upward spiraling of anxiety, to the point of a panic experience.

Quite apart from the discussion of repression, the positive feedback sequence I have described seems characteristic of certain clinical syndromes. For example, severely agoraphobic individuals will often report that when they wander too far from their experienced safe base (most frequently home) they not only experience the expected anxiety but also become anxious about being anxious and about the danger of an intensification of this anxiety. Of course, the anxiety about being anxious brings about precisely what is feared, namely, an intensification of the original anxiety. In short, in contrast to a negative feedback system (of which successful defense is an example), in which the initial anxiety triggers a mechanism that serves to dampen the anxiety, we see in this example the operation of a "runaway" positive feedback system in which the initial anxiety triggers a response that intensifies the initial anxiety and generates further anxiety.

It should be noted that the positive feedback system is not limited to situations in which anxiety is elicited by mental contents (ideas, wishes, and desires) that have come to be associated with the particular "danger situation" of parental disapproval and punishment. *Any mental content that for any reason comes to be associated with danger and anxiety may result in a positive feedback system if some means is not found to keep the anxiety from becoming amplified and intensified.* Banishing the mental content from conscious experience is one obvious means of preventing such intensification. In addition to the specific mechanism of repression, other means of accomplishing this goal are possible, including avoidance, denial, suppression, intellectualization, and tolerance for experiencing a given level of anxiety. Most people find some way of avoiding a chronic preoccupation with anxiety provoking thoughts that would keep one at a chronically high, or even spiraling level of anxiety.

I believe that quite apart from the specifics of Freud theory, it is in the preceding considerations that the adaptive or "normal" aspects of repression and repressive-like processes and the maladaptive aspects of failure of repression lie. That is, processes or "mechanisms" that enable one, under the appropriate conditions, to inhibit anxiety-provoking thoughts and feelings, and thereby prevent anxiety or keep it from spiraling may have adaptive functions: the failure of such processes and mechanisms may have clear maladaptive consequences. These conclusions hold whether or not one accepts particular aspects of Freudian theory (e.g., that certain sexual contents are associated with anticipated punishment and are therefore repressed).

There are many situations that illustrate the preceding conclusions. Consider, for example, the symptoms of fear of heights. Many people with this symptom report that when they are at a high height, they are "assailed" by thoughts of jumping (and, on occasion, urges to jump). Such thoughts, patients often report, seem to have a life of their own and cannot easily be

banished or inhibited by a voluntary attempt at suppression. Whatever their source or dynamic meanings, frequently accompanying fear of heights are these anxiety-inducing thoughts that cannot be inhibited or suppressed. That is, such individuals cannot stop thinking about or banish these ideas from consciousness when they are at a high height. In a sense, then, the fear-of-heights syndrome represents a failure of an inhibitory, repression-like mechanism that would enable the individual to stop thinking anxiety-laden thoughts.

There are many potentially anxiety-laden situations in which a kind of "not thinking" is an adaptive coping strategy. Consider as an example of the adaptive function of "not thinking" athletic situations in which winning or losing a championship game depends on the success or failure of an athlete's action, for example, making or missing a foul shot in a basketball game. The common wisdom is that the athlete must not think about what is riding on making or missing the foul shot. Indeed, a common tactic for the opposing team is to call a time out, either before the first foul shot is taken or between two foul shots, in order to give the foul shooter from the opposing team time to think about the importance of the upcoming shot and perhaps to "choke up." Indeed, what is meant by "choking up" is becoming anxious in situations where a great deal is riding on one's performance, with the result that one's performance is compromised. Such choking up implies that an excessive awareness or thinking about what is at stake and the anxiety it generates are directly implicated in compromising one's performance. What is necessary for optimal performance in the athletic situation is a background awareness, rather than a focal awareness, of the reality of the situation combined with an ordinary focus on carrying out the task— rather than on the extraordinary importance of the task or the extraordinary implications of one's success or failure at the task. In short, one must fine-tune a combination of background awareness and inhibition of certain anxiety-inducing thoughts.

The preceding examples raise the larger issue of when avoidant, denial, self-deception, and repression-like processes are adaptive, and when they are maladaptive. The psychoanalytic, certainly the Freudian, theory of psychopathology and treatment, as well as its underlying value system, partly rests on the assumption that awareness is liberating and curative, and that any limitation on awareness is inherently restrictive and, in many circumstances, pathogenic. However, there is a large nonpsychoanalytic literature suggesting that the real story is far more complex, and that the adaptive or maladaptive nature of what one might call awareness-restricting versus awareness-enhancing processes, is not at all a simple matter. I will return to the issue briefly later in the article.

Let us now return to the specific issue of repression and briefly recapitulate the two related questions I have been addressing: one, in what way repression is a normal adaptive process, and, two, in what way the return of the repressed (and the failure of defense that it implies) is pathological. To summarize the earlier discussion of these two points, certain mental contents have come to be associated with anxiety, and insofar as successful repression removes these contents from consciousness, it keeps anxiety in check. When repression is not successful, these anxiety-inducing mental contents cannot be entirely kept from consciousness and signal anxiety threatens to become traumatic anxiety. A partial solution is found in the formation of neurotic symptoms, which represent a compromise between the repressed mental contents and repressing forces. In that sense, neurotic symptoms constitute "a secondary defense" and "protective measures" (Freud, 1896: 172). Neurotic symptoms constitute "protective measures" in a number of ways. They are protective insofar as they entail partial (and disguised) discharge of excitation and thereby prevent a buildup of potentially damaging excessive excitation. But, in the context of a hydraulic model a "full" rather than a partial return of the repressed would even *better accomplish this "draining away" or discharge of excitation. If repression is pathogenic (partly) because it may lead to the buildup of excessive exaltation, then surely the failure of repression cannot be pathogenic for the same reason.* For it would seem that if repressed impulses gained entry to consciousness and access to motility and possibility of action, the likelihood of discharge of excitation would be increased and the consequent risk of excessive excitation decreased. Other considerations must be involved that lead to the conclusion that failure of repression is pathological.

One such consideration is that if the repressed contents reached consciousness (and access to motility), the anxiety that would be elicited by these contents (because of their association with the "danger situations" of loss of object, and the like) would entail a far greater level of excitation than the sum of excitation that is the result of repression. Implied in this latter view are (1) the famil-

iar idea that repression would not be necessary in the first place were it not for the fact that "the cultural development imposed on mankind . . . necessitates the restrictions and repression of the sexual instinct" (Freud, 1913: 209), and (2) the idea that the return of the repressed would not be pathological were it not for the fact that it elicits strong anxiety.

Repression and the Inherent Antagonism Between Id and Ego

According to the preceding account, because repression would not be necessary were it not for a particular kind of socialization, there would be no question of return of the repressed were it not for a particular type of cultural development. However, this scenario does not help one understand why, in some of his writings, Freud (as well as Anna Freud) suggests that there is an *inherent* antagonism between instinctual impulses and the ego, quite independent of forms of socialization, and why, therefore, the ego needs to defend itself against instinctual impulses, again quite independently of forms of socialization. As early as 1896, Freud refers to the danger of the ego being "overwhelmed" (Freud, 1892–1899: 227). He also refers to the "psychical helplessness" of the ego in the face of instinctual danger (Freud, 1926: 166). Finally, in *The Ego and the Id*, Freud (1923) writes that the ego's "fear is of being overwhelmed or annihilated" by external and "libidinal danger" (p. 57). Anna Freud (1966) explicitly refers to "the ego's primary antagonism to instincts" (p. 157). In the course of their work, both Freud and Anna Freud discuss the possibility of the ego being overwhelmed by the sheer quantitative strength of instinct. The implication is that the sheer intensity of instinct may represent a threat to the ego, independent of social prohibitions (although the latter may add to the threat by virtue of restriction on discharge of instinctual impulses).

In what ways does instinct represent an inherent threat to the ego? There are a number of answers to that question. The most general metapsychological one, based on Freud's constant principle, is that insofar as instinct entails an increase in the sum of excitations, it *places a demand on the ego, to find a way to decrease the level of excitation.* When the demand is too great, or the ego's capacity inadequate to the intensity of the demand, there is the danger of the ego being overwhelmed. One might say that the threat constituted by any demand on the ego is always relative to the ego's capacity. Thus, a demand that is experienced as a threat by someone with a relatively "weak" ego will likely be experienced as quite manageable by someone with a "strong" ego.

How, according to the logic of Freudian theory, would the condition of the ego being overwhelmed by instinct manifest itself in behavioral and clinical terms? Some possibilities include engaging in bizarre and destructive actions that appear to be "driven" and beyond the individual's control; a relative failure of secondary process thinking and the predominance of "drive organization" or primary process organization of cognition (Holt, 1967; Rapaport, 1967), as evidenced by various kinds of thought disorders; a relative incapacity to delay and to tolerate frustrations, as evidenced by impulsive and addictive behaviors; poor affect regulation; and inability to distinguish between reality and fantasy or wish, as evidenced by hallucinatory experiences and delusional thinking.

From an ego psychology perspective, all the preceding manifestations share in common a relative failure of ego functions and of primary and secondary ego autonomy. Furthermore, if one thinks of the ego as a controlling, delaying, and channeling structure, one can say that in all the disturbances just cited, the demands are too great for the ego to carry out its controlling, delaying, and channeling functions adequately. In addition to the various clinical manifestations previously referred to, one can get a more general feel for the idea of the ego being overwhelmed by instinctual demand by thinking of individuals who cannot seem to tolerate, and who become disorganized by, any experience or potential experience of intense affect.

What does repression—the main focus of this entry—have to do with the preceding discussion of the overwhelming of the ego by instinctual demand and the question of "weak" versus "strong" ego? One plausible hypothesis is that some individuals—those with weak egos—are so prone to feeling overwhelmed by intense affect or excitation of any kind that they engage in massive repression. However, since massive repression is difficult to maintain and itself puts a great strain on ego capacity, such individuals are also especially prone to failure of repression and return of the repressed. Note that according to this hypothesis, repression may be deployed not only against wishes and ideas that have been associated with punishment, but also, insofar as they also constitute dangers, the experience of intense

affect and excitation and wishes and ideas that elicit intense affect and excitation. In such situations, the failure of repression and the return of the repressed would be manifested not only in the experience of "incompatible" ideas and wishes whose specific contents are associated with punishment and anxiety, but also (or for certain individuals, primarily) in the experience of being overwhelmed by the sheer intensity of feeling and of level of excitation.

The fear and anticipation of being overwhelmed would lead to anxiety at the very prospect of experiencing intense affect; the anxiety is contained when intense affect can be avoided (partly through repression) and is fully experienced when intense affect cannot be avoided (failure of repression). When the latter occurs, the individual experiences an unmanageably increased level of arousal (is subjectively experienced as anxiety) from two sources: the intense affect that could not be successfully avoided, and the anxiety attendant upon that failure of repression. The individual most likely also relies on other defensive means to forestall the experience of intense excitation, such as the avoidance of situations and interactions that are likely to entail intense accumulation and strong affect, the isolation of affect, pedantry, overconformity, and ego restrictions and inhibitions.

Repression and Dissociation

Some discussion of the relation between repression and dissociation is relevant here. Freud's early account of hysteria relied heavily on such dissociation like concepts as "hypnoid states," "double conscience" (dual consciousness), "splitting of consciousness," and the "formation of a second psychical group." Along these lines, Breuer and Freud (1893–1895) wrote in their *Preliminary Communications* "that the splitting of consciousness . . . is present to a rudimentary degree in every hysteric, and that a tendency to such a dissociation and with it the emergence of abnormal states of consciousness . . . is the basic phenomenon of the neurosis" (p. 12). As we know, Freud soon relinquished dissociation accounts when he turned to repression—defined as the motivated banishment of "incompatible" mental contents from consciousness—as the "cornerstone" of psychoanalysis. However, Freud (1938) returned indirectly to the issue of dissociation when he wrote *Splitting of the Ego in the Process of Defense*, one of his last papers. Freud's return to the question of the "splitting of the ego" anticipates the primacy of "splits in the ego" in Fairbairn's (1952) formulations of psychopathology, and parallels, in certain respects, the contemporary preoccupation with dissociative mechanisms and phenomena, as for example, Kernberg's (1975) emphasis on splitting in borderline conditions, interest in posttraumatic stress disorders, the revival of interest in multiple personality, and concern with sexual abuse. In all these areas, dissociation plays a far more central role than the concept of repression. Indeed, it is my strong impression that one finds far more frequent references to dissociation them to repression in contemporary psychoanalytic literature.

Is it meaningful and useful to draw a distinction between repression and dissociation, and if so, what is the basic nature of that distinction? Some commentators (e.g., Erdelyi, 1990) have argued not only that Freud did not distinguish between repression and dissociation, but that "there is no formal distinction" between them (p. 11). I do not agree with this point of view and believe that it is useful to examine the distinction between repression and dissociation, although one should keep in mind that even if one distinguishes between the two, there is no sharp dichotomy between repression and dissociation. There are various ways to approach this issue. One can take the position, as some theorists do (including, at certain points, Freud) that dissociation is the generic term for processes that result in the failure to integrate mental contents into one's memory, conscious awareness, and/or unified sense of personal identity, and that repression is one form of this general process. This view, however, still leaves one with the task of distinguishing repression from other processes that result in failure of integration of mental contents. In addition, referring to dissociation as a generic process and the consequent failure to distinguish it adequately from repression overlooks certain historical realities, such as Freud's turn from dissociative concepts (e.g., hypnoid states, dual consciousness) to repression. The result of this turn was that whereas the development of psychoanalytic theory and treatment came to be increasingly linked to the psychoneuroses (in which repression was presumably central), the development of the nonpsychoanalytic theories of such figures as Janet and Morton Prince (e.g., 1906) came to be increasingly concerned with dissociative pathology (e.g., fugue states, amnesia, multiple personality). The "return" of psychoanalysis to the concept of dissociation was occasioned by an interest in the more severe pathologies of schizoid (Fairbairn, 1952) and borderline conditions (Kernberg, 1975).

In the context of discussing such topics as splitting of the ego, fetishism, disavowal, repression, and the different roles of the ego in neuroses and psychosis, Freud implicitly offers some useful and insightful distinctions between repression and dissociation. In discussing "splitting of the ego," Freud (1940) observes that "it is indeed a universal characteristic of neuroses that there are present in the subject's mental life, as regards some particular behavior, two different attitudes, contrary to each other and independent of each other" (p. 204). "In the cases of neuroses," he goes on to observe, "one of these attitudes belongs to the ego and the contrary one, which is repressed, belongs to the id" (p. 204). Despite the language of "splitting of the ego," it is clear that Freud is describing an interstructural conflict or "split" (i.e., between ego and id) rather than primarily an intrastructural split, that is, rather than a splitting of the ego. In psychosis, however, Freud describes "two psychical attitudes," one in which the ego is detached from external reality—because "reality has become intolerably painful"—and the other attitude that, to however minimal a degree, takes account of reality (p. 201). What mainly determines the diagnostic category to which the individual belongs is the relative strength of these contradictory attitudes. In psychosis, the ego's detachment from external reality is predominant and its taking account of reality is minimal and frequently virtually absent. According to Freud, there are also other psychological conditions, such as fetishism and reactions to severe loss, that are characterized by both the acknowledgment of an external reality (e.g., the danger of castration; the fact that women do not have a penis; a loved one is dead) and the *disavowal* of it. Freud (1927) describes reactions to the death of a loved one in which the death is both disavowed and acknowledged—both attitudes exist side by side (pp. 155–156). In these cases, the disavowal of reality is not psychotic because it is balanced by the equally strong presence of acknowledgment. We now know that one of the typical reactions to death of a loved one includes a stage of numbing and denial. Were such denial not balanced by some awareness of the reality, or were the denial excessively prolonged, or were such denial to take place in a different context, it would not be easily distinguished from psychosis.

There are a number of comments to be made regarding these observations. One, repression and neurosis always involve a "disavowal" of the individual's inner world of instinctual wishes, whereas in psychosis it is mainly (an "intolerably painful") external reality that is disavowed. Two, there exist a set of psychological conditions, which do not constitute either neurosis or psychosis, that involve both disavowal and acknowledgment of a piece of difficult reality. It seems to me that implied in Freud's account is that these latter conditions are characterized by nonpsychotic dissociative mechanisms and constitute a model of the operation of such mechanisms. That is, dissociation involves splitting of the ego's reality-testing (and also memory) function so that both disavowal and acknowledgment of an experience of a (traumatic) piece of reality, the representations of that experience, and the attitudes that correspond to disavowal and acknowledgment exist side by side. In extreme dissociation, the disavowal and acknowledgment and their accompanying attitudes may form "separate psychical groups" associated with separate personalities (i.e., multiple personalities).

It seems to me that Freud's observation as well as other considerations suggest relatively clear distinctions between dissociation and repression. Both historically and continuing into the present, the concept of dissociation is generally invoked in reference to *external trauma*, whereas repression is generally brought up in relation to *inner conflictual wishes*. That is, Breuer and Freud (1893–1895) noted, repression is a motivated attempt to banish from consciousness a mental content that is "incompatible" with (an already established) ego (and self-concept), whereas dissociative reactions "automatically" occur in response to traumatic events that overwhelm the individual's (or the ego's) normal coping capacity.

The use of repression as a defense implies an already developed and relatively intact ego that is able to keep mental contents inimical to it from reaching consciousness, and from threatening one's sense of who one is. Thus, when repression is successful, one's identity and consciousness remain unified, uninvaded by radically threatening and discrepant mental contents. This is so largely because threatening, ego-alien repressed material is kept from reaching consciousness, and from being directly experienced. Further, such material remains unconscious and inaccessible to conscious experience or is experienced in a partial and disguised way. This is what is meant by the idea of a horizontal barrier between conscious and unconscious, as seen in the diagram in Figure 1.

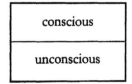

Figure 1. The horizontal barrier.

Although, as the horizontal line suggests, repression implies some kind of split in the mind, insofar as one's ego identity is equivalent to that which is conscious, one's sense of a unified consciousness and of a stable ego identity remain relatively undisturbed in successful repression. Furthermore, even when repression fails, as in the outbreak of neurosis, the threats to the unity of consciousness and to ego identity are limited to circumscribed "pockets" of ego-alien experiences to the form of neurotic symptoms that do not seriously compromise one's overall sense of unity of personality.

In contrast to repression, dissociation does entail a threat to one's experienced unity of consciousness itself and to the unity of personality. This is seen in a number of ways. Whereas repression keeps material from consciousness, in dissociation traumatic material reaches and "invades" consciousness, leading to experiences that are radically alien to one's normal state, with the result that the unity of consciousness is disturbed. Sullivan's (1953) concept of "not me" experiences comes to mind. When consciousness is "invaded" by massive ego-alien experiences that cannot be assimilated by one's existing structures, one's very sense of who one is (i.e., the unity of one's personality) becomes compromised. Furthermore, the "splits" that occur are not limited to subtle splits between conscious experience and unconscious mental contents, but include splits in consciousness itself—thus, Breuer and Freud's frequent references to "splits in consciousness," and "double conscience" when they understood hysteria in terms of dissociative mechanisms and processes. One may sum up much of this description by saying that whereas repressed material does not have *direct* access to consciousness (even when there is a partial failure of repression, the individual consciously experiences anxiety or neurotic symptoms rather than the directly repressed material itself), dissociated material *does* have access to consciousness, to alternative states of consciousness in the case of severe dissociation exemplified in so-called multiple personality (Hilgard, 1977). For whatever reasons, in dissociation the split-off segments of the personality achieve the same level of consciousness (and at times, the same level of personal ownership), as does the "normal" personality. Indeed, in severe dissociation, it may be not always easy to identify the normal personality. Thus, whereas in repression one speaks of one state of consciousness and one ego organization from which the repressed material is banished, in severe dissociation one finds alternate states of consciousness and different ego organizations. (This is what is meant by a vertical rather than a horizontal split.) As we have seen, in his early work Freud employed the terms "dual consciousness" ("double conscience"), and "the formation of second psychical groups" to capture these latter phenomena.

In contemporary psychoanalytic theorizing, Kernberg (1975) has attempted to make a clear distinction between repression and splitting in the context of discussing borderline personality organization and conditions. According to Kernberg, early in development "good" and "bad" object and self-representations (and their accompanying affects of love and hate) are not integrated into stable and unified representations. Also, according to Kernberg, in borderline personality organization these split good and bad representations either have not yet been integrated or there is a regressive use of defensive splitting. That is, good and bad representations are kept apart, with the result that the borderline individual alternates between primitive idealization and derogation (e.g., of the therapist). Note that Kernberg is essentially describing a dissociative process in which self-representations, object representations, and corresponding affects alternate with each other, a process very similar to "dual consciousness" and "the formation of second psychical groups." Note also that this dissociative process is clearly different from repression. Thus, when derogating the object, the individual does not repress the idealization—the idealization may be remembered. It is simply that the remembered idealization has minimal impact on the individual's current cognitive and affective state. Nor, when the individual is idealizing the object, does the memory of derogation have much impact on his or her cognitive and affective state. According to Kernberg, repression is a more developmentally advanced defense, requiring relatively stable and unified self and object representations.

Kernberg's description of splitting is very similar in certain respects, as are other descriptions of dissociative processes, to the phenomena of state-dependent learning, cognition, and memory. There is evidence from a variety of sources that in both animals and humans, what one learns in what one might call "one state of consciousness"—manipulated by or defined in terms of induced mood, type of drug administered, or some other means—is best remembered in that same state of consciousness and less well remembered in a different state of consciousness. For example, Bower (1990) has report-ed that when a depressed mood is induced (by hypnosis), individuals tend to recall sad and unpleasant events, a finding unsurprising to anyone who has observed depressed people. The point to be made in the present context is that when one is gripped by a particular mood or affect, cognitions and memories that are congruent with that mood or affect are recruited to one's conscious experience, with the result that much of one's state of consciousness is organized in a distinctive way, one different from one's state of consciousness when in a very different mood or experiencing a different affect.

This is similar to Rapaport's (1967) concept of drive organization of cognition. Although Rapaport focused on primary process versus secondary process thinking, the concept has broader application. Compare, for example, one's selective perception of the world—the affective tone of one's percepts and representations as well as one's state of consciousness—when one is ravenously hungry as compared with a state of satiety. Similarly, compare a state of sexual tension and desire versus a state of sexual release and gratification. Recognition of the capacity of sexual desire to influence strongly one's percepts, cognitions, representations, judgments, and decisions underlies the mature distinction between lust and love and the risks entailed in making long-term decisions based primarily on the former.

I have been struck with what one might call "the dissociations of everyday life." I venture to describe a personal experience because I have been told by others that it is a common enough experience. I wake up in the morning absolutely certain that I will eat carefully and will not "nosh" in the evening. During the day and through dinner, I am able to carry out my intention admirably. However, some time before going to bed, as I become increasingly tired and as I feel the need for some goodies or rewards with which to end a hard-working, tiring day, my resolve weakens and I "find myself" at the refrigerator door. I have made no conscious decision to annul my morning decision, yet there I am, noshing away. I am sure that I can recall my morning resolve—it has not been repressed—nor have I consciously decided to reverse or annul it. It simply has little influence on my current set of actions or my current state of consciousness. In subtle ways, I am a somewhat different person than I was in the morning. I strongly suspect that variations of the sort of phenomenon I am describing are ubiquitous throughout the biological and psychological rhythms of one's daily life. I refer to these phenomena as dissociations of everyday life because they involve subtle, nonpathological variations in the complex of affects, selective perceptions, attitudes, motives, desires, and so on that constitute one's state of consciousness.

Of course, if variations in motives, attitudes, and states of consciousness are widely discrepant from or even at odds with each other, then one is no longer talking about nonpathological dissociations of everyday life, but is describing pathological dissociation. In the variations that I have described as the normal dissociations of everyday life, there is a relatively stable core that is common to all these variations. Pathological dissociation, by contrast, is characterized by the relative absence of such a common stable core. This, I believe, is a critical difference between pathological and nonpathological dissociation. An obvious, extreme example of the relative absence of a common stable core of personality attributes is found in the case of multiple personality, particularly when the different personalities are markedly discrepant from and at odds with each other with regard to motives, values, desires, moral attitudes, and the like. A less extreme example of the relative absence of a common stable core is seen in the primitive splitting referred to earlier. The alternation of idealization and denigration is not compatible with a set of common core representations that are relatively stable across situations, time, and different affective and need states.

We generally insist on some minimal degree of stability of attributes in order to view someone as a reasonably intact person. From the point of view of a modular theory of mind, a minimal degree of relative stability also suggests reasonable success in the integration of different modules or conflicting structures, with the result that one is a relatively integrated and intact "unit." From this point of view, and as Spiegel (1993) points out, the so-called multiple personality is *not more than* but rather *less than* a single stable personality. For to be a single stable personality means that the various modules or constituents that make up a person have been integrated into, so to speak, a single, even if a very complex, unit. This integration the multiple personality has not achieved. Rather, modules or constituent parts, what Freud (1894) referred to as "separate psychical groups" (p. 49), have remained outside of and unintegrated into that hierarchical organization that we refer to as a single, intact personality.

As noted earlier, there is some evidence that dissociative processes are especially associated with experiences of severe external trauma, including sexual abuse. The experience of a chaotic and traumatic life may lead to a compartmentalization that makes it possible to go on with one's life despite the existence of chaos and trauma. As one patient diagnosed as multiple personality put it, the dissociations allowed her to "survive and go on with my life. . . . It was all just too much for one person" (Finnegan, 1993: 23). Thus, in the present context, dissociative processes can be understood not only as a failure of integration, but also as an adaptive attempt to "exclude painful realities from normal waking consciousness and allow psychic development to proceed, although in a manner not without compromise" (Finnegan, 1993: 27).

REFERENCES

Bower, G. (1990). Awareness, the unconscious, and repression: An experimental psychologist's perspective. In J. L. Singer (ed.). *Repression and Dissociation*. Chicago: University of Chicago Press.

Breuer, J., and Freud, S. (1893–1895). *Studies on Hysteria*. S.E. 2: 1–305.

Eagle, M. (1981). Interests as object relations. *Psychoanalysis and Contemporary Thought*, 4: 527–565.

——. (1982). Interests as object relations. In J. Masling (ed.). *Empirical Studies in Analytic Theory*. Hillsdale, N.J.: Erlbaum.

——. (1997). Attachment and psychoanalysis. *British Journal of Medical Psychology*, 70: 217–229.

——. (1998). The scientific status of psychoanalysis. *Psychoanalytic Psychology*, 15 (2): 281–310.

Ellenberger, H. (1970). *The Discovery of the Unconscious*. New York: Basic Books.

Erdelyi, M. H. (1990). Repression, reconstruction, and defense. History and integration of the psychoanalytic and experimental frameworks. In J. L. Singer (ed.). *Repression and Dissociation*. Chicago: University of Chicago Press.

Fairbairn, W. R. D. (1952). *Psychoanalytic Studies of the Personality*. London: Tavistock.

Finnegan, P. (1993). On multiple personality. Paper presented on May 12 to Toronto Psychoanalytic Society.

Freud, S. (1893). On the psychical mechanism of hysterical phenomena: A lecture. S.E. 3: 25–39.

——. (1892–1899). Extracts from the Fliess papers. S.E. 1: 175–280.

——. (1894). The neuro-psychoses of defense. S.E. 3: 43–70.

——. (1896). Further remarks on the neuro-psychoses of defense. S.E. 3: 163–185.

——. (1913). On psycho-analysis. S.E. 12: 207–211.

——. (1914a). On the history of the psycho-analytic movement. S.E. 14: 2–66.

——. (1914b). On remembering, repeating, and working-through (further recommendations on the technique of psychoanalysis II). S.E. 12: 143–156.

——. (1915). Repression. S.E. 14: 146–158.

———. (1920). *Beyond the Pleasure Principle.* 18: 1–64.

———. (1926). *Inhibitions, Symptoms, and Anxiety.* S.E. 20: 77–174.

———. (1927). Fetishism. S.E. 21: 149–157.

———. (1930). *Civilization and Its Discontents.* S.E. 21: 57–145.

———. (1937). Analysis terminable and interminable. S.E. 23: 209–253.

———. (1938). Splitting of the ego in the process of defense. S.E. 23: 271–278.

———. (1940). *An Outline of Psycho-Analysis.* S.E. 23: 141–207.

———. (1950). Extracts from the Fliess papers: Draft K. The neuroses of defense. (January 1, 1896). S.E. 1: 220–229.

Hilgard, E. R. (1977). *Divided Consciousness: Multiple Controls in Human Thought and Action.* New York: Wiley Interscience.

Holt, R. R. (1967). The development of the primary process. *Psychology Issues,* 5: 345–400. (Monograph 18/19). New York: International Universities Press.

Janet, P. (1889). *L'Automatisme Psychologique.* Paris: Alcan.

Kernberg, O. (1975). *Bordeline Conditions and Pathological Narcissism.* New York: Aronson.

Kohut, H. (1984). *How Does Analysis Cure?* Chicago: Chicago University Press.

Rapaport, D. (1967). *The Collected Papers of David Rapaport,* (ed.). M. M. Gill. New York: Basic Books.

Spiegel, D. (1993). Letter, May 20, 1993, to the Executive Council for the Study of Multiple Personality and Dissociation. *News, International Society for the Study of Multiple Personality and Dissociation,* 11 (4): 15.

Sullivan, H. S. (1953). *The Interpersonal Theory of Psychiatry.* New York: Norton.

Szalai, J. D., and Eagle, M. (1994). The role of deployment of attention in the overlearning reversal effect (ORE) with agressive and non-aggressive stimuli. *Psychoanalytic Review,* 72: 1195–1201.

MORRIS EAGLE

Research on Psychoanalysis

Freud considered psychoanalysis to be a unique form of inquiry that permitted observation of the unconscious. He further thought of free association, in particular, as a method not requiring external validation, or what has come to be known as "extraclinical demonstration" of its reliability. Despite his disavowal of the need for extraclinical validation of psychoanalytic hypotheses, in the second half of the twentieth century, the United States and Germany, especially, have produced a large corpus of research on psychoanalysis. Investigators have used extraclinical methods to study videotapes of psychoanalytic exchanges and sessions. There are also now computer-based studies of the interactions that occur in an analysis, computer-sorting approaches, and correlational studies carried out in accord with various models of treatment.

Current research focuses on the *process* of psychoanalysis, usually carried out on single sessions, or parts of sessions, of prerecorded analyses; *outcome studies* of psychoanalytic treatment with pre- and postanalytic measurement; and, finally, the *testing of psychoanalytic propositions,* especially through the direct observation of infants and children as they progress on the path to adulthood. There are a number of established centers where this work has been carried out and where formulations of new methods have been elaborated. The Ulm group in Germany, under the leadership of Thoma and Kachele, has gathered a very large tape library of analytic and psychotherapeutic sessions, as have Dahl and Teller in New York, Luborsky in Philadelphia, M. Horowitz, and Weiss and Sampson in San Francisco, to mention a few. These tapes have been open to critical reevaluation by scientists using different methods of study, and many of the extant studies are on a specific segment of the analysis of a patient known as "Mrs. C." The Mrs. C. file represents a completed, clinically successful analysis of some one thousand hours, conducted by an experienced analyst, that was subsequently transcribed and partially computer coded. It also has been scored with a variety of measures ranging from speech patterns to number of interventions and the like.

One of the earliest empirical research teams, Weiss and Sampson, tested the rival hypotheses of higher mental functioning (HMFH), where the patient tests beliefs with the therapist, and that of automatic functioning hypotheses (AFH), where repression is lifted by the interpretive process, as the means of change. They demonstrated that the HMFH provided a better account of the clinical facts than the conventional theory (AFH).

In another study, however, Caston and Martin (1993) failed to replicate their findings. This discrepancy is looked at as a demonstration of the efficacy of extraclinical, scientific approaches to testing psychoanalytic hypotheses, rather than as a simple inconsistency of findings, i.e., empirical testing shows that a psychoanalytic model can be disconfirmed, thereby indicating that the theory of change is amenable to extraclinical study.

Teller and Dahl note that the ultimate goal of any empirical inquiry is to develop a unified measure capable of identifying psychopathology, assessing the nature of the analytic process, and measuring the outcome of psychoanalytic treatment. Thoma and Kachele in turn seek to develop an empirically based theory of the process. None who do this work disavow that psychoanalysis studies subjectivity, but they do seek to translate idiosyncratic linguistic forms into public language. Mardi Horowitz, in turn, has examined the maladaptively repetitive elements in a patient's behavior, and has introduced the term "mental schemes." He seeks ultimately to formulate the shifting grounds of personality structure using this approach, while Enrico Jones, using classical Q-sort techniques employing judges, wishes to establish a basic language to classify interventions.

Each student of the psychoanalytic process has introduced his or her own carefully defined methodological stance. Luborsky uses a construct that sorts out core critical relationship themes (CCRTs). Horowitz has isolated what he calls a "role relationship" model, or RRM. And Dahl and Teller identify the recurrent structured sequences of events, representing wishes and beliefs manifested in actions, thoughts, perceptions, and emotions of the patient (fundamental repetitive and maladaptive emotion structures [FRAMES]). FRAMES are further based on the dual-code model of mental representation, as is Bucci's approach to psychoanalytic observation and research. In fact, Bucci proposes that there are three types of processing in analysis: a dominant nonverbal system, a system using verbal domination, and a referential process, which brings the two former moieties together in a therapeutic interpretive interaction.

Bucci and her colleagues describe the referential activity (RA) of the patient in terms of these multiple systems of reference, and trace the psychoanalytic process in relation to their fluctuations in cycles. The final, or referential, phase leads to the dominance of insight and making the representations precise in language.

The approaches of Dahl, Luborsky, and Horowitz are closely related. Careful scrutiny of each of these methods shows that each system is ordered in such a way that the subject and an object are viewed to be in interaction in a more or less stable structure in the mind of the patient. Horowitz's scheme designates the parties involved in what he calls "conflicted interaction." Each of the students of inner schemes concentrates on small units of observation and applies a specific reliable method of inquiry at various phases in the treatment, to ascertain the invariant repetitive interactions in an analysis. These patterns are thought to reflect an individual's plan or intention to code the world in a reproducible manner.

Enrico Jones has employed the Q-sort approach in analyzing data. He alerts us, however, to the error of averaging, suggesting that all of these methods can be used to examine cases in depth. Each observer also allows for observation from outside the clinical session, while acknowledging the constant possible intrusive effects of using a tape recorder. Thus, all hope that empirical observation will permit warranted scientific and even causal judgments about how the psychoanalytic process unfolds without taking a stand on the issue of whether hermeneutic and scientific approaches are in conflict.

Caston, armed with the observation that clinical senior analysts did not agree on a formulation following presentation of a clinical case, ventured to test whether there was something common in the language of psychoanalysis and the language of research, that might provide what he called a "mannequin" to serve as a basic confound in any observational scheme common in all empirical approaches. He found that the most common redundant construct was that of transference. To achieve reliability, each of these investigators insists upon having the coding done by unbiased observers and on some external validation for the outcomes measures employed.

The Ulm group has attempted to demonstrate how each method of analysis works, rather than finding a uniform approach to the process. They have introduced the idea of an *unconscious bargaining process* that takes place between the participants in an analysis. This leads easily to the matter of *outcome research* in psychoanalysis and psychodynamic psychotherapy, since Judy Kantrowitz, a Boston investigator, found that patient-analyst match has a significant effect on analytic outcome.

The most rigorous and complete evaluation of psychoanalytic outcomes is reported by Robert Wallerstein's study, *42 Lives.* Half of the patients studied were in psychoanalysis and half in expressive and supportive analytic psychotherapy at the Menninger Foundation. The study contains a number of surprises that can only arise in empirical work, for example, that structural change can be reached not only by insight but by supportive therapeutic modes, and even there with great emphasis on noninterpretive and supportive approaches.

The broadly conceived Columbia Records project, providing one of the largest database studies of psychoanalytic outcomes, including 1,575 adult patients treated at the psychoanalytic clinic between 1945 and 1971, was regrettably ahypothetical and does not offer firm con-

R

clusions. Nonetheless, the figures indicate a high rate of improvement with about one-fourth to one-third showing great improvement and more than half of those treated achieving good outcomes.

Lester Luborsky and his team's research centers on the core conflictual relationship theme (CCRT) and its use in treatment but also covers measurement of outcome and the use of CCRTs in the measure of transference. He also has completed a study of subjects with serious drug addictions and showed that dynamic therapy is efficacious in the population studied. Recent work by Kernberg and his colleagues on dynamic treatment of borderline conditions also represents a new foray into outcome research. They have developed adequate measures for establishing the reliability of interpretive methods and have further used these methods to study outcome.

Psychoanalysis may be said to have influenced research on child development most extensively insofar as the earliest proposals about the importance of mothering and caretaking have been tested by Spitz and others to demonstrate the Darwinian necessity of a continuous and sensitive parent for survival. Spitz's study of anaclitic depression in the early years is but a small example of empirical research on pathology that grew out of psychoanalytic propositions. Similarly, Spitz's genetic field theory provided the basis for observations of the biodevelopmental shift that gives rise to the observation of the social smile at six weeks of age. Observations on separation anxiety and stranger response have led immutably to a large area of empirical work on separation as a paradigm for attachment. The Ainsworth "strange situation" model based on Bowlby's attachment model has been enormously fruitful in defining secure and insecure attachments of eighteen-month-olds and the persistence of these early attachment effects into later years, defining the beginnings of psychopathology.

Further infant research initiated by Dan Stern, Robert Emde, and others has permitted a sounder investigative base for such concepts as maternal-child attunement, social referencing, and the careful sequencing of social and psychological landmarks as the child advances through the developmental process. Further empirical approaches to the study of moral judgment and conscience have been stimulated by psychoanalytic theorizing concerning structuralization around the Oedipus complex and formation of the superego, with recent work by Emde demonstrating that children as young as three show rudimentary to firm internalized ethical and moral judgment.

Early cross-cultural studies on latency have indicated that some cultures are much more permissive in regard to the expression of polymorphously perverse sexuality. Nonetheless, there does seem to have been another shift in orientation during this period based upon cognitive, emotional, Oedipal, neurodevelopmental lines, all converging to create what Erickson has called "the age of industry" (Shapiro and Perry, 1976).

Similarly, research in adolescence has shifted away from the early psychoanalytic belief that this is necessarily a period of chaos rather than a period in which personality is consolidated around identity and sexual integration (Hauser et al., 1991). Thus empirical research on the psychoanalytic method and the testing of psychoanalytic propositions has converged to create firmer bases for proposals that derive from clinical methods. Moreover, the introduction of new computer techniques and a tape library of psychoanalytic case material will continue to provide data for future creative investigation.

REFERENCES

Bucci, W. (1993). The development of emotional meaning in free association: A multiple code theory. In A. Wilson and J. Gedo (eds.). *Hierarchical Concepts in Psychoanalysis: Theory, Research, and Clinical Practice.* New York: Guilford Press, pp. 3–47.

Caston, J., and Martin, E. (1993). Can analysts agree? The problems of consensus and the psychoanalytic mannequin. Vol. 2. The empirical tests. *Journal of the American Psychoanalytic Association*, 41: 513–548.

Dahl, H. (1988). Frames of Mind. In H. Dahl, H. Kachele, and H. Thoma (eds.). *Psychoanalytic Process Research Strategies.* New York: Springer, pp. 51–66.

———. (1993). The discovery of FRAMES: Fundamental repetitive and maladaptive emotion structures. Charles Fisher Memorial Lecture, New York Psychoanalytic Society, January 26, 1993.

Fonagy, P., Steel, M., Moran, G., et al. (1993). Measuring the ghost in the nursery: An empirical study of the relation between parents' mental representations of childhood experiences and their infants' security of attachment. *Journal of the American Psychoanalytic Association*, 41: 957–989.

Hauser, S. T., Powers, S., and Noam, G. G. (1991). *Adolescents and Their Families.* New York: Free Press.

Horowitz, M., Milbrath, C., Jordan, D., Stinson, C., Ewert, M., Redington, D., Fridhandler, B., Reidbord, S., and Hartley, D. (1994). Expressive and defensive behavior during discourse on unresolved topics: A single case study. *Journal of Personality*, 62: 527–563.

Jones, E., and Windholz, M. (1990). The psychoanalytic case study: Toward a method for systematic inquiry. *Journal of the American Psychoanalytic Association*, 61: 395–402.

Kantrowitz, J., Katz, A. L., and Paolitto, F. (1990). Follow-up of psychoanalysis five to ten years after termination: vol 3. The relation of the transference neurosis to the patient-analyst match. *Journal of the American Psychoanalytic Association*, 38: 655–678.

Luborsky, L. (1990). A guide to the CCRT method. In L. Luborsky and P. Crits-Christoph (eds.). *Understanding Transference—The CCRT Method.* New York: Basic Books, pp. 15–36.

Shapiro, T., and Emde, R. N. (eds.) (1995). *Research in Psychoanalysis: Process, Development, Outcome.* New York: International Universities Press.

Shapiro, T., and Perry R. (1976). Latency revisited: The significance of age 7 ± 1. *Psychoanalytic Study of the Child*, 31: 79–105.

Spence, D. P., Dahl, H., and Jones, E. (1993). Impact of interpretation on associative freedom. *Journal of Consulting and Clinical Psychology*, 61, 395–402.

Wallerstein, R. S. (1986). *Forty-two Lives in Treatment: A Study of Psychoanalysis and Psychotherapy.* New York: Guilford Press.

Weiss, J., and Sampson, H. (1996). *The Psychoanalytic Process: Theory, Clinical Observation and Empirical Research.* New York: Guilford Press.

THEODORE SHAPIRO

Resistance

The resistant patient has never been able to confront the reality of just how disappointing her infantile objects really were. Instead, she protects herself against the pain of her grief by clinging to defenses that enable her to avoid dealing with her disappointment. These defenses constitute the patient's resistance and reflect her refusal to let herself know the truth about her objects. In the final analysis, the patient's resistance results from her refusal to grieve.

In the resistant patient there is conflict between (1) healthy (but anxiety-provoking) forces that would impel her in the direction of progress were such forces given free rein and (2) unhealthy (but anxiety-assuaging) counterforces, mobilized in response to the first set of forces, that impede her forward movement.

How do these resistive counterforces get played out in the treatment situation? The patient's need for her objects to be other than who they are gives rise to transference—both positive (in which the patient experiences the therapist as the "good" parent she never had) and negative (in which the patient experiences the therapist as the "bad" parent she did have). As a consequence, there is tension between (1) the patient's healthy ability to acknowledge the reality of who the therapist is and (2) her transferential need to experience the therapist as someone the therapist is not—be it a good parent or a bad parent. In other words, there is conflict within the resistant patient between her capacity to know the truth about the therapist and her defensive need not to know.

More generally, there will always be tension within the resistant patient between (1) her capacity to accept the truth about her objects and (2) her defensive need to deny that truth and to instead to insist that her objects be other than who they are; there will then be tension between their knowledge of reality (informed by her observing ego) and their experience of reality (informed by her experiencing ego). The internal tension created through the patient's awareness of that discrepancy will provide, ultimately, the impetus for therapeutic change.

As part of the working-through process, patient and therapist must both recognize the existence of the patient's defenses; appreciate the patient's investment in having them (the "gain"); and understand the price the patient pays for holding on to them (the "pain").

With respect to the gain, the patient must come to see that she is invested in maintaining her defenses because they serve to protect her against the pain of knowing the truth about her infantile objects. But within the context of safety provided by the relationship with her therapist, the patient will have an opportunity to achieve belated mastery of the parental failures. The patient will be able to do now what she could not possibly do as a child—that is, she will have an opportunity to grieve. As she begins to confront the reality of who her parents really were and as she starts to let herself feel the pain and the outrage against which she has spent a lifetime defending herself, the defenses (around which the resistance has organized itself) will become less necessary.

With respect to the pain, the patient must also come to feel the full impact of just how costly her refusal to know the truth about her infantile objects has actually been. As she begins to recognize the price she has paid for refusing to know, the defenses (to which she had once clung in order to ease her anxiety) will become themselves a source of anxiety. As the defenses become increasingly anxiety provoking, such defenses will no longer serve the patient as they once had and will become less adaptive.

As the defenses are gradually relinquished, the resistance will be overcome. The patient will let go of her infantile attachments—of her relentless pursuit of infantile gratification from her therapist (positive transference) and her compulsive need to re-create the early-on traumatic failure situation in the here-and-now engagement with her therapist (negative transference). She will now be free to experience her objects as they are, no longer needing them to be otherwise. Need will have been transformed into capacity, as the patient's need to experience reality in ways determined by her past is transformed into a capacity to know and to accept reality as it is.

At this point, the positive forces that had been held in check by the resistive counterforces will be liberated and, now unchecked, will fuel the patient's forward movement. The process will be accompanied by transformation of her infantile hope into mature hope (Searles, 1979). Mature hope will arise as the patient confronts the reality of her early-on disappointments and losses, as she grieves those heartbreakingly painful realities and discovers that she can survive the experience—sadder perhaps but certainly wiser and more solidly grounded. No longer held back by the infantile need for her objects (both past and present) to be different, the patient will now be open to experiencing reality as it is and able to direct herself toward the actualization of her realistic hopes and dreams.

REFERENCES

Searles, H. (1979). The development of mature hope in the patient-therapist relationship. In H. Searles, *Countertransference and Related Subjects: Selected Papers.* New York: International Universities Press, pp. 479–502.

Stark, M. (1994a). *Working with Resistance.* Northvale, N.J.: Jason Aronson.

———. (1994b). *A Primer on Working with Resistance.* Northvale, N.J.: Jason Aronson.

———. (1999). *Modes of Therapeutic Action: Enhancement of Knowledge, Provision of Experience, and Engagement in Relationship.* Northvale, N.J.: Jason Aronson.

MARTHA STARK

Return of the Repressed

Return of the repressed is a psychic process characterized by perplexing symptoms or ideas that symbolically express previously repressed traumatic memories, or covertly indulge a previously fended-off and prohibited gratification. Psychoanalysis of the process may culminate in recovery of memories.

Freud's first usage of the term "return of the repressed" appeared in 1896 (Freud, 1896). He posits the collapse of a psychical mechanism of unconscious defense against a distressing *sexual* idea opposed by the ego and originating in a prepubertal sexual trauma. The previously repressed material that now commands the attention of the psyche is the content of "the return of the repressed." In the same paper, Freud further proposes his general theory that symptoms are compromises between repressed material and repressing forces. Thus, symptoms represent a relative failure of the repressing force and function as a first stage in the return of the repressed. When perplexing symptoms arise, the analyst is advised to infer the recent collapse of a previously successful defensive repression that was an earlier developmental achievement.

Freud offers the clinical illustration of a boy of eleven who had been seduced in his bed by a servant girl when he was a younger child. The return of the repressed takes the pathway of obsessional rituals to fend off the seducer, walling his bed around with obstacles, kicking in his sleep, and confessing unrelated peccadillos to his mother.

"Return of the repressed" should be distinguished from a related term in the literature, "de-repression." The latter term ordinarily refers to the recovery of repressed material in a purposeful fashion, as a result of psychoanalytic work. In contrast, "return of the repressed" connotes an involuntary process, due to the failure of the unconscious but purposeful defensive process opposing emergence of the repressed material.

The mechanism of the "return of the repressed" must also be differentiated from the mechanism of character development. According to Baudry (1989, p. 655), what distinguishes character development from the mechanism of neurosis is the absence of any miscarriage of repression. In character development, repression either does not come into action or smoothly achieves its end.

The construct of "return of the repressed" has retained clinical currency across the many theoretical developments since its first appearance. The term occurs twenty-six times in Freud's papers, and is found in four hundred seventy-eight articles in the PEP/CD-ROM database of major psychoanalytic journals up to 1994 (about 1.5 percent of all articles).

One fruitful application of this construct has been the treatment of adult survivors of childhood incest

(Greer, 1994: 545–561). Analysts have used the concept, when formulating analytic reconstructions, to explain the analysand's multiple symptomatology, thus assisting the analysand to develop a meaningful personal narrative linking past abuse and present reality. A notable form of the "return of the repressed" frequently observed in trauma survivors is "remembering in the body," i.e., "return of the repressed" through perplexing, medically unexplainable bodily sensations. Two clinical examples of "return of the repressed" via bodily sensations are (1) gagging during adult sexual relations as a bodily memory of forced oral sex during childhood, or (2) repetitive abdominal cramping as a bodily memory of forced enemas.

REFERENCES

Baudry, F. (1989). Character, character type, and character organization. *Journal of the American Psychoanalytic Association*, 29: 655–686.

Brenner, C. (1957). The nature and development of the concept of repression in Freud's writings. *Psychoanalytic Study of the Child*, 12: 19–46.

Fenichel, O. (1932). Outline of clinical psychoanalysis. *Psychoanalytic Quarterly*, 121–165.

———. (1933). Outline of clinical psychoanalysis. *Psychoanalytic Quarterly*, 292–562.

———. (1934). Outline of clinical psychoanalysis. *Psychoanalytic Quarterly*, 545–652.

Freud, A. (1963). The concept of developmental lines. *Psychoanalytic Study of the Child*, 18: 245–265.

Freud, S. (1896). Further remarks on the neuro-psychoses of defense. S.E. 3: 163–188.

Greer, J. M. G. (1994). Return of the repressed in the analysis of an adult incest survivor: A case study and some tentative generalizations. *Psychoanalytic Psychology*, 11: 545–561.

Loewald, H. (1973). On internalization. *International Journal of Psychoanalysis*, 54: 9–18.

Niederland, W. (1965). Panel: Memory and repression. *Journal of the American Psychoanalytic Association*, 13: 619–633.

Rizzuto, A. (1976). Freud, God, the Devil, and the theory of object representation. *International Review of Psychoanalysis*, 3: 165–180.

Shengold, L. (1982). Anal erogeneity: The goose and the rat. *International Journal of Psychoanalysis*, 331–346.

Waelder, R. (1951). The structure of paranoid ideas: A critical survey of various theories. *International Journal of Psychoanalysis*, 32: 167–177.

JOANNE MARIE GREER

Reviews of Freud's Works

See RECEPTION OF FREUD'S IDEAS.

Rorschach Test See PROJECTIVE TECHNIQUES.

Russia/Soviet Union, and Psychoanalysis

R

Psychoanalysis has had sharply fluctuating fortunes in Russia, where the World War I and massive upheaval brought Communists to power in 1917. At the time a population of one hundred seventy million, most of them peasants or new industrial workers, had approximately three hundred specialists to serve their needs in "neuropathology and psychiatry." For that hard-pressed profession, psychoses and institutional care were of far greater concern than neuroses and psychotherapy; therefore psychoanalysis had scant practical appeal. But a psychoanalytical movement had emerged in prerevolutionary Russia, and the translation of Freud's works into Russian was under way. The leading organizers, N. E. Osipov (1877–1934) and I. D. Ermakov (1875, date of death unknown), promoted not only the clinical practice of psychoanalysis but even more the extension of Freudian doctrine into cultural studies. That broad tendency continued in the Soviet period, when Osipov and Ermakov emigrated, but among those who stayed, including I. V. Kannabikh (1876–1939) published on the clinical practice of psychoanalysis and included it in his ecumenical *History of Psychiatry* (1928). The vision of Marxism as a fusion of all worthy elements in the human sciences, including Freud's doctrine, captivated some young enthusiasts of the revolution, most eminently A. R. Luria (1902–1977), who founded a psychoanalytical society in 1921. He was also a disciple of L. S. Vygotsky (1896–1934), a literary scholar who became a major psychologist. As they rose to leading positions in Soviet psychology, they quietly abandoned the Freudian cause, for the ideological establishment had turned against it.

To explain the modest Soviet support that psychoanalysis enjoyed until the mid-1920s some speculation has focused on Leon Trotsky, the most important Communist after Lenin in the early years of the Russian Revolution. During Trotsky's prerevolutionary exile in Vienna, he had attended some meetings of Freudians, and, in his postrevolutionary outpouring of cultural commentary, he offered a brief speculation concerning the discordant efforts to create a science of mind or psyche. Trotsky pictured psychoanalysis and Pavlov's doctrine as complementary approaches, the former working "from the top down," the latter "from the bottom up."

Pavlov disdained to comment in public, while privately condemning psychoanalysis, a judgment that would weigh heavily against it when the Soviet ideological establishment exalted Pavlov's doctrine in the 1930s.

A major Soviet "Freudo-Marxist" was A. B. Zalkind (1888–1936), a Communist physician who championed "psychohygiene," as the Soviets called their version of a mental health movement. By warning Soviet activists against the excessive strain and extreme self-denial that had been exalted during the heroic early years after the revolution, this movement provoked a backlash from bosses who wanted no excuses for weaklings and slackers. "Psychohygiene" of any doctrinal form perished in "the great break," as Soviet dictator Joseph Stalin called the peak of forced industrialization and collectivization in 1929–1932, when he insisted that there were no limits on what Bolsheviks could achieve, "if we but nerve ourselves to it." Freudian doctrine invited especial hostility from the ideological establishment for the notion that normal and neurotic are not an either-or distinction between healthy and sick but a more-or-less variation within the common human condition, a kinship in illness that transformation of social relations cannot change.

Such issues were not debated at a profound level, whether in psychology or philosophy. The Russian Psychoanalytical Society had only about thirty members at its peak in the 1920s, when signs of official disapproval mounted toward anathema. Until the 1940s, a distinction between Freudian theory and psychoanalytic therapy permitted a vestigial continuation of psychoanalysis. The theory was reviled for its alleged pessimism, its emphasis on adaptation of suffering people to existing society rather than transforming society to remove the causes of suffering. The therapy was conceded to be of some benefit, though the medical services offered no support for it, and official condemnation of the theory was so heavy-handed as to crush the distinction. Already in 1929, when Wilhelm Reich visited Moscow and defended psychoanalytic theory at the Communist Academy, the cause was virtually lost. He implicitly acknowledged that psychotherapy could have little value in a backward country, but argued that the Five-Year Plan and the collectivization of agriculture would soon create a prosperous society that would need the services of psychoanalysts. None of his audience expressed agreement; even Zalkind responded with hostility. The series of Russian translations of Freud's works had come to a halt, not to be resumed until the collapse of the Soviet system sixty

years later. The interest of literary intellectuals, most notably the group surrounding the critic Bakhtin, found its last notable expression in *Freudianism: A Critical Essay* (1927), by V. N. Voloshinov (1895–1936).

Driven underground in the 1930s, psychoanalysis began to resurface during the post-Stalin era after 1953. The concept of the unconscious was repeatedly called to the attention of psychiatrists and intellectuals at large, most notably by a 1978 conference in the Georgian Republic. An impressive international array of scholars generated two massive volumes of papers: *The Unconscious: Nature, Functions, Methods of Study.* But that remained an isolated sign of a possible thaw, which became significant as Soviet reformer and leader Mikhail Gorbachev's policy of glasnost (openness) eased censorship in the late 1980s. A. I. Belkin renewed the publication of Freud's works in Russian—prefaced by a reminiscence of clandestine psychoanalysis in the forbidden years—and started an annual periodical of psychoanalytical papers. At first the ideological stance was Marxist; the long taboo on Freud and his views was attributed to a totalitarian regime, which was declared to be at odds with genuine Marxism. But the sudden transformation of reform into systemic collapse brought total abandonment of such distinctions. Marxism in any form has been dismissed or reviled, while Freudian doctrine has been embraced, along with varieties of religious thought, as a replacement for the all-embracing world view that suffered collapse. Today advocates of Freudian theory in Russia tend to present it uncritically, as a grand vision that is supposed to make sense of human experience in its entirety. There is so far scant awareness of the complex currents in Western discussions of Freud's doctrines.

Speculation concerning national character is a persistent though marginal aspect of psychoanalysis. Freud occasionally ventured into that area, for example, in describing "the Wolf Man," a famous patient who was Russian, as closer to "the psychic life of primitive races" than "we," meaning Germans. (Freud's turn to speculation about "us," meaning Jews, as distinguished from "them," meaning gentiles, in *Moses and Monotheism* [1939] was a belated response to Nazi "race science.") At the start of the Cold War, Geoffrey Gorer and Margaret Mead contrasted "us" Westerners and "them" Russians, who are fated, to swing from extreme subservience to extreme anarchy, unable to stay at the golden mean of democracy, as "we" do. Recently Daniel Rancour-

Laferriere has found the "slave soul" of Russia with Freudian analysis. Most scholars, and even popular pundits and political leaders, avoid talk of that sort, whether Freudian or not, after a century of unprecedented mass violence, much of it justified by assignment of special qualities to particular nationalities.

REFERENCES

Belkin, A. I. (1989). Zigmund Freid: vozrozhdenie v SSSR? In A. I. Belkin (ed.). Z. Freid (S. Freud), *Izbrannoe*. Moscow: Vneshtorgizdat, pp. 5–35.

Etkind, A. (1993). *Eros nevozmozhnogo: istoriia psikhoanaliza v Rossii*. St. Petersburg: Meduza. Transl. *Eros of the Impossible: Psychoanalysis and Russian Culture*. Boulder: Westview.

Joravsky, D. (1989). *Russian Psychology: A Critical History.* Oxford: Blackwell.

Rancour-Lafferiere, D. (ed.) (1989). *Russian Literature and Psychoanalysis*. Amsterdam: John Benjamins.

Rice, J. L. (1993). *Freud's Russia: National Identity in the Evolution of Psychoanalysis*. New Brunswick, N.J.: Transaction.

Rossiiskii psikhoanaliticheskii vestnik. (1991). Moscow: Assotsiatsiia. Annual publication. A. I. Belkin (ed.). Includes important historical articles and bibliographies.

Volshinov, V. N. (1995). *Filosofiia i sotsiologiia gumanitarnykh nauk*. St. Petersburg: Asta-press. Includes his 1927 essay on Freudianism (also available in English translation) and an introduction by N. L. Vasilev, which analyzes Bakhtin's role.

DAVID JORAVSKY

R

S

Sachs, Hanns (1881–1947)

One of the most loyal and devoted of Freud's followers, Hanns Sachs exerted a huge influence on the development of psychoanalysis during the first half of the twentieth century as an esteemed teacher and training analyst both in Berlin and later in Boston, and as a stalwart member of Freud's inner circle. He also made a large number of contributions to the field of applied psychoanalysis through his many published books and papers. Furthermore, he is one of the first psychoanalysts who did not possess a medical qualification, thus ushering in the possibility of "lay analysis."

Born in Vienna on January 10, 1881, Sachs trained originally as a lawyer, obtaining a legal degree from the University of Vienna in 1904. Shortly after graduation, he happened to read Sigmund Freud's *Die Traumdeutung (The Interpretation of Dreams)*, and this experience revolutionized his life completely. Sachs subsequently attended Freud's Saturday evening lectures at the psychiatric clinic of the University of Vienna, and thereafter, although he practiced law without much enthusiasm, he devoted as much of his life as he could to the field of psychoanalysis and the development of the psychoanalytical movement.

His formal relationship with Freud did not begin in earnest until 1910, through an introduction from his friend Otto Rank. Apparently, Sachs had impressed Freud with his translations of the "Barrackroom Ballads" poems by Rudyard Kipling; and by 1912, Freud had presented him with a ring, inviting him to become a member of his special secret committee, along with Karl Abraham, Sándor Ferenczi, Ernest Jones, and Otto Rank. As a nonmedical analyst, Sachs joined forces with

Otto Rank, another of the early "lay" analysts, to concentrate on the development of applied psychoanalysis and on psychoanalytical studies of art and literature. To this end, Rank and Sachs became joint editors of the journal *Imago* from 1912 onward; together, they authored *Die Bedeutung der Psychoanalyse für die Geisteswissenschaften (The Significance of Psychoanalysis for the Mental Sciences)*, which appeared in 1913.

In 1918, while attending the Fifth International Psycho-Analytical Congress in Budapest, Sachs began to cough up blood (hemoptysis), and this symptom developed into an attack of pulmonary tuberculosis. Sachs abandoned his vestigial legal career and moved to the mountains of Switzerland, where he hoped to recuperate from his illness. He eventually established a psychoanalytical practice in Zürich, in spite of some reservations expressed by medically qualified colleagues in Switzerland. In 1920, he emigrated to Berlin, accepting an offer to train future psychoanalysts.

As a training analyst at the Poliklinik für Psychoanalytische Behandlung Nervöser Krankheiten, later renamed the Berlin Psycho-Analytical Institute in 1924, he treated many talented younger colleagues, large numbers of whom became influential psychoanalytical practitioners and theoreticians in their own right. His many training patients included Franz Alexander, Alice Balint, Michael Balint, Robert Fliess, Karen Horney, Hans Lampl, Rudolph Loewenstein, Barbara Low, Fritz Moellenhoff, Carl Müller-Braunschweig, Sylvia Payne, and Ella Freeman Sharpe, to name but a few. He also psychoanalyzed Annie Winifred Ellerman, known as Bryher, a writer and close friend of the poet Hilda Doolittle, who had herself undergone a period of psychoanalysis with Freud.

His principal publications during his years in Berlin include a psychoanalytically oriented book-length study of the emperor Caligula, entitled *Bubi, die Lebensgeschichte des Caligula*, which appeared in 1930, no doubt influenced by the increasingly visible presence of National Socialism in Germany; he also authored many articles on dream analysis and on the application of psychoanalysis to works of literature, in particular the plays of William Shakespeare. Throughout the 1920s until his death, Sachs wrote powerfully about numerous other topics as well, notably, the genesis of perversions, the formation of the superego, the contagious psychoses, obsessional rituals and happiness, not to mention psychoanalytical portraits of Napoléon Bonaparte, Julius Caesar, Benvenuto Cellini, Friedrich Schiller, Arthur Schnitzler, and August Strindberg, among others.

As the years unfolded, Sachs became increasingly independent in his work, though ever loyal to Freud. He ended his relationship with Otto Rank in 1924, presumably over Rank's growing interest in birth trauma; and in 1927, Sachs resigned from important committee work within the International Psychoanalytic Association. In 1932, Sachs emigrated to Boston, Massachusetts, one of the first psychoanalysts to flee from the growing Nazi menace in Germany, and he took up an offer to serve as a training analyst for the developing psychoanalytical movement in the Boston area. During his remaining years in the United States, he became one of the most influential and sought-after practitioners, in view both of his contributions and of his close relationship to Freud. His creativity flourished during this period; he became a teacher at the Boston Psychoanalytic Institute and an instructor at the Harvard Medical School, one of the first nonmedically trained faculty to be honored with such an appointment. Sachs wrote many books, including the landmark tome *The Creative Unconscious: Studies in the Psychoanalysis of Art*, as well as the affectionate memoir *Freud: Master and Friend*. He also founded the journal *American Imago* in 1939, based on the Viennese publication *Imago*, devoted to psychoanalytical studies of the arts, which still flourishes today.

In his final years, he remained devoted to Freud and even had the opportunity for a farewell visit with him in London in July 1939, only months before Freud's death. When Fritz Moellenhoff, a psychoanalyst who chaired one of Sachs's lectures at Black Mountain College, North Carolina, in 1936, asked the venerable Viennese analyst how he wanted to be introduced to the audience, Sachs replied humbly, "Do not say anything but that I have worked with Professor Freud." This attitude summarizes Sachs's position within the early history of psychoanalysis. Sachs himself died rather suddenly, after complications from lung disease, on January 10, 1947, on the very morning of his sixty-sixth birthday.

REFERENCES

Jones, E. (1946). Hanns Sachs. *International Journal of Psycho-Analysis*, 27: 168–169.

Loewenstein, R. M. (1947). Hanns Sachs: 1881–1947. *Psychoanalytic Quarterly*, 16: 151–156.

Moellenhoff, F. (1966). Hanns Sachs. 1881–1947: The Creative Unconscious. In Franz Alexander, Samuel Eisenstein, and Martin Grotjahn (eds.). *Psychoanalytic Pioneers*. New York: Basic Books, pp. 180–199.

Sachs, H. (1942). *The Creative Unconscious: Studies in the Psychoanalysis of Art*. Cambridge, Mass.: Sci-Art Publications.

———. (1944). *Freud: Master and Friend*. Cambridge, Mass.: Harvard University Press.

BRETT KAHR

Sadism See MASOCHISM AND SADISM; PERVERSIONS.

Sadomasochism See MASOCHISM AND SADISM; PERVERSIONS.

Schizophrenia

As early as *On Psychotherapy*, Sigmund Freud (1905) hoped for a psychoanalytic psychotherapy for schizophrenia. Freud maintained this guarded hopefulness to the end of his life (1940). E. Bleuler reported that discharges at Burgholzli tripled after the introduction of Freudian understanding (Federn, 1943).

Most influential in the United States in developing psychotherapeutic treatment for schizophrenia were Harry Stack Sullivan, Frieda Fromm-Reichmann, and their students. In England, Kleinian analysts routinely treated borderline and psychotic individuals. Winnicott, Fairbairn, and Guntrip (1969) also contributed to the treatment of schizophrenia. Benedetti (1987) has had a profound influence in this area in Switzerland and Italy. Benedetti and Furlan (1987) reported a series of fifty severe cases treated with psychoanalytic therapy (two to five sessions per week) for three to ten years by supervisees, with very good outcomes in 80 percent of the cases.

In the United States, contemporary contributors include Boyer, Eissler Giovacchini, Grotstein, Kernberg,

Ogden, Searles, Spotnitz, Volkan, and Wexler. Karon (Karon and VandenBos, 1981; Karon and Teixeira, 1995) described technique and a controlled randomized study that found that psychoanalytic therapy, as compared with medication, dramatically improved the thought disorder, led to a more human way of life, earlier discharge, less rehospitalization, and dramatically lower costs over a four-year period. Most effective was psychotherapy without medication, or with medication reduced as rapidly as the patient could tolerate.

Schizophrenics are widely varied human beings, using drastic techniques of adjustment. "The difference between neurotic, borderline, and psychotic is sick, sicker, sickest. But the mechanisms are the same" (Brenner, personal communication). E. Bleuler's (1911/1950) primary symptoms of the disorder include autism, withdrawal from people; the thought disorder, an inability to think logically when they want to; and, mistakenly, an absence of affect, or inappropriate affect. But massive chronic terror blanches out lesser affects and gives the impression of affective flatness. Inappropriate affect may only be inappropriate in the eyes of an external observer. Schizophrenics may develop hallucinations, delusions, catatonic stupor, or other severe symptoms. Every symptom is a manifestation of or defense against chronic terror—"anxiety" is too mild a term. (*DSM-IV* [1994] strangely omits any reference to anxiety.)

The worse one's early life, the less current stress it takes to become schizophrenic, e.g., Freud's "complemental series." It is the meaning of a stress that determines its severity.

There are always destructive experiences in the lives of schizophrenics. In most cases, but not always, experiences with parents (or the lack of experiences, i.e., deficit) have contributed to their vulnerability.

The problems of schizophrenics usually begin in the relationship between mother and child in the early oral period. But the same psychological battles are fought successively on the oral, anal, and genital battlegrounds. When their life situation, as given meaning by conscious and unconscious fantasy structures, gives rise to a terror against which patients cannot defend except by gross distortions of reality, hallucinations, paranoid delusions, becoming mute, etc., they become blatantly psychotic.

An unfortunate childhood may make a child feel worthless and unlovable. But to be unlovable means that mother will not love you, that she will abandon you, and,

to the infant, this means pain and death. This infantile terror lurks behind the schizophrenic symptoms.

The child denies the "bad" mother, but the more "ideal" the rejecting mother, the more unlovable the child. The child tries to find something wrong to explain the rejection. But, when he or she changes, the rejection remains. The only solution is never to change or to attempt to change something unchangeable. In either case one can maintain the reassuring (false) belief that if one did change, everything would be all right. The child also looks around for a second "mother"—turning to father, to siblings, to others—but the schizophrenic symptoms are evidence that the schizophrenic never succeeded in finding a "good" mother in these other persons.

Three misconceptions about schizophrenics are:

1. There are no repressions and no unconscious. But their unconscious is *not* conscious; schizophrenics have a consciousness that is dominated by the unconscious, the way that the manifest content of a dream is dominated by the unconscious, but it is not the raw unconscious itself.
2. There is no transference. In fact, much of the psychopathology of schizophrenia is nothing but transference to the world at large.
3. There is no affect. But the affect is terror.

Catatonic stupor was first described by Fromm-Reichmann (1939/1947) as including a conscious fear of dying "if I move." Experimental studies (Ratner, Karon, VandenBos, and Denny, 1981) confirm that catatonic stupor is an adaptive terror state in animals threatened by hungry predators, increasing the survival chances of the individual and the species.

Hallucinations are wide-awake dreams, caused by intense motives, and are understandable and interpretable by the same psychoanalytic principles as sleeping dreams, except that while hallucinations may occur in any sensory modality, auditory hallucinations ("voices") are almost always present, because schizophrenia is an interpersonal disorder.

Withdrawal from others, or "autism," is clearly a defense against the anxiety engendered by interpersonal encounters, but it prevents the growth processes that are dependent on interactions with others, including corrective identifications. Isolation has been shown to increase hallucinations.

S

Four principles account for most delusions (Karon, 1989):

1. Transference to the world at large.
2. Defenses against pseudo-homosexual anxiety, as described by Freud (1911), using the defenses of projection, reaction formation, displacement, etc.
3. The teaching by a particular family of peculiar concepts or meanings to words, which the patient then erroneously believes the rest of the world shares.
4. The need to make sense out of one's world and experiences, even if one's actual life experiences and symptomatic perceptions are bizarre, and therefore require unusual explanations.

The therapist must create a therapeutic alliance by providing sufficient protection and gratification to overcome the patient's *conscious* resistance. The possibility that the therapist will take away the psychotic symptoms, which are the best psychodynamic solutions of which the patient is capable, stirs up intolerable terror, except for the protection the therapist also provides. Every therapeutic intervention that reduces terror reduces other symptoms.

The therapist must repeatedly distinguish between thoughts and feelings versus actions. Only actions have consequences.

The role of insight is the same as in any psychoanalysis: making the unconscious conscious, changing the defenses in part by awareness, making the connection between the past and the present. Understanding the transference is central. The more severely disturbed the patient, the more obvious the transference reactions. Schizophrenics are constantly trying to solve their problems, but they are too frightened to deal with the real problems directly; they deal with symbols. Only when the symbolic act (or symptom) and the original traumatic experience are reconnected in consciousness can the person overcome it.

Internalized fantasy structures are changed by the internalization of the therapist as a benign superego, as a model for the ego, and as a model for relationships with others.

REFERENCES

American Psychiatric Association (1994). *Diagnostic and Statistical Manual of Mental Disorders.* (4th ed.). Washington, D.C.

Benedetti, G. (1987). *Psychotherapy of Schizophrenia.* New York: New York University.

Benedetti, G., and Furlan, P. M. (1987). Individual psychoanalytic psychotherapy of schizophrenia. In G. Benedetti (ed.). *Psychotherapy of Schizophrenia.* New York: New York University, pp. 198–212.

Bleuler, E. (1950). *Dementia Praecox, or the Group of the Schizophrenias.* New York: International Universities Press. (Original work published 1911).

Federn, P. (1943). Psychoanalysis of psychoses I. *Psychiatric Quarterly,* 17(1): 3–19.

Freud, S. (1905). On psychotherapy. S.E. 7: 255–268.

———. (1911). Psycho-analytic notes on an autobiographical account of a case of paranoia (dementia paranoides). S.E. 12: 1–84.

Fromm-Reichmann, F. (1947). Transference problems in schizophrenia. In S. S. Tomkins (ed.). *Contemporary Psychopathology.* Cambridge, Mass.: Harvard University Press. (Original work published 1939).

Karon, B. P. (1989). On the Formation of Delusions. *Psychoanalytic Psychology,* 6(2): 169–185.

Karon, B. P., and Teixeira, M. A. (1995) Psychoanalytic therapy of schizophrenia. In J. Barber and P. Crits-Christoph (eds.). *Dynamic Therapies for Psychiatric Disorders (Axis I).* New York: Basic Books, pp. 84–130.

Karon, B. P., and VandenBos, G. R. (1981). *Psychotherapy of Schizophrenia: The Treatment of Choice.* New York: Aronson.

Ratner, S. G., Karon, B. P., VandenBos, G. R., and Denny, M. R. (1981). The adaptive significance of the catatonic stupor in humans and animals from an evolutionary perspective. *Academic Psychology Bulletin,* 3, 273–279.

BERTRAM P. KARON
MICHAEL A. TEIXEIRA

Schopenhauer, Arthur (1788–1860)

Arthur Schopenhauer was a German philosopher and one of the major inheritors of the Kantian tradition. After a disappointed attempt at academic life, Schopenhauer removed himself from the academic community and, supported by independent wealth, devoted himself to reading voraciously (in seven languages) and writing. Schopenhauer's notable pessimism was at least partly the result of a bitterly unhappy relationship with his mother, whose fame as a novelist overshadowed him for many years. His father is likely to have committed suicide.

Schopenhauer produced his only major work while still in his twenties, *The World As Will and Representation* (1819). He never departed from the substance of this work, though he added a second volume to it in a second edition in 1844 (all references will be to this edition in the original pagination), and published a third volume of essays carrying the argument further in 1851, *Parerga and Paralipomena*. Prior to the publication of these essays and despite producing a masterpiece as a young man, Schopenhauer had been ignored. With the publication of these essays, he became one of the most widely read authors in the German-speaking world and beyond. This fame continued for the next fifty years or so.

The World As Will and Representation begins with the observation that the world is a representation, that is, that one "does not know a sun and an earth, but only an eye that sees the sun, a hand that feels an earth; . . . the world . . . is there only as representation" (1844, p. 3). For Schopenhauer, this is one of the two fundamental perspectives. The other, which is more important to us here, is the will. The will is fundamental; it underlies and animates everything that we would call the objective world. We can know something of this will by being aware of our own volition. Our volition is a limited manifestation of the same will from which the entire objective world arises.

Schopenhauer's analysis of the will reveals a remarkably sophisticated insight into human psychology. The will, which is largely unconscious, manifests itself most notably in sexual desire; sexual drive "springs from the depths of our nature" (1844, p. 511):

> The sex-relation . . . is really the invisible central point of all action and conduct, and peeps up everywhere in spite of all the veils thrown over it. It is . . . the basis of the serious and the aim of the joke, the inexhaustible source of wit, the key to all allusions . . .; it is the daily meditation of the young and often the old as well, the hourly thought of the unchaste, and even against their will the constantly recurring imagination of the chaste, the ever ready material for a joke, just because the profoundest seriousness lies at its root. (1844, p. 513, translation slightly modified)

We see here a deep-running anticipation of Freud's views on the universality of sexuality in human motivation. Again like Freud, Schopenhauer claimed that this influence is for the most part unrecognized.

Schopenhauer also anticipated Freud in his view of the relationship between the unconscious will and the intellect. The will creates the intellect to serve its interests. The intellect is therefore secondary and subordinate to the will and has no motives of its own. Indeed, the intellect "must surprise the will in the act of expressing itself, in order merely to discover its real intentions" (1844, p. 210).

Schopenhauer's argument for the existence of the unconscious also anticipates Freud. Like Freud, he argued that consciousness is fragmentary. If so and if mental life has coherent psychological causes at all, these causes must be unconscious. Such observations led him to a strikingly original reevaluation of the importance of consciousness in general.

Anticipations of Freud can also be found in Schopenhauer's reflections on the causes of madness. He himself applied his account to what we would now call psychosis or severe affective disorder. As an account of the etiology of major psychiatric illness, it is not very plausible. Taken as a theory of neurosis, however, it anticipates Freud's first theory of neurosis in the most remarkable way. Schopenhauer locates the source of madness not in a simple inability to connect to reality but rather in memory (1819, p. 192). He bases this view on some real empirical evidence. For many years, he visited insane asylums to observe and talk to the patients. He found that in some of these patients, memory is preserved, but in others "the thread of memory" is broken by traumas. Where the trauma has been strong enough to destroy an individual, the mind defends itself by destroying the thread of memory and "fills up the gaps with fictions" (1819, p. 193).

Thus, not only did Schopenhauer anticipate Freud's view that "hysterics suffer from reminiscences," he also saw the essentials of what Freud later came to call defense mechanisms, the mechanisms that troubled people use to deal with memories. Indeed, we can recognize both repression and resistance in Schopenhauer's discussion; he even used the German terms for them. And behind his picture is another prescient idea: that madness is not the result of neurological breakdown; it is a motivated though unconscious technique for coping.

We can find other anticipations. Schopenhauer takes the first steps toward the clinical insight that it is therapeutic to bring unconscious thoughts to consciousness, arguing that they are thereby deprived of their power. He also developed a detailed theory of dreams that has extensive parallels with Freud's later account, and urged that following trains of associations is a valuable technique for restoring the thread of recollection. Finally, there is Schopenhauer's argument that the behavior of the mad is analogous to everyday psychological mechanisms for banishing unpleasant thoughts. Thus, Schopenhauer even had insights into the "psychopathology of everyday life."

These anticipations naturally lead one to ask about the nature and extent of Schopenhauer's influence on Freud. The answer is not entirely clear. Prior to 1914, Freud made a few references to Schopenhauer, especially in *The Interpretation of Dreams* (1900), but not many. In 1914, having been shown a passage from Schopenhauer by Rank, Freud explicitly acknowledged Schopenhauer as a forerunner of psychoanalysis but claimed that he had read him only late in life:

> The theory of repression quite certainly came to me independently of any other source; I know of no outside impression which might have suggested it to me and for a long time I imagined it to be entirely original, until Otto Rank . . . showed us a passage in Schopenhauer's *World as Will and Representation* in which the philosopher seeks to give an explanation of insanity. What he says there about the struggle against accepting a distressing piece of reality coincides with my concept of repression so completely that once again I owe the chance of making a discovery to my not being well read. (1914, p. 15)

Even if is true that Freud did not read Schopenhauer until late in life, the cultural milieu in which Freud grew up had been saturated with Schopenhauerianism. Freud could no more have escaped Schopenhauer's influence than someone working in psychology today could escape Freud's influence, reading him or not. Moreover, Freud's most influential teachers knew Schopenhauer well, and a book that Freud is known to have studied carefully, Von Hartmann's *Philosophy of the Unconscious*, was devoted to developing Schopenhauer's psychological insights. In addition, Freud belonged to the *Leseverein der Deutschen Studenten Wiens* (Reading Society of the German Students of Vienna). Along with Wagner and Nietzsche, Schopenhauer was a prime topic of conversation. In short, the evidence that Schopenhauer had an early influence on Freud is strong, whatever Freud said later.

REFERENCES
Ellenberger, H. (1970). *The Discovery of the Unconscious: The History and Evolution of Dynamic Psychiatry.* New York: Basic Books.
Freud, S. (1900). *The Interpretation of Dreams.* S.E. 4–5: 1–621.
———. (1914). *On the History of the Psycho-Analytic Movement.* S.E. 14: 7–66.
Gardiner, P. (1963). *Schopenhauer.* London: Penguin Books.
Gardiner, S. (1999). Schopenhauer, will, and the unconscious. In C. Janaway (ed.). *The Cambridge Companion to Schopenhauer.* Cambridge: Cambridge University Press, pp. 375–421.
Gupta, R. (1980). Freud and Schopenhauer. In Michael Fox (ed.). *Schopenhauer: His Philosophical Achievement.* New Jersey: Barnes and Noble.
Hartmann, E. V. (1869). *Philosophy of the Unconscious: Speculative Results According to the Inductive Method of Physical Science.* New York: Harcourt, Brace, 1931.
Kaiser-Al-Safti, M. K. (1987). *Der Nachdenker: Die Entstehung der Metapsychologie Freuds in ihrer Abhängigkeit von Schopenhauer und Freud.* Bonn: Bouvier Verlag Herbert Grundmann.
Magee, B. (1989). *The Philosophy of Schopenhauer.* New York: Oxford University Press.
McGrath, W. (1986). *The Politics of Hysteria: Freud's Discovery of Psychoanalysis.* Ithaca, N.Y.: Cornell University Press.
Proctor-Greg, N. (1956). Schopenhauer and Freud. *Psychoanalytic Quarterly,* 25: 197–214.
Schopenhauer, A. (1819). *The World As Will And Representation,* vol. 1. Trans. E. F. J. Payne. New York: Dover, 1969.
———. (1844). *The World As Will And Representation,* vol. 2. Trans. E. F. J. Payne. New York: Dover, 1966.
———. (1851). Essay on spirit seeing and everything connected therewith. In *Parerga and Paralipomena,* vol. 1. Trans. E. F. J. Payne. Oxford: Clarendon Press, 1974.
Young, C., and Brook, A. (1994). Schopenhauer and Freud. *International Journal of Psychoanalysis,* 75: 101–118.

CHRISTOPHER YOUNG
ANDREW BROOK

Schreber, Daniel Paul (1842–1911)

Daniel Schreber was born July 25, 1842, in Leipzig, the third child of Moritz (1808–1861) and Pauline Schreber, née Wenck (1815–1907). He died April 14, 1911, in the Leipzig-Dösen Asylum. His father, a physician who developed active exercise therapy for musculoskeletal disorders, with and without appliances, attained world fame with his 1855 *Medical Indoor Gymnastics,* which became a forerunner of modern rehabilitation medicine. During the last decade of his life, Schreber's father suffered from depression and wrote many books on child rearing; after his death in 1861, he was immortalized in the eponymous Schrebergarten, a city allotment garden. His first son, Gustav (born 1839), suffered from tertiary syphilis with mental complications and shot himself in 1877. The line continued through the descendants of Moritz's second child, Anna Jung (1840–1944).

Daniel Paul Schreber graduated from Leipzig University and became a doctor of law and a judge in Saxony (in present-day Germany). His marriage in 1878 to Sabine Behr (1857–1912), daughter of an opera director, remained childless after six miscarriages, the last in 1892. In 1884, Schreber became depressed after losing an election campaign and was successfully treated at Leipzig University Psychiatric Hospital, headed by Paul Flechsig (1847–1929), better known as neuroanatomist than psychiatrist. Schreber was readmitted to Flechsig's hospital as a voluntary patient in November 1893, following a psychotic depression rooted in conflicts about career and marriage. The second illness began as a prodrome, with dreams of his former illness returning as he fantasized that "it must be rather pleasant to be a woman succumbing to intercourse." After Schreber served six weeks as Senatspräsident at the Superior Court of Appeals in Dresden, his illness erupted with sleeplessness, agitation, suicide gestures, and hypochondriacal and nihilistic delusions. In March 1894, Schreber began "his contact with God," experiencing supernatural phenomena, visions, and voices, feeling persecuted by Flechsig, who allegedly seduced God to take part in a plot to "commit soul murder on him: [1] the surrender of his soul to another person, after his nervous illness had been assumed to be incurable [and 2] unmanning, i.e., his body transformed into a female body for sexual misuse and simply left to rot." This dread of impending soul murder made him feel that the world was coming to an end. Also at that time, owing to money disputes, his wife petitioned the court to have Schreber declared mentally incompetent; moreover, his replacement by another judge was announced in a newspaper. Still depressed, he was transferred in June to Sonnenstein Asylum, where Superintendent Guido Weber (1927–1914) diagnosed incurable chronic paranoia, resulting in Schreber's permanent incompetency and involuntary status. Since his persecutory feelings toward Flechsig were but a transient phase of the major depression, Schreber rightly claimed that his illness was not paranoia, i.e., legally defined insanity, but a mood disorder and a "nervous illness," the latter making him susceptible to supernatural influences. While never disputing that he was seriously ill until 1896, Schreber disagreed with psychiatrists that his hallucinations were merely pathological, regarding them as "his inner spiritual life," albeit clothed in terms of an intricate fantastic cosmology and religion. Thus, in time, God turned from malevolent to benevolent and

bad unmanning into good unmanning, ordaining Schreber to cultivate soul-healing "sensuous pleasure (voluptuousness) and femininity." This Schreber achieved by the use of "fancy" and "imagination" and by practicing minor cross-dressing to create an "illusion" of being a woman, thus returning, now without guilt, to his original fantasy of becoming a woman in intercourse and regaining his lost capacity for pleasure.

By 1897, Schreber came out of his delusional depression and was lucid and rational, but his wishes to be discharged were thwarted by Weber's diagnosis, the incompetency and involuntary status, and his wife's hesitation to take him home. Even though during his trial to rescind the incompetency, Schreber still claimed that his continuing "hallucinations" were proof that he "was dealing with God and divine miracle," the judges gave him his freedom and the right to his "religious beliefs." He expounded these beliefs with great acuity and eloquence in his famous book (from which all the above quotations are taken), *Memoirs of My Nervous Illness* (1903; the title in the original was *Reflections of a Nervous Patient*), written in the asylum, a masterpiece that has inspired scholars in diverse fields. As of 1902, he functioned normally, raising with love an adopted daughter, Fridoline (1890–1981). In 1907, after his mother died and his wife had a stroke, he became terminally psychotically depressed, dying of cardiopulmonary complications, after having spent some thirteen years of his life in asylums.

Freud endorsed Weber's view of Schreber's religious paranoia and reformulated it as a homosexual paranoia. Already by 1908, Freud had in place his famous dynamic formula that homosexual desire and conflict, and the resulting libidinal detachment, cause persecutory paranoia, first clinically described by Sándor Ferenczi (1911). Learning about Schreber's book from C. G. Jung in 1910, Freud used his limited formula to interpret selected passages while conceding he "was not acquainted with the society in which Schreber moved and the small events of his life . . . to trace back innumerable details of his delusions to their sources." Assuming a negative Oedipal constellation, Freud based his fictional pathogenesis of Schreber's entire second illness on an unproved and historically wrong premise: that Schreber's core conflict was a passive homosexual wish toward Flechsig, manifest already in the prodromal fantasy about what a woman feels in intercourse, i.e., *before* he set eyes on Flechsig for the second time. Moreover, the "soul murder" incident, which occurred months *after* admission, was interpreted as a sexual transformation of that desire for Flechsig into a delusion of persecution rather than seeing it for what it was, i.e., a reaction to Flechsig's actions toward Schreber. This theory also misses the fact that there are many paranoias and many homosexualities. Freud's was thus an exercise in applied, formulaic psychoanalysis, creating a myth that Schreber was paranoid and homosexual to validate and generalize his theory. Freud published his own clinical cases of women presenting this dynamic in 1896, 1915, and 1920, and of men in 1922, advancing other theories about the genesis of hallucinations and delusions, but he did not use them on Schreber. Subsequent generations of commentators extended Freud's theory to a canonical formulation of schizophrenia. The first to claim that Schreber was schizophrenic was Gross (1904), copied by authorities like Jung, Bleuler, and Jaspers, but without a differential diagnosis of a mood disorder. Freud's libido theory of paranoia and schizophrenia was challenged by Melanie Klein and her followers, Macalpine and Hunter (1953), and Arlow and Brenner (1969), to name a few. It is to Freud's credit that he saw Schreber's symptoms as an effort of self-healing, which applies more to the feminine fantasies than to the end-of-the-world delusions.

The second myth, that Paul Schreber's second illness of 1893 was caused by his father's abuse at age three to four by means of his alleged "torture machines" (i.e., orthopedic appliances), was created in 1959 by Niederland and popularized by Schatzman (1973). However, Niederland (1963) did express this caveat: "I do not claim that the data so far accumulated throw light on the nature of Schreber's psychosis . . . some of them appear . . . to make the hitherto incomprehensible aspects of Schreber's delusional system accessible to further investigation." Niederland's readings of Schreber were part formulaic and part historical.

While of inestimable heuristic value, these myths have not stood the test of historical research. The first to present a clinical case study of Paul Schreber was the psychoanalyst and psychiatrist Baumeyer in 1955, stressing the role of aggression. An important documentary contribution was made by Devreese (1981). In 1989, Israels published the first full biographical documentation of the Schreber family, arguing that the father was unduly demonized (Freud had a good opinion of the father, too). However, Israels did not deal with the many meanings of Schreber's fantasies or consider Schreber as

a thinker in his own right. Starting in 1989 with the historical research of his predecessors, in 1992 Lothane presented Schreber, a life, based on new materials and a close reading of the *Memoirs* in their entirety, to show that Schreber's fears of sexual abuse were a result of the psychotic process rather than its cause; that his conflicts were heterosexual and rooted in an identification with his mother, not mentioned by Freud at all, and resulting in a dependent transference onto his wife, who did not fulfill his sex, love, and progeny needs; that issues of gender identity (Lothane, 1993), better understood today than a century ago, played a decisive role in Schreber's fantasies. A forensic analysis of the case, offered for the first time, showed that "soul murder" was Schreber's term for his persecution by a psychiatry that had lost its soul: the betrayal of his trust by Flechsig and the removal to a public asylum that doomed his legal career, and the long incarceration by Weber, a continuous traumatic state that kept reverberating in symptoms such as bellowing. Moreover, Lothane elaborated on the role of love and loss of love in the genesis of Schreber's depressive illnesses in 1884, 1893, and 1907. It was the losses preceding 1893 that awakened Schreber's creativity and led to the writing of his immortal *Memoirs*, a continuing inspiration for future commentators.

REFERENCES

Arlow, J. A., and Brenner, C. (1969). The psychopathology of the psychoses: A proposed revision. *International Journal of Psychoanalysis*, 50: 5–14.

Baumeyer, F. (1955). Der Fall Schreber. *Psyche*, 9: 513–536. Reprinted in *International Journal of Psycho-Analysis*, 37: 61–74.

Devreese, D. (1981). Schreber-Dokumente I. *Psychoanalytische Perspektieven* (Gent), 1: 3–164.

Ferenczi, S. (1911). Über die Rolle der Homosexualität in der Pathogenese der Paranoia. *Jahrbuch Psychoanal. Psychopathol. Forsch.*, 3: 101–109.

Freud, S. (1911). Psycho-analytic notes on a case of an autobiographically described case of paranoia (dementia paranoides). S.E. 12: 9–79.

Gross, O. (1904). Ueber Bewusstseinzefall. *Monatschr. Psych. Neurol.*, 15: 46–51.

Israels, H. (1989). *Schreber Father and Son*. Madison, Conn.: International Universities Press.

Lothane, Z. (1989a). Schreber, Freud, Flechsig and Weber revisted: An inquiry into the methods of interpretation. *Psychoanalytic Review*, 79: 203–262.

———. (1989b). Vindicating Schreber's father: Neither sadist nor child abuser. *Journal of Psychohistory*, 16: 263–285.

———. (1992). *In Defense of Schreber: Soul Murder and Psychiatry*. Hillsdale, N.J.: The Analytic Press.

————. (1993). Schreber's feminine identification: Paranoid illness or profound insight? *International Forum of Psychoanalysis,* 2: 131–138.

Macalpine, I., and Hunter, R. A. (1903). Translators' analysis of the case. In *Memoirs of My Nervous Illness,* see Schreber (1903).

Niederland, W. G. (1963). Further data and memorabilia pertaining to the Schreber case. *International Journal of Psychoanalysis,* 44: 201–207.

————. (1974). *The Schreber Case/Psychoanalytic Profile of a Paranoid Personality.* New York, Quadrangle/New York Times, 2d ed., Hillsdale, N.J.: Analytic Press, 1984.

Schatzman, M. (1973). *Soul Murder Persecution in the Family.* New York: Signet.

Schreber, D. P. (1903). *Denkwürdigkeiten eines Nervenkranken.* Leipzig: Mutze. Trans. *Memoirs of My Nervous Illness,* Cambridge, Mass., Harvard University Press, 1988.

ZVI LOTHANE

Scientific Tests of Freud's Theories and Therapy

We review here the scientific data relevant to the validity of Freud's major theories and the soundness of his therapeutic paradigm. Since he regarded his own enterprise as a scientific one, it seems reasonable to evaluate his ideas on the basis of research data. The interminable debates regarding the soundness of his work are typically phrased in strongly held doctrinaire opinions. We base our evaluations entirely upon research findings.

It is widely assumed that little solid data exist bearing on the validity of Freud's assertions. In two previous volumes (Fisher and Greenberg, 1985; 1996), we were able to harvest and critique 2,500 research publications directly pertinent to testing Freud's formulations. We discovered that these formulations are not a monolithic structure, but rather factor into minitheories. The Freudian structure does not stand or fall as one totality. We were able to demonstrate that certain of Freud's minitheories hold up well to the research evidence and others do not. While the research studies we assembled vary in quality, they do overall compare well with the accumulated studies relevant to most other major sectors of psychology. It is paradoxical that while a massive quantity of scientific information has accumulated with respect to Freud's theories, they are still often depicted as untested, or even untestable.

In assessing Freud's formulations, it is necessary to state them as propositions that can be put to the test. The following emerged as amenable to scientific appraisal:

Etiology of depression
Etiology of paranoia
Anal character
Dream theory
Oral character
Oedipal dynamics
Psychoanalysis as therapy

We will outline the major questions relating to these topics and briefly sketch what the aggregate relevant research has to say about each (for further details, see Fisher and Greenberg, 1985; 1996).

Etiology of Depression

Freud's account of the etiology of depression is diffusely retiform but has a basic core. In essence, he proposed that depression is typically triggered by suffering the loss of a significant person, value, or role. Presumably the vulnerability to such loss is increased if the individual's mode of relating to others is unusually introjective. The term "introjective" in this context refers to identifying closely with lost objects, making them part of the self, entertaining conflicted ambivalent feelings (e.g., love and hate) toward them, and in the course of that confused process also channeling destructive (depression-inducing) hostility toward oneself. Freud believed that the more intense the self-critical orientation and the greater the inclination to be dependently (orally) oriented, the greater the probable susceptibility to depression.

The extensive research literature concerned with depression reveals a moderately good match between Freud's formulations and the multiple findings. While the evidence does not support Freud's idea that early loss is the anlage for depression, it does indicate that present loss, in the context of significant early loss, increases the likelihood of becoming depressed.

The evidence reinforces, too, Freud's theorizing concerning the roles of dependence (orality) and self-criticism (turning hostility against self) in vulnerability to depression. Multiple studies have shown significant connections between a dependent attitude and the development of depression. Further, measures of intropunitive tendencies based on projective or special situational responses (but not questionnaires) do indicate real trends for those susceptible to depression to be unusually self-attacking.

Particularly striking is the research support for Freud's assumption of a basic ambivalence toward the lost "introjected" object: the positive taking in of (identification

S

with) that object and the subsequent attack on it after becoming part of the self-territory. Freud considered this brand of ambivalence to be one of the prime "preconditions" for depression. Congruently, there are data indicating that the parents of the depressed behaved, early on, in unusually contradictory ways (being simultaneously nonnurturantly distant and overly closely controlling). In the same vein, studies actually find that the depressed obtain elevated scores on objective measures of ambivalence. This represents an impressive match with Freud's focus on how ambivalence toward the "introjected" object initiates a sequence leading to depression.

Etiology of Paranoia

One of Freud's most pinpointed theories relates to the origin of paranoid psychopathology. He proposed that paranoid distortions and delusions represent defensive efforts to deny unacceptable homosexual impulses. He portrayed both male and female paranoids as having experienced unusually intense (Oedipal) conflicts with the parent of the same sex that result in heterosexual difficulties and therefore initiate a regressive need for a homosexual bond with that parent. Presumably, though, this desire for homosexual closeness arouses anxiety of catastrophic intensity and therefore requires a defensive sequence of denial ("I do not love that parent." "I hate that parent." "That parent hates me."); that is, the dilemma is resolved by means of projection.

Research concerning this theory has largely centered on presenting (e.g., tachistoscopically) stimuli with homosexual connotations and measuring the degree to which such stimuli arouse anxiety and also repression or other defensive strategies. The findings have quite consistently, in both males and females, supported Freud's position.

Anal Character

Freud depicted a personality type, the so-called anal character, that presumably evolves in the course of learning to restrain anal impulses and wishes. He proposed three major defensive anal "character-traits" (orderliness, parsimony, obstinacy) that help the individual to maintain control and to block unconscious besmirching anal imagery threatening to break through into awareness. He suggested that some individuals have an exceptional sensitivity to anal sensations, but that they must, in the course of socialization, learn to repress their anal focus. They are said to emerge as preoccupied with main-

taining control, being in balance, and preventing self-contamination.

A progression of studies has supported Freud's anal character concept. These studies (often based on factor analyses) have shown, first of all, that there is, indeed, a cluster of traits corresponding to Freud's description of the anal character. This cluster includes such variables as stinginess, orderliness, punctuality, concern about money, interest in collecting things, rigidity, retentiveness, hoarding, and attention to detail.

In addition, it has been shown that an anal orientation is associated with the three specific traits (orderliness, parsimony, obstinacy) that Freud postulated to be basic to the defense strategy for avoiding loss of control.

Finally, the anal character paradigm has proven to be useful in explaining selective responses to stimuli with anal connotations, selective reactions to anal humor, and preferences for certain defense mechanisms. Overall, the anal character concept has turned out to be one of the best empirically validated among Freud's formulations.

Dream Theory

In his *Interpretation of Dreams*, Freud offered a theory concerning the dreaming process. He conceptualized the dream as a camouflaged way of concealing threatening desires beneath its surface. Dream images are presumably camouflaged "manifest" representations of "latent" wishes. Freud regarded the dream as having a sleep-preserving function insofar as it allows threatening unconscious impulses to filter into (and gain outlet through) dream figures not sufficiently alarming to be sleep-disruptive.

Analysis of the extensive investigative literature concerned with dreaming indicates little support for Freud's ideas about the nature of the dream. First, abundant data demonstrate that the manifest content of the dream is not simply a form of camouflage. Indeed, it is full of meanings relatively easy to access. The so-called latent content of the dream has proved to be a vague notion. The use of free association to define this latent component has been shown to be unreliable. Second, Freud's view of the dream as primarily a vehicle for expressing unconscious tensions has not stood up well. The accumulated research portrays the dream process as having rather a more general adaptive purpose analogous to thinking and problem solving. Studies clearly show that dreams can diversely facilitate complex learning, neutralize stress, enhance signal detection powers, and foster creativity.

The only way in which the research findings agree with Freud's overall dream theory is in the general sense that he recognized an underlying adaptive intent in dream construction. One should add that recent findings suggest that Freud may have been correct in his speculation that dreaming has sleep-preserving functions—but not in the specific sense that he originally thought.

Oral Character

Although the concept of the oral character was first developed by Abraham (1968), he did so by analogy with Freud's model of the anal character, and we know that Freud approved of this derivation. For that reason, we chose to appraise it as an accepted part of the original corpus of psychoanalysis. The oral character is represented as one who was unable to master the difficulties of the oral phase and who consequently was fixated on issues of special prominence during that phase. It was theorized that the existence of unsatisfied oral wishes produced a character structure dedicated to indirect (camouflaged) ways of expressing oral tensions and also repressive defenses for holding them in check. One could reduce the elements of the oral character orientation to the following:

- Intense concern with issues of giving-taking (nurturance-succorance)
- Conflict about dependence-independence
- Concern with issues of closeness distance (being alone versus attaching)
- Special susceptibility to depression
- Heightened needs to utilize oral channels for satisfaction or defensive denial (e.g., too much versus too little eating)

The research directed at testing the oral character formulations established the following:

There exists an empirical cluster (e.g., need to affiliate, passivity, extremes of optimism versus pessimism) of attitudes and attributes that match the oral character paradigm.

An oral orientation is accompanied by strong motivation to invest in relationships that guarantee dependence and freedom from loneliness.

Pessimism and depression occur with increased frequency in the oral character.

The orally oriented are especially likely to search for oral forms of gratification (e.g., overeating, smoking).

These findings, based largely on the use of objective psychological measures (e.g., questionnaires, perceptual responses), provide excellent support for the prime elements of the oral character concept.

Oedipal Dynamics

Freud's Oedipal theory has a number of constituents. It is a complex structure and we deal only with its most basic aspects. Freud portrayed the Oedipal phase of development as beginning around the age of four or five. Presumably the essence of the Oedipal dilemma is that the child becomes sexually attracted to the parent of the opposite sex and competitively jealous of the parent of the same sex. Freud offered different versions of how males and females cope with the Oedipal struggle.

Thus, the little boy is depicted as yearning for mother and the elimination of father. This is said to create the potential for disturbing rival encounters with father. However, balancing forces are described as coming into play. One of the major forces presumably derives from the male child's concern that the sexual rivalry for mother will stir father into castrating him. This anxiety is depicted as playing a large role in the male child's development of superego (conscience). Presumably, as part of the boy's repudiation of "evil" sexual impulses toward mother and as a maneuver to avoid father's wrath, he identifies with father (shifts to father's side) and introjects his rules and prohibitions. This resolves the Oedipal struggle and the boy enters a latency period during which sexual aims are repressed. Presumably, only at puberty does sexuality resurge and lead to adult heterosexual relationships. The inability to resolve Oedipal conflicts satisfactorily is said to be the source of later psychopathology.

Freud's account of the Oedipal course for the female assumes she initially adopts mother as her major love object; but when she discovers males have a penis, she assumes she has lost hers and that this marks her as inferior. For this reason and others she is said to blame her mother for her deficiencies. This motivates her to pull away from mother and to shift her love to father.

Presumably, up to this point, her clitoris was her primary source (through masturbation) of sexual gratification, but when she learns she has an "inferior organ," she shifts her interest away from the phallic clitoris and focuses instead on the passive receptive vagina. At the same time, said Freud, she evolves fantasies that her new love object, father, will impregnate her via the vagina and she will present a child to him. The child produced in this context has a reparative meaning, the acquisition of a penis equivalent. This was labeled "the penis-baby equation."

Freud assumed that the girl resolves her Oedipal rivalry (with mother) more gradually and less decisively than the male (with father). Since she has less need (because she does not have to cope with intense castration anxiety) to introject parental prohibitions against her Oedipal fantasies sharply, she supposedly develops a less definite, less severe superego. Following the Oedipal period, she is said to move into a latency phase, and at puberty her sexual aims revive.

Let us examine how well the spectrum of Oedipal hypotheses has fared in the research literature. Multiple studies affirm the most basic Oedipal proposition that boys and girls do adopt different attitudes toward the same- and opposite-sex parents. Boys have been shown to be more positive toward mother and more negative toward father; and the equivalent reverse pattern holds true for girls. The supporting data derive not only from systematic parent reports of their encounters with their offspring but also objectively measured projective fantasies obtained from children.

There is no empirical verification of the proposition that the male child adopts his father's superego values as part of a process based on fear (castration anxiety). His identification with father has been shown not to stem primarily from fear. Robust data indicate that a boy is more likely to identify with a father who is nurturant rather than fear-inspiring. Freud did not sufficiently recognize the power of positive motivations in shaping the boy's superego values.

Freud's assumption that the male superego is more articulated and stringent than the female's has recruited no empirical backing. Multiple studies refute Freud's view. There may even be trends for the female superego to be slightly more severe than the male's.

Freud's concept that the mature pattern of sexual development for females is to shift from preference for clitoral sexual arousal to vaginal arousal has also not fared well. A series of studies found no association between vaginal preference and measures of personality maturity, psychopathology, or anxiety level. There are even indications that those with a clitoral preference may be less psychologically maladjusted than those with a vaginal orientation.

Freud's formulation concerning the penis-baby equation (intuitively one of his most improbable) is sup-

ported by a network of data. As noted earlier, this formulation states that women normally resolve their sense of bodily inferiority (because they do not possess a penis) and their anger toward mother (whom they blame for their inferiority) by fantasizing that father will impregnate them and the resultant baby will provide a compensatory penis substitute. Thus, their inferior state would presumably be remedied. Research studies have shown, as would be predicted from this paradigm, that pregnant women are unusually preoccupied with phallic images, that subliminal pregnancy messages result in increased phallic imagery in nonpregnant women (but not in men), and that there are shifts in phallic imagery during menstruation as a function of intensity of motivation to become pregnant.

The research literature has validated some aspects of Freud's complex Oedipal theories and not others. In the same vein, there are segments of the larger Freudian corpus that are well substantiated and others that simply lack empirical integrity. Most important, we have demonstrated that it is feasible to appraise and revise Freud's fundamental ideas on the basis of tangible, quantitative evidence.

Psychoanalysis as Therapy: Outcome and Process

Empirically the study of psychoanalysis as a method of psychotherapy has proven difficult. Obstacles stem not only from the traditional hesitation of psychoanalysts to involve themselves in research utilizing conventional scientific methods (which protect against the biases of the participants) but also from ambiguity about what constitutes psychoanalysis as therapy. Freud was quite hesitant to describe the details of his technique. Drawing an analogy between chess and psychotherapy, he stated that only some of the opening and closing moves could be known, with the remainder left to the application of intuitive guidelines. It has been speculated that Freud's reticence to publish details of his technique sprang from reluctance to permit his patients to know too many of the specifics of his approach, his feeling that analysts should not be constrained by rigid rules, and his conviction that the analyst's personal analysis and clinical experiences were more important than reading books for the development of psychoanalytic therapy skills.

Freud's failure to be more specific about the implementation of his approach to treatment may be an important factor in promoting disagreements among psychoanalysts evidenced in the research literature. Study after study documents the difficulty psychoanalysts display in trying to reach consensus about almost any issue. Research focusing on analyst reliability demonstrated considerable disagreement about such matters as treatment techniques, case conceptualizations, goals for treatment outcomes, and the types of cases most suitable for psychoanalysis. One group of analysts in Chicago met periodically for three years in an unsuccessful attempt to develop a method that would yield agreement among them in formulating cases. In the end, they felt their efforts were undermined by an overreliance on intuitive impressions, without systematic checks on objectivity or the need to account for discrepant data.

Thus, any overview of the results of psychoanalysis as a therapy must focus on treatments as conducted by a diverse group of practitioners who to varying degrees diverge from conducting therapy as Freud might have practiced it. Incidentally, our conclusions about Freud's treatment results, based on an analysis of all the cases he wrote about, indicated that his track record as a therapist was not particularly good. In total, Freud mentioned briefly 133 minor cases and provided extensive discussion of only 12 cases. Examining the written record concerning the few patients Freud actually saw himself and wrote about at length reveals that only one seemed to benefit significantly. This is Freud's only published record of an apparently successful analysis. It is both odd and remarkable that Freud was able to market the usefulness of psychoanalysis as therapy through the presentation of largely failed treatments.

The restricted nature of the sample of patients Freud wrote about also clouds the generalizability of his pronouncements. Patients predominately came from the upper class, were mostly women, and were almost all between ages twenty and forty-four. Furthermore, at variance with the common perception regarding which patients are most suitable for psychoanalysis, Freud's reported cases tended to be severely disturbed. Many would be diagnosed as either borderline or schizophrenic according to contemporary standards.

It is notable that Freud's enthusiasm about the outcome of psychoanalytic therapy dampened toward the end of his career. For example, in his *New Introductory Lectures* he commented that Lourdes might provide more effective outcomes. Similarly, in his essay *Analysis Terminable and Interminable*, he stated that it might ultimately turn out that the differences in behavior between analyzed and nonanalyzed people might not be as significant as he once expected. We should mention, too, that Freud's writings drifted over time from concerns about treatment outcome to an emphasis on how his patients' productions could be used to construct and verify hypotheses about personality dynamics and the development of psychopathology.

Empirical research supports the conclusion that psychoanalytic treatment produced results superior to no treatment for patients with chronic problems (Fisher and Greenberg, 1985; 1996). However, comparisons with alternative treatments fail to reveal any consistent differences in outcome. Surprising to some is the finding that orthodox psychoanalysis (with more frequent treatment sessions and greater duration) is not superior in outcome to less intensive psychoanalytically oriented treatment. This has been so even though the patients receiving psychoanalysis have been more select in terms of prognostic desirability. Overall, though, these conclusions need to be viewed as tentative because of the lack of methodological rigor in all the reported investigations. In fact, it is possible to challenge the results of all existing studies because of compromised or contaminated data.

The scientific literature also justifies some determinations about the active ingredients in the process of psychoanalytic therapy. For Freud, the attainment of insight was a primary task of the treatment. Increasing patient awareness of underlying motivations and repressed memories (or "making the unconscious conscious") was central to Freud's beliefs about how change was to come about. He proposed that verbal interpretations would play a key role in helping patients forge links between past traumatic events and distortions of current perceptions. Increased awareness, it seemed, would lead automatically to decreased symptoms and patient benefit. At the same time, to support his developing personality theories, Freud wanted to promote the material produced by patients as data untainted by analyst influence. He, therefore, declared that analyst suggestion or persuasion played little role in psychoanalytic treatment results.

How have these conceptions fared empirically? Despite acknowledged difficulties in developing adequate measures, evidence now indicates that development of conscious insight is not as necessary for patient improvement as Freud initially assumed. Findings show that patients often demonstrate a level of change that is discordant with their level of insight. Also, in contrast to

S

Freud's statements, suggestion and persuasion have been found to be important elements in the treatment process, even in psychoanalytic therapy. Of particular significance, research has revealed the treatment relationship to be perhaps the most potent element in promoting change. Therefore, while therapist neutrality is important, Freud's portrait of the advantages of a distant therapist who is "emotionally cold" and "opaque" seems to be off the mark. On the other hand, the speculation that people display repetitive and characteristic patterns of relating to others, reminiscent of their relationship with parental figures (i.e., transference), has received research support. However, treatment gains appear to stem more from patients learning to experience the therapy alliance as different from past malignant relationships than from repeated, pointed, verbal transference interpretations that have unexpectedly demonstrated potentially harmful effects.

Though several of Freud's specific ideas about psychotherapy have not been substantiated by research, his pioneering speculations regarding the value of a talking cure for emotional problems remain basic to the practice of most clinicians and continue to inspire an increasingly sophisticated array of modern investigations.

Final Comment

We would reiterate that the scientific data bearing on Freud's creations are diverse with reference to whether or not they are validating. His theories and therapy can, indeed, be evaluated in an empirically differentiated fashion. We are now in a position to appraise his theories in a reasonable scientific manner. Those who would dismiss the total Freudian body of work as passé must reckon with myriad findings that declare the evaluative process cannot be global, but rather needs to be attuned to individual islands of data—varying in how much support, if any, they for Freud's constructions. Freud, like most of us, was right about some things and wrong about others.

REFERENCES

Abraham, K. (1968). The influence of oral erotism on character formation. In A. Brown and A. Strachey (eds.). *Selected Papers on Psychoanalysis.* New York: Basic Books, pp. 383–406.

Fisher, S., and Greenberg, R. (1985). *The Scientific Credibility of Freud's Theories and Therapy.* New York: Columbia University Press.

———. (1996). *Freud Scientifically Reappraised: Testing the Theories and Therapy.* New York: Wiley.

SEYMOUR FISHER
ROGER P. GREENBERG

Screen Memories

The term "screen memory" was introduced by Freud in 1899 in an article with that title (Freud, 1899), elaborated in his *Psychopathology of Everyday Life*, Chapter IV, "Childhood Memories and Screen Memories," and further elaborated in papers published in 1904, 1907, 1910, and 1924. Freud returned repeatedly to the subject of childhood memories. In the 1899 paper, he described the screen memory as an early memory that was rediscovered to serve as a screen against conflicts arising in the adolescent period. However, in his 1901 paper, he stated that the screen memory concealed conflicts arising at the time the memory is formed, or earlier.

In 1901, Freud questioned the trustworthiness of childhood memories: "[O]f the childhood memories that have been retained a few strike us as perfectly understandable while others seem odd or unintelligible. If the memories that a person has retained are subjected to an analytic inquiry it is easy to establish that there is no guarantee of accuracy. Some of the mnemonic images are certainly falsified, incomplete or displaced in time and place. Any such statement by the subjects of the inquiry that their first recollection comes from about their second year is clearly not to be trusted."

Freud thought, as do most authors writing today, that childhood verbal memories could not occur before the age of two and one half to three years: "It may indeed be questioned whether we have any memories at all from our childhood; memories relating to our childhood may be all that we possess. Our childhood memories show us our earliest years not as they were but as they appeared in the later years when the memories were recovered" (1901, pp. 46–47).

In commenting on childhood memories, Freud further concluded that ". . . one is faced by various considerations to suspect that in the so-called earliest childhood memories we possess not the genuine memory-trace but a later revision of it, a revision which may have been subject to the influence of a variety of later psychical forces. Thus the 'childhood memories' of individuals come in general to acquire the significance of 'screen memories' and in doing so offer a remarkable analogy with the childhood memories that a nation preserves in its store of legends and myths" (1901, pp. 447–448).

In view of the current controversy about the accuracy of memories of childhood sexual abuse, including those recalled in psychotherapy settings and under hypnosis, it is most important that those interested in the subject of early childhood memories become familiar with Freud's original papers on the subject (Rosenbaum, 1998).

REFERENCES
Freud, S. (1899). Screen memories. S.E. 3: 301–322.
———. (1901). *The Psychopathology of Everyday Life.* S.E. 6: 1–279.
Rosenbaum, M. (1998). Childhood screen memories—Are they forgotten?, *Psychosomatics*, 39: 68–71.

MILTON ROSENBAUM

Secret Committee See COMMITTEE, THE SECRET.

Seduction Theory

For a brief period during the years 1895–1897, Freud believed he had discovered that psychoneuroses occurred exclusively as a consequence of the repression of memories of sexual molestation in early childhood. By late 1897, he had considerable doubts about the theory and within a short time he abandoned it. He subsequently asserted that the infantile sexual experiences he had uncovered were generally unconscious fantasies.

In 1896, Freud published three papers in which he presented the thesis that all cases of psychoneurosis resulted from repressed memories of premature sexual experiences (1896a; 1896b; 1896c). By the "psychoneuroses," he had in mind specifically hysteria, a condition in which patients exhibit somatic symptoms having no apparent organic origin, and obsessional neurosis. He claimed that, utilizing his new technique of psychoanalysis, he had corroborated his thesis by uncovering, in all his current patients, repressed memories of sexual molestations from early childhood. However, within two years he lost faith in his theory, and when he subsequently referred to the episode, he asserted that the infantile "sexual scenes" he had uncovered at that time were mostly unconscious fantasies. It is generally considered that the seduction theory and its abandonment marked a crucial stage in the development of psychoanalysis, leading to Freud's theories of infantile sexuality. But traditional accounts of the episode have relied almost exclusively on his own retrospective reports, which in some important respects are discrepant with the seduction theory papers of 1896 (Cioffi, 1974; Schimek, 1987; Israëls and Schatzman, 1993). To ascertain what actually occurred, it is necessary to scrutinize not only the origi-

nal papers, but also the contemporaneous letters Freud wrote to his confidant Wilhelm Fliess. Additional information relating to Freud's current clinical methodology is contained in *Studies on Hysteria*, published jointly by Freud and Josef Breuer in 1895. The account that follows is based on these three sources.

To understand the precise nature of the claims made in the seduction theory papers, it is essential to have a knowledge of Freud's clinical practice in the period in question, details of which are given in *Studies on Hysteria*. Central to his methodology was the "pressure technique," developed from a procedure he had seen used by Hippolyte Bernheim (1895, pp. 109–110, 270–272). Freud believed that somatic symptoms he regarded as hysterical were caused by repressed memories of traumatic experiences, and that the therapeutic task was to induce the patient to bring these memories to conscious awareness. At such times that relevant thoughts were not forthcoming, he placed his hand on the patient's forehead and encouraged him or her to report any images or ideas that came to mind. In the event that nothing occurred to the patient, Freud took this as a sign of resistance and repeated the pressure on the forehead while insisting that a picture or an idea would emerge. In this manner he endeavored to set in motion a chain of associations that he believed would point to the direction for further investigation, and lead eventually to the pathogenic idea (pp. 270–272). The ideas and scenes obtained from the patient by this procedure generally emerged in a piecemeal fashion, with the essential elements missing (pp. 281–282). The task of the physician was "to put these [fragments] together once more into the organization which he presumes to have existed"; that is, to piece together the fragments to produce a coherent narrative, rather like the process of solving a picture puzzle (p. 291).

Even when the patients had been convinced of the logical coherence of the proposed solution, they often failed to recognize the ideas derived from the greatest depth, those that formed "the nucleus of the pathogenic organization" (p. 300). "[T]he climax of [the pressure procedure's] achievement in the way of reproductive thinking," Freud wrote, was that "it causes thoughts to emerge which the patient will never recognize as his own, which he never *remembers*, although he admits that the context calls for them inexorably" (p. 272).

Arriving at the solution, however, was not an automatic process, and required guidance from the physician. To

S

facilitate the emergence of appropriate associations, Freud wrote, it was "of use if we can guess the way in which things are connected up and tell the patient before we have uncovered it" (p. 295). And even more explicitly, in regard to "the things that we have to insist upon to the patient," he stated: "The principal point is that I should guess the secret and tell it to the patient straight out" (p. 281).

The therapeutic solution therefore involved both acknowledged and unacknowledged material. The logical consistency, and the interconnection between its various parts, justified Freud's confidence in the solution at which he arrived (pp. 300–301). At each stage he looked to the occurrence of "tension and signs of emotion" in the patient's face as indicators of emerging recollections (p. 281). He also claimed that when the patient gave utterance to the pathogenic memory, the symptom diminished, or even temporarily vanished, and that the "working-over" of the pathogenic material resulted in its complete disappearance (pp. 296–297).

In spite of his frank admission that it was his custom to propose the essential elements in his solution to the patients, and that they frequently initially resisted his suggestions, Freud insisted that he was not able to force erroneous ideas onto them. Had he done so, he argued, it would have been betrayed eventually by some contradiction in the material. For this reason the physician "need not be afraid of telling the patient what we think his next connection of thought is going to be" (p. 295).

At this stage Freud had not reported that any of his patients had been sexually abused in infancy. The thesis that the symptoms of hysteria and obsessional neurosis resulted exclusively from repressed memories of sexual molestations in early childhood was first put forward in letters he wrote to Wilhelm Fliess in October 1895. Specifically, he conjectured that hysteria was the consequence of "presexual sexual shock," and obsessional neurosis the consequence of "presexual sexual pleasure" (Masson, 1985: 141, 144). On November 2, 1895, he reported a case that "strengthened [his] confidence in the validity of [his] psychological constructions," though he acknowledged there was "disputed material" (p. 149).

No other cases were reported to Fliess at this time, though on January 1, 1896, Freud sent him an early draft of one of the seduction theory papers (pp. 162–169). The first public announcement of the theory appeared in two papers sent off to their respective publishers on February 5, 1896: *Heredity and the Aetiology of the Neu-*

roses, published in a French journal on March 30, and *Further Remarks on the Neuro-psychoses of Defense*, published May 15. In these papers Freud stated that he had carried out a complete psychoanalysis of all his thirteen cases of hysteria (two men, eleven women), and that in each of them he had uncovered repressed memories from early childhood of sexual experiences involving excitation of the genitals, occurring mostly before the age of five (1896, pp. 152, 163, 165). These were *passive* experiences, "submitted to with indifference or with a small degree of annoyance or fright" (p. 155). He also wrote that the events were "represented either by a brutal assault committed by an adult or by a seduction less rapid and less repulsive, but reaching the same conclusion" (p. 152). Seven of the patients, Freud wrote, had been victims of a slightly older boy (generally a brother). Other culprits were nursemaids, governesses, domestic servants, and teachers (pp. 152, 164). In his six cases of obsessional neurosis the incidents occurred at a slightly later age and were *active* pleasurable experiences; and in each of these cases there had occurred an earlier passive sexual experience (pp. 155, 168–169).

The third seduction theory paper (*The Aetiology of Hysteria*), originally delivered as a lecture on April 21, 1896, contained a more detailed presentation of Freud's thesis. In his introductory remarks he wrote of his methodology that, just as physicians can discover the cause of a symptom or injury in the absence of information from the patient, "In hysteria, too, there exists a similar possibility of penetrating from the symptoms to a knowledge of their causes." He explained that his procedure utilized Breuer's discovery that "*the symptoms of hysteria . . . are determined by certain experiences of the patient's which . . . are being reproduced in his psychical life in the form of mnemic symbols*" (pp. 191–192, Freud's emphasis). In one of the earlier papers he had illustrated his application of this notion in explaining an obsessional patient's bedtime ritual: for instance, the patient's compulsion "to kick both legs out a certain number of times" represented his "kick[ing] away the person who was lying on him" (pp. 172, 172–173 no. 1).

The number of cases of hysteria for which Freud reported that infantile "scenes" had been uncovered had increased to eighteen (six men and twelve women), and the culprits now included adult strangers and close relatives in addition to the older brothers and other categories listed in the previous papers. Moreover, most of the patients had experienced sexual traumas at the hands of two or more such culprits (pp. 207–208). However, Freud reported that "[b]efore they come for analysis the patients know nothing about these [sexual] scenes. They are indignant as a rule if we warn them that such scenes are going to emerge. Only the strongest compulsion of the treatment can induce them to embark on a reproduction of them." Further, having "no feeling of remembering the scenes" they are induced to reproduce, they "assure [Freud] . . . emphatically of their unbelief" (p. 204). A similar description occurs in *Heredity and the Aetiology of the Neuroses*: "these patients never repeat these stories spontaneously, nor do they ever in the course of a treatment suddenly present the physician with the complete recollection of a scene of this kind. One only succeeds in awakening the psychical trace of a precocious sexual event under the most energetic pressure of the analytic procedure, and against an enormous resistance. Moreover, the memory must be extracted from them piece by piece" (p. 153).

Although Freud's words elsewhere seem to imply that specific "scenes" were "reproduced" by patients in the form of mental images (Borch-Jacobsen, 1996: 25), the latter passage quoted above suggests that any ideas or pictures the patients were induced to reproduce were generally fragmentary and did not constitute complete images of sexual scenes. Some sketchy reports relating to later experiences with specific patients were given in letters Freud wrote to Fliess after the publication of *The Aetiology of Hysteria*. One particular case is instructive in that it illustrates the means by which Freud may have arrived at his findings. In the case of a patient, Miss G. de B., who had commenced treatment only a month before, he described what he called the "circumstantial evidence" for his diagnosis of infantile sexual abuse. This included his attributing the origin of symptoms of eczema and lesions around the mouth to an early experience of "sucking on [her father's] penis." Having inferred this scene, he then "thrust the explanation at her," and reported that "she was at first won over." However, after confronting her father she changed her mind, and Freud responded by threatening "to send her away" in order to obtain her compliance (Masson, 1985: 220).

As in *Studies on Hysteria*, Freud used two main arguments for the authenticity of the "scenes" arrived at by his clinical procedure. When the patients were, as he supposed, bringing these infantile experiences to consciousness, they exhibited violent sensations, which testified to the scenes being "a reality which is being felt with distress

and reproduced with the greatest reluctance" (1896c, p. 204); and a "stronger proof" of their authenticity was that the scenes were "indispensable supplements to the associative and logical framework of the neurosis" (p. 205). However, there are considerable grounds for doubting that such arguments suffice to justify Freud's claims that he had uncovered unconscious "sexual scenes." Among these are (1) the indications that Freud's conviction was based primarily on his symbolic interpretation of symptoms that "correspond to the sensory content of the infantile scenes," and that "make themselves heard as witnesses to the history of the origin of the illness" (1896c, pp. 192, 214), and (2) the extraordinarily short time between his alighting on the seduction theory and his claiming to have "traced back" to such scenes for no fewer than sixteen patients (pp. 151, 152, 155–156, 163, 168–169). In addition, it is apparent that, as indicated in the previous paragraph and elsewhere (1896a, pp. 153, 204; 1898, p. 269), Freud's clinical procedure at that time entailed his pressuring his patients to "reproduce" material that would provide him with evidence for the requisite sexual experiences.

Since Freud never published clinical details for the patients in question, we have very little knowledge of the specific material that he believed justified his claims. It is evident, however, that the conjecture that a repressed memory of infantile sexual molestation was a precondition for the development of psychoneuroses preceded his claiming to have uncovered such memories, and that the patients did not themselves report recollections of having been sexually abused in early childhood. Close scrutiny of the seduction theory papers, in conjunction with knowledge of Freud's current clinical procedure, points rather to the conclusion that "the knowledge of [the] original trauma, whether considered an unconscious memory or fantasy, was based on Freud's interpretation and reconstruction; it was not directly revealed by the patient" (Schimek, 1987: 960). This is consistent with one of Freud's historical accounts of his early psychoanalytic experience, in which he reported that the material provided by his patients "did not bring up what had actually been forgotten, but it brought up such plain and numerous hints that, with the help of a certain amount of supplementing and interpreting, the doctor was able to guess (or reconstruct) the forgotten material from it" (1924, pp. 195–196).

The above account of the seduction theory episode, based on the contemporary documents, differs from the traditional version, which asserts that Freud postulated the seduction theory because most of his early female patients reported that they had been sexually abused in early childhood by their father. It remains, therefore, to give some indication of how this latter account came to be almost universally accepted in spite of the fact that it is not consistent with Freud's own original reports in several key respects.

Freud made no mention of fathers as the primary culprits in his first two retrospective accounts of the seduction theory episode. In the first of these he wrote unspecifically that he had "learned to explain a number of phantasies of seduction as attempts at fending off memories of the subject's *own* sexual activity (infantile masturbation)" (1906, p. 274). The account given eight years later in *On the History of the Psychoanalytic Movement* was more detailed:

> Influenced by Charcot's view of the traumatic origin of hysteria, one was readily inclined to accept as true and etiologically significant the statements made by patients in which they ascribed their symptoms to passive experiences in the first years of childhood—to put it bluntly, to seduction. When this aetiology broke down under the weight of its own improbability and contradiction in definitely ascertainable circumstances, the result at first was helpless bewilderment. Analysis had led back to these infantile sexual traumas by the right path, and yet they were not true. . . . If hysterical subjects trace back their symptoms to traumas that are fictitious, then the new fact that emerges is precisely that they create such scenes in *phantasy*. . . . This reflection was soon followed by the discovery that these phantasies were intended to cover up the auto-erotic activity of the first years of childhood, to embellish it and raise it to a higher plane. (1914, pp. 17–18)

In 1924 Freud reread the seduction theory papers in preparation for their reprinting, and their influence is apparent in the account of the episode he gave in *An Autobiographical Study* (1925):

> Under the influence of the technical procedure which I used at that time, the majority of my patients reproduced from their childhood scenes in which they were sexually seduced by some grown-up person. With female patients the part of the seducer was almost always assigned to their father. I believed these stories, and consequently supposed that I had discovered the roots of the subsequent neurosis in these experiences of sexual seduction in childhood. . . . I was at last obliged to recognize that these scenes of seduction had never taken place, and that they were only phantasies which my patients had made up or which I myself had perhaps forced on them. (1925, pp. 33–34)

The acknowledgment that his forceful technique at that time had played a role in his supposed findings, and that he may have imposed the sexual scenes on the patients, reflects the contents of the 1896 papers. However, he went on to assert: "I do not believe even now that I forced the seduction phantasies on my patients, that I 'suggested' them." Significantly, no reason was given for his rejection of this possibility.

In his final reference to the episode, in *New Introductory Lectures on Psycho-Analysis* (1933), the role of fathers was again emphasized:

> In the period in which the main interest was directed to discovering infantile sexual traumas, almost all my women patients told me that they had been seduced by their father. I was driven to recognize in the end that these reports were untrue and so came to understand that hysterical symptoms are derived from phantasies and not from real occurrences. It was only later that I was able to recognize in this phantasy of being seduced by the father the expression of the typical Oedipus complex in women. (1933, p. 120)

The 1925 and 1933 accounts are the sources of the traditional story of the seduction theory episode. As demonstrated above, an examination of the original papers reveals that these retrospective accounts do not accurately reflect what Freud reported at the time. However, one particular item of evidence not yet mentioned has always been taken as confirmation of the traditional version, and this remains to be examined.

In a letter to Fliess on September 21, 1896, Freud confessed that he no longer believed in the seduction theory. Among the reasons he gave for his loss of faith he wrote: "Then the surprise that in all cases, the *father*, not excluding my own, had to be accused of being perverse?" (Masson, 1985: 264). ("Dann die Überraschung, dass in sämtlichen Fällen der *Vater* als pervers beschuldigt werden musste, mein eigener nicht ausgeschlossen" [Masson, 1986: 283]). This statement has always been taken as supporting the accounts Freud gave in 1925 and 1933, in which fathers were the prime seducers of the female patients. That it is inconsistent with the reported culprits in the original papers has been explained by presuming Freud had concealed the truth for reasons of discretion. However, there are several grounds for maintaining that such a view entails a misconstrual of the sentence in question (Esterson, 1998: 9–10). Freud did not write that fathers *had been* accused, but that they *had to be* accused (presumably for his clinical findings to conform to recent theoretical developments [Masson, 1985: 212, 228; Makari, 1998: 642]). (The first mention of the conjectural notion of seduction by the father occurred in a letter to Fliess dated December 6, 1896, prior to which there is no indication in any of Freud's writings in the seduction theory period of fathers as the putative culprits.) On May 31, 1897, Freud had reported his interpretation of a dream as indicating "the fulfillment of my wish to catch a *Pater* as the originator of neurosis" (p. 249), a statement that would make no sense if he had regularly been identifying fathers as the assailants prior to this time. Further, his expression of surprise indicates that he was not saying that fathers had been the culprits all along, for he could scarcely, at such a late stage, have been experiencing surprise about findings obtained for the most part more than eighteen months before. Finally, fathers were implicated by Freud in only a minority of the cases reported in letters to Fliess after the publication of the seduction theory papers, which is again inconsistent with the construal of the sentence in question as his asserting that "in all cases" fathers had been accused.

The above analysis of the episode, and of his methodology during this period, indicates that the infantile "sexual scenes" were initially analytically inferred by Freud and were not patients' recollections. A very different account is that associated with the name of Jeffrey Masson (1984), who contends that Freud was wrong to renounce the seduction theory, and that in doing so he capitulated to fierce opposition from his medical colleagues. Though this idea was not new (it had previously been put forward by at least two authors), Masson was the first to provide a comprehensive case. However, there is no evidence either of the widespread hostility toward Freud that Masson presumes (Decker, 1977; Sulloway, 1979: 448–467), or that the views of his colleagues played a significant role in Freud's abandonment of the theory. More important, Masson's account of Freud listening sympathetically to his female patients' stories of childhood sexual abuse (albeit remembered reluctantly and communicated with difficulty) (ibid, p. 9) relies heavily on Freud's retrospective reports. These, as demonstrated above, are discrepant with the original seduction theory papers, and cannot serve as the basis of an accurate account of the episode. Though it has been widely disseminated, Masson's version of events is not substantiated by the documentary evidence (Esterson, 1998).

There has still to be considered why Freud abandoned the seduction theory. In his letter of September 21, 1897, he listed his failure to bring a single case to a successful conclusion; his doubt that, given the frequent occurrence of hysteria, there could be such widespread perversions against children; the fact that "one cannot distinguish between truth and fiction that has been cathected with affect"; and the consideration that even "in the most far-reaching psychosis the unconscious memory does not break through" (Masson, 1985: 264–265). However, in his published accounts he provided rather different explanations, and the reasons for his abandonment of the theory remain a matter of debate (Israëls and Schatzman, 1993: 47–58); Kupfersmid, 1993; Macmillan, 1991: 636–640).

REFERENCES

Borch-Jacobsen, M. (1996). Neurotica: Freud and the seduction theory. *October 76*, October Magazine and MIT, spring 1996, pp. 15–43.

Breuer, J., and Freud, S. (1895). *Studies on Hysteria*. S.E. 2: 19–305.

Cioffi, F. (1974). Was Freud a liar? *The Listener*, 91: 172–174. Reprinted in *Freud and the Question of Pseudoscience* (1999), Chicago: Open Court: 199–204.

Decker, H. S. (1977). *Freud in Germany: Revolution and Reaction in Science, 1893–1907*. New York: International Universities Press.

Esterson, A. (1998). Jeffrey Masson and Freud's seduction theory: A new fable based on old myths. *History of the Human Sciences*, 11, no. 1: 1–21.

Freud, S. (1896a). Heredity and the aetiology of the neuroses. S.E. 3: 143–156.

———. (1896b). Further remarks on the neuro-psychoses of defence. S.E. 3: 162–185.

S

———. (1896c). The aetiology of hysteria. S.E. 3: 191–221.

———. (1898). Sexuality in the aetiology of the neuroses. S.E. 3: 261–273.

———. (1906). My views on the part played by sexuality in the aetiology of the neuroses. S.E. 7: 271–279.

———. (1914). *On the History of the Psycho-Analytic Movement*. S.E. 14: 7–66.

———. (1924). A short account of psychoanalysis. S.E. 19: 189–209.

———. (1925). An autobiographical study. S.E. 20: 7–74.

———. (1933). *New Introductory Lectures on Psycho-Analysis*. S.E. 22: 5–185.

Israëls, H., and Schatzman, M. (1993). The seduction theory. *History of Psychiatry*, 4: 23–59.

Kupfersmid, J. (1993). Freud's rationale for abandoning the seduction theory. *Psychoanalytic Psychotherapy*, 10, no. 2: 275–290.

Macmillan, M. (1991). *Freud Evaluated: The Completed Arc*. Amsterdam: North-Holland. Rev. ed., Cambridge, Mass.: MIT Press, 1997.

Makari, G. J. (1998). Between seduction and libido: Sigmund Freud's masturbation hypotheses and the realignment of his etiologic thinking, 1897–1905, *Bulletin of the History of Medicine*, 72: 677–694

Masson, J. M. (1984). *The Assault on Truth: Freud's Suppression of the Seduction Theory*. New York: Farrar, Straus and Giroux.

———. (1985). Trans. and ed. *The Complete Letters of Sigmund Freud to Wilhelm Fliess 1887–1904*. Cambridge, Mass.: Harvard University Press.

———. (1986). (ed.). *Sigmund Freud: Briefe an Wilhelm Fliess 1887–1904, Ungekürzte Ausgabe*. Frankfurt am Main: S. Fischer.

Schimek, J. G. (1987). Fact and fantasy in the seduction theory: A historical review. *Journal of the American Psychoanalytic Association*, 35, no. 4: 937–965.

Sulloway, F. (1979). *Freud: Biologist of the Mind*. New York: Basic Books.

ALLEN ESTERSON

Self-Analysis

The idea of self-analysis is controversial. Some analysts believe that there is no such thing as self-analysis, while others believe that without self-analysis there can be no psychoanalysis. Some of this dispute is definitional—as in many analytic controversies. Self-analysis and psychoanalysis with an actual analyst are necessarily different.

Self-analysis has been defined by Laplanche and Pontalis (1973, p. 413) as the investigation of oneself by oneself, conducted in a more or less systematic fashion and utilizing certain techniques of the psychoanalytic method, such as free association, dream analysis, and the interpretation of behavior. Some analysts consider that self-analysis becomes possible only after psychoanalysis, that the experience of being analyzed, with the internalization of the analyst, the analytic method, and theoretical ways of understanding, forms the necessary basis of self-analytic capacity. If, however, insight into previously unconscious wishes, fears, fantasies, memories, and means of defense is a crucial ingredient and result of psychoanalytic work, then self-analytic work can yield such psychoanalytic results, and not only in the hands of psychoanalysts or other previously analyzed persons. Writers, artists, philosophers and other psychologically talented people have been capable of insights into such processes and meanings in themselves and others long before psychoanalysis was invented.

Indeed, the invention of psychoanalysis involved self-analysis from the beginning. The treatment of Anna O., "the first analytic patient," was chiefly a case of self-analysis assisted by Josef Breuer. Interpretation by Breuer played a very small role. Freud's self-analysis, mainly via dreams and correspondence with Fliess and in synergistic interaction with his discoveries from his treatment of patients, led to the development and understanding of many basic psychoanalytic concepts, among them free association, the recognition of infantile sexuality, the role of unconscious drive impulses, repression leading to distortions of memory, and the function of screen memories. Nevertheless, Freud remained ambivalent about the possibility and usefulness of self-analysis. "My self-analysis is the most essential thing I have at present and promises to become of the greatest value to me if it reaches its end" (letter to Fliess, October 15, 1887, in Masson, 1985). "My self-analysis remains interrupted. I have realized why. I can analyze myself only with the help of knowledge obtained objectively (like an outsider). True self-analysis is impossible; otherwise there would be no [neurotic] illness" (letter to Fliess, November 14, 1887, in Masson, 1985). "One learns psychoanalysis on oneself, by studying one's own personality. This is not quite the same thing as what is called self-observation. . . . Nevertheless, there are definite limits to progress by this method. One advances much further if one is analyzed oneself by a practiced analyst" (Freud, 1916–1917: 19).

Freud recognized a serious difficulty with self-analysis, namely the unconscious nature of resistance, often masked by self-satisfaction with the results. "But in self analysis the danger of incompleteness is particularly great. One is too soon satisfied with a part explanation, behind which resistance may easily be keeping back something that is more important perhaps" (Freud, 1935: 234). Freud advised writing down associations to help put aside self-criticism in self-analysis.

Already in 1910 Freud noted, "We have become aware of the 'counter-transference,' which arises in [the physician] as a result of the patient's influence on his unconscious feelings, and we are almost inclined to insist that he shall recognize this counter transference in himself and overcome it. . . . We have noticed that no psychoanalyst goes further than his own complexes and internal resistances permit; and we consequently require that he shall begin his activity with a self analysis and continually carry it deeper while he is making his observations on his patients. Anyone who fails to produce results in a self analysis of this kind may at once give up any idea of being able to treat patients by analysis."

With the current stress on countertransference, enactments, inter-subjectivity, the interactive field between the analyst and patient, there is an even greater demand for self-observation and self-analytic work as part of ordinary analytic functioning. Consequently, the psychoanalytic literature increasingly contains examples of analysts' attempts at self-observation and self-analysis, often in the context of the presentation of clinical process and individual technique, i.e., what actually goes on between the patient and the analyst and within the analyst.

While within the acute analytic interaction the results of earlier analytic work may be available for use, often what the analyst knows about him- or herself and can discern through immediate self-observing capacities will have to serve at the moment, with more intense self-analytic work reserved for later. Different analysts have different routes via associative links to their unconscious conflicts stirred up by clinical work. Among these are: thoughts, affects (e.g., boredom, anger, irritation, hatred, disgust, anxiety, depression, discouragement, guilt, intense interest, pleasurable anticipation, excitement, loving feelings), visual images, hearing words or music, kinesthetic sensations, impulses, fantasies, memories, tendencies to activity or passivity, dreams, and parapraxes, occurring within or outside the analytic setting and found to be related to a patient. The particular timing, content, or wording of interpretations may also catch the analyst's attention as requiring investigation. Many analysts have found that writing down these observations and the associations to

them is vital to overcoming the lack of a second relatively more objective or disinterested observer, to overcome the tendency to repress or otherwise defend against unpleasant or unacceptable associative trends, and to help with self-objectification. Some have noted that even self-analysis occurs with witnesses, significant internalized figures from the past, and that all trends within the analyst, ideals, superego prohibitions, criticisms, self-punitive trends, impulses, wishes, character traits, defenses, including those against narcissistic injury, unconscious fantasies, theoretical predispositions, and so on, manifest themselves not only in the content, but also the shape and form of self-analytic endeavors. A danger stressed frequently is that of being too easily satisfied with rediscovering what one already knows, covering what may be more unacceptable or narcissistically wounding. The developmentally achieved capacity to bear negative affect partly determines self-analytic capacity. For some analysts, the analysand's increasing ability to use analytic methods to analyze him- or herself is one significant sign of analytic progress and almost a prerequisite for considering termination.

Besides clinical work, expectable adult crises and conflicts may also stimulate self-analytic work, for all analysands whose formal psychoanalysis is over. While some analysts routinely pursue self-analytic activities, others call upon them only under feelings of necessity. In the latter cases especially, and particularly at times of personal crises, self-analytic work may more easily assume the driven quality, accompanied by regression, that brings it closer to therapeutic psychoanalytic experiences, rather than the routine conscious or preconscious monitoring of one's "analytic toilette," an activity perhaps closer to ordinary introspection. Genuine self-analysis requires work, overcoming discomfort, to lead to genuine insights and inner change.

REFERENCES

Freud, S. (1910). The future prospects of psycho-analytic therapy. S.E. 11: 141–151.
———. (1916–1917). Introductory Lectures on Psycho-Analysis. S.E. 15–16: 9–496.
———. (1935). The subtleties of a faulty action. S.E. 22: 233–235.
Laplanche, J., and Pontalis, J. B. (1973). The Language of Psychoanalysis. New York: Norton.
Masson, J. M. (ed.) (1985). The Complete Letters of Sigmund Freud to Wilhelm Fliess, 1887–1904. Cambridge, Mass.: Harvard University Press.

HERBERT L. GOMBERG

Self-Deception

The term "self-deception" (German, *Selbsttäuschung*) does not appear in Freud's writings; yet under the topics of repression, defense and resistance, disavowal, fantasy ("phantasy" in the *Standard Edition*), and splits in the ego, closely related phenomena are central to his view of the mind. In his early *Studies on Hysteria*, Freud writes: "The hysterical patient's 'not knowing' was in fact a 'not wanting to know.'" Freud goes on to say that the path to consciousness may lie through the patient's associating to memories of which he or she has remained aware, or having his or her attention drawn to connections now forgotten, or calling up and arranging "recollections which have been withdrawn from association for many years" (Breur and Freud, 1895: 269–272).

"Disavowal" (*Verleugnung*) comes to the fore in Freud's discussion of sexuality (1923a; 1925; 1927). On his view, the boy's discovery of the anatomical differences between the sexes reinforces his fears of castration; the girl's discovery makes her feel inferior, already "castrated." A psychotic defense against an unwelcome idea or perception would typically deny it altogether, whereas disavowal acknowledges the perception but minimizes its importance, ignores its implications, or invests another object with its significance. (Described by him as "bad faith," Sartre's example [1957, p. 55–56] of a woman who gives sexual encouragement to a man by allowing him to hold her hand while telling herself the gesture is insignificant instances the phenomenology Freud has in mind.)

Though Freud's views about the universality and importance of early castration fears are no longer widely shared by psychoanalysts, many agree with him that disavowal characterizes the sexual perversions. Grossman describes the "perverse" attitude toward reality as the distracting of one's attention from unwelcome perceptions "in order to avoid challenging cherished fantasies" (Grossman, 1996: 510). For example, a male transvestite may dress as a woman, which he knows he is not, so he can tell himself that sensory evidence can be misleading. The pathology, on this view, is the license the patient gives himself not to test certain of his beliefs.

In his earliest discussion of fantasy, Freud writes: "The aim [of the symptoms, memories, psychical structures] seems to be to arrive back at the primal scenes. In a few cases this is achieved directly, but in others only by a roundabout path, via phantasies" (1950 [1892–1899], p. 248). Fantasies are a kind of visionary wish fulfillment of specifically conflicted wishes, often originating in different periods of the person's life. For example, in the fantasy that a child is being beaten, the child represents a sibling rival for the father's love; then, because of the guilt she later came to feel for her incestuous wishes, the fantasizer is herself the child who is being beaten (Freud, 1919). Implicit in the concept of fantasy are two of Freud's most fundamental ideas: that unconscious, wish-fulfilling imaginings are among the springs of action (Wollheim, 1984); and that such wishes may not only conflict with each other, but also with the agent's own occurrent perceptions, mature goals, and realistic assessments of how to achieve them. For example, Freud's patient the Rat Man engages in a ritual the meaning of which is that his father is alive and watching him, though the man knows that his father is dead (Freud, 1909).

In his later writings Freud expands on an idea he first suggested in connection with fetishism: the splitting of the ego (1940 [1938]a and 1940[1938]b). The fetishist's half-acknowledgment of an unwelcome idea is a compromise that is achieved, Freud says, "at the price of a rift in the ego. . . . The whole process seems so strange to us because we take for granted the synthetic nature of the processes of the ego. But we are clearly at fault in this. The synthetic function of the ego, though it is of such extraordinary importance, is subject to particular conditions and is liable to a whole number of disturbances" (1940 [1938]b, p. 276).

Freud is on to the fact that such self-reflexive attitudes as self-knowledge, self-discovery, and self-deception reflect ambiguities in the concept of the self. His use of the term—"*das Ich*," (the ego), with which Descartes and later continental philosophers invoked a special, unitary, mental "subject," is misleading, since Freud views the mind—self—as a set of interlocking structures. Some contemporary philosophers propose that we think of the mind as an elaborate network of ideas, connected to one another by varying degrees of closeness, and that, as Freud suggests, in irrationality the mind may be partitioned or divided (Davidson, 1982; Pears, 1984; Rorty, 1991; Cavell, 1993).

The concept of the unconscious does not itself resolve the puzzles implicit in the ideas of either self-deception or repression; for whether we call the self-deceiving (or repressing) censor conscious or unconscious, we impute to it the very unity of knowing and not knowing that generates the puzzles in the first place. So Freud himself acknowledges when, articulating the structural theory (according to which mental functioning is seen in terms of id, ego, and superego), he says that important processes in the ego itself, the source of both perception and censorship, are unconscious (1923b). Nevertheless, Freud's theory as a whole suggests strategies for dealing with the puzzles.

First, he draws our attention to the fact that what we call self-deception spans a spectrum. At one end are more or less conscious attempts to avoid acknowledging what one believes or wants; at the other are mental processes that have a more mechanical character. Second, whereas "self-deception" tends to imply the presence of fully formed propositional attitudes that are both avowed and denied, "repression" and "disavowal" often connote ideas that have not yet become full-fledged beliefs and desires but have more the character of isolated mental images. Third, the puzzles of self-deception arise from our considering it analogous to deceiving others, in which case we assume the unity of the deceiver as agent, and we hold his or her self-deceptions to be intentional. As indicated above, however, the sorts of "self-deception" that interest Freud are typically not fully intentional, and they suggest that "the unity of the self" may be an achievement rather than a metaphysical given.

REFERENCES

Breuer, J., and Freud, S. (1895). *Studies on Hysteria.* S.E. 2: 19–305.

Cavell, M. (1993). *The Psychoanalytic Mind, from Freud to Philosophy.* Cambridge, Mass.: Harvard University Press.

Davidson, D. (1982). Paradoxes of irrationality. In R. Wollheim and J. Hopkins (eds.). *Philosophical Essays on Freud.* Cambridge: Cambridge University Press, pp. 289–306.

Freud, S. (1909). Notes upon a case of obsessional neurosis. S.E. 10: 155–318.

———. (1919). "A child is being beaten": A contribution to the study of the origin of sexual perversions. S.E. 17: 179–204.

———. (1923a). The infantile genital organization: An interpolation into the theory of sexuality. S.E. 19: 141–145.

———. (1923b). *The Ego and the Id.* S.E.19: 12–59.

———. (1925). Some psychical consequences of the anatomical distinction between the sexes. S.E. 19: 248–258.

———. (1927). Fetishism. S.E. 21: 147–158.

———. (1940 [1938]a). *An Outline of Psychoanalysis.* S.E. 23: 144–207.

———. (1940 [1938]b). Splitting of the ego in the process of defence. S.E. 23: 271–277.

———. (1950 [1892–1899]). Extracts from the Fliess papers. S.E. 1: 173–282.

Grossman, L. (1996). "Psychic Reality" and reality testing in the analysis of perverse defences. *International Journal of Psychoanalysis,* 77: 509–517.

Pears, D. (1984). *Motivated Irrationality.* Oxford: Oxford University Press.

Rorty, R. (1991). Freud and Moral Reflection. In R. Rorty (author). *Essays on Heidegger and Others, Philosophical Papers, vol. 2.* Cambridge: Cambridge University Press.

Sartre, J. P. (1957). *Being and Nothingness, An Essay on Phenomenological Psychology.* Trans. Hazel Barnes. London: Methuen.

Wollheim, R. (1984). *The Thread of Life.* Cambridge, Mass.: Harvard University Press.

MARCIA CAVELL

Self Psychology

Psychoanalytic self psychology consists of the theoretical and clinical modifications introduced into psychoanalysis by Heinz Kohut (1913–1981) and his colleagues. These modifications evolved initially from an effort by Kohut to define more precisely the field of psychoanalytic science and to examine the relationship between mode of observation and theory (Kohut, 1959). Data collection methods delimit scientific fields. Differentiating from and excluding *physical* phenomena when the essential ingredient of observational methods includes the senses (and their extension by instruments), Kohut defined "phenomena" as *mental* or *psychological* when the essential ingredient is introspection and empathy, the latter defined as *vicarious introspection.* Thus psychoanalysis is the science of complex mental states accessed systematically through introspection and empathy. A clinical psychoanalytic approach based on this fundamental view stresses the pivotal importance of empathically derived data (Kohut, 1968).

Kohut locates a psychological structure, the *self,* at the center of his reconceptualization of psychoanalytic theory. The self manifests its presence as a cohesive, balanced, and energetic structure by providing the subject with a sense of self and a feeling of well-being characterized by healthy self-esteem. A self that lacks cohesion or whose constituents are out of balance or lacking in vital energy will tend toward disorganization (called *fragmentation*), i.e., the subject likely will experience anxiety or depression with a sense of seeming to fall apart. Various *defensive* or *compensatory* reactions may come into play in an attempt to restore an experience of a more vital self, often by way of *acting out.* Neonates are born

S

preadapted to an environment that provides not only for physiological needs but for psychological needs as well. There is a hunger for sensory stimuli that the brain orders into information. Speaking subjectively, there is a need for experiences that yield meaning.

A self comes into being during the early months after birth. Certain environmental inputs impinge on inherent structures resulting in the formation of a self, i.e., certain experiences evoke a sense of self: *those experiences that are needed to establish and to maintain a cohesive self-experience are called "selfobject" experiences*. Six types of essential selfobject experiences have been described. *Mirroring* experiences recognize and affirm the subject as highly valued, perhaps even admired; *idealizing* experiences are needed to link or merge the subject with an admired, calm, wise, beautiful, and strong other who possesses these valued characteristics that the subject lacks; *alter-ego* (twinship) experiences enhance the subject's self by demonstrating that it is all right to be like the other; *adversarial* selfobject experiences allow the subject to be antagonistic without evoking injurious responses, and are needed to open a path for healthy self-assertion, negativism, and anger in the service of strengthening the self; and *vitalizing* selfobject experiences consisting of cross-modal affective attunements by the caregiving other (cf. Stern, 1985) are an essential ingredient for the emergence of a cohesive self, as are *efficacy* selfobject experiences that authenticate the self by enabling it to decisively affect and alter some aspect of the other.

Individuals need selfobject experiences throughout life but their predominant form changes as the subject grows older. While the infant needs the selfobject experience in a close and intimate relationship to a concrete human other, the older child, to some extent, and the adult, largely, as a rule may have selfobject experiences that are more distant, more diffusely emanating from many individuals and groups. Finally, selfobject experiences associated to symbols representative of the earlier ones with the initial caregivers become central for the mature individual. Among these symbolically meaningful selfobject experiences, one may find some created by the arts, music, drama, literature, religion, and the like that convey the essence of the earlier needed experiences. Together, these construct a *developmental line* of selfobject experiences and the self (Wolf, 1980).

Disorders of the self result from faulty, deficient, or absent selfobject experiences. The normally needed

appropriate selfobject milieu may become traumatically distressful during the time before the first emergence of a self with a resulting *deformed* self, usually one that is severely damaged, as in the psychoses and borderline personalities. Injury endured during the time between the first emergence of the self and the final consolidation of a cohesive self is usually not as disabling and results in a *fragile* self, perhaps with a narcissistic personality or behavior disorder. *Unfulfilled* selves are manifested mostly as disorders of later life, often around a midlife crisis with much anxiety and depression, when a person is confronted with the finiteness of life and with having deviated from a life plan that was laid down at the time that the self had consolidated into a final cohesive form.

People with deformed, fragile, or unfulfilled selves come into psychoanalytic treatment because they suffer the symptoms of a weakened or disorganized self. The goal of treatment is to strengthen the self. Many less seriously injured selves whose pathology consists mostly of arrested development do well in the milieu created by an empathic understanding supplemented by explanatory interpretations that illuminate the etiologic link between trauma and symptoms. The analyst is experienced as an understanding other who provides needed recognition and is available for idealizing, alter-ego, adversarial, vitalizing, and efficacy selfobject experiences. It is a frequent misunderstanding of self psychology to conclude that the self psychologist merely dispenses sympathy or compassion. Rather often the facilitation of such an *ambient* therapeutic process requires limit setting within a framework of realistic expectations. However, most analysands require more. Inevitable disruptions in the therapeutic process lead to experiences of mutual disaffection that must be accepted without placing blame. The therapist must understand, explain, and discuss these disruptions with a view toward restoration of the treatment compact. Both participants in the therapeutic dialogue will then emerge with a better understanding of each other. This disruption-restoration sequence is the most important path to healing the injured selves of both patient and therapist, but it is particularly important for strengthening the analysand's self.

REFERENCES

Kohut, H. (1959). Introspection, empathy, and psychoanalysis. *Journal of the American Psychoanalytic Assosication*, 7: 459–483.
———. (1968). The psychoanalytic treatment of narcissistic personality disorders. *Psychoanalytic Study of the Child*, 23: 86–113.

Stern, D. (1985). *The Interpersonal World of the Infant.* New York: Basic Books.

Wolf, E. (1980). On the developmental line of selfobject relations. In A. Goldberg (ed.). *Advances in Self Psychology.* New York: International Universities Press, pp. 117–130.

———. (1994). Selfobject experiences: Development, psychopathology, treatment. In S. Kramer and S. Akhtar (eds.). *Mahler and Kohut: Perspectives on Development, Psychopathology, and Technique.* Northvale, N.J.: Jason Aronson, pp. 65–96.

———. (1988). *Treating the Self.* New York: Guilford Press.

ERNEST S. WOLF

Sexology

The term "sexology" was coined by Elizabeth Osgood Goodrich Willard in 1867, who, believing sex was a loathsome thing, was unhappy that people were born as a result of such an activity that was so easily abused. In spite of her hostility, the term came to be used to describe those who engage in the study of sex, although many prefer the term "sexual scientist."

Serious study of sex began in the nineteenth century, primarily in German-speaking lands where there was a conflict between the Napoleonic code, which determined whether certain sexual activities were illegal or not according to the two concepts of age and consent, and traditional Roman law. If the person was of age and consented to the activity, including homosexual activity, then according to the Napoleonic code, no crime was committed. The legal code in other parts of German-speaking Europe was based on traditional Roman law, which prohibited certain forms of conduct such as homosexuality because they were considered contrary to nature. The conflict between the two codes was a major factor in encouraging many scholars to engage in serious study of sexuality, and by the end of the nineteenth century there were specialized journals devoted to the subject. Some specific groups arose, devoted to disseminating information about sex. The German Iwan Bloch (1872–1922) was particularly influential because of his advocacy of *Sexualwissenschaft* (sexual science) as a new discipline based not only on biological and psychological data but on cultural, social, and historical materials as well.

Three men dominated sexology during the early years of the twentieth century: Magnus Hirschfeld (1868–1935), Havelock Ellis (1849–1939), and Sigmund Freud (1856–1939). All had been trained as physicians, and although Hirschfeld and Ellis collected and analyzed much more data on the topic, it was Freud, the new system maker, who became the model for much of the medical community, particularly in the United States. Because of the influence of Freud in the United States, psychoanalysts tended to dominate the explorations of sexual behavior in America, and this dominance was not challenged until the 1940s. Much of Hirschfeld's work remained untranslated, and while his name was known, few Americans read him. Havelock Ellis was more easily available to English-speaking peoples, but he lacked the kind of disciples that Freud had. Much of the German-language research was either temporarily lost or destroyed and all the sex organizations in Germany were disbanded as a result of the Hitler period (1933–1945). This gave further emphasis to Freud, who had many disciples in the United States.

Much of the research into sex shifted to the United States beginning in the 1920s largely through the efforts of Katherine Bement Davis (1860–1935), who persuaded John D. Rockefeller Jr. to organize and fund the Committee for Research in the Problems of Sex (CRPS). Several of her own studies were funded by Rockefeller, including one on female sexuality that found that women in the 1920s were far more sexually responsive than was popularly believed. Also influential on the American scene was Robert Latou Dickinson (1861–1950), a gynecologist who, like Davis, emphasized the sexuality of women.

Initially much of the research sponsored by the CRPS was in endocrinology, and this resulted in major breakthroughs on the influence of hormones and an understanding of the menstrual cycle. The CRPS also conducted much research into the sexuality of primates. It was not until 1940 that the CRPS began to support large-scale survey research into human sexual activity, and it was then that Alfred Kinsey (1894–1956) received his first grant from the group and he soon took a major share of its resources. It was Kinsey who challenged the medical and psychiatric dominance in the study of sex and encouraged biological and physiological research as well as research of the social scientists. Building upon the pathbreaking works of Kinsey was the research of William Masters and Virginia Johnson, particularly their work on the physiology of the sexual response.

Some indication of changing attitudes was the establishment of professional societies in the sex field, first the Society for the Scientific Study of Sex (SSSS) in 1960 and the American Association of Sex Educators and Counselors (and later Therapists) (AASECT) in 1967. Other organizations followed including international ones.

Few graduate programs in sexology were established, however, because by definition sexology was and still remains a multidisciplinary field, so that interdisciplinary graduate work is difficult to accomplish. Inevitably most sexologists specialize in one discipline; psychology is probably dominant right now, but sociology, anthropology, and one of the many areas of biology are also important. Many in the field still come from medicine, some from law, a few from history, and a handful from the various humanities. The interdisciplinary nature of sexology makes an individual sexologist particularly dependent upon the work of colleagues outside of his or her own discipline and encourages both collaboration and a real effort to go beyond narrow specialization. Its very weakness as a solid academic discipline becomes its strength because of the diversity of approaches and the need for individuals in the field to explore other disciplines and collaborate with other specialists.

REFERENCE

Bullough, V. L. (1994). *Science in the Bedroom: A History of Sex Research.* New York: Basic Books.

VERN L. BULLOUGH

Sexual Instinct See DRIVE THEORY.

Sexual Stages See DEVELOPMENTAL THEORY; LIBIDO THEORY; OEDIPUS COMPLEX.

Sexual Symbolism See SYMBOLISM.

Shame

Various theories have been advanced to explain Freud's relative neglect of shame in his writings. One is that guilt took priority in Freud's theories because of its relationship to the Oedipus complex and because of its role in his structural theory as a primary affect or function of the superego. Another explanation involves an inherent aspect of shame: shame seeks concealment. When experiencing acute shame, people avert their gaze and bow their heads. This natural defense of concealment in response to shame has led some to suggest that for Freud and for many other theorists, shame is difficult to recognize and to study (Lewis, 1971).

Shame was observed and discussed by Freud primarily in his early work. In an 1895 letter to Wilhelm Fliess, Freud proposed that shame, along with morality and disgust, was a cause for repression of sexual experience. In this same letter, Freud introduced the possibility of gender differences relating to shame. He suggested that in males there is a relative absence of shame, while on the other hand young girls are "seized by a non-neurotic sexual repugnance . . . the flood of shame which overwhelms the female" (Freud, 1892–1899: 270). Freud (1930) suggested that shame is a result of man's assuming an upright posture, thereby exposing the genitals. In 1933, he related shame to the desire for concealment of genital deficiency, and he suggested that shame be considered "a feminine characteristic par excellence" (p. 132).

Freud thus identified the association of shame with a sense of exposure. In Letter 66 (Freud, 1892–1899) to Fliess, Freud mentioned dreams in which an individual was wandering among strangers undressed, ashamed, and anxious. In *The Interpretation of Dreams*, he further described dreams of being naked as characterized by "a distressing feeling in the nature of shame and in the fact that one wishes to hide one's nakedness, as a rule by locomotion, but finds one is unable to do so" (Freud, 1900: 242).

In *Three Essays on the Theory of Sexuality*, Freud (1905) related the theme of exposure and shame to exhibitionism. He identified shame as the source of resistance to the wish to exhibit and suggested that it "impeded the course of the sexual instinct" (p. 177). Subsequent literature continued to explore the relationship between shame and exhibitionism. Fenichel (1945) defined shame as one of four intolerable affects and suggested that shame was a motive for defense against exhibitionism. He expanded that concept to include the relationship of shame to urethral eroticism and to feelings of inferiority. Nunberg (1955) introduced the idea that shame is a reaction formation against the wish to exhibit, and these concepts were expanded by Wurmser (1981).

In *On Narcissism*, Freud (1914) also laid the groundwork for subsequent thinking about the role of shame in self-esteem regulation. He introduced the concept of the ego ideal and related the ego ideal to maintaining self esteem. He viewed the ego ideal as invested with narcissism derived from the original experience of perfection. Piers and Singer (1953) differentiated the ego ideal from the superego and the ego. Like Freud, they identified the ego ideal as deriving from the infantile experience of omnipotence and perfection. When the sense of omnipotence is not adequately modified, shame results from the intolerable tension between the grandiose ego ideal and the ego.

Lewis (1971) initiated the contemporary study of shame and identified its role in symptom formation. She suggested that shame is "about the whole self," and delineated inherent difficulties in processing shame. These relate to the inability to tolerate shame, which triggers an immediate need for defense and concealment. Therefore the shame and its source are not expressed, examined, and resolved. The inevitable shame, anger, or humiliated fury that are consequences of shame perpetuate shame, while simultaneously restricting its expression. Shame and guilt set up self-perpetuation cycles that prevent resolution. Through microanalysis of psychotherapy sessions, Lewis identified processes associated with shame in treatment and suggested that unidentified shame can be a source of the negative therapeutic reaction and treatment failure.

Current work on shame has focused particularly on the relationship of shame to the development of the self with regard to narcissism (Thrane, 1979; Broucek, 1982; Kinston, 1983; A. Morrison, 1983; Nathanson, 1987). Andrew Morrison (1989) identified shame as the primary affect of narcissism and integrated the dynamics of shame with Kohut's theories of self. He suggested that a tension-generating dialectic occurs between narcissistic grandiosity and desire for perfection and the sense of the self as flawed that results from the recognition of dependency and loss of merger. The self is confronted with a desire for an absolute independence and autonomy and a desire for perfect merger. Thus states of shame and states of narcissistic grandiosity alternate and contribute to conflicts between desires for autonomy and for merger.

Other work has explored additional ways in which shame participates in development. Lewis (1981) referred to shame and guilt as universal affects that had as their function repairing lost affectional bonds and maintaining affiliation. This role complements the roles of shame in socialization (Schore, 1994) and in the differentiation of the self associated with the formation of autonomy and identity (Lynd, 1958; Severino et al., 1987). Shame thus contributes to the observing abilities of the self and to the establishment of morality (Schneider, 1977; N. Morrison and Severino, 1997).

Gender-related differences in the experience and management of shame are complex. Freud (1933) regarded shame as a feminine characteristic related to the awareness of genital deficiency. Lewis (1981) also suggested gender influences based on differences of field dependence, more common in women, and field independence, more common in men. She postulated that women are more prone to experience shame and men are more prone to experience guilt. Others suggest that men and women are equally prone to experience shame, but because of cultural, biological, and developmental differences, men and women will process and express shame differently (Krugman, 1995).

Schore (1994) presents the current understanding of the neurobiology of shame. At eighteen months, a child exhibits moral prosocial altruistic behavior by showing an attempt to comfort a distressed other. This suggests that the child is beginning to regulate his or her own negative affect and is capable of reading the affect of another. This primarily visual process is thought to relate to the development of the right hemispheric orbitofrontal cortex.

REFERENCES

Broucek, F. (1982). Shame and its relationship to early narcissistic developments. *International Journal of Psychoanalysis*, 65: 369–378.

Fenichel, O. (1945). *The Psychoanalytic Theory of Neurosis*. New York: Norton.

Freud, S. (1892–1899). Extracts from the Fliess papers. S.E. 1: 175–280.

———. (1900). *The Interpretation of Dreams*. S.E. 4–5: 1–621.

———. (1905). *Three Essays on the Theory of Sexuality*. S.E. 7: 125–243.

———. (1914). On narcissism: An introduction. S.E. 14: 69–102.

———. (1930). *Civilization and Its Discontents*. S.E. 21: 57–146.

———. (1933). *New Introductory Lectures on Psycho-Analysis*. S.E. 22: 3–182.

Kinston, W. (1983). A theoretical context for shame. *International Journal of Psychoanalysis*, 64: 213–226.

Krugman, S. (1995). Male development and the transformation of shame. In R. F. Levant and W. S. Pollack (eds.). *A New Psychology of Men*. New York: Basic Books.

Lewis, H. B. (1971). *Shame and Guilt in Neurosis*. New York: International Universities Press.

———. (1981). Shame and guilt in human nature. In S. Tuttman, C. Kaye, and M. Zimmerman (eds.). *Object and Self*. New York: International Universities Press, pp. 235–265.

Lynd, H. M. (1958). *On Shame and the Search for Identity*. New York: Harcourt, Brace and World.

Morrison, A. P. (1983). Shame, the ideal self, and narcissism. *Contemporary Psychoanalysis*, 19: 295–318.

———. (1989). *Shame: The Underside of Narcissism*. Hillsdale, N.J.: Analytic Press.

S

Morrison, N. K., and Severino, S. K. (1997). Moral values: Development and gender influences. *Journal of the American Academy of Psychoanalysis*, 25 (2): 255–275.

Nathanson, D. L. (1987). *The Many Faces of Shame*. New York: Guilford Press.

Nunberg, H. (1955). *Principles of Psychoanalysis*. New York: International Universities Press.

Piers, G., and Singer, M. B. (1953). *Shame and Guilt*. Springfield, Ill.: Thomas. Reprinted, 1971, New York: Norton.

Schneider, C. D. (1977). *Shame, Exposure and Privacy*. Boston: Beacon Press.

Schore, A. N. (1994). *Affect Regulation and the Origin of the Self: The Neurobiology of Emotional Development*. Hillside, N.J.: Lawrence Erlbaum Associates.

Severino, S. K., McNutt, E. R., and Feder, S. L. (1987). Shame and the development of autonomy. *Journal of the American Academy of Psychoanalysis*, 15, no. 1: 93–106.

Thrane, G. (1979). Shame and the construction of the self. *Annual of Psychoanalysis*, 7: 321–341. New York: International Universities Press.

Wurmser, L. (1981). *The Mask of Shame*. Baltimore: Johns Hopkins University Press.

NANCY K. MORRISON
SALLY K. SEVERINO
EDITH R. MCNUTT

Sleep

The problem of sleep was, for Freud, a physiological problem, and therefore something that fell outside his primary area of scientific interest (Freud, 1900: 6; 1916–1917: 88). Nevertheless, sleep was a necessary precondition for dreaming—and dreaming was of course a psychological issue of very great interest to Freud. He therefore tackled the problem of sleep by characterizing it in metapsychological terms, as the set of functional conditions that must prevail in the mental apparatus for dreams to occur.

On this basis, Freud took the view that the state of sleep consists fundamentally in a shift of the dynamic relations between the two major functional divisions of the mind—the discharge-seeking drives and the discharge-inhibiting ego—in favor of the drives (1900, pp. 526, 576; 1907, pp. 62–63). This shift explained the foremost psychological characteristic of dreams: the "important fact that the psi *primary processes*, such as have been biologically suppressed in the course of psi development, are daily presented to us during sleep" (1950, p. 336). Freud believed that the shift occurred as a result of a fundamental alteration in the state of the ego: it was the ego

that went to sleep at night (1923, p. 17), not the drives (1900, p. 555). Indeed, the sleeplessness of the drives was the primary cause of dreams (1917, p. 225; 1916–1917, p. 419). Thus, although Freud did occasionally acknowledge that sleep was encouraged by drive satisfaction (1950, p. 336), and indeed by nocturnal reduction in external stimuli (1921, p. 130), the decisive characteristic of sleep itself was consistently conceptualized by him as a change in the state of the ego itself: "the dominant system withdraws into a *wish to sleep*, realizes that wish by bringing about modifications which it is able to produce in the cathexes within the psychical apparatus, and persists in that wish throughout the whole duration of sleep" (1900, p. 570).

For Freud, the essence of sleep, then, consisted in a withdrawal by the ego into a wish to sleep (1900, p. 590), which in turn produced a range of modifications in the cathexes within the psychical apparatus. The latter consisted in the following four (primarily economic) modifications: (1) a partial suspension of secondary process thought activity—that is, a withdrawal of cathexis from the preconscious system itself (1900, pp. 554, 573) (This excludes the "wish to sleep" itself—and "the day's residues," which oppose the wish to sleep [Freud, 1950: 336; 1900, pp. 554–555; 1917, p. 224; 1916–1917, p. 89].); (2) a partial withdrawal of inhibitory anticathexis from the repressed (1900, p. 526) (This excludes the superego function of "censorship."); (3) a withdrawal of attentional precathexis from the perceptual system (1950, p. 337) (this facilitates regression [Freud, 1900: 544, 573; 1917, p. 234].); and (4) a withdrawal of tonic activation from the motor system (1950, p. 337).

The first and second of these modifications were theoretically contradictory, in that a withdrawal of inhibitory anticathexis necessarily released drive pressures that should be incompatible with the wish to sleep. The solution to this apparent contradiction was to be found in the fourth modification of the sleeping ego—the decathexis of the motor system, which rendered the disinhibited drives harmless by making it impossible for them to gain access to motility (1900, p. 568; 1901, p. 679; 1925, p. 44).

The saving in mental effort that these modifications implied reflected Freud's conception of the essential psychological *purpose* of sleep, namely, respite from the relentless stimuli to which the waking ego was subjected, which required it by day to tolerate a constant level of tonic activation—the hallmark of its normal inhibitory

S

function (1950, p. 336; 1900, pp. 575, 577; 1915, p. 151; 1916–1917, pp. 88–89; 1921, p. 130).

With the development of the concept of narcissism, Freud further elaborated this conception of the restitutive function of sleep (together with his conceptions of a relaxation of the secondary process and a withdrawal of perceptual precathexis) with the idea that sleep involved a withdrawal of object libido back into the ego. That is, according to this formulation, sleep entailed a return to the blissful self-sufficiency of intrauterine existence: a regression to absolute narcissism (1914, p. 83; 1917, pp. 222–223, 225; 1916–1917, p. 417; 1940, p. 166). This last conceptualization of the metapsychology of sleep enabled Freud to reinforce the theoretical links that he had always drawn among dreaming, regression, and psychotic symptom formation.

Modern neuroscience has cast fresh light on the physiology of sleep, and thereby (indirectly) tested some aspects of Freud's metapsychological conceptualization of it. We still have no way of accessing the neural correlates of so subtle a mental state as "the wish to sleep," but we are now in a position to comment pertinently on some of the contingent range of "modifications in the cathexes within the psychical apparatus" that Freud hypothesized were characteristic of the state of sleep. These were (1) partial suspension of secondary process thought activity (withdrawal of cathexis from the preconscious system itself); (2) partial withdrawal of inhibitory anticathexis from the repressed; (3) withdrawal of attentional precathexis from the perceptual system; and (4) withdrawal of tonic activation from the motor system.

The last of these functional modifications (having a simple external manifestation) is easiest to assess neurophysiologically. Freud's hypothesis that "sleep is characterized by *motor paralysis (paralysis of the will)*," which he attributed to the fact that "the spinal tonus is in part relaxed" (1950, p. 137), has been confirmed directly and repeatedly by various methods. During the REM phase of sleep (which is when most dreams occur), the final common path motor neurons in the spinal cord are inhibited. This level of motor inhibition is probably mediated by brain stem mechanisms (Pompeiano, 1967), but recent studies (Braun et al., 1998; Solms, 1997) have suggested that the "paralysis of the will" that Freud referred to might also be mediated by a decathexis of the executive portion of the motor system (the dorsolateral frontal lobes of the brain). (Here the metapsychological term "cathexis" is used synonymously with the neuro-

physiolgical term "activation," since they seem to be functionally equivalent.)

The same finding accounts for the hypothesized partial suspension of secondary process thought activity (withdrawal of cathexis from the preconscious system). In Freud's (1900) model, the system *Pcs.* was situated at the "output" end of the mental apparatus, just behind the motor system itself, over which the *Pcs.* exercised executive control. The dorsolateral frontal convexity is similarly situated and exercises the same function (Luria, 1980; Passingham, 1993). Modern neuroscientific investigators are unanimously of the view that this part of the brain mediates the "delayed response" function, which lies at the heart of the secondary process. Leading neuroscientific dream theorists (Braun et al., 1998; Hobson et al., 1998) now suggest that dorsolateral frontal deactivation during REM sleep accounts for the bizarre and delusional nature of dream mentation, and contributes to dream amnesia. (They suggest further that this explanation of dream bizarreness contradicts Freud's hypothesis of an active dream "censorship." However, the latter inference ignores the fact that the *ventromesial* frontal region, which is fundamentally implicated in critical self-awareness, is highly activated during REM sleep. This finding, it seems, is consistent with Freud's hypothesis that secondary process activity is *partially* suspended in dreams.)

Freud's third hypothesized modification (withdrawal of attentional precathexis from the perceptual system) finds an interesting counterpart in the discovery that the primary sensory cortices of the brain are almost entirely inactive during dreaming sleep (Braun et al., 1998; Solms, 1997).

We are not in a position to comment pertinently from the neuroscientific viewpoint on Freud's remaining hypothesis, to the effect that the repressed is relatively disinhibited during sleep. We have insufficient knowledge of the neural correlates of repression. Nevertheless, the striking increase in limbic system activation (and the concomitant decrease in neocortical activation) that characterizes dreaming sleep might be interpreted as lending indirect support to this hypothesis.

REFERENCES

Braun, A., Balkin, T., Wesensten, N., Carson, R., Varga, M., Balwin, P., Selbie, S., Belenky, G., and Herscovitch (1998). Regional cerebral blood flow throughout the sleep-wake cycle. *Brain*, 120: 1173–1197.

Freud, S. (1900). *The Interpretation of Dreams.* S.E. 4–5: 1–621.

———. (1901). On dreams. S.E. 5: 629–714.

———. (1907). *Delusions and Dreams in Jensen's Gradiva.* S.E. 9: 1–96.

———. (1914). On narcissism: An introduction. S.E. 14: 67–104.

———. (1915). Repression. S.E. 14: 141–158.

———. (1916–1917). *Introductory Lectures on Psycho-Analysis.* S.E. 15–16: 9–496.

———. (1917). A metapsychological supplement to the theory of dreams. S.E. 14: 217–236.

———. (1921). *Group Psychology and the Analysis of the Ego.* S.E. 18: 65–144.

———. (1923). *The Ego and the Id.* S.E. 19: 1–62.

———. (1925). An autobiographical study. S.E. 20: 1–74.

———. (1940). *An Outline of Psycho-Analysis.* S.E. 23: 139–208.

———. (1950). *Project for a Scientific Psychology.* S.E. 1: 281–387.

Hobson, J. A., Stickgold, R., and Pace-Schott, E. (1998). The neuropsychology of REM sleep dreaming. *Neuroreport,* 9: R1–R14.

Luria, A. (1980). *Higher Cortical Functions in Man,* 2d ed. New York: Basic Books.

Passingham, R. (1993). *The Frontal Lobes and Voluntary Action.* Oxford: Oxford University Press.

Pompeiano, O. (1967). The neurobiological mechanisms of the postural and motor events during desynchronized sleep. *Proceedings of the Association for Research of Nervous Mental Disorders,* 45: 351–423.

Solms, M. (1997). *The Neuropsychology of Dreaming: A Clinico-Anatomical Study.* Mahwah, N.J.: Lawrence Erlbaum Associates.

                                    MARK SOLMS

Slips, Theory of

As with several of Freud's claims, his view of slips of the tongue was at first widely accepted in psychology, then ignored and even debunked, and now has come to be accepted again—at least in part. Among other factors, the more recent endorsement may be attributed in large measure to laboratory research performed in the late 1970s and early 1980s yielding empirical support for some of Freud's notions of slips.

Freud viewed slips of the tongue as a window to the mind, believing that slips manifest repressed thoughts and other features of the speaker's personality (Freud, 1901). In effect, the Freudian view is that slips are distortions of a speaker's intended utterance caused by dimensions of his or her private cognitive state that are semantically independent of the intended utterance. The interference yields an error utterance that is closer in meaning (or other linguistic form) to the hidden state than to the original target utterance.

Anecdotal evidence of Freudian slips is abundant—a lover calling out the wrong name during the heat of passion, an applicant whose introduction to a job interview competitor produced, "It's a pleasure to *beat* you," a man whose compliment on a woman's translucent blouse took the form, "I like your *broust*," and so forth. Indeed, some Freudian analysts will claim manifestation of suppressed or repressed cognitions even in more ostensibly "innocent" slips, such as *sweet streeper* for *street sweeper,* "I can't cut my *meef*" for "I can't cut my *meat/beef,*" "scratch and *stiff snickers*" for scratch and *sniff stickers,*" and so forth. Such interpretations are consistent with Freud's view that *all* slips manifest hidden cognitions.

An opposite view—that *no* slips are "Freudian"—was popular in the 1960s and 1970s. Psycholinguistics, the study of the cognitive processes responsible for speech and language production and reception, was in its infancy, and early psycholinguistic models of speech production were incompatible with Freud's views. In essence, it made no sense that the semantic, lexical, syntactic, phonological, or motor components involved in the production of an utterance can receive interference from any cognition that is not somehow an essential part of the intended utterance itself.

This is not to say that psycholinguists ignored the obvious fact that speech errors do occur. Indeed, slips of the tongue were studied closely by some. Fromkin (1973a; 1973b) in particular performed linguistic analyses on a very large corpus of slips collected in a wide variety of natural settings. Interpretations were far from Freudian, however. Rather, the slip research provided evidence for and against purely *linguistic* processes being debated in cognitive theories of speech production.

The view of Freudian slips that emerged during the early years of psycholinguistic research—including research on slips—was simply that there is no such thing. Freud's view of slips was dismissed primarily on two grounds. For one, within the existing theories of speech production, there was no mechanism—that is, no known mechanism or operation by which cognitive factors linguistically independent of an intended utterance can influence the vocal output of the utterance (much less exert enough influence to create error output). For another, there was no clear empirical evidence of Freudian slips. Anecdotal evidence via "suspicious" slips (e.g., the above "... pleasure to *beat* you," "... like your *broust,*" etc.) was dismissed as a statistical fluke; that is, with the hundreds of slips we witness in a given period, it stands to reason that by chance some small proportion will appear suspiciously Freudian even though their origin is purely linguistic.

The absence of empirical evidence created something of an impasse with respect to scholarly views of Freudian slips. There were, on the one hand, those who readily accepted Freud's views without empirical evidence; on the other hand, a larger group of psycholinguists and cognitive psychologists dismissed Freud's views for lack of empirical support. Paradoxically, those who would have liked to have seen Freud's views supported were themselves not empiricists (for the most part), and were thus an unlikely source of empirical evidence. The empiricists, on the other hand, were an unlikely source as well. Most were not particularly interested in testing Freud's claims, being occupied instead with testing more contemporary theories of the day. But the impasse was exacerbated by another problem: Even for those who might have been inclined to empirically test Freud's view of slips, there was no method with which to do so.

A direct empirical test of Freud's theory of slips would require a reliable way to elicit accidental slips of the tongue (preferably under laboratory conditions), a way to know subjects' hidden cognitive state with reasonable certainty (or better yet, to manipulate the cognitive state), and a way for the cognitive state to be manifested convincingly via the form and frequency of presumably related slips. Methods for eliciting accidental slips under laboratory conditions began to be developed during the mid-1970s, originally for testing purely linguistic variables and, by the end of the decade, were recognized as a way to test Freud's theory of slips.

The standard method for generating laboratory slips produced spoonerisms—the type of verbal slip in which two phonemes (speech sounds) or phoneme clusters trade places between the target utterance and error utterance (e.g., intended *barn door* → *darn bore, mad dash*→ *dad mash*, etc.). The method requires subjects to watch a screen on which word pairs are flashed at approximately one-second intervals. They are instructed to read the word pairs silently until they hear a cue (buzzer), in which case they are to speak aloud the preceding (no longer exposed) word pair. Slips are promoted (unbeknown to subjects) by preceding each target word pair with "interference" word pairs. The most effective form of interference precedes the target word pairs with word pairs more phonologically similar to the predicted error than

to the intended target. For example, preceding the cued target *rage wait*, there would be one or two word pairs with the /r/ and /w/ reversed to match the predicted spoonerism (*wage rate*), such as *red wig* and *rough weather* (e.g., Motley and Baars, 1976a). One of several variations used semantic interference—word pairs more similar in meaning to the predicted error than to the target utterance. For example, the target *rage wait* (→ *wage rate*) might be preceded by *salary scale* and *pay bracket* (e.g., Motley and Baars, 1976b). Typical studies include about twenty to forty error-prediction targets, i.e., targets with interference, balanced with several control word pairs cued without interference. Subjects make accidental spoonerisms on about 30 percent of the targets on which slips are predicted. This 30 percent yield was sufficient to test a large number of psycholinguistic hypotheses, always with the dependent variable being slip frequency, and usually with the independent variable being the linguistic form of the error—e.g., lexically legitimate versus lexically anomalous, syntactically legitimate versus syntactically anomalous, and so on (e.g., Baars, Motley, and MacKay, 1975; Motley and Baars, 1975).

All that was needed to apply the laboratory slip methodology to Freud's theory was to induce a given cognitive state (as the independent variable) to design target word pairs so that their predicted errors would reflect the cognitive state, and to compare error frequencies (as the dependent variable) against those of control subjects in whom the relevant cognitive state was not induced. The first such study induced a fear-of-electric-shock state by asking subjects to perform the slip-eliciting task while one hand was attached to electrodes they believed would deliver an electric shock at some random point in the study. A control group performed the same task on the same stimulus list without fear of electric shock (i.e., no electrodes present). Subjects in the fear-of-shock group made far more slips of the type, *worst cottage* → *cursed wattage, varied colts* → *carried volts* than the control group (Motley and Baars, 1979). In a companion study, the same basic design was retained, but with mild sexual arousal as the independent variable. For one group of male college student subjects, the laboratory-slip task was administered by a confederate experimenter—an attractive and provocatively attired college-age female. For a matched control group, the task was administered by a male professor. The sexual-arousal group made more slips of the type *past fashion* → *fast passion, share boulders* → *bare shoulders*, and so forth than the control group (Motley and Baars, 1979).

S

These studies provided the first empirical support, by behavioral-science standards, for Freud's theory of slips—at least in its weaker form. It was apparent that undisclosed cognitions (e.g., fear of the shock, or attention to the sexy female) that are irrelevant to one's intended utterance can promote slips of the tongue semantically related to those cognitions. Stronger versions of Freud's views are more difficult to test, but a notable effort is presented in a study by Motley, Camden, and Baars (1979). Again, subjects were male college students with a cognitive-state manipulation of sexual arousal via an attractive and provocatively attired female. But in this study, the primary independent variable was sexual guilt (e.g., Mosher, 1966). As before, subjects encountering the female confederate made more sex-related errors than a male-experimenter control group. More important, sex-related slips (e.g., *ate grass* → *great ass, Brent* → *Wallace went braless*, etc.) were significantly more frequent for subjects with higher levels of sexual guilt than for those with lesser levels. To a reasonable degree, these results supported Freud's notion that cognitions at lower levels of consciousness, including repressed states, can influence slips of the tongue (Motley, 1980).

The explanatory mechanism in these studies was based on theories of "spreading activation" (e.g., Collins and Loftus, 1975) by which the language user's lexicon, or "mental dictionary," is thought to contain a spider-web-like network of connections between its various words, these connections being based not only upon semantic relationships (synonyms, opposites, etc.) but also upon world-view organization (e.g., *uncle* might be linked to *aunt, brother*, etc.; *airplane* to *sky, fly*, etc.), phonological similarity (e.g., *sky* to *fly, sigh, ski*, etc.), and perhaps syntactic function as well (e.g., Motley, 1974). Spreading-activation theory was originally conceived as an account of cognitive processing during language recognition. The idea was that when a word is heard, corresponding locations or "nodes" in the "web" are activated. This activation presumably spreads to associated nodes, then spreads with weakened diffusion to their associated nodes, and so forth, yielding the original word's meaning as a composite of all activated nodes (Collins and Loftus, 1975).

As an explanation for Freudian slips, the spreading-activation model was simply converted from speech recognition to speech production. Word-choice output during speech was imagined to be largely a matter of "automatically" selecting the node receiving the highest level of activation when all nodes relevant to the message are activated. Freud's theory had always been that factors independent of the intended spoken message can influence the output of the message. Within a spreading-activation model, this simply means that while some nodes are being activated by the semantic (and syntactic) parameters of the intended utterance, other nodes may be activated by cognitions not related to the intended message. Ordinarily, we would expect one of the message-related nodes to receive the highest overall activation, and then to be output in an error-free utterance. In Freudian slips, however, an *error* node apparently has received the highest activation, presumably as a result of partial activation via the intended-message network, plus partial activation of the "hidden cognition" network, these summing to a higher overall activation than for other nodes, message-related or otherwise. Thus, for example, in the above "pleasure to meet you → . . . beat you" error, nodes for *meet*, [make your] *acquaintance, know* [you], etc., would receive relatively high activation; their phonological relatives (including for *meet* → *beat, eat, seat*, etc.) would receive lesser levels of activation, and so on. But at the same time, nodes associated with the example's job competition would be activated as well, most likely including, among others, *defeat, win, beat*, and so on, and their spreading-activation relatives. Presumably, if the "hidden cognition" is strong enough, the cumulative multiple activation on the *beat* node might exceed that of the target *meet* node, and trigger the "pleasure to *beat* you" error (Motley, 1985a).

This reasoning would predict that double entendres operate in much the same way, quite consistent with Freud's explanation. In double entendres, the suspicious output is not an error as is the case with slips, but rather appears suspicious owing to an ostensible relationship to a suspected cognitive state (sometimes in combination with being an intuitively low-probability word choice for the given message). While Freud considered double entendres to be additional evidence of hidden cognitive states, skeptics have considered them to be coincidental flukes. Laboratory studies have supported a weak version of Freud's view (with a spreading-activation explanation), by showing that males in the threat-of-shock and arousal-via-sexy-confederate manipulations mentioned above are much more likely than control subjects to fill in the blank of stimulus sentences with related double entendres (Motley and Camden 1985; Motley, Camden, and Baars, 1983). For example, a sentence like "Tension mounted toward the end, as the symphony reached its ———" is much more likely to be completed aloud with *climax* by subjects experiencing mild sexual arousal than by control subjects (for whom *finale, conclusion, climax,* and *ending* are more probable). The spreading-activation explanation for double entendres is that the selected node (the double entendre) has received more activation than its competing nodes because it has been activated by both the message (e.g., *finish → finale, conclusion, climax,* etc.) and by the cognitive state (e.g., *sex → body, intercourse, climax,* etc.). The relatively straightforward empirical support for a spreading-activation account of double entendres has been interpreted as strengthening the spreading-activation account of Freudian slips (Motley, 1985b).

Thus, by the early 1980s, the essential reservations about Freud's theory of slips had begun to erode. The theory was no longer viewed as untestable, empirical support for Freud's explanation of slips had been provided, and an explanatory mechanism—one consistent with accepted psycholinguistic theory—had been suggested. But while several studies had demonstrated that slips of the tongue can be Freudian, several other studies had shown that some slips have more purely linguistic, non-Freudian origins. A series of slip studies had suggested—sometimes directly, sometimes obliquely—that virtually every kind of linguistic decision a speaker makes in selecting the components and sequence of his or her message involves competition among candidate choices, and that slips tend to occur when these competitions are—for whatever reasons—unresolved by the time the utterance is articulated.

Thus, for example, a slip like "this motor is too groily" would be interpreted as an unresolved *lexical-selection* competition between *greasy* and *oily*. Unresolved *word-order* competitions yield slips like *Spench* and *Franish* (*French and Spanish* versus *Spanish and French*). Unresolved *modifier options*, i.e., the decision to include or omit a potential adjective or adverb modifier, appear to generate errors such as *roon mock* (*moon rock* versus *rock*) and *dad mash* (*mad dash* versus *dash*). *Phrase sequence* competitions can yield errors as well, such as "*Brush your bed*" (*Brush your teeth and make your bed* versus *Make your bed and brush your teeth*). A few other variations on the slips-via-linguistic-competitions theme have been identified, as well (Motley, 1985a). There is a sense in which Freudian slips may be viewed as the result

of encoding competitions also, with the source of competition being linguistic nodes activated by hidden cognitions. For example, for the professor who told an attractive coed that her paper needed "more *orgasmic unity*" (intended: *organic unity*), the message intent and the physical attraction presumably instigated unresolved competition between *organic* and *orgasm*, both of which activated *orgasmic* (one phonetically, one semantically), with *orgasmic* "winning" the activation competition.

One way to look at the total body of work on verbal slips is to deny the rather strong evidence of linguistic competition as the source of some slips, and to insist that all slips are Freudian. The author once witnessed a debate, for example, where one scholar interpreted a child's slip, "I can't cut my *meef,*" as a simple competition blend of *meat* versus *beef,* while another scholar insisted that the error manifested the child's repressed sexual attraction to her father, with *meat* being a euphemism for *penis,* etc., etc. At the other extreme, one can deny the empirical evidence of Freudian influences on slips of the tongue. The author has witnessed more than one instance of the claim (technically correct, perhaps) that the empirical studies supporting Freud's theory do not flush out all the depths of repressed cognitions that Freud discussed. While there are still those who represent one or the other pole of these extremes, the more common view by far seems to be one that combines Freud's discussion of slips with more recent attention to slips: Not all slips, but almost certainly some slips, are indeed Freudian.

REFERENCES

Baars, B. J., Motley, M. T., and MacKay, D. G. (1975). Output editing for lexical status in artificially elicited slips of the tongue. *Journal of Verbal Learning and Verbal Behavior,* 14: 382–391.

Collins, A. M., and Loftus, E. F. (1975). A spreading-activation theory of semantic processing. *Psychological Review,* 82: 407–428.

Freud, S. (1901). *Psychopathology of Everyday Life.* S.E. 6: 1–279.

Fromkin, V. A. (1973a). *Speech Errors as Linguistic Evidence.* The Hague: Mouton.

———. (1973b). Slips of the tongue. *Scientific American,* 229: 110–117.

Mosher, D. L. (1966). The development and multitrait-multimethod matrix analysis of three measures of three aspects of guilt. *Journal of Consulting and Clinical Psychology,* 30: 25–29.

Motley, M. T. (1974). Verbal conditioning—Generalization in encoding: A hint at the structure of the lexicon. *Speech Monographs,* 41: 152–162.

534   Sociobiology, and Psychoanalysis

534   SOCIOBIOLOGY, AND PSYCHOANALYSIS

—. (1980). Verification of "Freudian Slips" and semantic prearticulatory editing via laboratory-induced spoonerisms. In V. A. Fromkin (ed.). *Errors in Linguistic Performance.* New York: Academic Press, pp. 133–147.

—. (1985a). Verbal slips. *Scientific American,* 253: 116–126.

—. (1985b). The production of verbal slips and double entendres as clues to the efficiency of normal speech production. *Journal of Language and Social Psychology,* 4: 275–293.

Motley, M. T., and Baars, B. J. (1975). Encoding sensitivities to phonological markedness and transitional probability: Evidence from spoonerisms. *Human Communication Research,* 2: 351–361.

—. (1976a). Laboratory induction of verbal slips: A new method for psycholinguistic research. *Communication Quarterly,* 24: 28–34.

—. (1976b). Semantic bias effects on the outcome of verbal slips. *Cognition,* 4: 177–187.

—. (1979). Effects of cognitive set upon laboratory induced verbal (Freudian) slips. *Journal of Speech and Hearing Research,* 22: 421–432.

Motley, M. T., Camden, C. T., and Baars, B. J. (1979). Personality and situational influences upon verbal slips: A laboratory test of Freudian and prearticulatory editing hypotheses. *Human Communication Research,* 4: 195–202.

—. (1983). Polyseantic lexical access: Evidence from laboratory-induced double entendres. *Communication Monographs,* 50: 193–205.

Motley, M. T., and Camden, C. T. (1985). Nonlinguistic influences on lexical selection: Evidence from double entendres. *Communication Monographs,* 52: 124–135.

MICHAEL T. MOTLEY

Sociobiology, and Psychoanalysis

"Sociobiology" was established as a term describing modern Darwinism by Edward O. Wilson's book of that title, published in 1975. Wilson declared that "psychoanalytic theory appears to be exceptionally compatible with sociobiological theory" (Wilson, 1977: 135), and David Barash was among the first to explore the extensive overlap between Freud's discoveries and sociobiology (Barash, 1979).

Sociobiology could be described as a synthesis of Darwinism and modern genetics and is characterized by the so-called selfish-gene view of evolution (Dawkins, 1978). This synthesis resolved numerous contradictions and fallacies in evolutionary thinking by showing that natural selection acts ultimately on individual genes. For example, suicidal self-sacrifice became fully intelligible to Darwinists for the first time. In a paradigmatic paper,

W. D. Hamilton advanced a mathematical model showing that self-sacrifice could evolve by natural selection if the benefit to genes shared by the donor and the recipient was greater than the cost to those same genes in the donor (Hamilton, 1964). This revealed the fallacy in "survival of the fittest" by showing that it was not survival of the individual organism that ultimately mattered to natural selection, but the survival of the individual's genes. As David Barash put it, "much of being human consists of contributing to the success of our genes just as being a kangaroo, or even a dandelion, involves contributing to the success of kangaroo and dandelion genes. Freud was right, much of our behavior has to do with sex" (Barash, 1979: 40).

An early attempt to interpret psychoanalytic findings in the light of evolution and ethology had been made by John Bowlby. In particular, Bowlby popularized his concept of "attachment" as a fundamental biological factor. However, sociobiology was to cast doubt on this when Robert L. Trivers persuasively argued that conflict between parents and offspring was unavoidable, irresolvable, and rooted in genetics (Trivers, 1974). He credited Freud with coming upon "sexual overtones in parent-offspring conflict" (Trivers, 1985: 146–147) and suggested an evolutionary rationale for Freudian findings such as regression and repression (Trivers, 1981).

More recently, it has been argued that such oral behavior as compulsive sucking independent of hunger is likely to be the child's response to the birth of a sibling within the first four years of an existing child's life, since that birth is the single greatest threat to it in primal hunter-gatherer and modern Third World conditions. Persistent stimulation of the mother's nipples inhibits her sexual cycles for about three years after giving birth and can be seen as a classical Darwinian adaptation that evolved to safeguard the life of such an existing child. In a similar way, Oedipal behavior, primal scene anxiety, penis envy, and other aspects of so-called infantile sexuality can be interpreted as episodes in parent-offspring conflict over parental investment (Badcock, 1994).

More generally, the relevance of psychoanalytic findings to sociobiology and its more recent derivative, evolutionary psychology, has been assessed by Lloyd and Nesse (Lloyd and Nesse, 1992). Attempts have also been made to interpret sociobiology in a way compatible with post-Freudian, objection-relations theory (Slavin and Kriegman, 1992), and with communicative psychotherapy (Langs, 1995).

In the 1980s, geneticists discovered that, even though everyone inherits a complete set of genes from each parent, some genes are expressed only if they come from one parent, rather than the other (Ohlsson et al., 1995). Such "genomic imprinting" is found in mammals and flowering plants where there is a major asymmetry in the investment of the parents. In mammals, for example, the father contributes nothing beyond his genes, whereas the mother makes a vast contribution of resources to the offspring during gestation and lactation. Consequently, genes that are active only when inherited from the father tend to motivate consumption of the mother's resources for growth and development, whereas those active only when inherited from the mother tend to the converse. This is because, in contrast with the father's, the mother's genes are certain to be present in all her offspring and so have a vested interest in conserving her resources (Haig and Graham, 1991). In 1995, it was found that in mice (and almost certainly in humans too) only paternal genes build the limbic, or "emotional" brain, whereas only maternal genes construct the "executive" brain, or neocortex (Allen et al., 1995; Keverne et al., 1996). The limbic brain is known to be primarily concerned with motivation, instinct, and appetite, and to contain the primary pleasure and anxiety centers (hypothalamus and amygdala). The cortex supports all higher cognitive functions such as speech, consciousness, and reason, and has direct access to external reality through the senses. In this context, it is tempting to see the Freudian id as the psychological agency of paternal genes and the ego as that of maternal ones, especially in view of the fact that a major attribute of the neocortex is its ability to inhibit and repress the primitive responses of the limbic brain. This way of looking at the mind provides a genetic and anatomical basis for Freud's basic discovery: the existence of an unconscious, repressed, infantile self, fixated on the mother, addicted to gratification and in conflict with the conscious, reality-aware ego.

At the very least, the new discovery suggests that the conflict may be built into the human brain long before birth and that the mind may be fractured from top to bottom. If so, Freud's persistent, but unsuccessful, attempts to ground psychoanalytic metapsychology on opposed instincts of various kinds might find a final solution. It may simply be that genetic conflict is mentally institutionalized in the ego and the id. Indeed, sociobiological insights suggest that the driving force behind the extraordinary expansion of the human brain in recent history could turn out to be an evolutionary arms race between parental genes, competing for control of growth, development, and behavior—a much more Freudian view of human evolution than might ever have seemed possible in the past.

REFERENCES

Allen, N. D., Logan, K., Lally, G., Drage, J. D., Norris, M. L., and Keverne, B. (1995). Distribution of parthenogenetic cells in the mouse brain and their influence on brain development and behavior. *Proceedings of the National Academy of Sciences, USA*, 92: 10782–10786.

Badcock, C. (1994). *PsychoDarwinism: The New Synthesis of Darwin and Freud.* London: HarperCollins.

Barash, D. (1979). *Sociobiology: The Whisperings Within.* London: Souvenir Press.

Dawkins, R. (1978). *The Selfish Gene*, 1st ed. Oxford: Oxford University Press.

Haig, D., and Graham, C. (1991). Genomic imprinting and the strange case of the insulin-like growth factor II receptor. *Cell*, 64: 1045–1046.

Hamilton, W. D. (1964). The genetical evolution of social behaviour. *Journal of Theoretical Biology*, 7: 1–16, 17–52.

Keverne, E. B., Fundele, R., Narasimha, M., Barton, S. C., and Surani, M. A. (1996). Genomic imprinting and the differential roles of parental genomes in brain development. *Developmental Brain Research*, 92: 91–100.

Langs, R. (1995). *The Evolution of the Emotion-Processing Mind.* London: Karnac Books, 1995.

Lloyd, A., and R. Nesse. (1992). The evolution of dynamic mechanisms. In J. Barkow, L. Cosmides, and J. Tooby (eds.). *The Adapted Mind: Evolutionary Psychology and the Generation of Culture.* Oxford: Oxford University Press.

Ohlsson, R, Hall, K., and Ritzen, M. (eds.) (1995). *Genomic Imprinting: Causes and Consequences.* Cambridge: Cambridge University Press.

Slavin, M., and Kriegman, D. (1992). *The Adaptive Design of the Human Psyche: Psychoanalysis, Evolutionary Biology and the Therapeutic Process.* New York: Guilford Press.

Trivers, R. (1974). Parent-offspring conflict. *American Zoologist*, 14: 249–264.

———. (1981). Sociobiology and politics. In E. White (ed.). *Sociobiology and Human Politics.* Toronto: Lexington.

———. *Social Evolution.* Menlo Park, Calif.: Benjamin Cummings.

Wilson, E.O. (1977). Biology and the social sciences. *Daedaleus*, 106: 127–140.

CHRISTOPHER BADCOCK

Soviet Union, and Psychoanalysis

See RUSSIA/SOVIET UNION, AND PSYCHOANALYSIS.

Spielrein, Sabina (1885–1941/42)

Interest in Sabina Spielrein, one of the earliest women psychoanalysts, was sparked in 1980 when, after their discovery by chance in the basement of the Department of Psychology and Education of the University of Geneva, her diary and correspondence with Carl Gustav Jung and Sigmund Freud were partially published in Italian and rapidly translated in other languages. Those papers revealed that Spielrein had been Jung's lover after having been his patient (Carotenuto, 1982; definitive expanded edition, 1986). Emphasis on Spielrein as the victim of male manipulation in the interests of psychoanalytic politics (Cremerius, 1987), sensationalist exploitation of the affair, and the erroneous view that it played the key role in the break between Jung and Freud (Kerr [1993] is the latest proponent of these views) are counteracted by studies on Spielrein's life and work in their own right (Cifali, 1988; Lothane, 1996; Van Waning, 1992; Vidal, 2001), as well as by the publication of her (mainly German) writings (Spielrein 1987; Italian translation: Spielrein, 1986).

Spielrein made pioneering contributions to the psychoanalytic study of the child and is seen as a precursor of Freud's "death instinct." Yet, although her work is of great historical interest, it is the drama of her life, and the way it partly illustrates the libidinal dynamics of the early psychoanalytic movement, that remain the focus of wide attraction. Fictionalized in 1994 in a well-documented and successful biographical novel by the Norwegian writer Karsten Alnaes (*Sabina*, translated into German and French, but not into English), it inspired in 1996 an off-Broadway play, and films about it are being planned.

Sabina Spielrein, born in 1885 in Rostov-on-Don (Russia), was the eldest daughter of well-to-do and cultivated Jewish parents who emphasized their children's education and learning foreign languages. Early behaviors (such as feces retention and masturbation) worsened after age fourteen, when her young sister died. Other symptoms then appeared: visual and auditory hallucinations, night fears, phobias, fits of laughter, screaming, and crying, and depression. In August 1904, she entered the Burghölzli clinic in Zürich (directed by Eugen Bleuler), where she was treated by Jung. Jung told Freud he used the psychoanalytic method (letter of October 23, 1906); in "The Freudian Theory of Hysteria" (1907), he described her illness as a "hysterical psychosis." Spielrein's clinical record and Jung's 1905 report to Freud about her (both in Minder, 1994) disclose that she experienced sexual arousal as a reaction to actual, witnessed, announced, or imagined corporal punishment. Never-

theless, the claim that she was sexually abused by her father and that she was an "incest survivor" is as injurious as it is unfounded (Wackenhut and Willke, 1994).

Spielrein was discharged from the Burghölzli in June 1905, and began medical studies. The love affair with Jung probably started in 1906; it has been therefore suggested (but without evidence) that the therapy with Jung was merely a screen for their relationship. Jung, a married man and father of two girls, interrupted it in 1909 in a particularly dishonest and humiliating manner. Spielrein sought Freud's support; Freud gave it to Jung.

Spielrein's 1911 thesis, "On the Psychological Content of a Case of Schizophrenia," takes up a topic that was a Burghölzli specialty, and is among the earliest uses of Bleuler's terminology. It reflects Jung's interests (e.g., in the mythological interpretation of schizophrenic productions), but Jung acknowledges his indebtedness to it in *Symbols and Transformations of the Libido*. While in Vienna from October 1911 to March 1912, Spielrein presented her ideas about the "destructive" component of the reproductive instinct to the Vienna Psychoanalytic Society (November 29, 1911). In *Beyond the Pleasure Principle* (1920) Freud mentioned her 1912 paper "Destruction as a Cause of Coming Into Being" as an instructive yet somewhat unclear anticipation of his own speculations about the death instinct. "Destruction" is now considered Spielrein's most important article (see *Journal of Analytical Psychology* 39, 1994, 156–186 for an English translation). Paul Federn (1913), however, disdainfully considered it as an example of "mystical thought."

In 1912, Spielrein married Pavel Scheftel, a Russian physician; a daughter, Renate, was born in 1913. Almost nothing is known of Spielrein's later life. In 1920, after living in Berlin and Munich, she moved to Geneva, where she became an informal member of the Jean-Jacques Rousseau Institute, an institution for child research and progressive education that also was a major transmitter of psychoanalytic ideas in the French-speaking world. When Jean Piaget (1896–1980) joined the Institute in 1921, he was psychoanalyzed by Spielrein, and the two planned collaborative research on symbolic thought in children and in the subconscious (Vidal, 2001). The years she spent in Geneva (1920–1923) were her most productive.

In 1923, Spielrein returned to Russia. She first lived in Moscow, working as a child physician and psychoanalyst, and was active in psychoanalytic institutions. The following year, she rejoined her husband in Rostov-on-Don;

a second daughter, Eva, was born in 1925. As did millions of others, Spielrein and her family suffered under the Soviet system. After years of being under attack, psychoanalysis was forbidden in 1936. Spielrein's husband died of a heart attack in 1937; her three brothers (Jan, a mathematician, Isaac, a psychologist, and Emil, a biologist) disappeared in the Stalinist purges of 1935–1937. Spielrein and her two daughters were killed with the city's other Jews during one of the two German occupations of Rostov-on-Don, in 1941 or 1942.

Starting in 1912, Spielrein's most important work dealt with children, and emphasized the study of symbolic thought, language, and birth and sexual fantasies. Her last known article (on children's drawings) appeared in *Imago* in 1931. Spielrein always remained loyal to Freud's thought and was published in official psychoanalytic journals. Nevertheless, her vocabulary, approaches, and interpretations demonstrate that she was more interested in the "subliminal" or the "subconscious" than in the unconscious in the Freudian sense.

REFERENCES

Carotenuto, A. (1982). *A Secret Symmetry. Sabina Spielrein Between Jung and Freud*. Trans. A. Pomerans, J. Shepley, and K. Winston. New York: Pantheon.

———. (1986). *Tagebuch einer heimlichen Symmetrie. Sabina Spielrein zwischen Freud und Jung*. Freiburg-im-Breisgau: Kore.

Cifali, M. (1988). Une femme dans la psychanalyse. Sabina Spielrein, un autre portrait. *Le Bloc-notes de la psychanalyse* 8, 253–265.

Cremerius, J. (1987). Sabina Spielrein: ein frühes Opfer der psychoanalytischen Berufspolitik. *Forum der Psychoanalyse*, 3: 127–142.

Federn, P. (1913). Review of "Sabina Spielrein, 'Die Destruktion als Ursache des Werdens.'" *Internationale Zeitschrift für ärtzliche Psychoanalyse*, 1: 92–93.

Freud, S. (1920). *Beyond the Pleasure Principle*. S.E. 18: 1–66.

Jung, C. G. (1907). The Freudian Theory of Hysteria. In Adler, G. and Hull, R. F. C. *Collected Works of C. G. Jung*. Vol. 4. Princeton, N.J.: Princeton University Press, 1970.

Kerr, J. (1993). *A Most Dangerous Method. The Story of Jung, Freud, and Sabina Spielrein*. New York: Knopf.

Lothane, Z. (1996). In defense of Sabina Spielrein. *International Forum of Psychoanalysis*, 5: 203–217.

Minder, B. (1994). Sabina Spielrein. Jungs Patientin am Burghölzli. *Luzifer-Amor. Zeitschrift für Geschichte der Psychoanalyse*, 7 (14): 55–127.

Spielrein, S. (1986). *Comprensione della schizofrenia e altri scritti*. Various translators. Naples: Liguori.

———. (1987). *Sämtliche Schriften*. Freiburg-im-Breisgau: Kore.

Van Waning, A. (1992). The works of pioneering psychoanalyst Sabina Spielrein. "Destruction as a cause of coming into being." *International Review of Psycho-Analysis*, 19: 399–414.

Vidal, F. (2001). Sabina Spielrein, Jean Piaget—going their own ways. *Journal of Analytic Psychology*, 46: 139–153. Special Issue on Spielrein.

Wackenhut, I., and Willke, A. (1994). *Sabina Spielrein. Missrauchüberlebende und Psychoanalytikerin*. Unpublished medical dissertation, Medizinische Hochschule Hannover.

FERNANDO VIDAL

Splitting of the Ego

A term used by Freud to denote the coexistence in the ego of two contradictory attitudes toward external reality. One accepts the reality while the other disavows it. The two attitudes persist side by side without influencing each other. Fetishism and psychoses are two cardinal examples of this phenomenon.

The concept of splitting has a long and complex history in psychiatry and psychoanalysis. The phenomenological tradition of the late nineteenth and early twentieth centuries made much use of such ideas as "dissociation of psychological phenomena," "split personality," "double conscience," and the like. Later, similar notions were elaborated within psychoanalysis.

Freud used the term "splitting" in many different ways over the course of his writings. In 1893, along with Breuer, he employed the term "splitting of consciousness" to denote the separation of a particular group of mental contents from the dominant mass of ideas in the individual's mind. He also used "splitting of personality" to describe alternating states of behavior in hysterical patients and "splitting of the mind" to describe the simultaneous existence of conscious and unconscious ideation. Freud felt that splitting was a pathological counterpart of synthesis, used defensively to avoid conflict: "In this way a transformation was effected which enabled the patient to escape from an intolerable mental condition" (Breur and Freud, p. 166).

As his emphasis shifted from the hysterical disturbances of consciousness and the related topographic model of the mind (conscious-preconscious-unconscious) to the more complex mental operations and the structural model (id-ego-superego) of the mind, Freud (1924) introduced the term "splitting of the ego." Freud maintained that the male child reacts to his first awareness of the absence of a penis in females with distress. This psychological discomfort mobilizes a denial of his perception. Such denial is reinforced by ascribing an imaginary penis to females and, with this accomplished, the child comes to accept the reality of genital distinction between sexes. A fetishist is one who persists in two contradictory attitudes of acknowledging and disavowing the absence of penis in women by his use of the fetish object, and this is referred to as "splitting of the ego."

Still later, Freud broadened the concept to explain that withdrawal from reality in psychoses is almost always partial. He noted the existence of two contradictory attitudes here: "one, the normal one, which takes account of reality, and another which under the influence of instincts detaches the ego from reality" (1940, p. 202). Thus in both fetishism and psychoses, the existence of two contradictory attitudes regarding reality forms the essential basis of Freud's concept of splitting. It is also to be noted that Freud's emphasis is upon a rupture *within* the ego rather than *between* the ego and other psychic structures (id and superego). It is precisely because of this aspect of splitting that no compromise formation between the two attitudes can occur and they continue to exist side by side in consciousness.

While Freud's usage of the term "splitting" is the focus here, it might not be out of place to add that the concept of splitting has been expanded and modified by subsequent psychoanalysts, especially Donald Winnicott, Melanie Klein, W. R. D. Fairbairn, Margaret Mahler, and Otto Kernberg. These investigators employ the term "splitting" to denote the separation of true and false selves in the schizoid individual and/or the defensive compartmentalization of the gratifying and frustrating aspects of the views of oneself and others by the developing child who seeks to avoid ambivalence. While the use of this mental mechanism is normal during early childhood, its persistence, to a considerable degree, in adulthood suggests psychopathology. Splitting then is associated with an inability to tolerate mixed feelings toward self and others, marked oscillation of self-esteem, impaired decision making, ego-syntonic impulsivity, and intensification of affects. This group of phenomena is usually seen in borderline, narcissistic, schizoid, paranoid, antisocial, and other severe personality disorders.

In sum, the term "splitting" has been described in many different ways. The contemporary trend is to focus upon its use in connection with severe personality disorders, especially as outlined in the works of Otto Kernberg. However, the fact remains that the original usage of the term "splitting of the ego" by Freud was intended

to designate the coexistence of two contradictory attitudes regarding reality in fetishism and psychoses.

REFERENCES

Akhtar, S., and Byrne, J. P. (1983). The concept of splitting and its clinical relevance. *American Journal of Psychiatry*, 140: 1013–1016.

Breuer, J., and Freud, S. (1893). *Studies on Hysteria*. S.E. 2: 1–252.

Freud, S. (1924). Neurosis and psychosis. S.E. 19: 149–156.

———. (1940). *An Outline of Psycho-Analysis*. S.E. 23: 141–207.

Kernberg, O. (1967). Borderline personality organization. *Journal of the American Psychoanalytic Association*, 15: 641–685.

Lichtenberg, J., and Slap, J. W. (1973). Notes on the concept of splitting and defense mechanism of splitting of representations. *Journal of the American Psychoanalytic Association*, 21: 722–787.

SALMAN AKHTAR

Stekel, Wilhelm (1868–1940)

Wilhelm Stekel, a flamboyant personality and one of Freud's early collaborators, was among the first to join the fledgling psychoanalytic movement at the beginning of the twentieth century. It was Stekel who suggested to Freud that the group, then very small, should have regular meetings; in 1902 these became the Wednesday Evening Society, renamed in 1908 the Vienna Psychoanalytic Society. Stekel, who had journalistic experience, became coeditor, together with his friend Alfred Adler, of the first psychoanalytic journal, the *Zentralblatt für Psychoanalyse*. There were disagreements, however, over the theoretical orientation of the journal and, for this and other reasons, Stekel's tenure in the society proved brief. He resigned in 1912 over differences with Freud, a year after Adler and a year before C. G. Jung left the fold, and pursued an independent course as a psychoanalytic psychotherapist. He wrote a great deal and formed his own group, which was active in Vienna between the two world wars. Yet, he is remembered mainly as one of the early "deviationists" from psychoanalysis. Today, his writings are largely unread and his contributions forgotten.

Born in one of the eastern provinces of the Austro-Hungarian Empire (later Romania), Stekel studied medicine in Vienna, where he opened a general practice. A photo of Stekel taken at this time shows a dapper, debonair, man-about-town with a short, pointed beard and a handsome mustache. As a physician, he had experience with a wide range of cases and with the physical manifestations of emotional disorders, which became a central interest of his.

Stekel's foremost contribution was as a psychoanalytic psychotherapist. He considered himself a psychoanalyst, even after he broke with Freud, but his brand of psychoanalysis differed markedly from that of Freud and his followers. Stekel was interested, indeed a specialist, in what later came to be known as psychoanalytic psychotherapy but that he regarded as an alternate form of psychoanalysis. Stekel found Freud's psychoanalysis too rigid, ritualized, and theory-bound, whereas he preferred a much freer, looser, intuitive, and active style. He saw no special merit in the use of the couch—the analyst sitting behind the patient was "like a hidden god." He liberally used suggestion, advice, and manipulation of the transference. He did not (in those early days, prior to the structural theory) spend much time analyzing defenses, preferring instead to make quick, intuitive, penetrating interpretations of what he perceived as the patient's central current conflict. He aimed at rapid symptom removal and his treatment approach was characteristically brief. Stekel was impatient with lengthy treatment (his own "analysis" with Freud lasted eight sessions) and with the management of difficult resistances. He strongly recommended the use of the "trial week" to test the rigidity of the patient's defenses and his or her motivation for treatment. One of his clinical dicta was that the analyst's principal task during the initial session is to determine the patient's "willingness to be cured." He would ask a patient that did not seem "ripe" for treatment to return at a later date. He practiced analytic psychotherapy in the style of the general practitioner who does not lance an abscess if it is not yet fluctuant and ready to be incised.

Stekel was not interested in what gradually became a major goal of psychoanalysis—the reconstruction of the personality and the integration of the present with its genetic past. He dealt with conflicts as they presented themselves in the present; he had great intuitive ability to grasp the core of the neurotic struggle and to interpret it to the patient. His stance toward the patient's difficulties and his own therapeutic accomplishments was optimistic and inclined to be boastful: the word "cure," which psychoanalysts use sparingly if at all, occurs with some frequency in his writings. Stekel often speaks of his own therapeutic victories with a touch of naive self-satisfaction, which undoubtedly did not endear him to

Freud and to his other colleagues in the psychoanalytic circle.

Ernest Jones in his biography of Freud admits that Stekel was exceptionally intuitive; Freud also credits him in this way and indicates that certain symbols in dreams were first clarified for him by Stekel. Other aspects of Stekel's personality—his boastfulness, his independence (Jones says that Stekel was the only one in the psychoanalytic circle who addressed Freud by name instead of calling him, as was protocol, "Herr Professor"), and, most important, his casualness with facts (the suspicion that he was not beyond inventing clinical material when it suited him)—made him increasingly unwelcome to his colleagues. Many Stekel stories circulated that made him the butt of jokes and a source of amusement. One example suffices. At meetings of the Wednesday Evening Society, Stekel often contributed to the topic under discussion by making reference to a patient he had seen that very morning who presumably proved or disproved the point of the presentation. Given the frequency of this occurrence, the other members came to speak jokingly of "Stekel's Wednesday morning patient."

Stekel wrote voluminously, and with great ease, more than a dozen books that contain a profusion of case material. Perhaps he wrote too much; it might have been better had he taken more time to review and prune his productivity. But that was not his style. In any case, his writings should not be ignored. He wrote on dreams, analytic psychotherapy, treatment of anxiety, sexual disturbances in men and women, masturbation, sadomasochism, obsessive-compulsive states. His best works probably are *Conditions of Nervous Anxiety and their Treatment* (German-language edition, 1912; English-language edition, 1950) and *Technique of Analytical Psychotherapy* (German-language edition, 1938; English-language edition, 1950). His *Autobiography* (English-language edition, 1950) also is of special interest.

His achievements include his standing as a pioneer, along with Georg Groddeck and Paul Schilder, in the discipline that later became psychosomatic medicine. More important, he was a creative innovator and a gifted contributor to the field of analytic brief psychotherapy. He introduced the concept of "bipolarity," which was later renamed "ambivalence" by Eugen Bleuler and remains in current usage under the latter name. His work undoubtedly stimulated Sándor Ferenczi and Otto Rank to experiment with shortening the length of analysis and with more "active" forms of treatment. In 1946, when

Franz Alexander and Thomas French published their landmark contribution, *Psychoanalytic Therapy*, it was seen as both highly innovative and controversial, yet it clearly echoed Stekel's earlier work. His name, however, was nowhere mentioned.

When Germany annexed Austria in 1938, Stekel and his wife managed to escape to safety in England. Tired, discouraged, and ill, he struggled with poorly controlled diabetes and a painful vascular disability of the foot. He committed suicide, at age seventy-two, in a London hotel room.

REFERENCES

Gay, P. (1955). *Freud. A Life for Our Time*. New York: Norton.

Jones, E. (1955). *The Life and Work of Sigmund Freud*, vol. 2. New York: Basic Books.

Nunberg, H., and Federn, E. (1906–1918). *Minutes of the Vienna Psychoanalytic Society*, vols. 1–4. New York: International Universities Press, 1962–1974.

Stekel, W. (1912). *Conditions of Nervous Anxiety and Their Treatment*. New York: Liveright, 1950.

———. (1938) *Technique of Analytical Psychotherapy*. New York: Liveright, 1950.

———. (1950). *The Autobiography of Wilhelm Stekel*. New York: Liveright, 1950.

PIETRO CASTELNUOVO-TEDESCO

Strachey, James (1887–1967)

Born in London in 1887, James Strachey belonged to one of the most illustrious intellectual families of those years. He studied classics at Trinity College of Cambridge University without great success and worked for a while as a sort of freelance writer at the periodical *The Spectator*. Together with his famous brother, Lytton, he belonged to the so-called avant-garde group of Bloomsbury, which during the first two decades of the twentieth century had quite an impact in trying to create a new cultural "taste" in Great Britain, although being, rather prudently, open to the new cultural ideas and experiences coming from the Continent.

Strachey started becoming interested in Freud's work through the work of F. Meyers, the founder of the Society of Psychical Research in Cambridge, who incidentally had been the first to mention Freud's work in Great Britain in 1896. Immediately after World War I, after marrying Alix Sargeant Florence and with a rudimentary knowledge of German, he contacted Ernest Jones because he wanted to become a psychoanalyst.

Having appreciated his literary talents, Jones managed to put Strachey and his brother Lytton in contact with Freud. From 1920 until 1922, both brothers simultaneously undertook an analysis with Freud in Vienna.

It was during this analysis that Strachey started translating Freud's work into English, sending his translations, which were checked by Freud himself, to Ernest Jones, who had started his own first project of collecting Freud's works and translating them into English. When Strachey returned to London, he got more and more involved with his wife, Alix, Joan Riviere (who had also been in analysis with Freud), and others in translating, editing, and publishing Freud's work, under Jones's control. Strachey was part of the group that in 1924 published the first glossary of Freud's technical terminology in English.

It was when he was in Vienna in analysis with Freud that Strachey, with the approval of Jones and in some ways also of Freud, created some of the famous terms that were adopted even later on in the *Standard Edition*, for instance, "cathexis" for the German word "*Besetzung*," "anaclitic" for the German "*Anlehnung*," and so on. It must nevertheless be stressed that terms like "ego" (for "*ich*") and "superego" were not Strachey's invention. They were imposed on him by Ernest Jones, who had planned the translation of Freud into English bearing in mind the monosemic language of the medical and hard sciences of that time. In Jones's view, psychoanalysis had to have a similar technical language to be respected by the scientific and cultural environment of Great Britain, as well as to counteract what Jones and his colleagues felt was the rather approximate way of translating Freud done at that time in the United States by Abraham Brill. Strachey at times disagreed with Jones, but in the end accepted his ideas. Freud, on the other hand, supported Strachey as his preferred translator into English.

Working part-time as a training analyst, Strachey translated most of the papers that were then published in five volumes during the 1920s and 1930s as *Sigmund Freud's Collected Papers*, by the Hogarth Press in London founded by Leonard and Virginia Woolf, who of course were personal friends of the Strachey brothers owing to their links with the Bloomsbury group. Strachey played quite a part in helping Melanie Klein come to London for her first series of lectures, after having heard about her from Alix, who in 1924 had gone to Berlin to undertake a second analysis with Karl Abraham.

After Freud's death in 1939, Jones contacted Strachey to consider the possibility of publishing the complete works of Freud in English. There were many difficulties at that time because of World War II and the financial situation in Great Britain. But after the war ended in 1945, with the great support of Freud's daughter Anna, who would check all Strachey's translations as she had already done in the 1920s, and with the financial support of the Americans and the Institute of Psychoanalysis in London, and owing also to the great enthusiasm of Leonard Woolf of the Hogarth Press, the complete translation of Freud's work into English, under the leadership of Strachey, was then called *The Standard Edition* of Freud's work, and its complete publication started to become a reality.

With financial support from the Institute of Psychoanalysis in London, Strachey and his wife retired to the English countryside and dedicated themselves to the translation, but also to the editing and critical annotation of Freud's psychoanalytic work. Because of the wishes of Anna Freud, Strachey did not include in the *Standard Edition* Freud's important preanalytical neurological work. The first volume of the *Standard Edition* was published by Strachey in 1953 and the last one, the twenty-third volume, in 1966, one year before his death. A twenty-fourth volume was published in 1974, edited by A. Harris; it contains all sorts of corrections and the general index, using material partially belonging to Strachey.

The *Standard Edition* has become the standard reference text for all psychoanalysts, although with the passage of time, many have raised doubts and criticisms about it. As happens with every translation and work of this kind, Strachey's magnum opus reflects his personality, the psychological status of Freud's original work in German as known at that time, and the cultural and sociopolitical context in which the work was conceived and eventually published. In this case, one has to consider that Strachey acted on decisions on how to translate Freud that were made by Jones, Strachey himself, and others in the 1920s. If one compares the glossary of Freud's technical terms published by Jones in 1924 with the glossary published by Strachey in the first volumes of the *Standard Edition* in 1953, one can easily see that no changes were made for a period that had lasted for thirty years. Strachey in fact used the same technical terminology he had inherited from Jones and had himself created with Jones's approval in the 1920s except for minor details and clarifications.

There is no doubt, therefore, that Strachey, supported by Jones, Anna Freud, and others, gave a particular interpretation of Freud's work to which he and his colleagues remained loyal for the rest of their lives. Even the famous five clinical cases translated by Strachey and his wife in the 1920s were republished in the *Standard Edition* with only minor corrections and further standardization of the language.

Because of the historical and sociopolitical vicissitudes of the Central European and German-speaking psychoanalysts who had to leave Germany and Austria because of Nazi persecution during the 1930s, English, rather than German, became and is still the hegemonic and official language of psychoanalysis. It is no wonder, therefore, that in spite of his at times questionable "medicalization" and "scientificization" of Freud's technical language, despite the aristocratic British rigidities of style of this translation, Strachey's work has become the unavoidable reference point even for those who have tried to translate and critically annotate Freud in their own language.

Besides his work as a translator of Freud, Strachey was also an interesting theoretician and clinician. He wrote some of the wisest comments on how to deal with tradition and change in psychoanalysis that have ever been written during the Anna Freud–Melanie Klein controversies of 1941–1945. Furthermore, under the influence of the work of Klein besides that of Freud, Strachey wrote what even today is still considered a classic paper on technique in psychoanalysis, "The Nature and Therapeutic Action of Psychoanalysis," published in 1934 in *The International Journal of Psychoanalysis* (vol. 1, pp. 127–186).

RICARDO STEINER

Structural Factors See METAPSYCHOLOGY; STRUCTURAL THEORY.

Structural Theory

The term "structural theory" customarily designates a model of the mind that Freud introduced in the 1923 monograph *The Ego and the Id* and elaborated in subsequent publications.

This model of the mind is usually understood to consist of three systems or agencies called "ego," "id," and "superego." The terms "id" and "superego" were

S

introduced in 1923; the term "ego" already had a long history in Freud's work. Behavior, both mental and motoric, is to be explained as the outcome of interaction of the three systems. Each agency consists of certain mental functions grouped together on the basis of their roles in mental conflict. Mental functions (for example, defenses) may operate synergistically in a situation of mental conflict and in opposition to other groups of mental functions. In conflict situations, the outcomes are known as "compromise formations." Ego functions may also operate in concert with drive derivatives, facilitating their expression in the relative absence of conflict. "Conflict" here means mental or intrapsychic conflict, not social conflict.

Freud's Early Models of the Mind

The 1923 structural theory is best understood in the context of the overall development of Freud's ideas on mental functioning. The structural theory was, in fact, the fourth general model of the mind that he proposed. In each of these models, there are components that are structures and other components that activate the structures, in rough analogy to bodily anatomy and physiology, especially that of the nervous system. The purpose of each model of the mind is to account for emotional, cognitive, and behavioral phenomena of human beings in a comprehensive scheme.

Freud's first model of the mind was *prepsychoanalytic* and, in fact, *protopsychological*, that is, not intended to be analogous to brain functioning but rather conceptualized directly as brain functioning (Breuer and Freud, 1895; Freud, 1950 [1895]). In this theory, the basic structures were "neurones" and the energizing factor was "Q," for quantity or quantity of excitation, where "excitation" meant, literally, neuronal excitation. Different neuronal groupings, activated by Q, were responsible for different psychological functions. The pre-1900 papers on the defense neuroses (1894; 1896) and Aktual neuroses (1895a; 1895b) were written within this general framework of mental functioning, although the model was not made explicit. In fact, it was published only posthumously in 1950.

Freud's second model of the mind comprised the "*topographic model*" (1900) and the classical theory of *instinctual drives* (1905 [1905–1920]). The topographic model is psychological and the prototypical psychoanalytic model. From this point on, Freud understood mental phenomena as the outcome of mental conflict. About

each model one may ask, "Which element(s) of the model is (are) proposed to be in conflict with which other element(s)?" Structures and energies are now *analogous* to physical structures and neuronal excitation, and only analogous. In this topographic model, the structures—or agencies or systems—are designated as the *Ucs., Pcs.,* and *Cs-Pcpt.,* formulas that Freud used to indicate the unconscious, preconscious, and conscious-perceptual as systems, rather than as descriptive qualities. For description, he employed the ordinary adjectival forms "unconscious," "preconscious," and so on. This model, consisting of stratigraphic (layers), rather than topographic (contours), is intended to explain human mental and physical behavior on the basis of *conflict* between the systems *Ucs.,* on the one side, and *Pcs.-Cs.-Pcpt.,* on the other. The drives that energized these structures were introduced as oral, anal, genital (phallic), exhibitionistic—voyeuristic and sadomasochistic (1905), later grouped as the sexual drives and contrasted with the ego or self-preservative drives (1915). The mind is conceptualized as having a reality-oriented, perceptual surface, with which consciousness is closely connected, and an underlying portion that largely subsumes the instinctual drives as they emanate from the body. Contents of the *Ucs.* are understood to reach consciousness only against resistance, or never to reach consciousness at all. The *Ucs.* contents are dynamically unconscious in the sense that other forces in the mind oppose their entry into awareness. The *Pcs.* is an intermediate realm. Contents of the *Pcs.* are accessible to consciousness without the interference of dynamic factors.

From 1910 to about 1921, Freud gradually introduced a third model of the mind, not generally recognized as such, which may be called the "*libido-narcissism model.*" In this model, the structures (systems) are the "ego," the "object," and the "ego ideal." The dynamic or energizing factor is "libido," which is transferred among the three types of structures (1914). Conflict, in this model, occurs between object libido and ego libido. The "libido theory," in the sense of an explicit set of closely related propositions, is part of this model. It was not articulated by Freud until 1915 (1905 [1915]), and is to be differentiated from the instinctual drive theory. "Libido" is a name for a hypothetical mental energy common to all the sexual drives. The libido-narcissism model temporally overlapped both the topographic-instinctual drive model and the subsequent "structural theory." Compatibility with its predecessor and successor is not clear, however. The "ego" of this model is a repository of libido. It does not seem to be conceptually the same as the ego of the previous model, where "ego" meant whatever appeared to serve self-preservative functions, nor that of the 1923 model, where "ego" means mental functions that operate synergistically in situations of conflict. The same questionable compatibility is true of the "object" and the "libido." Freud repeatedly recognized these complications in later years (e.g., 1924, p. 203).

During the period of time in which the libido-narcissism theory was expanded, Freud was working with new kinds of patients, who presented with schizophrenia, depression, or homosexuality. This work, in conjunction with the massive aggression on the battlefields of World War I, exposed problems in the topographic and libido-narcissism models that eventually led to a major restructuring of his hypotheses. Until 1920, there was no real provision for human aggression in Freud's theories. Aggression or hatred had been recognized only indirectly as something different from love, manifested in attitudes that Freud called "ambivalence," and in sadomasochistic expressions of the sexual drive. Aggression, directed toward others or toward oneself, now seemed to Freud to be equally as prominent and important as sexual and loving motivations and to deserve an equal place in his theories. There also had been no systematic provision in the earlier models for moral functions (conscience), although the concept of the "ego ideal" served this purpose, in some degree, for ideals.

A third major problem of the previous models of the mind was of a more technical nature. In the topographic model, conflict was hypothesized to exist between the system *Ucs.* and the system(s) *Cs.-Pcpt.* Descriptively, ideas in the system *Ucs.* were unconscious and prevented from becoming conscious by forces within the opposing system(s). Clinical work with all types of patients, however, revealed that the forces that prevented wishes and other ideas from becoming conscious were themselves unconscious and accessible to consciousness only with great effort. These opposing forces had been designated as *defenses* for many years (1894) and were recognized clinically in the form of vigorous resistance to the analytic work. Now it became clear to Freud that the defenses themselves were unconscious and effort by the analyst was required to bring them to the patient's attention. This necessitated the theoretical clumsiness of providing for an unconscious aspect of the system *Cs.*—descriptively and dynamically, an unconscious consciousness.

Freud had to find a place for aggression in mental conflict and to make his model of the mind correspond more closely to clinical phenomena, in which the prominence of guilt and related trends was increasingly obvious. The solution was to abandon systemic categorization according to the quality of consciousness/unconsciousness and to look for groupings that more penetratingly reflect alignments of mental functions in psychic conflict. For reasons that need not concern us here, Freud altered the concept of libido to refer to an expression of an omnicellular life instinct and found a source for aggression in a corresponding, omnicellular death instinct. He also molded and fortified an old concept, "ego," and introduced two new terms, "id" and "super-ego," both of which had conceptual predecessors. It is helpful to consider that a fourth construct, "reality," is a necessary part of this and the earlier models. Freud used this term regularly, though he never recognized it as a formal constituent. "Reality," for Freud, means essentially everything outside the organism, including both material objects (animate and inanimate) and social phenomena.

The Elements of the Structural Theory

Id. The "id" subsumed the systemic unconscious and the closely related concept of the mental "representation" of instinctual drives (1933, pp. 73–75). The id contains the passions, as opposed to reason and common sense, and operates exclusively according to the pleasure principle and the primary process (1923, p. 125). Its "sole prevailing quality is that of being unconscious" (1940, p. 163). Also:

> The id, cut off from the external world, has a world of perception of its own. It detects with extraordinary acuteness certain changes in its interior, especially oscillation in the tension of its instinctual needs, and these changes become conscious as feelings in the pleasure-unpleasure series. It is hard to say, to be sure, by what means and with the help of what sensory terminal organs these perceptions come about. But it is an established fact that self-perceptions—coenaesthetic feeling and feelings of pleasure-unpleasure—govern the passage of events in the id with despotic force. The id obeys the inexorable pleasure principle. (1940, p. 198)

S

Ego. Prior to 1919, Freud's published work contained a number of scattered hypotheses concerning the "ego" but little systematic exposition of a systemic ego. The nature of the concept remained unclear and contained contradictory elements (discussed above). The "warding-off" or defensive aspects of the ego were introduced prior to 1900 (1894; 1896). Ego functions other than opposing unconscious ideas were mentioned, including reality testing, censorship between psychical systems, perception, consciousness, memory, judgment, action, and thinking (1900; 1911). In the years from 1915 to 1919 Freud added as ego functions control over motility; and institution of secondary gain from illness. "Ego functions" were postulated to undergo development and to be subject to fixation and regression, just as drives were (1915).

In 1919, a more integrated concept of the ego appeared:

> A picture of obscure instinctual forces, organic in origin, striving towards inborn aims, and, above them, of an agency comprising more highly organized mental structures—acquisitions of human evolution made under the impact of human history—an agency which has taken over portions of the instinctual impulses, has developed them further, or has even directed them towards higher aims, but which in any case binds them firmly and manipulates their energy to suit its own purposes. This higher organization, however, which is known to us as the ego, has rejected another portion of the same elementary instinctual impulses as being unserviceable. (1919, pp. 259–260)

Because conflict was thought to occur fundamentally between sexual drives, on the one side, and ego or self-preservative drives, on the other, ego functions were thought to be energized by the ego drives. The term "ego drives," however, also had fluctuating meanings. In 1920, Freud traced his own uses of the term "ego drives":

> To begin with, we applied that name to all the instinctual trends which could be distinguished from the sexual instincts directed towards an object; and we opposed the ego instincts to the sexual instincts. . . . Subsequently we . . . recognized that a portion of the ego instincts is

also of a libidinal character and has taken the subject's own ego for its object . . . narcissistic self-preservative instincts. . . . The opposition was transformed into one between ego instincts and object instincts, both of a libidinal nature, but in its place a fresh opposition appears between the libidinal (ego- and object-) instincts and others which must be presumed to be in the ego . . . destructive instincts. (p. 61, fn.)

Hunger and thirst are the primary examples of ego drives or, more properly, their derivatives.

The 1923 monograph, *The Ego and the Id*, is the major statement of Freud's revision of the structure of psychoanalytic theory. Here Freud integrated the new ideas he had been gradually introducing.

There were several characterizations of the ego as a systemic concept: "We have formed the idea that in each individual there is a coherent organization of mental processes, and we call this his *ego*." This coherent organization controls motility, exercises dream censorship, carries out defensive operations, and supervises its own constituent processes. Consciousness is "attached" to it. The recognition of this ego and the antithesis between it and the repressed that is split off from it is an "insight into the structural conditions of the mind" (1923, p. 17). Probably the term "structural theory" was derived from this phrase. As we have noted, however, the 1923 model was neither more nor less structural in its elements than previous models.

The logical relations between the elements of this model, the ego and its mental co-agencies, are not always easy to discern. We shall consider these relations in terms of elements of the core concept, the formation of structural components, relations of the structured systems, energics, and differentiable meanings of the term "ego."

Elements of the Core Concept

Besides being a coherent organization of mental processes, the ego is centered around perception (of both external and internal stimuli) and consciousness (including preconsciousness) (1923, p. 23). These qualities imply a close relation to surfaces, that is, the surfaces of the body. "The ego is first and foremost a bodily ego" (pp. 25–26). In terms of the structural conditions of the mind, a distinction is to be made between the ego, which is largely unconscious, and the other part of the mind, the id, which is entirely unconscious (p. 23). A second distinction is that there is a grade or differentiation within the ego called the "ego ideal" or "superego," again largely but not entirely unconscious (p. 28).

Formation of Structural Components

Freud offered ontogenetic and phylogenetic hypotheses or speculations about how the systems of the mind are formed. His statement that "the ego is that part of the id which has been modified by the direct influence of the external world through the medium of the *Pcpt.-Cs.*; in a sense it is an extension of the surface differentiation" (p. 25) probably refers to phylogenetic development. Ontogenetically, aside from growth and maturation, the process of identification—being or becoming like another person in one or more aspects—is the crux of ego development: "The character of the ego is a precipitate of abandoned object cathexes" (p. 20)—that is, of identifications. This means that emotional (sexual and aggressive) investment in the mental correlates of other people (object cathexes) does not simply disappear but is rather replaced by becoming like the other person in some respect—an identification. Identifications then remain as building blocks for ego functions and for the modification of existing ego functions. These identifications may become so numerous and powerful that disruption of the ego may occur if they are incompatible with one another (p. 30). Conflicts between identifications may also occur without pathological consequences (p. 31).

Relations of the Structural Systems

The data suggesting the concepts of psychic structures are the clinical manifestations of conflict in which opposing forces in the mind can be discerned. Freud also postulates that the structures work synergistically. The superego may, for example, be allied with either the ego or the id in situations of mental conflict. Moral values may enhance the expression of aggression toward others who do not share the same moral or religious values. Moral values may prohibit the expression of unconscious sexual desires and thus activate or reinforce defensive operations against such drive derivatives (wishes or impulses). The ego may influence the id by transforming object cathexes into ego structures (i.e., identifications) (p. 55). On the other hand, the powers or functions of the ego may be viewed as being at the behest of "three masters": the external world, the superego, and the id.

Energics

Within the framework of the classical metaphors of psychoanalysis, a legitimate system must have a source of energy and, preferably, its own kind of energy. Prior to 1910 the source of energy for the ego was unclear or unspecified. From 1910 until 1920 the source of energy was the ego- or self-preservative-drives. Subsequently, Freud stated that the ego, via the process of identification and perhaps in other ways, is able to alter other forms of psychic energy (libidinal and aggressive energy) to a form of neutralized energy with which it operates.

Differentiable Meanings of the Term

Several meanings of the term "ego," other than the systemic meaning, are apparent in Freud's usages. These include the person or "self" or "own body"; a mental representation that may receive cathexes like an object representation; a subjectively experienced sense of oneself; and a general designation for discussing a subject as opposed to others—that is, objects or the world external to the organism.

Superego. In Freud's structural model, an epigenetically unfolding group of instinctual drives and a number of mental functions (such as perception and memory) were inborn or genetically determined. Differentiation of the mind into an ego and an id began shortly after birth. The third major system in mental conflict, the superego, is different in this respect, itself a product of mental conflict, a compromise formation arising as a structured piece of conflict resolution. The superego, "a differentiating grade in the ego," is "the heir to the Oedipus complex." The formation and integration of a set of identifications of a unique nature brings to an end the fluorescence of infantile sexuality. These are identifications with the moral and ideal values of parents—that is, with aspects of the superego of each parent. *Moral* here means, approximately, "ought not," and ideal means "ought to." The superego enters situations of mental conflict as an independent factor, once formed, and may be aligned with either the ego or the id. It plays a major role in the channeling of aggression toward oneself or the external world, and is a central factor in self-esteem regulation.

The relation of the superego concept to the earlier concept of ego ideal is complex because Freud used "ego ideal" in different senses at different times. In 1914, when the concept was introduced, Freud placed the ego ideal in direct continuity with infantile narcissism and specifically distinguished it from conscience. In 1921 ego ideal and conscience are condensed and together called "ego ideal." In 1923, "superego" was introduced and "ego ideal" was used synonymously. In 1932 the two concepts were again differentiated: one of the functions of the superego was called "*Idealfunktion*"—"the holding up of ideals," and the superego was said to be "the vehicle of the ego ideal." This last sense, in which the ego ideal is seen as a substructure of the psychical system superego, is probably the most widely accepted meaning of the term.

REFERENCES

Breuer, J., and Freud, S. (1895). *Studies on Hysteria.* S.E. 2: 19–305.

Freud, S. (1894). The neuro-psychoses of defense. S.E. 3: 41–61.

———. (1950 [1895]). *Project for a Scientific Psychology.* S.E. 1: 281–397.

———. (1895a). On the grounds for detaching a particular syndrome from neurasthenia under the description "anxiety neurosis." S.E. 3: 85–117.

———. (1895b). A reply to criticisms of my paper on anxiety neurosis. S.E. 3: 119–139.

———. (1896). Further remarks on the neuropsychoses of defense. S.E. 3: 157–185.

———. (1900). *The Interpretation of Dreams.* S.E. 4–5: 1–621.

———. (1905 [1905–1920]). *Three Essays on the Theory of Sexuality.* S.E. 7: 123–243.

———. (1910). The psychoanalytic view of a psychogenic disturbance of vision. S.E. 11: 209–218.

———. (1911). Formulations on the two principles of mental functioning. S.E. 12: 213–226.

———. (1914). On narcissism: An introduction. S.E. 14: 67–102.

———. (1915). Papers on metapsychology. S.E. 14: 166–204.

———. (1919). Preface to Reik's Ritual: Psychoanalytic studies. S.E. 17: 257–263.

———. (1920). *Beyond the Pleasure Principle.* S.E. 18: 1–64.

———. (1921). *Group Psychology and the Analysis of the Ego.* S.E. 18: 65–143.

———. (1923). *The Ego and the Id.* S.E. 19: 1–59.

———. (1924). A short account of psychoanalysis. S.E. 19: 191–209.

———. (1933). *New Introductory Lectures on Psychoanalysis.* S.E. 22: 5–185.

———. (1940 [1938]). *An Outline of Psychoanalysis.* S.E. 23: 139–207.

Strachey, J. (1974). Editorial annotations to "*The unconscious.*" S.E. 14.

ALLAN COMPTON

Sublimation

"Sublimation" is the cathartic transformation of an impulse that causes an intrapsychic conflict into socially acceptable and productive activity. This indirect catharsis allows the ego to defend against the impulse without directly experiencing the adverse consequences associated with direct impulse expression.

In 1897, Freud first used the term "sublimation" in a letter to Wilhelm Fliess discussing the nature of fantasies in hysterics: "They are protective structures, sublimations of the facts, embellishments of them, and at the same time serve for self-exoneration" (Freud, 1897). After this initial use of the term, however, Freud did not elaborate on sublimation until he gave us the definition with which we are now familiar in his *Three Essays on the Theory of Sexuality*: "historians of civilization appear to be at one in assuming that powerful components are acquired for every kind of cultural achievement by [the] diversion of sexual instinctual forces from sexual aims and their direction to new ones—a process which deserves the name of sublimation" (Freud, 1905). Thus, Freud saw sublimation as the process by which sexual instincts are changed or redirected toward targets that are more socially appropriate. In the same essay, Freud suggests that sexual instincts can "be diverted [sublimated] in the direction of art, if its interest can be shifted away from the genitals onto the shape of the body as a whole" (Freud, 1905).

In *Character and Anal Erotism* (1908), Freud linked sublimation to anal eroticism. He thought that sublimation was integral to orderly psychosexual development, but that orderly, parsimonious, and obstinate behavior was characteristic of those for whom sexual instincts were focused on the anus. He called this "anal eroticism." Freud suggested, however, that some people avoid anal fixation, partly through the process of sublimation: "the amounts of excitation coming in from these parts of the body [e.g., the anus] do not all undergo the same vicissitudes—only part of them is made use of in sexual life; another part is deflected from sexual aims and directed towards others—a process which deserves the name of sublimation" (Freud, 1908).

Freud saw the defense mechanism of sublimation as originating in the phallic period prior to the latency period of psychosexual development. In both his *Three Essays on the Theory of Sexuality* (1905) and *Character and Anal Erotism* (1908), sublimation was depicted as a mechanism for redirecting sexual instincts away from erotogenic zones and toward alternative objects resulting in nonsexual manifestation. Sublimation is one of the few defense mechanisms that Freud specifically indicated could lead to healthy outcomes, although neurotic outcomes could still result (Freud, 1905). Sublimation was considered a mechanism by which the ego could transform instincts into noble virtues: "[Sublimation] enables excessively strong excitation from particular sources of sexuality to find an outlet and use in other fields, so that a not inconsiderable increase in physical efficiency results . . . the multifarious perverse sexual disposition of childhood can accordingly be regarded as a source of a number of our virtues" (Freud, 1905).

REFERENCES

Freud, S. (1897). Letter 61. S.E. 1.
———. (1905). *Three Essays on the Theory of Sexuality.* S.E. 7: 130–243.
———. (1908). Character and anal erotism. S.E. 9: 169–175.
MICHAEL WM. MACGREGOR
KARINA DAVIDSON

Suggestion

Freud was deeply concerned with how it is that patients can be influenced by psychotherapists through essentially irrational means. He argued that influence by means of suggestion was intrinsic to all forms of psychotherapy, including psychoanalysis.

Prior to his creation of psychoanalysis, Freud practiced hypnotherapy and translated two of Bernheim's texts on the subject into German. Between 1887 and 1889, he used Bernheim's approach of prohibitory suggestion, and in 1889 he began to use Breuer's method of using hypnosis to assist the recall of pathogenic experiences. This was transformed into the method of pressing and insisting in 1891. Freud did not abandon the use of *intentionally* suggestive measures until the mid-1890s. He regarded suggestive therapy as having limited applicability, as having transitory and capricious therapeutic effects, and as vulnerable to symptom substitution (Freud, 1916). Freud found that the therapeutic effects of suggestive therapy were highly dependent on the relationship to the therapist: "If that relation was disturbed, all the symptoms reappeared, just as though they had never been cleared up" (Freud, 1923: 237).

Freud (1921) regarded the term "suggestion" as unacceptably vague and welcomed efforts to fix its usage more definitely. He also believed it incorrect to treat suggestion as "an irreducible, primitive phenomenon," and he protested that "suggestion, which explained everything, was itself to be exempt from explanation" (p. 89). Freud believed that suggestion is often invoked in a scientifically irresponsible way to explain human behavior. There is an "all too ready acceptance" of the explanatory value of the concept of "the catchword 'suggestion'" (Freud, 1909: 102).

"Nobody knows and nobody cares what suggestion is, where it comes from or when it arises,—it is enough that everything awkward in the region of psychology can be labelled 'suggestion'" (ibid.).

Even after abandoning hypnotic and quasi-hypnotic methods, Freud continued to regard suggestion and suggestibility as important psychological processes requiring psychoanalytic explanation. Following Ferenczi (1909), Freud argued that suggestibility stems from positive transference onto the physician. Suggestive therapies cultivate and manipulate the transference to induce patients to make desired changes in their thinking and behavior.

"Hypnotic treatment seeks to cover up and gloss over something in mental life; analytic treatment seeks to expose and get rid of something. The former acts like a cosmetic, the latter like surgery" (Freud, 1916: 450).

In hypnotic induction, the hypnotist skillfully manipulates the patient's positive transference.

"The hypnotist avoids directing the subject's conscious thoughts towards his own intentions, and makes the person upon whom he is experimenting sink into an activity in which the world is bound to seem uninteresting to him; but at the same time the subject is in reality unconsciously concentrating his whole attention upon the hypnotist, and is getting into an attitude of *rapport*, of transference onto him" (Freud, 1921: 126).

Freud recognized that insofar as positive transference is present in psychoanalysis, psychoanalytic treatment inevitably involves a measure of suggestion. In fact, Freud stated at a meeting of the Vienna Psychoanalytic Society that psychoanalytic patients give up their resistances "to please us" (Nunberg and Federn, 1962: 88–89). Positive transference makes the patient submissive to the therapist (Freud, 1920).

"Psycho-analytic procedure differs from all methods making use of suggestion, persuasion, etc., in that it does not seek to suppress any mental phenomenon that may occur in the patient. . . . In psycho-analysis the suggestive influence which is inevitably exercised by the physician is diverted onto the task assigned to the patient of overcoming his resistances, that is, of carrying forward the curative process" (Freud, 1923: 250–251).

The psychoanalyst must take care to refrain as much as possible from suggestive influence by means of "the prudent handling of the technique" (p. 251).

The analyst respects the patient's individuality and does not seek to remold him in accordance with his own—that is, according to the physician's personal ideals; he is glad to avoid giving advice and instead to arouse the patient's power of initiative" (ibid.).

As a form of positive transference, suggestion is driven by sexuality. In dealing directly with the causal underpinnings of suggestibility, "it becomes possible for us to derive an entirely fresh advantage from the power of suggestion; we get it into our hands" (Freud, 1916: 451).

Although positive transference provides the motive for the patient's acceptance of the analyst's interpretations, the psychoanalyst must in the end interpret the positive transference itself. The analyst's avoidance of intentional suggestion conjoined with the strategy of interpreting the positive transference itself demarcates psychoanalytic treatment from the suggestive therapies. The striving to avoid suggestive influence in psychoanalysis became known as the rule of "neutrality," a term that Freud himself never used (Ventham, 1997).

Freud (1916) was aware that the inevitable role of suggestion in psychotherapy might impugn the objective validity of psychoanalytic theories. He held that this criticism could be neutralized by the fact that psychoanalysts analyze and eliminate the positive transference itself. This argument has been critically scrutinized by Grünbaum (1984).

REFERENCES

Ferenczi, S. (1909). *Introjection and Transference. Sex in Psychoanalysis.* Trans. Ernest Jones. New York: Basic Books.

Freud, S. (1910). Analysis of a phobia in a five-year-old boy. S.E. 10: 5–149.

———. (1916–1917). *Introductory Lectures on Psycho-Analysis.* S.E. 15–16: 9–496.

———. (1920). *Beyond the Pleasure Principle.* S.E 18: 7–64.

———. (1921). *Group Psychology and the Analysis of the Ego.* S.E. 18: 69–143.

———. (1923). Two encyclopaedia articles. S.E. 18: 235–259.

Grünbaum, A. (1984). *The Foundations of Psychoanalysis: A Philosophical Critique.* Berkeley: University of California Press.

Nunberg, H., and Federn, E. (1962). *Minutes of the Vienna Psycho-Analytical Society*, vol. 1. New York: International Universities Press.

Ventham, B. (1997). "The Role of Neutrality in Contemporary Psychoanalysis" M.A. diss.

DAVID LIVINGSTONE SMITH

Suicide

Freud published only one short paper on suicide (1910), but he made scattered comments on the subject in other writings. In his 1910 paper, *Contributions to a Discussion on Suicide*, he begins by introducing a discussion that took place in a meeting of the Vienna Psycho-Analytical Society in April of that year. The subject was suicide among adolescents. In his concluding remarks, he raises the question of how it becomes possible, in cases of suicide, for the extraordinarily powerful life instinct to be overcome and whether this can come about only with the help of a disappointed ego or whether the ego can renounce its instinct for self-preservation for its own motives. He concludes that, at the time of the discussion, he has no adequate means of approaching the question, but he also suggests that, at some later date, he will take as a starting point for his analysis the condition of melancholia and a comparison between it and mourning (p. 232).

Freud returns to this starting point in his better-known paper *Mourning and Melancholia* (1917 [1915]), where he develops his comparison between melancholia (including states of depression) and mourning (which typically involves a certain type of reaction to the loss of a loved person or ideal). Both conditions, Freud notes, possess many of the same psychological features including a profoundly painful dejection, cessation of interest in the outside world, loss of a capacity to love, and an inhibition of all activity; but there are also several important differences. In melancholia alone is there a lowering of self-esteem, resulting in a tormenting of one's self, and an unawareness of what has been lost—not necessarily a lack of knowledge of the identity of the lost object (i.e., the person who has been lost) but of what the object-loss means to the loser: "This would suggest that melancholia is in some way related to an object-loss which is withdrawn from consciousness, in contradistinction to mourning, in which there is nothing about the loss that is unconscious" (Freud, 1917 [1915]: 245). A third important difference is that in melancholia, but not in mourning, the self-tormenting signifies "a satisfaction of trends of sadism and hate" (p. 251); this sadism relates to the lost object, but it is turned around and directed at the subject's own self. It is this sadism, Freud contends (p. 252), that solves the riddle of the tendency to suicide and that makes melancholia so dangerous: "The analysis of melancholia now shows that the ego can kill itself only if . . . it can treat itself as an object—if it is able to direct against itself the hostility which relates to an object and which represents the ego's original reaction to objects in the external world" (p. 252).

It is not clear how far Freud wants to extend his explanation of suicide. He notes at the outset of his (1917 [1918]) paper that some forms of melancholia appear to have somatic rather than psychological causes; partly for this reason, he drops any claim to general validity. Moreover, it is not clear that he intends his hypothesis to explain cases of suicide where somatic causes are not implicated but neither is the agent suffering from depression or any form of melancholia.

Post-Freudian Psychodynamic Formulations of Suicide

Aside from Freud's brief remarks on the subject, there is nothing that constitutes *the* psychoanalytic theory of suicide. There are, however, widely accepted accounts, loosely based on Freud's psychodynamic principles, that conceptualize suicide in terms of deficiencies in a person's self-regulatory system. On these psychodynamic theories, individuals vulnerable to suicide are usually unable to maintain an adequate sense of self-worth, a sense of internal composure, and an ability to moderate extremes of rage without exterior sustaining resources (Maltsberger, 1986). Developmental psychologists influenced by Freud have held that the deficiency in a person's self-regulatory system likely derive from psychopathological ego development. This means that such individuals have not yet formed a healthy psychological structure or an integrated self. At the present moment, no one can be sure about the cause of such a psychopathological development. Many clinicians believe, however, that the disintegration of one's family, the divorce of one's parents, disruption in mother-child or father-child relationships, early emotional abandonment, unempathetic treatment, and physical or sexual abuse would most probably result in a deficiency in one's self-regulatory system. Individuals who are lacking self-regulatory capacity are frequently confined to conditions of self-contempt, intolerable states of feelings of abandonment, anxiety (aloneness), and murderous rage (mania) if they are deprived of the essential exterior sustaining elements. To compensate for such a deficient self-regulatory capacity, one can sometimes depend on the regulatory capacity of other people; a codependence situation is usually a by-product in such a case. The other way to compensate is to rely on valued work, or on intellectual, physical, or sexual gratification. In this sort of case, the loss of work, skill, intellectual capacity, or any other means of gratification can trigger a suicidal crisis.

The Psychoanalytic Prevention of Suicide

Based on the above-mentioned psychodynamic formulation of suicide, the first priority in preventing suicide is a careful examination of the high-risk individual's developmental history. The purpose is to identify his or her exterior sustaining resources essential for the preservation of emotional integrity, and to assess the nature and intensity of emotional disruption when these resources are cut off. The next step is to determine the extent of the person's self-contempt, feelings of abandonment, anxiety, and the depth and quality of emotional disruptions that the individual experiences in the here-and-now situation. Once the emotional disruptions or feelings are identified, it is important to clarify what the emotional complications mean to the individual. Once these feelings are understood, it is essential to make sure that the individual at risk of suicide personally acknowledge these feelings. Such individuals tend to ward off their feelings as they are usually undergoing painful experiences. Therefore, they should be encouraged to take responsibility for their feelings, and they should be reinforced for ventilating feelings directly and personally. Finally, after their feelings have been identified, clarified, and acknowledged, a good rapport can easily be built up. Further explorations of the individual can then be carried on without too much difficulty; suggestions can also be made concerning desirable behavior, such as adopting other options besides suicide for solving problems.

In Maltsberger's (1988) psychodynamic study of suicide in women, he concluded that an individual's emotional disruptions can be related to her exterior sustaining resources, and the likelihood of suicide can be estimated by assessing the availability or elimination of these essential resources, and her capacity for obtaining or using them.

In crisis situations, a high-risk suicidal boy or girl is very likely to ignore all the available external resources. Therefore, the next priority is to assess how much the individual has invested in his or her external environment as contrasted with his or her delusional world. The more investment in the real world, the lower the risk of suicide; the more investment in one's imaginary world, the stronger the intention that he or she will try to unite with the next world by committing suicide. Reality testing, consequently, is an essential step to follow in preventing suicide.

REFERENCES

Freud, S. (1910). Contributions to a discussion on suicide. S.E. 11: 231–232.

———. (1917 [1915]). Mourning and melancholia. S.E. 14: 237–258.

Maltsberger, J. (1986). *Suicide Risk: The Formulation of Clinical Judgment.* New York: New York University Press.

———. (1988) Suicide risk: The formulation of suicide in women. San Francisco: Suicide Education Institute of Boston, San Francisco Symposium.

ALEXANDER C. LO

Sullivan, Harry Stack (1892-1949)

Harry Stack Sullivan is regarded as the seminal figure in the early development of the American school of interpersonal psychoanalysis. Born and reared in rural upstate New York, Sullivan spent most of his professional life in Washington, D.C., and New York City. During his lifetime, he was famed as a gifted, intuitive clinician and brilliant supervisor, teacher, and theoretician. His pioneering interpersonal approach to the understanding and treatment of schizophrenia is considered to have been revolutionary in its impact on the psychoanalysis of severe problems in living.

Sullivan never referred to himself as a psychoanalyst, preferring the term "psychiatrist"; but his thinking and sensibility were broadly psychoanalytic in nature. Sullivan initially framed his ideas within a Freudian lexicon (see, for example, his early paper on "The oral complex" [1925]); but he soon began to develop an original interpersonal psychoanalytic theory of personality, with a language of its own, that rivals Freud's theory in its comprehensiveness, theoretical elegance, and clinical sophistication. Though employing fundamental Freudian concepts—such as psychic determinism, unconscious conflict, the emotional significance of early experience, transference, and anxiety and resistance—Sullivan's theoretical and clinical conceptions uniquely reflect the American ethos of pragmatism, pluralism, and egalitarianism within which they were developed.

For Sullivan, psychoanalysis, or, in his term, psychiatry, is first and foremost the study of interpersonal relations. Sullivan rejected Freud's libido concept and bio-instinctivism as well as the classical Freudian view of the analyst as a "blank-screen"—a nonparticipant-observer. Sullivan's ideas played a pivotal role in the interpersonal turn in psychoanalysis—the broad movement from a drive to a relational metapsychology, and from an impersonal to interpersonal and personal models of praxis. Sullivan shares with British object relations theorists (e.g., Winnicott, Klein, Fairbairn) and Freudian ego psychologists (e.g., A. Freud, Hartmann, Reich) a common analytic focus on adaptation, reality, defense, resistance, the self, character analysis, and the modification of technique for analysis of the severely disturbed, the so-called narcissistic neuroses. However, unlike these theorists, Sullivan did not retain metapsychological ties with Freudian orthodoxy. Instead, he created his unique theory of interpersonal relations, which features a relational theory of human development, anxiety, and psychopathology; a new interactive conception of intrapsychic life; an emphasis on the centrality of the social field and actual experience in psychological functioning and fantasy; a radical clinical focus on the transactive nature of psychoanalytic experience; and a rigorous empiricism and operationist methodology marked by simple, specific, and verifiable concepts.

For many, Sullivan's complex and subtle turn of mind, coupled with his dense and digressive style of expression and his unique terminology, has made his ideas, as outlined in his *Conceptions of Modern Psychiatry* (1940) and the posthumously published *Interpersonal Theory of Psychiatry* (1953), *Psychiatric Interview* (1954), and *Clinical Studies* (1956), seem recondite or idiosyncratic, too difficult to understand or unrelated to mainstream psychoanalytic ideas. Yet many of his ideas, particularly his therapeutic conceptions, have been, almost secretly, assimilated into mainstream Freudian psychoanalysis. Sullivan's broad influence extends beyond psychoanalysis, in fact, to include the wider fields of psychiatry, psychology, and psychotherapy, as well as the related fields of anthropology, sociology, and even political science.

Though Sullivan's contributions to the development of psychoanalytic theory are important, his more enduring legacy may lie in his contributions to clinical theory and the practice of psychoanalysis. Many now common themes of freer and more active neoclassical technique find roots in the clinical and therapeutic conceptions of Sullivan and his cultural-interpersonal coevals (e.g., Fromm, Fromm-Reichmann, Horney, and Thompson). This has been particularly true in the treatment of the severely disturbed neurotic or "narcissistic personality," as well as that of the so-called borderline and the psychotic patient. Central among Sullivan's seminal conceptions that have presaged modern developments in post-Freudian psychoanalysis are his notion of anxiety and the self as interpersonal processes and his definition of the analytic situation as an interpersonal field (formulated by Sullivan as the clinical principle of participant observation).

For Sullivan, the self is a social product, the sum of reflected appraisals by significant others. This representational self finds its interpersonal origins in the human need for security from social disapproval and anxiety. Sullivan, unlike Freud, viewed anxiety as an inherently interpersonal process, originally transmitted by empathic contagion. For Sullivan, the self—the personified "good-me" and "bad-me"—is circumscribed by one's experience with anxiety in interpersonal relations, with severe anxiety, or horrifying, uncanny emotion, dissociated as "not-me" experience. In Sullivan's formulations, anxiety, or interpersonal self-threat, forms the major disjunctive force in psychic life, the social source of all analytically relevant discontinuities in experience and distortions in living. Consequently, for Sullivan, the psychic dimension of the interpersonal self, the interpersonal need for esteem, becomes the central, and most crucial, area of analytic inquiry. Sullivan's clinical focus, like that of his theoretical emphasis, was on the study of the interpersonal self, on the analytic play of the universal human need for approval and affirmation. It is this same dimension of the psyche that Kohut years later, working broadly within the Freudian tradition, studied as narcissism or self-object relatedness (see Fiscalini, 1993).

Central to Sullivan's interpersonal formulation of psychoanalytic inquiry is his concept of the analyst as a participant observer who is, inextricably, an integral part of the observational field. In this view, patient and analyst are seen as integrated in an intersubjective field of experience in which understanding of the patient inevitably involves an understanding of the patient-in-relation-to-the analyst, and vice versa. This interpersonal concept of the analytic situation has become so broadly assimilated in post-Freudian psychoanalysis that it no longer appears as revolutionary as it, in fact, once was. Contemporary interpersonalists, such as Edgar Levenson (1972) and Benjamin Wolstein (1959), have, however, extended Sullivan's participant observer principle in modern, more radical concepts of analytic *co-participation* that call for a more radical approach to transference and countertransference analysis and a more radical use of analysts' and patients' selves. These contemporary inter-

personal conceptions, like those of Sullivan, inform, in important ways, emerging interpersonal directions in Freudian psychoanalysis.

REFERENCES

Fiscalini, J. (1993). The psychoanalysis of narcissism: An interpersonal view. In J. Fiscalini and A. L. Grey (eds.). *Narcissism and the Interpersonal Self.* New York: Columbia University Press, pp. 315–348.
Levenson, E. A. (1972). *The Fallacy of Understanding.* New York: Basic Books.
Sullivan, H. S. (1925). The oral complex. *Psychoanalytic Review,* 12: 30–38.
———. (1940). *Conceptions of Modern Psychiatry.* New York: Norton.
———. (1953). *The Interpersonal Theory of Psychiatry.* New York: Norton.
———. (1954). *The Psychiatric Interview.* New York: Norton.
———. (1956). *Clinical Studies in Psychiatry.* New York: Norton.
Wolstein, B. (1959). *Countertransference.* New York: Grune and Stratton.

JOHN FISCALINI

Superego

The superego develops out of the ego. The ego processes all experience, responds to all conflicts and needs, and is the filter through which the significant objects in the child's world are passed. In this sense, the superego is clearly a product of the ego. However, in many of the ways it operates, the superego gives the appearance of being more closely related to the id than to the ego. One obvious example is when the superego demands the immediate paying out of rather absolute and even, at times, draconian punishments (which is why Freud once described it as, despite being a subset of the ego, functioning as if it were a pure culture of the death instinct).

Structuralization of the superego is usually thought of as a developmental achievement. In mainstream analysis, the superego is often described as "the heir to the Oedipus complex" because, although many of its contents and functions are present at earlier developmental periods, it does not begin to become structuralized as a separate mental agency until the Oedipus complex approaches resolution. Different analytic schools have suggested other timetables for superego development (the Kleinians, for example, set the establishment of the superego in the first six months of life). There is also some disagreement about the differences between *superego precursors* and the structured mental agency itself. Concepts such as "talion law" or "the maternal superego" suggest *superego precursors*; that is, superego-like operations not yet fully internalized by the child. Despite these differences, most analysts are in general agreement about the psychic operations that are primarily organized by the superego.

One of the most important functions of the superego is to serve as the mental agency in which one's morals and ethics are both established and enforced. This aspect of the superego grows out of an internalization of the combined superegos of the child's parents, and includes both the conscious and the unconscious value systems held by the parents. Over time, it also can encompass the value systems of the wider, surrounding culture (for example, the way a teacher can take over the moral authority of the parents during latency, or the way new values are established in late adolescents undergoing military training and indoctrination). Lacunae or deformations in parental superego functioning may also be reproduced in the child, creating parallel (although not necessarily identical) superego pathologies.

The superego also contains our aspirations, mainly in the subsystem known as the ego ideal. Aspirations in the ego ideal are based on wishes and on identifications that may have started out with a very high instinctual charge but that have been somewhat toned-down by the ego. Unless they can be (moderately) tamed by the ego before internalization into the superego, they, too, can be a source of superego pathology (for example, instead of having realistic aspirations, one might long to reach heights that can be achieved only by the typical superheros of latency, or that are believed to exist only in the fantasized "omnipotent" mother of earliest infancy; or one might aspire to parental identifications that are themselves tied up with pathological aspects of the parents' superegos, areas of pathology in which mastery of their own instinctual life has not been sufficiently accomplished; or one might aspire to be like pathological objects, for example, criminals, purely for defensive reasons).

The final thrust of superego structuralization occurs in response to castration anxiety and to other fears generated primarily, but not exclusively, in the Oedipus complex. Control of dangerous, incestuous wishes is the central problem of the phallic stage. The ability to inhibit such wishes toward one's childhood objects, whether through fear or through mastery, is the key to the process of aim-inhibited identification (which is absolutely central to superego functioning). For example, one must be able to modify the wish to be in an actively romantic relationship with a parent; to alter the wish to be erotically stimulated and gratified by a parent; and to temper the wish to remove and replace a parent. The ideal method of modifying such highly instinctualized wishes is to substitute identification in the place of the demand for satisfaction (this is what Freud meant when he described identifications as abandoned object cathexes). In this way, the wish for sexual love is replaced by the establishment of affectionate love, and the wish to kill and supersede is replaced by admiration and the child's desire to emulate. The term "aim inhibition" refers then to the transformation of wishes—it does not suggest a renunciation of the object, it simply changes one's relation to the object. This achievement is, dynamically, the very hallmark of early superego organization. Aim inhibition also suggests that there is a particular durability, an autonomy, to such identifications. When the actual presence of the parents (and their responses to the child) are withdrawn, the internal representation of the parents becomes sufficient to inhibit unacceptable impulses. The child has internalized and made his or her own the prohibitions; that is, the child has established an independent moral principle in the superego. Such transformations are the dynamic marker of superego structuralization, and they provide the superego with the resources to engage in further levels of structuralization. This capacity, to form aim-inhibited identifications, is equally critical in moving the child from the phallic stage (which is dominated by the conflicts associated with the Oedipus complex) into the (comparatively conflict-free) setting of latency.

In early analytic theory, women were thought to have weaker and less autonomous superegos than men. This was based on the idea that, because they are less subject to castration anxiety, they develop fewer incestuous inhibitions and, consequently, fewer aim-inhibited identifications in the superego. This has not been confirmed by clinical experience. Superego development in females is now considered to be every bit as strong as it is in males; it is prompted, however, by different forces (by prephallic as well as by phallic/Oedipal genital anxieties and, also, by reaction formations first developed in response to anal-erotic wishes that are then concentrated into phallic/Oedipal superego dynamics), and there are some dissimilarities of content (primary identifications being with the good, clean mother rather than with the potentially punitive father).

RICHARD LASKY

Sweden, and Psychoanalysis

To some degree, Freud's thought was anticipated in Sweden at the end of the nineteenth century in the work of the famous Swedish playwright and novelist August Strindberg, who wrote penetrating dramas, novels, and short stories about religious doubt, the relationship between the sexes, and the father and his position in the family. Strindberg studied bigotry, destructive forces, and unconscious motivations of men and women at the turn of the century.

Freud's name, together with those of Breuer, Janet, and Charcot, appeared for the first time in a Swedish medical journal in 1893. The article, which addressed the traumatic neuroses, was written by Frithiof Lennmalm, professor of neuropathology.

In a note added in 1923 to *On the History of the Psycho-Analytic Movement* (Freud, 1914), Freud wrote: "At the present time Scandinavian countries are still the least receptive" (p. 34). Psychoanalysis had indeed been introduced in Sweden in an ambiguous way. Two pioneers, Emanuel af Geijerstam, who worked in Gothenburg between 1898 and 1928, and Poul Bjerre, active in Stockholm and its immediate vicinity during the first five decades of the twentieth century, were united in a common ambivalent attitude toward it.

Geijerstam was a conscientious scientist and psychotherapist who felt a kinship to Alfred Adler and Carl Gustav Jung. He had already written about Freud in 1902, but after 1916 he consistently pointed out that so-called anagogue analysis must be regarded as an improvement of Freud's method.

Poul Bjerre met Freud in 1910. The following year, he presented a selection of Freud's ideas to the Swedish Society of Physicians, and in 1924 he translated and published some of Freud's articles. Already after their first meeting, Bjerre was preoccupied with the notion that his own ideas were more important than those of Freud. He believed that Freud's allegedly mechanistic views led to his not understanding the significance of so-called psychosynthesis.

Thus, during the first three decades of the twentieth century, Freud was introduced in Sweden by two physicians both of whom, in spite of mutual differences, were incapable of or unwilling to embrace Freud's theory as a whole.

There were additional sources of opposition to Freud. In the Society of Physicians, the influential psychiatrists Bror Gadelius (1862–1938) and Olof Kinberg (1873–1960) set the tone. The following statement by Gadelius is an example:

> Freud has exaggerated the importance of sexuality, and he has reached his views because his clientele in a world city like Vienna are, in a specific way, predisposed to such exaggerations. It cannot be emphasized too strongly that, aside from the sexual complexes, the importance of which in the etiology of hysteria I certainly do not deny, other and in a different way affect-laden complexes create neuroses and hysteria, and these ideational complexes are related to the 'Ich-Triebe.' (Svenska läkarsällskapet, 1913: 470)

Later, Gadelius saw merits in Freud's work. In his textbook of psychiatry, *Det mänskliga själslivet" (The Life of the Human Mind)*, he wrote: "during the last decades, the importance of the sexual drives for our mental life has received far greater attention, primarily through the work of Freud and his school" (Gadelius, 1921–1924 [1989]: 339).

As the interest in psychoanalysis developed in Sweden at the end of the 1920s and the beginning of the 1930s, so did the resistance against it. This was evident in connection with Bjerre's attempt to publish his lecture "The Psychoanalytic Method," in which he had presented his most positive evaluation of psychoanalysis and responded to objections that others had raised against it. Normally lectures at the Society of Physicians were published in the journal *Hygiea*. But Bjerre's contribution was rejected under the pretext that it was too long. In 1934, Gadelius organized his critique of psychoanalysis in the book *Tro och helbrägdagörelse, jämte en kritisk studie av psykoanalysen (Faith and Healing, and a Critical Study of Psychoanalysis)*.

In the second half of the 1920s, psychoanalysis was also discussed in *Clarté*, a socialist literary journal that was part of the international Clarté movement. Intellectual champions of psychoanalysis published their contributions in this journal, impassioned with the idea that psychoanalysis could be an element of a radical political theory and an instrument for social change.

An interest in psychoanalysis in literary circles in the 1930s was seen in a new journal, *Spektrum*. Not only modernist poetry and prose were published there, but also translations of works by psychoanalytic writers such as Anna Freud, Erich Fromm, and Wilhelm Reich. One of the editors was Pehr Henrik Törngren, who also published psychoanalytic contributions of his own. During this period parts of Freud's *The Interpretation of Dreams* and the complete *The Future of an Illusion* and *Civilization and Its Discontents* were translated into Swedish.

In August 1931, a group of Nordic clinicians interested in psychoanalysis met to discuss the establishment of a psychoanalytic society. Sigurd Naesgaard from Denmark, Harald Schelderup from Norway, Vriö Kulovesi from Finland, and Alfhild Tamm from Sweden took part in these discussions. Two groups were formed. Tamm, Sweden's first female psychiatrist and a member since 1926 of the Psychoanalytic Society in Vienna, became chairperson of the Finnish-Swedish Psychoanalytical Society. In the spirit of enlightenment, Tamm countered prejudice about masturbation. She also had a special interest in speech disorders. However, she appears to have been too isolated to develop a forceful Swedish branch of psychoanalysis.

In the early 1930s, psychoanalysts trained in Central Europe, foremost in Vienna, started arriving in the Scandinavian countries. Ludwig Jekels, a pupil of Freud's, stayed in Stockholm for almost three years. He experienced this time as wearing and difficult, and he left Sweden with a sense of defeat. During the same period, Scandinavians traveled to Vienna, Berlin, and Zürich to be in analysis with August Aichhorn, Helene Deutsch, Paul Federn, Eduard Hitschmann, Oskar Pfister, et al.

While the Nordic psychoanalysts were educating and organizing themselves according to the post-1926 standards of the International Psychoanalytic Association, alternative psychotherapeutic organizations were established in the Scandinavian countries. These organizations tended to reject tenets of psychoanalysis such as the theories of infantile sexuality and dreams. In 1932, the Nordic Psychoanalytical Association (Nordisk Psykoanalytisk Samfund) was founded in Norway with, among others, Poul Bjerre from Sweden and Sigurd Naesgaard from Denmark as members. In Denmark a society called the Psychoanalytical Association (Psykoanalytisk Samfund) was established in 1933, again, by Bjerre and Naesgaard, as well as Irgens Strømme from Norway.

In connection with the growth of Nazism and World War II, the Dutch psychoanalyst René de Monchy, who had married the Swedish psychoanalyst Vera Palmstierna

in Vienna, where she was in analysis with Freud, came to Sweden and settled in Stockholm. A key person in Dutch psychoanalysis with personal contact with Freud, de Monchy played a dominant role during his eight years in Sweden. He was the analyst of Ola Andersson as well as of the Hungarian psychologist Lajos Szekely. The latter had arrived in Sweden as a Jewish refugee together with his wife, Edith, also a psychoanalyst. Szekely had started his analytic training in Holland and completed it in Sweden. For five decades, he played an important role for Swedish physicians and psychologists in psychoanalytic training. He published articles on creativity and the unconscious in English, French, German, Hungarian, and Swedish.

Stefi Pedersen (1908–1980) started her psychoanalytic training at the Psychoanalytic Institute in Berlin. Her first analysis was with Otto Fenichel, whom she followed to Oslo 1933. In 1943, she continued her escape from the Nazis over the high mountains in northern Scandinavia with a group of Jewish children. Her second analysis was with de Monchy. Pedersen became active in what had become the Swedish society—the Swedish and Finnish psychoanalytic groups became independent societies in 1943—and took the position of an independent outsider. She had an intellectual kinship and maintained personal ties with such seemingly different psychoanalytic thinkers as Alexander Mitscherlich and Margaret Little. Pedersen published articles and books in German, English, Norwegian, and Swedish on narcissism and humiliation and the psychological consequences of political terror.

In August 1943, Tor Ekman (1887–1971) returned to Sweden after almost twenty years in Leipzig and Berlin. In Leipzig, he had held a position as lecturer at the university. Ekman was trained by Therese Benedek and was close to Tamm. Until his death he had an influential position in the Swedish Psychoanalytical Society. His publications, however, were few.

A similarly prominent position in the Swedish society was held by Carl Lesche, a philosopher of science who was born in Finland and moved to Sweden in the early 1950s. Lesche was influenced by the philosophies of Husserl, Dilthey, and Apel. A primary focus of his work was the nature of psychoanalysis as a scientific discipline. Lesche delineated what, in his view, made psychoanalysis a hermeneutical discipline in contrast to a natural scientific one, and he considered it important to differentiate psychoanalysis from psychotherapy.

Anna-Stina Rilton is another clinician and teacher of the same generation as Szekely, Pedersen, and Lesche who played an important role in the training of Swedish psychoanalysts in the postwar years. Bo Larsson and Andras Pöstenyi represent the second generation of philosophically minded Swedish psychoanalysts influenced by Lesche and who in turn played an important role as teachers of new generations of Swedish psychoanalysts. In addition to those already mentioned, Birgitta Ejve, Imre Szecsödy, and Ulf Tidén (who died in 1997) represent the second postwar generation of influential psychoanalytic teachers and leaders of the Swedish society and institute.

Historically, relatively few Swedish contributions to psychoanalytic thought have had an international impact. Outstanding exceptions to this are Ola Andersson's doctoral dissertation, "Studies in the Prehistory of Psychoanalysis," in 1962 and the historian Gunnar Brandell's essay "Freud and His Times." Andersson uncovered the historical and philosophical context of the development of Freud's ideas until 1896, that is, to the point when psychoanalysis started to take form as an independent discipline. He demonstrated Herbart's influence on Freud, and he also carried out original research leading to the verification of the true identity of Freud's patient, Emmy von N. Andersson and Brandell had participated in seminars organized by Wilhelm Sjöstrand at the Department of Education at Uppsala University. During this period Michel Foucault worked at the same university.

Many Swedish psychoanalysts have been engaged in psychiatry, public health, and preventive medicine. In the 1950s, a group of psychoanalysts led by Thorsten Sjövall worked as consultants to an abortion clinic in Stockholm. Eventually the needs of the counselors—mainly social workers—at the clinic led to the establishment of a psychoanalytically oriented training program in psychotherapy, the first of its kind in the country. As legislation was liberalized during the 1960s and 70s, and psychological consultations prior to abortions ceased to be mandatory, the clinic's services were modified and its name changed first to the Bureau for Mental Health and subsequently to the Stockholm County Council Institute of Psychotherapy. Psychotherapy training at the institute is currently integrated with a graduate program offered by the Department of Psychotherapy at the Karolinska Institutet medical school.

Other psychoanalysts who have been influential in Swedish psychiatry and shaping social policy in recent years, who are also writers in fields of applied psychoanalysis, are Johan Cullberg and Clarence Crafoord. Cullberg, who was awarded a personal professorship from the Swedish government, has written best-selling textbooks in psychiatry and coordinated psychoanalytically informed academic research in recent decades. Profits from his books have been directed to a fund that supports psychodynamic research. Another foundation that promotes psychoanalytic projects is the Gunnar Wennborg Memorial Foundation in Gothenburg.

In 1934, a child psychotherapeutic clinic named Ericastiftelsen (Erica Foundation) was founded by Hanna Bratt, a teacher. Eventually, a psychoanalytically oriented program was offered to child psychiatrists and psychologists who wished to learn child psychotherapy. An early leader of the clinic was Gunnar Nycander, who was trained in the Swedish-Finnish Psychoanalytic Institute. Another psychoanalyst, Gösta Harding, who trained in Stockholm, headed the Erica Foundation after 1945. Harding's successors have all been psychoanalysts.

Since the late 1960s, the membership of the Swedish Psychoanalytic Society has grown steadily. In 1982 and 1986, the respective presidents of the Swedish Psychoanalytical Society, Bo Larsson and Birgitta Ejve, asked the International Psychoanalytic Association to provide consulting visits. The background of this request was a sense of deadlock and diminished creativity within the society. The consultations strengthened the society's democratic organization as well as provided a more open intellectual climate. One aspect of this development was an increased openness toward the public. In the last two decades the Swedish society has organized a range of lectures and seminars on psychoanalytic topics. In 1991, it hosted a highly successful European Congress of Psychoanalysis, and in 1998 the European Conference of Child Psychoanalysis took place in Stockholm.

Since its inception the orientation of the Swedish Psychoanalytical Society has been mainstream Freudian. However, in the late 1970s, a group of Swedish psychoanalysts invited Herbert Rosenfeld of London to lead clinical seminars in Stockholm, which inspired a wave of interest in Kleinian thought among Swedish psychoanalysts. The only significant previous link between Melanie Klein and Sweden was that her husband, Arthur Klein, moved to the provincial town of Säffle in western Sweden in 1920, after the establishment of a Communist dictatorship in Hungary in 1919, to work for the large paper mill Billeruds AB.

According to Grosskurth (1986), both Arthur and Melanie Klein became Swedish subjects at this time!

When Ann-Marie Sandler, a representative of the contemporary Freudian group in the British Psychoanalytical Society, concluded her years as a supervisor to groups of Swedish psychoanalysts in the mid-1980s, she was followed by Irma Brenman-Pick, a "modern Kleinian." Like Sandler, Brenman-Pick is a child analyst, and a Kleinian influence is particularly noticeable today in the Child and Adolescent Psychoanalytic Clinic within the Swedish society. This clinic was started in 1987 by Johan Norman, a former president of the society, and Agneta Sandell, who is currently president.

In 1988, Lars Sjögren and Ludvig Igra—the latter a member of the non-IPA Swedish Society for Holistic Psychoanalysis and Psychotherapy (now the Swedish Psychoanalytical Association, see below) as well as of the Swedish Psychoanalytical Society—translated and published a selection of texts by Melanie Klein. Sjögren subsequently published a biography of Freud. Together with Clarence Crafoord and Bengt Warren (a member of the association), Sjögren in 1996 launched the largest psychoanalytic publication project in Sweden yet, an authorized and carefully edited translation of Freud's collected works, published by Natur och Kultur.

As in other countries, Swedish university departments of psychology and psychiatry are rarely oriented toward psychoanalysis. A notable exception is the department of applied psychology at Lund University. In the 1940s, a "percept-genetic" methodology for psychological testing was developed there. This technique exploits subliminal perception to study anxiety and psychological defense mechanisms. Professors Gudmund Smith, Ulf Kragh, and Alf Nilsson are the most prominent exponents of this tradition. They have published books and articles internationally, as well as in psychoanalytic journals (cf. Kragh and Smith, 1970).

In light of the pervasive antipsychoanalytic sentiment in academic life in Sweden in general, it is perhaps a paradox that a number of psychoanalytically informed doctoral dissertations have been defended by psychoanalysts at Stockholm University and the Karolinska Institute during the last decade. Professor Per Vaglum of Oslo recently named this phenomenon the "Stockholm tradition." Within the field of psychotherapy research, the work of Rolf Sandell, a psychoanalyst and a professor of psychology at the new Linköping University, is also internationally acknowledged.

In 1968, one of the members of the Swedish Psychoanalytic Society, Margit Norell, who was critical of the way its training was organized, left the society and formed the aforementioned Swedish Society for Holistic Psychoanalysis and Psychotherapy. Norell was subsequently expelled from the Holistic Society and continued to work as an independent clinician and supervisor. One of her students, Barbro Sandin, has achieved international fame through her psychotherapeutic work with psychotic patients at Säter, a mental hospital in central Sweden.

The Holistic Society found ideological support in the work of neo-Freudians such as Erich Fromm, Frieda Fromm-Reichmann, and Harry Stack Sullivan. Until his death in 1976, Harold Kelman of New York, who was close to Karen Horney, was an important figure for the holistic group, which joined the non-IPA International Federation of Psychoanalytic Societies in 1972. In recent years, the Holistic Society has oriented itself toward the British object-relations schools, Klein, Bion, and then back to Freud. After a period of collaboration on scientific matters with the Swedish Psychoanalytical Society, the Holistic Society has changed its name to Swedish Psychoanalytical Association and applied to the International Psychoanalytic Association for membership. It currently has the status of study group in the IPA and expects to be upgraded to provisional society at the international congress of psychoanalysis in Nice in 2001.

An interest in recent years in Jaques Lacan and French psychoanalysis among university departments in the humanities was preceded by the translation into Swedish of French structuralist philosophers and social thinkers. Only a small part of Lacan's own writings have been translated. A selection of his *Ecrits* was edited by Iréne Matthis and published in 1989. Matthis, a member of the Swedish Psychoanalytical Society, is an influential writer whose widely read writings combine psychoanalysis with other theoretical perspectives such as semiotics and, more recently, neuroscience.

In Gothenburg, Sweden's second-largest city, psychoanalysts from the United States and Latin America worked for shorter periods of time during the 1970s and 1980s offering training in psychoanalytically oriented psychotherapy. In 1974, the Göteborg Psychotherapy Institute was founded by Angel and Dora Fiasché, who had previously worked with, among others, Leon Grinberg and Enrique Pichon-Rivière. The Göteborg Psychotherapy Institute, which is not affiliated with the

International Psychoanalytic Association, has an official socialist orientation.

Largely inspired in the early 1970s by Nils Nielsen, an influential Swedish training analyst who worked in Copenhagen from 1949 to 1955 then moved to Malmö, a group of psychoanalysts has emerged in the Malmö-Lund region in southern Sweden (Skåne) during the last decades. Many of these members and candidates, who were trained or are in training in Copenhagen, are members of both the Swedish and the Danish Psychoanalytical Societies. They are active in the Danish Psychoanalytical Institute as well as in their own informal Skåne Psychoanalytical Society.

At the end of the twentieth century, in Sweden as elsewhere, psychoanalysis was exposed to a renewed onslaught of criticism. In light of this as well as Freud's downhearted reflection about psychoanalysis in Scandinavia in 1923, the strength of psychoanalysis in Sweden and the endurance of its followers are an intriguing inconsistency.

REFERENCES

Andersson, O. (1962). *Studies on the Prehistory of Psychoanalysis.* Stockholm: Svenska Bokförlaget.

Brandell, G. (1970). *Freud och hans tid (Freud and His time).* Stockholm: Bonniers

Freud, S. (1914). *On the History of the Psychoanalytic Movement.* S.E. 14: 7–66.

Gadelius, B. (1989). *Det mänsliga själslivet (The Life of the Human Mind)*, vols. 1–4. Stockhom: Hugo Gebers förlag. Originally published 1921–1924.

Grosskurth, P. (1986). *Melanie Klein: Her World and Her Work.* New York: Knopf.

Kragh, U., and Smith, G. (1970). *Percept-Genetic Analysis.* Lund: Gleerups.

Lennmalm, F. (1893). Om de så kallade traumatiska neuroserna (On the So-Called Traumatic Neuroses). Stockholm: *Hygiea.*

Svenska Läkarsällskapet. (1913). Förhandlingar vid Svenska Läkarsällskapet (Minutes of the Swedish Society of Physicians).

PER MAGNUS JOHANSON
DAVID TITELMAN

Symbiosis

A term used variously in psychoanalytic self-theory and object relations theory to describe the phenomenology of the self in its relation to others—in particular, the subjective experience of *oneness* that occurs either as (1) a normative stage occurring prior to self-other differentiation (early infancy), or (2) as a state of self-other fusion that occurs (a) as a consequence of pathological regressions in the face of unendurable affect or distress, or (b) as normatively encountered self-regulated regressions occurring within contexts of positive/adaptive intimacy. Over the course of psychoanalysis's mid- and late-twentieth-century development, the term has had both theoretical (metapsychological) importance and clinical (therapeutic) importance.

The concept of symbiosis recurs throughout psychoanalytic theoretical writings (see, for example, Benedek, 1949; Greenacre, 1959), but, contemporaneously, largely in reference to Margaret Mahler's codification of it in her theory of separation individuation development. Mahler applied the term in the context of her views concerning ego and object-relational development (Mahler, 1952; Mahler et al., 1975; see also Greenberg and Mitchell, 1983; Mitchell, 1988). Mahler's theory was quite derivative, though it constituted a useful consolidation of terms and concepts appropriate to the domain of self and object differentiation and development. Her framework offered constructs that were theoretically congenial to a more structurally framed ego-centered psychology, and clinically congenial to the phenomenologies of various psychopathological states. As such, Mahler's theory of developmental and structural transformations along the line of separation individuation preserved Freud's core principle that the experiencing ego exists at the interstice of converging internal (drives) and external (caregiving/maternal) forces (Freud, 1911).

Mahler assigned the term "symbiosis" both to a specific developmental phase in infancy in which the inchoate self feels one with the world (more precisely, the mother) and to adult states in which regressions to the infantile state are presumed to have occurred. Symbiosis is the earliest formation of a cohesive self (without a sense of identity) that coalesces following the initial phase of non-self feeling, a phase Mahler termed "normal autism"—a disastrous coinage of terminology when viewed in relation to the condition of actual autism (see Peterfreund, 1978). Affected by and newly perceptive of external events and conditions, the symbiotic infant forms mental representations of the self that are nevertheless undifferentiated with respect to the self and others. Symbiotic states in infancy are undifferentiated self states.

Symbiotic object relations in older children and adults are therefore analogous to what followers of Kohut (e.g., 1971) term "self-object relations," or to what classic psychoanalytic authorities have termed "narcissistic object relations" (see Mitchell, 1988; Blanck and Blanck, 1979, especially Chapters 4 and 5).

From both a developmental and a clinical perspective, Mahler's use of the term "symbiosis" is primarily (and therapeutically) metaphorical, a loose, pseudoscientific borrowing from the terminology of biology. It bears little effective conceptual or technical relationship to the term "symbiosis" as used in descriptive biology. (In biology, the term arches over a set of group or dyadic configurations of organisms defined, respectively, by specific [functional] dependencies and interdependencies, e.g., commensalism, mutualism, parasitism—see Horner [1992] for a survey of the term's uses in biology and psychoanalysis, as well as for his application of the term "synsitism" to the biological symbiosis of infant and mother in humans). In psychoanalysis, it is used primarily to refer to affects and their mental representational correlates that are normatively generated by closeness (intimacy) with and distance (alienation/abandonment) from others, respectively. The term has positive connotations when it refers normatively to momentary (felt) fusions and correlative losses of self-other distinctions (see, for example, Pine's moments of symbiosis, 1985, pp. 38ff.); it has negative (psychopathological) meanings when it refers to primitive defensive adaptations made in the face of emotional or situational distress (see, for example, Masterson, 1976).

The antecedents of the symbiosis concept as employed by Mahler to deal with separation individuation phenomena are to be found in Freud and, before Freud, in German romanticist literature and philosophy, specifically the Idealist philosophical writings of Fichte, von Schelling, and Hegel, where the problem of self (being) in relation to the universe was at times preoccupying. Reliance on psychoanalytic writings alone to trace the prepsychoanalytic history of the symbiosis concept rarely allows this historico-literary connection to be made, as nineteenth-century romanticist authors have been rarely cited by psychoanalytic writers. Familiarity with the German romanticist foundations of science and art in the nineteenth century, however, helps one to see this historical connection.

Thus, the writings of Fichte and Hegel in particular are preoccupied with the ontology of the self both in individual and in generalized terms. One cannot read many passages in Hegel's *The Phenomenology of Mind* (1807; 1967) and *Philosophy of Mind* (1830; 1971), or, for that matter, in Fichte's *Foundations of the Entire Science*

of Knowledge (1794–1802; 1982) or *Outline of the Distinctive Character of the Theory of Scientific Knowledge* (1795; 1988), without bringing instantly to mind Freud's (and subsequently Mahler's) structural-dynamic theory of self-object differentiation as delineated, for example, in Freud's *Formulations on the Two Principles of Mental Functioning* (1911) or in Mahler's *The Psychological Birth of the Human Infant* (Mahler et al., 1975). (See in this regard especially Hegel's *Philosophy of Mind*, [pp. 94ff.], wherein the subjective states of the actual infant and mother are employed by Hegel to delineate and to illustrate the development of self-feeling in the individual!)

Although Freud maintained an outward tone of derision toward nineteenth-century romanticist-Idealist philosophers, (see, for example, Freud, 1933: 177ff.), his implicit intellectual indebtedness to them is unmistakable to the historian of philosophy.

REFERENCES

Benedek, T. (1949). The psychosomatic implications of the primary unit: Mother-child. *American Journal of Orthopsychiatry.*

Blanck, G., and Blanck, R. (1979). *Ego Psychology II: Psychoanalytic Developmental Psychology.* New York: Columbia University Press.

Fichte, J. G. (1792–1802). *The Science of Knowledge.* Trans. P. Heath and J. Lachs. New York: Cambridge University Press.

———. (1795). *Outline of the Distinctive Character of the Theory of Scientific Knowledge.* Trans. D. Breazeale. In D. Breazeale (ed.). *Fichte: Early Philosophical Writings.* New York: Cornell University Press, 1994.

Freud, S. (1911). Formulations on the two principles of mental functioning. S.E. 12: 215–226.

———. (1933). *New Introductory Lectures on Psychoanalysis.* S.E. 22: 1–182.

Greenacre, P. (1959). Focal symbiosis. In L. Jessner and E. Pavenstedt (eds.). *Dynamic Psychopathology in Childhood.* New York: Grune and Stratton.

Greenberg, J. R., and Mitchell, S. A. (1983). *Object Relations and Psychoanalytic Theory.* Cambridge, Mass.: Harvard University Press.

Hegel, G. W. F. (1807). *The Phenomenology of Mind* (1807). Trans. J. B. Baillie. New York: Harper and Row, 1967.

———. (1830). *Philosophy of Mind.* Trans. W. Wallace. Oxford: Clarendon Press,1894.

Horner, T. M. (1992). The origin of the symbiotic wish. *Psychoanalytic Psychology,* 9: 25–48.

Kohut, H. (1971). *The Analysis of the Self.* New York: International Universities Press.

Mahler, M. (1952). On child psychosis and schizophrenia: Autistic and symbiotic infantile psychoses. *Psychoanalytic Study of the Child,* 7: 286–305.

Mahler, M., Pine, F., and Bergman, A. (1975). *The Psychological Birth of the Human Infant.* New York: Basic Books.

Masterson, J. F. (1976). *Psychotherapy of the Borderline Adult: A Developmental Approach.* New York: Brunner/Mazel.

Mitchell, S. A. (1988). *Psychoanalytic Concepts in Psychoanalysis: An Integration.* Cambridge, Mass.: Harvard University Press.

Peterfreund, E. (1978). Some critical comments on psychoanalytic conceptualizations of infancy. *International Journal of Psychoanalysis*, 59: 427–441.

Pine, F. (1985). *Developmental Theory and Clinical Process.* New Haven, Conn.: Yale University Press.

THOMAS M. HORNER

Symbolism

Webster's dictionary defines symbolism as "the practice or art of using symbols, as by investing things with a symbolic meaning or by expressing the invisible, intangible, or spiritual by means of visible or sensuous representations, specifically traditional signs."

Moore and Fine, in their *Psychoanalytic Terms and Concepts* (1990, p. 191), define symbolization as "a uniquely human psychic process in which one mental representation stands for another, denoting its meaning not by exact resemblance, but by vague suggestion or in some accidental or conventional relation. In a broad sense, therefore, symbols encompass all substitutes for words representing an idea, quality or totality. . . . In psychoanalysis, however, two types of such indirect representation are distinguished. In the case of the conscious *sign* or token . . . what is signified is arbitrary and dictated by conventional agreement (as in the case with most words)." In this sense symbolism conforms to the general meaning of the term defined earlier. "The *symbol*, on the other hand, has a conscious manifest form but also latently represents unconscious mental content, and the relationship between the symbol and its referent is not arbitrary but is based on . . . some perceived similarity or analogy" (Moore and Fine, 1990: 191).

Jones (1916) notes that "the term symbolism has come to have many meanings in language and popular literature. It refers, in its broadest sense, to the metaphoric or allegorical significance of a term, a thought or an object." Although many symbols seem to be universal, and generally mean the same thing in different cultures, to different people, and to the same person at different times, they may also reflect the influence of diverse cultures and thus have different meanings in different circumstances.

Freud considered symbols as one paradigm in understanding the manifestation of unconscious material and applied it to dreams, fantasies, parapraxes, neurotic symptoms, psychotic manifestations, and the like. As with any element, the use of a symbol in dreams must be considered from several aspects: (1) whether it is to be viewed from a positive or negative standpoint, (2) whether it is to be viewed historically, or (3) whether it is to be based on the word used for the symbol. Furthermore, sexual symbols may stand for aggression (or the reverse); heterosexual material may be used to disguise homosexual content (or the reverse); symbols of activity may represent passivity.

In all instances, the individual's associations must be considered before one uses an ad hoc symbolic interpretation. Freud insisted that a dream element should be interpreted symbolically only as an *auxiliary method* for understanding the dreamer's associations. Otherwise one risks engaging in reductionism and being charged with arbitrariness. In those instances where the thread of associations does not appear to lead to any significant understanding of a dream or fantasy, symbolic interpretation may be used. Such an approach frequently facilitates the metaphoric understanding of the dream or fantasy as an expression of the individual's concerns. This allows for the emergence of other valuable considerations that ultimately lead to the understanding of some repressed material.

Generally speaking, in analytic work, subjects expressed in symbolic terms in dreams and fantasies offer a means of communicating with the patient's unconscious. In this connection, "symbolism" refers to a significant list of subjects that deals primarily with the most intimate aspects of life. These include the individual's relationship to various important figures of autobiographical significance. Many symbols represent the body as a whole or as specific parts, as well as its functioning.

If one takes all dreams into account, a majority of symbols in dreams are of a sexual nature. Most often the genitals themselves appear symbolically rather than realistically, with more symbols of the male genital than any other symbol (Jones, 1916). Concerns about the genitals lead to an expression of sexual problems (such as castration anxiety)—current problems or those from an earlier time in the individual's development. In addition, various symbols can readily be used to refer to menstruation, pregnancy, and childbirth. It should be stressed that a single symbol can stand for a host of references to the body's physical appearance as well as its functioning.

Symbols can also often refer to other matters of great importance to individuals in their current life situations, as well as such subjects as aging and death.

REFERENCES

Blum, H. Symbolism. (1995). In B. Moore and B. Fine (eds.). *Psychoanalysis: The Major Concepts.* London: Yale University Press, pp. 149–154.

Freud, S. (1900). *The Interpretation of Dreams.* S.E. 4–5: 1–621.

———. (1915–1916). A connection between a symbol and a symptom. S.E. 14: 339–340.

———. (1923 [1922]). Remarks on the theory and practice of dream-interpretation. S.E. 19: 109–121.

Grinstein, A. (1983). *Freud's Rules of Dream Interpretation.* New York: International Universities Press.

Jones, E. (1916). The theory of symbolism. *British Journal of Psychology*, 9: 181–229.

Moore, B., and Fine, B. (eds.) (1990). *Psychoanalytic Terms and Concepts.* London: The American Psychoanalytic Association and Yale University Press.

ALEXANDER GRINSTEIN

T

Taboo

Also "*tabu*," *taboo* refers to a strong social prohibition, accompanied by anxiety that it may be violated (intentionally or not) and that the violator (or others) will be punished, perhaps by supernatural forces. In *Totem and Taboo*, a series of essays first published in 1912 and 1913, Freud attempted to explain various institutions of "savage society" using dynamic principles derived from his study of neurotics. It is generally agreed that his analysis of taboo is more useful than the discussion of totemism, which relies on an unverified historical hypothesis (the "primal crime" of parricide). For the fullest treatment of *Totem and Taboo*, its history and relation to Freud's later thought, see Wallace (1983).

At the core of each taboo, Freud argues, lies *ambivalence*: conflict between a social prohibition and the unconscious desire to violate that prohibition. Against those who viewed incest taboos as instinctive, Freud insisted that it would be unnecessary to prohibit or to severely punish actions that were not desired. Furthermore, such arguments ignore the emotional dimension of taboo. His psychological model for these social institutions was the compulsive neuroses in which protective rituals were devised by individuals: "The neuroses are social structures; they endeavor to achieve by private means what is effected in society by collective effort" (1913, p. 73; on the renunciations demanded by religion, see Freud, 1930: 32).

The significance of the incest taboo continues to be a contentious issue in psychoanalysis, especially as it relates to the Oedipus complex. Thus, it is in his treatment of the "taboo upon the dead" that Freud's understanding of the psychic mechanisms involved may be most clearly illustrated. Why, he asks, do people fear the spirits of the dead and attempt to dispatch them to another world by funerary rites and exorcisms? It seems strange that "a dearly loved relative at the moment of his death changes into a demon . . . against whose evil desires they must protect themselves by every possible means," for it is the closest relatives who are the most threatened by the spirits of the dead. Freud's theory is that survivors *project* their unconscious hostility toward the deceased onto his or her spirit. Thus the fear of ghosts and ritual restrictions imposed on mourners are due to emotional ambivalence: "The taboo upon the dead arises . . . from the contrast between conscious pain and unconscious satisfaction over the death that has occurred" (1913, p. 61; see Bock, 1999: 31–34). Love and hate, approach and escape, the desire to eat and not to eat, to see and not to see, are found in all taboos, while the prohibition of suicide would be the result of the desire "to be [and] not to be."

Menstrual taboos are also quite widespread and appear to follow from beliefs about the polluting effects of menstrual blood. Women may be forbidden to have contact with men, male food, or hunting implements during their periods. In many societies, menstruating women are spatially isolated and required to undergo ritual purification before rejoining the group, though stringent taboos are limited to a few geographic areas (Bock, 1967). Pragmatic, symbolic, and even biochemical explanations have been offered for the distribution of menstrual taboos, but these fail to provide reasons for the highly emotional reactions of people to this universal condition. Again, Freud's emphasis on the ambivalent feelings attached to female fertility and to the periodic bleeding that signals both its onset and the absence of conception is surely at the base of widely divergent attitudes and practices, including menstrual huts, purifying baths, and ads for tampons or vaginal deodorants (Freud, 1930: 46n.; also Bettelheim, 1962).

Indeed, emotional attitudes toward animal and human blood reveal the combination of fascination and repulsion that suggests a taboo, whether in the hospital operating room or at the site of a car crash. In his book on the history of the Spanish bullfight, Mitchell (1991, p. 166) argues persuasively that one of the adaptive traits of human culture "lies in its paradoxical ability to strengthen taboos by providing for their transgression in carefully designed collective formats of one kind or another." This applies equally to Roman gladiatorial combats, Spanish bullfights, and Las Vegas boxing matches, where the violation of the blood taboo is socially sanctioned. Similarly, in tabloids or on television, the theme of incest attracts special attention. The myth of Oedipus continues to fascinate us in music or drama, and although his transgression was unintended (i.e., unconscious), he is as much a figure of sympathy as of fear or demonization.

Contemporary studies of taboo tend to deconstruct the category or to give less dynamic explanations for the phenomenon. For example, materialists explain taboos by the alleged biological, dietary, or ecological consequences, while symbolic structuralists see taboos as "an aspect of coding social attitudes by dramatizing contrasts in social identity" (Slater, 1966: 1282). Perhaps rules of endogamy or sumptuary laws yield to such analyses, but these approaches fail to account for the highly emotional reactions to violations of, for example, incest prohibitions that, according to some research, have negligible genetic effects even at the level of first cousins. Here, Freud's observation (1933, p. 32) that "in neurotic anxiety . . . what one fears is obviously one's own libido" seems a better key to the meaning of taboo.

REFERENCES

Bettelheim, B. (1962). *Symbolic Wounds*. New York: Collier.
Bock, P. K. (1967). Love magic, menstrual taboos, and the facts of geography. *American Anthropologist*, 69: 213–217.
———. (1999). *Rethinking Psychological Anthropology*, 2d ed. Prospect Heights, Ill.: Waveland.
Freud, S. (1912–1913). *Totem and Taboo*. S.E. 13: 1–161.
———. (1930). *Civilization and Its Discontents*. S.E. 21: 64–145.
———. (1933). *New Introductory Lectures on Psychoanalysis*. S.E. 22: 5–185.
Mitchell, T. (1991). *Blood Sport: A Social History of Spanish Bullfighting*. Philadelphia: University of Pennsylvania Press.
Slater, M. (1996). Taboo. In D. Levinson and M. Ember (eds.). *Encyclopedia of Cultural Anthropology*, vol. 4. New York: Henry Holt.
Wallace, E. R., IV (1983). *Freud and Anthropology: A History and Reappraisal*. New York: International Universities Press.

PHILIP K. BOCK

Tausk, Victor (1879–1919)

Tausk's life ended tragically by an extraordinary suicide: He simultaneously shot and hanged himself on the very day of his planned marriage to a former patient. He managed this feat by shooting himself after fastening the rope around his neck; he was hanged fragments of a second later.

Originally a lawyer, Tausk was part of the circle around Freud during the last ten years of his life (1908–1919). He had wide cultural interests, and was especially fond of literature, including drama, prose, and poetry. After a broken marriage Tausk went to Berlin in 1907 where he tried to establish himself as a journalist and critic. He found the work degrading, and after some time he collapsed and was admitted to a sanatorium. When recuperating from his crisis, Tausk decided to try something entirely new and sought out Freud who immediately saw his intellectual potential. Tausk commenced studies in medicine financially aided by Freud. He finished his studies in 1914 and was then one of the few psychiatrists in Freud's circle. He worked at the psychiatric clinic at the University of Vienna headed by Julius Wagner-Jauregg (1859–1940). During World War I, Tausk served as a military psychiatrist and distinguished himself by showing great courage. After the war, Tausk sought analysis by Freud but Freud choose to refer him to Helene Deutsch (1884–1982), another young psychiatrist in the circle who worked at the same clinic as Tausk. Deutsch was an analysand of Freud. After some time, Freud found that this triangular constellation disturbed Deutsch's analysis and required that further analysis of Deutsch was possible only if she broke off her analysis of Tausk. During his time in the milieu around Freud, Tausk was also an intimate of Lou Andreas-Salomé (1861–1937).

The restlessness and turbulence of Tausk's life has been interpreted as illustrative of the typical personal characteristics of some of Freud's early followers. Posterity has clearly been more preoccupied with Tausk's life at the expense of his work. Interest in Tausk was significantly boosted by the publication of Paul Roazen's book

T

Brother Animal: The Story of Freud and Tausk (1969). Roazen implied that Freud was somehow partly to blame for Tausk's suicide by not giving him the recognition he deserved and by not accepting him for analysis. Kurt Eissler (1971) gives a radically different interpretation of the biographical facts, defending Freud against Roazen's allegations. A debate focusing on interpretations of Tausk's biography followed. *American Imago* devoted an issue to Victor Tausk in 1973 and Kurt Eissler published another book, *Victor Tausk's Suicide* (1983).

All of Tausk's estate was destroyed as he had requested in his will. His collected psychoanalytic papers were published in English as *War, Sexuality, and Schizophrenia* (1991) facilitating an evaluation of his theoretical work. Perhaps symptomatically his interests in psychoanalysis were wide and multifaceted. Tausk was especially interested in the philosophical foundations of psychoanalysis and regarded Nietzsche and Schopenhauer as important precursors of psychoanalysis. His philosophical orientation represents a marked contrast to Freud. Also in contrast to Freud and most of the other members of his circle, Tausk had substantial experience as a psychiatrist and published papers on severe psychological malfunctioning, like alcoholic psychoses and war psychoses. Tausk's most important article is "On the Origin of the Influencing Machine in Schizophrenia" (1919), containing the case study "Miss Natalija A." The Vienna Psycho-analytical Society devoted two of its meetings in January 1918 to a discussion of this article, which is a pioneering effort at a psychoanalytic understanding of the psychoses. Tausk sees the psychotic patients' delusions of being influenced by an advanced machine as a projection of the patients' impulses and as a defense against regression to primary narcissism. This article was published posthumously in the very issue of *Internationale Zeitschrift für Psychoanalyse* that also contained Freud's eulogy of Tausk.

Tausk published on ego-borders, identity, impotence, masturbation, deserting soldiers, parapraxes, melancholy, the relation of psychoanalysis to philosophy, as well as the interpretation of literature. He also analyzed the dreams of his own children. This diversity can be said to mirror the restlessness of his life. Tausk divided his interests on a wide array of subjects, and did not build a comprehensive theory. His writings contain many worthwhile interpretations, but it may also be fair to say that the expectations aroused by reading single papers will not be fulfilled by surveying his total production. His writings also contain some quite extreme biological interpretations of phenomena at the expense of sociocultural explanations, typical of early psychoanalysis. Tausk is also characterized by a propagandistic bent and by a kind of excessive loyalty to Freud that may have hampered the development of his own thought.

Tausk had problems developing lasting and harmonious relationships with people. His relationships with women were Don-Juanistic. He was obviously very intelligent and had a sometimes irresistible personal charm, but was also known as a difficult and unpredictable person who with his sarcastic and aggressive way of expression contributed to distancing him from others. Within the early psychoanalytic milieu, Tausk was treated with respect sometimes bordering on fear. Freud is reputed to have uttered "He is going to kill me!" (Roazen, 1990: 17) in regard to the prospect of analyzing Tausk.

Tausk's turbulent life lends itself easily to myth and speculation and has a potent symbolic meaning in regard to themes characteristic of modernism and postmodernism. Posterity has also been more interested in his life than in his work, a situation that may be more balanced after the publication of Tausk's collected papers in 1991.

In his eulogy, Freud (1919) applauds Tausk for his studies on the philosophical base of psychoanalysis and his studies on the psychoses. An ambivalence is quite obvious: "His passionate temperament found expression in sharp, and *sometimes too sharp* criticisms, which however were combined with a brilliant gift for exposition. These personal qualities exercised a great attraction on many people, *and some too, may have been repelled by them.* No one, however, could escape the impression that here was a man of importance . . . (Freud, 1919. Emphasis mine). Freud's letter to Lou Andreas-Salomé presents a very different evaluation: "I confess *I do not really miss him: I had long taken him to be useless, indeed a threat to the future.* . . . [I] would long since have dropped him had *you* not so boosted him in my esteem. . . . I never failed to recognize his significant gift, but it was prevented from being translated into correspondingly valuable achievements. (Freud to Andreas Salomé, August 1, 1919. First emphasis mine, second emphasis in original.)

REFERENCES

American Imago. (1973). Tausk issue, vol. 27.

Eissler, K. R. (1971). *Talent and Genius. The Fictitious Case of Tausk contra Freud.* New York: Quadrangle Books. 1971.

———. (1983). *Victor Tausk's Suicide*. New York: International Universities Press.

Freud, S. (1964 [1919]). Letter to Lou Andreas-Salomé. August 19. 1919. In Andreas-Salomé: *The Freud Journal.* Trans. Stanley A. Leavy. London: Quartet Books.

———. (1919). Victor Tausk. S.E. 17: 273–275.

Roazen, P. (1969). *Brother Animal: The Story of Freud and Tausk*. New York: Knopf. Edition with new foreword. London: Transaction Publishers, 1990.

Tausk, V. (1919). On the origin of the influencing machine in schizophrenia. *Internationale Zeitschrift für Psychoanalyse.*

———. (1991). *Sexuality, War and Schizophrenia. Collected Psychoanalytic Papers of Victor Tausk*. Edited and with an introduction by Paul Roazen. Trans. Eric Mosbacher et al. London: Transaction Publishers, 1991. English version (1933). *Psychoanalytic Quarterly*, 2, 519–556.

KIM LARSEN

Telepathy See OCCULT, AND FREUD.

Theism See RELIGION, AND PSYCHOANALYSIS.

Thematic Affinity

See MEANING, AND PSYCHOANALYSIS.

Thematic Apperception Test

See PROJECTIVE TECHNIQUES.

Therapeutic Alliance

Freud did not use the term "therapeutic alliance," but the concept of the analyst and patient joining forces to work together was described very early in his work. However, the concept of an analytic pact did not appear in Freud's publications until 1937, in *Analysis Terminable and Interminable*, and a few years later in the *An Outline of Psycho-Analysis* (1940). Freud said (1940, p. 173): "The ego is weakened by the internal conflict and we must go to its help. The physician is like that in a civil war which has to be decided by the assistance of an ally from outside. The analytic physician and the patient's weakened ego, basing themselves on the real external world, have to band themselves together into a party against the enemies, the instinctual demands of the id and the conscientious demands of the superego. We form a pact with each other."

Freud goes on to say, "The sick ego promises us the most complete candour—promises, that is, to put at our disposal all the material which its self-perception yields it; we assure the patient of the strictest discretion and place at its service our experience in interpreting material that has been influenced by the unconscious. Our knowledge is to make up for his ignorance and to give his ego back its mastery over lost provinces of his mental life. This pact constitutes the analytic situation." Freud states that a pledge to obey the fundamental rule of analysis is necessary and the patient must say everything even if it is "disagreeable," "unimportant," or "actually nonsensical." He acknowledged the significance of transference impinging on the pact. In 1912, he wrote of the unobjectionable positive transference, and he saw this aspect of transference as essential for the success of the treatment.

In Freud's earlier work, many references relate to an alliance between patient and analyst. For example, he states, "compliance enough to respect the necessary conditions of the analysis" (1914, p. 154); "the ego which is our collaborator" (1916–1917, p. 437); "the analytic situation consists in our allying ourselves with the ego of the person under treatment. . . . The ego, if we are able to make such a pact with it, must be a normal one" (1937, p. 235)

Sterba (1934) introduced the concept of "a therapeutic split in the ego" that is between the experiencing and the observing ego. Zetzel (1956) introduced the term "therapeutic alliance" and Greenson (1965) the term "working alliance." Zetzel emphasized the significance of the mother-child relationship as being recapitulated in the analysis and as an important part of the therapeutic alliance. Greenson stressed humanistic understanding as being very significant for the analyst's work and for his or her participation in the therapeutic alliance. Kanzer (1981) reviews the components of Freud's analytic pact and stresses the importance of the superego in the alliance. Meissner (1992) outlines elements of the therapeutic alliance: empathy, the therapeutic framework, responsibility, authority, freedom, trust, autonomy, initiative, and ethics.

Some analysts, such as Curtis (1979) and Brenner (1979), raise important objections to the concept of therapeutic alliance. Curtis expresses his concern about the alliance being seen as therapeutic in its own right, and he also emphasizes, contrary to Zetzel's mother-child view, that the alliance rests on mature, realistic aspects of the relationship and on mature ego functions. Brenner's primary criticism relates to his view of the overriding importance of transference in the therapeutic

T

process. He concludes: "it is neither correct nor useful to distinguish between transference and therapeutic or working alliance."

Despite such criticisms, most analysts consider the therapeutic alliance to be a necessary, fundamental part of the analytic process. Hanley (1994), for example, sees it as a necessary condition for therapeutic change, although he also emphasizes the importance of interpretation in the analytic process: "interpretation is both a necessary and a sufficient condition." The therapeutic alliance is especially significant in the opening phase of the analysis, setting the stage for the collaborative efforts of the analyst and patient, to help the patient gain understanding of his or her problems and character structure. The analyst's intuitive phrases, such as "let us look at that" and "we need to understand," signify and underline the collaboration that is beginning and will develop as the analysis proceeds. The more the alliance is consolidated, the more it helps the analyst and patient in the middle phase, the working through phase of analysis, especially when the negative and positive transference may become very strong. At this point deep and significant resistances occur when patients may threaten to leave the analysis, when there may be significant acting out, and when the analyst may be hard put to deal with the intensity of the patient's strongly erotic or hostile, destructive feelings. Here the therapeutic alliance is a bulwark that sustains collaboration in the face of the complexities of this phase.

The analytic pact enunciated by Freud has remained the cornerstone of analytic work with its evolution into the therapeutic alliance, which today has shifted from Zetzel's earlier formulations and which now is used synonymously with other terms such as the "working alliance" of Greenson. Of course, the therapeutic alliance is subject to many of the vicissitudes that impinge and relate to all other aspects of the analysis. It may be used in a defensive, overly compliant fashion, and it may also be used in an oppositional struggle against the analysis. Transference, as well as the analyst's countertransference, play important roles in the functioning of the alliance.

REFERENCES

Brenner, C. (1979). Working alliance, therapeutic alliance, and transference. *Journal of the American Psychoanalytic Association*, 27: 137–157.

Curtis, H. (1979). The concept of therapeutic alliance: Implications for the "widening scope." *Journal of the American Psychoanalytical Association*, 27: 159–192.

Freud, S. (1912). The dynamics of transference. S.E. 12: 99–108.

———. (1914). Remembering, repeating, and working-through. S.E. 12: 147–156.

———. (1916–1917). *Introductory Lectures on Psycho-Analysis.* S.E. 15–16: 9–496.

———. (1937). Analysis terminable and interminable. S.E. 23: 216–253.

———. (1940). *An Outline of Psycho-Analysis.* S.E. 23: 144–207.

Greenson, R. R. (1965). The working alliance and the transference neurosis. In R. R. Greenson (author). *Explorations in Psychoanalysis.* New York: International Universities Press (1978), pp. 194–264.

Kanzer, M. (1981). Freud's "analytic pact": The standard therapeutic alliance. *Journal of the American Psychoanalytic Association*, 29: 60–87.

Meissner, W. (1992). The concept of the therapeutic alliance. *Journal of the American Psychoanalytic Association*, 40: 1059–1087.

Sterba, R. (1934). The fate of the ego in analytic therapy. *International Journal of Psychoanalysis*, 15: 117–126.

Zetzel, E. (1956). The concept of transference. In E. Zetzel (author). *The Capacity for Emotional Growth.* New York: International Universities Press, pp. 168–181.

PHILIP J. ESCOLL

Therapy, Psychoanalytic

See CHILD PSYCHOANALYSIS;
PSYCHOANALYTIC TECHNIQUE AND PROCESS;
PSYCHOANALYTICALLY ORIENTED PSYCHOTHERAPY.

Toilet Training

As understood by psychoanalytic developmental psychology, toilet training is an interaction between parent and child that not only results in the child's ability to comfortably control elimination processes but also stimulates adaptive intrapsychic attitudes and capabilities toward self and others.

During the second and third year of life, the toddler develops the capacity to open and close, at will, the anal and urethral musculature. These actions are highly enjoyable and the toddler has no innate interest in regulating them. That demand comes from the parents. Increasingly, awareness of parental power and importance stimulates a conflict between the infantile pleasures associated with the freedom to wet and soil and the parental demands for cleanliness. Eventually, the desire to grow up and the need for parental approval and love override the pleasures associated with the freedom to wet and soil, and the child is trained.

From Wetting and Soiling to Bowel and Bladder Control

Anna Freud (1965, pp. 72–75) described the developmental line "From Wetting and Soiling to Bowel and Bladder Control" to offer a technique for toilet training and to describe the intrapsychic changes that take place as a result of the process. The developmental line is divided into four phases.

The first, beginning at birth and continuing until the toilet training process is initiated, is characterized by the complete freedom to wet and soil.

The second phase, active toilet training, begins at approximately age two because by then the child has the ability to understand what is expected and the mental and physical capacity to comply. Anna Freud described the parental attitudes that facilitate the toilet training process as follows: "If she succeeds in remaining sensitive to the child's needs and as identified with them as she is usually with regard to feeding, she will mediate sympathetically between the environmental demands for cleanliness and the child's opposite anal and urethral tendencies; in that case toilet training will proceed gradually, uneventfully and without upheavals" (1965, p. 74).

Phase three, the acceptance by the child of the parental demands for controlled urination and defecation, may occur quickly or emerge gradually over many months. As the child internalizes the parental expectations, the result is far-reaching intrapsychic change: "the child accepts and takes over the mother's and the environmental attitudes to cleanliness and through identification, makes them an integral part of his ego and superego demands; from then onward, the striving for cleanliness is an internal, not an external, percept, and inner barriers against urethral and anal wishes are set up through the defense activity of the ego, in the well known form of repression and reaction formation" (p. 74). At this point, the child experiences the typical disgust toward urine and feces found in all older children and adults, and demonstrates an increased ability to control powerful feelings, particularly aggression.

During phase four, bowel and bladder control becomes wholly secure, an autonomous ego function disconnected from its environmental origins. At this point, usually during the early elementary school years, lapses in control no longer occur, even at times of stress, and elimination functions are completely disconnected from parental knowledge or direction.

The Mechanics of Toilet Training

Toilet training should be an active process, initiated by the primary caregivers. After explaining the expectation to the toddler, all diapers are removed and replaced by training pants. This change, along with consistent parental involvement by taking the child to the toilet at regular intervals, conveys the parental expectations and focuses the child's attention on the mechanics of urination and defecation. The use of a potty-chair is recommended because it allows the toddler to sit comfortably, thus dissipating concerns about falling or balancing.

Some children comply quickly while others resist mightily for months. In either event, compliance should be responded to with praise, and resistance with the nonpunitive expectation of compliance in the future.

If the ideas contained in Anna Freud's developmental line are understood, the adults involved will realize that the goals of physical compliance and intrapsychic mastery can be achieved only over a period of years. In most instances, consistent control of bowel and bladder functions, day and night, are achieved between ages three and four and complete autonomy by ages seven or eight.

The successful completion of toilet training and the engagement of the major issues and conflicts of the anal stage of development have a profound effect upon personality development and result in the internalization of highly adaptive character traits. As Anna Freud notes, "Disgust, orderliness, tidiness, dislike of dirty hands guard against the return of the repressed; punctuality, conscientiousness, and reliability appear as by-products of anal regularity; inclinations to save, to collect, give evidence of high anal evaluation displaced to other matters. In short, what takes place in this period is the far-reaching modification and transformation of the pregenital anal drive derivatives which—if kept within normal limits—supply the individual personality with a backbone of highly desirable, valuable qualities (74–75).

REFERENCE

Freud, A. (1965). *Normality and Pathology in Childhood: Assessments of Development.* New York: International Universities Press.

CALVIN A. COLARUSSO

Topographic Point of View
See METAPSYCHOLOGY.

Transference

Every human being has formative experiences that determine the individual: Parental love, displeasure, discipline, sibling rivalry, loss, as well as anger, certain fantasies and wishes, for example, to be loved and needed. Conflict, too, can be experienced, for example, when one wishes to be the favorite child. Wishes and experience must be reconciled and integrated in the interest of psychological stability. This process of personal integration produces a unique personality with beliefs, wishes, and characteristic ways of reacting to stimuli and events.

Put another way, each individual transfers to new situations ways of responding based upon past experience. These characteristic ways of believing, feeling and reacting, created out of formative experiences, are referred to in psychoanalysis as "transference."

Transferences—expressive displacements from the past into the present—are universal. Transferences may be considered the current living syntheses of past experiences, wishes, desires, prohibitions, inhibitions, and conflicts, accounting for why some individuals are friends and others enemies, why some are attractive, or why some are needed. Transferences are who we are.

For most people, the transference mixture of expectation and need is adaptive. For others, however, the transference mixture of needs, wishes, and desires is maladaptive, particularly in their intimate and creative lives, and may lead to distressing conflicts and painful psychological symptoms. Individuals who find their transferences maladaptive are sometimes motivated to pursue analytic relief.

"Transference" is also used in the specific sense in psychoanalysis, in which it occupies a special position and has particular functions. Transference as the repository for the currently alive elements of past experience contains the information needed to understand the life of the analysand. When enhanced, focused, and examined psychoanalytically, it facilitates transformation. The general transferences brought to psychoanalysis will tend to be complex and impassioned, creating a special environment within analytic work. The psychoanalytic situation is specifically constructed to facilitate the development, expression, and identification of transferences as the best available means to achieve access to the patient's formative experiences. In every analysis, there are both positive and negative transferences. Positive transferences, such as compliant, even adoring tendencies, complement the aggressive and malevolent qualities of the negative transference. If the analysis proceeds well, there develops a special form of the transference unique to psychoanalysis, the transference neurosis. This special, analytically created aspect of transference consists in an intense form of transference focused on the analyst in which particularly strongly felt wishes and needs are expressed. It is referred to as a transference "neurosis" because in it are expressed the most conflicted and symptom-creating wishes and needs, analogous to a neurosis.

As mentioned earlier, the psychoanalytic environment is designed to maximize the expression of transference, so that it may be observed by both the patient and the analyst and utilized therapeutically. For example, the recumbent position, in which the patient lies down facing in a direction away from the analyst, encourages internal looking and free associating by minimizing distractions. Additionally, the frequency of analysis, typically four sessions weekly, fosters an intense but familiar, intimate, and emotionally supportive working connection necessary for transference expression.

While Freud coined the term "transference," he was not the first to utilize transferences. Transference dispositions had long been manipulated in commercial, political, religious, and healing enterprises to sell products, create influence and power, gain converts, and produce "cures" by inducing emotional catharsis. Freud was, however, the first to recognize the importance of the transference as a general phenomenon and its special importance in the treatment of psychological illnesses. The path to this discovery, however, was not direct. Each step along the way investigated an additional aspect of the transference. Because the history of the discovery and utility of the transference illustrates many of its functional characteristics, we will discuss the process within a historical context.

Freud's Development of the Concept and Technique of Transference
Freud's shift from neurology to psychoanalysis began with his studies at the Salpetriere under Charcot (Freud, 1886), where he was astonished by the phenomenon of hypnotism and intrigued with the prospect of scientifically investigating hysteria and neurosis through hypnosis. After

returning to Vienna, Freud employed hypnotism as a curative method. As he was not an adept hypnotist, he used other means to approximate hypnotic states through suggestion (Breuer and Freud, 1895). Collaborating with Breuer, he modified his use of suggestion to make it more exploratory. He suggested that patients could and would trace the pathway of their symptoms back through their memories to the traumatically repressed moment when an overwhelming experience had to be stifled leading to "strangulated" feelings and repressed memories. It was postulated that recovering the memory and releasing the feelings would relieve the patient's symptoms. This process became the "cathartic method" of Breuer and Freud. Both hypnotism and the cathartic method are important for our exploration of transference because both depend upon using transference, which has been heightened by the office setting and hypnotic or other techniques, to suggest symptom relief. An important difference between hypnotism and the cathartic method, however, is that the latter, while still heavily dependent on suggestion, requires the active participation of the patient in reporting layers of memories instead of passively recovering them while in a trance.

In some instances the transferences elicited by the cathartic method were unexpectedly intense. Breuer found these experiences unsettling and gradually abandoned his interest in such psychological phenomena. At this critical juncture, Freud found the transferences scientifically fascinating rather than off-putting. Part of his genius lay in gradually recognizing that while transferences possessed a life of their own, they could be facilitated, studied, and understood.

In "The Psychotherapy of Hysteria" (Freud, 1895: 255–305), the last chapter of Breuer and Freud's *Studies on Hysteria*, transference was first mentioned in something like the analytic sense. Freud noted that the patient might frequently link "distressing ideas" with the person of the doctor. Despite this observation, the significance of the phenomenon was not yet appreciated. Freud felt that, "Transference onto the physician takes place through a *false connection*" (p. 302).

Freud struggled for years to gain an appreciation of the fundamental nature of transference. In his famous "Dora" case (1905a), the analysis of the adolescent girl terminated prematurely because Freud underestimated her transference. He commented, "that portion of the technical work which is the most difficult never came into question with the patient; for the factor of 'trans-ference,' . . . did not come up for discussion during the short treatment" (1905a, p. 13). From our current vantage point, we understand that the transference was not absent but rather not noticed. Always able to learn from his failures, however, Freud commented in an appendix that the "productive powers of the neurosis . . . are occupied in the creation of a special class of mental structures . . . 'transferences' [which are] . . . new editions . . . of the impulses and phantasies . . . aroused and made conscious during . . . analysis." (1905a, p. 116). He acknowledged that the premature termination of treatment was made almost inevitable by his failure to appreciate and analyze Dora's transference.

Freud realized through his work with "Dora" that transferences "*replace* some earlier person by the person of the physician. To put it another way: a whole series of psychological experiences are revived, not as belonging to the past, but as applying to the person of the physician at the present moment." More important, the experience taught him that transference is an "inevitable necessity" (p. 116).

Transference After Two Decades: The Technical Papers

After "Dora," Freud was relatively silent about transference until the publication of his "technical" papers, spanning the years 1911 to 1915 (S.E. 12: pp. 85–171). These papers contained the fruits of twenty years of clinical experience and outlined Freud's evolving psychoanalytic technique. These papers illustrate the definitive turn from the preanalytic methods of hypnosis and catharsis to psychoanalysis since they recognize the essential nature of transference, define the task of psychoanalysis as understanding the transference, and describe transference and resistance as inseparable.

Although it is difficult to select from the richness of the technical papers, *The Dynamics of Transference* (1912a), *Remembering, Repeating and Working-Through* (1914), and *Observations on Transference-Love* (1915) are essential. Freud conceptualized transference as the "specific method" each individual has acquired "in his conduct of his erotic life," which stands as a "stereotype plate" to be imposed on the analyst. Phrased differently, the analyst will be introduced "into one of the psychical 'series' that the patient has already formed" (1912a, pp. 99–100). By giving the analyst a specific role to play as mother, father, loved one, or hated one, the transference insinuates the analyst into the inner life of the patient.

The analyst is assigned the roles of persons important to the patient and becomes enmeshed in the patient's characteristic ways of loving and hating.

Transference and Transference-Resistance

As noted above, transference and resistance are inseparable. In fact, they may be considered opposite sides of the same coin, the one side "expressive" and the other "protective." On the expressive side, the transference gives voice and life to the patient's loves and hates in the freest way available at the moment. At the same time, on the protective side, the transference hides deeper layers, or more uncomfortable aspects of the patient's feelings. Not uncommonly, for example, transferential angry feelings will be used to cover tender ones or erotic feelings to cover angry ones.

In 1912, Freud observed the link between the transference and resistance as follows, "the transference-idea has penetrated into consciousness in front of any other possible associations *because* it satisfies the resistance" (1912a, p. 103). In Freud's view, transference satisfied resistance by helping protect unconscious portions of infantile libidinal complexes. On a broader conceptual plane, Freud felt that "Every single association, every act of the person under treatment must reckon with the resistance and represents a compromise between the forces . . . striving towards recovery and the opposing ones" (1912a, p. 103). Freud also noted, "in analysis transference emerges as *the most powerful resistance* to the treatment" (1912a, p. 101), and "the part transference plays in the treatment can only be explained if we enter into its relations with resistance" (1912a, p. 104). Transference is sufficiently closely linked to resistance as to itself become a resistance.

These seemingly conflicting ideas are of paramount importance and not easily grasped by those without direct analytic experience. On the one hand, transference is the vehicle for carrying forward the essential elements of thought and feeling from formative experiences, bringing them to life in the analysis. On the other hand, transference is the means by which the patient disguises other vital means of thinking and feeling. In other words, since the psyche is complex and multilayered, material expressed at one level may be shielding or protecting material at another. Every association or enactment is to be regarded as having an expressive component, which manifests itself with the most freedom possible at a given moment, and a defensive component, which uses that very expression to conceal other wishes, desires, and feelings. Since every transference will have elements of resistance and every resistance elements of transference, it is most useful to think of them, as noted above, as opposite sides of the same coin.

The Development of Freud's Psychoanalytic Technique: Relationship to Transference and Resistance

We can use Freud's own words to describe the development of his technique. The first part of the quote is a review of material we have already examined but serves as an introduction to Freud's later thinking. In 1914 Freud wrote, as follows:

> In its first phase—that of Breuer's catharsis— . . . [technique] consisted in bringing . . . into focus the moment at which the symptom was formed, and in . . . endeavoring to reproduce the mental processes involved . . . in order to direct their discharge along the path of conscious activity. . . . Next, when hypnosis had been given up, the task became one of discovering from the patient's free associations what he failed to remember. The resistance was to be circumvented . . . by making its results known to the patient. . . . Finally, there was evolved the consistent technique . . . in which the analyst . . . [studies] whatever is present . . . on the surface of the patient's mind, and . . . employs the art of interpretation mainly for the purpose of recognizing the resistances which appear there, and making them conscious to the patient. (1914, p. 147)

To the question of how the analyst knows when a resistance is present, Freud responded that it is when actions within the analysis replace productive remembering. In his words, "the patient does not *remember* anything of what he has forgotten and repressed, but *acts* it out. He reproduces it not as a memory but as an action; he *repeats* it, without . . . knowing that he is repeating it . . . the patient . . . cannot escape from this compulsion to repeat; and in the end we understand that this is his way of remembering" (1914, p. 150).

The patient does not act in a random way, but rather within the template of the transference. The patient acts in—loving, hating, rebellious, secretive, and so on—ways toward the analyst without remembering, for example, that he was rebellious and secretive toward his father possibly out of guilt for Oedipal wishes. As Freud noted,

> What interests us most . . . is . . . the relation of this compulsion to repeat to the transference and to resistance. We soon perceive that the transference is itself only a piece of repetition. . . . The part played by resistance, too, is easily recognized. The greater the resistance, the more extensively will acting out (repetition) replace remembering. (1914, p. 151)

The more unwilling the patient is, for example, to let himself or herself recognize guilty Oedipal wishes, the more likely is there to be unconscious enactments of those wishes with the analyst. Although the terms "transference," "resistance," and "enactment" may at times sound pejorative, nothing could be further from the truth. In reality, the expressive and defensive components of transference, resistance, and enactment are essential to advance the analysis and the analysand's subsequent transformation. As Freud noted,

> We render the compulsion [to repeat] harmless, indeed useful, by giving it the right to assert itself in a definite field. We admit it into the transference as a playground in which it is allowed to expand in almost complete freedom and in which it is expected to display . . . everything . . . that is hidden in the patient's mind . . . we regularly succeed in giving all the symptoms of the illness a new transference meaning and in replacing his ordinary neurosis by a "transference-neurosis" of which he can be cured by the therapeutic work. (1914, p. 154)

The "transference-neurosis" that we referred to earlier and that Freud introduces in this passage is a product of the psychoanalytic work. It consists of a distilled and concentrated version of the transference focused within the analysis on the analyst in which the essential conflicts of the neurosis come intensely alive. At this point, the patient is ideally free of neurotic symptoms and behaviors in his or her life because their conflicts are focused within the analysis. In addition to the intensity,

the transference neurosis has qualities or currency and immediacy—it is "real time."

If everything essential to the neurosis becomes active and alive during the analysis, then we are not analyzing the past but the living present. As Freud commented,

> We have . . . made it clear . . . that the patient's state of being ill cannot cease with the beginning of his analysis, and that we must treat his illness, not as an event of the past, but as a present-day force. . . . Repeating, as it is induced in analytic treatment according to the newer technique . . . implies conjuring up a piece of real life. (pp. 151–152)

When the neurosis comes alive in the transference with immediacy and vitality, the patient develops an appreciation and respect for the illness's power, scope, pervasiveness, and the fact that it is interwoven with much that is vital and valuable as well as constricting and ill. Freud observed that transferences existed in an "intermediate region between illness and real life through which the transition from one to the other is made" (1914, p. 154).

It is through the explication of the expressive aspects of the transference and the curiosity about its resistive side that the most significant aspects of the neurosis come into play and into awareness. As Freud commented,

> It cannot be disputed that controlling the phenomena of transference presents the psychoanalyst with the greatest difficulties. But it should not be forgotten that it is precisely they that do us the inestimable service of making the patients' hidden and forgotten erotic impulses immediate and manifest. For when all is said and done, it is impossible to destroy anyone *in absentia* or *in effigie*. (1912a, p. 108)

To state the analytic paradox concisely, neurosis was created by the patient's formative experiences but must become part of the vital present if it is to be analyzed and cured. The medium through which this occurs is the transference, the process of relating to the analyst according to the dictates of the neurosis. For every element of the neurosis that is revealed by a transference enactment, another is hidden by the resistance so that the analyst, Janus-like, is always looking for both what is expressed and what is repressed. These processes come to culmination in the transference neurosis, in which the neurosis becomes alive and immediate with the analyst as its focus.

Transference and Countertransference

We cannot leave the subject of transference and resistance without considering another of Freud's significant and related discoveries, the countertransference. "Countertransference" refers to the analyst's transferential response to the patient's transference and has significance for the discussion of transference and resistance. Countertransference represents the analyst's reactions to the patient's productions and actions. The requirement that analysts be psychoanalyzed as a part of their training serves to minimize the possibility of complicating countertransferences, which may become a serious impediment to their work. For example, if the patient's resistance is made operational by falling in love with the analyst, the analyst might augment that resistance by reciprocally falling in love with the patient. It goes almost without saying that such reciprocity immeasurably complicates the analytic work.

Conclusion

Since Freud, psychoanalysts have thought of transference as an ubiquitous part of the human experience representing the synthesis of past experience into an emotional template patterning our perceptions and reactions. More specifically, analytic transferences, and especially the transference neurosis, are analytically enhanced and clarified versions of the more general transference phenomenon. The analytic experience is structured in such a way as to facilitate full expression and consolidation of the transference.

The history of the concept and of the use of transference in psychoanalysis has followed an evolutionary path. Transference was used, but not analyzed, during the hypnotic and cathartic periods. Despite a more consolidated idea of transference represented in the "Dora" paper of 1905a, it was with the publication of his technical papers beginning in 1911 that Freud laid the substantive foundation of transference in psychoanalysis proper. In summary form, it was the means for enabling the conflicts of the neuroses to come alive in the present to allow the possibility of resolution.

As Freud solidified his concept of transference as the present-day, real-time vehicle for expressing neurotic conflicts, he also gained an appreciation of the multilayered character of the psyche and the relationship of transference to resistance. Transference and resistance are two concepts often paired in psychoanalysis, and are often described as though in opposition, as in transference versus resistance: e.g., transference as the vehicle that carries the analysis and resistance as the barrier that impedes it. Actually, the distinction between the expressive side—transference—and the protective side—resistance—is not easily made. These terms actually represent complementary concepts, enhancing one another. "Transference" refers to those mental and physical actions of the patient in relationship to the analyst through which certain wishes, fantasies, and beliefs are expressed; "resistance" refers to those aspects of the same mental and physical actions that simultaneously deny expression to other wishes, fantasies, and beliefs. In other words, the process of expressing one set of wishes, fantasies, and beliefs impedes the expression of another, and both transference and resistance operate simultaneously. This synergy is expressed by speaking of the transference-resistance. Part of the art and science of clinical psychoanalysis is to decide which process requires more attention at a particular time. At any given moment, it becomes a matter of experience, skill, technique, and even art, to decide whether it is more advantageous to treat a certain phenomenon as an aspect of transference or of resistance.

To further enrich the analytic concept of transference, Freud delineated the concept of countertransference, the analyst's reaction to the patient's transference. It was both the intensity of the patient's transference, especially in the transference neurosis, and the countertransference that made it so essential that the analyst himself or herself be analyzed.

The psychoanalytic process has as its essential components the establishment of an analytic environment in which transference can flourish, the recognition of the resistance (defensive) aspects of transference, the development of the vital aspects of the transference neurosis, and relative freedom from confounding countertransference.

REFERENCES

Breuer, J., and Freud, S. (1895). *Studies on Hysteria.* S.E. 2: 19–305.

Freud, S. (1886). Report on my studies in Paris and Berlin. S.E. 1: 3–15.

———. (1905a). Fragment of an analysis of a case of hysteria. S.E. 7: 3–122.

———. (1905b). *Three Essays on the Theory of Sexuality*. S.E. 7: 123–243.

———. (1911). The handling of dream-interpretation in psychoanalysis. S.E. 12: 90–96.

———. (1912a). The dynamics of transference. S.E. 12: 97–108.

———. (1912b). Recommendations to physicians practicing psycho-analysis. S.E. 12: 109–120.

———. (1913). On beginning the treatment. S.E. 12: 121–144.

———. (1914). Remembering, repeating and working-through. S.E. 12: 145–156.

———. (1915 [1914]). Observations on transference-love (Further recommendations on the technique of psychoanalysis, III). S.E. 12: 57–171.

JOHN K. MEYER
BRENDA BAUER

Trauma See WAR NEUROSIS.

Traumatic Neurosis

Traumatic neuroses eluded nosological integration until the late nineteenth century. In the preceding century, they were regarded as purely organic conditions and were included in Cullen's neuroses. The term "psychic trauma" was introduced by Eulenberg in 1878. It referred to emotional shock leading to molecular concussion of the brain, analogous to the *commotio cerebri* characteristic of actual head trauma. The neurological basis of psychological trauma was further advocated by the German neurologist Oppenheim (1889), particularly in regard to railway accident trauma. Opponents of the concept of posttraumatic conditions emphasized simulation, secondary gain, and compensation neurosis, recurring themes throughout twentieth-century psychiatry.

A crucial attempt to bridge the posttraumatic psychosomatic divide was made by Charcot (1889), whose dynamic ideas were the basis of the revolutionary notions of Janet and Freud. Charcot found traumatic neurosis frequently indistinguishable from hysteria. It affected men as well as women, followed civilian as well as military trauma, and manifested the same symptoms as hysteria including paralyses, contractures, anesthesias, and melancholia. Its etiology was seen in fright, and he ascribed a pathogenetic role to specific posttraumatic ideas, e.g., his patient LeLog's fear he would be run over by a car, which led to a paralysis below the line where he thought the wheels would have hit him. Charcot termed this "hystero-traumatic paralysis."

Janet, who was invited by Charcot to work at the Salpêtrière, advanced the role of ideas in the development of traumatic neurosis (1919, 1925), drew attention to the frequently subjective nature of trauma, included hereditary factors, and regarded posttraumatic hysteria and psychasthenia (present-day anxiety and obsessional disorders) as a subset of their parent neuroses. He was particularly active in pursuing the dissociative model. Under the influence of powerful emotions, traumatic memories are dissociated as subconscious fixed ideas, reemerging as posttraumatic reexperiencing phenomena, e.g., automatisms. These are the accidental symptoms of posttraumatic hysteria.

Breuer and Freud (1893–1895) similarly linked traumatic reactions with hysteria. They initially described dissociative inaccessibility of traumatic memories and personality functions due to the psychological impact of emotions such as anxiety or shame. Freud subsequently developed the category of defense hysteria based upon repression (1894). He replaced his trauma-seduction theory of neurosis by the Oedipal conflict model (1905). However, he and his followers still gave some credence to the etiologic significance of trauma. War trauma, for example, was seen by Abraham (1919) as activating latent psychosexual processes. In *Beyond the Pleasure Principle* (1920), Freud emphasized psychosomatic disruption in response to fright. The subject is unable to bind the posttraumatic influx of excitation, and is prevented from emotional discharge or psychological working through. Instead, there is compulsive repetition, particularly in dreams. Freud believed that common ground between traumatic and transference neuroses was to be found in their childhood determinants. In *Inhibitions, Symptoms and Anxiety* (1926), he claimed that it was unlikely that neurosis could result only from external danger without activation of deeper psychological levels.

Psychiatric interest in war neurosis (see WAR NEUROSIS) peaked during and just after World War I (1914–1918), and again in World War II (1939–1945). Psychoanalytic contributions to traumatic neurosis, however, waned. In his 1933 article "Confusion of Tongues Between Adults and the Child," Ferenczi bemoaned the neglect of the role of sexual abuse; there were no major analytic developments in traumatic neurosis until the post–World War II era. European émigré analysts to the United States then developed traumatic neurosis as a spectrum concept. It has since referred to the initial shock and subsequent emergence after an incubation period of the neurosis (Laplanche and Pontalis, 1973). At one end, trauma is a precipitating factor revealing a preexisting neurotic structure. At the other, trauma is a decisive factor and refers to extreme experience that cannot be assimilated and that leads to shock. Subsequent conceptual advances in traumatic neurosis have not emanated from psychoanalysis. Krystal (1978) felt that Freud never resolved the problem of traumatic neurosis, ultimately leaving us with two separate psychoanalytic models of trauma: the unbearable situation model and the unacceptable impulse model.

Conceptual reappraisal of traumatic neurosis awaited simultaneous studies of combat reactions in American Vietnam War veterans and contemporaneous child abuse in the domestic civilian arena. The diagnostic category of posttraumatic stress disorder emerged from studies of the former, and dissociative disorders, seen by some as a complex form of posttraumatic disorder, from the latter. These disorders were incorporated into *DSM-III* (1980), but psychodynamic factors were excluded from it and its successor *DSM-IV* (1994). Contemporary dynamic approaches to traumatic neurosis tend to conflate dissociation and repression, and the field is still marred by lack of conceptual clarity (Singer, 1990).

REFERENCES

Abraham, K. (1919). Zur psychoanalyse der Kriegsneurosen: Zweites Korreferat. In S. Ferenczi et al. (eds.). *Zur Psychoanalyse der Kriegsneurosen*. Leipzig: Internationaler Psychoanalytischer Verlag, pp. 31–41.

Breuer, J., and Freud, S. (1893–1895). *Studies on Hysteria*. S.E. 2: 19–305.

Charcot, J. M. (1889). *Clinical Lectures on the Diseases of the Nervous System*, vol. 2. London: New Sydenham Society.

DSM-III. (1980). *Diagnostic and Statistical Manual of Mental Disorders*, 4th ed., Washington, D.C.: American Psychiatric Association.

DSM-IV. (1994). *Diagnostic and Statistical Manual of Mental Disorders*. 4th ed., Washington, D.C.: American Psychiatric Association.

Eulenberg, A. (1878). *Lehrbuch der Nervenkrankheiten*. Berlin: August Hirschwald.

Ferenczi, S. (1930). The principle of relaxation and neocatharsis. *International Journal of Psychoanalysis*, 11: 428–443.

Freud, S. (1894). The neuro-psychoses of defense. S.E. 3: 49–61.

———. (1905). *Three Essays on the Theory of Sexuality*. S.E. 7: 125–243.

———. (1920). *Beyond the Pleasure Principle*. S.E. 18: 3–64.

———. (1926). *Inhibitions, Symptoms and Anxiety*. S.E. 20: 87–172.

Janet, P. (1919). *Les Médications Psychologiques*. Paris: Alcan. English ed.: *Psychological Healing*. Trans. E. and C. Paul. New York: Macmillan, 1925.

Krystal, H. (1978). Trauma and affects. *Psychoanalytic Study of the Child*, 33: 81–116.

LaPlanche, J., and Pontalis, J. B. (1973). *The Language of Psychoanalysis*. London: Hogarth Press, pp. 470–473.

Oppenheim, H. (1889). *Die traumatischen Neurosen*. Berlin: August Hirschwald.

Singer, J. L. (ed.) (1990). *Repression and Dissociation: Implications for Personality Theory, Psychopathology, and Health*. Chicago: Chicago University Press.

PAUL BROWN
ONNO VAN DER HART

U

Unconscious, The

From 1895 onward, Freud held that mental states are essentially unconscious in nature. Freud's specific propositions about the nature of unconscious mental activity form the cornerstone of psychoanalytic theory and are intimately bound up with his views on the nature of consciousness, the mind-body problem, the cognitive role of language, and several other topics that lie at the conceptual heart of psychoanalytic thought.

Historical Background

The concept of unconscious mental processes grew out of the failure of traditional Cartesian psychology to successfully confront challenges posed by scientific developments in the mid- to late nineteenth century. Although many nineteenth-century neuroscientists, philosophers, psychologists, and psychiatrists spoke of "unconscious" or "subconscious" mental events, Freud's conception of the unconscious was distinct from and far more intellectually radical than most of the views of his contemporaries and predecessors.

Early in the seventeenth century, René Descartes elegantly formalized a conception of the relationship between mind and body and between mind and itself. Descartes proposed that mind and body are irreducibly separate. Bodies are made of material substances while minds are composed of immaterial substances, and human life is best conceptualized in terms of the interaction between body and mind. He also held that the mind is entirely conscious, and that one is automatically and incorrigibly aware of the contents of one's mind. By implication, he held that introspection is a sound tool for psychological research (Lyons, 1986). Although there were grave problems inherent in Descartes' formulations, most notably his failure to explain how an immaterial mind could causally interact with a material body, the broad features of dualistic Cartesian thinking set the horizons for psychological thinking for almost four hundred years. During the latter part of the nineteenth century, when the sciences of mind and brain were taking shape, it was almost universally believed that all mental states are conscious states, that introspection is the most appropriate method for psychological research, and that mind and body are radically distinct (Smith, 1999).

Although these dualistic intuitions were very prevalent, they conflicted with developments in the sciences. In physics, the discovery of the law of the conservation of energy by Meyer, Helmholz, and Joule in 1847 effectively ruled out Cartesian body-mind interactionism. Darwin's research demolished the dualist dichotomy between animals and human beings, and suggested that the human mind is a product of strictly physical selection pressures. The discipline of neuroscience, which became established in the nineteenth century, demonstrated that mental events are causally dependent on the brain, and that the brain is itself a purely physical system. Furthermore, the study of organic mental disorders produced by brain lesions, such as the aphasias and agnosias, sharply contradicted the essentially commonsensical dualist conception of mind. The resurgence of interest in mesmerism, or hypnotism as it came to be called, allowed experimenters to demonstrate that behavior can be influenced by suggestions of which the subject is unaware. It was this intellectual milieu that Freud entered when he enrolled in the University of Vienna, and which deeply affected his thinking during the formative years of his scientific career.

Historians of psychology have rightly underscored the fact that concepts of the unconscious were widely accepted in nineteenth-century philosophical and scientific circles (Ellenberger, 1970; Whyte, 1979). However, these writers generally pay scant attention to precisely what was meant by the term "unconscious" in nineteenth century discourse. Almost without exception, nineteenth and early twentieth century thinkers were constrained by the dualist paradigm, that is, they had to find some way to reconcile their observations and inferences with neo-Cartesian dualist metaphysics. At first glance, this would appear to be a hopeless prospect. How can the existence of an unconscious mind be squared with the claim that mental states are intrinsically conscious? One option was to affirm that the phenomena in question are truly mental, but to deny that they are intrinsically unconscious. This *dissociationist* model held that although minds are entirely conscious, they are also *divisible*. Once a single mind has been split or "doubled," perhaps in response to some trauma, both portions remain fully conscious but neither has direct introspective access to the other's mental states. Advocates of the dissociationist approach included Paul and Pierre Janet, Azam, Ribot, Binet, and Taine in France, and James and Prince in the United States.

A second option was to affirm that the states in question are intrinsically unconscious but deny that they are genuinely mental. This *dispositionalist* approach asserted that so-called unconscious mental events are actually nothing more than neurophysiological dispositions that, under the right circumstances, realize their causal powers to produce conscious mental phenomena. In the words of psychophysicist Gustav Fechner:

> Sensations, ideas, have, of course, *ceased actually to exist* in the state of unconsciousness, insofar as we consider them apart from their substructure. Nevertheless something persists within us, i.e., the body-mind activity of which they are a function, and which makes possible the reappearance of sensation, etc. (Fechner, cited in Brentano, 1874: 104).

Champions of the dispositionalist model included Brentano in Austria, Fechner in Germany; and Mill, Carpenter, Jackson, and Maudsley in England.

The dissociationists claimed that "unconscious" mental states are unintrospectable because they are excluded from the subject's primary consciousness, and

that the study of these states is the province of psychopathology. For the dissociationists, on the other hand, "unconscious" states are unintrospectable as a consequence of their not being mental at all, and they held that the study of these states properly comes under the disciplinary umbrella of neuroscience. All parties tended to view the idea of a truly mental state that is intrinsically unconscious as a contradiction in terms. Thus in James Mark Baldwin's monumental *Dictionary of Psychology and Philosophy* (1902), Baldwin defines mind as "The individual's conscious process, together with the dispositions and predispositions which condition it" (p. 83). In the same volume, Titchner defines "unconscious" as "not conscious, not mental, not possessed of mind or consciousness" (p. 724).

In the early years of his career Freud, too, wholeheartedly embraced the neo-Cartesian approach. Prior to 1896, his published writings only occasionally include the term "unconscious," and on the rare occasions when it is used, it is in a rather loose, descriptive sense. By the same token, his early writings contain endorsements of both dissociationist and dispositionalist models. The former is most evident in Breuer and Freud's work on hysteria, which describes the disorder as caused by a splitting of consciousness:

> The longer we have been occupied with these [hysterical] phenomena the more we have become convinced that the splitting of conscious which is so striking in the well-known classical cases . . . is present to a rudimentary degree in every hysteria, and that a tendency to such a dissociation, and with it the emergence of abnormal states of consciousness . . . is the basic phenomenon of this neurosis (Breuer and Freud, 1893: 12).

An example of Freud's invocation of dispositionalism can be found in his paper on *The Neuro-psychoses of Defence* (1894), which describes the displacement of affect as occurring "without consciousness" and as "perhaps . . . not of a psychical nature at all, they are physical processes whose psychical consequences present themselves as if what is expressed by the terms 'separation of the idea from its affect' and 'false connection' of the latter had actually taken place" (p. 53).

Freud began to question the value of these theories in March, 1895 (Smith, 1999). Later in the same year, while composing the *Project for a Scientific Psychology* (Freud, 1950 [1895]), he rejected them in favor of the philosophically radical notion that all cognitive processes are intrinsically unconscious and simultaneously jettisoned the prevailing body-mind dualism for the materialist theory of mind/brain identity. The mind, or "mental apparatus," is a physical system that functions in conformity with the laws of physics and is to be studied like other natural things: introspection is described as providing "neither complete nor trustworthy" (1950 [1895]: 308) knowledge of the neurophysiological processes that instantiate mental states.

Freud's *Project* makes a fundamental distinction between perception and memory. Memory is understood as the modification of neural firing thresholds caused by the passage of information through the apparatus. Perception, on the other hand, requires neurons that quickly recover from stimulation and return to their normal state after being stimulated. Freud therefore distinguished between two functional systems within the mental apparatus designated ϕ and ψ, and corresponding to perception and memory respectively.

The model described by Freud in the *Project* is what is nowadays called a connectionist model. As such it describes cognition as a function of the passage of information through the vast, ramifying network of massively interconnected neurons in the brain. As Freud was to eloquently put it a few years later:

Thoughts and psychical structures in general must never be regarded as localised in organic elements of the nervous system but rather, as one might say, between them, where resistances and facilitations provide the corresponding correlates. Everything that can be an object of our internal perception is *virtual*. (Freud, 1900: 611)

Within Freud's model, then, the ψ system does double-duty as a memory system, where information is laid down, and as a cognitive processing system. Freud identified consciousness with a third neurophysiological system, the ω system. By "consciousness," Freud meant the experience of what he called "psychical qualities" and what contemporary philosophers call "qualia." Freud's "consciousness" consists, to use a distinction introduced by Owen Flanagan (1992), of states of experiential rather than merely informational sensitivity. Qualia are "the ways it feels to see, hear and smell, the way it feels to have

a pain; more generally, what it's like to have mental states" (Block, 1995: 514).

Within Freud's model, then, cognition takes place in a different system than consciousness. Thoughts only become conscious when the ψ system transmits information to ω. Even then, consciousness is entirely passive. In fact, Freud's account of the relationship between consciousness and cognition is neatly captured by the contemporary cognitivist metaphor of the computer. The ψ system is analogous to the processing unit, where information is laid down and where incoming information is processed. The ω system, on the other hand, is analogous to the monitor, which merely displays information.

The movement of information from ϕ to ω is the basis of conscious perception. Information proliferating from ψ to ω, on the other hand, brings about awareness of thoughts and affects. Freud understood affects as essentially qualitative, and thus perfectly adapted to the receptive capabilities of ω. But what about thought? How can nonsensory thoughts, which contain abstractions, relations, and logical operators such as "and" "or" and "if . . . then" be represented in the concrete, sensory modes of consciousness? Freud's proposed solution to this problem, to which he adhered throughout the rest of his career, is crucial to his theory of the unconscious. The *Project* advances what is nowadays called a "sententialist" theory of thinking, that is, the view that cognitive activity is the silent manipulation of a language-like propositionally structured neural code, an idea which he may have borrowed from the linguist Berthold Delbrück (Greenberg, 1997).

In order for thoughts to be represented in consciousness, they must be expressed through some qualitative, sensory medium; they must be, in Freud's words, "reinforced by new qualities" (Freud, 1915a: 202) which is also a propositionally ordered system of symbols structurally homologous with the brain's own neural code. Freud believed that language fulfills both of these requirements. Language is both richly symbolic and propositionally ordered and also richly sensory, possessing auditory, visual and kinaesthetic dimensions. In order for an unconscious thought to become conscious, it must activate the mental representation of a sentence capable of expressing it. In the *Project* these "verbal presentations" or "verbal residues" are specifically described as *motor* representations. Conscious thought, then, involves silently talking to oneself, a hypothesis that anticipated Lashley's idea of thought as subvocal speech by almost half a century (Lashley, 1923).

It is clear from the above discussion that Freud believed that, strictly speaking, thoughts *never* become conscious, they merely produce conscious *effects*. Representations do not *move* from ψ to ω, they cause effects in ω: so-called conscious mental processes are actually conscious representations of unconscious information structures. Freud's striking claim that "mental processes are in themselves unconscious" (1915a, p. 171) anticipated Lashley's (1956) identical claim by sixty years.

If cognition and consciousness are activities of entirely distinct mental modules, and thoughts can only enter consciousness by means of the proliferation of information from the first system to the second one, it is possible that information may be excluded from consciousness or repressed. In order for a mental content to be repressed, it need only be prevented from activating linguistic representations. Although he rarely used the term "repression" in the *Project*, Freud makes it clear that the process is driven by the primal tendency of the mind to avoid experiences of unpleasure. Repressed ideas are invariably "representatives" of the instinctual drives, and are kept out of (pre)consciousness because of the feelings of unpleasure that they would otherwise generate. It is perhaps useful to note at this juncture that Freud believed that only thoughts can be repressed. Affects cannot be repressed because they are sensory and nonpropositional in nature and do not therefore require translation into language in order to participate in the qualitative structure of consciousness.

Freud's Topographical Models

Freud began to refer to this theoretical conception of the unconscious in publications from 1896 onward, which coincided with his introduction of the term "psychoanalysis." It was the formulation of the concept of the unconscious that gave birth to the distinctively psychoanalytic conception of the mind.

Freud's first systematic discussion of the unconscious appears in *The Interpretation of Dreams* (1900) and is developed in a host of later publications, most notably his paper *The Unconscious* (1915a). Until 1923, his discussions of the unconscious were articulated in the context of what is known as the first topographical model of the mind, which is in many respects a restatement of his reflections in the then unpublished *Project*, although expressed in psychological rather than neuroscientific language. However, it also contains several innovations. The model conceives of the mind as divided into three functional units: consciousness (*Cs.*), system preconscious (*Pcs.*) and system unconscious (*Ucs.*). Consciousness is described as an organ for sensing mental qualities, as it was in the *Project*. Although "descriptively unconscious," preconscious mental contents are able to enter consciousness if attention is turned in their direction, as they are linked to verbal representations.

For many years, Freud held contradictory views about the nature of system unconscious. He usually described its contents as consisting of thoughts that have been excluded from or denied access to system preconscious by the operation of a filtering mechanism called the "censorship." This "repressed" or "dynamic" unconscious is described as operating under the sway of the pleasure principle and the primary process, and as being fundamentally illogical and irrational in nature. Although in *The Interpretation of Dreams* Freud claimed that the dreaming mind is unable to *represent* logical relations (presumably as a consequence of its lack of access to language), by the time he wrote *The Unconscious* (1915a), Freud argued that the system unconscious is in itself illogical and irrational, listing five distinctive characteristics of unconscious cognition that differentiate it from preconscious thinking: exemption from mutual contradiction, exemption from negation, displacement, condensation, timelessness, and disregard for reality. However, Freud also accepted the seemingly contradictory observation that system unconscious is able to make sophisticated psychological inferences about other minds (Freud, 1912a; 1912–13; 1913; 1915a).

This tension in his theorizing about the unconscious was not resolved until the publication of *The Ego and the Id* (Freud, 1923), which rejected the model of the three systems (*Cs,. Pcs.* and *Ucs.*) in favor of what is known as the "structural model" or "second topography," consisting of the three "agencies" (*Instanzen*) of id, ego, and superego. From this point onward, the term "unconscious" is no longer used to denote a mental system, but is now used *descriptively* to denote a *property* of mental events or systems. The unconscious id takes the place of the irrational side of the old system unconscious, and Freud describes it as possessing the five characteristics formerly attributed to *Ucs.*, stating that "the logical laws of thought do not apply in the id" (Freud, 1923). The rational and logical components of unconscious mental functioning are gerrymandered into the ego, that mental module which represents "reason and common sense" (Freud, 1923: 25) but which is nonetheless in part unconscious. The older distinction between "unconscious" and "preconscious" was for the most part replaced by "unconscious id" and "unconscious ego," respectively.

Freud's Justifications for the Unconscious

Freud's justification for postulating the unconscious was primarily philosophical. This is made inevitable by the fact that any evidence for the existence of unconscious mental processes could also be interpreted as evidence in favor of the dispositionalist or dissociationist theses. Freud's philosophical arguments were thus used to differentially support his conception of the unconscious over and against its rivals.

Many of Freud's contemporaries rejected the idea of unconscious mental events on purely semantic grounds, that is, they held that the meaning of the term "mental" is such that it is incompatible with the term "unconscious." Freud derided this objection as a "trifling matter of definition" (1905) and "a matter of convention" (1940a). He objected to the idea that scientific discourse should be constrained by the conventions of ordinary language (Freud, 1905; 1912; 1913; 1916–1917; 1923; 1925; 1940a).

Freud used a powerful philosophical argument against the dispositionalist theory, which I refer to as the "Continuity Argument" (Smith, 1999). The continuity argument appears at many points in Freud's writings (e.g., Freud, 1912, 1913, 1915a, 1926a, 1926b, 1940a, 1940b). The argument is based on the observation that the stream of consciousness is phenomenologically discontinuous. It is riddled with "gaps," such as the dramatic daily occurrence of sleep. During sleep, our normal conscious mental life ceases, and yet is restored with no loss of coherence or identity when we awaken. Another example, singled out by Freud, is the experience of giving up work on a seemingly intractable intellectual problem and putting the problem out of mind only to have the answer later occur to one "out of the blue." There are many examples of this phenomenon recorded in the literature on scientific creativity (Hadamard, 1949). A particularly fine one was provided by the French mathematician/physicist, Henri Poincaré, who described how he abandoned research on a mathematical problem in order to go on vacation. Although Poincaré had consciously laid the problem aside, he had apparently not done so unconsciously, for he records that:

Having reached Coustances, we entered an omnibus to go some place or other. At the moment I put my foot on the step the idea came to me, without anything in my former thoughts seeming to have paved the way for it, that the transformations I had used to define the Fuchsian functions were identical to those of non-Euclidian geometry. I did not verify the idea; I should not have had time, as, upon taking my seat in the omnibus, I went on with a conversation already commenced, but I felt a perfect certainty. On my return to Caen, for conscience's sake I verified the result at my leisure. (Poincaré, 1913: 383–384)

In this example, there was a temporal gap between Poincaré's final moments of conscious work on the problem (at time T_1) and the experience on the omnibus (at time T_2). On a dispositionalist interpretation, the unconscious events that occurred between T_1 and T_2, and that secured the continuity between them, were neurophysiological but nonmental. This way of understanding the sequence of events entails the absurd conclusion that no cognitive work was done on the problem during the interval, and that it was therefore entirely fortuitous that the answer occurred to Poincaré when it did. Unless one is determined to reject the notion of unconscious cognition at all costs, it is obvious that truly mental, cognitive processes supplied the continuity between the event at T_1 and the event at T_2. It is equally obvious that they were unconscious, and that truly mental unconscious processes rather than mere neurophysiological dispositions were the cause of Poincaré's revelation in Coustances. As Freud (1905, p. 158) put it, if we confine ourselves to the conscious dimension we find "broken sequences" that are "obviously dependent on something else." More explicitly:

1. *There are gaps in the continuity of conscious mental events.* In the example given above, there is a gap in conscious mental continuity between Poincaré's work on the mathematical problem at T_1 and the idea that suddenly entered his mind while on vacation in Coustances at T_2.
2. *Only mental processes can provide mental continuity.* We say that there are "gaps" in conscious mental continuity when there are *semantic* discontinuities in the flow of conscious thought. The

principle that the possession of intentionality distinguishes mental from nonmental phenomena entails that semantic continuity is supplied only by mental processes. Nonmental processes do not possess semantic content and therefore cannot provide semantic continuity.

3. *All mental events are caused.* This is a special case of the view that all nonquantum-level events are caused and is, of course, an expression of Freud's doctrine of psychical determinism.

4. *In cases where a conscious mental event at T_1 is followed by:*

   a. *a period of conscious mental activity semantically discontinuous with it, or a period during which conscious mental activity has ceased entirely, and*

   b. *which is in turn followed by the involuntary occurrence of a conscious mental event at T_2 the content of which provides a solution to the problem addressed at T_1, which*

   c. *cannot reasonably be attributed to any cause other than the subject's own mental activity, then:*

   d. *the subject's unconscious mental activity is a necessary cause for the event at T_2.*

   In the Poincaré example, the thought at T_2 that the transformations he had used to define the Fuchsian functions were identical to those of non-Euclidian geometry could not reasonably be attributed to any cause other than his own cognitive activity. We are therefore justified in concluding that Poincaré unconsciously thought about the problem during the interval between T_1 and T_2.

5. *Therefore, unconscious mental states can be occurrent.*

Freud (1915a, 1940b) also introduces a metaphysical consideration. The dispositionalist restriction of mental states to consciousness is motivated by a desire to preserve the Cartesian distinction between mental and neuropsychological processes, and fails to address the old Cartesian problem of how physical states of the nervous system can possibly interact with nonphysical mental states. Freud also rejected the metaphysical doctrine of psychophysical parallelism, and used the continuity argument to infer that unconscious mental activity is realized by some of the neurophysiological processes occurring during the gaps in conscious mental life. Whereas the dispositionalists were tied to an unsatisfactory dualism, psychoanalytic theory insisted on the materialist alternative that neurophysiological processes instantiate cognitive states.

A different argument was required to refute the dissociationist theory that, if applied to the example above, would lead to the conclusion that Poincaré's consciousness had split itself into a part that was unconcerned with the mathematical problem (his "primary" consciousness) and a part that continued to work on the problem (his "secondary" consciousness). Freud raised several objections to the dissociationist thesis of an "unconscious consciousness." His first objection was that there is something incoherent about the notion of "a consciousness of which its own possessor knows nothing" (1915a, p. 170) which seems to violate the most basic definitional criterion for consciousness. It might be argued that Freud is here resorting here to the same kind of semantic argument that he found so objectionable in the writings of his detractors. However, it is logically possible for a mental state to lack the property of consciousness, but there is no possible world in which a conscious state can, at the same time, be unconscious. The idea of an unconscious consciousness is thus not merely a violation of linguistic convention, it is blatantly self-contradictory. The only support for the dissociationist thesis is the logically and evidentially unjustified *axiomatic* equation of mind with consciousness, the "preconceived belief that regards the identity of the psychical and the conscious as settled once and for all" (1923, p. 16n). Second, the idea of unconscious consciousness requires us to multiply entities needlessly, particularly in light of the fact that it allows us to "assume the existence not only of a second consciousness, but of a third, fourth, perhaps of an unlimited number of states of consciousness, all unknown to us and to one another" (1915a, p. 170). Finally, Freud (1915) claimed that irrational unconscious mental processes are in many ways so dissimilar to what we know to be conscious mental processes that the extrapolation from the latter to the former loses force. Although Freud regarded the final consideration as the weightiest of the three, this is clearly not the case as, unlike the previous two, which are theoretically neutral, it derives its credibility from the credibility of specifically psychoanalytic hypotheses about the nature of the unconscious mind.

Yet another alternative to the idea of unconscious mental events is the notion that these are best explained by *gradations* in consciousness, like Leibnitz's *petites perceptions*. Perhaps Poincaré was only dimly aware—but nonetheless conscious—of his continuing preoccupation with the mathematical problem. Freud retorts that the bare fact that there are gradations in consciousness is irrelevant to the question of the existence of unconscious mental states. It "has no more evidential value than such analogous statements as 'There are so very many gradations in illumination . . . therefore there is no such thing as darkness at all'" and adds that:

> Further, to include "what is unnoticeable" under the concept of "what is conscious" is simply to play havoc with the one and only piece of direct and certain knowledge that we have about the mind. And after all, a consciousness of which one knows nothing seems to me a good deal more absurd than something mental that is unconscious. (1923, p. 16n)

The Freudian Unconscious and the Cognitive Unconscious

The field of psychology has undergone three major transformations in its short history. For much of its early history, psychology was the study of conscious mental phenomena. However, after the spectacular failure of introspectionism in the early twentieth century, behaviorism became the dominant paradigm. The behaviorists dealt with the scientific unreliability of introspective reports by ignoring mental states altogether. During the latter decades of the twentieth century, the preeminence of behaviorism was successfully challenged by cognitivism, which understands the mind largely in terms of nonconscious information processing. Of the three consecutive concepts of psychology as the science of consciousness, the science of behavior, and the science of unconscious information processing, the latter would seem prima facie to be more hospitable to Freudian concepts.

It is true that there is some convergence between Freudian and cognitive scientific ideas insofar as cognitivists routinely invoke unconscious mental processes for explanatory purposes. There are also more specific overlaps. For example, Freud's theory of consciousness bears some striking similarities to recent work in cognitive neuroscience and cognitive linguistics (Smith, 2000). However, these conceptual and theoretical linkages should not be taken to imply that specific Freudian claims about the

unconscious have been validated or even supported by contemporary research in cognitive science. Although Freud's unconscious is indeed cognitive in nature, and it is true that Freud described *all* cognitive processes as intrinsically unconscious, the type of items characteristically described by Freud as unconscious are rather different from those characteristically invoked by cognitive scientists (Eagle, 1987). Cognitive scientists typically refer to unconscious processes and contents that are (a) distant from affective life, and (b) incapable of even in principle of becoming conscious, whereas Freud's chief concern was with affectively significant unconscious thoughts that can at least in principle be admitted into consciousness. Although at present the gap between cognitivist and psychoanalytic conceptions is a large one, this may be partially due to the fact that it is only very recently that cognitive science has begun to investigate affectively significant mental phenomena.

REFERENCES

Baldwin, J. M. (ed.) (1902). *Dictionary of Psychology and Philosophy*, vol. 1. London: Macmillan.

Block, N. (1995). On a confusion about a function of consciousness. *Behavioral and Brain Sciences*, 18: 228–287.

Brentano, F. (1874). *Psychology from an Empirical Standpoint*. London: Routledge and Kegan Paul, 1973.

Breuer, J., and Freud, S. (1893). The psychical mechanism of hysterical phenomena: Preliminary communication. S.E. 2: 3–17.

Darwin, C. (1859). *The Origin of the Species*. London: Penguin, 1968.

———. (1871). *The Descent of Man, and Selection in Relation to Sex*. London: John Murray.

Eagle, M. N. (1987). The psychoanalytic and the cognitive unconscious. In S. Stern (ed.). *Theories of the Unconscious and Theories of the Self*. Hillsdale, N.J.: Analytic Press.

Ellenberger, H. F. (1970). *The Discovery of the Unconscious: The History and Evolution of Dynamic Psychiatry*. New York: Basic Books.

Flanagan, O. (1992). *Consciousness Reconsidered*. Cambridge, Mass.: Bradford/MIT.

Freud, S. (1894). The neuro-psychoses of defence. S.E. 3: 45–61.

———. (1900). *The Interpretation of Dreams*. S.E. 4–5: 1–621.

———. (1905). *Jokes and their Relation to the Unconscious*. S.E. 8: 3–237.

———. (1912a). A note on the unconscious in psycho-analysis. S.E. 12: 260–266.

———. (1912b). Recommendations to physicians practicing psycho-analysis. S.E. 12: 111–120.

———. (1912–1913). *Totem and Taboo*. S.E. 13: 1–161.

———. (1913). The claims of psycho-analysis to scientific interest. S.E. 13: 165–190.

———. (1916-1917). *Introductory Lectures on Psycho-analysis.* S.E. 15–16: 9–496.

———. (1915a). The unconscious. S.E. 14: 166–215.

———. (1915b). Repression. S.E. 14: 146–158.

———. (1923). *The Ego and the Id.* S.E. 19: 1–59.

———. (1925). The resistances to psycho-analysis. S.E. 19: 213–222.

———. (1926a). *Inhibitions, Symptoms and Anxiety.* S.E. 20: 87–172.

———. (1926b). *The Question of Lay Analysis.* S.E. 20: 183–258.

———. (1940a). *An Outline of Psycho-Analysis.* S.E. 23: 139–207.

———. (1940b). Some elementary lessons in psycho-analysis. S.E. 23: 281–286.

———. (1950 [1895]). *Project for a Scientific Psychology.* S.E. 1: 281–397.

Greenberg, V. D. (1997). *Freud and His Aphasia Book: Language and the Sources of Psychoanalysis.* Ithaca, N.Y.: Cornell University Press.

Hadamard, J. (1949). *The Psychology of Invention in the Mathematical Field.* Princeton, N.J.: Princeton University Press.

Lashley, C. (1923). The behavioristic interpretation of consciousness, II. *The Psychological Review*, 30(5): 329–353.

———. (1956). Cerebral organization and behavior. In H. Solomon, S. Cob, and W. Penfield (eds.). *Brain and Human Behavior.* Baltimore: Williams & Wilkins.

Lyons, W. (1986). *The Disappearance of Introspection.* Cambridge, Mass.: Bradford/MIT.

Poincaré, H. (1913). *Last Essays.* Trans. J. W. Bolduc. New York: Dover, 1963.

Smith, D. L. (1999). *Freud's Philosophy of the Unconscious.* Boston: Kluwer Academic Publishers.

———. (2000). Freudian science of consciousness: then and now. *Neuropsychoanalysis*, 2(1): 45–47.

Whyte, L. L. (1979). *The Unconscious Before Freud.* London: Julian Friedman.

DAVID LIVINGSTONE SMITH

United States, and Psychoanalysis

Psychoanalysis has enjoyed immense popularity in the United States both in psychiatry and in the general culture. The momentous impact and long-term effect of Freud's lectures at Clark University in Worcester, Massachusetts, in 1909, in which he brought to the United States his theory and methodology of understanding and utilizing the unconscious mind, is well documented. Those in attendance included many of the then current and future leaders of American professional life, such as G. Stanley Hall, president of Clark University and founder of the American Psychological Association, who organized the event and issued the invitations; Edward Tichener, a famous introspective and experimental psy-

chologist; William James, the philosopher; Franz Boas, the noted anthropologist; A. A. Brill, an important translator of Freud who came to play a key role in organized psychoanalysis in this country; Ernest Jones, one of Freud's inner circle and author of the definitive three-volume biography of Freud; James J. Putnam, a famed neurologist; Adolf Meyer, a leading figure in American psychiatry between the two world wars; and Emma Goldman, a "notorious" feminist, anarchist, and proponent of free love (Rosenzweig, 1992: 132–134).

After the Clark University lectures, published in English as *Five Lectures on Psychoanalysis* (Freud, 1910), the psychoanalytic movement in the United States began as a loosely knit corps of self- or European-trained psychiatrists and neurologists, many of whom went to Vienna or Berlin for personal analysis by Freud or one of his followers. However, formal training requirements gradually evolved in the 1920s and 1930s as the field became professionalized as an increasingly medical discipline and subspecialty of psychiatry. Brill, though an important popularizer of psychoanalysis, was also a key proponent of medicalization and the exclusion from the training and practice of psychoanalysis by psychologists, social workers, and other nonphysician mental health professionals. Brill was at odds with Freud on this score despite his role as a promulgator of psychoanalytic thought and as an important translator of Freud's works. Freud clearly favored the admission of gifted nonphysicians, and he deplored the medicalization of psychoanalysis in the United States—fearing its absorption and dilution by psychiatry.

A formal training structure under the American Psychoanalytic Association (founded in 1911) was established and solidified as many European refugee analysts fleeing Nazism came to the United States. Some of these individuals strengthened the orthodoxy of organized psychoanalysis, but because the group included a number of distinguished nonphysicians, their arrival also resulted in the formation of splinter groups, such as the one founded by Theodore Reik in New York. Other refugee nonphysician analysts were accepted into the ranks of component societies of the American Psychoanalytic Association, but they needed a special waiver and were accorded limited voting rights. However, the door was firmly closed to American-trained nonphysicians from psychology and other professions when the American Psychoanalytic Association was given unique regional status under the International Psychoanalytic Association (IPA), and was thus able to maintain its exclusionary policies without interference. This occurred in 1939, the year of Freud's death, as World War II was breaking out in Europe.

While the professionalization of psychoanalysis was occurring between the world wars, there was a concomitant popularization of Freud's ideas in the general culture and particularly in the literary culture of major eastern seaboard cities. Psychoanalysis also infused the mental hygiene movement of that era, as well as the fields of education and criminology. There appears to have been a uniquely American enthusiasm for psychoanalysis in the cultural and intellectual life of many literate Americans. Karl Menninger's popular books, beginning with *The Human Mind* in 1930, fostered and reflected both America's enthusiasm and optimism for psychoanalysis and its applications. This was in stark contrast to Freud's growing cynicism about these American developments. His dislike of the United States and of psychoanalytic applications by Americans paralleled his dislike of the medicalization of analysis within psychiatry and coincided with his growing pessimism about therapeutic results, at a time when enthusiasm for psychoanalytic treatment and applications in the United States was increasing. However, he shared the ideal that psychoanalysis might become a panacea for many of society's ills, while deploring what he felt was its absorption, dilution, and distortion in the United States. Freud reports his initial pleasure over his American reception and his developing disenchantment in his autobiographical study (Freud, 1925: 52). In Europe, psychoanalysis had been largely excluded by the medical community, and it also failed to gain the general popularity enjoyed in the United States from both the Clark University lectures and its seeming utility in understanding the human tragedies of World War I (Hale, 1995: 16). This popularity reached its zenith, however, during and after World War II, when psychoanalysis dominated psychiatry and mental health for decades, and psychoanalytic practice was at its height.

In those years, psychoanalysis in the United States developed a significant orthodoxy through the contributions of European émigrés who elaborated Freud's tripartite model of the mind—id, ego, and superego. The joint publications of Heinz Hartman, Ernst Kris, and Rudolph Lowenstein on psychic structure and ego psychology dominated psychoanalytic theory (Hartman, Kris, and Lowenstein, 1964). Kurt Eissler's classic 1953

paper delineating a "basic model technique" became most analysts' idealized goal of how analysis should be conducted (Eissler, 1953).

However, in the 1960s and 1970s, a new wave of theoretical diversity began with the work of Heinz Kohut of Chicago, who introduced a special emphasis on narcissism as an independent line in human development (Kohut, 1971). He eventually became the founder of a new theoretical branch of psychoanalysis known as self-psychology. Many mainstream analysts were affected in their thinking and analytic technique by Kohut's ideas, although they eschewed formal adherence to self-psychology. Nevertheless, his theory and corresponding technical differences gained notable interest and adoption in other psychoanalytic centers. Also, self-psychology has remained under the umbrella of organized psychoanalysis (the American Psychoanalytic Association) and did not result in an institute "split" in Chicago as has occurred in other cities on various theoretical and technical grounds. This contrasts with Freud's day, when deviant theorists such as Adler, Jung, and Rank left or were expelled from the Freudian fold, because Freud would not tolerate their challenge to his official theoretical position.

During this same time of ferment in American psychoanalysis, the works of Melanie Klein from England began to take root in Los Angeles. Klein focused on primitive object relations with a new set of concepts and terms heretofore considered heretical by most American-trained analysts (Klein, 1948). A Kleinian group succeeded in forming their own independent organization, eventually gaining recognition by the International Psychoanalytic Association outside the purview of the American Psychoanalytic Association. Independent IPA membership became possible as a result of a lawsuit by a group of Ph.D. psychologists against both the American and the International Psychoanalytic Associations filed in the mid-1980s. The terms of its settlement included the right of independent training organizations in the United States to apply for International Psychoanalytic Association membership. As a result, there are now five such "independent" IPA institutes in the United States— three in Los Angeles and two in New York. Additional results of the lawsuit included a mechanism for the admission for training of Ph.D. psychologists to institutes of the American Psychoanalytic Association—a direction in which the association was headed by the time the suit was filed. Subsequently, there has been further liberalization of admission to training by member institutes to include nurse practitioners and psychiatric social workers. Thus, the growing theoretical pluralism has been accompanied by rapid, multidisciplinary changes in the ranks of organized psychoanalysis.

Psychoanalysis and psychoanalytic therapy have declined in popularity in the United States in recent decades for a number of reasons. Advances in biological and pharmacological psychiatry that offer cheaper and easier remedies, combined with the fact that psychoanalysis was oversold in the post–World War II era, are among them. However, during this period of decline, its institutional, multidisciplinary, multitheoretical identity has blossomed. Theoretical and disciplinary diversity has led to a proliferation of new books and journals with an emphasis on interpersonal, interactional, and relational considerations of the analyst-patient dyad. Mainstream orthodoxy has declined, and many mainstream practitioners have been influenced to some extent by the burgeoning new theoretical "schools."

Another noteworthy psychoanalytic development in the United States has been the growth of psychoanalytic research in general, and particularly research in the field of infant and child observation begun by Margaret Mahler in New York and by René Spitz in Denver. New knowledge about the beginning and development of the human psyche has enriched the working hypotheses of analysts of adult patients, as well as of child analysts (Mahler et al., 1975). Many of the findings are seen as congruent with Kohut's work and that of other developmentalists who have focused on relational and interactional issues in treatment. Hence, there has been a greater emphasis in theory and technique on factors in the mother-infant dyad that parallel the adult situation of analyst and patient. While this constitutes a shift in emphasis away from the centrality of the Oedipus complex postulated by Freud, many mainstream analysts view it as an enrichment of factors affecting the still central Oedipal conflicts of adult neurotic patients.

Practicing analysts have had a sharp increase in the incidence of a less purely neurotic and of more seriously characterologically disturbed patients in their practices. These include severe narcissistic and borderline personality disorders, about which a spate of literature has developed. This is highlighted by the work of Otto Kernberg, who retains a classical theoretical position, while developing new clinical concepts and techniques that he considers to constitute a special type of psychoanalytic

psychotherapy (Kernberg, 1975). His work and that of others weds classical concepts with those of object-relations theory derived from Klein, Kohut, Mahler, and the like. Most of the adherents of the "schools" alluded to above (interpersonal, self-psychology, relational, and interactional) take the position that they still practice psychoanalysis, as opposed to derivative psychotherapy. Classical analysts tend to differ about this.

While these developments have centered in the United States, other "schools," such as that of Jacques Lacan in France as well as those of Jung, Adler, and Rank, have had relatively little impact in this country. Melanie Klein's influence and that of her followers has become more widespread as time goes by. The same is true for the work of Donald Winnicott, a British pediatrician-psychoanalyst who represents the British middle school, positioned between the official Freudian and official Kleinian groups in that country.

The infusion of psychoanalytically influenced mental health professionals and layworkers into the fields of education, criminology, and mental hygiene is exemplified by the work of Benjamin Spock, an analyzed pediatrician. His fundamentally psychoanalytic point of view has had an immense influence on child rearing for generations of post–World War II parents. Spock's *Common Sense Book of Baby and Child Care* has outsold every book but the Bible in the United States (Spock, 1946). The influence of Spock and others has persisted, although with the general decline in the popularity of psychoanalysis, there has been a reversion to a more conservative, often behavioristic, and biological point of view in psychiatry and in the lay community as well.

Psychoanalytically oriented mental health professionals are now organizing in community efforts to reestablish a new awareness of the value of their field. Those who were not physicians and had formerly been denied psychoanalytic training continued to practice psychoanalytically informed psychotherapy, as well as serving educational, legal, and other social institutions with a psychoanalytic perspective. Now that these individuals have access to full psychoanalytic training, there are many more nonphysician analytic practitioners, despite a waning psychoanalytic influence in social and educational institutions. This paradox occurs from the advances in biological and pharmacological psychiatry that now dominate psychiatry and a lag in the influence of the swelling ranks of psychoanalytic practitioners on the social institutions where they formerly held sway. In addition, there has been a proliferation of nonmedical therapists with varying degrees of psychoanalytic training and sophistication. They all belong to an enlarging psychoanalytic community, often organized under local institutes and societies both inside and outside the American Psychoanalytic Association (APA). Thus psychoanalytic community "outreach" is again gaining strength.

Additionally, profound changes in the field of psychiatry have led most medical school departments of psychiatry to shift from a predominately post–World War II psychoanalytic orientation to an eclectic or exclusively biological and pharmacological orientation. Few fully trained psychoanalysts have held full-time academic posts in recent times, whereas in the 1950s and 1960s, most chairs of psychiatry departments were held by psychoanalysts. Analysts have continued, however, to provide courses and supervision to psychiatry residents and to maintain a presence in university psychiatric residency programs.

Concurrent changes in health-care delivery in the United States have also encroached on psychoanalytic practice, as managed care gains ascendancy. Many analysts and analytically oriented therapists find managed care incompatible with any kind of psychoanalytic therapy, because of the resulting intrusions on privacy. Further changes in the direction of corporate- or government-operated medicine are anticipated—discouraging many young people from seeking psychoanalytic carers, and thus adversely affecting psychoanalytic training programs. Nevertheless, there appears to be a surprising resurgence of interest after an initial setback in enrollment, and the numbers of patients or clients in individual psychoanalytic therapy of one kind or another are increasing again (Hale, 1995: 378).

An ongoing debate in the halls of psychoanalytic organizations in the United States concerns the minimum number of sessions per week necessary to qualify a psychoanalytic therapy as psychoanalysis proper. The institutes of the American Psychoanalytic Association (APA) require a minimum of four and recommend an optimum of five sessions per week, while three or fewer are the standard frequency in some other organizations. This bears importantly on the definition of a "psychoanalytic process" in which there is sufficient intensity for the development and analysis of the patient's relationship with the analyst from past images, known as transference, a key conceptualization that distinguishes psychoanalysis from other therapies. The concept of transference

itself is a mainstay of most therapies designated as "psychoanalytic," but the need or desirability of its resolution by interpretation and insight has become an issue. The managed care phenomenon and other economic considerations constitute pressures toward less frequent sessions, but psychoanalysis proper is usually still defined as requiring four or more sessions per week utilizing the analytic couch. Modifications are common, however, among many practicing psychoanalysts despite the policies of the APA. Also, the William Alanson White Institute, a prominent group outside the APA, requires three weekly sessions. It has been denied affiliation with the International Psychoanalytic Association principally for this reason.

Scientific validation of this controversy and others, concerning such matters as the importance of reconstruction of the patient's childhood in psychoanalysis, is difficult to gauge by empirical research. Still, there is a marked increase in such research in a number of psychoanalytic centers in the United States, most notably in New York, Philadelphia, and San Francisco. Psychoanalytic research of all types, including infant observational studies and outcome studies, has accordingly received increasing attention in the psychoanalytic literature.

The issue of whether psychoanalysis constitutes a science, and if so what kind, has been debated at great length by philosophers of science as well as by analysts themselves. Changing paradigms of science since Freud's day have supported the general abandonment of psychoanalysis as a positivistic set of laws analogous to nineteenth-century physics and biology upon which Freud attempted to anchor his theories and practice (Freud, 1895). Nonetheless, the validity of psychoanalysis as a scientific theory as opposed to a hermeneutic discipline like history or literature has held sway in America, despite recent support for the hermeneutic position by prominent writer-practitioners such as Roy Schafer (Schafer, 1976) and Donald Spence (Spence, 1982). Without doubt, however, Freud's postulates of a metapsychological overview of psychoanalytic theory has been generally abandoned in the United States after its heyday promulgation by David Rappaport, a famous Hungarian-born psychoanalyst of the Menninger Clinic in Topeka, Kansas, in the late 1940s and 1950s (Rappaport and Gill, 1959). Robert Holt, Roy Schafer, George Klein, Merton Gill, and other students and colleagues of Rappaport became the principal antagonists and spokespersons against an overarching, clinically distant metapsychology, while

U

developing their own individual emphases on clinical theory. Gill's reflective account of these and other developments are discussed in his monograph published just before his death (Gill, 1994).

Despite the widespread questioning by psychoanalysts of Freud's metapsychology and the assaults of his critics, there are signs that the pendulum is beginning to swing back. These include the more dynamic Freudian teaching in psychiatric residency programs at U.S. medical schools, the development of new research programs in psychoanalysis (see RESEARCH ON PSYCHOANALYSIS), recent findings in neuroscience that appear to support parts of Freudian theory (see BRAIN SCIENCE, AND PSYCHOANALYSIS; and SLEEP), and the continuing vibrancy of psychoanalytic traditions in countries around the world.

REFERENCES

Eissler, K. (1953). The effect of structure on the ego and psychoanalytic technique. *Journal of the American Psychoanalytic Association*, 1: 104–143.

Freud, S. (1950 [1895]). *Project for a Scientific Psychology*. S.E. 1: 281–392.

———. (1910). *Five Lectures on Psychoanalysis*. S.E. 2: 9–55.

———. (1925). *An Autobiographical Study*. S.E. 20: 7–74.

Gill, M. (1994). *Psychoanalysis in Transition. A Personal View*. Hillsdale, N.J.: Analytic Press.

Hale, N. (1971). *Freud and the Americans. The Beginnings of Psychoanalysis in the United States*. New York: Oxford University Press.

———. (1995). *The Rise and Crisis of Psychoanalysis in the United States (1917–1985)*. New York: Oxford University Press.

Hartman, H., Kris, E., and Lowenstein, R. (1964). Papers on psychoanalytic psychology. In *Psychological Issues*, v. 4, no. 2, monograph 14. New York: International Universities Press.

Kernberg, O. (1975). *Borderline Conditions and Pathological Narcissism*. New York: Jason Aronson.

Klein, M. (1948). *Contributions to Psychoanalysis*. London: Hogarth Press.

Kohut, H. (1971). *The Analysis of the Self*. New York: International Universities Press.

Mahler, M., Pine, F., and Bergman, A. (1975). *The Psychological Birth of the Human Infant*. New York: Basic Books.

Menninger, K. (1930). *The Human Mind*. New York: Knopf.

Rappaport, D., and Gill, M. (1959). The points of view and assumptions of metapsychology. *International Journal of Psychoanalysis.*, 40: 153–162.

Rosenzweig, S. (1992). *The Historic Expedition to America (1909)*. St. Louis: Rona House.

Spence, D. (1982). *Narrative Truth and Historical Truth: Meaning and Interpretation in Psychoanalysis*. New York: Norton.

Spock, B. (1946). *Common Sense Book of Baby and Child Care*. New York: Dutton, 1985.

GEORGE H. ALLISION

V

Vaginal and Clitoral Orgasm

In his *Three Essays on the Theory of Sexuality* (1905), Freud mistakenly proposed that little girls' genital sexuality was solely clitoral and masculine until puberty, when, in order to become feminine, they had to transfer their "erotogenic susceptibility to stimulation . . . from the clitoris to the vaginal orifice" (p. 221). Over the next twenty years, he made additions and modifications but never altered this thesis. In fact, subsequently his view of the development of sexuality in women (1925, 1931, 1933 [1932]) was even more adamant. A product of patriarchal fin de siècle Vienna, his particular sociocultural milieu, his gender, and his specific intrapsychic conflicts, Freud was unable (possibly unwilling) to understand women except from a phallocentric perspective (Horney, 1926; Jones, 1927; Fliegel, 1973, 1986; Gay, 1988; Young-Bruehl, 1990; Makari, 1991). Unfortunately his seminal contributions to our understanding of human sexual development often have been discredited because his theories about female development have been disproved.

Freud deduced that as the clitoris was homologous to the male glans penis, the sexuality of little girls was wholly masculine and that libido in men or women was "invariably and necessarily of a masculine nature" (1905, p. 219). Dismissing the reports of others, Freud (1931; 1933 [1932]; 1940) maintained that girls had no early vaginal sensations and were ignorant of their vaginas until puberty. "The occurrence of early vaginal excitations is often asserted. But it is most probable that what is in question are excitations in the clitoris—that is, in an organ analogous to the penis" (1940, p. 154n). Therefore, he concluded that there was no possibility of dis-

tinguishing the autoerotic activity between the two sexes until after puberty, when girls first became aware of the vagina. Equating the clitoris to a small, "atrophied" penis (1933 [1932], p. 65), he assumed little girls' masturbatory pleasure was inadequate compared with that of boys, which caused girls to feel deficient, inferior, and envious of boys (1905, 1925, 1931, 1933 [1932]). These misconceptions led to the fallacious idea that penis envy formed the foundation for female development. Thus, realizing the futility of competing with boys, girls replace their wish for a penis with a wish for a child. With this in mind, first they transfer their affections from their mothers to their fathers. Next, with their discovery of the vagina at puberty, as prerequisite for femininity, they inhibit their childish, masculine clitoral masturbation and transfer their primary erotogenic zone to the vaginal introitus.

From the beginning, Freud's ideas on female sexuality were disputed (Horney, 1924; 1926; 1933 [1932]; Jones, 1927, 1935; Muller, 1932). Even Freud (1927) acknowledged the sparseness of his data, the need for further research to amend or refute his ideas, and his lack of understanding of women, as well expressed in his comment (1926): "We know less about the sexual life of little girls than of boys. But we need not feel ashamed of this distinction; after all, the sexual life of adult women is a 'dark continent' for psychology" (p. 212, also see 1925, pp. 243–245). He did not recognize that, although the clitoris is small (unlike the small, immature male child's penis), throughout a woman's life the clitoris is capable of arousing very intense pleasure and orgasm. We now know not only that female infants and little girls are aware of their vaginas, but that little girls' masturbatory pleasure—whether it be clitoral, vaginal, or a combination—can be very intense and pleasurable, and can result in orgasm (Bornstein, 1953; Kramer, 1954; Barnett, 1966; Kestenberg, 1968; Fraiberg, 1972; Kleeman, 1976; Chehrazi, 1986; Frenkel, 1993, 1996). Furthermore, Masters and Johnson (1966) have shown that anatomically and physiologically clitoral and vaginal orgasms are not distinct entities regardless of the area and means of stimulation (p. 66, also see summary by Wiedeman, 1995: 341). Despite marked variations in intensity and duration, all orgasms always have vaginal contractions. Even in the neonatal period female infants have rhythmic vaginal lubrication (Kleeman, 1976: 19). Regardless of how orgasm occurs, the subjective experience does not necessarily correlate with physiologic measurements, and there are marked variations in the intensity and duration of orgasms (Glenn and Kaplan, 1968: 557).

While Freud wrote extensively about genital sexuality, there are only 20 occurrences of the word "orgasm" and only one reference to a woman's capacity for multiple orgasms (Guttman et al., 1984). In view of the mistaken emphasis formerly placed on women analysands to shift their primary source of genital pleasure to the vagina, it is noteworthy that there are no references at all in Freud to vaginal or clitoral orgasm. Of the twenty-one citings, three are from his correspondence with Fliess, two referring to a woman with hysterical symptoms and one to the woman who had multiple orgasms. Breuer used the term "orgasm" twice in the *Studies on Hysteria*. One was attributed to Ruth Mac Brunswick equating anger after an enema to orgasm, and three referred to nocturnal emissions. In these and the remaining twelve citings, Freud does not clearly differentiate physiologic from psychologic responses, and at times he seems to contradict himself. Thus, in his introductory *Lectures on Psycho-Analysis* (1917), he wrote: "In children orgasm and genital excretion are scarcely possible; their place is taken by hints which are once more not recognized as being clearly sexual" (p. 321). Yet in an earlier discussion of these hints of infantile sexuality, he noted (1905) that thumb sucking or "sensual sucking involves a complete absorption of the attention and leads either to sleep or even to a motor reaction in the nature of orgasm" (p. 180). Ironically, while Freud discovered the importance of orgasm to women (with his proposal that premature sexual experience was etiologic for hysteria), throughout his writings he implies that, in child or adult, female genital arousal and satisfaction is less intense and inferior to male genital pleasure.

REFERENCES

Barnett, M. C. (1966). Vaginal awareness in the infancy and childhood of girls. *Journal of the American Psychoanalytic Association*, 14: 129–141.

Bornstein, B. (1953). Masturbation in the latency period. *Psychoanalytic Study of the Child*, 8: 65–78.

Chehrazi, S. (1986). Female psychology. *Journal of the American Psychoanalytic Association*, 34: 141–162.

Fliegel, Z. O. (1973). Feminine psychosexual development in Freudian theory: A historical reconstruction. *Psychoanalytic Quarterly*, 42: 385–408.

———. (1986). Women's development in analytic theory: Six decades of controversy. In J. Alpert (ed.). *Psychoanalysis and Women; Contemporary Reappraisals*. Hillsdale, N.J.: Analytic Press, pp. 3–31.

Fraiberg. S. (1972). Genital arousal in latency girls. *Psychoanalytic Study of the Child*, 27: 439–475.

Frenkel, R. S. (1993). Problems in female development: Comments on the analysis of an early latency-age girl. *Psychoanalytic Study of the Child*, 48: 171–192.

———. (1996). A reconsideration of object choice in women: Phallus or fallacy. *Journal of the American Psychoanalytic Association*, 44/Suppl.: 133–156.

Freud, S. (1905). *Three Essays on the Theory of Sexuality*. S.E. 7: 130–243.

———. (1916–1917) *Introductory Lectures on Psychoanalysis*. S.E. 15–16: 9–496.

———. (1925). Some psychical consequences of the anatomical distinctions between the sexes. S.E. 19: 248–258.

———. (1926). *The Question of Lay Analysis*. S.E. 20: 183–258.

———. (1927). *The Future of an Illusion*. S.E. 21: 5–56.

———. (1931). Female sexuality. S.E. 21: 225–243.

———. (1933 [1932]). *New Introductory Lectures on Psycho-Analysis*. S.E. 22: 3–182.

———. (1940). *An Outline of Psycho-Analysis*. S.E. 23: 144–207.

Gay, P. (1988). Woman, the dark continent. In P. Gay (author). *Freud: A Life for Our Time*. New York: Norton, pp. 501–522.

Glenn, J., and Kaplan, E. H. (1968). Types of orgasm in women. *Journal of the American Psychoanalytic Association*, 16: 549–564.

Guttman, S., et al. (eds.) (1984). *The Concordance to the Standard Edition of the Complete Psychological Works of Sigmund Freud*. New York: International Universities Press.

Horney, K. (1924). On the genesis of the castration complex in women. In H. Keyman (ed.) *Feminine Psychology*. New York: Norton, 1967, pp. 37–53.

———. (1926). The flight from womanhood: The masculinity complex as viewed by men and women. *International Journal of Psychoanalysis*, 7: 324–339.

———. (1933). The denial of the vagina. Contribution to the problem of the genital anxieties specific to women. *International Journal of Psycho-Analysis*, 14: 57–70.

Jones, E. (1927). The early development of female sexuality. *International Journal of Psychoanalysis*, 8: 459–472.

———. (1935). Early female sexuality. *International Journal of Psychoanalysis*, 16: 262–273.

Kestenberg, J. S. (1968). Outside and inside, male and female. *Journal of the American Psychoanalytic Association*, 16: 457–520.

Kleeman, J. A. (1976). Freud's view of early female sexuality in the light of direct child observation. *Journal of the American Psychoanalytic Association*, 24 (suppl.): 3–27.

Kramer, P. (1954). Early capacity of orgastic discharge and character formation. *Psychoanalytic Study of the Child*, 9: 128–141.

Makari, G. J. (1991). German philosophy, Freud, and the riddle of the woman. *Journal of the American Psychoanalytic Association*, 42: 183–213.

Masters, W., and Johnson, V. (1966). *Human Sexual Response.* Boston: Little, Brown.

Muller, J. (1932). A contribution to the problem of libinal development of the genital phase of girls. *International Journal of Psycho-Analysis*, 13: 361–368.

Wiedeman, G. H. (1995). Sexuality. In B. Moore and B. Fine (eds.). *Psychoanalysis: The Major Concepts.* New Haven: Yale University Press, pp. 334–345.

Young-Bruehl, E. (1990). *Freud on Women.* New Haven, Conn.: Yale University Press.

RHODA S. FRENKEL

Venezuela, and Psychoanalysis

The true history of psychoanalysis in Venezuela did not begin until the decade of the 1950s (Olivares, 1984), when several Venezuelan doctors left the country to be trained as psychoanalysts. The first ones to return were G. Teruel and H. Quijada, and in 1961 the first psychoanalytical group was constituted, when M. Kizer, W. Hobaica, A. García, F. Acuña, and J. Araujo returned. Then others also returned, once they had fulfilled their foreign training: C. Ottalagano, J. Aray, H. Dominguez, J. Olivares, H. Voss, N. Cupello, and A. Briceño. All of them requested their formal acceptance as a Study Group by the International Psychoanalytic Association (IPA). This membership was formalized in 1965, at the Congress of Copenhagen. At that moment, with the exception of the Argentinean, the Latin American societies had been founded for a very short time, and all of them had been influenced by the Argentinean group (the so-called "older sister") (Zambrano, 1987).

At the same time (1960), Fernando Rísquez also returned from Canada and Europe and founded a dynamic psychiatry and clinical psychology postgraduate course, which then became an important quarry of psychoanalysts and psychotherapists in Venezuela.

In 1969, the study group of Venezuela was promoted to provisional association, and some members came to

didactic category, which started the Teaching Institute. Then followed an intense and fruitful exchange with the Latin American societies. In 1971, the Teaching Institute was approved as a Component Society of the IPA at the Vienna Congress. With all of this, the Venezuelan psychoanalytical movement received strong international support, especially from Latin Amercan organizations, which at that moment were rapidly developing. In 1973, the first group of analysts were graduated from the Institute.

At that moment, the Association was very young and its members had received dissimilar training in diverse countries. The Association was subjected to various pressures and was intensely dedicated to spreading psychoanalysis through courses and scientific meetings for the community and for students. The number of applicants to the group grew steadily, and many of the members of the Association became professors of postgraduate university courses. In this dynamic climate, the first institutional growth crisis occurred, with the formation of two rival groups who attempted to control the Association. The rivalry only partially had to do with theoretical matters. It was a fight for power. The authorities of IPA intervened in the Association, and after an arduous process they achieved the reunification of the two groups. This forced integration was neither simple nor devoid of pain, but in the long run it turned out to be beneficial.

The students, whose training was indefinitely interrupted by the conflict, suffered the most. They had requested the collaboration of the Colombian Institute, which agreed to come to Caracas to provide the seminars of the interrupted program. In this manner, nine members of the second class were graduated in 1978.

This increase in membership had a positive impact at the beginning, because the young members worked actively for the institution and soon took directive responsibilities. But what had seemed a promising sign degenerated after several years into a new crisis: the growing confrontation of those former students with their old professors. The crisis was settled in 1989, and although today there are still certain visible traces of it, the preponderance of new members who did not experience it ensures institutional stability. Since then, the Venezuelan Association of Psychoanalysis has earned a reputation as a solid and serious institution.

The members who resigned in 1989 requested the IPA to immediately accept them as a study group with teaching capacity. This petition was granted (1990) and,

V

in due course, the group became the Psychoanalytical Society of Caracas. This group of former members of the Venezuelan Association demonstrated great activity at all levels. They were driven by the necessity of establishing themselves as a new psychoanalytic institution, and they accepted the largest number of candidates to augment their membership.

The schools of psychoanalysis that influenced the Venezuelan analysts the most were the Kleinian, through the founders in Argentina and England, and the French. This "polarization," however, has progressively diminished, and the tendency nowadays is to integrate diverse theoretical postures. The French influence was evidenced in the creation of the Lacanian "Freudian School" (1980), which received strong support from J. Lacan. They received support from diverse private and cultural institutions in Caracas. However, it did not displace in prestige the two societies belonging to the IPA.

The followers of Jung also have their place, through the Center of Jungian Studies, and F. Risquez's "School of Deep Psychology." All the institutions discussed here are in Caracas, but several psychoanalysts are working in other cities, and candidates in the provinces presently attend seminars in Caracas, which ensures the expansion of psychoanalysis throughout the country.

The first psychoanalytic candidates were doctors, accepted for training as psychologists. Today, candidates come from other fields as well. Psychoanalysis has become established in Venezuela and is making creative contributions to the theoretical as well as clinical practice throughout the profession.

REFERENCES

Olivares, J. A. (1984). Breve reseña histórica de la Asociación *Venezolana de Psicoanálisis, Psicoanalisis*, vol. 1. Caracas: Asovep.

Zambrano de N., N. (1987). Caracteristicas del desarrollo psicoanalítico latinoamericano. *Correio da Fepal (Edición especial del I Simposio de Fepal)*. Sao Paulo: Fepal.

ALFONSO GISBERT S.

Vienna, and Psychoanalysis

The significance of Vienna as the site of the foundation and development of psychoanalysis is evident: from 1859 until 1938, Sigmund Freud (1856–1939) lived and worked in Vienna. His prominence has nurtured the illusion of a one-time, ahistoric development of psycho-

analysis. Interest in supporters, students and contributors has generally been marginal or limited to only the most well-known representatives. Similarly, the institutional framework, the form in which these individuals cooperated scientifically, and their exchanges with other social structures, have received little attention. The production of scientific findings seen as a social process, where internal and external factors are in a constant exchange, does not minimize the part of the founder of the new science of the unconscious in its beginning, but it destroys the illusion of a single ahistoric discovery. The economic and political situation, as well as cultural and sociohistorical connections, influence the theoretical, practical, and organizational developments of a discipline and are part of the production of knowledge. In the history of psychoanalysis, studies in the area of Freud biography and the pre- and early history of psychoanalysis dominate. These studies mainly deal with Freud's fin de siècle Vienna, and a special interest has been focused on Freud's Jewish identity and the relationship between Judaism and psychoanalysis.

Psychoanalysis developed in Vienna until 1918 during the Habsburg monarchy, in the "Red Vienna" of the First Republic until 1934, and then in Vienna during Austro-fascism until 1938 under different sociopolitical and sociocultural circumstances, from which various scientific and organizational developments benefited or were impeded. Austria's annexation by Germany in 1938 led to the destruction of psychoanalysis and the exodus of almost all psychoanalysts from Austria. The establishment of psychoanalytic organizations and psychoanalysis's representation in popular and intellectual culture were reestablished slowly and under difficult circumstances after World War II. Scientific traditions had been broken and tendencies of anti-enlightenment, especially clerical prejudices, had continued from the time of Austro-fascism and National Socialism.

The psychoanalytic movement was in its first heyday in the years before World War I. Bourgeois society and European modernity experienced significant crises in the Vienna of the fin de siècle. On a sociopolitical level, the multinational state tended to foster a search for a renewal that included different forms of living. During the period 1890 to 1910, extraordinary achievements in the areas of music, literature, art, and science were made and were fundamentally influential for new developments in observation and thought in the twentieth century. The following factors are descriptive of the potential of this creativity: (1) the rise of new cultural founding figures of the liberal bourgeousie; (2) the influence of the Jewish intelligentsia and the upward mobility of immigrants from the Austro-Hungarian empire; (3) the resistance against political constraints, bureaucracy, and repression of the church and censorship; and (4) the cultural networks established with other centers and the import of foreign ideas as well as the intellectual exchange between the regions and countries of the monarchy (Nautz and Vahrenkamp, 1993; Rabinbach, 1992).

Freud's science of the unconscious, with its topics of "subjectivity" and the "scientific empirical method," can be interpreted as a characteristic product of the Vienna modernity, as were Zionism and Austrian Marxism. The extraordinary role of the Jewish intelligentsia is reflected in the members of the "Psychological Wednesday Society" (*Psychologische Mittwoch-Gesellschaft*), the pioneer group of the psychoanalytic movement (Mühlleitner, 1992; Mühlleitner, Reichmayr, 1997). Many projects of the Vienna modernity would see their realization in the social-democratic "Red Vienna." After the Habsburg monarchy fell and revolutionary changes failed to materialize, Red Vienna became the democratic model of the antibourgeois modern age. In a time of experimentation, the "new human being" could be created without constraint but rather through education. In the new era, observation, description, and social change would take place on the basis of scientific findings in the so-called "laboratory of modernity." Because it attributed a special importance and idealization to science in general, psychoanalysis could benefit as well (Gruber, 1991). On the level of mutual understanding, the relationship between psychoanalysis and social democracy was extended to institutional and public levels.

For its adherents and other interested groups, psychoanalysis in Red Vienna represented an attractive and fascinating enterprise as the science of the unconscious; from this point on, psychoanalysis developed internationally. It had already undergone diverse applications and had helped shape the profile of new professions. In addition, psychoanalysis opened new possibilities for scientific discovery. Through the activity of its publishing house, founded in 1919, the work done at the outpatient clinic of the Vienna Psychoanalytic Society, which opened in 1922, and the Psychoanalytic Training Institute, founded in late 1924, an intensive atmosphere of research and study prevailed that extended into the members' social life. The theoretical developments and

practical applications in several specific projects and general areas of inquiry, such as the research of children and adolescents and the psychotherapy of psychoses, are examples.

With the advent of a totalitarian state in Austria in 1934, psychoanalytic work lost its cultural and intellectual ground, and the illegalization of the social democratic political movement, and its large number of cultural, scientific, and educational institutions, prompted the emigration of a number of important leftist Freudians. Freud distanced himself from the publication of his critical theory of religion in *Moses and Monotheism* because he did not want to risk the outlawing of psychoanalysis. In the authoritarian Catholic-dominated Austria, his theories on religion could easily be considered a criticism of the state. Freud's political attitude and fears were decisive and determined the degree of conformity and the dimensions of concessions to the government as well as the distancing from the left. The attacks of clerical and fascist opponents pushed psychoanalysis into professional self-diminishment and cultural-political isolation. The "fear of politics" can be verified from various sources within the ranks of Viennese psychoanalysts, and it led even to the denial of social reality in the formulation of psychoanalytic theory.

With Hitler's seizure of power in Germany in 1933 and the consolidation of the National Socialist dictatorship, psychoanalysis, which became an object for fascist and racist propaganda, was branded an atheistic-materialistic, enlightenment-oriented, and "Jewish" science.

The history of psychoanalysis in Austria after 1933 is one of emigration. With the installment of fascism, one of psychoanalysis's fiercest enemies, the Catholic church, gained great influence. Nonetheless, for a short period between 1933 and 1938, Vienna again became the center of the psychoanalytic movement, taking over the role Berlin had played before. But the consolidation of the Austrian fascist system had grave consequences for psychoanalysis. The destruction of intellectual freedom and the establishment of the authoritarian corporative state (*Ständestaat*) proceeded rapidly, and the final exodus of psychoanalysis was effected by the Nazis in 1938.

Following the German occupation of Austria, the Board of the Vienna Psychoanalytic Society held a meeting on March 13, 1938. A consensus was soon reached and a resolution passed that urged psychoanalysts to leave the country and to move the seat of the society to the city in which Freud would settle. The majority of the

Viennese psychoanalysts left occupied Austria between the middle of May and the middle of June 1938 (Mühlleitner and Reichmayr, 1995). On June 4, 1938, Sigmund Freud and his family left Vienna for exile in London.

The flight of fifty established psychoanalysts, as well as many others still in training, meant the end of psychoanalysis in Vienna. The result of this rupture is still obvious and remains a factor in the history of Austrian psychoanalysis after 1945. The postwar truce between the Social Democrats and the Catholic camp had the unfortunate consequence of ensuring a continuity of the opposition to psychoanalysis, including its anti-Semitic undercurrents.

Five of the former members of the Vienna Psychoanalytic Society had stayed in Vienna. August Aichhorn, who was able to practice privately during the Nazi rule and World War II, had organized a group of analysts and individual psychologists who were concerned with keeping their independence, and they refused as much as possible to conform. Officially, the group was affiliated with the Institute for Psychological Research and Psychotherapy of the German Reich. The majority of them formed the core of the new Vienna Psychoanalytic Society in 1946, but its rebuilding suffered from enormous difficulties, and psychoanalysis remained an alien element in Austria after 1945. The rupture created by the previous exodus of Viennese psychoanalysts had created a situation tantamount to beginning totally anew. Among the general public and the official authorities, there was virtually no more interest in Freudian psychoanalysis.

It was under the rubric of "depth psychology," a concept more common in postwar Austria, that it became possible once again to discuss Freudian psychoanalysis. Yet it remained exposed to arbitrary revisions, simplifications, reductions, and interpretations in keeping with the Christian worldview. Psychoanalysis was employed mainly to supplement eclectic psychotherapies. Psychoanalysis and its symbols became important general cultural icons and were stylized as effective trademarks used in advertisements for tourism and the cultivation of the Austrian image. The numerous phenomena of the vacuous popularization of psychoanalysis are rather a symptom of the fact that, until today, the spirit of psychoanalytic thinking has hardly taken root in the post-war culture of Vienna.

REFERENCES

Gruber, H. (1991). *Red Vienna: Experiment in Working-Class Culture, 1919–1934.* New York: Oxford University Press.

Huber, W. (1977). *Psychoanalyse in Österreich seit 1933.* Vienna: Geyer.

Mühlleitner, E. (1992). *Biographisches Lexikon der Psychoanalyse. Die Mitglieder der Psychologischen Mittwoch-Gesellschaft und der Wiener Psychoanalytischen Vereinigung 1902–1938.* Tübingen: Edition Diskord.

Mühlleitner, E., and Reichmayr, J. (1995). The exodus of psychoanalysts from Vienna. In F. Stadler and P. Weibel (eds.). *Vertreibung der Vernunft. The Cultural Exodus from Austria,* 2d ed. Vienna: Springer-Verlag, pp. 98–121.

———. (1997). Following Freud in Vienna. Development and structure of the Wednesday Psychological Society and the Viennese Psychoanalytical Society 1902–1938. *International Forum of Psychoanalysis,* 6: 73–102.

Nautz, J., and Vahrenkamp, R. (eds.). (1993). *Die Wiener Jahrhundertwende. Einflüsse, Umwelt, Wirkungen.* Vienna: Böhlau Verlag.

Rabinbach, A. (1992). *The Human Motor. Energy, Fatigue, and the Origins of Modernity.* Berkeley: University of California Press.

ELKE MÜHLLEITNER
JOHANNES REICHMAYR

Virginity

Freud wrote only one paper explicitly devoted to virginity and defloration. However, in one of his early writings (Freud, 1893), he makes several references to the connection between "virginal anxiety" (the "first encounter with the problem of sex") and hysteria in girls. In *A Fragment of an Analysis of a Case of Hysteria*, Freud (1905) interprets Dora's two famous dreams as reflecting her wishes and fears about defloration. According to Freud, one unconscious meaning of the first dream was "I must flee from this house for I see that my virginity is threatened here" (p. 85). Freud deduces a fantasy of defloration, that of a man forcing his way into the female genitals, in the second dream. He notes that Dora's fantasy was represented from a male's point of view, that is, she wished to be the penetrator. Thus ideas about virginity led to Freud's important insights about bisexual identification and homosexuality in hysteric patients. Freud also describes Dora's need for revenge against all the men in her life. This is the earliest representation of his idea that women desire revenge in connection with threatened loss of virginity.

This theme of revenge became the cornerstone of Freud's major contribution about virginity in his paper *The Taboo of Virginity* (1918). Here Freud notes that in primitive cultures defloration of girls is frequently performed by surrogates. He attributes men's avoidance of deflowering women to their horror of blood and menstruation as well as to their sadistic fantasies. Additionally, this avoidance reflects neurotic anxiety about dangers associated with new undertakings. Freud links frigidity in women with anxiety about defloration. Destruction of the hymen leads to "narcissistic injury." Frigidity also reflects the Oedipal wishes or fixations in which the father is unconsciously perceived as the rightful lover/deflowerer and the husband as the resented substitute. Finally, frigidity derives from envy and aggression toward the husband/deflowerer. In this discussion, Freud also describes a common childhood fantasy of the "perpetual virgin" in which the sexuality of the mother is denied. Earlier Freud had observed the presence of this fantasy in Dora's fascination with the Sistine Madonna, an important association to one of her dreams.

Throughout his writings, Freud delineates common symbols for virginity and defloration in dreams or symptoms. Among these are flowers, breaking of glass, the color red, blood, and so on. For example, Freud (1900, pp. 374–375) describes a prudish but neurotic woman who had to postpone her marriage. She dreamed of a table with a floral centerpiece made up of precious lilies of the valley. For this woman, the table represents a woman's body and the flowers, her genitals. He interprets the dream as expressing the idea of "the overvaluation of virginity," a fear of the violence of defloration, and feminine masochistic character traits. In a later case, Freud (1917) utilizes his understanding of dream symbolism to decode the meaning of a compulsive symptom, an attempt to cover up a stain symbolizing blood, which expressed a woman's shame that her husband was unable to deflower her on her wedding night.

Freud suggests that castration anxiety and fear of blood and menstruation are important ubiquitous elements in the unconscious conflicts and experiences associated with the ideas of the loss of virginity, for both men and women. Freud's contemporaries, Abraham, Deutsch, Bonaparte, and Horney, concur with and elaborate his major points. They reaffirm the psychological connections between first menstruation and defloration, virginal blood and injury and death. Yates (1930) distinguishes the differing fantasies of men and women about defloration. Horney (1935) and others have enhanced the understanding of the meaning of the loss of virginity in terms of the broader social context.

Anzieu (1986) discerns an underlying metaphor of defloration in many of Freud's writings, in his language in describing femininity, in the content of a screen memory (1899), and in his countertransference in clinical reports. For example, Freud writes of the case of Dora: "Frankly, I had no desire to penetrate more deeply at this point" (1905, p. 113). Anzieu interprets Freud's famous dream depicting an examination of a woman patient's nose and throat ("The Specimen Dream of Psychoanalysis" or "Irma's Injection," 1900, pp. 96–121) as a disguised gynecological examination that represents a defloration. Anzieu points out that in general Freud's new discoveries carried a metaphoric meaning of defloration; he was the first to explore the unconscious.

Holtzman and Kulish (1997) reaffirm the conflict-based origins of sadomasochistic Oedipal/castration anxieties for both males and females, but they elaborate the meanings for women. Drawing upon contemporary psychoanalytic thinking about female sexuality and development, they suggest that separation issues and losses are central to women's psychic experience of loss of virginity. They comment on what has been called Freud's phallocentric bias and errors in the emphasis on rage and aggression on the part of the woman toward the male/deflowerer, and disagree with his attribution of obligatory masochistic tendencies in the female. They also suggest that Freud missed the importance of the loss of virginity as a major developmental milestone in young adolescent girls' lives.

Although Freud was constrained by the social context of his times as well as his gender and omitted the conceptualization of the female as something other than sexual object, he made brilliant major contributions in clarifying the importance of the first sexual experiences in clinical cases and in dreams and the effect of the unconscious on this aspect of sexuality. He was a pioneer in his "penetrating the veil of secrecy" surrounding this topic. Much of what he had described and theorized about virginity has an enduring validity.

REFERENCES

Anzieu, D. (1986). *Freud's Self-Analysis.* New York: International Universities Press.

Breuer, J., and Freud, S. (1893–1895). *Studies on Hysteria.* S.E. 2: 19–305.

Freud, S. (1899). Screen memories. S.E. 3: 301–322.

———. (1900). *The Interpretation of Dreams.* S.E. 4–5: 1–621.

———. (1905). Fragment of an analysis of a case of hysteria. S.E. 7: 3–122.

———. (1916–1917). *Introductory Lectures on Psychoanalysis.* S.E. 15–16: 9–496.

————. (1918). *The Taboo of Virginity (Contributions to the Psychology of Love, III)*. S.E. 11: 191–208.

Holtzman, D., and Kulish, N. (1997). *Nevermore, the Hymen, and the Loss of Virginity*. Northvale, N.J.: Jason Aronson.

Horney, K. (1935). The problem of feminine masochism. *Psychoanalytic Review*, 22: 214–233.

Yates, S. L. (1930). An investigation of the psychological factors in virginity and ritual defloration. *International Journal of Psychoanalysis*, 11: 167–184.

DEANNA HOLTZMAN
NANCY KULISH

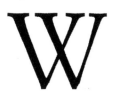

War Neurosis

Honigmann (1907) was probably the first to consider war neuroses as a special case of the traumatic neuroses (see entry on "Traumatic Neurosis"). Although they have been noted since antiquity—e.g., in the report by Herodotus of the Spartan commander Leonidas's enlightened approach to his troops' combat reactions at the Battle of Thermopylae—systematic study awaited the development of military psychiatry during World War I. The vast numbers of psychological casualties then made comprehensive description possible. Nomenclature subsequently varied with the prevailing symptom cluster, itself dependent upon the type of war engagement and sociopolitical context, and on variations in contemporaneous psychiatric thought.

World War I was characterized by static trench warfare. It led to nostalgia, neurasthenia, and quasi-neurological acute mental states known as shell shock, typified by fear, dissociation, and what used to be called "hysterical conversion reactions" (MacCurdy, 1918); recent research indicates that the latter reactions are more properly termed "somatoform dissociative symptoms" (Nijenhuis, 1999). By way of contrast, World War II was a war of movement, and the gradual development of anxiety, psychosomatic reactions, and fatigue was known as combat exhaustion (Grinker and Spiegel, 1945).

The prevalence of these acute and chronic war neuroses was well documented. Feudtner (1993) quoted followup studies demonstrating chronic war neurosis in 60 percent of those suffering from shell shock after World War I. Swank and Marchand (1946) noted that following five weeks of sustained combat, 98 percent of combatants manifested war neuroses. Nevertheless, interest

in them waned between the world wars and after World War II, largely because of denial of psychological war trauma within the military system, by the psychiatry profession, and within society in general. War neuroses were diagnosed as gross stress reactions in *DSM-I* (APA, 1952) and omitted from *DSM-II* (APA, 1968).

Combat reactions during the Vietnam War included traumatic reexperiencing, homesickness, and restricted psychological functioning. The complexities of this war neurosis and post-traumatic states in general were included (Young, 1993, felt that they were "re-invented") under the rubric of post-traumatic stress disorder in *DSM-III* (APA, 1980), with additional acute stress disorder in *DSM-IV* (APA, 1994). However, MacCurdy (1918) believed that the war neuroses differed from civilian reactions to trauma in regard to the specificity of the war stressor, the anticipatory arousal of the instinct of self-preservation, and the mostly diminished contribution of psychosocial (and psychosexual) factors.

With regard to psychoanalytic approaches, by the turn of the twentieth century, Freud and his followers had begun to play down environmental factors. Interest in the war neuroses surfaced toward the end of World War I, but the Budapest Symposium at the Fifth Psychoanalytic Congress in 1918 came too late to make an impact. Simmel, Abraham, and Sándor Ferenczi, also military physicians, noted the balance of endogenous and exogenous contributions to the war neuroses. In his introduction to the Symposium (1919), Freud focused on the conflict between the psychosexual parameters of the peacetime ego and its "parasitic double," the war ego. Employing libido theory, he attempted to conceptually unify war neuroses with those of peacetime. He compared the narcissistic gratification of flight into traumatic

595

neurosis under the threat of war with psychotic withdrawal under the "traumatic" threat of libidinal arousal of narcissistic neuroses, and to a lesser degree, neurotic decompensation under the "traumatic" threat of libidinal frustration of transference neuroses. These themes were further advanced in *Beyond the Pleasure Principle* (1920), where war trauma was explained as due to the impact of the massive liberation of sexual excitation on the unprepared ego, and to the intrapsychic conflicts consequently engendered. Freud felt that although no complete explanation had been given for either the war neuroses or the traumatic neuroses of peace, neither condition appeared to contradict the pleasure principle or its modifier, the reality principle (1920).

Freud believed that when hostilities ceased, the "neurotic conditions of war" would vanish. Chronic and delayed cases seemingly escaped his purview. Psychoanalysis, however, made a significant and humanizing contribution to psychiatric treatment during and after both world wars. Brown (1918) and Simmel (1919) found psychological abreaction (see ABREACTION) to be an effective therapeutic technique, and this was subsequently combined with chemical approaches by military psychiatrists. These abreactive techniques shared the goals of ventilating trauma affects, working through war trauma and reactivated earlier traumas, and reintegration of the personality. These and subsequent psychoanalytic contributions to the therapy of post-traumatic stress disorder were theoretically wanting. Conscious suppression and subconscious dissociation of traumatic memory appear to be more applicable than unconscious repression.

Clearly war neuroses have not vanished as Freud expected. The military analyst Gabriel (1986) held that war neurosis is the reaction of the sane to insane circumstances, and that war in the twentieth century had become so lethal and intense that despite psychological screening, all combatants eventually succumb.

REFERENCES

Brown, W. (1918). The treatment of cases of shell shock in an advanced neurological centre. *Lancet*, pp. 197–200.

DSM-I. (1952). *Diagnostic and Statistical Manual of Mental Disorders*, 1st ed., Washington, D.C.: American Psychiatric Association.

DSM-II. (1968). *Diagnostic and Statistical Manual of Mental Disorders*, 2d ed., Washington, D.C.: American Psychiatric Association.

DSM-III. (1980). *Diagnostic and Statistical Manual of Mental Disorders*, 3d ed., Washington, D.C.: American Psychiatric Association.

DSM-IV. (1994). *Diagnostic and Statistical Manual of Mental Disorders*, 4th ed., Washington, D.C.: American Psychiatric Association.

Feudtner, C. (1993). Minds the dead have ravished: Shell shock, history, and the ecology of disease systems. *History of Science*, 31: 377–420.

Freud, S. Introduction to psycho-analysis and the war neuroses. S.E. 17: 205–210.

———. (1920). *Beyond the Pleasure Principle.* S.E. 18: 3–64.

Gabriel, R. A. (ed.) (1986). *Military Psychiatry: A Comparative Perspective.* New York: Greenwood Press.

Grinker, R. R., and Spiegel, J. P. (1945). *Men under Stress.* New York: McGraw Hill.

Honigmann, G. (1907). Neuroses of military men after a campaign. *Lancet*, June 22: 1740.

MacCurdy, J. T. (1918). *War Neuroses.* Cambridge: Cambridge University Press.

Nijenhuis, E. R. S. (1999). *Somatoform Dissociation: Phenomena, Measurement, and Theoretical Issues.* Assen, Netherlands: Van Gorcum.

Simmel, E. (1919). Zur psychoanalyse der Kriegsneurosen: Zweites Korreferat. In S. Ferenczi et al., (eds.). *Zur Psychoanalyse der Kriegsneurosen.* Leipzig: Internationaler Psychoanalytischer Verlag, pp. 42–60.

Swank, R. L., and Marchand, W. E. (1946). Combat neuroses: Development of combat exhaustion. *Archives of Neurology and Psychiatry*, 55: 236–247.

Young, A. (1993). *The Harmony of Illusions: Inventing Post-traumatic Stress Disorder.* Princeton, N.J.: Princeton University Press.

ONNO VAN DER HART
PAUL BROWN

Wednesday Society

In the history of science, the actors, supporters, and contributors of a scientific discipline are seen as major forces in its development. This applies to an even greater degree to psychoanalysis, because its representatives saw themselves as protagonists of a new scientific movement. The first expression of the formation of the psychoanalytic movement is considered to be the weekly conferring assembly, which began in late 1902, and was known as the Psychological Wednesday Society (*Psychologische Mittwoch-Gesellschaft*). In this circle, psychological knowledge was brought into a new light and addressed those questions that would become relevant to psychological thinking in the twentieth century. Sigmund Freud (1856–1939) invited the first participants via postcard to his apartment in Vienna's Berggasse 19. The founding members of the Psychological Wednesday Society were four Jewish medical doctors who were, on average, ten years younger than Freud: Alfred Adler (1870–1937), Max Kahane (1866–1923), Rudolf Reitler (1865–1917) and Wilhelm Stekel (1868–1940). The gatherings were arranged every Wednesday night at 8:30 P.M.

Adler and Stekel were general practitioners in Vienna; Stekel had experienced psychoanalytic treatment with Sigmund Freud for a short period. Reitler and Kahane ran private clinics in Vienna, offering mainly physical therapy. The older doctors who joined the circle were familiar with physical-physiotherapeutic methods, concepts that were person- as opposed to sickness-oriented in their private practices and sanatoriums. There was ample opportunity to examine patients more thoroughly over a longer period at these institutions. Having experienced the limited nature of these methods, these physicians were at the same time searching for new methods of treatment, which led them to psychoanalysis. The first participants became interested in Freud's discoveries and achievements from having attended his lectures at the University of Vienna (from 1886–1887 onward) and were invited to the discussions held in Freud's home. Some of the early members were representatives of social medicine, a discipline of socially oriented doctors who worked toward the modernization of health with medical services, preventive medicine, and social reforms (Adler, Adolf Deutsch, Alfred Bass, Kahane). Hardly any of the early followers were psychoanalyzed, and the conditions for training analysis were not yet defined. Reitler was the first to begin practicing psychoanalysis in Freud's footsteps (Jones, 1953–1957).

Otto Rank (1884–1939), the first paid secretary of the group sessions, who began taking minutes in 1906, compiled the first membership list for that year: Seventeen men had been continuous participants in the rounds of discussion (Mühlleitner and Reichmayr, 1997). The professional and religious backgrounds of the early members (Klein, 1981), as well as their value systems, were studied by the group (Rose, 1992).

The minutes of the Vienna Psychoanalytic Society for the period from 1906 to 1918 (Nunberg and Federn, 1962–1975) illustrate how the establishment of psychoanalysis as an independent scientific discipline and its further practical and theoretical development proceeded, as well as showing how its organizational establishment by Sigmund Freud led to a mutual exchange with a larger group. In 1907, Freud himself dissolved the group and asked its members to reaffirm their membership in the Wednesday Society. The minutes show a list

with twenty-one members. Despite the increasing number of followers, Freud remained fairly isolated with his ideas in his circle of Viennese doctors. Contact with Carl Gustav Jung (1875–1961), assistant medical director under Eugen Bleuler (1857–1939) at the renowned university psychiatric clinic Burghölzli in Zürich, Switzerland, in the spring of 1906 brought Freud his first taste of international recognition. In 1907, the Berlin psychiatrist Max Eitingon (1881–1943), who had received psychiatric training in Zürich, was the first foreign participant in the society.

On April 27 and 28, 1908, exemplifying the expansion of psychoanalysis, an international meeting took place in Salzburg, the First Congress for Freudian Psychoanalysis (participants: 26 Austrians, 6 Swiss, 5 Germans, 2 English, 2 Hungarians, 1 American); in the same month, the Wednesday Psychological Society was registered in Vienna and officially confirmed in 1910 as the Vienna Psychoanalytic Society (*Wiener Psychoanalytische Vereinigung*). The increasing awareness of psychoanalysis, internationally a field that had appeared to emerge from Zürich, now showed its effects in Vienna. Guests came from abroad to participate in the discussions of the Wednesday Society and/or to undergo analysis. Between 1909 and 1910, membership almost doubled, from twenty-three to forty-three. In April 1910, the first female member, the Viennese physician Margarete Hilferding (1871–1942), was accepted into the group. Before formulation of the statutes, new members were generally advised or introduced through registration at the secretary; generally, in the following session, decisions regarding acceptance were made. In 1910, the society's mandates on membership were set.

REFERENCES

Klein, D. B. (1981). *Jewish Origins of the Psychoanalytic Movement*. New York: Praeger.

Jones, E. (1953–1957). *The Life and Work of Sigmund Freud*, vols. 2 and 3, New York: Basic Books.

Mühlleitner, E., and Reichmayr, J. (1997). Following Freud in Vienna. Development and structure of the Wednesday Psychological Society and the Viennese Psychoanalytical Society 1902–1938. *International Forum of Psychoanalysis*, 6: 73–102.

Nunberg, H., and Federn, E. (eds.) (1962–1975). *The Minutes of the Vienna Psychoanalytic Society*. New York: International Universities Press.

Rose, L. (1992). The moral journey of the first Viennese psychoanalysts. *Psychoanalytic Quarterly*, 31: 590–623.

ELKE MÜHLLEITNER
JOHANNES REICHMAYR

Wish See DRIVE THEORY; REPRESSION.

Wish Fulfillment See DREAMS, THEORY OF.

Wolf Man

The Wolf Man is the best-known, and most followed-up of all Freud's cases. In February 1910 (Freud, 1918: 3), the wealthy, twenty-three-year-old Russian aristocrat Sergey Pankejeff came to Freud with a number of serious psychological symptoms. His health had deteriorated after he contracted a gonorrheal infection approximately five years previously. He was entirely dependent upon, and traveled with, his own physician and companion. He had already seen two of the most prominent European psychiatrists of that time: Theodor Ziehen in Berlin and Emil Kraepelin in Munich. Both had given up on him. Freud's analysis lasted until July 1914, when he considered the case completed. It was probably his longest analysis.

The case history does not deal with the patient's current illness, but, as the title *From the History of an Infantile Neurosis* indicates, the case deals with a neurosis that occurred between the ages of four and ten. The purpose of focusing on the infantile neurosis was to respond to the criticisms of Jung and Adler about the role of infantile sexuality, particularly witnessing the primal scene, in subsequent pathological conditions. Both Jung and Adler disagreed with Freud's emphasis on the role of infantile sexuality. To prove his point, Freud relied on the reconstruction of a dream that supposedly had taken place almost twenty years earlier when the Wolf Man was four years old. The dream referred to an event that had occurred when the patient was one and a half years old and had witnessed his parents having sexual intercourse.

The early history Freud elicited from the Wolf Man included precocious sexual activities initiated by his sister, who was two years older than he, and threats of castration by his nanny when he approached her for sexual play. Because of castration anxiety, the Wolf Man retreated from a phallic stage to anal sadism and masochism. The anal sadism manifested itself in sadistic behaviors toward small animals. His father became his sexual object, and he provoked his father to beat him to fulfill his own masochistic wishes.

Then, just before his fourth birthday, the Wolf Man had the wolf dream (hence his name): he was in his bed facing a window. Suddenly, the window opened and he saw six or seven white wolves with long, foxlike tails and pricked-up ears sitting on the branches of a big walnut tree. In great anxiety about being eaten by the wolves, he woke up screaming. Six months later, he had a full-fledged obsessional neurosis. The dream was interpreted again and again over the years.

Associations to the dream suggested to Freud a primitive, deep-seated fear of the father and a wish for sexual gratification with the father that led to castration fears. The Wolf Man fantasized that he had to become a girl to satisfy his father. Because the dream was so detailed, Freud suspected that a distorted piece of reality had been reproduced. Using the principle of reversal in the dream work, Freud thought that the stillness of the wolves suggested that the Wolf Man had seen an agitated scene. Passively, the Wolf Man concurred with the suggestion that he must have woken up to such a scene. Freud asserted that the dream referred to an actual event: the Wolf Man's seeing his parents having sexual intercourse. In addition, Freud was specific about the details: the incident occurred when the patient was one and a half years old; he witnessed his parents having sex three times, including at least once a tergo, from behind, which gave him a view of both of his parents' genitals. Although quite assertive about the actual events that the dream referred to, Freud showed some caution about his interpretations. He wondered whether the copulating that the Wolf Man had seen was not necessarily that of his parents, but that of animals, which he then generalized to his parents. In a curious statement that sounded as if Freud was agreeing with his antagonist Jung, Freud indicated that memories of witnessing primal scenes, seductions, and castration threats were undoubtedly inherited. He stressed that whether these events were fantasies or reality, their effects were the same, that these real events or fantasies about them occurred in the past and influenced subsequent development. They were not, as Jung asserted, current events that had been extended to the past.

In his technique in the Wolf Man's case, Freud appears to have been an active therapist, although less forceful and less suggestive than he was with the Rat Man, whose analysis ended two years before the start of this one. The most important technical contribution of this case was the analyst's forced termination of it. Although the Wolf Man was intelligent, he was passive and did not allow the analysis to touch him emotionally. To push him to become more engaged with the analysis,

Freud set a date for termination, a year hence. Freud would not waver from that decision, and when they terminated treatment, both Freud and the Wolf Man were satisfied with the results.

Their optimism about the results was not borne out by subsequent events. The Wolf Man lost his wealth after the Russian Revolution of 1917. In 1919, he returned to Vienna where Freud and other analysts helped him financially, and he briefly reentered analysis with Freud. In 1926, Freud referred him to Ruth M. Brunswick, who saw him for about five months for a somatic delusion (Brunswick, 1948). The Wolf Man settled in Vienna, working in a mid-level bureaucratic job. Subsequently, he had a number of physical and psychological illnesses and participated in writing a book about himself (Gardiner, 1971). The Wolf Man died in Vienna in 1979 at age ninety-two (Gardiner, 1983).

REFERENCES

Brunswick, R. M. (1948). A supplement to Freud's *History of an Infantile Neurosis*. In R. Fliess (ed.). *The Psychoanalytic Reader*. New York: International Universities Press, pp. 65–103.

Freud, S. (1918). From the history of an infantile neurosis. S.E. 17: 3–122.

Gardiner, M. (1971). *The Wolf-Man by the Wolf-Man*. New York: Basic Books.

———. (1983). The Wolf-Man's last years. *Journal of the American Psychoanalytic Association*, 31: 867–897.

GEORGE A. AWAD

Women, Psychology of See FEMINISM, AND PSYCHOANALYSIS.

Working Alliance See THERAPEUTIC ALLIANCE.

Working Through

Freud used the term "working through" to refer to the process by which insight develops into enduring change. Freud viewed working through as a phase of analysis that followed insight, but many analysts have found that the same factors that promote change after insight are important in the analytic process even before insight occurs. As a result, the concept of working through is used by some to refer only to processes subsequent to insight, while others use it to refer to all change processes in analysis other than interpretation and insight, regardless of when these occur in the analytic process. Analysts who feel that interpretation and insight are sufficient to account for all analytic change believe that the concept of working through is redundant and possibly misleading. There is some support for each position in Freud's writing on the subject.

In view of the integral place of working through in the description of the psychoanalytic process, it is surprising that the term is used only two times in the entire standard edition of Freud's works. It first appears in *Remembering, Repeating, and Working Through* (Freud, 1914), and again in *Inhibitions, Symptoms, and Anxiety* (1926 [1925]). In *Remembering, Repeating, and Working Through*, Freud was still using the topographic model to understand his clinical material. In this model, the aim of analysis was making the unconscious conscious, and the bulk of the paper describes the analytic process that leads to the patient's remembering previously unconscious pathogenic experiences and fantasies. During the analysis, the patient resists remembering by unconsciously repeating the childhood experiences in the transference to the analyst. By interpreting to the patient that these are repetitions, the analyst can help the patient remember in a way that is emotionally convincing. This is the basic action of psychoanalysis.

Almost as an addendum to the paper, Freud says that the first step in overcoming the resistance (the repetition in the transference) is the analyst's uncovering of it (recognizing it and pointing it out), thereby acquainting the patient with it, but that change rarely occurs at this point in the treatment. Not only does the resistance not vanish (the repetition does not stop) at this point, but it often becomes more insistent and the situation more obscure. However, this is entirely predictable, and begins the next phase of the analysis: working through. Freud writes:

> One must allow the patient time to become more conversant with this resistance with which he has now become acquainted, to *work through* it, to overcome it, by continuing, in defiance of it, the analytic work according to the fundamental rule of analysis. Only when the resistance is at its height can the analyst, working in common with his patient, discover the repressed instinctual impulses which are feeding the resistance; and it is this kind of experience which convinces the patient of the existence and power of such impulses. The doctor has

nothing else to do than to wait and let things take their course, a course which cannot be avoided nor always hastened. (1914, p. 155)

He goes on to say:

This working-through of the resistances may in practice turn out to be an arduous task for the subject of analysis and a trial of patience for the analyst. Nevertheless it is a part of the work which effects the greatest changes in the patient and which distinguishes analytic treatment from any kind of treatment by suggestion. From a theoretical point of view one may correlate it with the 'abreacting' of the quotas of affect strangulated by repression—an abreaction without which hypnotic treatment remained ineffective. (1914, pp. 155–156)

The second reference to working through, in *Inhibitions, Symptoms, and Anxiety*, was written after the development of the structural model. The aim of the analytic process is conceptualized in this model as the changing of impulses that are automatically and unconsciously controlled by the id, into activities under ego control. However, the basic structure of the treatment is the same. The patient free-associates and invariably resists undoing the repression by repeating in the transference his or her characteristic ways of avoiding the recognition of id impulses. The analyst first makes the resistance (the avoidance) conscious, and then brings forward logical arguments against it, demonstrating the greater security and gratification that will come from letting go of the resistance. Eventually, with the help of the unobjectionable positive transference to the analyst, the patient's ego is persuaded. However, the situation is more complicated. Freud writes:

For we find that even after the ego has decided to relinquish its resistances it still has difficulty in undoing the repressions; and we have called the period of strenuous effort which follows after its praiseworthy decision, the phase of 'working through.' The dynamic factor which makes a working-through of this kind necessary and comprehensible is not far to seek. It must be that after the ego's resistance has been removed the power of the compulsion to repeat—the attraction exerted by the unconscious prototype upon the repressed instinctual process—has still to be overcome. There is nothing to be said against describing this factor as the *resistance of the unconscious*. (1926 [1925], p. 159)

In both instances, where Freud uses the concept of working through, it is clear that he was responding to two related clinical observations. The first was that it takes longer than one would initially expect for lasting change to occur in analysis. The second observation was that frequent repetition of interpretation and insight are necessary to create change, and that pathological repetitions and actions continue even after their resistant function is genuinely understood. Although the observations themselves are not questioned by any analysts, a minority believe that "working though" is not a useful descriptive term. Brenner (1987) believes that it is simply a fact about analysis that overcoming resistance takes time and requires repetition. We do not really know why this is so, he says, but working through is simply the interpretive work of analysis; it is the analysis of psychic conflict in all its aspects and the idea of a separate phase following insight is mistaken. Insight is a sufficient explanation for change in psychoanalysis, and there is no need for the term "working though."

Brenner uses the first quotation above (Freud, 1914) to substantiate his view. In it, Freud states that it is only when the resistance has been recognized for what it is, yet is at its height of intensity, that the instinctual impulses behind it can be discovered. Brenner considers all of this to be nothing more than the full analysis of the transference. It is only after the ego resistances are recognized that the underlying impulses can be effectively interpreted, and all this takes time. Brenner also uses Freud's analogy of abreacting with working through to support his view. Since abreacting is a process that liberates bound libido, when Freud says that working through, like abreacting, must be done bit by bit, he seems to be saying that time is necessary to redeploy the libido that is being freed up in the analytic process, and that the redeployment (working through) is necessary for enduring change. For Brenner, this is again simply part of the basic work of analysis, a natural outgrowth of repeated interpretation and insight. Brenner emphasizes that the analysis of conflict is sufficient to account for analytic change, and that no other techniques are required. Insofar as working through has been read as implying that other processes are involved and other techniques may be needed in analysis he believes it is a misleading concept and a misreading of Freud's intent.

The majority of analysts, on the other hand, have read Freud's use of the concept of working through as an indication that he believed that more goes into analytic change than interpretation and insight. However, they disagree about precisely what else it refers to. A number of analysts have taken the term "working through" as describing the processes that go on within the patient as insight is developed into enduring change. The support for this reading comes from the second quotation cited above. Freud says there that this part of the analysis is an "arduous task for the subject of analysis," and it is the "part of the work which effects the greatest changes in the patient." Although the description of what the patient does during working through depends upon the theoretical orientation of the analyst, in general the focus has been on the necessity of the patient utilizing his or her new understanding to act differently. Insight makes new actions possible, but the patient has to engage in them to actually change. This includes trying new actions and refraining from old, habitual repetitions. Since the patient has a new openness to the meanings of events and relationships as a result of the preceding insight, these actions now result in new experiences that lead to new learning and new development. The reevaluation of reality that comes about through the new experiences leads to new, less distorted expectations, the development of realistic self-esteem and an internal reorganization of a new self and world view. All of this takes time, is a necessary part of analysis, and, for many analysts, this constitutes the process of working through. A similar view of working through from drive theory is that working through is the process of developing new discharge paths and new modes of gratification to replace the old ones that have been relinquished as a result of insight.

Others believe that Freud used the term working through not just to highlight what occurs within the patient during analysis as a result of insight, but also to indicate that more needs to go on in the analytic process itself than just insight and interpretation. Part of the support for this comes from Freud's analogizing working through to abreaction. Although Brenner reads this as supporting the view that insight is all that is necessary and that the redeployment of the libido follows automatically from insight, others read this as indicating that

Freud never viewed insight as sufficient; there was always an additional process (abreaction) that was necessary and was separate from insight. The additional process in Freud's later model was working through. These analysts have likened the working through process to mourning, a kind of abreaction, and have focused on the necessity of affectively grieving the lost self and the lost fantasies as a necessary part of consolidating change.

Most of the support for the view that working through requires more than insight comes from the third citation above. By associating a particular resistance, id resistance, with the necessity for working through, Freud seems to imply that this particular resistance does not yield to insight. There is further support for this reading in some of Freud's later writings on id resistance. For Freud, id resistances generally included psychical inertia, fixation of the libido, adhesiveness of the libido, the attraction of the unconscious, and the repetition compulsion. These terms are closely related but are not always identical in his writing. In *Analysis Terminable and Interminable* (1937, pp. 240–242), Freud distinguished between the adhesiveness of the libido and psychical inertia. He mentioned that adhesiveness of the libido could be greatly exaggerated in some patients, perhaps on a constitutional basis, and make the analytic process much slower. This implies that working through could become particularly problematic in some analyses regardless of the patient's openness to insight. Freud then goes on to specifically distinguish psychical inertia from id resistance. He makes the interesting observation that in some people there is a marked hesitation before an impulse enters a path that has been newly opened up for discharge. He says that we call this resistance of the id, but that this may not be correct. He connects the hesitation instead with psychical inertia. Although he says no more about this in the paper, he seems to be relating psychical inertia to an unmotivated, biologically built-in reluctance to change that may have to be addressed.

Some analysts have viewed overcoming the reluctance to change, whether on the basis of psychical inertia or adhesiveness of the libido, as an act of will and not as an automatic result of insight, and have described the part of the analytic process that enables the patient to overcome this reluctance (id resistance) as working through. They believe that the development of new ego structures is often necessary to enable the patient to turn insight into new actions and enduring change. These ego structures include the ability to master anxiety and other painful affects, to tolerate frustration, to control impulses, and to develop object constancy. These are felt to come from the experiences with the analyst in the analytic process, and not from the interpretations per se. Karush (1967), for example, has focused on the importance of the analyst as an example, rather than as an interpreter, for providing the new experiences that lead to the patient overcoming the compulsion to repeat and using insight in order to change. In his view, this can go on silently and without the analyst doing anything other than the traditional activity of interpretation and clarification. However, for him the concept of working through highlights the recognition that it is factors in the analytic situation other than insight that are responsible for the changes taking place.

However, other analysts have pointed out that "nontraditional" activities may be necessary to promote working through. For some this has simply amounted to a different interpretive focus, like a focus on the lack of will to change (Valenstein, 1983), or on the difficulty maintaining the alliance during the height of the transference neurosis (Greenson, 1965), or a focus on specific reconstructions of particular traumatic experiences (Greenacre, 1956). Greenson also says that the analyst may have to actively promote psychosynthesis that, in some patients, can involve technical modifications such as having them sit up for a time. Others, such as Frank (1993), have gone further in suggesting technical modifications that the analyst may have to use to help some patients develop the ego capacities needed for utilizing insight. Frank includes the encouragement to act differently as a possible analytic intervention, stating that action can often lead to insight, not only the other way around. An additional aspect of this argument is the idea that working through does not necessarily follow insight, but, insofar as working through relates to curative factors other than interpretation and insight, it is often a necessary precursor to useful insight. Stewart (1963) agrees that the patient's experience of the analyst that helps to develop necessary ego capacities is equally important prior to insight, and helps make true insight possible. For other analysts working through, by definition, follows insight and refers only to making effective use of it.

The fact the Freud referred to working through only twice has left the concept with a lack of specificity that supports these different understandings. What everyone agrees upon is that "working through" refers to the need for time and some kind of process in order for repeated analytic insight to lead to enduring change. The differences are in conceptualizing what goes on during that time and in that process: whether working through automatically follows insight or requires other analytic experiences and/or interventions to promote it, and whether the processes involved in working through only come into play after insight. Many have thought of "working through" as a term that functionally takes the place of an analytic theory of learning, and the different ways of understanding working through may simply reflect the ongoing attempt to articulate a comprehensive analytic theory of learning and change.

REFERENCES

Brenner, C. (1987). Working through: 1914–1984. *Psychoanalytic Quarterly*, 56: 88–108.

Frank, K. (1993). Action, insight, and working through: An integrated approach. *Psychoanalytic Dialogues*, 3: 535–577.

Freud, S. (1914). Remembering, repeating and working-through (Further recommendations on the technique of psychoanalysis, II). S.E. 12: 145–156.

———. (1926 [1925]). *Inhibitions, Symptoms and Anxiety.* S.E. 20: 75–172.

———. (1937). Analysis terminable and interminable. S.E. 23: 216–253.

Greenacre, P. (1956). Re-evaluation of the process of working through. *International Journal of Psychoanalysis*, 37: 439–444.

Greenson, R. (1956). The problem of working through. In Max Schur (ed.). *Drives, Affects, and Behavior, Vol. 2, Essays in Memory of Marie Bonaparte.* New York: International Universities Press, pp. 277–314.

Karush, A. (1967). Working through. *Psychoanalytic Quarterly*, 36: 497–531.

Novey, S. (1962). The principle of "working through" in psychoanalysis. *Journal of the American Psychoanalytic Association*, 10: 658–676.

Ornstein, A. (1991). The dread to repeat: Working-through process in psychoanalysis. *Journal of the American Psychoanalytic Association*, 39: 377–398.

O'Shaughnessy, E. (1983). Words and working through. *International Journal of Psychoanalysis*, 64: 281–290.

Schmale, H. (1966). Panel: Working through. *Journal of the American Psychoanalytic Association*, 14: 172–182.

Sedler, M. (1983). Freud's concept of working through. *Psychoanalytic Quarterly*, 52: 73–98.

Shane, M. (1979). The developmental approach to "working through" in the analytic process. *International Journal of Psychoanalysis*, 60: 375–382.

Stewart, W. (1963). An inquiry into the concept of working through. *Journal of the American Psychoanalytic Association*, 11: 474–499.

Valenstein, A. (1983). Working through and resistance to change: Insight and the action system. *Journal of the American Psychoanalytic Association*, 31: 353–374.

MARK LEVEY

INDEX

Page numbers in boldface refer to the main entry on the subject.

A

A la recherche du temps perdu (Remembrance of Things Past) (Proust), 277
Aalto, Alvar, 206
Aberastury, Arminda, 34
Abraham, Hilda, 1
Abraham, Karl, **1–4**, 26, 225, 317, 393
  Alix Strachey analyzed by, 540
  Andreas-Salomé and, 22
  British analysts and, 243
  character problems, 72
  depression, 145
  Deutsch analyzed by, 147
  development of oral character, 511
  Eitingon and, 173
  genitality theory, 235
  Glover analyzed by, 239
  Horney analyzed by, 261
  identification, 273
  Klein analyzed by, 303
  loss of virginity, 593
  member of the Berlin Psychoanalytical Training Institute, 235
  move to Berlin, 235
  quarrel with Rank, 227
  Reik analyzed by, 472
  secret committee member, 97, 225, 445
  war neurosis, 572
  and war neurosis, 595
abreaction, **4–5**, 29, 482
  therapeutic technique for war trauma, 68, 596
  working through compared to, 601
Abse, D. W., 268
abstinence, rule of, **5**
Acerboni, Anna Maria, 285
acting out, **6–7**
  and neuroses, 367
activation-synthesis hypothesis, 56
active technique of Ferenczi, 202, 469
Acton, William, 311

Functions and Disorders of the Reproductive Organs, 177
actual neuroses, 29, 276, 361, 437, 542
  distinguished from psychoneuroses, 363
Acuña, F., 589
Adelman, Janet, 265
Adler, Alfred, **7–9**, 224
  Andreas-Salomé and, 22
  criticism of infantile sexuality, 598
  defection of, 445
  Freud and, 15
  influence in the United States, 584
  and Nietzsche, 369
  "On the Psychology of Marxism," 329
  and Rank, 461
  and Stekel, 538
  and Wednesday Society, 597
  and *Zentralblatt für Psychoanalyse*, 225
Adler, Viktor, 368
adolescence, 89–90, 150, 151
  research on, 494
Adorno, Theodor, 236, 330
  Authoritarian Character, The, 231
aesthetics and psychoanalysis, **9–10**
Aetiology of Hysteria, The (Freud), 440, 516
affect, **10–12**
  distinguished from psychic energy, 30
  obsessional symptoms associated with affective disorders, 393
  repression preventing discharge of, 481
  used interchangeably with anxiety, 29
Africa and psychoanalysis, **12–15**
aggression, **15–16**, 114, 164, 543
  clinical theory, 93–94
  infantile aggressive impulses, 306
  Jones and, 294
  paranoia and, 409
"Agressivity in Psychoanalysis" (Lacan), 316
Aichhorn, August, 218
  in Austria during World War II, 592
  Eissler and, 172
  Scandinavians in analysis with, 554
aim. *See* drive theory
aim inhibition, 552
Ainsworth, Mary D. S., 13
  anaclitic depression, 17

Ainsworth (*continued*)
  developmental theory, 151
  "strange situation" model, 494
Aiza, Víctor, 342, 343
Ajase complex, 291
Akhtar, Salman, 20, 276
Alayza, Fernando, 413
alchemical tradition, Jung's work on, 299
Alexander, Franz, 202, 261
  in Berlin, 236
  and Ferenczi, 204
  Psychoanalytic Therapy, 540
  training patient of Sachs, 501
Alexandris, Athina, 244
Allende Navarro, Fernando, 83
Allison, R. B., 352
Allport, Gordon, 253
Alnaes, Karsten, 536
Altamirano, Noel, 413
  Neruda, a Psychoanalytical Reading, 414
Althusser, Louis, 86
Althusserean-Lacanian model, 86
altruistic surrender, 219
ambivalence, **16–17**, 539
  taboo and, 561
Amenhotep IV (Abraham), 3
American Anthropologist, 26
American Association of Sex Educators and Counselors
    (Therapists), 526
American Imago (journal), 13, 457. *See also Imago*
  founded by Sachs, 502
  issue devoted to Victor Trausk, 563
American Institute for Psychoanalysis, 261
American Journal of Psychoanalysis, 261
American object relations theory
  and conflict, 105
  different from British school, 386
American Psychiatric Association, 433
  and diagnoses, 460
American Psychoanalytic Association (APA), 65, 167, 582
  and American Psychiatric Association, 433
  Fromm suspended by, 231
  Jones and, 242, 293, 445
  prohibition of inclusion of lay analysts, 466
American Psychopathological Association, 445
American Society for Psychical Research, 396
anaclitic, term created by Strachey, 540
anaclitic depression, 17–18
  studied by Spitz, 494
anaclitic object, **17–18**, 388
anal character, **18–19**
  scientific tests of, 510
anal stage of development, 162, 321
  anal-sadistic stage, 99
  and development of orderliness, parsimony and obstinacy,
    464
"'Anal' und 'Sexual'" (Andreas-Salomé), 22
analysis
  analyst's forced termination, 598–599
  beginning phase, 448–449, 565
  end phase, 449–450

middle phase, 449, 565
  pretermination phase, 450
  trial period of, 20
  working through as phase of, 599
Analysis of a Phobia in a Five-Year Old Boy (Freud), 326
*Analysis of the Sexual Impulse, Love and Pain, The Sexual
    Impulse in Women* (Ellis), 177
Analysis Terminable and Interminable (Freud), 228, 247,
    248, 447–448, 513
  analytic pact, 564
  id resistance, 601
Analytical Psychology: Theory and Practice (Jung), 299
analyzability, **19–21**
Anderson, John, 419
Andersson, Ola
  analyzed by Monchy, 554
  "Studies in the Prehistory of Psychoanalysis," 555
Andreas, Freidrich Karl, 21
Andreas-Salomé, Lou, **21–23**, 225
  Anna Freud and, 218
  letter from Freud on Tausk, 563
  Nietzsche and, 370
  Tausk and, 562
anger, paranoia and, 409
Anna Freud Centre, 81
Anna Freud Foundation, 172
Anna O., 4, **24–25**, 88, 197, 336, 364, 436, 437
  hallucinations, 251, 252
  regression, 468
  repression, 478–479
  self-analysis, 520
  termination of treatment, 446, 449
Annual Book of Psychoanalysis (Delgado, ed.), 414
Ansbacher, H. L., 8
Ansbacher, R. R., 8
Anthony, E. J., 269
anthropology and psychoanalysis, **25–28**, 264
antisocial personality disorder
  Anna Freud's developmental model of, 115
  and splitting, 538
"Antisocial Tendency, The" (Winnicott), 115
anxiety. *See also* anxiety neurosis
  basic anxiety of Horney, 263
  of child, 305
  and defense, **28–31**, 484
  and ego, 443–444
  and formation of neurosis, 103, 364–366
  and primal scene, 424
  Rank on, 462
  revision of the theory of, 148
  Sullivan on, 551
  and World War II, 595
anxiety neurosis, 29, **31–32**, 334, 361, 365, 367, 437
Anzieu, D., 593
Apel, Karl Otto, 554
aphasia, **33–34**
  hysterical, 77
"Apples of Cézanne, The" (Schapiro), 121
Araujo, J., 589
Aray, J., 589
Arche, Die (journal), 245

Architecture of Cognition, The (Anderson), 419
Argentina
    persecution of Argentinean psychoanalysts, 330
    Peruvian psychoanalysts in, 414
    and psychoanalysis, 34–35
Argentine Psychoanalytic Association, 34–35
Argentine Psychoanalytic Society, 342
Arlow, Jacob A., 129–130, 133, 134, 453, 508
Aron, Raymond, 241
art. *See also* aesthetics and psychoanalysis; cinema and
    psychoanalysis
    Freud's interest in, 111
    and psychoanalysis, 87, 121
Art and Artist (Rank), 462
"Art of Cameo Engraving during the Renaissance"
    (Kris), 312
Artist, The (Rank), 461
Aryan Christ: The Secret Life of Carl Jung (Noll), 299
"as if" identification, 147
Associação Brasileira de Psicanálise, 59
association. *See* free association
Association for the Advancement of Psychoanalysis, 467
Association Freudienne de Belgique, 45
Association of Belgian Psychoanalysts, 44
Association of Child Psychoanalytical Psychotherapy, 414
Association of Psychoanalytical Psychoterapists (Chile),
    83
Association Psychanalytique de France, 209
associationism, 44
Associationprincip in der Aesthetik, Das (Fechner), 194
associative rectification, 481–482
atheism of Freud, 419
attachment, test of, 151
attachment, theory of (Bowlby), 150–151, 494, 534
"Attachment and Loss" (Bowlby), 115
Attentats aux moeurs, Les (Brouardel), 269
Auden, W. H., 345
Aufreiter, Gottfriede, 65
Aufreiter, Johann, 65
Aulagnier, Piera, 211
Auletta, Irene, 413
Australia and psychoanalysis, **35–36**
Australian Psychoanalytic Society, 36
Authoritarian Character, The (Adorno), 231
autism, 503
Autobiographical Study, An (Freud), 97, 435, 445
    1935 postscript, 227
    autoerotism, 38
    myths, 353
    seduction theory, 518
Autobiography (Stekl), 539
autoerotism, **36–38**, 89, 385
    and infantile sexuality, 277
Auto-erotism (Ellis), 176–177
Automatisme psychologique, L' (Janet), 287
autonomy, **38–40**
    of patient, 181
avoidance, 485
    and phobic neuroses, 366
Ayala, Jaime, 342
Azam, E., 576

B

Baars, B. J., 532
Bachofen, Johann, 26
Bachrach, H. M., 20
Baginsky, Adolf, **41–43**, 222
    Freud's training with, 301, 302
Bahia, Alcyon, 58
Baistrocchi, Marta, 34
Bak, Robert, 204
Baker, Grace, 65
Bakhtin, Mikhail, 498
Balagtas, Francisco, 417
Baldwin, James, Mark, 576
Balint, Alice, 501
Balint, Michael, 36, 203, 238, 243
    and Ferenczi, 204, 390
    as object relations theorist, 386
    pursuing Ferenczi's work, 469
    training patient of Sachs, 501
Bandura, Albert, 96
Barajas, Rafael, 341, 342
Baranger, Willy, 34, 413
Barash, David, 534
Barber, C. L., 265
Bartlett, Frederic, 27
Basch, Michael Franz, 119
Bateson, Gregory, 25
battle trauma. *See* war neurosis; war trauma
Baudry, F., 496
Bauduin, A., 45
Bauer, Ida. *See* Dora
Baumeyer, F., 508
Beard, George Miller, 361
    Sexual Neurasthenia, 437–438
"Beating Fantasies and Daydreams" (A. Freud), 22, 218
Beauvoir, Simone de, 195
Becker, Ernest, 462
Beer-Hofmann, Richard, 472
behavioral implosion therapy, catharsis in, 68
behaviorism
    dominance in China, 84
    and psychoanalysis, **43–44**
Belgian Psychoanalytical Society, 45
Belgian School of Jungian Psychoanalysis, 45
Belgian School of Psychoanalysis, 45
Belgian Society for Analytic Psychology, 45
Belgium and psychoanalysis, **44–45**
Belkin, A. I., 498
Benedek, Therese, 554
    in Berlin, 236
    and Ferenczi, 204
Benedetti, G., 502
Benedict, Ruth, 25, 264
Benova, Marie, 137
Beratis, Stavroula, 244, 245
Bergson, Henri, 395
Berlin
    discussion on Freud and Marx in, 330
    Klein in, 302–303
    psychoanalytic movement in, 445

Berlin (*continued*)
  Sachs in, 501
  Scandinavians in, 554
Berlin Psycho-Analytical Institute, 235, 238
  Denichel teaching at, 200
  Deutsch and, 147
  Eitingon and, 173
  Glover's training at, 239
  Horney founding member of, 261
  polyclinic opened by, 2, 236
  Reich training analyst at, 471
  Reik and, 472
  Sachs as training analyst at, 501
Berlin Psycho-Analytical Society, 1
  Eitingon and, 172, 173
Bernard, Claude
  influence on Freud, 418–419
  Studies in Experimental Medicine, 418
Bernay, Jacob, 68
Bernays, Martha, 195, 221
Bernays, Minna, 224
Bernfeld, Siegfried, 33, 199, 329
  in Berlin, 236, 330
  identifying Freud as patient in "Screen Memories," 229
  and politics, 236
  "Sisyphus or the Boundaries of Education," 331
Bernheim, Hippolyte, 223, 515
  Freud's study with, 439
  texts translated by Freud, 547
Bernstein, D., 174
Bernstein, P., 383
Besetzung, translation of, 70
Bettelheim, Bruno, 390
Between the Myth and History, Psychoanalysis and Its Andean Past (Lemlij, ed.), 414
"Beyond Good and Evil" (Nietzsche), 375
Beyond Psychology (Rank), 462
Beyond the Pleasure Principle (Freud), 103, 164
  agression as an independent drive, 475
  conflicting drives, 419
  death instinct, 423
  mentioning Spielrein, 536
  principle of constancy, 481
  repetition compulsion, 226
  war trauma, 572, 596
"Beyond the Pleasure Principle" (Freud), 2, 4
Bhandari, Prakash, 276
Bibring, Edward
  and Anna Freud, 218
  and depression, 146
Bibring, Grete, 218
Bick, Ester, 59
Billroth, Theodor, 62, 295
binding, **45–47**
Binet, Alfred, 78, 289
  and dissociationist model of the unconscious, 576
Binswanger, Ludwig, 33, 182, 225, 266, 370
biography and psychoanalysis, **47–48**, 264–265, 457, 458, 502
biology and psychoanalysis, **48–52**
Bion, Wilfred R., 59, 238, 243, 309
  influence in India, 276

influence in Italy, 285
  influence in Mexico, 342
bipolar self (Kohut), 358
bipolarity. *See* ambivalence
Birth of Tragedy Out of the Spirit of Music, The (Nietzsche), 368
birth trauma, 30
  challenging primacy of Oedipus complex, 461
bisexuality, 311, 322, 592
  early concept of, 260
  Fliess and, 207
Bjerre, Poul, 22, 553, 554
Björk, Stig, 205
Black Hamlet: The Mind of an African Negro Revealed by Psychoanalysis (Sachs), 13
Blacky Test, 67, 405, 428
Blatt, Sidney, 17
Bleuler, Eugen, 421, 502, 539, 597
  Abraham and, 1
  Eitingon and, 172
  Jung and, 298
  and occult phenomena, 395
  on schizophrenia, 503
  and term ambivalence, 16
Bloch, Iwan, 525
Bloom, Harold, 265
Blos, Peter, 218
Blum, G. S., 19, 405
B'nai B'rith, Freud and, 224, 295
Boas, Franz, 582
Bock, Philip, 25
body-ego, 168
Boehm, Felix
  after World War II, 237
  Nazis and, 236
Bollas, C., 101
  as object relations theorist, 386
Bonaparte, Marie, **52–53**, 209, 228
  and Greek psychoanalytic study group, 244
  on loss of virginity, 593
  in South Africa, 13
Bondy, Theresa, 136
Bonomi, C., 302
Book of Hours (Rilke), 22
Book of the It, The (Groddeck), 227, 246
borderline disorders
  and splitting, 488, 490, 538
  treatment by Sullivan, 550
  treatment of, 584
Borecky, Miroslav, 137
Bornstein, Berta, 81
  in Berlin, 236
Bornstein, Steff, 136
  in Berlin, 236
Bornstein-Windholz, Steffi, 136
Bose, Girindrasekhar, 275
Boss, Medard, 182, 266
Boston Psychoanalytic Institute, 502
bound energy. *See* binding
bound energy, physics concept of, 45
Bourdon, Jean, 45
Bourgeois Experience, The: Victoria to Freud (Gay), 265

Bourneville, Désiré-Magloire, 76
Bouvet, Maurice, 209
Bower, G., 490
Bowlby, John, 114, 390
    attachment theory, 150–151, 494, 534
    criminality, 115
    developmental theory, 150–151
    Horney and, 263
    and Preu, 412
Boyer, Bryce, 27
    and Mexico, 342
    treatment of schizophrenia, 502
Boza, Charo, 414
Braatøy, Trygve, 384
brain science and psychoanalysis, 45, **53–57**
Brandell, Gunnar, 555
Braun, A. R., 56
Braun, B. G., 351
Braun, Heinrich, 220
    and Nietzsche, 368
Brazil and psychoanalysis, **57–59**
Bredenkamp, J., 120
Breger, Louis, 229
Brenman-Pick, Irma, 556
Brenner, Charles, 103, 129–130, 133, 134, 146, 247, 448, 453, 508
    conflict theory, 105
    defense theory, 105
    objections to the concept of therapeutic alliance, 564–565
    working through, 600–601
Brentano, Franz, **59–61**, 132, 182, 221
    dispositionalist approach of the unconscious, 576
    Freud student of, 371, 418
    influence on cognitive psychologists, 95
    influence on Freud, 95, 118, 378–379, 438
Breuer, Josef, 45, **61–63**, 88, 102, 117, 221, 296, 364, 436
    abreaction, 4
    affect, 10–11
    and Anna O., 24–25, 33, 68, 78, 437
    and Charcot's traumatic hysteria, 76
    Freud's interest to publish with, 436
    Hartmann analyzed by, 254
    reinterpretation of Anna O. case, 437
    tonic excitation, 46
    transference, 568
    traumatic reactions linked to hysteria, 572
Briand, Aristide, 52
Briceño, A., 589
Brief, M., 136
Brief, Otto, 136
Brill, Abraham A., 71, 225, 227, 540
    at Freud's lectures at Clark University, 582
    Jones and, 293
    and medicalization of psychoanalysis, 582
British Journal of Delinquency (British Journal of Criminology), 240
British Journal of Medical Psychology, 4
British Psycho-Analytical Society
    Glover and, 239
    Jones and, 242, 293, 445
    and Klein, 304
Broca, Paul, 76

Bröder, A., 120
Brother Animal: The Story of Freud and Tausk (Roazen), 562–563
Brouardel, Paul, 269
Brouillet, André, 78
Brown, W., 68
    and war neurosis, 596
Brown, William, 4
Brücke, Ernst, 62, 221, 418
Brunswick, Ruth M., 599
Buber, Martin, 231
Bubi, die Lebensgeschichte des Caligula (Sachs), 502
Bucci, W., 493
Buckle, Henry Thomas, 26
Budapest
    Marxist psychoanalysts in, 330
    psychoanalytic movement in, 203, 304, 445
Budapest Psychoanalytic Society
    Ferenczi founder of, 203
    Klein member of, 304
Bugacov, Mario, 34
Bühler, Karl, 172
Buie, D., 448
Bulletin of the International Psychoanalytic Association, 239
Bullitt, William C., 227, 228
Bürgholzli Mental Clinic
    Jung at, 298
    Spielrein patient at, 536
Burke, Mark, 58
Burke Kenneth, 265
Burlingham, Dorothy, 218

C

Caecilia M., 33, 223
Caesar, George, 101
Cage, John, 346
California law on confidentiality, 101
Camden, C. T., 532
Canada
    Indian psychoanalysts in, 276
    and psychoanalysis, **65–66**
Canadian Psychoanalytic Society, 66
Canale, Juan, 34
Caplansky, Matilde de, 413
Cárcamo, Celes, 34
Carmichael, Hugh, 65
Carnap, Rudolf, 420
Carpelan, Henrik, 205
Carpenter, William Benjamin, 576
Carrington, Hereward, 396
Carus, Carl Gustav, 376, 379
Castellaro de Pozzi, María Aidé, 34
Caston, J., 492, 493
Castoriano, Alex, 414
castration anxiety, 66, 365, 402. *See also* castration complex
    reinterpreted in context of phallic stage, 234
    Wolf Man and, 598
castration as a medical procedure, 41
castration complex, **66–68**, 410. *See also* castration anxiety
    feminine genital castration complex, 149
catatonic stupor, 503

Catechism, A, or Examination of Human Physiology (Fechner), 193
Catechism on Logic or the Laws of Thought, A (Fechner), 193
catharsis, **68–69**
cathartic method, 61, 117, 437, 568
cathexis, **69–72**, 426
  term created by Strachey, 540
Catholic Church. *See* Roman Catholic Church
Caudill, William, 25
Cavell, Stanley, 266
Center of Jungian Studies (Venezuela), 590
Central Institute for Psychic Illnesses, 237
Centre for the Development of Psychoanalysis in Peru, 412
Césarman, Fernando, 342, 343
Cesio, F., 34
Cézanne, Paul, 121
character, **72–73**
  analysis, 74
Character and Anal Erotism (Freud)
  reaction formation, 464, 465
  sublimation, 546
"Character and Anal Erotism" (Freud), 72
character development, 496
character disorders. *See* character neurosis
character neurosis, **73–75**, 366
  distinguished from neurotic symptom, 73
  psychoanalytic classification, 72
  versus symptom neurosis, 363
character resistance
  distinguished from transference resistance, 73–74
"Characteranalyse" (Character Analysis) (Reich), 471
characterological masochists, 332
Charcot, Jean-Martin, 41, **75–79**, 287, 289, 364
  Freud and, 87–88, 222, 436, 567
  investigation of occult phenomena, 395
  traumatic neurosis, 572
  treatment of hysteria, 42, 437
Chasseguet-Smirgel, Janine, 245, 357
Chavafambira, John, 13
Chentrier, Theodore, 65
Chessman, Caryl, 53
Chestnut Lodge, 204
Chewra Pschoanalytih b'Erez Israel, 172, 173
Chicago Psychoanalytic Institute, 261
Child, I., 67
child abuse. *See* child sexual molestation; seduction theory
"Child Analysis in the Analysis of Adults" (Ferenczi), 202
Child Is Being Beaten, A (Freud), 234, 260
  and masochism, 331–332
child observation, 218, 584, 585
child psychoanalysis, **79–82**, 218
  in the Netherlands, 361
  Spielrein and, 536
  training in Mexico, 342
child psychology, 313
child psychotherapy, 555
child sexual molestation
  Abraham on, 2
  memories of, 514–515
  and multiple personality, 351
  and psychoneuroses, 515

childhood memories, 514–515
childhood neurosis, **82**
childhood sexuality. *See* infantile sexuality
children. *See also* child sexual molestation; infantile sexuality
  denial as age-appropriate defense, 143
  early Oedipal phantasies of Klein, 305
  Freud's study of cerebral palsy in, 301
  Piaget on, 421
  as pre-operational, 393
  and projection, 427
  psychoanalysis contraindicated, 80–81
Children of Oedipus (Lapuz), 417
Children's Apperception Test, 428
Chile and psychoanalysis, **83–84**
Chilean Psychoanalytical Association, 83, 84
China and psychoanalysis, **84–86**
Chinese-German Academy for Psychotherapy, 85
Chiozza, L., 34
Chodorow, Nancy, 198
Chomsky, Noam, 44
Chrobak, Rudolf, 62
Churchland, P. M., 46
Cifuentes, Abdón, 83
cinema and psychoanalysis, **86–87**, 266
  feminist film studies, 198
  Lacan's "gaze" and "imaginary" used in film studies, 266
Cioffi, F., 429, 430, 431
Civilization and Its Discontents (Freud), 15, 25, 27, 227, 296
  and Freud's view on religion, 474–475
  influence of Nietzsche on, 375
  nationalism and curbing of human agression, 457
  objections to, 476
  reference to Klein in, 305
Civin, M., 424
Cixous, Hélène, 197, 198
Claparède, Edouard, 421
Clark, Ronald, 229
Clark University (Worcester, Mass.)
  Freud at, 225, 582
  Jung at, 299
Clarté (journal), 553
Claus, Carl, 221
Cleckley, H., 114
"Clinical Diary" (Ferenczi), 469
clinical ethics. *See* ethics, clinical
Clinical Papers and Essays on Psycho-Analysis (Abraham), 2
Clinical Studies (Sullivan), 550
clinical theory, **87–94**
  Sullivan and, 550
Cobb, Stanley, 147
cocaine, use of, 409
  by Freud, 221, 222
cognition. *See* cognitive psychology, and psychoanalysis; preconscious unconscious
cognitive psychology
  influence of Brentano on, 95
  and psychoanalysis, **94–97**
  and theory of slips, 531
  and unconscious, 119, 581
Cognitive Psychology (Neisser), 96

coitus interruptus, neurasthenia and, 361, 362, 437
Collected Works (Nietzsche), 183
collective unconscious, 299
Collomb, Henri, 13
Colombian Institute, 589
Coltart, N., 20
Columbia Records project, 493
committee, the secret, **97–98**, 99, 225, 445
    Eitingon and, 173
    Ferenczi and, 203
    Rank and, 461
    Sachs and, 501
Committee for Research in the Problems of Sex (CRPS), 525
Committee for the Promotion of Psychoanalysis in Greece
        and Yugoslavia, 244
Common Sense Book of Baby and Child Care (Spock), 584
Communication (Liberman), 34
communicative psychotherapy, 534
compatibilism of free will and determinism, 215, 435
Compendium of Papers in Psychoanalysis (Windholz, ed.), 136
"Complexes familiaux dans la formation de l'individu, Les"
        (Lacan), 316
compulsion and obsession, **99–100**. *See also* obsessive-
        compulsive
    Fenichel on, 459
compulsion to repeat. *See* repetition compulsion
Concept of Repression (Bose), 275
Conceptions of Modern Psychiatry (Sullivan), 550
condensation, 159, 160
    and overdetermination, 406
Conditions of Nervous Anxiety and their Treatment (Stekel), 539
confidentiality, **100–102**, 181–182
conflicts, theory of, **102–106**
    conflict as structural, 389
    ego and, 168
    and formation of neurosis, 103
    Freud's evolving theory of, 102–103
    importance of id in, 272
Confrontations with Myself (Deutsch), 148
"Confusion of Tongues between Adults and the Child: The
        Language of Tenderness and of Passion" (Ferenczi),
        203, 227, 572
    publication in English, 204
Congress of Psychoanalysis of Children and Adolescents, 414
connectionist models of mental functioning, 46
conscience. *See* superego
conscious processes
    double attribute theory of, 108–109, 343
    preconscious and, 423
consciousness, **107–109**, 578
    cognitive psychology and Freud, 95
    ego and, 168, 544
    Freud's interest in, 55
    threshold of, 377
constancy principle, 4, 422, 481
constructivist hermeneutics, 257
Contingency, Irony, and Solidarity (Rorty), 266
"Contraindications to the 'active' technique" (Ferenczi), 202
"Contribution One" (Freud), 311
"Contribution to the Psychogenesis of Manic-depressive
        States, A" (Klein), 243

Contributions to a Discussion on Suicide (Freud), 548
Controversial Discussions (1943–1944), 218, 239, 243, 304
    Jones and, 294
    Strachey's comments on, 541
Conty, Ricardo Díaz, 342
"Convergences and Divergences in Contemporary
        Psychoanalytic Technique" (Kernberg), 133
conversion, **109–111**
    and neuroses, 367
    symptoms, 483
Cooper, A. M., 74
COPSI (magazine), 413
Corona, Carlos, 342
Counteridentification (Grinberg), 34
countertransference, 447, 451, 571. *See also* transference
Cox, D. N., 114
Crafoord, Clarence, 555, 556
Crapanzano, Vincent, 13
Crawley, Ernest, 264
Creation of Woman (Reik), 473
*Creative Unconscious, The: Studies in the Psychoanalysis of
        Art* (Sachs), 502
Creative Writers and Day-Dreaming (Freud), 225
creativity, **111–113**
Cremerius, Johannes, 237
Crews, Frederick, 229
Crick, F., 96
"Criminal Tendencies in Normal Children" (Klein), 306
criminality
    multiple personality and, 352
    and psychoanalysis, **113–117**
"Criminals From a Sense of Guilt" (Freud), 113
criminology and psychoanalysis in the United States, 583, 584
Crisanto, Carlos, 412, 413
criticism of psychoanalysis. *See* critique of psychoanalysis;
        experimental evidence, Freudian; pseudoscience, and
        psychoanalysis
critique of psychoanalysis, **117–136**
cryptomnesia, 380
Cuadernos de Psicoanálisis (journal), 342
Cullberg, Johan, 555
Cullen, William, 363
cultural evolutionism, 26
culture
    cross-cultural studies on latency, 494
    cultural adaptations of Oedipus complex, 291, 310
    psychoanalysis as cultural theory, 237, 497
    and psychoanalysis in Norway, 383
    and psychoanalysis in Philippines, 417–418
    psychoanalytic theory and Western culture, 120–122
Cupello, N., 589
Curtis, H., 564
Czech Psychoanalysis Association, 137
Czech Republic and psychoanalysis, **136–138**

D

Dahl, H., 492, 493
Dai, Bingham, 85
Daly, Mary, 196
Damasio, Antonio, 96

Danger of Words, The (Drury), 266
Danish Psychoanalytic Society, 144
Danish Psychoanalytical Institute, 557
Danish-Norwegian Psychoanalytic Society, 200
Darwin, Charles, 575
   influence on Freud, 26
"Das Es" borrowed from Groddeck, 271
"Das Ich," translation of, 253
Daudet, Alphonse, 75
David, M., 285
"David Strauss, the Confessor and the Writer" (Nietzsche), 368
Davidson, Donald, 266, 420
Davis, Katherine Bement, 525
Dawkins, Richard, 323
Daybreak (Nietzsche), 369, 374
De la psychose paranoïaque dans ses rapports avec la personnalité (Of Paranoid Psychosis in Its Relations with the Personality) (Lacan), 315
De locis affectis (Galen), 268
De Mijolla, A., 285
De Wind, Eddy, 361
death instinct (Thanatos), 164, 226, 423, 443, 477
   linked with Freud's theory of agression, 114
   used interchangeably with destructive aggression, 15
Decker, H., 156, 157
deep psychology
   in Austria, 592
   Janet's contribution to, 288
   in Venezuela, 590
defense mechanisms, 31, **139–141**
   adaptive repression, 484–486
   Anna Freud on complexity of, 218–219
   and binding, 46
   of child, 305
   conflict and, 103
   ego and, 168
   Horney and, 262–263
   intellectualization as secondary defense, 279
   isolation, 283–284
   Klein on, 242
   and neuroses, 365, 367
   and psychoanalytically oriented psychotherapy, 455
   and reaction formation, 465
   Schopenhauer anticipating, 505
defense neuroses, 542
defensive or compensatory reaction in self psychology, 523
defiance, paranoia and, 409
Delboeuf, J. R. L., 68, 78, 290
Delbrück, Berthold, 577
Deleuze, Gilles, 317
Delgado, Gustavo, 413, 414
Delgado, Honorio, 411
delusions, **141–142**
   projective identification and, 307
Delusions and Dreams in Jensen's "Gradiva" (Freud), 225
denial, 139–140, **142–143**, 485
   distinguished from repression, 480
Denial of Death, The (Becker), 462
Denmark
   and psychoanalysis, **143–145**
   Reich in, 471

depression, **145–146**
   Abraham on manic-depression, 2
   anaclitic depression, 17–18, 494
   introjective depression, 18
   narcissism and, 355
   neurasthenia now diagnosed as, 362
   scientific tests of etiology of, 509–510
   use of pharmacologic agents for treatment, 460
depressive position of Klein, 304, 306, 307–308
de-repression, 496
Deri, Frances, 200
Derrida, Jacques, 208
   on Freud, 346, 347
   postmodernism of, 345
Descartes, René, 434, 575
Design of Experiments (Fisher), 192
Design Within, The: Psychoanalytic Approaches to Shakespeare (Faber, ed.), 265
Dessoir, Max, 395
"Destruction as a Cause of Coming Into Being" (Spielrein), 536
destructive instinct, used interchangeably with death instinct, 15
determinism, 419
Deutsch, Felix, 147, 227
   Dora and, 154
Deutsch, Helene, **147–148**, 329
   analyzed by Abraham, 2
   critique by Marie Bonaparte, 53
   and loss of virginity, 593
   Scandinavians in analysis with, 554
   Tausk analyzed by, 562
Deutscher Reichsverband für Proletarische Sexualpolitik (German Association for Proletarian Sexual Politics—Sexpol), 471
Development of Psychoanalysis, The (Ferenczi and Rank), 202, 227, 461
developmental psychology, 95–96
   studies from a psychoanalytic perpective, 13
   on suicide, 549
developmental theory, **148–152**. *See also* Oedipus complex
   Abraham and pregenital phases, 2
   autonomy and developmental processes, 39
   child psychological dysfunction as deviation in, 80
   cognitive psychology and Freud, 95–96
   developmental lines, 219
   Freud's theory of early development, 387
   Hartmann and theory of normal development, 253
   research on child development, 494
   and sexual drive, 162
   stages of, 405
"Devil as a Father-Substitute, The" (Freud)
   and ambivalence, 16
Devresee, D., 508
Di Chiara, G., 285
Diagnostic and Statistical Manual of Mental Disorders, 115, 349, 460, 573, 595
Diagnostic Association Studies (Jung), 298
"Dialektischer Materialismus and Psychoanalyse" (Dialectic Materialism and Psychoanalysis) (Reich), 471
Dickinson, Robert Latou, 525
Dicks, Henry V., 350

Dictionary of Psychology and Philosophy (Baldwin), 576
Dictionnaire de la psychanalyse (De Mijolla, ed.), 285
Dilman, Ilham, 192
Dilthey, Wilhelm, 256, 554
Dinnerstein, Dorothy, 197–198
"Direction of the Treatment and the Principles of Its Power,
      The" (Lacan), 316
disavowal, 488, 522
Discovery of the Unconscious, The (Ellenberger), 120, 266
displacement, 140, **152–153**
      overdetermination, 406
      phobic neuroses and, 366
"Disposition to Obsessional Neurosis, The" (Freud), 37
dissociation, **153–154**, 573. *See also* multiple personality;
      splitting
      and hysterical neuroses, 267, 367
      Janet and, 290, 350
      repression and, 487–491
Dissociative Identity Disorder. *See* multiple personality
Dissolution of the Oedipus Complex, The (Freud), 274
      criticism of Rank, 227
Dodes, L., 100
Dolto, Françoise, 209
      and child psychoanalysis, 210
Dominguez, H., 589
Don Juan Legend, The (Rank), 461
Doo-Young, Cho, 310
Dora, **154–157**, 189–190, 224, 345
      attempt to describe the disorder, 459
      end of analysis, 446, 449
      fascination with the Sistine Madonna, 593
      Freud's choice of name, 155
      interpretations of her dreams, 592
      mother of, 392, 393
      overdetermination in case of, 407
      and presentation of psychoanalytic technique, 188
      and regression, 469
      and transference, 568
Dostoyevsky, Fyodor, Freud's psychobiography of, 47–48, 326
Dosuzkov, B., 136
Dosuzkov, Theodor, 136–137
Dosuzkov-Fischer, Eugenia, 137
Double, The (Rank), 461
double entendres, 532–533
Doyle, Iracy, 58
"Dr. Mises." *See* Fechner, Gustav Theodor
Dräger, Käthe, 237
Draguns, J. G., 140, 141
Drapier, Willy, 45
"Dream of the Botanical Monograph" (Freud), 55, 56
dreams, 56–57
      cognitive psychology and Freud, 96–97
      corroboration dreams, 161
      Freud's interest in, 55
      Hartmann on, 253
      Linder and, 377, 378
      and reality testing, 466
      resemblance to jokes, 292
      similarity to neurotic symptoms, 442
      and symbolism, 559
dreams, theory of, 90–91, **157–161**, 188, 213, 447

adaptive function of dreaming, 159, 160, 161
      critique of, 128–130
      dream censorship, 158, 159
      dream construction, theory of, 158
      dream processes similar to delusions, 141
      dreams as point of access to a patient's unconscious wish
            and fantasies, 160
      and genetics, 233
      Schopenhauer, 505
      scientific tests of, 510–511
"Dreams and Myths" (Abraham), 3
Dreams and Telepathy (Freud), 396
Drei Briefe an Einen Knaben (Andreas-Salomé), 21
*Drei Motive und Gründe des Glaubens, Die (The Three
      Motives and Grounds of Faith)* (Fechner), 194
drive theory, 100, **161–165**, 387, 542
      and affect, 11
      aggressive drives and theory of conflicts, 102–103
      aim of drives, 163
      as distinguished from object relations theory, 387
      ego and, 168
      Freud's definition of drive, 163
      libido theory part of, 323
      object of drives, 163, 165
      pressure, 163, 164, 165
      sleeplessness of the drives, 528
      source of drives, 163, 165
drives according to Nietzsche, 368
Drury, M. O'C., 266
Du Bois-Reymond, Emil, 221, 378, 439
      "On the limits of our understanding of nature," 438
dual instinct theory, 15, 443
      and concept of narcissism, 356
Duchenne de Boulogne, Guillaume Benjamin, 75
Dugautiez, Maurice, 44
Dührssen, Annemarie, 237
Dundes, Alan, 264
Durell, L., 247
Dutch Psychoanalytical Association, 360
Dutch Psychoanalytical Institute, 360
Dutch Society of Psychoanalysis, 359
Duyckaerts, Françoise, 45
Dworkin, Andrea, 196
dynamic unconscious, theory of, 271
Dynamics of Transference, The (Freud), 568

E

Eagle, Morris, 119, 133–134
      and experimental evidence, 185
Earl, James W., 265
early models of the mind, 542–543
East Germany. *See* Germany
Ebbinghaus, Hermann, 376
Ecce Homo (Nietzsche), 369–370
Eckstein, Emma, 197, 207, 223, 229
École de la Cause Freudienne, 45, 211
École Freudienne de Paris, 45, 209, 318
Economic Problem of Masochism, The (Freud), 332
Écrits (Lacan), 318
Edel, Leon, 48

Edelson, Marshall, 127–128, 131–132, 191
   Psychoanalysis: A Theory in Crisis, 133
Edinger, Dora, 24, 25
education
   and analysts, **167–168**
   of juvenile delinquents, 114
   and psychoanalysis in the United States, 583, 584
"Effect on Women of Pre-mature Ejaculation in Men, The"
   (Ferenczi), 201
ego, **168–169**, 443, 477, 544–545. *See also* ego ideal
   adaptation, 168, 170
   antagonism with id, 486–487
   anxiety, 30, 443–444
   compared to Schopenhauer's intellect, 374 tab. 2
   consciousness as, 107
   defense mechanisms, 139
   effects of choice of Latin name, 390
   Herbart on, 255
   id distinguished from, 272
   of infant according to Klein, 307
   Lacan on, 315–316
   in the libido-narcissism model of the mind, 542
   line of development of, established by Anna Freud, 219
   and morality, 348
   multiple meanings of, 545
   observing ego and neuroses, 367
   overwhelmed, 486
   pleasure principle and, 423
   preconscious and, 423
   regression, 469
   and sleep, 528
   strength of, 92
   superego product of, 551
Ego and the Id, The (Freud), 16, 103, 139, 164, 170, 226,
   271, 544
   appropriation of *das Es*, 247
   dissociations of hysteria, 350
   guilt, 114
   introducing structural theory, 541
   narcissism, 356
   on overwhelmed ego, 486
   and process of ego development, 273
   and unconscious, 578
Ego and the Mechanism of Defense, The (A. Freud),
   139, 218
   displacement not mentioned in, 152
   reviewed by Kris, 312
"Ego Development and the Comic" (Kris), 312
ego drives, fluctuating meanings of, 544
ego ethics, 348
ego ideal
   formation of, 356
   in the libido-narcissism model of the mind, 542
   and narcissism, 357, 526
   superego and, 545–546
ego libido *versus* object libido, 443
ego psychology, 38–39, 133, **169–171**, 467
   character concept, 72
   emergence of, 149
   Hartmann school of, 253, 312, 313
   interpretation of free association, 214

   in Mexico, 342
   order of interpretation, 452
   repression, 487
   Sullivan and, 550
ego-percept, 168
ego-syntonic, 73
Ehrenzweig, Anton, 112
Eickhof, Fridrich Wilhelm, 137
Eissler, Kurt, **172**, 563, 583
   on Freud, 229
   isolation, 284
   treatment of schizophrenia, 502
Eitingon, Max, 136, **172–174**, 224
   Andreas-Salomé and, 23
   Berlin Polyclinic, 2, 236
   and Indian Psychoanalytic Institute, 275
   Schmideberg analyzed by, 303–304
   secret committee member, 97, 99, 225, 445
   and Vienna Psychoanalytic Society, 597
Ejve, Birgitta, 555
Ekman, Tor, 554
*El valor del Psicoanálisis en Policlínico (The Value of
   Psychoanalysis in the Out-Patient Clinic)* (Allende
   Navarro), 83
"Elasticity of Psychoanalytic Technique, The" (Ferenczi), 202
Electra complex, **174–175**
electrotherapy, 213
Elementary Textbook on Electromagnetism, An (Fechner), 193
Elemente der Psychophysik (Elements of Psychophysics)
   (Fechner), 192, 194, 376
Elhers, W., 140, 141
Eliot, T. S., 346
Elizabeth von R., **175–176**
   and repression, 479
Ellenberger, Henri, 300, 375, 442
   and Anna O., 25
   Discovery of the Unconscious, The, 120, 266
   on Fechner, 193
Ellerman, Annie Winifred (Bryher), 501
Ellis, Havelock, **176–178**, 310, 441, 525
   compared to Krafft-Ebing, 311
   invited to Australia, 35
   and term "autoerotism," 37
   and term "narcissism," 355
Embirikos, Andreas, 244
Emde, Robert N., 494
   and developmental theory, 151
Emmy von N., 33, 223, 478, 555
   and hallucinations, 251, 252
emotions
   cognitive psychology and Freud, 96
   Freud's interest in, 55
empirical studies
   of developmental theory, 149
   on recovery of unconscious memories vie free association, 213
Enciclopedia Italiana Treccani, 285
Enckell, Mikael, 205
Encyclopédie Française, 316
Engelbrecht, Hilke, 413
England. *See* Great Britain
English School of Psychoanalysis, 197

English Society for Psychical Research, 395
envy, **178–180**. *See also* penis envy
epiphenomenalist view of Freud, 343
epistemophilic instinct, 305
Eranos Conferences, 299
Erdelyi, Matthew H., 137, 213
    experiments on free association, 214
Erikson, Erik, 27, 171, 393
    basic mistrust, 263
    and developmental theory, 150, 151–152
    on Dora, 155
    Dorothy Burlingham and, 218
    ego development, 39
    ego ethics, 348
    identity, 169
    infantile stages of development, 148
    Martin Luther: A Study in History and Psychoanalysis, 457
    struggle for identity, 151
    studies of charismatic leaders, 48, 265
Erle, J., 20
Ermakov, I.D., 497
Eros. *See* life instinct
Erotic Symbolism, the Mechanism of Detumescence, the Psychic State of Pregnancy (Ellis), 177
Erotik, Die (Andreas-Salomé), 21
erotogenic zones, 321, 385
Escape from Freedom (Fromm), 231
Essence of Christianity, The (Feuerbach), 221
Etat mental des hystériques, L' (Janet), 287
Etchegoyen, Horacio, 34, 35, 59, 413
Etezady, M. H., 82
ethics
    clinical, **180–182**
    superego and, 552
ethnopsychoanalysis, 331
    Africa's influence on, 14
Ethos (journal), 25
"Etiology of Hysteria, The" (Freud), 223
Eulenberg, A., 572
European Conference of Child Psychoanalysis (1998, Sweden), 555
European Congress of Psychoanalysis (1991, Sweden), 555
European émigré psychoanalysts in the United States, 466, 582, 583
European Psychoanalytic Federation (EPF)
    Czech Republic and, 137
    Danish Psychoanalytic Society and, 145
    Dutch psychoanalysts and, 360
Evang, Karl, 383
evolutionary biology, 49–50
evolutionary psychoanalysis, 49
    and libido theory, 323–324
evolutionary psychology, 534
existentialism, **182–183**
Exner, Sigmund, 46
exogamy rules, Oedipal explanation of, 27
"Experiencing of Sexual Traumas as a Form of Sexual Activity, The" (Abraham), 2
experimental evidence, Freudian, **183–186**. *See also* research on psychoanalysis; scientific tests of Freud's theories and therapy

Experimental Physics (Biot), 193
experimental psychology, 192
expressive psychotherapies, 455–456
extraclinical theory, 339
extrasensory perception, Freud's interest in, 395
Eysenck, H. J., 67
    on Little Hans case, 327
Eysenck, Hans, 120, 121

F

Faber, M. D., 265
Fackel, Die (The Torch), 222
Faimberg, Heyde, 137
Fairbairn, W. R. D., 357, 388
    agression, 114
    coining term "object relations theory," 386
    conflict, 104
    on criminality, 115
    Horney and, 263
    no id, 390
    repression, 480
    splitting, 388, 487, 538
    treatment of schizophrenia, 502
Faith and Healing, and a Critical Study of Psychoanalysis (Gadelius), 553
Familienroman der Neurotiker, Der (Family Romances) (Freud), 187
family romance, **187–188**
Fanon, Frantz, 12
fantasy, **188–192**, 223, 522
    children and, 305
    primal scene fantasy, 425
Farah, Martha, 419
fear, 30, 365. *See also* anxiety
Fear of Freedom, The (Fromm), 467
Fechner, Gustav Theodor, 45, **192–195**, 379
    dispositionalist approach to the unconscious, 576
    Elements of Psychophysics, 376
    influence on Freud's pleasure principle, 422
    Nietzsche and, 368
Féder, Luis, 342
Federation of Psychoanalytic Societies, 556
Federn, Ernst, 290, 291
Federn, Paul, 136, 224, 329, 536
    Fenichel analyzed by, 199
    Kulovesi analyzed by, 205
    Reich analyzed by, 470
    Scandinavians in analysis with, 554
    Weiss analyzed by, 284
Fellner, Oscar (Herr E.), 223
female sexuality, 53, 512, 525, 593
    Freud's ideas disputed, 587
    Jones on, 294
    little girls' genital sexuality, 587
"Female Sexuality" (Freud), 174
Feminine Mystique, The (Friedan), 196
Feminine Psychology (Horney), 261
feminism
    critic of psychoanalysis, 87
    and Dora case, 156

feminism (*continued*)
    and psychoanalysis, **195–199**
    and word "hysteria," 268
feminist therapy centers and training institutes, 199
Fenichel, Otto, 58, 74, **199–200**, 329, 362
    in Berlin, 236, 330
    isolation, 284
    in Oslo, 383
    Pederson analyzed by, 554
    and politics, 236
    in Prague, 136
    on process of analysis, 448, 449, 450
    and psychopathology, 459
    Reich and, in Oslo, 471
    and secret circular letters, 330
    and Vienna Seminar for Sexology, 470
Ferenczi, Sándor, 149, 156, **200–205**, 225
    active technique, 202, 469
    Andreas-Salomé and, 23
    and Berlin Psychoanalytical Training Institute, 235
    on conversion, 110
    description of persecutory paranoia, 507
    Development of Psychoanalysis, The (with Rank), 461
    genitality theory, 235
    and Groddeck, 246
    and homosexuality, 259
    influence on Balint, 390
    influence on Klein, 390
    interest in occult, 395
    Jones analyzed by, 293
    Klein and, 243, 302
    Rank and, 461
    regression, 469
    secret committee member, 97, 99, 225, 445
    and "Statutes of the International Psychoanalytic
      Association," 98
    Stekel's influence on, 539
    on suggestibility, 547
    on war neurosis, 595
Ferrer, S., 34
Ferstel, Marie, 224
Fetal Psychism (Tascovsky), 34
fetishism
    Krafft-Ebing on, 311
    and splitting of the ego, 522, 537, 538
Feudtner, C., 595
Feuerbach, Ludwig
    Essence of Christianity, The, 221
    influence on Freud, 26, 473
Fiasché, Angel, 556
Fiasché, Dora, 556
Fichte, Johann Gottlieb, 558
film studies/criticism. *See* cinema and psychoanalysis
Fine, Bernard D., 392, 559
Fink, D., 352
Finland and psychoanalysis, **205–206**
Finnish Psychoanalytic Society, 205–206
Finnish Psychoanalytic Study Group, 205
Finnish-Swedish Psychoanalytical Society,
    205, 554
Firestein, S., 450

First Lines of the Practice of Physick (Cullen), 363
Fischelova, Vera, 137
Fischer, Rene, 137
Fisher, Charles, 214
Fisher, R. A., 192
Fisher, S., 67, 405
    and experimental evidence, 184, 185
Fishman, Carlos, 414
Five Lectures on Psycho-Analysis (Freud), 435, 582
fixation, 405
Flagey, Danielle, 45
Flanagan, Owen, 577
Flechsig, Paul, 409, 507, 508
Fleischl-Marxow, Ernst von, 221, 222
Fliess, Robert
    analyzed by Abraham, 2
    in Berlin, 236
    training patient of Sachs, 501
Fliess, Wilhelm, **206–208**, 269. *See also* Freud-Fliess
    correspondence
    Freud and, 222
    influence on Freud's view of infantile sexuality, 441
    numerical determinism, 222–223
    source of inspiration for book on jokes, 292
Fliess Papers, 361
Fliess-Freud correspondence. *See* Freud-Fliess
    correspondence
Florante at Laura (Balagtas), 417
Flournoy, Théodore, 298
    and occult phenomena, 395
    Piaget and, 420
Flying Saucers: A Modern Myth (Jung), 300
focal treatment, 455
Fonagy, Peter, 81, 113
Fontane, Theodor, 380
Forest, Izette de, 204
Formulations on the Two Principles of Mental Functioning
    (Freud), 9, 225
    pleasure principle and reality principle, 422
    and symbiosis, 558
Forrester, J., 33
Förster-Nietzsche, Elizabeth, 370
42 Lives (Wallerstein), 493
Forum, 238
Foucault, Michel, 317, 555
Foundation of Psychoanalytic Technique (Braatøy), 384
Foundations of the Entire Science of Knowledge (Fichte), 558
"Four Fundamental Concepts of Psycho-Analysis, The"
    (Lacan), 318
Fragment of a Great Confession (Reik), 473
Fragment of an Analysis of a Case of Hysteria (Freud), 110, 154
    interpretation of Dora's dreams, 592
France
    and psychoanalysis, **208–212**
    Rank in Paris, 461–462
Frank, Jan, 136
Frank, K., 602
Fränkel, Alexander. *See* Ferenczi, Sándor
Frankfurt Institute of Social Research, 236
    Fromm and, 231
Frankfurt Psychoanalytic Association, 137

Frankfurt Psychoanalytic Institute, 236
  Fromm and, 231
Frankfurt School of philosophy, 236
Frazer, James, 26, 264
free association, **212–214**, 283, 441, 449
  critique of, 124–127
  and psychical determinism, 435
  and psychotherapy, 455
free energy, physics concept of, 45
free will, **214–217**
  and psychical determinism, 435
Freidman, L., 248
  on free association, 449
Freidman, Otto, 136
Freie Bühne, Die (journal), 21
Freies Judisches Rehrhaus, 231
French, Thomas, 540
French school of psychoanalysis
  in Brazil, 59
  in Canada, 66
  in Venezuela, 590
Freud: A Life for Our Time (Gay), 436
Freud, Anna, 81, 98, 136, 197, **217–219**, 269,
    305, 329
  Andreas-Salomé and, 21, 22
  on antagonism of ego and id, 486
  checking Strachey's translations, 541
  description of identification with the aggressor, 140
  developmental theory, 115, 149
  displacement during puberty, 152–153
  ego, 171
  on Freud's view of telepathy, 396–397
  influence in Mexico, 342
  intellectualization, 279
  isolation, 284
  and Klein, 240, 303 (*See also* Controversial Discussions)
  Kris analyzed by, 312
  libido theory, 321
  obsessional neuroses, 392
  secret committee member, 99
  toilet training, 566
  translations in Swedish, 554
  visit to Greece, 244
Freud: Master and Friend (Sachs), 502
  on the secret committee, 97
Freud, Sigmund, **219–229**
  correspondence (*See* Freud-Andreas-Salomé; Freud-Ferenczi; Freud-Fliess; Freud-Pfister; Freud-Silberstein; Freud-Spielrein; Freud-Weiss)
  Deutsch analyzed by, 147
  Eitingon analyzed by, 173
  emigration, 592
  ethical commitments of his views, 419
  eulogy of Tausk, 563
  Ferenczi analyzed by, 201
  first psychohistorian, 456
  Freud, Anna, analyzed by, 218
  Hartmann analyzed by, 254
  rejection of free will, 214–215
  and religion, 295, 419, 473
  and roots of object relations theory, 386–387

self-analysis, 223, 441, 520–521
  Strachey, Alix and James, analyzed by, 243
Freud: The Mind of the Moralist (Rieff), 346
Freud and Anthropology: A History and Reappraisal (Wallace), 264
"Freud and His Times" (Brandell), 555
Freud and Honorio Delgado, Chronicle of a Breakaway (Rey de Castro), 414
Freud and Philosophy: An Essay on Interpretation (Ricoeur), 266
"Freud and the Future" (Mann), 228
"Freud and the Seduction Theory: A Brief Love Affair" (Eissler), 172
Freud archives. *See* Sigmund Freud Archives
Freud for Historians (Gay), 265
Freud Literary Heritage Foundation, 172
Freud or Jung? (Glover), 239
Freud-Andreas-Salomé correspondence, 563
Freud-Ferenczi correspondence, on extrasensory perception, 395
Freud-Fliess correspondence, 37, 61, 311
  edited by Marie Bonaparte, 52
  on female sexuality, 588
  on Freud's self-analysis, 441
  introduction by Kris, 312
  on Nietzsche, 369
  and notes of *Project for a Scientific Psychology*, 425, 439
  on paranoia, 409
  on philosophical knowledge, 371
  on primal scene, 424
  reference to King Oedipus, 397–398
  on role of sexuality in neuroses, 437
  on seduction theory, 440, 515, 516, 517, 518–519
  on shame, 526
  on sublimation, 546
  and use of word "metapsychology," 337, 338
"Freudian Heory of Hysteria, The" (Jung), 536
"Freudian School" (Venezuela), 590
"Freudian Thing, The, or the Meaning of the Return to Freud in Psychoanalysis" (Lacan), 316
Freudianism: A Critical Essay (Voloshinov), 498
Freud-Pfister correspondence, 416, 474
Freud's Collected Neuroscientific Writings (Solms, ed.), 117
Freud's family, **229–231**
"Freud's Psycho-analytic Procedure" (Freud), 19
Freud-Silberstein correspondence, 60, 378
Freud-Spielrein correspondence, 536
Freud-Weiss correspondence, on thought transference, 396
Freund, Otto von, 226
Friedan, Betty, 196
Friedjung, Karl Josef, 329
Friedländer, Saul, 48
Friedman, Michael, 130
Friedman, S. M., 67
Frijling-Schreuder, E. C. M., 360, 361
Frischauf-Pappenheim, Marie, 471
From the History of an Infantile Neurosis (Freud), 598
From Thirty Years with Freud (Reik), 473
Fromkin, V. A., 530
Fromm, Erich, 200, **231–232**, 262, 330
  and Adler, 8
  in Berlin, 236, 330

Fromm, Erich (*continued*)
  ego ethics, 348
  Fear of Freedom, The, 467
  and Ferenczi, 204
  on Ferenczi and Groddeck, 246
  at Frankfurt Psychoanalytical Institute, 236
  and Horney, 262, 263
  Man for Himself, 467
  in Mexico, 341
  and Swedish Holistic Society, 556
  translations in Swedish, 554
Fromm-Reichmann, Frieda, 142
  in Berlin, 236
  description of catatonic stupor, 503
  at Frankfurt Psychoanalytical Institute, 236
  and Swedish Holistic Society, 556
  treatment of schizophrenia, 502
  and William Alanson White Institute, 231
Fuchs, S. H. (Foulkes), 236
"Function and Field of Speech and Language in
    Psychoanalysis" ("Rome Discourse") (Lacan), 316
functional psychoses, 366
Functions and Disorders of the Reproductive Organs (Acton), 177
"Funktion des Orgasmus, Die" (The Function of Orgasm)
    (Reich), 470
Furlan, P. M., 502
Further Remarks on the Neuro-psychoses of Defense (Freud), 516
Future of an Illusion, The (Freud), 25, 27, 227, 296, 416
  and Freud-Pfister correspondence, 474

G

Gabriel, R. A., 596
Gadamer, H. G.
  conceptualization of hermeneutics, 257
  Truth and Method, 256–257
Gadelius, Bror, 553
Galen of Pergamon, 267
  De locis affectis, 268
Galenson, E., 151
Gallo, Beatriz, 34
Gallwey, P., 116
Galvez, Javier, 414
García, A., 589
Garma, Angel, 34
  analyzed by Reik, 412
  in Berlin, 236
  and Mexico, 341
Garza, César, 342
Gay, Peter, 297
  Bourgeois Experience, The: Victoria to Freud, 265
  Freud: A Life for Our Time, 229, 436
  Freud for Historians, 265
Gay Science, The (Nietzsche), 369, 374
"Gehirn" (*The Brain*) (Freud), 343, 344
Geijerstam, Emanuel af, 553
gender
  bias in Freud's writings, 86
  and differences in shame, 527
  Ferenczi sensitivity to inequity, 201
Genetic Psychology (Rank), 462

genetics and psychoanalysis, **233–234**
genital stage of development, 162. *See also* developmental
    theory
genitality, theories of, **234–235**
Georg Groddeck Gesellschaft, 248
George, Stefan, 241
German Psychoanalytic Association, 238
  under Nazi regime, 236
German Psychoanalytic Society, 238
  under Nazi regime, 236
  Reich member of, 471
German Radio Propaganda, The (Kris and Speier), 312
German Society for Psychoanalysis, Psychotherapy,
    Psychosomatics and Depth Psychology, 238
German Society for Psychoanalysis and Depth Psychology, 237
Germany. *See also* Berlin
  disbanding of sex organizations under Hitler, 525
  Indian psychoanalysts in, 276
  and psychoanalysis, **235–239**
  research on psychoanalysis in, 492
Gerö, George, 200
Gesammelte Werke (Freud), 52
Gheiler, Marcos, 413
Gill, Merton M., 103, 455, 585, 586
  analysis of transference, 451
  and conflict, 105
  and metapsychology, 338, 339
Gillespie, Sadie, 14
Gillespie, William, 243
  and origin of homosexuality, 261
Gilligan, Carol, 198
Gilman, Sander, 229
Gilovich, Thomas, 123
Giovacchini, Peter L., 502
Glasser, M., 116
Glossary Committee, 293
Glossary of Psychoanalytic Terms and Concepts (Moore and
    Fine), 392, 559
Glover, Edward, **239–241**
  analyzed by Abraham, 2
  beginning phase of analysis, 448
  criminality, 115
  interpretation, 452
  review of Klein, 303
  Schmideberg analyzed by, 303–304
Glymour, Clark, 420
Goethe, Johann Wolfgang von
  Freud's psychobiography of, 47
  influence on Freud, 235
  Reik's study of, 472
Goethe Prize, **241–242**
Goldberg, D., 20
Golden Notebook, The (Lessing), 196
Goldman, Emma, 582
Goldwasser, Alberto, 414
Gombrich, E. H., 467
Gongsun, Zhang, 84
González, Avelino, 342
González, José Luis, 342
Gorbachev, Mikhail, 498
Gorer, Geoffrey, 498

Göring, M. H., 236
Göteborg Psychotherapy Institute, 556–557
Gradiva (Jensen), 147
  Freud's analysis of, 112
Graf, Max, 225
grandiosity
  narcissism and, 355
  paranoia and, 409
Great Britain
  diagnosis in, 460
  Indian psychoanalysts in, 276
  Klein's early lectures in London, 303
  little use of projective techniques in, 428
  Peruvian psychoanalysts in, 414
  and psychoanalysis, **242–244**
  psychotherapeutic treatment for schizophrenia, 502
Greece and psychoanalysis, **244–245**
Greek Society for Psychical Research, 396
Green, André, 59
Greenacre, Phyllis, 114
  and origin of homosexuality, 261
Greenberg, Clement, 467
Greenberg, Harvey, 266
Greenberg, J. R., 7, 8
Greenberg, R., 67
  and experimental evidence, 184, 185
Greenson, R. R., 448
  compassionate (benevolent) neutrality, 180
  on therapeutic alliance, 565
  and working through, 602
Gregory, Ian, 348
Greve, Germán, 83
Grief and English Renaissance Elegy (Pigman), 265
Griesinger, Wilhelm, 363
Grieve, Patricia, 414
Grinberg, Léon, 34, 35
  in Sweden, 556
Grinstein's Index of Psychoanalytics Writings, 247
Groddeck, Georg, **245–249**
  in Berlin, 236
  concept of the id, 226–227
  Das Es, 271
  Ferenczi and, 201
  and Frankfurt Psychoanalytic Institute, 231
  and psychomatic medicine, 539
Groen, Jan, 360
Groen-Prakken, H., 360
  in Prague, 137
Grombich, C. H., 312
Gross, Alfred, 236
Gross, Otto, 330
  and Schreber as schizophrenic, 508
Grosskurth, P., 556
Grossman, L., 522
Grotjahn, M., 247
Grotstein, James S., 502
Group A, 236, 237
Group for Psychoanalytic Studies of Monterrey (Mexico), 342
group psychology, 322, 388–389
  group analysis in Brazil, 59

Group Psychology and the Analysis of the Ego (Freud), 25, 27, 179, 226, 331, 388–389
  analysis of army and church, 457
  destructiveness of envy, 115
  identification, 273
Grünbaum, Adolf, 257, 345, 420, 548
Grygier, T., 19
Guiler, Hugh, 462
guilt, **249–250**
  narcissism and, 355
  unconscious as cause of crimes, 114–115
Guntrip, Harry S.
  Horney and, 263
  as object relations theorist, 386
  treatment of schizophrenia, 502
Gupta, Tapasi, 276
Guzder, Jaswant, 276

H

Haas, Ladislav, 137
Habermas, Jürgen, 131, 256
Hale, N., 312
Hall, G. Stanley, 71, 225, 582
  and investigation of occult phenomena, 395
Hallowell, Alfred, 26
hallucinations, **251–252**
  projections as, 427
  projective identification and, 307
  and schizophrenia, 503
Halsmann Case, 113–114
Hamilton, W. D., 534
Hamlet (Shakespeare)
  Freud on, 112, 265
  psychoanalytic criticism of Oliver's Hamlet, 87
Hamlet and Oedipus (Jones), 265, 294
Hammerschlag, Samuel, 296
Hampstead Clinic, 218
Handbuch der Schul-Hygiene (Baginsky), 41
Hansen, Finn, 384
Harding, Gösta, 555
Hare, R. D., 114
Harmon, Robert, 17
Hartmann, Heinz, 133, 148, 248, **252–254**, 467, 583
  adaptation as major ego function, 171
  autonomous ego function, 104
  clinical ethics, 180
  and Kris, 312
  and Mexico, 341
  and term ego psychology, 38–39
Hartocollis, Peter, 244, 245
Haunting Melody, The (Reik), 473
Hauptmann, Gerhart, 21
Haus, Das (Andreas-Salomé), 21
Hauslexicon (Fechner, ed.), 193
Hayman, Anne, 14
Hazari, A., 19, 392
health insurance and psychoanalysis, 36, 433
  and confidentiality of analysis, 101–102
  in Denmark, 144
  in Germany, 237–238

health insurance and psychoanalysis (*continued*)
 government subsidization in Holland, 360
 in the United States, 585
Hegel, Georg Wilhelm Friedrich, 316, 376, 558
 Lacan and, 266
 and unconscious, 324
Heidegger, Martin, 182, 256
 influence on Lacan, 266
Heilbron, Hanna, 136, 200
Heilbrun, Erich, 13
Heimann, Paula, 243
 influence on Peruvian psychoanalysis, 412
Heinroth, Johann Christian August, 247
Hellenic Study Group, 244
Hellman, Ilse, 243
Helmholtz, Hermann von, 45, 221, 378, 379
 and unconscious inference, 118, 119, 575
Hentschel, U., 140, 141
Herbart, Johann Friedrich, **254–256**, 371
 influence on Freud, 376–378, 379–380, 381
 Nietzsche and, 368
 topographical model of the mind, 442
Heredity and the Etiology of the Neuroses (Freud), 516, 517
 and term psychoanalysis, 117, 223
heredity of psychopathological conditions. *See* genetics and
 psychoanalysis
Hering, Ewald, 62
Hermann, Imre, 193
 and Ferenczi, 204
hermeneutics
 history of, 256–257
 Italian psychoanalysis and, 285
 and psychoanalysis, **256–257**, 334–335
Hernández, Max, 412, 413, 414
Herskovits, Melville, 26
heterosexuality as anaclitic, 17
Hilferding, Margarethe, 329, 597
Hinkle, Beatrice, 299
Hinojosa, José Rubén, 342
Hirschfeld, Magnus, 525
Hirschmüller, Albrecht, 25
history. *See also* psychohistory
 myths and, 353
 and psychoanalysis, 264–265
History of Psychiatry (Kannabikh), 497
history of psychoanalysis. *See* psychoanalysis, origin and
 history of; psychoanalytic movement
History of the Psychoanalytic Movement (Ellis), 177, 178
History of the Psycho-Analytic Movement (Freud), 127
Hitschmann, Eduard
 Kulovesi analyzed by, 205
 Scandinavians in analysis with, 554
Hobaica, W., 589
Hobson, J. Allan, 96–97
Hoffer, A., 243, 248
Hoffer, Willi, 238, 243, 329
Hoffman, Ernst, 44
Hogarth Press, 293, 294, 540
holding environment, 182
 Ferenczi and, 201
Holland, Norman, 265

Holmström, Reijo, 205
Holstijn, Westerman, 360
Holt, Robert R., 19, 46, 339, 585
Holter, Peter Andreas, 384
Holtzman, D., 593
Holtzman Inkblot Test, 428
Holzman, Philip, 134
homosexuality, 322, 415, 592. *See also* lesbianism
 Ellis on, 176
 Hartmann on, 253
 Krafft-Ebing on, 311
 as narcissistic, 17
 origin of paranoia in repressed, 409–410, 507, 510
 psychoanalytic theory of, 198, **258–261**
 study of, 459
Honigmann, G., 595
Horizon, 240
Horkheimer, Max, 236, 330
 Fromm and, 231
Horney, Karen, 53, **261–264**, 330, 593
 and Adler, 8
 analyzed by Abraham, 2
 and Association for the Advancement of Psychoanalysis, 467
 in Berlin, 236
 on Deutsch, 147
 and Ferenczi, 204
 influence on Freud's views on women, 195
 on loss of virginity, 593
 Neurotic Personality of Our Time, The, 467
 penis envy, 411
 Schmideberg analyzed by, 303–304
 training patient of Sachs, 501
Horowitz, Mardi J., 351, 492, 493
House-Tree-Person Test, 428
Hug-Hellmuth, Hermine, 218, 303, 305
 first child psychoanalyst, 81
Hughlings Jackson, John, 76, 293
 influence on concept of repression, 468
 influence on Freud, 438, 442
Human, All Too Human (Nietzsche), 369, 374
Human Mind, The (Menninger), 583
Human Potential Movement, 68
humanities and psychoanalysis, **264–267**
Hume, David, 26
humiliation, narcissism and, 355
Hungarian Psychoanalytical Association, 302
Hunter, R. A., 508
Hurst, Arthur, 268
Husserl, Edmund, 59, 60, 182, 554
Hyatt-Williams, A., 116
Hygiea (journal), 553
hypercathexis. *See* cathexis
hypnosis, 568, 575
 Charcot and, 76, 77
 Freud and, 223
 Janet and, 287
 as mode of therapy, 439
 posthypnotic suggestions, 252
 to recall pathogenic experiences, 547
 to recover unconscious material, 213
Hypnotism (Forel), 395

hypochondriasis, narcissism and, 355
Hyppolite, Jean, 317
hysteria, 29, **267–270**
 Breuer and Freud on, 161, 351–352
 Charcot and, 76
 defense hysteria, 479–480, 572
 description and classification, 458
 fantasies, 188–189
 Freud *versus* Janet, 478, 480
 hallucinations, 252
 hypnoid hysteria, 479
 and identification, 273
 Janet on, 288, 290, 480
 neuropsychic conception of, 42
 physiological basis of, 78
 and repression, 478, 515
 retention hysteria, 479
 role of genitals in, 41–42
 sexual origin of, 437, 515
 symptom formation, 87, 90
 as trauma theory, 88, 572
 and virginal anxiety, 592
"Hysteria" (Freud), 268
hysterical neuroses, 365, 367
hysterical paralysis, 436
 Charcot and, 78
Hysterical Phantasies and Their Relation to Bisexuality
 (Freud), 189
hysteriform, 268
hysteroid, 268

I

Ian, Marcia, 265
id, **271–272**, 443, 477, 543
 compared to Schopenhauer's Will, 373 tab. 1
 and ego, 170, 486–487
 resistance, 601
identification, **272–273**, 388, 389, 509
 with the aggressor, 140, 219
 narcissism and, 356
 projective identification, 307, 427
identity, 344
 adolescent struggle for, 151
ideo-motor action, theory of, 78
Igra, Ludvig, 556
Ikonen, Pentti, 205
"Illusion of a Future, The" (Pfister), 416, 474
Im Zwischenland (Andreas-Salomé), 21
imagery, Freud's interest in, 55
Imaginary Signifier, The (Metz), 266
Imago (journal), 22, 226. *See also American Imago*
 Kris editor of, 312
 Pfister published in, 416
 Rank and Sachs joint editors of, 457, 461, 501
 Servadio published in, 285
 Spielrein published in, 537
"Importance of Symbol-Formation for the Development of
 the Ego, The" (Klein), 306
In der Schule bei Freud (Andreas-Salomé), 22
In re: Lifschutz, 101, 102

In Sachen des Psychophysik (Fechner), 194
Inability to Mourn, The (Mitscherlich-Nielsen), 237
incest, **273–275**
 Oedipal explanation of, 27, 113
 taboo, 561
Incest Theme in Literature and Legend, The (Rank), 461
incompatibilism of free will and determinism, 216–217
incorporation. *See* identification
India and psychoanalysis, **275–276**
Indian Psychoanalytic Institute, 275
Indian Psychoanalytic Society, 275
individuation psychology, literary studies and, 265
infant research, 494
Infantile Genital Organization, The (Freud), 234
infantile narcissistic object, 387–388
infantile neurosis. *See* childhood neurosis
infantile sexuality, 148, 234, **276–278**, 306, 323, 441
 autoerotism, 37
 criticism by Jung and Adler, 598
 mocked by Ellis, 178
 and neuroses, 416
 and perversions, 415
inhibition, and concept of binding, 46
Inhibitions, Symptoms and Anxiety (Freud), 8, 82, 100, 170,
 283, 392, 599, 600
 criticism of Rank, 227
 traumatic neuroses, 572
Insel, T. R., 392
insight, role of, in therapy, **278–279**, 513–514
 Freud's promotion of conscious insight, 68
 and treatment of schizophrenia, 504
instinct, sex as an, 414, 443
instincts, theory of. *See* drive theory
Instincts and Their Vicissitudes (Freud), 163, 226, 380
 ambivalence, 16
 autoerotism, 37–38
Institute for Children's Diseases (Vienna) (Erstes
 Öffentliches Kinder-Krankeninstitute), 222, 301
Institute for Psychological Research and Psychotherapy
 (German Reich), 592
Institute for Psychotherapy (Germany), 237
Institute for the Study and Treatment of Delinquency
 (ISTD), 240–241
Institute für Sexualökonomische Lebensforschung (Institute
 for Sexual Economic Life Research), 471
Institute of Psychoanalysis (Mexico), 342
insurance. *See* health insurance
intellectualization, **279–280**, 485
 in neuroses, 367
 in obsessive-compulsive neuroses, 366
internal censor, 163
International Journal of Psychoanalysis (Psycho-Analysis),
 204, 242, 541
 founded by Jones, 293
 Kris published in, 312
International Psychoanalytic Congresses
 1908, Salzburg, 225, 597
 1910, Nuremberg, 97, 225
 1911, Weimar, 22, 225
 1918, Budapest, 595
 1920, The Hague, 359

International Psychoanalytic Congresses (*continued*)
    1924, Salzburg, 227
    1927, Innsbruck, 471
    1965, Copenhagen, 225
    1971, Vienna, 589
    1999, Santiago, 84
    in Bad Homburg, 173
    in Germany, 235
    in Holland, 360
    in Rome, 285
International Psychoanalytic Library, 294
International Psychoanalytical Association (IPA), 136
    Abraham and, 1–2
    and Brazil, 58
    and China, 85
    and Czech Republic, 137
    democratization of, 59
    and Denmark, 144
    and Dutch psychoanalysts, 360
    and education of analysts, 167
    Eitingon president of, 173
    Ferenczi and, 203
    founding of, 225
    Fromm dropped from membership of, 231
    Hartmann president of, 254
    influence of Freud's political views on, 330
    Jones and, 293, 294, 445
    Lacan denied admission as a teacher to, 209
    and Mexico, 342
    modernization of, 59
    and Netherlands, 359
    and Norway, 383–384
    and persecution of Argentinean psychoanalysts, 330
    and Peru, 412, 413
    Reich excluded from, 471
    and Sweden, 554
    and United States, 582–583
    and Venezuela, 589
    and World War II, 467
International Society for Medical Psychotherapy, 299
Internationale Zeitschrift für Psychoanalyse, 225
    Fenichel editor of, 200
    Hartmann editor of, 254
    Tausk in, 563
Internationaler Psychoanalytischer Verlag
    Eitingon director of, 173
    Marie Bonaparte and, 52
interpersonal psychologists, 39
interpersonal school of psychoanalysis
    Horney as inspiration of, 263
    Sullivan and, 550
Interpersonal Theory of Psychiatry (Sullivan), 550
interpretation, **280–282**, 452
    clinical method of, 157
Interpretation of Dreams, The (Freud), 55, 61, 88, 220, 223, 224, 226, 443, 447
    binding, 46
    different concepts of regression in, 468
    displacement, 152
    ego, 170
    elements of psychoanalytical methodology implicit in, 188

    endopsychic perception, 252
    and Freud's readings of philosophical literature, 371
    influences on, 442
    Millian form of argument in, 418
    myths, 353
    overdetermination, 406
    primal scene, 424
    psychoanalysis as postmodernist enterprise, 345–346
    Rank's "Dream and Myth" included in editions from 1914 to 1922, 461
    reference to King Oedipus, 397
    references to Schopenhauer, 506
    and Sachs, 501
    shame and dreams of being naked, 526
    topographical model of the mind, 107, 438, 442
    unconscious, 578
    von Hartmann cited in, 376
intersubjectivism, 257
Introduction to the Neuro-Scientific Works of Sigmund Freud, An (Solms), 118
Introductory Lectures on Psychoanalysis (Psycho-Analysis) (Freud), 208, 226
    on artists, 112
    autoerotism, 38
    free will, 215
    homosexuality, 260
    infantile sexuality, 588
    Marie Bonaparte and, 52
    obsessional behavior, 190
    perverted sexuality, 277
    reception in the United States, 466
    transference, 442
    translation in Chinese, 85
introjection. *See* identification
"Introjection and Transference" (Ferenczi), 201
inversion, 258. *See* homosexuality
"invert," 258
involutional depression. *See* depression
Irigaray, Luce, 197
    on Freuds views on sexual differences, 196
Irma dream, 223, 302, 335
irrationality, **282–283**
    drive-theory model, 283
    reasons-explanation model, 282–283
Isaacs, Susan S., 243
    "Nature and Function of Phantasy, The," 306
Isakower, Otto, 453
isolation, 140, **283–284**
Israels, H., 508
It, the, 245
Italian Association of Psychoanalysis, 285
Italian Psychoanalytical Society, 284, 285
Italy and psychoanalysis, **284–286**

J

Jackson, Earl, Jr., 576
Jackson Nursery (Vienna), 218
Jacobs van Merlen, Therese, 45
Jacobson, Edith, 146, 200, 386
    in Berlin, 236, 330

object relations, 357
  and politics, 236
Jaffe, Aniela, 300
Jaffe v. Redmond, 102
Jahrbuch, 238
*Jahrbuch für psychoanalytische und psychopathologische
    Forschungen*, 225
James, William, 225, 298
  and dissociationist model of the unconscious, 576
  on Fechner, 193
  at Freud's lectures at Clark University, 582
  Jung and, 299
  and occult phenomena, 395
Janet, Paul, 287, 395, 576
Janet, Pierre, 68, 222, **287–290**, 298, 364, 488
  child development, 421
  disaggregation, 153
  dissociationist model of the unconscious, 576
  experiments on telepathic suggestion, 395
  on hysteria, 267, 350, 437, 478, 480
  and traumatic neuroses, 572
Japan and psychoanalysis, **290–292**
Japanese Psychoanalytic Society, 291
Jaspers, Karl, 131, 334
  General Psychopathology, 335
jealousy, relationship with paranoia and homosexuality, 260
Jekels, Ludwig, 554
Jelgersma, Gebrandus, 359
Jensen, Wilhelm, 147
Jerusalem, Wilhelm, 379, 380
"Jesus der Jude" (Andreas-Salomé), 21–22
Jetmalani, Narain, 276
Jewish intelligentsia, and early psychoanalysis, 591
Joffe, Adolf, 330
Joffe, Max, 14
Joffe, W. G., 100, 393
Joffe, Wally, 14
Johnson, Allen, 264
Johnson, Virginia, 177, 525, 588
jokes and humor, **292–293**
Jokes and Their Relationship to the Unconscious (Freud),
    112, 205, 224
  written simultaneously with *Three Essays*, 292
Jokipaltio, Leena-Maija, 205, 206
Jones, Enrico, 493
Jones, Ernest, 13, 26, 35, 36, 62, 97, 177, 225, 242, **293–294**, 445
  analyzed by Ferenczi, 204
  on Anna O., 25
  biography of Freud, 222, 228
  and Brazil, 58
  and Canada, 65
  and Danish-Norwegian society, 383
  and Ferenczi, 203
  on Freud-Fliess correspondence, 269
  at Freud's lectures at Clark University, 582
  and genetics, 233
  Hamlet and Oedipus, 265
  head of the psychoanalytic movement, 445
  on Herbart's influence on Freud, 254
  and Indian Psychoanalytic Society, 275
  influence on Freud's views on women, 195

  and *International Zeitschrift für Psychoanalyse*, 225
  Klein and, 303
  Life and Work of Sigmund Freud, The, 436
  member of the Berlin Psychoanalytical Training Institute, 236
  and Mexico, 341
  and Nietzsche, 369, 370
  on penis envy, 411
  and Rank, 227, 461, 462
  on the secret committee, 98–99
  secret committee member, 97, 225
  on Stekel, 539
  Strachey and, 540
  on symbolism, 306, 559
  and translation, 70
Jong, Erica, 325
Joseph, Betty, 243
Journal for Psychology and Sexual Economy, 471
Journal of Psychoanalytic Anthropology, 25
Journal of Psychological Anthropology, 25
Journal of the American Psychoanalytic Association, 137
Joyce, James, 325, 346
Judaism, and Freud, **294–298**
Juefu, Gao, 85
Jung, Carl Gustav, 4, 35, 47, 224, **298–300**
  Abraham and, 1
  and Anna O., 25
  autonomy of patient, 181
  at Clark University, 225
  criticism of infantile sexuality, 598
  defection of, 225, 445
  and Dutch psychiatrists, 359
  Eitingon and, 172
  Electra complex, 174
  Ferenczi and, 200
  and Freud, 26, 98, 225, 445
  influence in the United States, 584
  influence in Venezuela, 590
  influence on Freud, 26
  and *Jahrbuch für psychoanalytische and
      psychopathologische Forschungen*, 225
  and Nietzsche, 369
  Piaget and, 421
  president of International Psychoanalytical Association, 225
  and Reichsinstitut, 236
  and Schreber, 507
  Spielrein and, 536
  Vienna Psychoanalytic Society and, 597
Junova, Hana, 137

K

Kächele, H., 114, 238, 492
Kafka, Franz, 346
Kagan, Jerome, 134
Kahane, Max, 597
Kakar, Sudhir, 276
Kannabikh, I. V., 497
Kant, Immanuel, 271, 418, 419
Kantrowitz, Judy, 20, 493
Kanzer, M., 564
Kaplan, E. Ann, 87

Kaposi, Moriz, 62
Kardiner, Abram, 27, 262, 330
    and psychoanalysis, 264
Karminski, Hannah, 24
Karon, B. P., 503
Karpe, M., 136
Karpe, R., 136
Karush, A., 602
Kassowitz, Max, 222, 301
Kassowitz Institute, **301–302**
Katan, Annie, 218
Katan, Maurits, 360
    and Anna Freud, 218
Katharina case, 424
Kay, Ellen, 21
Keilson, Hans, 361
Kelman, Harold, 556
Kemper, Werner, 58
    in Berlin, 236
    and Central Institute for Psychic Illnesses, 237
Kenya, psychoanalysis in, 13
Kernberg, Otto F., 83, 116, 133, 238, 386, 413, 467, 584
    ambivalence, 16
    borderline conditions, 488, 494
    conflict, 104–105
    distinction between repression and splitting, 490
    influence in Mexico, 342
    masochism, 333
    narcissism, 358–359
    origin of homosexuality, 261
    splitting, 488, 538
    sponsor of Peruvian study group, 413
    treatment of narcissistic personalities, 452
    treatment of schizophrenia, 502
Kerrigan, William, 265
Khan, Masud, 276
    supervisor of Peña, 412
Kierkegaard, Søren, 182
Kim, Sung Hee, 309
Kinberg, Olof, 553
King, Pearl, 205
King Oedipus (Sophocles), 277, 397
Kinsey, Alfred, 177, 525
Kitcher, Patricia, 43
Kizer, M., 589
Kleimberg, León, 414
Klein, George, 191, 339, 585
    and role of the self, 105–106
Klein, H., 20
Klein, Melanie, 34, 81, 114, 191, 197, 218, 238, 242, **302–304**, 317, 386, 467. *See also* Controversial Discussions
    ambivalence, 16
    analyzed by Abraham, 2
    analyzed by Ferenczi, 204, 243
    and Brazil, 59
    criminality, 115
    depression, 146
    developmental theory, 149
    family romance, anticipating ideas of, 187
    Ferenczi's influence on, 390

Glover's struggle with, 239–240
    identification, 273
    influence in India, 276
    influence in the United States, 583, 584
    Jones and, 294
    object relations, 357
    and objects, 386
    on Schreber, 508
    splitting, 388, 538
    Strachey and, 540
    translations in Swedish, 556
Kleinian analysts, 309
    independent organization in the United States, 583
    treatment of borderline and psychotic individuals, 502
Kleinian theory, **304–309**
    in Canada, 66
    different from object relations theory, 386
    influence in Venezuela, 590
    in Mexico, 342
    in Sweden, 555, 556
Kline, Paul, 67, 429, 430
    and experimental evidence, 185
Kluckhohn, Clyde, 25, 26
Kluft, R. P., 351
Klüwer, Rolf, 137
Knapp, P., 20
Kneipp, Sebastian, 362
knowing *versus* acknowledging, 283
Koch, Adelheid, 58
Kocourek, Jiří, 137
Kohut, Heinz, 133, 146, 238, 467, 551, 557
    conflict theory, 106
    developmental theory, 151
    Ferenczi's influence on, 204
    Horney and, 263
    influence in Mexico, 342
    narcissism, 358
    psychoanalytic research and, 584
    repression, 480
    self psychology, 169, 523, 583
Koitta, Saida, 276
Kojève, Alexandre, 315, 316, 318
Koller, Carl, 221
"Komik und Humor" (Lipps), 292
Königstein, Leopold, 221
Kopp, Viktor, 330
Korchin, S. J., 213
Korea and psychoanalysis, **309–310**
Korean Academy of Psychotherapy, 310
Korean Association of Jungian Psychology, 310
Koren Psychoanalytic Study Group, 310
Kosawa Heisaku, 290, 291, 309
Kouretas, Demetrios, 244
Kouretas, Nikos, 245
Kovács, Vilma, 204
Kraepelin, Emil, 364, 460, 598
Krafft-Ebing, Richard, 176, 224, **310–312**
    on Freud's "Etiology of Hysteria," 223
    on homosexuality, 176
Kragh, Ulf, 556
Kramer, Robert, 462

Kraus, Karl, 222
Kris, A., 106
Kris, Ernst, 111, 206, 207, **312–314**, 467, 583
    and Anna Freud, 218
    and regression, 469
Kris, Marianne, 312
    and Anna Freud, 218
Kristeva, Julia, 197, 317
Kroeber, Alfred, 26, 264
Krohn, A., 269
Krystal, H., 573
Kubie, Lawrence S., 240
Kucera, Otokar, 137
Kuhn, Thomas, 184
    postmodernism of, 345
Kuipe, Piet, 238
Kulish, N., 593
Kulovesi, Vriö, 554
Kulovesi, Yrjö, 205
Kurz, O., 312
Kurzweil, Edith, 238

L

LaBarre, W., 268
Labarthe, Carmen, 414
Labyrinths of Madness (Delgado), 414
Lacan, Jacques, 45, 86, 133, 315–319, 346, 347
    on Dora, 155, 156
    founder of École Freudienne de Paris, 209
    in Greece, 244
    and Heidegger, 266
    influence on Mitchell, 197
    linguistic usage and choice of symptoms, 176
    notion of the gaze, 266
    notion of the imaginary, 266
    and the "passe," 210
    and phenomenologists, 266
    and Saussure, 266
    and Venezuela, 590
Lacanianism, 133, 210, 316
    in Brazil, 59
    in Canada, 66
    in Chile, 83
    in Mexico, 342
    in Sweden, 556
    transmitted primarily through spoken word, 318
    in the United States, 584
Laforgue, René, 12, 52, 209, 210
Lagache, Daniel, 209
Laing, R. D., 266
    Horney and, 263
Lalande, André, 421
Lamarck, Jean-Baptiste, 201, 338
Lampl, Hans
    in Berlin, 236
    reforming Dutch training program, 360
    training patient of Sachs, 501
Lampl-de Groot, Jeanne, 236, 237, 360, 361
    in Berlin, 236

on multiple personality, 350–351
    reforming Dutch training program, 360
Lancelet, 240
Landauer, Karl
    in Berlin, 236
    emigration to Holland, 360
    and Frankfurt Psychoanalytic Institute, 231, 236
    Fromm studying with, 231
Lange, Helene, 21
Langer, Marie, 34, 330
Langer, Susan, 10
Langer, William, 457
language. *See also* slips, theory of
    Freud's interest in, 55
    linguistic usage and choice of symptoms, 176
    medicalization of Freud's language, 293
    preconscious and, 423
Language and Thought of the Child, The (Piaget), 421
Lanzer, Ernst. *See* Rat Man
Laplanche, Jean, 317
    definition of self-analysis, 520
Lapuz, Lourdes, 417
Larsson, Bo, 555
Lashley, C., 577, 578
"Lasting Effects of Psychoanalytic Treatment"
    (Schjelderup), 384
latency, 149, 162.322
    cross-cultural studies on, 494
    reaction formation tied to, 465
latent dreams, 158
Latin American Psychoanalysis Journal, 413
Lawrence, D. H., 325
lay analysis, 227, 319–320, 433
    in Canada, 65
    in Greece, 244
    Jones and, 294
    in Mexico, 342
    Netherlands and, 360
    Reik's influence in the United States, 472
    in the United States, 466, 582, 584–585
Lazare, A., 19, 405
Lazar-Geroe, Clara, 35–36
Le Coultre, Rik, 360
Leaff, L. A., 20
Lebovici, Serge, 244, 413
Lechat, Fernand, 44
Leclaire, Serge, 210, 317
left-wing psychoanalysts
    emigration from Austria, 591
    international organizations of, 330
Legend of the Artist, The (Kris and Kurz), 312
*Lehrbuch der empirischen Psychologie als inductiver
    Swissenschaft* (Linder), 377
Lehrbuch zur Psychologie (Herbart), 376
Leibniz, Gottfried Wilhelm, 118, 581
Lemlij, Moisés, 413, 414
Lemmertz, José, 58
Lennmalm, Frithiof, 553
Leonardo da Vinci
    Eissler study of, 172
    Freud's psychobiography of, 47, 225, 259–260, 264, 326, 456

Leonardo da Vinci and a Memory of His Childhood (Freud),
    47, 225, 264, 326, 456
    and defensive functions of homosexuality, 259–260
lesbianism. *See also* homosexuality
    Deutsch's analysis of, 147
    lesbian theorists and Freud, 198
Lesche, Carl, 205, 554
Leseverein der Deutschen Studenten Wiens, 371, 506
Lessing, Doris, 196
Lethargy, Actual Neurosis and Somatic Manifestations (Cesio), 34
Levenson, Edgar, 551
Levi Bianchini, Marco, 284
LeVine, Robert A., 13, 27
Levinson, H., 247
Lévi-Strauss, Claude, 317
    influence on Lacan, 316
Lewis, H. B., 527
Liberman, David, 34, 35
libido, 542
    difference between somatic and psychic, 29
    divergence between Adler and Freud on, 9
libido theory, 148, 163, **321–324**
    infantile genital organization of, 234
    line of development established by Anna Freud, 219
    in post-Freudian psychoanalysis, 323
libido-narcissism model of the mind, 542–543
Lichtheim, Anna, 223
Liébault, Ambroise, 223
Lieben, Anna von. *See* Caecilia M.
Lieberman, E. James, 462
Lieberman, Herman, 147
Liepmann, Wilhelm, 1
Life and Work of Sigmund Freud, The (Jones), 294, 436
life instinct (Eros), 164, 323, 443, 477
Life of the Human Mind, The (Gadelius), 553
Lima Association of Psychoanalytical Psychotherapy, 413
Limentani, Adam, 244, 412, 413
    supervisor of Peña, 342
Linder, Gustav Adolf, 377
Linton, Ralph, 25
Lipiner, Sigfried, 368
Lipps, Theodor, 182, 292, 379, 442
Listener, 240
Listening with the Third Ear (Reik), 473
literary criticism and psychoanalysis, 265–266, 325–326
    in Denmark, 145
    in Sweden, 553
    in the United States, 583
literature and psychoanalysis, **324–326**, 502
Little, Margaret, 554
"Little Chanticleer, A" (Ferenczi), 201
Little Hans, 8, 29, 82, 208, **326–328**, 366
    castration complex, 66
    displacement, 140, 152
    irrationality, 282
    publication of case, 181
Little Herbert. *See* Little Hans
Lloyd, A., 534
Loewald, H., 104
    conflict, 105
    identification, 273
    linguistic tradition, 266

Loewenfeld, J., 136
Loewenstein, Rudolph, 209, 467, 583
    and Kris, 312
    training patient of Sachs, 501
Loftus, Elizabeth, 96
"Logical Time and the Assertion of Anticipated Certainty:
    A New Sophism" (Lacan), 316
Lombardi, K., 424
"Looking Glass Phase, The" (Lacan), 315
Lorand, Sándor, 136
    analyzed by Ferenczi, 204
Los Angeles Psychoanalytic Study Group, 200
lost object, 388
Lothane, Z., 508
love objects, anaclictic *versus* narcissistic choice of,
    356
Low, Barbara, 423, 501
Löwenfeld, Ludwig, 207, 334
Lowenfeld Mosaic Test, 428
Lowenthal, H. Luidpold, 137
Lubbock, John, 26
Luborsky, Lester, 184, 492, 493, 494
Lucy R.
    hallucinations, 251
    repression, 479, 483–484
Luria, A. R., 497
Lussier, André, 65

M

Macalpine, I., 508
McCormick, Harold, 299
McCormick, Medill, 299
MacCurdy, J. T., 595
McCurdy, John, 65
McDougall, William, 4
McGrath, W. J., 379
McGrath, William, 229
McHugh, P., 429, 430, 431
McLennan, John F., 26
Macleod, Alastair, 65
Maeder, Alphonse, 26
Magazine of Psychoanalysis, 34
magical thinking
    of children, 421
    in obsessive-compulsive neuroses, 366
Mahler, Gustav, Reik's study of, 472
Mahler, Margaret, 187, 238, 386, 393
    developmental theory, 150
    and Ferenczi, 204
    in Greece, 244
    infant and child observation, 584
    origin of homosexuality, 261
    splitting, 538
    symbiosis, 557–558
Mahler, Martin, 137
Main, Mary, 151
Major, René, 210
Malcolm, Norman, 420
Malinowski, Bronislaw, 26
    Sex and Repression in Savage Society, 264
Maltsberger, J., 549

Man and His Symbols (Jung), 300
Man for Himself (Fromm), 467
Mandler, George, 95
manic-depressive syndrome. *See* depression
manifest dream, 158
Mann, Thomas, 325, 370
    "Freud and the Future," 228
Mannheim, Hermann, 240
Mannoni, Maud, 317
Mannoni, Octave, 12, 317
Marchand, W. E., 595
Marcondes, Durval, 58
Marcus, S., 156
Marcuse, Herbert, 236, 330
marriage, object-relations view of, 388
Martin, E., 492
Martin Luther: A Study in History and Psychoanalysis
    (Erikson), 457
Martins, Cyro, 58
Martins, Mário, 58
Martins, Zaira, 58
Marui Kiyoyasu, 290, 291
Marx, Karl, 324
Marxism
    Fenichel and, 200
    and Freudianism, **392–331**
Masling, J. M., 405
Maslow, Abraham, 263
masochism and sadism, 331, **331–334**
    Ellis on, 177
    Freud on, 15, 16
    Krafft-Ebing on, 311
    narcissism and, 355
    paranoia and, 410
Masochism in Modern Man (Reik), 473
mass hysteria, 268
"Mass Psychology of Fascism, The" (Reich), 331
massage, to recover unconscious material, 213
Masson, Jeffrey Moussaieff, 196, 269, 364, 519
Mastalier, Joseph Johann, 301
master stories, 191
Masters, William, 177, 525, 588
masturbation
    childhood, 41, 441
    Ellis on, 177
    Krafft-Ebing on, 177
    and neurasthenia, 361, 362, 437
materialism of Freud, 434
materialists' view of taboos, 562
"matheme," 319
Matisse, Henri, 346
Matte Blanco, Ignacio, 83, 84
    bilogic of experience, 423
Matthis, Iréne, 556
Mattson, G., 205
Maudsley, Henry, 576
Maupassant, Guy de, 75
Mead, Margaret, 235, 498
    and psychoanalysis, 25, 26
meaning and psychoanalysis, **334–337**
Medawar, P. B., 229
media, psychoanalytical ideas and, 58

Medical Journal of Australia, 35
medicalization of Freud's language, 293
Médications psychologiques (Janet), 287
Meehl, Paul E., 134
Meghnagi, D., 293
Mehra, Baljeet, 276
Mehra, Kamal, 276
Mehta, Purnima, 276
"Mein Dank an Freud" (Andreas-Salomé), 22
Meinong, Alexix, 60
Meissner, W., 453
    on therapeutic alliance, 564
melancholia, psychopathology of
    according to Freud, 273
    versus mourning, 548
Melbourne Institute of Psychoanalysis, 36
Memoirs of My Nervous Illness (Schreber), 141, 507, 508
Memories, Dreams, and Reflections (Jung and Jaffe),
    300
memory
    chilhood memories, 514
    cognitive psychology and Freud, 96
    dreams and, 159, 160
    Freud's interest in, 55
    neural memory networks, 56
    Piaget's criticism of Freudian conception of memory,
        422
    screen *versus* genuine memories, 313
men
    and hysteria, 268
    and Oedipus complex, 402–403, 511
    and shame, 527
    superego of, 512, 552
Menaker, Esther, 462
Mendeleyev, Dmitry, 130
Meng, Heinrich
    in Berlin, 236
    and Frankfurt Psychoanalytic Institute, 231, 236
Menninger, Karl
    Human Mind, The, 583
    and Mexico, 341
Menninger Clinic (Topeka, Kansas), 81, 417, 585
Menninger Foundation, 493
Meno, The (Plato), 118
"Mensch als Weib, Der" (Andreas-Salomé), 21
menstruation
    psychological connection with defloration, 593
    taboos about, 561–562
mental energy. *See* binding; cathexis
mental entropy, law of, 51
mental health, defined by Hartmann, 253
mental hygiene movement, 583, 584
mental illness, Schopenhauer theory of, 372, 505
Mentzos, Stavros, 244, 245
metapsychology, **337–341**
    multiple agent theory of, 419
    narcissism and, 356
Metz, Christian, 266
Mexican Group for Psychoanalytic Studies, 342
Mexican Institute of Psychoanalysis, 231
Mexican Psychoanalytic Association, 342
Mexican Society of Neurology and Psychiatry, 341

Mexico
   Fromm in, 231
   and psychoanalysis, **341–343**
Meyer, Adolf, 582
Meyers, F., 540
Meynert, Theodor, 369, 379, 458
   cognitive neuropsychology of, 418
   Freud's conflict with, 222
   influence on Freud, 364
Mikota, Václav, 137
Mill, John Stuart
   dispositionalist approach of the unconscious, 576
   Freud's translations of, 60, 118, 221, 418
   influence on Freud, 418–419
Miller, Alice, 263
Miller, Emmanuel, 268
   and *British Journal of Delinquency*, 240
Miller, Henry, 325
   and Rank, 462
Miller, Jacques-Alain, 211, 318
Millones, Luis, 414
Milner, Marion, 412
Milton, John, psychoanalytic commentary of, 265
mind, Freud's view of. *See* early models of the mind;
      structural theory; topographical model of the mind
mind and body, **343–345**, 438
"mirror-stage," theory of, 86–87, 315, 316
Miss G. de B., 517
Mitchel, S. Weir, 361
Mitchell, Juliet, 197
Mitchell, S. A., 7, 8
Mitchell, T., 562
Mitchison, G., 96
Mitscherlich, Alexander, 237, 412, 554
Mitscherlich, Margarete, 237
Modern Education (Rank), 462
modernism, Freudianism and, **345–347**
Moellenhoff, Fritz, 501, 502
Moll, Albert, 441
Monchy, René de, 554
mood. *See* affect
Moore, B. E., 392, 559
Morales, Manuel, 414
Morales, Pedro, 413
Morales Galarreta, Julio, 414
morality and psychoanalysis, **347–349**
morals, superego and, 552
Mordell, Albert, 177
Moreira, Juliano, 57
Moreno, J. L., 68
Morgan, Lewis, 26
Morgenthaler, Fritz, 14
Morrison, Andrew, 527
Moser, Fanny. *See* Emmy von N.
Moses, Ralf, 137
Moses and Monotheism (Freud), 25, 27, 228, 296–297, 456, 475
   criticism of, 476
   myths, 353
   as psychobiography, 48
Moses of Michelangelo, The (Freud), 112, 225–226

mother-infant relationships, 59
mothering theorists, 198
Mothers of Psychoanalysis (Sayers), 148
Motley, M. T., 121, 532
mourning, 356
   depression similar to, 145–146
Mourning and Melancholia (Freud), 26, 226, 283, 548
   and anaclitic object, 388
   and identification, 272–273
Movies on Your Mind (Greenberg), 266
Müller-Braunschweig, Ada, 236
Müller-Braunschweig, Carl
   in Berlin, 236, 237
   training patient of Sachs, 501
multiple personality (dissociative identity disorder),
      115, 153, 154, **349–352**
Mulvey, Laura, 198
Munich, R. L., 392
Murray, Henry, 428
Musatti, Cesare, 284, 285
Myer, Adolph, 290
Myers, Charles, 4
Myers, D. Campbell, 65
Myers, Frederick, 298
   and investigation of occult phenomena, 395
Mystery on the Mountain (Reik), 473
Myth of the Birth of the Hero, The (Rank), 461
myths, **353–354**
*Mythus von der geburt des Helden, Der (The Myth of the
      Birth of the Hero)* (Rank), 187

N

Nacht, Sacha, 209
   and Mexico, 341
Naesgaard, Sigurd, 554
Nagel, T., 121, 122
Nandy, Ashis, 276
Nanna, oder über das Seelenleben der Pflanzen (Fechner),
      193–194
narcissism, 37, 322, **355–359**
   Adler's influence on, 9
   clinical theory and, 92–93
   line of development established by Anna Freud, 115, 219
   paranoia and, 409
   shame and, 355, 527
narcissistic neuroses, 363
   acting out in, 6
   and splitting, 538
   treatment by Sullivan, 550
   treatment of, 584
narrativity and literary studies, 266
narratology, Italian psychoanalysis and, 285
"Narzissmus als Doppelrichtung" (Andreas-Salomé), 22
national character, speculation concerning, 498
National Psychological Association for Psychoanalysis
      (NPAP), 472
Natterson, J. M., 473
naturalism of Freud, 434
"Nature and Function of Phantasy, The" (Isaacs), 306

"Nature and Therapeutic Action of Psychoanalysis, The" (Strachey), 541
Nazism, psychoanalysis and, 236–237, 591
Negation (Freud), 61, 279
negative transference, 450
Neisser, Ulrich, 96
Nelson, Marie, 13
neo-analysis, 237
neo-Darwinism. *See* selfish gene theory
Neruda, a Psychoanalytical Reading (Altamirano), 414
nervous system, Freud's theory of, 425–426
Nesse, R., 534
Netherlands
    and psychoanalysis, **359–361**
    Reik in, 472
Neu, Jerome, 264
neurasthenia, 31–32, **361–363**, 437
    and World War I, 595
neuropsychopharmacology, Freud as founder of, 118
Neuro-psychoses of Defense, The (Freud), 103
    dispositionalism in, 576
    on repression, 479, 480
neuroscience, 433, 575
    and clinical psychoanalysis, 55
    cognitive-emotional, 54, 56
    and sleep, 529
neuroses, **363–368**. *See also* actual neuroses; anxiety neurosis; character neurosis; childhood neurosis; narcissistic neuroses; obsessional neurosis; obsessive-cumpulsive neurosis; traumatic neurosis; war neurosis
    acting out in, 6
    and character neurosis, 73
    etiology of, 392
    Ferenci's work on, 202
    Hartmann and, 253
    Horney's model for the structure of, 262
    and infantile sexuality, 416
    Krafft-Ebing on, 311
    role of unconscious phantasies, 189
    and splitting of the ego, 488
Neuroses and Character Types (Deutsch), 147
Neurosis and Human Growth (Horney), 261
Neurosis and the Neurotic Character (Schjelderup), 384
Neurotic Personality of Our Time, The (Horney), 261, 262, 467
neutralization, 313
"Neutralization and Sublimation: Observations on Young Children" (Kris), 313
Névroses, Les (Janet), 288
Névroses et les idées fixes, Les (Janet), 288
New Informants, The: The Betrayal of Confidentiality in Psycho-analysis and Psychotherapy (Bollas and Sundelson), 101–102
New Introductory Lectures on Psycho-Analysis (Freud), 16, 73, 228
    id, 271
    outcome of therapy, 513
    psychoanalisis as modernist enterprise, 345
    seduction theory, 518
    telepathy, 396
    translation in Chinese, 85

two readings of "Wo es war, soll ich werden," 346–347
New Jung Scholarship, 300
"New Psychology, The" (Ellis), 178
New School for Social Research
    Ferenczi at, 204
    Reich at, 471
New Sydenham Society (London), 76
New Ways in Psychoanalysis (Horney), 261, 262
New York City
    Ferenczi at, 204
    Rank in, 462
    Reich in, 471
    Reik in, 472, 582
New York Psychoanalytic Institute, 231
New York Times, 240
"Next Assignment, The" (Langer), 457
Nichols, N. P., 68
Niederland, W. G., 508
Nielsen, Nils, 557
Nietzsche, Friedrich Wilhelm, 119, 182, 183, 324, 335, **368–370**
    Andreas-Salomé and, 21
    anticipating key ideas of Freud, 235
    influence on Freud, 26, 368, 374–375, 381, 419
    Tausk's view of, 563
Nietzsche in Seinen Werken (Andreas-Salomé), 21
Nilsson, Alf, 556
Nin, Anaïs, 325
    and Rank, 462
nineteenth-century precursors of Freud, **370–383**.
    See also specific precursors
nirvana principle, 423
Noble, Douglas, 65
Noll, Richard, 299
nonmedical analysis. *See* lay analysis
Nordic Psychoanalytic Society, 383
Nordic Psychoanalytical Association, 554
Norell, Margit, 556
Normality and Pathology in Childhood (A. Freud), 218
Norman, Johan, 556
Norway
    and psychoanalysis, **383–384**
    Reich in, 471
Norwegian Psychoanalytic Institute, 384
Norwegian-Danish Psychoanalytic Society, 384
"Note upon the 'Mystic Writing Pad,' A" (Freud), 61
"Notes on Some Schizoid Mechanisms" (Klein), 306
"Notes on the Development of Some Current Problems in Child Psychology" (Kris), 313
"Notes on the Theory of Agression" (Harmann, Kris and Loewenstein), 313
Nothnagel, Hermann, 221, 224, 301
not-me experience, 489, 551
Notturno, M., 429, 430, 431
Nousiainen, Tapio, 205
Novelletto, A., 285
Nunberg, H., 74
    on shame, 526
Nuñez Saavedra, Carlos, 83
Nycander, Gunnar, 555

O

Oberholzer, Emil, 416
object, **385–386**
  Freud on, 387–388
  in the libido-narcissism model of the mind, 542
object constancy, Hartmann and, 252
object relations theory, 39, 104, 133, **386–391**, 584.
    See also British object relations theories
  in Canada, 66
  character concept, 72
  criminology, 115
  feminist, 197
  in Germany, 238
  importance of actual mother, 386
  line of development of, established by Anna Freud, 219
  and neuroses, 367
  Rank and, 462
  sociobiology and, 534
  Sullivan and, 550
  symbiosis, 557
  theories of agression, 114
  in United States, 467
"object removal," 81
Observations on Transference-Love (Freud), 568
obsessional neurosis, 88, 99. *See also* obsessive-compulsive
    neurosis
  hallucinations in, 252
  Rat Man and, 462
  role of unconscious fantasies, 190
  sexual origin of, 437, 515
  symptom formation, 90
  treated pharmacologically, 392–393
  undoing in, 140
obsessional phenomena, **391–395**
obsessions
  description and classification, 458
  distinguished from obsessive-compulsive neuroses,
    392
Obsessions et la psychathénie, Les (Janet), 288
Obsessive Actions and Religious practices (Freud), 296
obsessive-compulsive neurosis, 18, 366, 367
obstinacy, 18–19, 464–465
  obsessional character and, 99
  paranoia and, 409
occult, Freud and, **395–397**
"Occult Significance of Dreams, The" (Freud), 396
O'Connnor, Noreen, 147
O'Connor, John Cardinal, 122
Oedipal triads, 401–402
Oedipe Africain (Ortigues and Ortigues), 13
Oedipus (Sophocles)
  Freud and, 398–400
  Nietzsche and Freud's references to, 369
Oedipus complex, 82, 277, 321–322, 323, **397–404**, 441
  and character development, 72
  dissolution of, 322
  evolutionary scenario for, 49
  and incestuous feelings, 274
  Klein's depressive position and, 308
  literature and, 325
  objections of feminists to, 196

reinterpreted in context of phallic stage, 234
resolution of, 91, 365
revised view in Japan, 291
revised view in Korea, 310
role of, 89
scientific tests of dynamics, 511–512
used to explain how civilization originiated, 456
Oedipus in the Trobriands (Spiro), 264
Oedipus Ubiquitous (Johnson and Price-Williams), 264
Of Love and Lust (Reik), 473
Ogden, T. H.
  as object relations theorist, 386
  treatment of schizophrenia, 503
Ohtsuki Kenji, 291
Okonogi Keigo, 291
Olden, K., 136
Olivares, J., 589
Oliveira, Walderêdo de, 58
omega system, 426
"On a Question Preliminary to Any Possible Treatment of
    Psychosis" (Lacan), 316
On Aphasia (Freud), 33, 222
  influence of John Hughlings Jackson, 438
  mental states identified with physical states, 419
  "object representation," 385
  parallelist view of mind-body, 343, 344
  regression, 468
"On Coca" (Freud), 221
On Narcissism (Freud), 226, 359
  autoerotism, 37
  development of psychoanalysis, 355
  ego, 170
  shame and self-esteem regulation, 526
"On Neurotic Exogamy" (Abraham), 1, 3
"On Psychoanalysis" (Freud), 35
"On Rationalization in Everyday Life" (Jones), 293
"On Some Vicissitudes of Insight in the Course of
    Psychoanalysis" (Kris), 314
On Suggestion (Bernheim), 223
On the Early Development of the Mind (Glover), 239
"On the Efficacy of Psychoanalysis" (Barach et al.), 127
On the Genealogy of Morals (Nietzsche), 375
  discussed by the Vienna Psychoanalytic Society, 369
  studied by Freud, 370
On the Highest Good (Fechner), 193
On the History of the Psychoanalytic Movement (Freud),
    7, 225, 435, 445
  mention of Scandinavian countries, 553
  reference to Chilean paper, 83
  and seduction theory, 518
"On the limits of our understanding of nature" (Du Bois-
    Reymond), 438
On the Method of Right and Wrong Cases (Fechner), 194
"On the Origin of the Influencing Machine in
    Schizophrenia" (Tausk), 563
"On the Psychological Content of a Case of Schizophrenia"
    (Spielrein), 536
"On the Psychology of Marxism" (Adler), 329
"On the Significance of Sexual Trauma in Childhood
    for the Symptomatology of Dementia Praecox"
    (Abraham), 2
"Open Letter to Biographers" (Ellis), 177

Ophuijsen, Johann H. W. van, 360
  secret committee member, 99
  in South Africa, 13
Oppenheim, H., 572
oral character, **405–406**
  scientific tests of, 511
oral stage of development, 162, 321
  Abraham, 308
  and schizophrenia, 503
orderliness, 18–19, 464–465
  obsessional character and, 99
Organisation Psychanalytique de Langue Française
    (Organization for French-Speaking Psychoanalysis),
    211
orgasm, vaginal and clitoral, **587–589**
orgone theory, 471
"Origins of Language and Freudian Psychology, The"
    (Triandagyllidis), 244
Origins of Psychoanalysis, The (Bonaparte, A. Freud and
    Kris), 409
Ornstein, P. H., 156
Ortigues, Edmond, 13
Ortigues, Marie-Cécile, 13
Osipov, Nikolai, 136, 497
Ottalagano, C., 589
Our Inner Conflicts (Horney), 261
outcome studies of psychoanalytic treatment, 492, 493,
    512–514, 585
Outline of Psychoanalysis, An (Freud), 228
  on analytic pact, 564
  on id, 271
  on neurotic conditions, 459
Outline of the Distinctive Character of the Theory of
    Scientific Knowledge (Fichte), 558
overdetermination, **406–407**

P

Palacios, Agustín, 342
Palmstierna, Vera, 554
Pan-American congresses, 34
Paneth, Joseph, 221
  and Nietzsche, 368, 369
Pankejeff, Sergei. See Wolf Man
"Papers on Psychoanalysis" (Jones), 294
Pappenheim, Bertha. See Anna O.
Paquet, Alfons, 241
paranoia, **409–410**
  delusions, 142
  hallucinations in, 252
  and homosexuality, 260
  projection in, 140
  scientific tests of etiology of, 510
  splitting, 538
paranoid-schizoid position of Klein, 304, 306, 307
parapraxes. See slips, theory of
Parell, Ernst. See Reich Wilhelm
Parerga and Paralipomena (Schopenhauer), 505
Parin, Paul, 14
Parin-Matthèy, Goldy, 14
Parkin, Alan, 65, 66
Parres, Ramón, 341, 342

parricide
  Oedipal theme and, 113
  in Totem and Taboo, 400, 456–457, 473
parsimoniousness, 18–19, 464–465
  obsessional character and, 99
Parsons, Talcott, 467
"passe," experiment of the, 210–211, 318
pathogenesis, 5
  and reality testing, 465
pathogenesis of narcissism, 357
patients
  autonomy of, 181
  of the early 2000s, 211–212
  suffering from malaise and neuroses, 467
Paul, Robert, 264
Pavlov, Ivan Petrovich, 498
Payne, Sylvia, 501
Paz de la Puente, María, 414
Peau noire, masques blancs (Fanon), 12
Pederson, Stefi, 554
Peña, Saúl, 412, 413, 414
Péndola, Alberto, 413, 414
penis envy, 66–67, 149, 402, **410–411**, 587
  reinterpreted in context of phallic stage, 234
  strategies to cope with, 179–180
penis-baby equation, 512
percept-genetic methodology of psychological testing, 556
perception, Freud's interest in, 55
perceptual consciousness, 109, 542
perceptual malfunction, denial as, 143
perceptual system, 107
Perestrello, Danielo, 58
Perestrello, Marialzira, 58
Perls, Fritz, 68
  in South Africa, 13
Perrier, François, 211
Perrotti, Nicola, 284, 285
Perry, R., 149
Persona (Bergman), psychoanalytic criticism of, 87
personal perception, 289
personality types, 96
Peru and psychoanalysis, **411–414**
Peruvian Institute of Psychoanalysis, 413
Peruvian Institute of Psychotherapy, Research, and
    Interdisciplinary Application of Psychoanalysis
    Sigmund Freud, 413
Peruvian Library of Psychoanalysis, 414
Peruvian Psychiatric Association, 412
Peruvian Psychoanalytical Society, 412, 413–414
perversions, 163, 321, **414–416**. See also fetishism
  and disavowel, 522
  as failures to achieve full genital primacy, 234
Peto, A., 468
Peto, Andrew, 36
Pfister, Oskar, 225, 246, **416**, 474, 475
  correspondence with Freud, 416, 474
  Piaget and, 421
  Scandinavians in analysis with, 554
phallic stage of development, 162, 234, 321–322, 403
phantasy. See fantasy
Pharmaceutisches Centralblatt, 193
phenomenology, 59

Phenomenology of Mind, The (Hegel), 558
Phenomenology of Spirit (Hegel), 316
phi system, 426
Philippines and psychoanalysis, **417–418**
philosophy and psychoanalysis, 266, **418–420**
Philosophy of Mind (Hegel), 558
Philosophy of the Unconscious (Von Hartmann), 375, 506
phobias
    description and classification, 458
    fear of heights, 485
    sexual origin of, 437
phobic neuroses, 366, 367
photography use at the Salpêtrière, 76
phylogenetics
    experience of birth, 29
    formation of the systems of the mind, 545
physicalism, 94–95
Piaget, Jean, 95–96, 393, **420–422**
    psychoanalyzed by Spierlrein, 536
Picasso, Pablo, 346
Pichler, Hans, 227
Pichón Rivière, Enrique, 34, 342
    in Sweden, 556
Pierloot, Roland, 45
Piers, G., 526–527
Pigman, G. W., 265
Pineda, Francisco González, 342
Pines, Dinora, 245
Pines, Malcolm, 14
Pirillo, N., 285
Planck, Max, 241
Plata, Carlos, 413
Plataforma, 330
Plato, 118
play therapy
    developed by Klein, 149, 303, 305, 309
    Freud on, 112
    in lieu of free association with children, 80
    use by Anna Freud, 149
pleasure principle, 387, **422–423**
    and affect, 11
    and conflicts, 102
    and infantile sexuality, 277
Poe, Edgar Allan, 53
Poetzl, Otto, 213
Poetzl Phenomenon, 214
Poincaré, Henri, 579
Poland, W., 448–449, 453
Poliklinik für Psychoanalytische Behandlung Nervöser
        Krankheiten. *See* Berlin Psycho-Analytical Institute
politics, psychoanalysis and, 58, 236
Pontalis, J. B., 317
    definition of self-analysis, 520
Popper, J., 177
Popper, Karl, 257, 420, 428–429, 432
Portman Clinic (England), 240–241
Pöstenyi, Andras, 555
post-Freudian psychoanalysis
    conceptualizations of conflict, 104–106
    critique of, 133–134
    views on crime, 115–116

post-Kleinian theories, 66
postmodernism, Freudianism and, **345–347**
    postmodernist feminists and psychoanalysis, 197
posttraumatic stress disorder, 351, 573, 595
    cathartic treatment of, 68
Potamianou, Anna, 244, 245
Prados, Miguel, 65
Prague Institute of Psychoanalysis, 137
preambivalence, 16, 17
preconscious, 107, **423–424**, 542, 578
    term introduced by Hartmann, 376
pregenital eroticism. *See* infantile sexuality
"Preliminaries to a Metapsychology" (Freud), 338
Preliminary Communications (Breuer and Freud),
        117, 124–125
    influence of Nietzsche on, 369
    and repression, 478, 479, 487
presentation, 60, 61
pressure technique, 223, 440, 441, 515, 547
    to recover unconscious material, 213
    used in case of Elizabeth von R., 175
Pribram, Karl, 420
Price-Williams, Douglass, 264
pride system (Horney), 263
Prihoda, Petr, 137
primal repression. *See* repression
primal scene, **424–425**
primary clinical model, formation of, 87–88
primary narcissism, 355, 387
Prince, Morton, 488
    and dissociationist model of the unconscious, 576
"Principles or Relaxation and Neocatharsis, The"
        (Ferenczi), 202
prohibitory suggestion, 547
Project for a Scientific Psychology (Freud), 48, 61, 70, 95,
        108, 223, 226, **425–426**
    ambiguity of terminology, 29
    connectionist model of the unconscious, 577
    displacement, 283
    distinction between perception and memory, 577
    ego, 169
    influence of Brentano on, 418
    materialist position, 434
    mental states identified with physical states, 419
projection, 140, **426–427**
    narcissism and, 355
    overused in paranoia, 409
    racism and, 141
projective techniques, **427–428**
"Propos sur la causalité psychique" (Lacan), 316
Prospero et Caliban: Psychologie de la colonization
        (Mannoni), 12
"Protocols of the Vienna Psychoanalytical Society," 97
Proust, Marcel, 346
    *A la recherche du temps perdu (Remembrance of
        Things Past)*, 277
Prunes, Celestino, 58
pseudoscience and psychoanalysis, **428–432**
psi system, 426
Psiche (journal), 285
Psyche, 238

Psychiatric Interview (Sullivan), 550
"Psychiatrie anglaise et la guerre, La" (Lacan), 316
Psychiatrist and the Dying Patient, The (Eissler), 172
psychiatry
    drug treatments, 392–393, 460
    effect of biological and pharmacological advances, 584, 585
    importance of diagnosis with introduction of drug
        treatments, 460
    interest in war neurosis, 572
    military, 595
    and psychoanalysis, **432–434**
    and use of term neuroses, 363
psychic energy, theory of, 434. *See also* cathexis
    distinguished from theory of affects, 30
psychic mechanism of Herbart, 255
psychic trauma, 572
psychical determinism, 104, 215, **434–345**
    and child psychoanalysis, 79
    as opposed to existentialism, 182–183
"Psychischer Kontakt und Vegetative Strömung" (Psychic
    Contact and Vegetative Flow) (Reich), 471
"Psychoanalyse in der Jungendbewegung, Die"
    (Psychoanalysis in the youth movement) (Bernfield), 199
psychoanalysis
    contemporary, 133, 243
    first use of the term, 439
    and growth of psychiatry, 433
    internationalization of, 224–225
    origin and history of, **435–444**
    as science, 51, 585–586
Psychoanalysis: A Theory in Crisis (Edelson), 133
"Psychoanalysis, Psychology of the Unconscious"
    (Kouretas), 244
Psychoanalysis (Glover), 239
Psychoanalysis and Feminism (Mitchell), 197
"Psychoanalysis and its relationship with child psychology"
    (Piaget), 421
Psychoanalysis and Moral Values (Hartmann), 253
Psychoanalysis and Shakespeare (Holland), 265
Psychoanalysis and Society (Peru), 414
Psycho-Analysis and Telepathy (Freud), 396
Psychoanalysis of Becoming Ill, The (Chiozza), 34
"Psycho-Analysis of Children, The" (Klein), 306
Psychoanalysis of Children (Aberastury, Garma, and Ferrer), 34
Psychoanalysis of Dreams (Garma), 34
Psychoanalysis of the Neuroses (Deutsch), 147
Psychoanalysis Technique (Racker), 34
Psychoanalytic Clinic (Mexico), 342
psychoanalytic cognitive neuroscience, 51–52
Psychoanalytic Confederation (Federation) of Latin
    America, 342
Psychoanalytic Explorations in Art (Kris), 312
psychoanalytic feminists, 197, 198
psychoanalytic movement, 435, **444–446**
    importance of women in, 197
*Psychoanalytic Notes on an Autobiographical Account of a
    Case of Paranoia (Dementia Paranoides)* (Freud), 260
Psychoanalytic Practice (Kächele and Thomä), 238
Psychoanalytic Quarterly, 453
    Fenichel editor of, 200
    Glover on editorial board, 239

Psychoanalytic Study of Society, 25
Psychoanalytic Study of the Child
    Glover on editorial board, 239
    Kris managing editor of, 312
Psychoanalytic Study of the Myth of Dionysius and Apollo, A
    (Deutsch), 147
psychoanalytic technique and process, **446–454**, 453
    analyst's role during free association, 212–213
    Freud's technique in Dora case, 155–156
    Kris on, 313
    number of sessions per week, 585
    personal variable of the practitioner, 281
    research on process of psychoanalysis, 492, 512–514
    Sullivan and, 550
    transference and resistance, 569–571
    used in the case of the Rat Man, 464
    in Wolf Man's case, 598
Psychoanalytic Theory of Neurosis, The (Fenichel), 200
    description of defense mechanism, 139
    mentioning Kulovesi, 205
Psychoanalytic Therapy (Alexander and French), 540
Psychoanalytical Association (Denmark), 554
Psychoanalytical Association of Buenos Aires, 35
Psychoanalytical Federation of Latin America, 34
Psychoanalytical Field, The (Baranger), 34
psychoanalytical sessions
    length of, 318
    number per week, 585
Psychoanalytical Society of Caracas, 590
*Psychoanalytical Study of Individual Personality as the Basis
    for the Development of Scientific Ideas, A* (Hermann), 193
psychoanalytically oriented psychotherapy, **454–456**
    Stekel and, 539
psychobiography. *See* biography and psychoanalysis
psychodynamics
    catharsis and, 68
    Herbart's influence on Freud, 255
psychohistory, 353, **456–458**
    Sachs' psychoanalytical portraits of historical figures, 502
psychohygiene, 498
psycholinguists, and theory of slips, 530, 531
Psychological Birth of the Human Infant, The (Mahler), 558
psychological mindedness, concept of, 20
Psychological Types (Jung), 299
Psychological Wednesday Society (*Psychologische Mittwoch-
    Gesellschaft*). *See* Vienna Psychoanalytic Society;
    Wednesday Society
Psychologie als Wissenschaft (Herbart), 193, 376
Psychology and Soul-Belief (Rank), 462
Psychology from an Empirical Standpoint (Brentano),
    59–60, 418
"Psychology of Daydreams, The" (Varendonck), 44
Psychology of Dementia Praecox, The (Jung), 298
Psychology of Fear and Courage, The (Glover), 239
Psychology of Sex Relations, The (Reik), 473
Psychology of the Unconscious, The (Jung, trans. Hinkle), 299
Psychology of Women, The (Deutsch), 147
Psychology of Women's Sexual Functions, The (Deutsch), 147
psychoneuroimmunology, 50–51
psychoneuroses, 361
    distinguished from actual neuroses, 363

psychoneuroses (*continued*)
   as failures to achieve full genital primacy, 234
   and repression, 484
Psychopathia Sexualis (Krafft-Ebing), 310, 311
Psychopathologie Africaine (journal), 13
psychopathology, **458–460**
   Anna Freud's developmental theory of, 115
   Freud *versus* Fenichel, 459
Psychopathology of Everyday Life, The (Freud), 130, 224, 396
   occult phenomena, 395
   overdetermination, 407
   term screen memories, 514
psychopathy, 114
psychopharmacology, 433, 460
psychoses, 363. *See also* paranoia; schizophrenia
   Freud on, 409, 459
   hallucinations and, 427
   reality testing, 465
   splitting of the ego, 488, 537, 538
psychosexual development. *See* developmental theory, libido
   theory; infantile sexuality
Psychosis (Pichón Rivière and Rolla), 34
psychosomatic medicine, 539
   Groddeck and, 245
Psychosomatic Medicine (Uexküll), 238
psychotics, analysis of
   in Brazil, 59
   Klein's influence on, 309
   treatment by Sullivan, 550
Psykiatriens Grundtraeek (An Outline of Psychoanalysis)
   (Vogt), 383
puberty, 322
Putnam, James J., 225
   and autonomy of patient, 181
   at Freud's lectures at Clark University, 582
Pynchon, Thomas, 346

Q

qualia, 577
queer theorists, 198
Question of Lay Analysis, The (Freud), 227, 320, 416
   written in defense of Reik, 472
Questionnement Psychanalytique, 45
Quijada, H., 589
Quine, Willard van Orman, 420

R

Racker, Enrique, 34, 342
Racker (E.) Investigation and Direction Center, 34
Radó, Sándor
   analyzed by Abraham, 2
   Fenichel analyzed by, 199
   and Ferenczi, 204
   Hartmann analyzed by, 254
Rainer Maria Rilke (Andreas-Salomé), 22
Ramanujam, B. K., 276
Ramírez, Santiago, 341, 342, 343
Rancour-Laferriere, Daniel, 498–499
Rangell, Leo, 412, 413

Rank, Otto, 26, 224, **461–462**
   defection of, 98, 445
   and *Imago*, 226
   influence in the United States, 584
   and *International Zeitschrift für Psychoanalyse*, 225
   member of the Berlin Psychoanalytical Training Institute, 236
   *Mythus von der geburt des Helden, Der (The Myth of the
      Birth of the Hero)*, 187
   and Nietzsche, 369
   quarrel with Abraham, 227
   quarrel with Jones, 227
   Sachs and, 501, 502
   secret committee member, 97, 98, 225, 445
   secretary of Wednesday Society, 597
   Stekel's influence on, 539
   and theory of creativity, 112
Rao, Dwarkanath, 276
Rao, Madhu, 276
Rapaport, David, 164, 376
   drive organization of cognition, 490
   ego psychology, 170–171
   genetic theory of development, 148
   metapsychology, 337, 338, 339, 585
   and Mexico, 342
   and Rubinstein, 205
Rapella, Diego, 34
Rascovsky, Arnaldo, 34, 342
   analyzed by Garma, 412
Rat Man, 99–100, 127, 128, 225, **462–464**
   attempt to describe the disorder, 459
   end of analysis, 449
   irrationality, 282
   post-Freudian analytic literature and, 100
   self-deception, 522
rationality, 282
reaction formation, 140, **464–465**
   in obsessive-compulsive neuroses, 366
reality principle
   Adler's influence on, 9
   and affect, 11
   codified in *Formulations on the Two Principles of Mental
      Functioning*, 422
reality testing, 61, 251, **465–466**
   narcissism and, 355
   and neuroses, 367
reception of Freud's ideas, **466–468**
Rechardt, Eero, 205, 206
Recherche (Piaget), 421
Reddy, Satish, 276
Redlich, Emil, 301
Rée, Paul, 21
Regnard, Paul, 76
regression, 140, **468–470**
   under the control of the ego, 313
   and hallucinations of dreaming, 251
   two types according to Kris, 314
Reich, Annie, 136, 200, 329, 471
Reich, Wilhelm, 68, 200, 329, 334, 384, **470–472**
   in Berlin, 330
   character problems, 72
   in Copenhagen, 144

influence in Norway, 383
"Mass Psychology of Fascism, The," 331
in Moscow, 498
and politics, 236
theory of genitality, 235
translations in Swedish, 554
treatment of patients resistant to classical analysis, 73–74
Reichsinstitut, 236
Reik, Theodor, 44, 227, 293, 319, **472–473**
analyzed by Abraham, 2
in Berlin, 236
emigration to Holland, 360
Fromm studying with, 231
Garma analyzed by, 412
Heimann analyzed by, 412
and interpretation, 452
in New York, 582
Sachs' training with, 13
training psychologists in the U.S., 467
Reisfeld, Pepa, 414
Reitler, Rudolf, 597
rejection, narcissism and, 355
relational analysts, 8
relational perspective, 257
religion
and delusions, 142
Freud's aversion toward religion, 295, 419
and obsessional phenomena, 393
and psychoanalysis, **473–477**
"Remarks on Laughter" (Kris), 312
Remembering, Repeating and Working-Through (Freud), 2, 283, 599
on transference, 568
Remembering the Phallic Mother (Ian), 265
Remus, Estela, 342
Remus, José, 342
reparation psychology of Klein, literary studies and, 265
Repertory of Experimental Physics (Fechner), 193
repetition compulsion, 90, 104, 226, **477–478**
Abraham and, 2
"Report on My Studies" (Freud), 42
Representing Shakespeare: New Psychoanalytic Essays (Faber, ed.), 265
repression, 90, 139, 441, **478–492**. *See also* return of the repressed
and affect, 11
critique of, 122–124
as defense, 31, 489
differentiated from dissociation, 350
differentiated from suppression, 140
ego as source of, 170
evolutionary scenario for, 49
and hysterical symptoms, 267
judgment as substitute for, 279
literature and, 325
and neuroses, 365, 366, 367
in obsessive-compulsive neuroses, 366
and overdetermination, 406
and pathology, 480–483
Schopenhauer and, 372
Repression (Freud), 163

research on psychoanalysis, **492–495**, 584, 585
resistance, 213, **495–496**
analysis method, 73–74
Ellis on, 178
Groddeck and, 245
and psychoanalytically oriented psychotherapy, 455
removal of, 447
and self-analysis, 520–521
transference and, 73–74, 569
return of the repressed, 483–484, 486, **496–497**
Revision der Hauptpunkte der Psychophysik (Fechner), 194
Revue Française de psychanalyse, 52
Rey de Castro, Alvaro, 413, 414
Reyes, Baltazar, 417
Ribot, Théodule, 287
and dissociationist model of the unconscious, 576
Nietzsche and, 368
Richer, Paul, 78
Richet, Charles, 287
Richter, Horst-Eberhard, 237
Rickman, John, 35, 243, 293
analyzed by Ferenczi, 204
Ricoeur, Paul, 130–131, 132, 256, 317, 476
Freud and Philosophy: An Essay on Interpretation, 266
Rie, Marianne. *See* Kris, Marianne
Rieff, Philip, 180
Freud: The Mind of the Moralist, 346
Triumph of the Therapeutic, The, 467
Rilke, Rainer Maria, 21, 22, 23
Rilton, Anna-Stina, 555
Riojas, Eduardo, 342
Rísquez, Fernando, 589, 590
Rittmeister, Johannes, 236
Ritual (Reik), 473
Riviere, Joan, 243, 293, 540
Rivista di Psicoanalisi, 285
Rizal, Jose, 417
Roazen, Paul, 148, 172, 239
Brother Animal: The Story of Freud and Tausk, 562–563
Rocha, Franco da, 58
Rockefeller, Edith, 299
Rockefeller, John D., Jr., 525
Ródinka (Andreas-Salomé), 21, 22
Rodríguez, César, 414
Rodríguez, Diego, 342
Rogerian therapy, catharsis in, 68
Rogers, Carl, 263
Róheim, Géza, 52, 264
analyzed by Ferenczi, 204
Roiphe, H., 151
Rolland, Romain, 475
Roman Catholic Church and psychoanalysis
in Austria, 591
in Chile, 83
in Italy, 285
in Philippines, 417
Roose, S., 137
Roots of Crime, The (Glover), 115, 239
Rorschach, Hermann, 427, 428
Rorschach Inkblot Test, 428
and oral character, 405

Rorty, Richard
    Contingency, Irony, and Solidarity, 266
    postmodernism of, 345
Rose, Gilbert, 112
Rosenblatt, B., 273
Rosenfeld, Herbert, 243, 309, 555
Rosenzweig, Franz, 231
Rostafinski, Michael J., 352
Rostworowski, María, 414
Rousseau Institute of Geneva, 421, 536
Rubinstein, B. R., 339
Rubinstein, Benjamin, 205
Ruddick, Bruce, 65
Rudnytdky, Peter, 229
Rundbriefe of Fenichel, 200
Russian Psychoanalytic Society, 330, 498
Russia/Soviet Union
    and psychoanalysis, 330, **497–499**
    Reich in, 471
Ruth (Andreas-Salomé), 21
Ryan, Joanna, 147
Rycroft, Charles, 412

S

Sachs, Hanns, 224, 461, **501–502**
    in Berlin, 2, 236
    British analysts and, 243
    Fromm studying with, 231
    Horney analyzed by, 261
    and *Imago*, 226, 457
    member of the Berlin Psychoanalytical Training Institute,
        236
    secret committee departure, 99
    secret committee member, 97, 98, 225, 445
    visit to Nietzsche's sister, 370
Sachs, Wulf, 13
Sacred Complex, The: On the Psychogenesis of Paradise Lost
        (Kerrigan), 265
Sadger, Isidor
    and homosexuality, 259
    Reich analyzed by, 470
sadism. *See* masochism and sadism
sadomasochism. *See* masochism and sadism
Safouan, Moustafa, 317
Sakellaropoulos, Panayotis, 244
Saling, M., 344
Salmon, Wesley, 125–126
Samiksa (journal), 275
Sampson, H., 492
San Francisco Psychoanalytic Society, 200
Sand, George, 53
Sandell, Agneta, 556
Sandell, Rolf, 556
Sandin, Barbro, 556
Sandler, Anne-Marie, 243, 245, 556
    in Prague, 137
Sandler, Joseph, 14, 19, 100, 243, 244, 392, 393
    and identification, 273
    in Prague, 137
Santiago, Virgilio, 417

Sapir, Edward, 26
Sarabhai, Kamalini, 276
Sarphatie, Herman R., 361
Sartre, Jean-Paul, 182
Saussure, Ferdinand de, 316
Saussure, Janice de, 244
Scandinavian Psychoanalytic Review, 145, 205–206
Schachtel, Ernest, 263
Schafer, Roy, 74, 103, 256, 585
    identification, 273
    layering of conflict and defense, 105
    and linguistic tradition, 266
    metapsychology, 340
    penis envy, 411
    psychoanalytics interpretation as re-narration,
        257
Schalin, Lars-Johan, 205
Schapiro, Meyer, 121
Scharff, D., 386
Scharff, J., 386
Schatzman, M., 508
Schelling, Friedrich Wilhelm von, 376, 558
    and unconscious, 324
Scherner, Albert, 177
Schilder, Paul, 392, 471
    and psychomatic medicine, 539
Schiller, Johann Christoph Friedrich von
    influence on Freud, 235
    Sachs psychoanalytical portrait of, 502
schizoid disorders, splitting and, 488, 538
schizophrenia, **502–504**
    diagnostic of Schreber, 508
    Freud on, 459
    hallucinations in, 252
    Sullivan and treatment of, 550
    thinking process in, 46
Schjelderup, Harald Krabbe, 383, 384, 554
Schleiermacher, Friedrich Daniel Ernst, 473
Schmideberg, Melitta, 240
    in Berlin, 236
    dissension with Klein, 303–304
Schmidt, Otto, 330
Schneider, Ernest, 231
Schnitzler, Arthur
    Reik's study of, 472
    Sachs psychoanalytical portrait of, 502
Schönberg, Ignaz, 224
Schopenhauer, Arthur, 119, 177, 369, 371–374, **504–506**
    anticipating key ideas of Freud, 235
    influence on Freud, 368, 381
    Nietzsche and, 368
    Tausk's view of, 563
    and the unconscious, 380, 505
Schore, A. N., 527
Schreber, Daniel Paul, 141–142, 225, 252, 409, **506–509**
    attempt to describe the disorder of, 459
Schultz-Hencke, Harald
    in Berlin after World War II, 237
    and Central Institute for Psychic Illnesses, 237
Schur, Max, 171, 228
    biography of Freud, 228

Schüttauf, K., 120, 121
Schwab, Sophie, 368
Schweitzer, Albert, 241
Schweninger, Ernst, 245
Scientific Proceedings of the Australian Psychoanalytic Society, The, 35
scientific tests of Freud's theories and therapy, **509–514**
    experiments on free association, 214
    outcome studies of psychoanalytic treatment, 492, 493, 512–514, 585
    personality test for anal character, 510
    personality tests for oral character, 405, 511
    projective tests, 428
    studies of castration complex, 67
    of theory of slips, 531–534
scientificization of Freud's language, 293
Scodel, A., 429–431
scopophilia, 463
Scott, Clifford, 65
screen memories, **514–515**
"Screen Memories" (Freud), 220–221, 514
    ego and, 169
Screen Memories (Greenberg), 266
Searle, J., 132
Searles, H., 142, 246
Sebek, Michael, 137
Second Sex, The (Beauvoir), 195
secondary consciousness, 289
secondary narcissism, 322, 355, 356, 387
secret committee. *See* committee, the secret
seduction theory, 389, 440, **515–520**
    repudiation of, 223
seduction theory papers, 516, 517
Seelensucher, Das (The Seeker of Souls) (Groddeck), 248
Segal, Hanna, 243, 309
Seguin, Carlos Alberto, 412
Selected Papers (Abraham), 2
Selected Problems of Adolescence (Deutsch), 147
self, Sullivan on, 551
self-analysis, **520–521**
    of Freud, 223, 441
Self-Analysis (Horney), 262
self-deception, 485, **522–523**
self-esteem
    and paranoia, 409
    shame and, 526
Selfish Gene, The (Dawkins), 323
selfish gene theory, 49, 534
self-motivation, 20
self-object experiences, 524
self-object relations
    similar to symbiotic object relations, 557
self-observation, 521
self-preservation, or ego, drives, 163, 542
self-psychology, 39, 133, 467, **523–525**, 583
    in Canada, 66
    development of, 116
    in Germany, 238
    Horney different from, 263
    and literary studies, 266
self-theory

and symbiosis, 557
Seligman, Charles, 26
"Seminar on 'The Purloined Letter,' The" (Lacan), 316
Senegal, psychoanalysis in, 13
Servadio, Emilio, 284, 285
Severn, Elizabeth, 204
Sex and Repression in Savage Society (Malinowski)
    and Oedipus complex, 264
sexology, **525–526**
    Freud's definition of sex, 414
sexual aberrations, 276–277
    narcissism and, 355
sexual drive, 162, 163, 443, 542
    conflict with self-preservation drives, or ego instincts, 162–163
Sexual Information (journal), 383
Sexual Inversion (Ellis), 176
Sexual Neurasthenia (Beard), 437–438
Sexual Selection in Man (Ellis), 177
sexuality, role of, 88–89
    and hysteria, 437
    and neurasthenia, 361
    Schopenhauer anticipating Freud, 505
    of symbolism in dreams, 559–560
Shakespeare, William
    psychonalytic literary criticism, 265
    Reik's study of, 472
    Sachs writing on, 502
Shakespeare's Personality (Faber, ed.), 265
Shakow, D., 376
Shamdasani, Sonu, 300
shame, **526–528**
    narcissism and, 355, 527
Shapiro, T., 149
Sharpe, Ella Freeman
    analyzed by Abraham, 2
    on interpretation, 280
    training patient of Sachs, 501
shell shock. *See* war trauma
Shengold, L., 100
Shizhao, Zhang, 85
Sigmund Freud Archives, 228
    founded by Eissler, 172
Sigmund Freud Institute (Frankfurt), 238
    support of psychoanalysis in Czechoslovakia, 137
Sigmund Freud's Collected Papers, 540
"Significance of Intermarriage Between Close Relatives, The" (Abraham), 1, 3
Significance of Psychoanalysis for the Mental Sciences, The (Rank and Sachs), 461, 501
Sikl, Zdenek, 137
Silberberg, William, 467
Silberstein, Eduard, 220
    correspondence with Freud, 60, 378
Sillanpää, Frans Emil, 205
Silove, D., 69
Silverstein, B., 343
Simenauer, Erich, 13
Simmel, Ernst, 173, 235
    in Berlin, 236
    and politics, 236
    on war neurosis, 595, 596

Simons, R. C., 333
Simonsen, Hjørdis, 384
Singer, N. B., 526–527
Singh Gill, Hawrant, 276
"Sisyphus or the Boundaries of Education" (Bernfeld), 331
Sjögren, Lars, 556
Sjöstrand, Wilhelm, 555
Sjövall, Thorsten, 555
Skinner, B. F., 43, 44
Slavney, Phillip R., 268
sleep, **528–530**
    REM sleep studies, 158–159, 529
slips, theory of, 213, **530–534**
Smith, G. J. W., 140, 141
Smith, Gudmund, 556
"Sobre psicología y psicoterapia de cierros estados angustiosos" (Greve), 83
Socarides, Charles W., 261
social criticism, psychoanalysis as, 237
social instinct, 389
social medicine, 597
social psychology of Fromm, 232
Socialist Society for Sexual Counselling and Sexual Research, 471
Sociedade Brasileira de Psicanálise, 58
Sociedade Brasileira de Psicanálise do Rio de Janeiro, 59
Sociedade Brasileria de Psycanálise de São Paulo, 58
Société de psychologie physiologique, 287
Société Française de Psychanalyse, 316, 317
Société Psychanalytique de Paris, 209
    Lacan breaking away from, 316
    Marie Bonaparte and, 52
    Sokolnicka and, 204
Society for Free Psychoanalytic Research, 225
Society for Psychical Research (London), 287
Society for the Scientific Study of Sex (SSSS), 525
Society of Psychical Research (Cambridge), 540
Society of Psychoanalysts in the Netherlands, 360
Society without the Father: A Contribution to Social Psychology (Mitscherlich), 237
sociobiology and psychoanalysis, **534–535**
Sokolnicka, Eugénie, 204
Solms, Mark, 14, 117, 118, 344
Solomon, G. F., 351
somatic convergence, 175
Some Additional Remarks on Dream Interpretation as a Whole (Freud), 396
Some Character-Types Met in Psycho-analytic Work (Freud), 458
Some Neurotic Mechanisms in Jealousy, Paranoia and Homosexuality (Freud), 260
"Some Practical Aspects of Psychoanalytical Treatment" (Jones), 35
Some Psychical Consequences of the Anatomical Distinction between the Sexes (Freud), 234–235
"Some Reflections on the Ego" (Lacan), 316
"Some Remarks on the Unconscious" (Freud), 271
Sorrows of Young Werther, The (Goethe), 401
South Africa, psychoanalysis in, 13
South African Psychoanalytic Society, 13
Soviet Union. *See* Russia
Spain, Peruvian psychoanalysts in, 414

"Specimen Irma Dream" (Freud), 129, 593
Spectator, The, 240, 540
speech apparatus, Freud's model of, 33
Speier, H., 312
Spektrum (journal), 553
Spellbound (Hitchcock), psychoanalytic criticism of, 87
Spence, Donald, 256, 585
    appraisal of the analytic interpretive process, 191–192
Spencer, Herbert, 26, 264
Spezielle Pathologie und Therapie, 301
Spiegel, D., 491
Spielrein, Sabina, **535–537**
    Piaget and, 421
Spinoza, Baruch, 419
Spiro, Melford, 264
Spitz, René, 237, 393
    anaclitic depression, 17, 494
    in Berlin, 236
    developmental theory, 150
    in Greece, 244
    infant and child observation, 584
split-consciousness theory, 479, 537
    abandonned by Freud, 107
    repression and, 481
    weakening of the personality, 482–483
splitting of personality, 537
splitting of the ego, 153–154, 388, 487, 488, **537–538**.
    See also dissociation
    different from repression, 350
Splitting of the Ego in the Process of Defense (Freud), 481, 487
splitting of the mind, 537
Spock, Benjamin, 584
Spotnitz, Hyman, 503
spreading-activation theory
    and double entendres, 533
    and theory of slips, 532
Sripada, Bhaskar, 276
"Stages in the Development of the Sense of Reality" (Ferenczi), 201
Stalin, Joseph, 498
Standard Edition of the Complete Psychological Works of Sigmund Freud (Strachey, ed.), 71, 130, 188, 228, 323, 541
Stärcke, August, 359
state of being in love, 388
State Psychoanalytic Institute (Moscow), 330
"Statutes of the International Psychoanalytic Association," 98
Stekel, Wilhelm, 224, **538–540**
    defection of, 445
    on masturbation, 362
    psychoanalytic study of telepathic dreams, 396
    and Wednesday Society, 597
    and *Zentralblatt für Psychoanalyse*, 225
Stengel, E., 33
Stephan, Achim, 132
Sterba, Editha, 218
Sterba, Richard, 13, 290
    and Anna Freud, 218
    on therapeutic split in the ego, 564
Stern, Daniel N., 494
    and developmental theory, 151
Stevenson, Robert Louis, 350

Stewart, W., 602
Stöcker, Helene, 21
Stockholm County Council Institute of Psychotherapy, 555
Stone, L., 180
Storr, Anthony, 132
Strachey, Alix, 293, 540
   analyzed by Abraham, 2
   analyzed by Freud, 243
   Klein and, 303
Strachey, James, 33, 188, 293, 294, 425, 445, 451, 452, **540–541**
   analyzed by Freud, 243
   and Anna O., 25
   discharge of affect, 481
   interpretation, 452
   introduction of word "ego," 253
   introduction to *The Ego and the Id*, 169
   and term cathexis, 69–70
   on term "object," 386
   and transference, 451
Strachey, Lytton, 540
Strange Case of Dr. Jekyll and Mr. Hyde, The (Stevenson), 350
Strenger, C., 257
stress trauma, coined by Kris, 313
Strindberg, August, 553
   Sachs psychoanalytical portrait of, 502
Strømme, Irgens, 554
structural model of the mind. *See* structural theory
structural theory, 443, 477, **541–546**
   affect, 11
   conflict, 103–104
   consciousness, 107–108
   defense, 103
   drives, 164
   ego in, 169, 170
   narcissism, 356
   and neuroses, 364–366
   unconscious, 578–579
   working through, 600
Stuchlik, J., 136
student movement of the 1960s, 330
Studies in Experimental Medicine (Bernard), 418
"Studies in the Prehistory of Psychoanalysis" (Andersson), 555
Studies in the Psychology of Sex (Ellis), 176
Studies on Hysteria (Breuer and Freud), 24, 42, 62, 148, 223, 436
   and case of Elizabeth von R., 175
   conversion, 110, 483
   orgasm mentioned in, 588
   overdetermination, 407
   primal scene, 424
   repression, 478, 479
   seduction theory, 515, 517
   self-deception, 522
   transference, 568
Study of Psychopathology, A (Lapuz), 417
Stumpf, Carl, 60
sublimation, 112, 139, **546–547**
Suffocating Mother: Fantasies of Maternal Origin in Shakespeare's Plays (Adelman), 265
suggestion, **547–548**
suicide, **548–550**

Sullivan, Harry Stack, 27, 142, 262, 467, **550–551**
   and Adler, 8
   Bingham Dai training under, 85
   and Ferenczi, 204
   not-me experience, 489, 551
   and Swedish Holistic Society, 556
   treatment of schizophrenia, 502
   and William Alanson White Institute, 231
Sulloway, Frank, 26, 223
   on Freud, 229
Sundelson, D., 101
superego, 91, 356, 443, 477, 545–546, **551–552**
   formation reinterpreted in context of phallic stage, 234
   id distinguished from, 272
   Klein and child's superego, 305
   line of development established by Anna Freud, 219
   and morality, 347–348
   and neuroses, 367
superego precursor, 552
supportive psychotherapies, 455–456
suppression
   different from repression, 140
   Ellis on, 178
Surprise and the Psychoanalyst (Reik), 473
surrealism, 325
Sutherland, J. D., 386
Swales, Peter, 224
   and Anna O., 25
Swank, R. L., 595
Sweden
   Danish psychoanalysis and, 144
   and psychoanalysis, **553–557**
   Reich in, 471
Swedish Psychoanalytical Association, 556
Swedish Psychoanalytical Society, 554, 555
Swedish Society for Holistic Psychoanalysis and Psychotherapy, 556
Swiss Medical Society for Psychoanalysis, 416
Swiss Society for Psychoanalysis, 416
   Piaget member of, 421
Swoboda, Hermann, 222
symbiosis, **557–559**
symbolism, 245, 247, **559–560**
   Freud and, 306
   Jones and, 294, 306
   Kelin and, 306
   myths and, 353
   Piaget's criticism of Freud, 422
   structuralists' view of taboos, 562
   for virginity and defloration, 593
Symbols and Transformations of the Libido (Jung), 536
symptom neuroses, 366
symptoms
   conversion, 483
   formation of, 90
   hysterical, 87, 90, 267
   linguistic usage and choice of symptoms, 176
   obsessional, 90, 393
   rapid removal of, 539
Szecsödy, Imre, 555
Szekely, Edith, 554
Szekely, Lajos, 554

T

taboo, **561–562**. *See also Totem and Taboo* (Freud)
   and obsessional phenomena, 393
Taboo of Virginity, The (Freud), 592–593
Taft, Jessie, 462
Tähkä, Veikko, 205
Taine, Hippolyte Adolphe
   and dissociationist model of the unconscious, 576
   Nietzsche and, 368
Talent and Genius (Eissler), 172
Talking Cures, The (Wallerstein), 455
Tamez, Rubén, 342, 343
Tamm, Alfhild, 205, 383, 554
taoistic psychotherapy, 310
Tarasoff v. the Regents of the University of California, 101
Tardieu, Ambroise, 269
Target, Mary, 81, 113
Tausk, Victor, 172, **562–564**
   Andreas-Salomé and, 22
   suicide of, 226
Tausk's Suicide (Eissler), 172, 563
Technique of Analytical Psychotherapy (Stekel), 539
Technique of Psychoanalysis (Rank), 462
telepathy
   experiments between Ferenczi, Freud and Anna Freud, 395
   Freud's first published endorsement of, 396
temporal regression, 468
Temptation of Saint Anthony, The (Flaubert), psychoanalytic
   dissertation on, 472
Teruel, Guillermo, 589
   sponsor of Peruvian study group, 413
testing of psychoanalytic propositions, 492
Teuns, Joseph P., 360
Texbook of Theoretical and Practical Chemistry (Thénard), 193
Thalassa (Versuch einer genital Theorie) (Ferenczi), 202
Thales of Miletus, 130
Thanatos. *See* death instinct
Thematic Apperception Test (TAT), 428
Theme of the Three Caskets, The (Freud), 353
Theory of Celestial Motions (Gauss), 194
Theory of Psychoanalysis (Jung), 174
therapeutic alliance, 448, 514, **564–565**
   Rank and emotional aspects of, 462
   and treatment of schizophrenia, 504
therapeutic integration, 4
therapy
   and homosexuality, 260
   psychoanalysis as, 512–514
thinking, modes of, 422
Thinking about 'Beowulf' (Earl), 265
Third Latin American Congress of Psychoanalysis
   (Santiago), 83
Thoma, H., 114, 238, 492
Thomas Woodrow Wilson: A Psychological Study (Freud and
   Bullitt), 227, 264
Thompson, Clara, 262, 467
   and Adler, 8
   and Ferenczi, 204
   and William Alanson White Institute, 231
Thorner, Hans, 59

thought-consciousness, 109
Three Essays on the Theory of Sexuality (Freud), 9, 15, 38,
   177, 224, 322
   ambivalence, 16
   "'Anal' aund 'Sexual'" (Andreas-Salomé) and, 22
   autoerotism, 37
   and Fliess's theory of bisexuality, 207
   genitality, 234
   homosexuality, 258–259, 259
   impact of anatomical distinction on boys and girls, 443
   infantile sexuality, 276
   introduction of term *Trieb*, 162
   on little girls' genital sexuality, 587
   pregenital stages of development, 443
   primal scene, 425
   reaction formation, 464, 465
   sex defined, 414
   sexual object *versus* sexual aim, 385, 414–415
   shame, 526
   Strachey's footnote about "object," 386
   sublimation defined, 546
   understanding of infant's needs, 389
   written simultaneously with *Jokes and Their Relation to
   the Unconscious*, 292
Ticho, E., 450
Tidén, Ulf, 555
Time Magazine, 371
Times (London), 240
   on Melanie Klein, 302
Titchener, Edward B., 582
   on unconscious, 576
toilet training, **565–566**
Tokyo Institute of Psychoanalysis, 291
Tomasi, Allessandra, 284
topographical model of the mind, 55, 387, 439, 542
   arising from clinical reflection of repetition, 477
   defense and, 103
   ego in, 169, 170
   influence of Hughlings Jackson, 438
   and neuroses, 364
   and preconscious, 422
   structural theory superimposed on, 389
   unconscious in, 578
   and working through, 599–600
Törngren, Pehr Henrik, 554
Torres, Enrique, 34
Totem and Taboo (Freud), 25, 26–27, 226, 296, 561
   incest, 274–275, 400
   myths, 353, 354
   overdetermination, 406
   rejection from anthropologists, 475–476
   religion and obsessive-compulsive disorders, 473
   reviewed by Kroeber, 26, 264
training analysis, concept of, 298
transference, 191, 442, 446, 451–453, 495, **567–572**
   analysis of, 447, 452
   critique of, 127–128
   in Dora's case, 156
   Groddeck and, 245
   mutative insights and, 279
   negative, 450

neurosis, 367, 567, 570
and number of sessions per week, 585
and psychoanalytically oriented psychotherapy, 455
Rank on, 462
regression and, 468
resistance distinguished from character resistance, 73–74
revival of preverbal experiences, 6
and schizophrenia, 503
and suggestibility, 547–548
therapeutic alliance and, 564
transference love, 5
Transformation and Symbols of the Libido (Jung), 299
"Transformations of Puberty" (Freud), 178
translations of Freud
by A. Brill, 293, 540
Besetzung, translation of, 70
in Chinese, 84–85
choice of Latin terminology, 390
in Danish, 145
"*Das Ich*," translation of, 253
in English, 70, 293, 540–541
Fenichel on committee for, 200
in Italian, 285
in Japanese, 291
Jones and, 70
by Marie Bonaparte, 52
in Russian, 497, 498
by Strachey, 70, 540–541
in Swedish, 553, 554, 556
Trauma of Birth, The (Rank), 227, 461
traumatic neurosis, **572–573**
Treurniet, N., 137, 361
Triandafyllidis, Manolis, 244
Triebe
Freud and Nietzsche's use of term, 368
Freud's introduction of term, 162
Trilling, Lionel, 467
Triology: Memoir of the Future (Bion), 59
Triumph of the Therapeutic, The (Rieff), 467
Trivedi, Dushyant, 276
Trivers, Robert L., 534
Trotsky, Leon, 330
and psychoanalysis, 497
Trotter, W. B. Louis, 293
truth, Freud's devotion to, 180
Truth and Method (Gadamer), 256–257
Truth and Reality (Rank, trans. Taft), 462
Tuovinen, Matti, 205
Turgenev, Ivan, 75
Two Encyclopedia Articles (Freud), 260
Tyler, Parker, 266
Tylor, Edward, 26, 264
typology of artistic, average and neurotic characters by Rank, 462
tyrannical shoulds of Horney, 263
Tzavaras, Nikos, 245

U

Über die Seelenfrage (Concerning the Soul) (Fechner), 194
"Über männliche Hysterie" (Freud), 268

"Über Sexualfragen in der Jugendbewegung "(On Sexual issues in the youth movement) (Fenichel), 199
Uexküll, Thure von, 37
Ulm group, 492, 493
"'Uncanny,' The" (Freud)
free will, 215
repetition compulsion, 226
unconscious, the, 542, **575–582**
continuity argument for, 579–580
difference between cognitive psychology and psychoanalysis, 119
dispositionalist approach, 576, 579–580
dissociationist model of, 576, 580–581
electrotherapy used to recover unconscious material, 213
Freud's interest in, 55, 107
Freud's justifications for, 579–581
Herbart and, 254–255, 376–377
and importance of confidentiality, 101
Leibniz and, 118, 581
literature and, 324–325
Piaget's criticism of Freud's concept of, 422
and schizophrenia, 503
Schopenhauer and, 380, 505
term linked to Hartmann, 376
Unconscious, The: Nature, Functions, Methods of Study, 498
Unconscious, The (Freud), 163, 226, 578
related to *On Aphasia*, 33
Undiscovered Self, The (Jung), 300
undoing, 140, 284
and neuroses, 367
in obsessive-compulsive neuroses, 366
United Kingdom. *See* Great Britain
United States. *See also* New York City
diagnosis in, 460
education of analysts in, 167
Indian psychoanalysts in, 276
Peruvian psychoanalysts in, 414
projective tests in, 428
and psychoanalysis, **582–586**
psychotherapeutic treatment for schizophrenia, 502, 503
reception of Freud's ideas in, 466–468, 582
research on psychoanalysis in, 492
Sachs in Boston, 501, 502
universal causal sufficiency, thesis of, 216
"Unlocking the Heart of Genius" (Ellis), 177
unpleasure, 422
designating anxiety, 29
distinguished from anxiety, 30
Untimely Meditations (Nietzsche), 368

V

Vackova, Bohumila, 137
vaginal and clitoral orgasm, **587–589**
Vaillant, G., 366, 367
Valdez, Gilberto, 414
Valdivia, Oscar, 412
Vallejo and the Poetry of the Body (Altamirano), 414
Vampyr (Dreyer), psychoanalytic criticism of, 87
Van der Hart, O., 68
Van der Kolk, B. A., 351

Van Emden, J., 359, 360
Van Ophuijsen, Johann H. W. *See* Ophuijsen,
     Johann H. W. van
Vannypelseer, Jean-Louis, 45
Varendonck, Julien, 44
Vatillon, A., 137
Vaughn, S., 137
Vegetti Finzi, S., 285
Venezuela and psychoanalysis, **589–590**
Venezuelan Association of Psychoanalysis, 589
Vergopoulo, Thalia, 245
Verlag für Sexualpolitik (Press for Sexual Politics), 471
vicissitudes of the instincts, 91–92
Victor Tausk's Suicide (Eissler), 172, 563
Viderman, S., 280
Vienna
     pedagogically oriented psychoanalysis in, 320–330
     and psychoanalysis, 445, **590–592**
     Scandinavians in, 554
Vienna Psychoanalytic Society, 7
     beginning of, 224
     and cases of apparent telepathy, 395
     debate of Marxism at, 329
     debate on masturbation, 362
     debates on Nietzsche, 369–370, 375
     decision to move out of Austria, 591–592
     Deutsch and, 147
     Eitingon and, 172
     Fenichel and, 199
     influence of Freud's political views on, 330
     minutes from 1906 to 1918, 597
     on "On the Origin of the Influencing Machine in
          Schizophrenia" (Tausk), 563
     outpatient clinic of, 591
     Rank and, 461
     Reich and, 471
     Reik and, 472
Vienna Psychoanalytic Training Institute, 591
     Deutsch first president of, 147
     Eissler trained at, 172
Vienna Youth Movement, 329
Vietnam War, and combat reactions, 595
Villarreal, Inga, 413
Virchow, Rudolf, 378
Virgin and St. Anne with the Infant Jesus (Leonardo
     da Vinci), Freud's analysis of, 112
virginity, **592–594**
Visual Agnosia (Farah), 419
Vocabulaire technique et critique de la philosophie
     (Lalande, ed.), 421
Vogt, Ragnar, 383
Volkan, Vamik, 503
Volkelt, Johannes, 379
Voloshinov, V. N., 498
Von Hartmann, Eduard
     influence on Freud, 368, 375–376
     Nietzsche and, 368
     Philosophy of the Unconscious, 506
Vorschule der Aesthetik (Fechner), 194
Voss, H., 589
Vulpain, Claude Bernard, 75

Vuoristo, Gunvor, 205
Vygotsky, L. S., 497

W

Waal, Nic, 383, 384
Waelder, Jenny, 218
Waelder, Robert, 72, 114
     and Anna Freud, 218
     editor of *Imago*, 312
     Santiago training under, 417
Wagner, Miguel, 414
Wagner-Jauregg, Julius, 172, 562
Wahl, François, 318
Waiting: The Whites of South Africa (Crapanzano), 13
Wallace, Edwin, 264
Wallerstein, Robert S., 446
     42 Lives, 493
     Talking Cures, The, 455
Wallon, Henri, 315
War, Sadism, and Pacifism (Glover), 239
War, Sexuality, and Schizophrenia (Tausk), 563
war neurosis, **595–596**. *See also* war trauma
     treatment of, 4
war trauma, 226, 572. *See also* war neurosis
     and hysteria of traumatized soldiers, 268
Warhol, Andy, 346
Warren, Bengt, 556
water immersion to recover unconscious material, 213
Wayward Youth (Aichorn), 218
     preface by Freud, 114
Weber, Alfred, 231
Weber, Ernst Heinrich, 193, 194
Weber, Guido, 507, 508
Wednesday Society, 224, **596–597**. *See also* Vienna
     Psychoanalytic Society
     influence of Jewish intelligentisia on, 591
Weininger, Otto, 207, 222
Weinshel, E., 452
     and transference, 451
Weiss, Edoardo, 284, 285
Weiss, J., 492
Wellhausen, Julius, 476
West Germany. *See* Germany
Westermarck, Edward, 264
Wexler, Bruce, 503
Wheeler, Richard, 265
White, William Alanson, 204
White, William Alanson, Institute, 585
     Fromm and, 231
Whiting, J., 67
Whitman, Walt, study by Marie Bonaparte, 53
Whole Journey, The: Shakespeare's Power of Development
     (Barber and Wheeler), 265
Why War? (Freud), 228
Widlöcher, Daniel, 412
Wiener Seminar für Sexuologie (Vienna Seminar for
     Sexology), 470
     founded by Fenichel, 199
wild analysis, 383, 446
     dangers of, 279

Wilhelm, Richard, 299
will. *See also* free will
    Schopenhauer's analysis of, 505
    will therapy of Rank, 462
Will Therapy (Rank, trans. Taft), 462
Willard, Elizabeth Osgood Goodrich, 525
William Alanson White Institute, 585
    Fromm and, 231
Wilson, E., 48
Wilson, Edward O., 534
Wilson, G. D., 67
Windholz, Emanuel, 136
Winn, Roy, 35
Winnicott, Donald W., 59, 182, 187, 197, 205, 243, 317
    agression, 114
    developmental theory, 149
    false self theory, 115
    Freud's influence on, 112
    Horney and, 263
    identification, 273
    influence in Mexico, 342
    influence in Peru, 412
    influence in the United States, 584
    Italy and, 285
    as object relations theorist, 386
    objects, 386
    primary omnipotence, 304
    splitting, 538
    supervisor of Peña, 412
    transitional space, 453
    treatment of schizophrenia, 502
Winson, J., 233
Witenberg, Wilhelm, 231
Wittgenstein, Ludwig, 266
Wittkower, Eric, 65
Wolf Man, 82, 226, 410, **598–599**
    attempt to describe the disorder, 459
    end of analysis, 449–450
    national character speculations, 498
    and primal scene, 425
Wolff, Moshe, 173
Wolstein, B., 155
Wolstein, Benjamin, 551
women. *See also* female sexuality
    and early psychoanalysis, 197
    Freud's psychology of, 227
    Freud's psychology of, modified by Horney, 261, 262
    and hysteria, 268
    and Oedipus complex, 402–403, 511–512
    and shame, 527
    superego of, 512, 552
Woolf, Leonard, 540, 541
Woolf, Virginia, 346, 540
    on Melanie Klein, 302
word associations, Jung and, 298
working alliance. *See* therapeutic alliance

working through, 495, **599–602**
World as Will and Representation, The (Schopenhauer), 504, 505
World Council for Psychotherapy, 14
World War I
    interest in war neurosis, 572, 595
    Tausk during, 562
World War II
    Holocaust sequelae work, 361
    and psychiatry, 433
    psychoanalysis in Vienna after, 590
    and war neurosis, 572, 595
Writings of Anna Freud, The, 218
Wundt, Wilhelm
    influence on Freud, 26
    Nietzsche and, 368
Wurmser, L., 526

Y

Yabe Yaekichi, 291
Yagnik, Dushyant, 276
Yates, S. L., 593
"Young Girl Diary, A" (Hug-Hellmuth), 81

Z

Zac, Joel, 35
Zalkind, A. B., 498
Zallenka, Hans, 154
Zallenka, Peppina, 154, 155
Zavitzianos, George, 65, 244
Zax, M., 68
Zeitschrift, 238
Zeitschrift für Sozialforschung, 231
Zela, Francisco de, 414
Zend-Avesta, Über die Dinge des Himmels und der Jenseits (Fechner), 194
Zentner, Marcel, 119
Zentralblatt für Psychoanalyse, 225
    Stekel and Adler co-editors of, 538
Zetzel, E., 448
    depression, 146
    therapeutic alliance, 564, 565
Ziegler, Leopold, 241
Ziehen, Theodor, 598
Zimmermann, David, 413
Zohar, J., 392
Zuan, Ding, 85
"Zum Typus Weib" (Andreas-Salomé), 22
Zur experimentellen Aesthetik (Fechner), 194
Zürich
    psychoanalytic movement in, 445
    Scandinavians in, 554
Zweig, Arnold, 228, 370

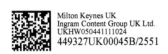

9 780415 762335